D1264928

ANTIBIOTICS IN LABORATORY MEDICINE

FIFTH EDITION

ANTIBIOTICS IN LABORATORY MEDICINE

Victor Lorian, M.D.
Professor of Laboratory Medicine, RET.
Albert Einstein College of Medicine
New York

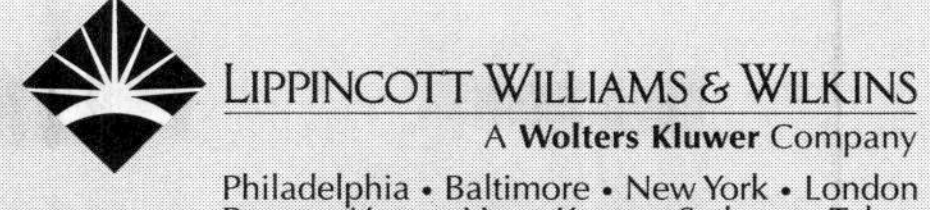

Philadelphia • Baltimore • New York • London
Buenos Aires • Hong Kong • Sydney • Tokyo

Acquisitions Editor: Frances Destefano
Developmental Editor: Mike Standen
Project Manager: Alicia Jackson
Senior Manufacturing Manager: Benjamin Rivera
Marketing Manager: Kathy Neely
Designer: Teresa Mallon
Production Service: TechBooks
Printer: Edwards Brothers

**530 Walnut Street
Philadelphia, PA 19106 USA
LWW.com**

Printed in the USA

Library of Congress Cataloging-in-Publication Data

Antibiotics in laboratory medicine / [edited by] Victor Lorian.—5th ed.
p. ; cm.
Includes bibliographical references and index.
ISBN 0-7817-4983-2
1. Microbial sensitivity tests. 2. Antibiotics—Analysis.
3. Drug resistance in microorganisms. I. Lorian, Victor.
[DNLM: 1. Microbial Sensitivity Tests. 2. Anti-Bacterial Agents—pharmacology. QW 25.5.M6 A629 2005]
QR69.A57A57 2005
615′.329—dc22

2004027260

Care has been taken to confirm the accuracy of the information presented and to describe generally accepted practices. However, the authors, editors, and publisher are not responsible for errors or omissions or for any consequences from application of the information in this book and make no warranty, expressed or implied, with respect to the currency, completeness, or accuracy of the contents of the publication. Application of this information in a particular situation remains the professional responsibility of the practitioner.

The authors, editors, and publisher have exerted every effort to ensure that drug selection and dosage set forth in this text are in accordance with current recommendations and practice at the time of publication. However, in view of ongoing research, changes in government regulations, and the constant flow of information relating to drug therapy and drug reactions, the reader is urged to check the package insert for each drug for any change in indications and dosage and for added warnings and precautions. This is particularly important when the recommended agent is a new or infrequently employed drug.

Some drugs and medical devices presented in this publication have Food and Drug Administration (FDA) clearance for limited use in restricted research settings. It is the responsibility of health care providers to ascertain the FDA status of each drug or device planned for use in their clinical practice.

10 9 8 7 6 5 4 3 2 1

To Marina Lorian, wife, companion, and friend, with love and appreciation. Her constant support and inspiration have made my career accomplishments possible and contributed to the realization of this work.

Contents

Preface

The antibiotic era is now 65 years old, and for the past 25 years *Antibiotics in Laboratory Medicine* has tracked the development of new compounds and classes of antimicrobial agents and presented detailed methods and approaches for evaluating the efficacy and the mechanisms of action and resistance of these compounds *in vitro* and *in vivo*.

In this, the fifth edition, the first of the new millennium, I am cognizant of the limited development of new antimicrobial agents, although I have witnessed the expansion of new classes of anti-infective compounds, namely, antifungal and antiviral agents. Increasingly, molecular methods, computer algorithms, and complex statistical programs are relied on for evaluating the potency of new and old drugs or comparing activity within classes of agents, selecting appropriate therapy, accurately identifying the genetic resistance of microorganisms, and tracking resistance trends locally, nationally, and internationally. All three—methods, algorithms, and programs—are included in this work.

Of the seventeen chapters that make up this volume, five are new contributions on recent subjects and concepts in this ever developing field. The remaining chapters, expanded and reworked, represent current science and practice. In addition, the large number of references, including citations of works published in 2004, will help relieve the reader of tedious literature searches and surveys.

Several aspects of the revised and newly added chapters are worth highlighting. In the opening chapter on breakpoint determination Drs. Wikler and Ambrose set the tone for this volume. It lays out a rationale for establishing breakpoints that is meaningful and acceptable to laboratorians and clinical practitioners. In Chapter 3, Dr. Daniel Amsterdam discusses the relevance and clinically predictive value of *in vitro* antimicrobial susceptibility testing. In my estimation, this is the first time that the issues covered are addressed in a monograph on this subject. Additionally, a new *in vitro* parameter, the MPC (mutant prevention concentration) is discussed, along with the impact of quorum sensing genes on antibiotic resistance. In Chapter 11, Dr. Magareta Ieven describes in great detail the latest methods for the detection of antibacterial resistance genes—methods applicable in the clinical laboratory. In an expanded and updated version of a chapter that appeared in the fourth edition, Dr. Charles Stratton discusses and interprets the molecular mechanisms of action for all antimicrobial classes, with particular emphasis on the newer effects of cell wall activity by aminoglycosides. His explanations are truly original and illuminating. The antivirogram, discussed by Dr. Pierre Dellamonica and colleagues in Chapter 13, is analogous to the antibiogram. It can be used to compare the potency of antiviral compounds against HIV and explain the molecular action mechanisms of antiviral agents. In Chapter 14, on disinfectants and antiseptics, Drs. Ascenzi and Favero present groundbreaking evidence and bring together the current state of knowledge of these compounds and their modes of action, strategies for use, spectrum of activity, and mechanisms of resistance. For the first time, the molecular link between these chemical disinfectants, sterilants, and antibiotics is established. Chapter 16, by Dr. David Bamberger and coauthors, discusses the level of antibiotics in most tissues and body fluids. It has been brought completely up to date and will be a vital resource for clinical practitioners. Lastly, the contribution of Drs. Thomas Fritsche, Helio Sader, and Ronald Jones describes the dynamic epidemiological patterns in antibiotic resistance regionally, nationally, and internationally. Regularly published data from several ongoing trending programs are presented.

During the past 25 years, I have often been reminded of the talented investigators who contributed to make the editions of this book scientifically sound and clinically meaningful. The fifth edition is authored by distinguished physicians and scientists who are experts in their particular areas, brilliant in their vision, and recognized worldwide. I am pleased to welcome the new authors and wish to thank them not only for their important contributions but for their patience and courteous response to my many requests and queries during the editing process.

It is fitting and appropriate that I express my gratitude and appreciation to those who have made my effort in completing this work truly rewarding. Of special note are the efforts and counsel of Dr. Daniel Amsterdam in discussions of the subject matter as well as his availability for resolution of several issues related to the preparation of this work. His contributions had a direct impact on the editing process. I also wish to acknowledge the interest, competence, and intense dedication of Mr. Mike Standen of Lippincott, Williams & Wilkins in the preparation of this manuscript for publication.

Victor Lorian, M.D.
New York

Contributing Authors

Paul G. Ambrose, Pharm. D.
Associate Research Professor
Pharmacy Practice
School of Pharmacy and Pharmaceutical Services
University at Buffalo
Amherst, NY

Daniel Amsterdam, M.D., Ph.D.
Professor, Department of Microbiology, Medicine and Pathology
School of Medicine and Biomedical Sciences
State University of New York at Buffalo
Buffalo, New York

D. A. Andes
University of Wisconsin School of Medicine
Madison, Wisconsin

Joseph M. Ascenzi, Ph.D.
Senior Manager, Regulatory Affairs
Advanced Sterilization Products
Irvine, California

David M. Bamberger, M.D.
Professor
Department of Medicine
University of Missouri–Kansas City
Kansas City, Missouri

Jan M. Bell, B.Sc.
Head, Antibiotic Research Laboratory
Women's and Children's Hospital
North Adelaide, South Australia

Robert A. Bonomo, M.D.
Infectious Diseases Section
Louis Stokes Cleveland Veterans Affairs Medical Center
Cleveland, Ohio

Darcie L. Bridwell
Assistant Professor
Department of Medicine
University of Missouri–Kansas City
Kansas City, Missouri

Vincent Calvez, M.D., Ph.D.
Professor of Virology
Department of Virology
Medical School of Pitié Salpêtriére
University of Pierre et Marie Curie
Paris, France

Pierre Dellamonica, M.D., Ph.D.
Professor of Infectiology
Department of Infectious Diseases
Director of Laboratory of Infectious Diseases
Medical School of Nice
University of Nice Sophia-Antipolis
Nice, France

Daniel J. Diekema, M.D., M.S.
Clinical Associate Professor
Department of Internal Medicine and Pathology
University of Iowa College of Medicine
Iowa City, Iowa

Stephen C. Edberg, Ph.D.
Professor, Department of Laboratory Medicine
Yale University School of Medicine
New Haven, Connecticut

George M. Eliopoulos, M.D.
Professor of Medicine
Harvard Medical School
Beth Israel Deaconess Medical Center
Boston, Massachusetts

Martin S. Favero, Ph.D.
Director, Scientific and Clinical Affairs
Advanced Sterilization Products
Irvine, California

John W. Foxworth
Associate Professor
Department of Medicine
University of Missouri–Kansas City School of Medicine
Kansas City, Missouri

N. Frimodt-Møller
Microbiological Research and Development
Statens Serum Institute
Copenhagen, Denmark

Thomas R. Fritsche, M.D., Ph.D.
Associate Director
The JONES Group/JMI Laboratories
North Liberty, Iowa

Dale N. Gerding, M.D.
Professor
Department of Medicine
Loyola University Chicago
Maywood, Illinois

David W. Hecht, M.D.
Professor of Medicine
Chief, Division of Infectious Diseases
Loyola University Stritch School of Medicine
Hines Medical Center
Maywood, Illinois

Margareta Ieven, M.D.
Associate Professor
Department of Medical Microbiology
University Hospital Antwerp
Antwerp, Belgium

Clark B. Inderlied, Ph.D.
Professor of Clinical Pathology
University of Southern California, Keck School of Medicine
Children's Hospital Los Angeles
Los Angeles, California

Ronald N. Jones, M.D.
Director, International Surveillance Programs
The JONES Group/JMI Laboratories
North Liberty, Iowa
Adjunct Professor
Department of Medicine
Tufts University School of Medicine
Boston, Massachusetts

Roger D. Klein, M.D., J.D.
Clinical Fellow in Microbiology and Virology
Department of Laboratory Medicine
Yale University School of Medicine
New Haven, Connecticut

Bruno Lina, M.D., Ph.D.
Professor of Virology
University of Claude Bernard
Deputy–Chief
Virology Laboratory of Hospices Civils of Lyon
Rockefeller University
Lyon, France

Anne-Geneviève Marcelin, Pharm.D., Ph.D.
Doctor of Virology
Department of Virology
Pitié-Salpêtrière Hospital
Medical School of Pitié-Salpêtrière
University of Pierre and Marie Curie
Paris, France

Marie-Christine Mazeron, M.D., Ph.D.
Laboratory of Virology/Bacteriology
Lariboisière Hospital
Medical School of Lariboisière Saint-Louis
University of Paris
Paris, France

Robert C. Moellering, Jr., M.D.
Herman L. Blumgart Professor of Medicine
Harvard Medical School
Physician-in-Chief and Chairman
Department of Medicine
Beth Israel Deacaness Medical Center
Boston, Massachussetts

Kevin A. Nash, Ph.D.
Assistant Professor
Department of Pathology
Children's Hospital Los Angeles
University of Southern California
Los Angeles, California

Terry O'Reilly, Ph.D.
Novartis Institute for Biomedical Research
Basel, Switzerland

Ch. Østergaard
Statens Serum Institute
Copenhagen, Denmark

Michael A. Pfaller, M.D.
Professor, Department of Pathology
Director, Department of Molecular Epidemiology and Fungus Testing Laboratory
University of Iowa College of Medicine and College of Public Health
Iowa City, Iowa

Satish K. Pillai, M.D.
Clinical Fellow in Medicine
Department of Medicine
Beth Israel Deaconess Medical Center
Harvard Medical School
Boston, Massachussetts

Didier Raoult, M.D., Ph.D.
Professor
Marseilles Medical School
Director of Rickettsia Unit
Marseilles, France

Louis B. Rice, M.D.
Case Western Reserve University School of Medicine
Chief, Infectious Diseases Section
Veterans Administration Medical Center
Cleveland, Ohio

Michael G. Rinaldi, Ph.D.
Professor of Pathology and Medicine
University of Texas Health Science Center at San Antonio
Director, Department of Veterans Affairs Mycology Reference Laboratory
Audie L. Murphy Memorial Veterans Hospital
San Antonio, Texas

Pierre-Marie Roger, M.D., Ph.D.
Doctor of Infectiology
Department of Infectious Diseases
Medical School of Nice
University of Nice Sophia-Antipolis
Nice, France

Jean-Marc Rolain, Pharm.D., Ph.D.
Unité des Rickettsies
Faculté de Médecine
Université de la Mediterranée
Marseille, France

Helio S. Sader, M.D., Ph.D.
Director, International Surveillance Program
The JONES Group/JMI Laboratories
North Liberty, Iowa
Professor
Division of Infectious Diseases
Federal University
Sao Paulo, Brazil

Christopher S. Shain, Pharm.D.
Assistant Professor in Clinical Pharmacology
University of Missouri–Kansas City
School of Medicine
Kansas City, Missouri

Charles W. Stratton, IV, M.D.
Professor
Departments of Pathology and Medicine
Vanderbilt University
Director, Clinical Microbiology Lab
Vanderbilt University Medical Center
Nashville, Tennessee

Albert Tran, M.D., Ph.D.
Professor in Hepato-Gastroenterology
Director of Hepato-Gastroenterology Federation
Medical School of Nice
University of Nice Sophia-Antipolis
Nice, France

John D. Turnidge, M.B.B.S., FRACP, FRCPA
Clinical Professor of Pathology and Pediatrics
University of Adelaide
Director, Microbiology and Infectious Diseases
Chief, Division of Laboratory Medicine
Women's and Children's Hospital
North Adelaide, Australia

Matthew A. Wikler, M.D.
Chief Medical Officer and Executive Vice President
Peninsula Pharmaceuticals, Inc.
Alameda, California
Chairholder, Subcommittee on Antimicrobial Susceptibility Testing
National Committee for Clinical Laboratory Procedures

ANTIBIOTICS IN LABORATORY MEDICINE

CHAPTER 1

The Breakpoint

Matthew A. Wikler and Paul G. Ambrose

WHAT IS A BREAKPOINT?

A breakpoint, in its simplest terms, represents the concentration of an antimicrobial that separates populations of microorganisms. Breakpoints are used in many ways, and so there may be more than one breakpoint for a specific antimicrobial-microorganism combination. It is also of interest that a breakpoint may change from time to time for a variety of reasons, as discussed later. In addition, breakpoints can vary from one country to another and from one official body to another (e.g., the National Committee for Clinical Laboratory Standards [NCCLS] versus the Food and Drug Administration [FDA]) within the same country. The determination of a specific breakpoint is not a black-and-white decision, as many factors must be considered when selecting breakpoints.

Breakpoints that are reported by clinical microbiology laboratories to assist physicians in selecting antimicrobial agents to treat patients are commonly referred to as antimicrobial susceptibility test interpretive categories. A result of "susceptible" implies that an infection due to the isolate may be appropriately treated with the dosage of an antimicrobial agent recommended for that type of infection and infecting species. A result of "resistant" implies that the isolate is not inhibited by the usually achievable concentrations of the agent with normal dosage schedules and/or falls in the range where specific microbial resistance mechanisms are likely and clinical efficacy has not been reliably attained in treatment studies. A result of "intermediate" implies that an infection due to the isolate may be appropriately treated in body sites where the drugs are physiologically concentrated or when a high dosage of the drug can be used. The category of "intermediate" is also used as a "buffer zone" to prevent small, uncontrolled technical factors from causing major discrepancies in interpretations (21).

WHY DO WE NEED BREAKPOINTS?

Ultimately, the purpose of breakpoints is to provide clinicians with vital information to assist in making decisions about antimicrobial treatments for patients with infections. Breakpoints serve many purposes, some of which are important for an individual patient, others for epidemiological reasons. If breakpoints did not result in better patient care, then there would be little need to determine them, other than as an academic exercise.

The remainder of this chapter focuses on breakpoints for bacteria, as these are currently the most advanced, and many of the principles apply to the setting of breakpoints for other types of microorganisms.

THE HISTORY OF BREAKPOINT SETTING

NCCLS has been setting standards for the testing of bacteria and breakpoints since 1975. Initially, breakpoints were set by examining scatterplots of the distributions of bacteria versus the results of susceptibility testing conducted with antibacterial agents. Such scatterplots would frequently divide the bacteria into two populations, one of which would appear to be more susceptible to the antibacterial being tested, the other less susceptible. The breakpoint would be the value separating the two populations. Setting breakpoints in such a manner is probably suitable for epidemiologic purposes, as it allows one to easily determine shifts in the populations of organisms and to identify the emergence of resistant populations. From a clinical perspective, however, such an approach does not take into account the clinical implications.

In an attempt to improve the manner of setting breakpoints, NCCLS put together a working group to develop a document to provide guidelines on how to determine breakpoints. The first version of this document was published in 1994 (19) and introduced the concept of looking at other types of data, including clinical data, in an attempt to correlate proposed breakpoints with what is likely to occur in the clinical setting. The most recent revision of this document was published in 2001 (20).

At the current time, so-called clinical breakpoints (antimicrobial susceptibility test interpretive categories) are determined by NCCLS utilizing the following types of information: microbiologic data, animal modeling data, pharmacokinetic (PK) and pharmacodynamic (PD) modeling data, and human clinical data. These data are all considered and compared one against the other. In an ideal world, these data would all correlate with one another so that a breakpoint could be determined with certainty.

The microbiologic data considered consist of distributions of organisms and their minimum inhibitory concentrations (MICs). Numerous distributions are evaluated including those for a broad spectrum of organisms against which the antimicrobial agent is likely to be utilized and those for select populations of organisms that have specific types of resistance mechanisms. As clinical studies are conducted with a new antimicrobial, the susceptibility patterns seen in actual patients enrolled in studies are also reviewed. By utilizing data of this type, one can gain a sense of the various populations of organisms that exist and their relative susceptibility to the antimicrobial agent. Clearly one would not want to set a breakpoint that bisects a large population of organisms.

Animal studies are quite useful in determining which targets one should be evaluating when trying to predict clinical efficacy. In the case of some of the more frequently used classes of antimicrobials, animal studies have demonstrated the ability to predict clinical efficacy by examining specific parameters (6). For example, it has been clearly demonstrated for β-lactam antibiotics that the most critical parameter predictive of clinical outcomes is the time that free drug plasma concentrations remain above the MIC of the causative organism (4,12,13). This is an example of a class of antibiotics where the predictive parameter is "time-dependent." For cephalosporin antibiotics and *Streptococcus pneumoniae,* it appears that clinical success is likely if the free drug concentration above the MIC of the causative organism is maintained for 40% to 50% of the dosing interval, while for penicillins the target appears to be 30% to 40% of the dosing interval (6).

The area under the drug-concentration time curve (AUC) is a measure of drug exposure. Mathematically, the AUC is calculated as the integral of the drug concentration-time curve. Response to drugs *in vivo* can usually be linked to the AUC. In some instances, the shape of the concentration-time curve can affect *in vivo* response to a drug, and thus other measures of exposure (e.g., C_{max}, C_{min}) can also be important. Fluoroquinolone antibiotics have been demonstrated in animal models to be "concentration-dependent"; that is, clinical outcomes can be predicted based on the ratio of AUC to MIC and/or by the ratio of the peak drug concentration to MIC. For such drugs, it appears that clinical success (3,7) depends on attaining a free drug AUC:MIC ratio of around 30 for Gram-positive organisms and around 100 for Gram-negative organisms (6,17).

Although these general targets tend to apply to many types of infections, one must keep in mind that levels obtained in certain tissues and body fluids may result in these targets not being predictive. For example, for drugs that are renally excreted and where active drug is concentrated in the urine, one would anticipate the ability to successfully treat organisms in the urinary tract with higher MICs. On the other hand, most drugs do not achieve high levels in the cerebrospinal fluid, and so one would anticipate that higher doses of an antimicrobial may be required to adequately treat an infection in that site. It would not be sufficient only to determine targets based on responses in animal models, and so it is important that the results of clinical studies be correlated with these targets. Such work has been done with β-lactam antibiotics and fluoroquinolones (3,5,6,16,17,23). Unfortunately, for new classes of antimicrobials, the correlations between the targets and the clinical outcomes in humans have yet to be well studied.

Once the target predicting clinical success has been identified, one can take PK data that have been developed for an antimicrobial and the MIC values likely to be of relevance for the infections to be treated and model numerous things. One of the best ways to conduct such an analysis is by using Monte Carlo techniques (8,10). Basically, the strategy is to take (a) the PK parameters along with anticipated variability and (b) the MIC values of organisms likely to cause an infection along with the proportion of time a specific MIC value is likely to be encountered and then model patients by randomly matching up PK profiles and MICs. By using such a technique, one can easily simulate 5,000 or 10,000 patients and make predictions as to what MICs one is likely to be able to treat successfully with various dosing regimens (1,11). Ideally, this process should be done in the earliest stages of drug development, as this allows one to determine the optimal dosing regimen likely to result in a successful clinical outcome while minimizing the potential for toxicity. Such modeling can also be utilized to justify the initial breakpoint for a new antimicrobial prior to the availability of a large amount of clinical data (2,9).

Ultimately, the purpose of breakpoints is to provide information to the clinician for the selection of optimal antimicrobial therapy. Because of this, it is critical to evaluate clinical data from well-designed clinical studies that allow the examination of the correlation of a breakpoint and the clinical outcomes. Unfortunately, this is far from an exact science, as there are many factors that determine clinical outcomes other than the antimicrobial used.

Consequently, clinical correlations are generally used to confirm susceptibility breakpoints predicted by the previously mentioned techniques and data.

For many reasons, the true limits of an antimicrobial are rarely tested in clinical studies conducted for the purpose of gaining regulatory approval. First, most of these studies exclude or discontinue patients whose infections are caused by organisms with an MIC above a tentative breakpoint. As a result, even if clinical studies could demonstrate a breakpoint, the probability of this happening is greatly reduced. In most cases, clinical studies can be ethically designed in a manner that would blind the investigator to susceptibility test results, allowing the decision to continue or discontinue therapy with the study drug to be determined by clinical and microbiological responses. Clinical studies so designed are more likely to aid in determining a clinical breakpoint. Another reason that breakpoints often fail to be determined by clinical data is that many of the newer antibiotics being developed are quite potent and only a small percentage of organisms will have MICs high enough to truly test their limits. In fact, few or no patients may be enrolled who have infections due to organisms with MICs at a sufficient level to uncover the limits of the antibiotic being evaluated.

SETTING BREAKPOINTS BY SITE OF INFECTION

It is sometimes necessary to consider the need for different breakpoints based on the site of the infection being treated. For example, the ability of a drug to get into the cerebrospinal fluid is frequently quite different from the ability of the same drug to get into the urine or into other tissues. As a result, it is reasonable to anticipate needing a different breakpoint for the treatment of meningitis or urinary tract infections than for the treatment of an infection in the lung.

As an example, consider the drug ceftizoxime. NCCLS has no breakpoint for this drug for *Pseudomonas aeruginosa* when the organism is isolated from sites outside of the urinary tract. On the other hand, the breakpoint for ceftizoxime for *P. aeruginosa* when isolated from the urine is listed as <8 μg/mL. In addition, NCCLS, in Table 1 of document M100, recommends that ceftizoxime be tested for urinary isolates of *P. aeruginosa* but does not recommend that this drug be tested when *P. aeruginosa* is isolated from any other site (22). Ceftizoxime is renally excreted as active drug into the urine, resulting in very high and long-lasting drug concentrations in the urine. Although ceftizoxime has limited activity against *P. aeruginosa,* the high concentrations of the drug in the urine are adequate to effectively treat infections in the urinary tract. NCCLS made this decision based on microbiological, PK/PD, and clinical data indicating that ceftizoxime is an effective drug for this use. Since similar data for the treatment of *P. aeruginosa* were unavailable to support its use for non-urinary-tract infections, no breakpoint was established for isolates obtained outside of the urinary tract.

SETTING BREAKPOINTS WHEN THERE ARE NO RESISTANT STRAINS

As previously noted, many of the newer antimicrobials being developed are very potent and few resistant strains exist. When there is a dearth of resistant strains, it is difficult to obtain animal or clinical data to determine the true breakpoint. In these circumstances, the breakpoint is generally set at one or two 2-tube dilutions above the known susceptible population of strains for that organism. In such a situation, a "susceptible" breakpoint is usually published, along with a notation that any strains isolated with a higher MIC should be sent to a reference laboratory to confirm the results. With time, a population of less susceptible strains will frequently emerge, and additional animal and clinical data may become available. At this point, it may become possible to establish a breakpoint reflective of the new situation.

CORRELATION BETWEEN MIC AND DISK ZONES

Many hospitals and laboratories do not do MIC testing but rather depend on disk diffusion susceptibility testing methods. In order to meet the needs of these institutions, breakpoints are set for disk diffusion methods by looking at correlations of MIC results and disk diffusion results. Once again, various types of distributions are looked at, including distributions for a broad spectrum of organisms against which the antimicrobial agent is likely to be used and for select populations of organisms that have specific types of resistance mechanisms. Statistical methods are generally utilized to determine the best correlation between disk zones and MICs. Once the disk zone breakpoint is statistically determined, the rates of discrepant results are evaluated (i.e., where one method predicts "susceptible" and the other predicts "resistant" or "intermediate"). The number of discrepancies that occur within one two-fold dilution of the "intermediate" MIC is less important than the number of discrepancies that occur at other MICs. After analysis of such discrepancies, the disk test may be adjusted to make it more predictive of the MIC test (i.e., by reducing the number of discrepancies). In some cases, it is impossible to develop a disk test that correlates with the MIC test. A recommendation is then made to not perform disk testing.

OVERRIDING THE BREAKPOINT

There are circumstances in which the breakpoint determined utilizing the standard methods is known to be inaccurate. When this occurs, the laboratory is instructed to override the results of the test and to adjust the report to the physician. For example, in recent years organisms that produce extended-spectrum β-lactamases (ESBLs) have started to emerge, and the standard testing methods could produce results indicating that the organism is "susceptible" to cephalosporins that are likely to be ineffective against such strains. As a result, NCCLS has developed methods to detect ESBL-producing strains. When such strains are detected, laboratories are instructed to override certain results (22). As new mechanisms of resistance develop, it is critical that organizations and agencies that produce standardized antimicrobial susceptibility testing methods and interpretive criteria be diligent in looking for circumstances where the results of such tests are not accurate.

THE USE OF SUSCEPTIBILITY TESTS OF ONE ANTIBIOTIC TO PREDICT ANOTHER

Laboratories often use testing systems developed by antimicrobial susceptibility testing manufacturers. Such testing systems may contain a panel of antibiotics that do not replicate the available agents in a particular hospital or within the formulary of a particular health care system. In such a case, a laboratory may wish to use the results for one antibiotic to predict the susceptibility of an organism to another similar antibiotic. This has been a common practice, for example, with various cephalosporin antibiotics. In Table 1 of NCCLS document M100 (22), there are suggestions as to when this may be possible. One must be aware that the correlations for certain types of organisms may be much better than for others within the same antibiotic class and that depending on one antimicrobial to predict another will invariably lead to some reporting errors. NCCLS will be evaluating such correlations to better characterize when such surrogate testing is appropriate.

WHY ARE THERE DIFFERENT BREAKPOINTS IN VARIOUS PARTS OF THE WORLD?

It is not uncommon to find that the clinical breakpoints for an antimicrobial-microorganism combination are different in different parts of the world. The reasons for this should become clear when one examines the variables involved in determining breakpoints. Breakpoints are set based on results achieved using a standardized testing method. If everyone used exactly the same testing method with good controls, the results would be expected to be similar. Unfortunately, testing methods are not currently standardized around the world, and thus there is the potential for different breakpoints to be established using different methods. Second, an antimicrobial might be used differently in different geographic areas. If it is customary to use an antimicrobial at a higher dose or to dose more frequently in one geographic area, the breakpoint will likely be higher in that area. Third, different microorganisms are encountered in different parts of the world. If resistant strains of bacteria have evolved in one geographic area but have not been seen or are not an issue in other areas, it may be necessary to adjust the breakpoints to ensure that the new resistant strains are being properly reported. There are also public health reasons why a breakpoint may vary. Public health authorities in one geographic area may want to avoid a resistance problem, deal with a resistance problem, or promote the use of certain antimicrobials over others. One way to impact antimicrobial use is to adjust breakpoints.

CURRENT EFFORTS TO DEVELOP STANDARDIZED METHODS AND BREAKPOINTS IN OTHER PARTS OF THE WORLD

Currently, efforts are being undertaken in various parts of the world to develop standardized methods for susceptibility testing. Ultimately, it would be ideal if one standardized testing method was accepted worldwide, as this would allow the direct comparison of results from one part of the world to another. The lack of harmonization of methods can create significant problems when evaluating epidemiologic trends. For example, suppose the goal is to examine the development of resistance for a particular organism and its spread in various parts of the world. The use of different methods makes it impossible to ascertain the true level of resistance. Even if one standardized testing method was accepted and utilized throughout the world, it is likely that there would still be different clinical breakpoints, for the reasons noted previously.

Another problem resulting from the lack of standardized methods for susceptibility testing concerns the development of new antibiotics. When conducting clinical trials and looking for correlations between outcomes and MICs or disk zones, it is necessary to use the same methods wherever the drug is tested.

The European Committee on Antimicrobial Susceptibility Testing (EUCAST) is a standing committee of the European Society of Clinical Microbiology and Infectious Diseases (ESCMID). EUCAST was set up to standardize susceptibility testing in Europe so that comparable results and interpretations would be produced. It has both a general committee, whose membership includes representatives from all European countries, from the pharmaceutical industry, and from the *in vitro* media and device industries, and an ESCMID-appointed steering committee, which consists of a chair, a scientific secretary, six National Breakpoint Committee representatives, and two representatives from the general committee. Decisions are made by the steering committee after consultation with the general committee (ESCMID website, www.escmid.org). Unlike the NCCLS, which develops only clinical breakpoints, EUCAST is in the process of developing both epidemiological and clinical breakpoints. Epidemiological breakpoints are breakpoints that differentiate the wild-type strains from strains that have developed resistance. Epidemiological breakpoints can be extremely valuable when one wants to evaluate the emergence of resistant populations of organisms. The methods used by EUCAST (14,15) are in general agreement with those of the NCCLS. EUCAST has been collecting MIC distribution data from worldwide sources for the purposes of establishing epidemiological breakpoints. This extensive database is available on the EUCAST website (www.eucast.org).

WHY THE BREAKPOINTS OF NCCLS AND THE FDA MAY DIFFER

At times, breakpoints contained in the FDA-approved package insert for an antimicrobial agent do not agree with the breakpoints published in NCCLS documents. There are many reasons why this may occur, including differences in the interpretation of data and differences in how the two organizations function. When a new antimicrobial agent is approved by the FDA, interpretive criteria utilizing the NCCLS standardized methods are approved and included in the product label. Most pharmaceutical sponsors will also submit a package of data to NCCLS within a year of a new drug approval requesting breakpoints. Although there is generally agreement between the FDA and NCCLS, at times there are differences based on interpretation of the data. It is common for differences to occur after an antimicrobial has been on the market for a few years, as new resistance mechanisms become apparent requiring a re-evaluation of the breakpoint. Unlike the FDA, NCCLS has the ability to review breakpoints for any antimicrobial when there appears to be a need to do so. As a result, NCCLS will make changes in single drugs or will frequently evaluate a class of drugs at the same time and make whatever adjustments seem necessary. Currently, the FDA generally considers a change in a breakpoint only when the sponsor submits a package to the FDA requesting a change. FDA staff participate in NCCLS meetings as members, advisors, and observers. Sponsors are encouraged to submit new data to the FDA to allow for updating the product label.

The natural question arising from this is which breakpoints will clinical laboratories in the United States use? When there are published NCCLS breakpoints, US laboratories use these breakpoints when testing organisms and providing reports to physicians. In fact, US laboratories are tested and accredited based on their compliance with NCCLS methods and interpretive standards.

THE IMPORTANCE OF QUALITY CONTROL

The ability of the laboratory to follow the standardized testing methods utilized for setting breakpoints and the ability of the automated testing system to replicate the results that would be obtained utilizing the standard methods are critically important. Clearly, if such methods are not followed and well controlled, then the MIC or disk zone reported may be inaccurate, potentially resulting in a misinterpretation and inaccurate reporting to the health care provider. For this reason, care must be taken in performing these tests, and proper quality control must be implemented. In order to help the laboratory, NCCLS and other organizations that produce documents outlining standardized methods provide quality control ranges for various standard bacterial strains tested against specific antibiotics. It is critical to ensure that the test performed on the quality control strains produces results that are within the accepted ranges. In addition, the laboratory must make certain that the breakpoints applied are those based on the methods that are being utilized. It is also critical that growth of the bacterial strain is sufficient for an accurate MIC or disk zone to be obtained. That is why it is necessary to have a control well or area on the test plate where the bacterial strain can grow uninfluenced by the antimicrobial agent.

HOW TO REPORT AND USE BREAKPOINTS

Although breakpoint information is valuable when used for a specific patient, it can also have an impact on antimicrobial selection for a much larger group of patients. Most antimicrobial use is empiric; that is, a patient appears with what seems to be a bacterial infection, and the physician prescribes an antimicrobial agent without knowledge of the causative organism or its susceptibility. If the laboratory periodically collects its susceptibility testing data, summarizes such data, and distributes them to its physicians, then physicians are in a better position to prescribe antimicrobials likely to be successful. Most hospitals publish an antibiogram once or twice a year just for this purpose. There are numerous things one must consider when constructing antibiograms, and NCCLS document M39-A (18) provides a guideline to help laboratories in developing them.

WHY DO BREAKPOINTS CHANGE?

Although epidemiological breakpoints tend to be static, clinical breakpoints are not. There are numerous reasons why a breakpoint may need to be changed, and many of them are outlined in NCCLS document M23 (20):

1. Strains less susceptible and/or more resistant to an antimicrobial agent may develop.
2. Organisms with new mechanisms of resistance may develop.
3. New dosages or formulations of an antimicrobial agent and/or new clinical uses may require a change.
4. New clinical and/or pharmacological data may suggest the need for reassessment.
5. Actions by and/or data from the FDA or other regulatory authorities, the CDC, the College of American Pathologists, or other sources may suggest the need for reassessment.
6. Changes in NCCLS-approved reference methods may have an impact on interpretive criteria and/or quality control parameters.
7. Other *in vitro* testing may suggest the need for reassessment.
8. Changes may also be made when public health concerns require action in situations where clinical information is limited.

PUBLIC HEALTH CONSIDERATIONS

The setting of breakpoints has an impact not only on individual patients but on public health. The breakpoints will determine how antimicrobials will be perceived to work against specific organisms. As a result, when a physician receives an antibiogram of the susceptibility patterns of the organisms in his or her hospital and/or the local community, the physician's antimicrobial use patterns may be affected. Since the vast majority of bacterial infections are treated empirically, physicians depend on the antibiogram to direct their selection of initial antimicrobial therapy. If a breakpoint is changed and the change results in a commonly used antimicrobial no longer appearing to be efficacious, this may lead physicians to alter their prescribing habits. As a result, one class of drugs may end up being substituted for another. This shift in antimicrobial use can have an impact on future resistance patterns in the hospital and the community. For example, the low MIC that currently defines resistance for penicillin against *S. pneumoniae* has led to a greater use of vancomycin. The increased use of vancomycin in hospitals seems to have led to an increase in the incidence of vancomycin-resistant enterococci. In addition, if a change in a breakpoint leads to the use of more expensive antimicrobials, there is an economic impact on the health care system. Clearly, there are important economic and health consequences when a breakpoint change results in the development of more problematic and difficult-to-treat organisms. These potential issues must be carefully considered when setting and/or changing breakpoints.

NEED FOR GREATER UNDERSTANDING OF BREAKPOINTS

As stated previously, the primary reason for breakpoints is to provide information to health care providers that will allow for the selection of antimicrobials likely to successfully treat infections. If a health care provider does not understand what the susceptibility report means, nor understands the assumptions that underlie the report, then the actions taken may not be optimal for the patient. For example, if the breakpoint is set based on a specific dose of an antimicrobial being used, and if the physician uses a lower dose, then the actual clinical result may not be as anticipated. It is critical that efforts be made to properly communicate to health care providers what breakpoints mean and the assumptions that go into these interpretive standards. Information concerning some of the assumptions made in selecting breakpoints is contained in the documents and tables developed by NCCLS and other standards-setting organizations. Unfortunately, this information rarely is communicated to physicians. If breakpoints are to be optimally utilized to maximize patient care, greater communication and education must occur. The education process could involve scientific publications that specifically discuss the decisions made by NCCLS and other standards-setting organizations and the rationale for the decisions and the assumptions made. Such publications would likely be of interest primarily to microbiologists, infectious disease physicians, and hospital epidemiologists. These health care professionals should then convey the information they acquire to physicians through local educational activities.

In summary, breakpoints allow microbiology laboratories to provide valuable information to clinicians for the optimal selection of antimicrobial therapies. Epidemiological breakpoints make it easier to detect the emergence of resistant populations of bacteria. Clinical breakpoints may vary due to differences in testing methods and in how antimicrobials are used in different parts of the world. Health care providers must be knowledgeable about the assumptions that go into the setting of breakpoints if they are to utilize such information to optimize patient care.

REFERENCES

1. Ambrose PG, Craig WA, Bhavnani BM, et al. Pharmacodynamic comparisons of different dosing regimens of penicillin G against penicillin-susceptible and -resistant pneumonococci. In: Program and abstracts of the 42nd Interscience Conference on Antimicrobial Agents and Chemotherapy; September 27–30; San Diego, CA. Abstract A-635.
2. Ambrose PG, Grasela DM. The use of Monte Carlo simulation to examine the pharmacodynamic variance of drugs: fluoroquinolones against Streptococcus pneumoniae. *Diagn Microbiol Infect Dis* 2000;38:151–157.

3. Ambrose PG, Grasela DM, Grasela TH, et al. Pharmacodynamics of fluoroquinolones against *Streptococcus pneumoniae* in patients with community-acquired respiratory tract infections. *Antimicrob Agents Chemother* 2001;45:2793–2797.
4. Andes D, Craig WA. In vivo activities of amoxicillin and amoxicillin-clavulanate against *Streptococcus pneumoniae:* application to breakpoint determinations. *Antimicrob Agents Chemother* 1998;2375–2379.
5. Bodey GP, Ketchel SJ, Rodriguez N. A randomized study of carbenicillin plus cefamandole or tobramycin in the treatment of febrile episodes in cancer patients. *Am J Med* 1979;67:608–616.
6. Craig WA. Pharmacodynamics of antimicrobials: general concept and applications. In: Nightigale CH, Murakawa T, Ambrose PG., eds. *Antimicrobial pharmacodynamics in theory and clinical practice.* New York: Marcel-Dekker, 2002:1–22.
7. Craig WA, Andes DR. Correlation of the magnitude of the AUC24/MIC for 6 fluoroquinolones against *Streptococcus pneumoniae* with survival and bactericidal activity in an animal model. In: Program and abstracts of the 40th Interscience Conference on Antimicrobial Agents and Chemotherapy; September Toronto, Canada. 2000;17–21.
8. Drusano GL. Antimicrobial pharmacodynamics: critical interactions between "drug and bug." *Nat Rev Microbiol* 2004;2:289–300.
9. Drusano GL, Preston SL, Hardalo C, et al. Use of preclinical data for selection of a phase II/III dose for evernimicin and identification of a preclinical MIC breakpoint. *Antimicrob Agents Chemother* 2001;45:13–22.
10. Dudley MN, Ambrose PG. Pharmacodynamics in the study of resistance and establishing in vitro susceptibility breakpoints: ready for primetime. *Curr Opin Microbiol* 2000;3:515–521.
11. Dudley MN, Ambrose PG. Monte Carlo simulation and new cefotaxime, ceftriaxone, and cefepime breakpoints for *S. pneumoniae,* including strains with reduced susceptibility to penicillin. In: Program and abstracts of the 42nd Interscience Conference on Antimicrobial Agents and Chemotherapy; September 27–30; San Diego, CA. Abstract A-1263.
12. Eagle H. Effect of schedule of administration on therapeutic efficacy of penicillin: importance of aggregate time penicillin remains at effective bactericidal levels. *Am J Med* 1950;9:280–299.
13. Eagle H, Fleischman R, Levy M. Continuous vs. discontinuous therapy with penicillin. *N Engl J Med* 1953;238:481–486.
14. EUCAST Definitive Document E. Def 2.1. Determination of antimicrobial susceptibility test breakpoints. *Clin Microbiol Infect* 2000;6:570–572.
15. EUCAST Definitive Document E. Def 3.1. Determination of minimum inhibitory concentrations (MICs) of antibacterial agents by agar dilution. *Clin Microbiol Infect* 2000;6:509–515.
16. Forrest A, Chodash S, Amantae MA, et al. Pharmacokinetics and pharmacodynamics of oral grepafloxacin in patients with acute exacerbation of chronic bronchitis. *J Antimicrob Chemother* 1997;40(suppl A):45–57.
17. Forrest A, Nix DE, Ballow CH, et al. Pharmacodynamics of ciprofloxacin in seriously ill patients. *Antimicrob Agents Chemother* 1993;37:1073–1081.
18. National Committee for Clinical Laboratory Standards. *Analysis and presentation of cumulative antimicrobial susceptibility test data.* Wayne, PA: National Committee for Clinical Laboratory Standards, 2002. NCCLS document M39-A.
19. National Committee for Clinical Laboratory Standards. *Development of in vitro susceptibility testing criteria and quality control parameters.* Villanova, PA: National Committee for Clinical Laboratory Standards, 1994. NCCLS document M23-A.
20. National Committee for Clinical Laboratory Standards. *Development of in vitro susceptibility testing criteria and quality control parameters.* Wayne, PA: National Committee for Clinical Laboratory Standards, 2001. NCCLS document M-23-A2.
21. National Committee for Clinical Laboratory Standards. *Methods for dilution antimicrobial susceptibility tests for bacteria that grow aerobically.* Wayne, PA: National Committee for Clinical Laboratory Standards, 2003. NCCLS document M7-A6.
22. National Committee for Clinical Laboratory Standards. *Performance standards for antimicrobial susceptibility testing: fourteen informational supplements.* Wayne, PA: National Committee for Clinical Laboratory Standards, 2004. NCCLS document M100-S14.
23. Preston SL, Drusano GL, Berman AL, et al. Pharmacodynamics of levofloxacin: a new paradigm for early clinical trials. *JAMA* 1997;279:125–129.

CHAPTER 2

Antimicrobial Susceptibility on Solid Media

John D. Turnidge and Jan M. Bell

Susceptibility testing on solid media is a widely used alternative to the traditional broth-based testing developed originally to measure minimum inhibitory concentrations. With rare exceptions, it relies on the use of agar as the solidifying agent and the nature of agar, which permits slow diffusion of chemicals through its three-dimensional matrix. There are now three formats for testing using solid media: agar dilution, disk diffusion, and gradient diffusion. Of these, the one that has proven most popular and adaptable to routine laboratory testing is disk diffusion. It has been the subject of excellent chapters in previous editions of this book (1,2).

FEATURES OF SOLIDIFYING AGENTS

Solidifying agents for susceptibility testing and culture media generally need the following features to be useful: (a) water solubility, (b) ability to remain solid above incubation temperatures (≤42°C), (c) ability to liquefy at higher temperatures to permit pouring and incorporation of additives, (d) chemical inertness, (e) relative transparency, and (f) resistance to bacterial degradative enzymes.

Agar

Agar is a natural product obtained from several red seaweeds from the Rhodophyceae class. It takes its name from the Malay word *agar-agar*, which describes these seaweeds. The most widely harvested and used are *Gelidium* species and *Gracilariopsis lemaneiformis*. Agar also has wide application in the food industry as thickening and emulsifying agents. Agar liquefies when heated to boiling and does not gel until cooled to 45°C–50°C. After gelling, it requires reheating to near boiling to liquefy again.

The principal components of agar are the polysaccharides agarose and agaropectin. Purified agarose has become one of the mainstays of electrophoretic analysis. As a natural product, agar is subject to lot-to-lot variation. Variation occurs in the presence of sulfate ions, which affect the overall negative charge of the polysaccharides, which in turn can affect diffusion of certain chemicals. Calcium, essential in small amounts to permit gelling, and other trace elements also affect the activity of certain antimicrobials and can also vary in content.

Other Solidifying Agents

A range of other gelling agents have been experimented with over the years, but none has yet displaced agar for susceptibility tests. In part this relates to cost but also to the daunting challenge of recalibrating endpoints (minimul inhibitory concentrations [MICs], zone diameters) for a very broad range of bacteria and drugs. Substances examined include Separan NP10, a polyacrylamide that allows smaller concentrations of agar to be used, Gelrite, a gellan gum formed from the fermentation products of a *Pseudomonas* species, and Neutra-Gel, a polyoxyethylene polymer that held the greatest promise when combined with a synthetic amino acid medium. Gelrite is the only one still available commercially (Merck & Co., Kelco Division, Rahway, NJ).

FEATURES AND CHOICE OF AGAR

The two main media used for conventional bacteria are Mueller-Hinton and Iso-Sensitest. Which medium is advocated depends on which side of the Atlantic is making the case. North America has preferred Mueller-Hinton, in large part because it was the medium selected for disk susceptibility testing when it was first standardized in the United States by Bauer et al. (17). Curiously, the medium was originally developed for the cultivation of *Neisseria* species. A large number of criticisms have been leveled at Mueller-Hinton over the years. Its problems include the possibility of different MIC values in broth versus the agar version, antagonism of tetracyclines, high levels of folate synthesis inhibitor antagonists, variation in performance between manufacturers due to difference in peptone sources, poor support for streptococcal species, and variable growth rates with Gram-positive bacteria generally (109). Almost of these problems have been overcome through the intensive efforts of investigators and manufacturers toward its standardization, including intensive quality control procedures (94) and the development of "golden pound" reference lots (101). The principal problem with Mueller-Hinton was the variability in the concentrations of Ca^{++} and Mg^{++} cations, which can have significant effects on the activity of aminoglycosides, especially against *Pseudomonas aeruginosa*. This has now been overcome during the manufacturing process, and the concentrations are adjusted to within an acceptable range specified by the National Committee for Clinical Laboratory Standards (NCCLS) (101). Nevertheless, Mueller-Hinton continues to be criticized by some (151).

Iso-Sensitest agar is a common choice in European countries, except in France and Germany, where Mueller-Hinton is favored. In an attempt to reach common ground, the European Committee for Antimicrobial Susceptibility Testing (EUCAST) of the European Society for Clinical Microbiology and Infectious Diseases has tentatively recommended Mueller-Hinton for agar dilution testing (54). Iso-Sensitest was developed by Oxoid from the original Diagnostic Sensitivity Test agar and then Sensitest agar and is designed to minimize the amount of variable nutrients and maximize the defined components. To a lesser extent, problems have been encountered over the years in the performance of Iso-Sensitest (137). PDM Antibiotic Sensitivity Medium, long recommended (along with Iso-Sensitest) by the Swedish Reference Group on Antibiotics (131), has recently been withdrawn from the market (A. Bolmström, personal communication, January 2004).

The medium recommended for anaerobe susceptibility testing is Brucella agar or Wilkins-Chalgren (5,94,102). Less attention has been paid overall to the suitability of different media for anaerobes. Recent studies by a number of investigators have shown that supplemented Brucella agar supports the growth of a wider range of anaerobes than other media (65,116,117) and is now recommended as the reference medium by NCCLS (102).

There are considerable differences in the formulas of different agars (Table 2.1).

FACTORS IN AGAR COMPOSITION

Antagonists of Folate Synthesis Inhibitors

Paraaminobenzoic acid (*p*-ABA) is a potent inhibitor of sulfonamides. Concentrations found in certain media such as peptone water and nutrient agar will virtually eliminate sulfonamide activity (145). Susceptibility testing agar used in any of the current published methods has minimal concentrations of *p*-ABA.

Thymidine and thymine in sufficient concentrations antagonize the dihydrofolate reductase inhibitors such as trimethoprim, increasing MICs and reducing zone diameters in agar diffusion tests. This nucleoside and its pyrimidine base possibly act by competing for the target enzyme. Thymidine is by far the more potent of the two, and methods to reduce or eliminate its presence in agar will restore DHFR inhibitor activity. Indeed, one common method is to use lysed horse blood, which is rich in the enzyme thymidine phosphorylase, which converts thymidine to thymine and 2-deoxyribose-1-phosphate. Further, most bacteria, except *Enterococcus faecalis,* cannot utilize thymine as a substrate (145). Some bacterial strains require thymidine for growth and will grow poorly or not at all on susceptibility testing agar. Because such strains are naturally DHFR inhibitor–resistant, no problems of testing occur when thymidine is added back into the medium.

Although Mueller-Hinton agar is purportedly low in thymidine and thymine, occasionally problems can arise. NCCLS has developed a quality control procedure to test for low thymidine content using either of two ATCC strains of *E. faecalis* and trimethoprim-sulfamethoxazole disks (105).

Calcium, Magnesium, and Zinc

The divalent cations of calcium (Ca^{++}) and magnesium (Mg^{++}) are well-known antagonists of aminoglycosides. The antagonism is complex and cannot simply be accounted for by the concentrations of the cations themselves (146). It appears to be affected to a large extent by other constituents such as sodium chloride and phosphate. The effects are most obvious when testing *P. aeruginosa* (43,113,144). The variability of concentrations in Mueller-Hinton agar in the past has been one reason that certain European countries have favored Iso-Sensitest agar, where the divalent cation concentrations are defined in the formulation. However, this is more an issue for broth than for agar, as agar is processed to remove free cations and anions (109), although recent studies have demonstrated that there can still be a wide range of calcium and magnesium concentrations in different batches of Mueller-Hinton agar (58). Further, this problem has been controlled to some extent by the manufacture of

TABLE 2.1

Formulations of Agar Media Used in Current Susceptibility Testing Methods

	Mueller-Hinton	Iso-Sensitest	Diagnostic Sensitivity Test	Sensitest	Wilkins-Chalgren	Brucella
Protein source	Dehydrated beef infusion 300 g/L (or similar) Hydrolysed casein 17.5 g/L	Hydrolysed casein 11 g/L Peptones 3 g/L	Proteose peptone 10 g/L Veal infusion solids 10 g/L	Hydrolysed casein 11 g/L Peptones 3 g/L	Tryptone 10 g/L Gelatin peptone 10 g/L	Peptone 10 g/L Dehydrated meat extract 5 g/L
Sugars		Glucose 2 g/L	Glucose 2 g/L	Glucose 2 g/L	Glucose 1 g/L	Glucose 10 g/L
Starch	1.5 g/L	1 g/L		1 g/L		
Sodium chloride		3 g/L	3 g/L	3 g/L		5 g/L
Buffers		Sodium acetate 1 g/L Disodium hydrogen phosphate 2 g/L	Sodium acetate 1 g/L Disodium phosphate 2 g/L	Buffer salts 3.3 g/L		
Calcium	Supplement after autoclaving	Calcium gluconate 0.1 g/L				
Magnesium	Supplement after autoclaving	Magnesium glycerophosphate 0.2 g/L				
Metal salts		Cobaltous sulfate 0.001 g/L Cupric sulfate 0.001 g/L Zinc sulfate 0.001 g/L Ferrous sulfate 0.001 g/L Manganous chloride 0.002 g/L				
Yeast extract					5 g/L	
Vitamins		Menadione 0.001 g/L Cyanocobalamin 0.001 g/L		Thiamine 0.00002 g/L	Menadione 0.0005 g/L Haemin 0.005 g/L	
Amino acids		L-Cysteine hydrochloride 0.02 g/L L-Tryptophan 0.02 g/L Pyridoxine 0.003 g/L Pantothenate 0.003 g/L Nicotinamide 0.003 g/L Biotin 0.0003 g/L Thiamine 0.00004 g/L	Aneurine 0.00002 g/L		L-Arginine 1 g/L Sodium pyruvate 1 g/L	
Nucleosides		Adenine 0.01 g/L Guanine 0.01 g/L Xanthine 0.01 g/L Uracil 0.01 g/L	Adenine sulfate 0.01 g/L Guanine hydrochloride 0.01 g/L Uracil 0.01 g/L	Nucleoside bases 0.02 g/L		
Agar	17 g/L (12–18 g/L)	8 g/L	12 g/L	8 g/L	10 g/L	15 g/L
pH	7.3 ± 0.2	7.4 ± 0.2	7.4 ± 0.2	7.4 ± 0.02	7.1 ± 0.2	7.5 ± 0.2

all Mueller-Hinton lots to a standard that ties their performance characteristics to a primary reference medium (101). In this reference standard, the concentration of divalent cations is not stipulated; rather the NCCLS disk diffusion method is used to compare the zones of a range of control bacterial strains generated with the newly manufactured lot to those of the primary reference medium and subsequently to those of a secondary reference medium. Other susceptibility test media have not been subject to control of their divalent cations, and the reproducibility of aminoglycoside results with different lots has not been examined. Calcium and magnesium concentrations can also affect the action of tetracycline against *Pseudomonas* species, although this of little importance, as tetracyclines are not considered clinically active.

The concentration of Ca^{++} is critical to the interpretation of daptomycin susceptibility (58). Daptomycin activity varies greatly with Ca^{++} concentration, and specified concentrations are required in the media (usually those seen physiologically). For this reason, daptomycin has not yet been completely standardized for tests in agar, and supplementation is required for broth testing (57).

High levels of zinc can reduce the *in vitro* activity of carbapenems (32). The effect is greatest with *P. aeruginosa,* but some other Gram-negatives are known to be affected to a minor extent. The zinc concentration is defined in the Iso-Sensitest formulation, and it is now controlled for in the manufacture of Mueller-Hinton lots by testing imipenem against *P. aeruginosa*.

Sodium Chloride

Less well known is the effect of sodium chloride concentration on the activity of aminoglycosides (22,93). As summarized by Waterworth (146), variations in NaCl can have quite significant effects: an increase in concentration from 22 to 174 mM can increase the MIC of gentamicin by as much as 32-fold. NaCl is not part of the Mueller-Hinton formulation, but the manufacture to a reference standard at least generates consistent results. NaCl is part of the Iso-Sensitest formulation, but viable amounts could also come from the hydrolyzed casein and peptones.

pH

Major variation in the pH of the medium can result in major changes in the activity of aminoglycosides, macrolides, and tetracyclines. Aminoglycoside activity is substantially increased in alkaline conditions and substantially inhibited in acidic conditions. Similar effects are observed with macrolides. Susceptibility testing agars are manufactured to performance standards of pH, and in some testing methods, such as those of NCCLS, it is recommended to confirm the pH in the cooled, prepoured state or with a surface pH meter after pouring, once the agar has been prepared from the dried powder in the routine laboratory.

The pH effect does become significant, however, when agar plates are incubated in increased concentrations of CO_2, such is recommended for streptococci and *Haemophilus* species in most methods. Rosenblatt and Schoenknecht have shown an increase in pH from 7.4 to 8.4 over a period of 24 hours when Mueller-Hinton blood agar plates are incubated in 5% to 7% CO_2 in air (120). Carbon dioxide is absorbed onto the surface during incubation, some of which will be converted to carbonic acid initially and then carbonate ions, first decreasing and later increasing the pH at the surface (120). Acidity is known to reduce the activity of macrolides in particular (including the azalides and ketolides) (20,45,62,78,114,129) and of aminoglycosides to some extent (115,139) while increasing the activity of tetracyclines (2). In agar-based tests, this effect will result in higher MICs and smaller zones for macrolides and aminoglycosides, as the pH at the surface will be more acidic at the critical time.

Additives

Some bacterial species require the addition of specific nutrients to ensure adequate growth. The most common of these is blood, usually sheep or horse blood, at a concentration of 5%. When testing sulfonamides, horse blood is preferred, as it is low in sulfonamide antagonists. Specific reagent additives are required for staphylococci when testing antistaphylococcal penicillins (in agar dilution but not disk diffusion), for *Haemophilus* species, and for *Neisseria gonorrhoeae* and in the NCCLS reference method for testing anaerobes. Specific details are given under the description of the methods below.

Defined Growth Supplement

One important additive, noted here and in NCCLS documents as *defined growth supplement*, is a complex mixture of vitamins, cofactors, and other nutrient substances. The two most recognizable and important brands are IsoVitaleX (Becton-Dickinson) and Vitox (Oxoid). These products contain 1.1 g L-cystine, 0.03 g guanine, 3 mg thiamine HCl, 13 mg *p*-ABA, 0.001–0.012 g vitamin B_{12}, 0.1 g cocarboxylase, 0.25 g NAD, 1.0 g adenine, 10 g L-glutamine, 100 g glucose, 0.02 g ferric nitrate, and 25.9 mg cysteine HCl per liter of water. It is most commonly used at a 1% concentration to ensure the growth of the fastidious organisms, especially *N. gonorrhoeae.*

PNPG and Other Antiswarming Agents

Paranitrophenylglycerol (PNPG) has been used among other techniques to prevent the swarming of *Proteus mirabilis* and *Proteus vulgaris* across agar surfaces. This is mostly a problem for agar dilution testing when multiple strains including strains of these two species are being tested on a single series of plates. As a result of the swarming, spots close to the *Proteus* species can be difficult or impossible to read. However, PNPG has been shown to affect the MIC results of a number of bacterial species and antimicrobials, especially *P. aeruginosa* (142,143).

A second antiswarming agent, Dispersol LN, has also been evaluated and shown to affect the activity of some antimicrobials (150). The addition of PNPG or another antiswarming agent is no longer recommended routinely in any method and should only be used if there are data to show that the agent does not interfere with the MICs of that organism-antimicrobial combination.

Higher concentrations of agar (e.g., 2%) can be used to inhibit swarming. None of the three options—use of PNPG, use of Dispersol LN, or increasing the concentration of agar—is now recommended.

Strains with Special Growth Requirements

Special problems arise with strains or species with unusual growth requirements. The so-called nutritionally variant "streptococci" *Abiotrophia defectiva* (*Streptococcus defectivus*) and *Granulicatella adiacens* (*Streptococcus adjacens, Abiotrophia adiacens*) require pyridoxal for growth. Media can be supplemented with pyridoxal (0.001%) and lysed horse blood to ensure growth of the strains (94,100,138,153) and allow interpretation of MICs at least (no breakpoints have been determined).

Occasionally, mutant strains of *Staphylococcus aureus* will depend on thiamine or menadione (vitamin K_3) for growth. These often exhibit small colonies on primary isolation. The addition of thiamine (2 mg/L) and menadione (0.5 mg/L) to susceptibility testing media will allow susceptibility (MIC) tests to be performed (3).

Strains of *Escherichia coli* and other Gram-negatives dependent on thymine for growth are sometimes encountered. They can be selected for during treatment with folate synthesis inhibitors (136).

AGAR DILUTION SUSCEPTIBILITY TESTING

Agar dilution susceptibility testing is the solid equivalent of broth dilution susceptibility testing, either in macro- or microbroth format. One advantage it offers over broth-based methods is that it allows the simultaneous testing of a large number of strains on a single agar plate, for example, 32 on a 90 mm plate using a Steers-Foltz or similar replicator (Fig. 2.1). It is therefore well suited to the rapid evaluation of new compounds or for large-scale centralized surveillance programs. The comparative disadvantages of this method are that it includes an additional variable (agar) in the medium and that, once prepared, the plates have a limited shelf life owing to degradation of the antimicrobial.

In the standard approach to determining MICs, the antimicrobial is incorporated into molten agar over a series of twofold dilutions, gently rotated to ensure even distribution of the antimicrobial, and then poured into plates. Detailed methods have been published, based on national standards (5,48,94,103), and these are outlined in Tables 2.6 and 2.7, which appear later in the chapter. With minor variations, the tentative European standard resembles the

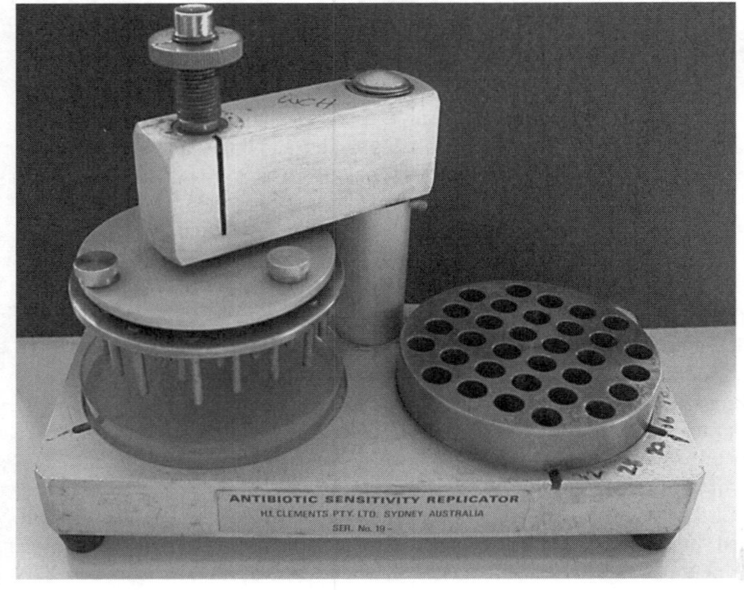

FIGURE 2.1 ● Replicator for agar dilution.

NCCLS standard (54). Each describes the crucial steps to achieving accurate and reproducible results. These are as follows.

Antimicrobial Powders

Antimicrobial powders should be obtained as "pure substance" from the manufacturer or from a reputable chemical supplier (e.g., Sigma Chemical Company). It is not acceptable to use powders found in vials for parenteral drug administration, as these may contain preservatives, surfactants, or fillers that interfere with the antimicrobial activity, and their contents may vary legally by as much as 10% above or below the label amount. Each powder should come with an expiration date and an indication of its potency and (sometimes) water content. It is vital that all these data be taken into account before preparation of stock solutions. Data should also be available from the manufacturer or another reliable source on choice of solvent and solubility before preparing stock solutions.

Powders should be stored as recommended by the manufacturer. If no instructions for storage are available, then store powders at −20°C in a desiccator, preferably under vacuum (103). This will ensure the product retains its potency for the maximum time.

Choice of Dilution Range

Before preparing stock solutions, it is essential that an appropriate dilution range be chosen. Suggested ranges for different species or bacterial types have been published (5). A full range is generally 10–12 doubling dilutions. Doubling dilutions are appropriate, as they provide the narrowest integer series on a logarithmic scale, and MICs for a single bug-drug combination are log-normally distributed in the absence of a resistance mechanism. Although any series could be used, the most widely accepted doubling dilution series is that of base 2. This implies that preferably the highest concentration (the concentration at the start) should be a power of 2 (e.g., $2^7 = 128$). Following this pattern will allow comparison with the majority of published data and MICs for published quality control strains.

Preparation of Stock Solutions

Stock solutions should be prepared by weighing out the *exact amount* of powder using a balance designed for milligram amounts. Ideally, amounts less than 100 mg should not be weighed out. Alternatively, an approximate amount can be weighed out, and using the formula below, the *exact volume* can be added. The amount weighed is calculated using the formula

$$W = \frac{V \times C}{P}$$

where W = weighted amount, V = volume of stock solution required, C = concentration of solution required, and P = potency in μg/mg. Usually, a potency value is provided. If not, it will need to be calculated from the values provided in the certificate of analysis. These values are purity (as measured, e.g., by HPLC), water content (as measured, e.g., by Karl Fisher analysis), and active fraction, which will be lower for salts than for free acids or bases.

$$\text{Potency} = \text{Purity} \times \text{Active Fraction} \times (1 - \text{Water Content } (\%))$$

The choice of final concentration will depend on whether the antimicrobial is being used immediately or whether it is intended for aliquotting and storage. Stock solutions for storage are best prepared as a tenfold concentration of the highest dilution being used. Concentration choices will also be determined by the solubility of the antimicrobial. Stock solutions should stored frozen at −20°C or lower and only thawed once before use; any unused thawed stock should be discarded.

Some antimicrobial agents require special solvents to achieve the high concentrations required in stock solutions. A comprehensive list of appropriate solvents and diluents is provided in Table 2.2.

Preparation of Dilution Range

In order to avoid compounding minor errors in pipetting that would occur if low volumes were used or with repeated dilution, dispensing and dilution schemes such as those recommended by NCCLS (103), the British Society for Antimicrobial Chemotherapy (BSAC) (5), EUCAST (54), and the Deutches Intitut für Normung (DIN) (48) should be followed. These are adaptations of the original dilution scheme proposed by Ericsson and Sherris (53). An antimicrobial-free control plate should be added to any dilution series for quality control (i.e., to ensure that the selected strains are indeed viable).

Agar Selection

The description of each method identifies which agar media to use for particular bacterial groups or species. As all subsequent interpretations depend on data generated from these media, the nominated media for each method must be used. The range of media specified for each method are listed in Table 2.3.

Preparation of Agar Plates

Mueller-Hinton or Iso-Sensitest agars are prepared from a dehydrated base following the manufacturer's instructions with regard to amounts of base, water, and autoclaving. After autoclaving, bottles should be cooled to 45°C to

(*text continues on page 17*)

TABLE 2.2

Solvents and Diluents Used for Stock Solution Preparation

Antimicrobial Agent (Form)	Solvent	Diluent
Amikacin	Water	Water
Amoxicillin (trihydrate)	Phosphate buffer, pH 6.0, 0.1 mol/L	Phosphate buffer, pH 6.0, 0.1 mol/L
or	Dimethyl sulfoxide	Water
or	Saturated $NaHCO_3$ solution	Water
Ampicillin (trihydrate)	Phosphate buffer, pH 8.0, 0.1 mol/L	Phosphate buffer, pH 6.0, 0.1 mol/L
or	Saturated $NaHCO_3$ solution	Water
Azithromycin (dihydrate)	95% ethanol	Broth media
or	Glacial acetic acid[a]	Water
Azlocillin	Water	Water
Aztreonam (anhydrous crystalline B form)	Saturated $NaHCO_3$ solution	Water
Carbenicillin (disodium)	Water	Water
Cefaclor	Water	Water
Cefadroxil	Phosphate buffer, pH 6.0, 0.1 mol/L	Water
Cefamandole	Water	Water
Cefazolin	Phosphate buffer, pH 6.0, 0.1 mol/L	Phosphate buffer, pH 6.0, 0.1 mol/L
Cefdinir	Phosphate buffer, pH 6.0, 0.1 mol/L	Water
Cefditoren	Phosphate buffer, pH 6.0, 0.1 mol/L	Water
Cefepime (dihydrochloride)	Phosphate buffer, pH 6.0, 0.1 mol/L	Phosphate buffer, pH 6.0, 0.1 mol/L
or	Water	Water
Cefetamet	Phosphate buffer, pH 6.0, 0.1 mol/L	Water
Cefixime	Phosphate buffer, pH 7.0, 0.1 mol/L	Phosphate buffer, pH 7.0, 0.1 mol/L
Cefmetazole	Water	Water
Cefonicid	Water	Water
Cefoperazone	Water	Water
Cefotaxime (sodium)	Water	Water
Cefotetan	Dimethyl sulfoxide	Water
Cefoxitin (sodium)	Water	Water
Cefpirome (sulfate)	Water	Water
Cefpodoxime (sodium)	0.10% (11.9 mmol/L) aqueous $NaHCO_3$	Water
Cefprozil	Water	Water
Ceftazidime (pentahydrate)	Sodium carbonate[b]	Water
or	Saturated $NaHCO_3$ solution	Water
Ceftibuten	1/10 volume of dimethyl sulfoxide	Water
Ceftizoxime	Water	Water
Ceftriaxone	Water	Water
Cefuroxime (sodium)	Phosphate buffer, pH 6.0, 0.1 mol/L	Phosphate buffer, pH 6.0, 0.1 mol/L
Cephalexin (hydrate)	Phosphate buffer, pH 6.0, 0.1 mol/L	Water
Cephalothin	Phosphate buffer, pH 6.0, 0.1 mol/L	Water
Cephapirin	Phosphate buffer, pH 6.0, 0.1 mol/L	Water

(continued)

TABLE 2.2 (Continued)

Solvents and Diluents Used for Stock Solution Preparation

Antimicrobial Agent (Form)	Solvent	Diluent
Cephradine	Water	Water
Chloramphenicol	95% ethanol	Water
Cinoxacin	1/2 volume of water, then add 1 mol/L NaOH drop by drop	Water
Ciprofloxacin (hydrochloride monohydrate)	Water	Water
Clarithromycin	Methanol	Phosphate buffer, pH 6.5, 0.1 mol/L
or	Glacial acetic acid[a]	Phosphate buffer, pH 6.5, 0.1 mol/L
or	Dimethyl sulfoxide	Water
Clavulanic acid	Phosphate buffer, pH 6.0, 0.1 mol/L	Phosphate buffer, pH 6.0, 0.1 mol/L
Clinafloxacin	Water	Water
Clindamycin (hydrochloride)	Water	Water
Cloxacillin (sodium monohydrate)	Water	Water
Colistin (sulfate)	Water	Water
Dirithromycin	Glacial acetic acid[a]	Water
Doxycycline (hydrochloride)	Water	Water
Enoxacin	1/2 volume of water, then add 0.1 mol/L NaOH drop by drop	Water
Ertapenem	Phosphate buffer, pH 7.2, 0.01 mol/L	Phosphate buffer, pH 7.2, 0.01 mol/L
Erythromycin	95% ethanol	Water
or	Glacial acetic acid[a]	Water
Fleroxacin	1/2 volume of water, then add 0.1 mol/L NaOH drop by drop	Water
Flucloxacillin (sodium)	Water	Water
Fosfomycin (calcium)	Water	Water
Fusidic acid (fusidate sodium)	95% ethanol	Water
Garenoxacin	Water with stirring	Water
Gatifloxacin	Water with stirring	Water
or	1/2 volume of water, then add 0.1 mol/L NaOH drop by drop	Water
Gemifloxacin	Water	Water
	Methanol	Water
Gentamicin (sulfate)	Water	Water
Grepafloxacin (hydrochloride)	1/2 volume of water, then add 0.1 mol/L NaOH drop by drop	Water
Imipenem (monohydrate)	Phosphate buffer, pH 7.2, 0.01 mol/L	Phosphate buffer, pH 7.2, 0.01 mol/L
or	MOPS buffer, pH 6.8, 1.0 mol/L	MOPS buffer, pH 6.8, 1.0 mol/L
Kanamycin (monosulfate)	Water	Water
Levofloxacin (hemihydrate)	Water	Water
Linezolid	Water	Water
Lomefloxacin	?	?

(continued)

TABLE 2.2 (Continued)

Solvents and Diluents Used for Stock Solution Preparation

Antimicrobial Agent (Form)	Solvent	Diluent
Loracarbef	Water	Water
Mecillinam	Water	Water
Meropenem (trihydrate)	Water	Water
Methicillin (sodium)	Water	Water
Metronidazole	Dimethyl sulfoxide	Water
or	Water	Water
Mezlocillin	Water	Water
Minocycline	Water	Water
Moxalactam	0.04 mol/L HCl and leave for 1.5 to 2 hours	Phosphate buffer, pH 6.0, 0.1 mol/L
Moxifloxacin (hydrochloride)	Water	Water
Mupirocin (lithium)	Water	Water
Nafcillin	Water	Water
Nalidixic acid	½ volume of water, then add 1 mol/L NaOH drop by drop	Water
Netilmicin (sulfate)	Water	Water
Nitrofurantoin	Phosphate buffer, pH 8.0, 0.1 mol/L	Phosphate buffer, pH 8.0, 0.1 mol/L
or	Dimethyl sulfoxide	Phosphate buffer, pH 8.0, 0.1 mol/L
or	Dimethyl formamide	Dimethyl formamide
Norfloxacin	½ volume of water, then add 0.1 mol/L NaOH drop by drop	Water
or	Water 1 mL + 10 μL glacial acetic acid[a]	Water
Ofloxacin	½ volume of water, then add 0.1 mol/L NaOH drop by drop	Water
Oxacillin (sodium)	Water	Water
Penicillin (benzyl, potassium)	Water	Water
Piperacillin (sodium)	Water	Water
Quinupristin-dalfopristin	Water	Water
Rifampin (crystalline)	Methanol to a maximum concentration of 640 μg/mL	Water with stirring
or	Dimethyl sulfoxide	Water
Roxithromycin	95% ethanol	Water
Sparfloxacin	Water	Water
or	½ volume of water, then add 0.1 mol/L NaOH drop by drop	Water
Spectinomycin (dihydrochloride pentahydrate)	Water	Water
Streptomycin (sulfate)	Water	Water
Sulbactam	Water	Water

(continued)

TABLE 2.2 (Continued)

Solvents and Diluents Used for Stock Solution Preparation

Antimicrobial Agent (Form)	Solvent	Diluent
Sulfonamides	½ volume of hot water and minimal amount of 2.5 mol/L NaOH	Water
Tazobactam	Water	Water
Teicoplanin	95% ethanol	Water
Telithromycin	Glacial acetic acid[a]	Water
or	Water 1 mL + 10 μL glacial acetic acid[a]	Phosphate buffer, pH 8.0, 0.08 mol/L
Tetracycline (hydrochloride)	Water	Water (do not freeze subsequently)
Ticarcillin (sodium)	Phosphate buffer, pH 6.0, 0.1 mol/L	Phosphate buffer, pH 6.0, 0.1 mol/L
or	Water	Water
Tobramycin (sulfate)	Water	Water
Trimethoprim (base)	0.05 mol/L lactic or hydrochloric acid, 10% of final volume	Water but may require heat
or	Glacial acetic acid[a]	Water
Trimethoprim lactate	Water	Water
Trospectomycin	Water	Water
Vancomycin (hydrochloride)	Water	Water

[a] Use ½ volume of water, then add glacial acetic acid drop by drop until dissolved. Maximum volume should be 2.5 μL/mL.
[b] Use anhydrous sodium carbonate at exactly 10% of ceftazidime. It is dissolved in most of the required water. The ceftazidime is then dissolved in the sodium carbonate solution, and the remaining water is added. Freeze or use within 6 h.

50°C by placing them in a water bath at this temperature. When the agar has reached this temperature, antimicrobial dilutions and supplements—and blood if required—are added aseptically.

Adequate mixing of the antibiotic in the molten agar is essential, and this is best achieved by mixing each antibiotic solution in a small decanted volume of molten agar and then mixing the result with the bottle of molten agar. If the antibiotic solution is added directly to the whole bottle of molten agar, the solution should be warmed to avoid small portions of agar solidifying around the solution as it is added. The antimicrobial solution is mixed into the molten agar by gentle swirling and inverting the bottle rather than by shaking so that frothing is avoided. Plates should be poured onto a level surface as soon as practical after mixing.

The pH of each batch of agar should be measured after preparation. An aliquot of molten agar can be poured into a beaker or cup over a suitably designed pH electrode and allowed to gel and reach room temperature. Alternatively, a surface electrode can be placed on an aliquot of agar poured into a Petri dish and allowed to reach room temperature. It is also possible to macerate a sufficient amount of set agar and submerge the tip of an electrode.

Agar plates are then poured from the cooled molten agar as soon as possible after mixing in order to minimize any impact on the antimicrobial concentration. There is no specified depth, but 20 mL of molten agar in a 90-mm plate is considered adequate. The volume is not critical, although the DIN method does specify volumes per plate depending on size (48). It is advisable to dry the plates, for instance, in a fan-assisted drying cabinet for 10 minutes (5) or in a 35°C to 37°C incubator inverted with the lids off (38), as moisture buildup is common if covers are placed over cooling agar in Petri dishes.

Preparation of Inoculum

Most standards offer the choice of two methods for the preparation of inocula: the "growth" method and the "direct" method. The direct method is often preferred for inocula prepared from fastidious organisms, as growth of these organisms in broth can be a little unpredictable. The solution for final suspension varies somewhat between standards and sometimes between groups or species being tested, but is generally either 0.85% to 0.9% sodium chloride,

TABLE 2.3

Agar Medium and Additives for Different Bacterial Species in Agar Dilution Tests

Species	Organization	Basal Agar Medium	Additive(s)
Enterobacteriaceae, *Pseudomonas* spp, *Staphylococcus* spp, *Enterococcus* spp	NCCLS	Mueller-Hinton	Nil except add 2% NaCl when testing the antistaphylococcal penicillins oxacillin, methicillin, and nafcillin
	BSAC	Iso-Sensitest	Nil
	CA-SFM	Mueller-Hinton	Nil except add 2–4% NaCl when testing the antistaphylococcal penicillin oxacillin
	DIN	Mueller-Hinton	Nil
Acinetobacter spp, *Stenotrophomonas maltophilia*, other nonfastidious glucose-nonfermenting bacilli	NCCLS	Mueller-Hinton	Nil
	BSAC	Not defined	Nil
	CA-SFM	Mueller-Hinton	
	DIN	Mueller-Hinton	
Bacillus anthracis, Vibrio cholerae	NCCLS	Mueller-Hinton	Nil
	BSAC	Not defined	
	CA-SFM	Not defined	
	DIN	Mueller-Hinton	Nil
Streptococcus spp	NCCLS	Mueller-Hinton	5% defibrinated sheep blood (use horse blood when testing sulfonamides)
	BSAC	Iso-Sensitest	5% defibrinated horse blood
	CA-SFM	Mueller-Hinton	5% defibrinated sheep blood (use horse blood when testing sulfonamides and/or trimethoprim)
	DIN	Mueller-Hinton	2% lysed horse blood and 15 mg/L NAD[a]
Haemophilus influenzae	NCCLS	Not defined	
	BSAC	Iso-Sensitest	5% whole horse blood and 20 mg/L NAD[a]
	CA-SFM	Chocolate or HTM[b]	Add defined growth supplement[c] to chocolate
	DIN	Mueller-Hinton	2% lysed horse blood and 15 mg/L NAD[a]
Moraxella catarrhalis	NCCLS	Not defined	(HTM[b] has not been calibrated in its agar form)
	BSAC	Iso-Sensitest	5% defibrinated horse blood
	CA-SFM	Not defined	
	DIN	Mueller-Hinton	2% lysed horse blood and 15 mg/L NAD[a]
Neisseria gonorrhoeae	NCCLS	GC	Defined growth supplement[c] (use cysteine-free supplement when testing carbapenems and clavulanate)
	BSAC	Iso-Sensitest	5% defibrinated horse blood
	CA-SFM	Chocolate	Defined growth supplement[c]
	DIN	Mueller-Hinton	2% lysed horse blood and 15 mg/L NAD

(*continued*)

TABLE 2.3 (Continued)

Agar Medium and Additives for Different Bacterial Species in Agar Dilution Tests

Species	Organization	Basal Agar Medium	Additive(s)
Neisseria meningitidis	NCCLS	Mueller-Hinton	5% defibrinated sheep blood (use horse blood when testing sulfonamides)
	BSAC	Iso-Sensitest	5% defibrinated horse blood
	CA-SFM	Mueller-Hinton	None
	DIN	Mueller-Hinton	2% lysed horse blood and 15 mg/L NAD[a]
Campylobacter spp	NCCLS	Mueller-Hinton	5% defibrinated sheep blood (this medium is still under development)
	BSAC	Not defined	
	CA-SFM	Mueller-Hinton	5% defibrinated sheep or horse blood
	DIN	Not defined	
Helicobacter pylori	NCCLS	Mueller-Hinton	5% aged (≥2 weeks) sheep blood
	BSAC	Not defined	
	CA-SFM	Not defined	
	DIN	Not defined	
Anaerobes	NCCLS	Brucella	5% laked sheep blood, 5 mg/L of hemin, and 1 mg/L of vitamin K_1
	BSAC	Wilkins-Chalgren	5% defibrinated horse blood
	CA-SFM	Wilkins-Chalgren or	5% defibrinated sheep or horse blood
		Brucella	1 mg/L vitamin K_1 and 5% defibrinated sheep or horse blood
	DIN	Wilkens-Chalgren or	
		brain heart dextrose	0.3 g L-cysteine HCl

[a] NAD, nicotinamide adenine dinucleotide.
[b] HTM, *Haemophilus* test medium: Mueller-Hinton agar with 15 mg/L NAD, 15 mg/L hematin, and 5 g/L yeast extract.
[c] Defined growth supplement = 1.1 g L-cystine, 0.03 g guanine, 3 mg thiamine HCl, 13 mg *p*-ABA, 0.012 g vitamin B_{12}, 0.1 g cocarboxylase, 0.25 g NAD, 1.0 g adenine, 10 g L-glutamine, 100 g glucose, and 0.02 g ferric nitrate per liter of water (IsoVitaleX, PolyViteX).

the same type of broth used in the agar, or phosphate-buffered saline (the recipe is at the end of Table 2.4).

Two standards, the French and the German, require that inocula be prepared from subcultures in order to ensure purity. This should also be the practice for all reference MIC work.

Calibration of Turbidity

Inocula are always calibrated to a turbidity standard, usually a McFarland turbidity standard, which employs particulate suspensions of barium sulfate. McFarland 0.5 is the commonest choice and can be prepared as described in various texts (38,103). Briefly it is a 0.5-mL aliquot of 1.175% w/v $BaCl_2 \cdot 2H_2O$ added to 99.5 mL of 1% w/v H_2SO_4 (103). Alternative turbidity standards made from other materials such as latex particles but optically equivalent to 0.5 McFarland are available commercially (e.g., Remel, Lenexa, and KS). Normally a visual comparison is made with the turbidity standard. It is important that this be done in good lighting and against a card with a white background and a contrasting black line. More recently there has been a move to use a nephelometer or photometer to achieve this calibration. For instance, at a wavelength of 550 nm, a 5-mL glass tube with 2 mL of inoculum suspension with an optical density of

(*text continues on page 28*)

TABLE 2.4

Features of the Different International Agar Dilution Standards by Bacterial Group or Species

Enterobacteriaceae	
NCCLS	
Medium	Mueller-Hinton agar
Inoculum	Growth method or direct colony suspension to reach a 0.5 McFarland standard
Inoculation	For 1-mm pin replicators, apply neat inoculum; for 3-mm pin replicators, dilute inoculum 1 in 10
Incubation	35°C, ambient air, 16–20 h, 24 h for *Yersinia pestis*
QC strains	*Escherichia coli* ATCC 25922; add *E. coli* ATCC 35218 if testing β-lactamase inhibitor combinations
BSAC	
Medium	Iso-Sensitest agar
Inoculum	Growth method or direct colony suspension to reach a 0.5 McFarland standard
Inoculation	Dilute inoculum 1 in 10 and apply 1–2 μL per spot
Incubation	35–37°C, ambient air, 18–20 h
QC strains	*E. coli* ATCC 25922 (NCTC 12241) or *E. coli* NCTC 10418
CA-SFM	
Medium	Mueller-Hinton agar
Inoculum	Growth method or direct colony suspension to reach a 0.5 McFarland standard in Mueller-Hinton broth or 0.9% saline
Inoculation	Dilute inoculum 1 in 10 and apply 1–2 μL per spot
Incubation	35–37°C, ambient air, 18–24 h
QC strains	*E. coli* ATCC 25922 (CIP 76.24) ± *Pseudomonas aeruginosa* ATCC 27853 (CIP 76.110) ± *Staphylococcus aureus* ATCC 25923 (CIP 76.25)
DIN	
Medium	Mueller-Hinton agar
Inoculum	Growth method or direct colony suspension to reach a 0.5 McFarland standard in phosphate-buffered saline[a]
Inoculation	Inoculate an area of 0.5 cm^2 with a replicator or micropipette
Incubation	35–37°C, ambient air, 16–20 h
QC strains	*E. coli* ATCC 25922 (DSM 1103), *E. coli* ATCC 35218 (DSM 5564), *Enterococcus faecalis* ATCC 29212 (DSM 2570). *P. aeruginosa* ATCC 27853 (DSM 1117), *S. aureus* ATCC 29213 (DSM 2569), *S. aureus* ATCC 43300 (DSM 13661)
Nonfastidious glucose-nonfermenting Gram-negative bacilli (including *P. aeruginosa,* other *Pseudomonas* species, *Acinetobacter* species, *Stenotrophomonas maltophilia*, *Burkholderia cepacia* complex [CA-SFM only], and other glucose-nonfermenters)	
NCCLS	
Medium	Mueller-Hinton agar
Inoculum	Growth method or direct colony suspension to reach a 0.5 McFarland standard
Inoculation	For 1-mm pin replicators, apply neat inoculum; for 3-mm pin replicators, dilute inoculum 1 in 10
Incubation	35°C, ambient air, 16–20 h
QC strains	*P. aeruginosa* ATCC 27853, *E. coli* ATCC 25922; add *E. coli* ATCC 35218 if testing β-lactamase inhibitor combinations
BSAC	
Medium	Iso-Sensitest agar
Inoculum	Growth method or direct colony suspension to reach a 0.5 McFarland standard

(continued)

TABLE 2.4 (Continued)

Features of the Different International Agar Dilution Standards by Bacterial Group or Species

Inoculation	Dilute inoculum 1 in 10 and apply 1–2 μL per spot
Incubation	35–37°C, ambient air, 18–20 h
QC strains	*P. aeruginosa* ATCC 27853 (NCTC 12934) or *P. aeruginosa* NCTC 10662
CA-SFM	
Medium	Mueller-Hinton agar
Inoculum	Growth method or direct colony suspension to reach a 0.5 McFarland standard in Mueller-Hinton broth or 0.9% saline
Inoculation	Dilute inoculum 1 in 10 and apply 1–2 μL per spot
Incubation	35–37°C, ambient air, 18–24 h
QC strains	*P. aeruginosa* ATCC 27853 (CIP 76.110) ± *E. coli* ATCC 25922 (CIP 76.24) ± *S. aureus* ATCC 25923 (CIP 76.25)
Medium	Mueller-Hinton agar
Inoculum	Growth method or direct colony suspension to reach a 0.5 McFarland standard in phosphate-buffered saline[a]
Inoculation	Inoculate an area of 0.5 cm^2 with a replicator or micropipette
Incubation	35–37°C, ambient air, 16–20 h
QC strains	*E. coli* ATCC 25922 (DSM 1103), *E. coli* ATCC 35218 (DSM 5564), *E. faecalis* ATCC 29212 (DSM 2570). *P. aeruginosa* ATCC 27853 (DSM 1117), *S. aureus* ATCC 29213 (DSM 2569), *S. aureus* ATCC 43300 (DSM 13661)
***Staphylococcus* species**	
NCCLS	
Medium	Mueller-Hinton agar; add 2% NaCl to plates containing oxacillin, methicillin, or nafcillin
Inoculum	Growth method or direct colony suspension to reach a 0.5 McFarland standard
Inoculation	For 1-mm pin replicators, apply neat inoculum; for 3-mm pin replicators, dilute inoculum 1 in 10
Incubation	35°C, ambient air, 16–20 h; 24 h for oxacillin, methicillin, nafcillin, and vancomycin
QC strains	*S. aureus* ATCC 29213; add *E. coli* ATCC 35218 if testing β-lactamase inhibitor combinations
BSAC	
Medium	Iso-Sensitest agar
Inoculum	Growth method or direct colony suspension to reach a 0.5 McFarland standard
Inoculation	Dilute inoculum 1 in 10 and apply 1–2 μL per spot
Incubation	35–37°C, ambient air, 18–20 h
QC strains	*S. aureus* ATCC 25923 (NCTC 12981) or *S. aureus* NCTC 6571
CA-SFM	
Medium	Mueller-Hinton agar
Inoculum	Growth method or direct colony suspension to reach a 0.5 McFarland standard in Mueller-Hinton broth or 0.9% saline
Inoculation	Dilute inoculum 1 in 10 and apply 1–2 μL per spot
Incubation	35–37°C, ambient air, 18–24 h; 24 h for oxacillin in hypersalted media or at 30°C for 24 h in non-salt-supplemented media
QC strains	*S. aureus* ATCC 25923 (CIP 76.25) ± *P. aeruginosa* ATCC 27853 (CIP 76.110) ± *E. coli* ATCC 25922 (CIP 76.24)

(continued)

TABLE 2.4 (Continued)

Features of the Different International Agar Dilution Standards by Bacterial Group or Species

DIN	
Medium	Mueller-Hinton agar
Inoculum	Growth method or direct colony suspension to reach a 0.5 McFarland standard in phosphate-buffered saline[a]
Inoculation	Inoculate an area of 0.5 cm^2 with a replicator or micropipette
Incubation	35–37°C, ambient air, 16–20 h
QC strains	*E. coli* ATCC 25922 (DSM 1103), *E. coli* ATCC 35218 (DSM 13661), *E. faecalis* ATCC 29212 (DSM 2570), *P. aeruginosa* ATCC 27853 (DSM 1117), *S. aureus* ATCC 29213 (DSM 2569), *S. aureus* ATCC 43300 (DSM 13661)
***Enterococcus* species**	
NCCLS	
Medium	Mueller-Hinton agar
Inoculum	Growth method or direct colony suspension to reach a 0.5 McFarland standard
Inoculation	For 1-mm pin replicators, apply neat inoculum; for 3-mm pin replicators, dilute inoculum 1 in 10
Incubation	35°C, ambient air, 16–20 h; 24 h for vancomycin
QC strains	*E. faecalis* ATCC 29212
BSAC	
Medium	Iso-Sensitest agar
Inoculum	Growth method or direct colony suspension to reach a 0.5 McFarland standard
Inoculation	Dilute inoculum 1 in 10 and apply 1–2 μL per spot
Incubation	35–37°C, ambient air, 18–20 h
QC strains	*E. faecalis* ATCC 29212
CA-SFM	
Medium	Mueller-Hinton agar
Inoculum	Growth method or direct colony suspension to reach a 0.5 McFarland standard in Mueller-Hinton broth or 0.9% saline
Inoculation	Dilute inoculum 1 in 10 and apply 1–2 μL per spot
Incubation	35–37°C, ambient air, 18–24 h
QC strains	No specific strain recommended; use *E. coli, P. aeruginosa,* or *S. aureus* control strain
DIN	
Medium	Mueller-Hinton agar
Inoculum	Growth method or direct colony suspension to reach a 0.5 McFarland standard in phosphate-buffered saline[a]
Inoculation	Inoculate an area of 0.5 cm^2 with a replicator or micropipette
Incubation	35–37°C, ambient air, 16–20 h
QC strains	*E. coli* ATCC 25922 (DSM 1103), *E. coli* ATCC 35218 (DSM 5564), *E. faecalis* ATCC 29212 (DSM 2570). *P. aeruginosa* ATCC 27853 (DSM 1117), *S. aureus* ATCC 29213 (DSM 2569), *S. aureus* ATCC 43300 (DSM 13661)
Streptococcus pneumoniae	
NCCLS	
No agar dilution method has been developed for this species.	

(continued)

TABLE 2.4 (Continued)

Features of the Different International Agar Dilution Standards by Bacterial Group or Species

BSAC	
Medium	Iso-Sensitest agar + 5% defibrinated sheep blood
Inoculum	Direct colony suspension to reach a 0.5 McFarland standard
Inoculation	Apply neat inoculum 1–2 μL per spot
Incubation	35–37°C, 406% CO_2, 18–20 h
QC strains	*Streptococcus pneumoniae* ATCC 49619
CA-SFM	
Medium	Mueller-Hinton agar + 5% defibrinated sheep blood (5% lysed horse blood for testing co-trimoxazole)
Inoculum	Direct colony suspension to reach a 0.5 McFarland standard in Mueller-Hinton broth or 0.9% saline
Inoculation	Dilute inoculum 1 in 10 and apply 1–2 μL per spot
Incubation	35–37°C, 5% CO_2, 18–24 h
QC strains	No specific strain recommended; use *E. coli, P. aeruginosa*, or *S. aureus* control strain (there is no ATCC equivalent)
DIN	
Medium	Mueller-Hinton agar + 2% lysed horse blood + 15 mg/L NAD + 5 g/L yeast extract
Inoculum	Growth method or direct colony suspension to reach a 0.5 McFarland standard in phosphate-buffered saline[a]
Inoculation	Inoculate an area of 0.5 cm^2 with a replicator or micropipette
Incubation	35–37°C, ambient air, 16–20 h
QC strains	*Haemophilus influenzae* ATCC 49247 (DSM 9999), *H. influenzae* ATCC 49766 (DSM 11970), *S. pneumoniae* ATCC 49619 (DSM 11967), *S. pneumoniae*, DSM 11865 (there is no ATCC equivalent), *Moraxella catarrhalis* ATCC 43617 (DSM 11994), *Neisseria gonorrhoeae* ATCC 49226 (DSM 9189).
Other *Streptococcus* species	
NCCLS	
Medium	Mueller-Hinton agar + 5% sheep blood (lysed horse blood when testing sulfonamides)
Inoculum	Direct colony suspension to reach a 0.5 McFarland standard
Inoculation	For 1-mm pin replicators, apply neat inoculum; for 3-mm pin replicators, dilute inoculum 1 in 10
Incubation	35°C, ambient air (CO_2 if necessary for growth), 20–24 h
QC strains	*S. pneumoniae* ATCC 49619
BSAC	
Medium	Iso-Sensitest agar + 5% defibrinated horse blood
Inoculum	Growth method or direct colony suspension to reach a 0.5 McFarland standard
Inoculation	Dilute inoculum 1 in 10 and apply 1–2 μL per spot
Incubation	35–37°C, ambient air, 18–20 h
QC strains	*S. pneumoniae* ATCC 49619
CA-SFM	
Medium	Mueller-Hinton agar + 5% defibrinated sheep blood (5% lysed horse blood for testing co-trimoxazole)
Inoculum	Direct colony suspension to reach a 0.5 McFarland standard in Mueller-Hinton broth or 0.9% saline

(continued)

TABLE 2.4 (Continued)

Features of the Different International Agar Dilution Standards by Bacterial Group or Species

Inoculation	Dilute inoculum 1 in 10 and apply 1–2 μL per spot
Incubation	35–37°C, 5% CO_2, 18–24 h
QC strains	No specific strain recommended; use *E. coli*, *P. aeruginosa*, or *S. aureus* control strain
DIN	
Medium	Mueller-Hinton agar + 2% lysed horse blood + 15 mg/L NAD + 5 g/L yeast extract
Inoculum	Growth method or direct colony suspension to reach a 0.5 McFarland standard in phosphate-buffered saline[a]
Inoculation	Inoculate an area of 0.5 cm^2 with a replicator or micropipette
Incubation	35–37°C, ambient air, 16–20 h
QC strains	*H. influenzae* ATCC 49247 (DSM 9999), *H. influenzae* ATCC 49766 (DSM 11970), *S. pneumoniae* ATCC 49619 (DSM 11967), *S. pneumoniae* (DSM 11865) (there is no ATCC equivalent), *M. catarrhalis* ATCC 43617 (DSM 11994), *N. gonorrhoeae* ATCC 49226 (DSM 9189).
Haemophilus influenzae	
NCCLS	
No agar dilution method has been developed for this species.	
BSAC	
Medium	Iso-Sensitest agar + 5% whole horse blood + 20 mg/L NAD
Inoculum	Direct colony suspension to reach a 0.5 McFarland standard in Mueller-Hinton broth or 0.9% saline
Inoculation	Apply undiluted inoculum at 1–2 μL per spot
Incubation	35–37°C, 4–6% CO_2, 18–20 h
QC strains	*H. influenzae* ATCC 49247 (NCTC 12699) or *H. influenzae* NCTC 11931
CA-SFM	
Medium	Chocolate agar with defined growth supplement or HTM agar
Inoculum	Direct colony suspension to reach a 0.5 McFarland standard
Inoculation	Apply undiluted inoculum at 1–2 μL per spot
Incubation	35–37°C, ambient air, 18–24 h
QC strains	No specific strain recommended; use *E. coli*, *P. aeruginosa*, or *S. aureus* control strain
DIN	
Medium	Mueller-Hinton agar + 2% lysed horse blood + 15 mg/L NAD + 5 g/L yeast extract
Inoculum	Growth method or direct colony suspension to reach a 0.5 McFarland standard in phosphate-buffered saline[a]
Inoculation	Inoculate an area of 0.5 cm^2 with a replicator or micropipette
Incubation	35–37°C, ambient air, 16–20 h
QC strains	*H. influenzae* ATCC 49247 (DSM 9999), *H. influenzae* ATCC 49766 (DSM 11970), *S. pneumoniae* ATCC 49619 (DSM 11967), *S. pneumoniae* (DSM 11865) (there is no ATCC equivalent), *M. catarrhalis* ATCC 43617 (DSM 11994), *N. gonorrhoeae* ATCC 49266 (DSM 9189).
Neisseria gonorrhoeae	
NCCLS	
Medium	GC agar + 1% cysteine-free defined growth medium

(*continued*)

TABLE 2.4 (Continued)

Features of the Different International Agar Dilution Standards by Bacterial Group or Species

Inoculum	Direct colony suspension to reach a 0.5 McFarland standard
Inoculation	For 1-mm pin replicators, apply neat inoculum; for 3-mm pin replicators, dilute inoculum 1 in 10
Incubation	35°C, 5% CO_2, 20–24 h
QC strains	*N. gonorrhoeae* ATCC 49226
BSAC	
Medium	Iso-Sensitest agar + 5% defibrinated horse blood
Inoculum	Direct colony suspension to reach a 0.5 McFarland standard
Inoculation	Apply undiluted inoculum at 1–2 μL per spot
Incubation	35–37°C, 4–6% CO_2, 18–20 h
QC strains	*N. gonorrhoeae* ATCC 49226 (NCTC 12700)
CA-SFM	
Medium	Chocolate agar with defined growth supplement or HTM agar
Inoculum	Direct colony suspension to reach a 0.5 McFarland standard in M/15 PBS (pH 7.2)
Inoculation	Apply undiluted inoculum at 10 μL per spot
Incubation	35–37°C, 5% CO_2, 18–24 h (36–40 h if growth insufficient after 1 d)
QC strains	No specific strain recommended; use *E. coli, P. aeruginosa*, or *S. aureus* control strain (there is no ATCC equivalent)
DIN	
Medium	Mueller-Hinton agar + 2% lysed horse blood + 15 mg/L NAD + 5 g/L yeast extract
Inoculum	Growth method or direct colony suspension to reach a 0.5 McFarland standard in phosphate-buffered saline[a]
Inoculation	Inoculate an area of 0.5 cm^2 with a replicator or micropipette
Incubation	35–37°C, ambient air, 16–20 h
QC strains	*H. influenzae* ATCC 49247 (DSM 9999), *H. influenzae* ATCC 49766 (DSM 11970), *S. pneumoniae* ATCC 49619 (DSM 11967), *S. pneumoniae* (DSM 11865) (there is no ATCC equivalent), *M. catarrhalis* ATCC 43617 (DSM 11994), *N. gonorrhoeae* ATCC 49266 (DSM 9189)
Neisseria meningitidis	
NCCLS	
Medium	Mueller-Hinton agar + 5% sheep blood (lysed horse blood when testing sulfonamides)
Inoculum	Direct colony suspension to reach a 0.5 McFarland standard
Inoculation	For 1-mm pin replicators, apply neat inoculum; for 3-mm pin replicators, dilute inoculum 1 in 10
Incubation	35°C, 5% CO_2, 24 h
QC strains	*N. gonorrhoeae* ATCC 49226
BSAC	
Medium	Iso-Sensitest agar + 5% defibrinated horse blood
Inoculum	Direct colony suspension to reach a 0.5 McFarland standard
Inoculation	Apply undiluted inoculum at 1–2 μL per spot
Incubation	35–37°C, 4–6% CO_2, 18–20 h
QC strains	No specific strain recommended

(*continued*)

TABLE 2.4 (Continued)

Features of the Different International Agar Dilution Standards by Bacterial Group or Species

CA-SFM	
Medium	Mueller-Hinton agar
Inoculum	Direct colony suspension to reach a 0.5 McFarland standard in M/15 PBS (pH 7.2)
Inoculation	Apply undiluted inoculum at 10 μL per spot
Incubation	35–37°C, 5% CO_2, 18–24 h
QC strains	No specific strain recommended; use *E. coli, P. aeruginosa,* or *S. aureus* control strain
DIN	
Medium	Mueller-Hinton agar + 2% lysed horse blood + 15 mg/L NAD + 5 g/L yeast extract
Inoculum	Growth method or direct colony suspension to reach a 0.5 McFarland standard in phosphate-buffered saline[a]
Inoculation	Inoculate an area of 0.5 cm^2 with a replicator or micropipette
Incubation	35–37°C, ambient air, 16–20 h
QC strains	*H. influenzae* ATCC 49247 (DSM 9999), *H. influenzae* ATCC 49766 (DSM 11970), *S. pneumoniae* ATCC 49619 (DSM 11967), *S. pneumoniae* (DSM 11865) (there is no ATCC equivalent), *M. catarrhalis* ATCC 43617 (DSM 11994), *N. gonorrhoeae* ATCC 49266 (DSM 9189).
Moraxella catarrhalis	
NCCLS	
No agar dilution method has been developed for this species.	
BSAC	
Medium	Iso-Sensitest agar + 5% defibrinated horse blood
Inoculum	Direct colony suspension to reach a 0.5 McFarland standard
Inoculation	Apply undiluted inoculum at 1–2 μL per spot
Incubation	35–37°C, ambient air, 18–20 h
QC strains	No specific strain recommended
CA-SFM	
No agar dilution method has been developed for this species.	
DIN	
Medium	Mueller-Hinton agar + 2% lysed horse blood + 15 mg/L NAD + 5 g/L yeast extract
Inoculum	Growth method or direct colony suspension to reach a 0.5 McFarland standard in phosphate-buffered saline[a]
Inoculation	Inoculate an area of 0.5 cm^2 with a replicator or micropipette
Incubation	35–37°C, ambient air, 16–20 h
QC strains	*H. influenzae* ATCC 49247 (DSM 9999), *H. influenzae* ATCC 49766 (DSM 11970), *S. pneumoniae* ATCC 49619 (DSM 11967), *S. pneumoniae* (DSM 11865) (there is no ATCC equivalent), *M. catarrhalis* ATCC 43617 (DSM 11994), *N. gonorrhoeae* ATCC 49266 (DSM 9189).
***Campylobacter* species**	
NCCLS	
Medium	Mueller-Hinton agar + 5% defibrinated sheep blood
Inoculum	Direct colony suspension to reach a 0.5 McFarland standard

(continued)

TABLE 2.4 (Continued)

Features of the Different International Agar Dilution Standards by Bacterial Group or Species

Inoculation	For 1-mm pin replicators, apply neat inoculum; for 3-mm pin replicators, dilute inoculum 1 in 10
Incubation	36°C for 48 h or 42°C for 24 h, 10% CO_2 + 5% O_2 + 85% H_2, or a microaerophilic atmosphere
QC strains	*Campylobacter jejuni* ATCC 33560

BSAC

No agar dilution method has been developed for this species.

CA-SFM

Medium	Mueller-Hinton agar with 5% defibrinated sheep or horse blood
Inoculum	Direct colony suspension to reach a 0.5 McFarland standard in Brucella broth or 0.9% saline
Inoculation	Apply undiluted inoculum at 2–5 μL per spot
Incubation	35–37°C, microaerophilic or anaerobic atmosphere, 18–24 h
QC strains	No specific strain recommended; use *E. coli, P. aeruginosa*, or *S. aureus* control strain

DIN

No agar dilution method has been developed for this species.

Helicobacter pylori

NCCLS

Medium	Mueller-Hinton agar + 5% aged (2 weeks) sheep blood
Inoculum	Direct colony suspension in saline to reach a 2 McFarland standard
Inoculation	Apply undiluted inoculum at 1–3 μL per spot
Incubation	35°C for 3 d, 10% CO_2 + 5% O_2 + 85% H_2, or a microaerophilic atmosphere
QC strains	*Helicobacter pylori* ATCC 43504

BSAC

No agar dilution method has been developed for this species.

CA-SFM

No agar dilution method has been developed for this species.

DIN

No agar dilution method has been developed for this species.

Anaerobes

NCCLS

Medium	Brucella agar + 5 μg/mL hemin + 1 μg/mL vitamin K_1 + 5% laked sheep blood
Inoculum	Growth method (in enriched thioglycollate broth without indicator) or direct colony suspension (in Brucella or other clear broth) to reach a 0.5 McFarland standard
Inoculation	Apply undiluted inoculum at 1–2 μL per spot
Incubation	35°C, anaerobic atmosphere with 4–7% CO_2, 42–48 h
QC strains	*Bacteroides fragilis* ATCC 25285, *Bacteroides thetaiotaomicron* ATCC 29741, *Eubacterium lentum* ATCC 43055

BSAC

No agar dilution method has been developed for this species.

(*continued*)

TABLE 2.4 (Continued)

Features of the Different International Agar Dilution Standards by Bacterial Group or Species

CA-SFM	
Medium	Wilkins-Chalgren agar + 5% defibrinated sheep blood or Brucella agar + 1 mg/L vitamin K_1 + 5% blood; add 1 mg/L of sodium bicarbonate or 5 mg/L hemin for certain species
Inoculum	For rapid growing strains, direct colony suspension to reach a 0.5 McFarland standard in Brucella or Schaedler broth; for slow-growing strains (>72 h), use a 1 McFarland suspension
Inoculation	Apply undiluted inoculum at 2–3 μL per spot
Incubation	35–37°C, anaerobic atmosphere, 48 h
QC strains	No specific strain recommended
DIN	
Medium	Wilkins-Chalgren agar or Brain Heart Dextrose agar with 0.3 mg/L cysteine HCl
Inoculum	Growth method: Rosenow broth or thioglycollate broth supplemented with 5 mg/L hemin and 0.1 mg/L vitamin K_1, or Schaedler agar supplemented with 5% sheep blood and 0.1 mg/L vitamin K_1; cultures should proceed for 24–48 h depending on the generation time of the species
Inoculation	From Rosenow broth, dilute 1 in 10 in thioglycollate or broth of test medium; from thioglycollate broth, dilute to McFarland 0.5; from solid media, dilute in thioglycollate broth or broth of test medium to McFarland 0.5; inoculate an area of 0.5 cm^2 with a replicator or micropipette
Incubation	35–37°C, anaerobic atmosphere, 40–48 h
QC strains	*B. fragilis* ATCC 25285 (DSM 2151), *B. thetaiotaomicron* ATCC 29741 (DSM 2255), *Clostridium perfringens* ATCC 13124 (DSM 756), *Peptostreptococcus anaerobius* ATCC 27337 (DSM 2949), *Prevotella bivia* ATCC 29303 (DSM 20514)

[a] Prepared by adding 8.5 g NaCl and 20 mL phosphate buffer stock (12.5 g/L $Na_2HPO_4 \cdot 12H_2O$ and 2.88 g/L KH_2PO_4 in de-ionized water) to 1 L of de-ionized water, adjusting pH to 7.2, and autoclaving for 15 min at 121°C (47).

0.1–0.12 approximates a 0.5 McFarland barium sulfate standard (38). Equally, at 625 nm and a light path of 1 cm, the standard has an optical density of 0.08–0.10 (103).

Barium sulfate standards are affected by light and heat, and hence they should be stored between uses in a dark place at room temperature. Their turbidity should be checked in a nephelometer or photometer monthly. They also require vigorous agitation at each use.

Growth Method

Usually two to five morphologically similar colonies are picked from a primary or subculture plate. The wire loop is used to touch each colony, and it is then immersed in about 5 mL of the recommended broth (e.g., tryptic soy broth in the NCCSL method). The broth is incubated at 35°C until it equals or exceeds the correct turbidity, generally 2–6 hours for rapidly growing pathogens. The broth is then diluted with a suitable sterile fluid such as broth, saline, or phosphate buffered saline (PBS) according to the instructions until 0.5 McFarland is reached.

Direct Colony Suspension Method

In this method two to five colonies are touched or picked up and suspended directly in the fluid of choice. Clearly, the turbidity should be adjusted subsequently as for the growth method. This method is acceptable in almost all situations, but it slightly more labor intensive. Hence it remains an option. The choice of growth versus direct method depends on laboratory workflow. Almost all standards prefer this method for fastidious organisms such as *Haemophilus* species and *N. gonorrhoeae*.

Plate Inoculation

In almost all circumstances, it is preferable to use a replicator apparatus to inoculate the agar plates. These are expensive items but last indefinitely. They generally come with 32 to 36 pins to deliver this number of strains to a 90-mm agar plate. The size of the pins is critical to decisions about how or whether the inoculum to be used for various species is to be further diluted. Prongs of 3 mm deliver approximately 2 μL to the plate surface, while prongs of 1 mm deliver around tenfold less (0.1–0.2 μL). Hence, some standards recommend dilution for some organism groups or species when using the 3-mm pins. The German standard also permits the use of a micropipette to inoculate plates (48).

There is considerable variation between standards regarding whether further dilution of the standardized inoculum prepared as outlined above should be performed and how it should be performed. The commonly stated intention is that each spot on the plate should contain around 10^4 colony-forming units (CFU). However, in preparing standardized inocula, there are considerable differences between species in the number of CFU per milliliter for a given turbidity (98).

Incubation

Temperature and Duration

Most organisms should be incubated at 35°C to 37°C. An incubator set at 36°C can generally operate within this range. The NCCLS method specifies 35°C for all bacteria. The duration of incubation depends on the species. For rapidly growing species such as the Enterobacteriaceae, the glucose-nonfermenting Gram-negative bacilli, *Enterococcus* species, and *Staphylococcus* species, overnight incubation for a minimum of 16 h is needed. Longer incubation is recommended for fastidious species (18–20 hours plus), for *Staphylococcus* species when testing against antistaphylococcal penicillins (24 hours), for *Campylobacter* species (24–48 h depending on the standard and incubation temperature), for *Helicobacter pylori* (NCCLS 3 days), and for anaerobes (42–48 h).

Atmosphere

Enrichment of air with CO_2 is recommended in most standards for a variety of fastidious species, including *Streptococcus pneumoniae, Haemophilus influenzae,* sometimes other *Streptococcus* species, and *N. gonorrhoeae*. The concentration is usually 5%, although some standards tolerate ranges of 4% to 6%. The effect on the activity of certain drugs under these circumstances is discussed earlier.

Campylobacter species and *H. pylori* demand incubation in a microaerophilic atmosphere, identical to that recommended for primary isolation. Commercial systems are available for generating the required microaerophilic environment.

Anaerobic bacteria should obviously be incubated in the standard anaerobic environment used for primary isolation of anaerobes. Either an anaerobic chamber or jar is acceptable.

Plate Stacking

The effect of stacking plates on the incubation temperature is not widely recognized. After placement in the incubator, plates in the middle of a stack will take longer to reach the desired incubation temperature than plates at the top and bottom (34,35). This is important because the incubation temperature can have a profound effect on the generation time of bacteria, which in turn will affect the endpoint determination. In general, no more than five plates should be used in a stack. Even then it can take up to 4 h for the center plate to reach the incubator temperature (35).

Reading

Plates should be read with optimum lighting, preferably on a dark, nonreflecting surface. For instance, in Fig. 2.2, growth has obviously occurred at some spots but not at others. The MIC is taken as the first concentration at which no growth occurs. Most standards recommend that the appearance of one or two colonies or a faint haze can be ignored. However, if there are one to two colonies at a number of concentrations rather than a single one above the putative MIC, then the MIC is that concentration at which no colonies are seen. If this is the case, the purity of the strain should be checked, as it may be an indication of contamination. The only significant exception to these reading rules occurs in the reading of the endpoints for folate synthesis inhibitors, where growth can diminish gradually over a range of concentrations. NCCLS recommends that the endpoint be read as that concentration resulting in 80% inhibition of growth (103). Other bacteriostatic drugs, such as chloramphenicol and

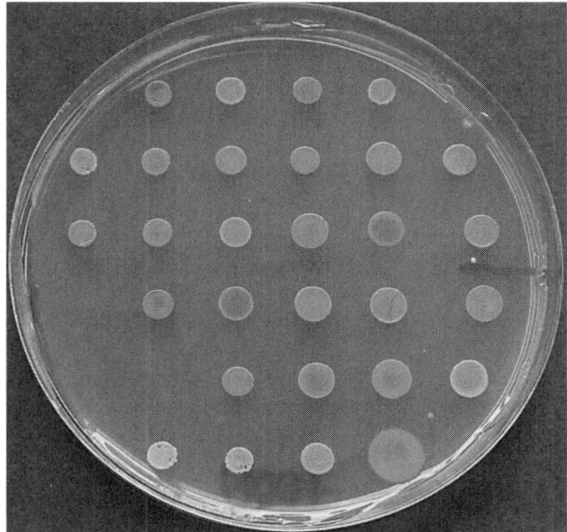

FIGURE 2.2 • Agar dilution plate after 24 hours of incubation. The medium is Mueller-Hinton agar. The strains are of *Staphylococcus aureus*. The last spot at bottom right is a control. Three strains have not grown at this concentration.

clindamycin, can exhibit the same phenomenon to a lesser degree.

Quality Control

Quality control procedures in the performance of agar dilution are designed to ensure the reproducibility of the test and to confirm the performance of the reagents and the persons conducting the test. Most importantly, it is designed to detect errors of concentration or dilution of the antimicrobials, a not infrequent hazard in agar dilution testing. It is assumed that the laboratory is using reagents and materials from trusted suppliers who undertake quality control checks during manufacture. Using a trusted supplier does not prevent problems that may develop during shipping and handling, and hence there is a need to have a quality control system at the laboratory level.

Quality Control Strains

The main component of quality control is the testing of reference quality control strains. The number tested varies between standards and with the type of strains being tested. Wherever possible, it is desirable to test a quality control strain of the same family, genus, and species as the strains under examination. The following ATCC reference strains have become almost universal as quality control strains for testing rapidly growing aerobic bacteria: *E. coli* ATCC 25922, *S. aureus* ATCC 29213, *P. aeruginosa* ATCC 27853, and *E. faecalis* ATCC 29212. Other strains recommended by different standards include *E. coli* ATCC 35218 (NCCLS for β-lactamase inhibitor combinations), *S. aureus* CIP 6525 (CA-SFM for methicillin and oxacillin), *H. influenzae* ATCC 49217 (NCCLS and BSAC), *H. influenzae* ATCC 49766 (NCCLS), *N. gonorrhoeae* ATCC 49226 (NCCLS and BSAC), *S. pneumoniae* ATCC 49619 (NCCLS and BSAC), *H. pylori* ATCC 43504 (NCCLS), *Campylobacter jejuni* ATCC 33560 (NCCLS), *B. fragilis* ATCC 25285 (NCCLS), *B. fragilis* NCTC 9343 (BSAC), *Bacteroides thetaiotaomicron* ATCC 29741 (NCCLS), and *Eubacterium lentum* ATCC 43005 (NCCLS).

The selection of quality control strains involves a compromise between the objective of getting strains with MICs close to the center of a dilution series of a range of antimicrobials (103), and the number of strains that would be required to achieve this objective. The strains commonly recommended have also been selected for their stability over long periods of time and repeated subculture. There is nothing to inhibit a laboratory from developing and using its own quality control strains.

Storage of Quality Control Strains

Stock cultures of the quality control strains should be maintained in the freezer below $-20°C$ (ideally at $-70°C$) in a suitable stabilizer such as fetal calf serum, glycerol broth, or skim milk or should be freeze-dried. Some workers recommend that two sets of stock cultures be stored, one set to create working cultures and the other as emergency backup. This will guarantee that the laboratory always has unaltered quality control strains. Working cultures should be stored on agar slants at $2°C$ to $8°C$ and subcultured each week for no more than 3 successive weeks. New working cultures are generated each month from frozen or freeze-dried stock and subcultured twice before use.

Frequency of Testing and Corrective Action

Each standard provides MIC quality control ranges for these strains against some or all of the antimicrobials of interest. The recommended quality control strains are included in each test run. When these strains fall within the quality control range, the test run is valid. When one or more results are out of this range, the test run must be considered invalid and be rerun.

Use in Routine Susceptibility Testing

Agar dilution can been adapted to routine susceptibility testing. Essentially, it is a truncated method that incorporates one or two selected concentrations of antimicrobial, usually at breakpoint values (so-called breakpoint susceptibility testing). It has been advocated as an option for routine testing by some authorities (153) but is slowly being supplanted by other methods. The advantages and disadvantages of this method have been described in detail by the British Society for Antimicrobial Chemotherapy (153). When testing multiple strains of Gram-negative bacteria that may include *Proteus mirabilis* and *P. vulgaris,* it is necessary to include an antiswarming agent, which, as discussed earlier, can affect result. The method offers specific challenges in terms of quality control, because the limited number of concentrations will only detect the grossest of preparation errors in standard quality control organisms and will often fail to detect the commonest error—a tenfold error in antibiotic dilutions. To overcome this, there are a number of options available: (a) assaying antibiotic dilutions prepared from stock solutions, (b) assaying agar plugs removed from a poured agar plate (56), and (c) assaying paper disks applied for a fixed interval to the surface of a poured agar plate (91). McDermott et al. provided a detailed analysis of two of these methods and recommended methods with high precision (91).

DISK DIFFUSION SUSCEPTIBILITY TESTING

Disk diffusion susceptibility testing has a long history, having evolved out of antibiotic diffusion from wells used for drug assay and susceptibility testing. The method in its various forms still has wide popularity owing to its ease of use and low cost compared with other methods. It has spawned many variants around the world. Unlike in dilution methods, an MIC value is not generated. Instead, in the development of the test, zone diameters must be compared with the MIC values of the same strains in order to determine which zone diameters predict which MIC values and hence what category of susceptibility.

Theoretical Aspects

All disk diffusion methods are based on the diffusion through agar of drug released from an impregnated disk. There are a large number of variables affecting this diffusion. Important features of antibiotic diffusion were worked out by Cooper and others in the 1950s (33–37,71). They have been clearly explained by Barry, who detailed the dynamics of zone formation and the "critical concentration," "critical time," and "critical population" (12,13).

When an antibiotic is placed in a well cut into agar or in a disk applied to the agar surface, the drug commences diffusion immediately and diffuses in a decreasing gradient of concentration from the edge of the well or disk. Over a number of hours, the height of this gradient deceases from very steep initially to quite shallow as the drug continues to diffuse (12). In disk susceptibility testing, disks are applied after the surface has been inoculated with bacteria. The formation of the zone edge is thus a contest between the diffusion of the drug and the growth rate of the bacterial inoculum, including any initial lag phase after incubation commences. The critical concentration is the concentration just capable of inhibiting growth, and it is also that concentration found at the zone edge at the critical time. It is similar but not identical to the MIC as measured by dilution methods. The critical time is the time it takes for the critical concentration to be reached at what ultimately becomes the zone edge. It is generally around 3–4 hours under standard test conditions. The critical population is the number of bacterial cells found at the critical time at the ultimate zone edge. The relationships between these parameters are as follows:

$$C_C = \frac{M}{4\pi D T_0 h} e^{\frac{r^2}{4DT_0}}$$

$$T_0 = L + G \log_2 \left(\frac{N'}{N_0} \right)$$

where C_C = critical concentration, M = disk content, T_0 = critical time, D = diffusion coefficient of drug, h = depth of agar, r = zone radius, L = lag time, G = generation time, N' = critical population at the critical time, and N_0 = number of viable cells at beginning of incubation. Although inaccurate, it is useful to simplify these relationships by imagining the zone of inhibition as a "cylinder" in which the drug is evenly distributed. The concentration of drug in this cylinder is thus the disk content (M) divided by the volume of the cylinder, namely $pd^2h/4$, where d is the zone diameter and h is the depth of the agar and therefore $d = \sqrt{4M/\pi hC}$. Thus the zone diameter increases in proportion to the square root of the disk content and decreases in proportion to the square root of the agar depth. This defines the essential relationships between zone size, disk content, and agar depth and how variations in these affect zone diameters.

Disk Production

Disks for almost all antimicrobials can be obtained commercially. Even drugs that are still under development are likely to have disks available for use in the laboratory and clinical development programs. From time to time, it may be useful for a laboratory to manufacture its own disks. Strict standards must be adhered to if this is done. The same stipulations in drug sourcing and preparation of stocks as have been described in the section on agar dilution apply. Paper disks should be obtained that adhere to the same standards that apply to commercial manufacturers. In the United States, the standard is 740-E (Schleicher and Schuell, Keene, NH), and the paper used should be 30 ± 4 mg/cm^2 (125).

Solvents used in disk manufacture are described in Table 2.5. This information comes from a previous edition (125).

Factors Influencing Zone Diameters

A large range of factors can influence the zone sizes produced. The most important are the disk content (also called *potency*, *mass*, or *strength*, namely, the amount of drug in the disk), the disk size, the diffusion characteristics of the drug, the depth of the agar, the growth rate of the bacterium (including the initial lag phase), the density of the inoculum, and the activity of the drug against the strain being tested. Other factors such as medium composition, pH, and the effect of additives are dealt with at the beginning of this chapter.

Disk Content

The amount of drug impregnated into the disc is somewhat arbitrary. Amounts are chosen that are likely to produce zones of moderate size (15–35 mm) under normal conditions. Different disk methods have often selected different disk contents based on early experience with the antibiotic during development and precedents set within antibiotic classes.

Disk contents will be subject to variation during manufacture, and regulators such as the FDA have set tolerances on the true amount in the disk in the range of 90% to 125% of the label. Such small errors will have a small effect on the zone diameter, because it is proportional to

TABLE 2.5

Solvents for Antimicrobials Used in the Manufacture of Susceptibility Test Disks

Antimicrobial Agent	Solvent	Antimicrobial Agent	Solvent
Amdinocillin	50% methanol	Furazolidone	DMF
Amikacin	50% methanol	Fusidic acid	Methanol
Amoxicillin	75% methanol	Gentamicin	50% methanol
Ampicillin	Methanol	Imipenem	1% PVP/isopropanol or 0.5 mol/L MOPS buffer
Apalcillin	Phosphate buffer	Isoniazid	Methanol
Azlocillin	Methanol	Josamycin	Methanol
Aztreonam	Methanol	Kanamycin	Water
Bacitracin	50% methanol	Lincomycin	Methanol
Carbenicillin	Methanol	Methacycline	Methanol
Cefaclor	2-Propanol/PVP	Methicillin	Methanol
Cefadroxil	Methanol	Metronidazole	Methanol
Cefamandole	2-Propanol/PVP	Mezlocillin	Methanol
Cefazolin	50% methanol	Minocycline	Methanol
Cefixime	50% methanol	Moxalactam	Heptane/sorbitan
Cefmenoxime	Methanol	Mupirocin	Phosphate buffer
Cefmetazole	Water	Nafcillin	Acetone
Cefonicid	75% methanol	Nalidixic acid	Methanol/NaOH
Cefoperazone	Methanol	Netilmicin	Water
Ceforanide	Phosphate buffer	Neomycin	Water
Cefotaxime	Methanol	Nitrofurantoin	DMF
Cefotetan	Methanol	Norfloxacin	50% methanol/NaOH
Cefotiam	Methanol	Novobiocin	60% methanol
Cefoxitin	Methanol	Oleandomycin	Methanol
Cefroxadine	5% acetic acid	Oxacillin	50% methanol
Cefsulodin	95% methanol	Oxolinic acid	50% methanol/NaOH
Ceftazidime	Phosphate buffer	Oxytetracycline	Methanol
Ceftizoxime	Methanol	Pefloxacin	50% methanol/NaOH
Ceftriaxone	Methanol	Penicillin G	50% methanol
Cefuroxime	75% methanol	Pipemidic acid	Methanol
Cephacetrile	75% methanol	Piperacillin	Methanol
Cephalexin	75% methanol	Piromidic acid	50% methanol/NaOH
Cephaloridine	75% methanol	Polymyxin B	60% methanol
Cephalothin	2-Propanol/PVP	Rifampin	Methanol
Cephapirin	75% methanol	Sisomicin	50% methanol
Cephradine	Methanol	Spectinomycin	Methanol
Chloramphenicol	Methanol	Streptomycin	50% methanol
Cinoxacin	Methanol/NaOH	Sulfachloropyridazine	50% methanol
Ciprofloxacin	75% methanol	Sulfadiazine	50% methanol
Clindamycin	Methanol	Sulfamethizole	Methanol
Cloxacillin	50% methanol	Sulfamethoxine	Methanol
Colistin	50% methanol	Sulfamethoxypyridazine	Methanol
Cyclacillin	Methanol	Sulfathiazole	Methanol
Demeclocycline	Methanol	Sulfisoxazole	Methanol
Dibekacin	Water	Teicoplanin	50% methanol/NaOH
Dicloxacillin	50% methanol	Temocillin	Methanol
Doxycycline	Methanol	Tetracycline	Methanol
Enoxacin	50% methanol/NaOH	Ticarcillin	Methanol
Erythromycin	Methanol	Tobramycin	50% methanol
Flucytosine	Methanol	Trimethoprim	DMF
Fosfomycin	50% methanol	Trimethoprim/sulfamethoxazole	DMF
		Vancomycin	40% methanol

DMF, dimethylformamide; MOPS, morpholinopropane sulfonate; PVP, polyvinylpyrrolidone the square root of the disk content, which means that the possible variation in the diameter ranges from about –5% to +12%.

The difference in zone diameters with different disk contents has been exploited to determine critical concentrations (12). When three or more disks with a range of antibiotic contents are used, the resulting zone diameters, when squared, are directly proportional to the logarithms of the disk contents. The results are subjected to linear regression, extrapolation of which to no zone yields the critical concentrations. These values will often be good approximations of the MICs as measured by other methods.

Disk Size

The extent of drug diffusion will obviously be affected by the width of the disk. Paper disks are now almost universally manufactured 6 mm wide. Further, the nature of the paper is subject to regulation, as different varieties of paper have been shown to affect the release characteristics of antibiotics (125). One disk method, that of Neo-Sensitabs produced by the Danish company Rosco Diagnostica A/S (30,119), uses 9-mm disks made from hardened inert "chalk-like" substances. These larger disks result in larger zones for the same disk content.

Diffusion Characteristics of the Drug

The two crucial properties of the drug molecules are size and charge. In general, larger molecules diffuse more slowly, and the zones formed as a consequence are smaller. Large molecules demonstrating this include the glycopeptides such as vancomycin and teicoplanin (31) and the polymyxins such as polymyxin B and colistin. Strongly cationic molecules will also be inhibited in their diffusion owing to interaction with acid or sulfate groups on the agar polymer. Polymyxins are cationic, and their diffusion is also reduced for this reason. Aminoglycosides are cationic to a lesser extent, and their diffusion is reduced slightly as a result (2).

Agar Depth

As noted, agar depth will naturally alter the size of the inhibition zone. Most methods have settled on a depth of 4 mm or a similar amount. This represents a balance between a smaller depth, which is likely to generate a reasonable zone size, and a larger depth, which is designed to reduce the zone size variation due to small variations in depth. A number of studies have demonstrated greater plate-to-plate variation in zone diameter when the agar depth is less than 3 mm (14,44).

Time between Inoculation and Disk Placement

The period of delay between the inoculation of the agar surface and the placement of the disks prior to incubation will have a significant effect on the ultimate zone diameter. This is a direct result of the concept of "the critical time" discussed earlier. Many bacteria are capable of initiating growth at room temperature, the temperature at which plates are usually inoculated. If the plates are preincubated at 35°C, the effect will be exaggerated. Studies examining this phenomenon have been used to elucidate the critical time (13). With two exceptions, disk diffusion methods recommend that the disks be applied within 15 minutes of plate inoculation (see Table 2.4). The exceptions are the Swedish SRGA method, which requires disk placement within 30 minutes, and the CDS method, which requires disk placement within 45 minutes. The Swedish method also requires a period of 30–60 minutes of prediffusion, during which the plates are left on the bench to allow adequate drug diffusion before "initiating" growth in the incubator.

Incubation Time

With rapidly growing bacteria, the zone diameter is formed within a few hours of commencing incubation (13). In theory, therefore, it is possible to read zone diameters when growth becomes visible. With further incubation—recommended for all organisms in all methods—there can be subtle changes in the zone diameter beyond the time when growth first becomes visible. These changes are the result of (a) delayed growth, (b) better visualization of partial inhibition, and/or (c) the delayed appearance of resistant variants. As zone diameter breakpoints are applied to species after specified incubation periods, it is not generally possible to use these values to determine susceptibility earlier. However, if the zone of inhibition is clearly in the resistant range, further incubation is only likely to make the zone smaller, and therefore it would be possible to categorize a strain as resistant when growth becomes visible. Incubation of the plate for a few hours longer than typically recommended (e.g., Enterobacteriaceae for 24 rather than 18 hours) will not usually significantly influence the interpretation.

Some bacteria need longer intervals of incubation than 24 hours, such as *H. pylori* (3 days) and some strains of *Yersinia pestis* (48 hours). The French CA-SFM method also allows the testing of anaerobes by disk diffusion and recommends 48 hours of incubation for this group (38).

A specific incubation duration of 24 hours is recommended in many methods for staphylococci when tested against the antistaphylococcal penicillins, usually represented by oxacillin or methicillin, and the glycopeptides, represented by vancomycin. In parallel with broth-based susceptibility testing methods, which can use 2% NaCl, this duration is used in order to maximize the expression of strains with heteroresistance. It must be used in consort with an incubation temperature of 35°C (and no greater). In the BSAC disk method, incubation at 30°C and the addition of 2% NaCl are also used, as these factors are known to enhance heteroresistance expression (8,11). Incubation for 24 hours is also recommended for enterococci when testing them against vancomycin in the NCCLS method (105).

Incubation Temperature

Incubation temperatures are designed to optimize the growth of the organisms under test. Most human bacterial pathogens are adapted to optimum growth at 37°C. Most methods therefore recommend growth at 35°C to 37°C. Incubation at 30°C is known to enhance the expression of heteroresistance to methicillin and other antistaphylococcal penicillins (8) and has been recommended as part of the recently developed BSAC disk susceptibility test (7).

Inoculum Density

Inoculum density probably has a greater effect on the ultimate zone diameter than any other variable. As described by Barry, the critical population is one of the three critical parameters in determining zone size. Higher inoculum densities will result in bacterial numbers reaching the critical population sooner, at a time when the critical concentration has diffused less than with lower inoculum densities (12). In the case of very dense inocula, it is likely that no zone at all will be formed, even if the organism is susceptible. Inoculum density is particularly important when the bacteria produce inactivating enzymes such as β-lactamases, especially if the enzyme requires induction, such as in the case of staphylococcal penicillinase. At low inoculum densities, the drug has the ability to kill the organism before sufficient enzyme is produced, and much larger zones will result.

In the development of different methods internationally, two approaches have been taken to the choice of inoculum density. Some methods have opted for simplicity and use inocula calibrated to a turbidity standard, almost always a McFarland 0.5 barium sulfate standard. This has been shown to result in quite different inoculum densities (in terms of cfus per milliliter) for different species (98). Hence methods some have chosen to vary the inoculum density by species or bacterial group, most notably the CA-SFM method (38,94). Denser inocula (i.e., those with higher turbidity) are required for selected species such as *Campylobacter* species and *H. pylori* to ensure prompt and adequate growth (119).

Zone Edge

The features of the zone edge will be determined, by the drug activity-species relationship, the resistance mechanism (if present) and occasional peculiarities of the species. Certain drug classes are notorious for producing "fuzzy" zone edges, where there is a gradual decrease in inhibition over a distance of 1–5 mm. This is a standard feature of sulfonamides and will be seen sometines with dihydrofolate reductase inhibitors and amphenicols. Most methods recommend that when a fuzzy zone is seen, the reader should make a judgment as to where approximately 80% inhibition occurs and define that as the zone edge. Judging 80% inhibition accurately and consistently takes practice.

A second phenomenon, a "heaped" zone edge, is seen occasionally, but it is a normal feature of penicillinase-producing *S. aureus*. It is recommended that a heaped edge be interpreted as showing that the strain is producing penicillinase.

P. mirabilis and *P. vulgaris* typically swarm up the disk even when susceptible to the drug. When the organism is susceptible, a thin film is observed inside a more or less distinct zone of inhibition. This film should be ignored when making zone diameter interpretations.

Disk Spacing

Although inappropriate disk spacing is a common problem, it has been little studied in critical way. The distance between individual disks will be determined principally by the disk contents and organism growth rate. Higher disk contents and slower growth produce larger zones. If zones are large enough, ones from adjacent disks can run into each other and reduce the chance of accurately determining the zone diameter. The NCCLS method, among others, specifies the distance between adjacent disks (24 mm from center to center) to minimize the chances of zone overlap. This limits to five the number of disks that can be placed on a 90-mm plate, a considerable inconvenience if six to eight drugs need to be tested, as the cost of large plates is often substantially more that the cost of the common 90-mm Petri plate. Other methods address the problem of disk spacing in different ways, and many allow up to six disks per 90-mm plate, relying to some degree on lower disk contents to avoid zone overlap.

Current Disk Susceptibility Testing Methods

Currently there are seven methods published internationally and are kept up to date through constant revision and the addition of new agents (Tables 2.6 and 2.7). Of these, the most widely applied is the NCCLS method. The French CA-SFM method is similar to the NCCLS method but differs in a small number of crucial aspects,

(*text continues on page 49*)

TABLE 2.6

Details of Current Disk Susceptibility Methods

Technical Detail	NCCLS (105)	CA-SFM (94)	BSAC (6,7)	DIN (43,46)	SRGA (132)	CDS (18,19)	Neo-Sensitabs (119)
Basic agar medium	Mueller-Hinton	Mueller-Hinton	Iso-Sensitest	Mueller-Hinton	Iso-Sensitest	Sensitest	Mueller-Hinton (or Iso-Sensitest or Danish Blood Agar)
Additional special media	HTM for *Haemophilus* spp; MH + 5% defibrinated sheep blood for *Streptococcus* spp; GC agar with 1% defined growth supplement for *Neisseria gonorrhoeae*	HTM or Chocolate PolyViteX for *Haemophilus* spp; Chocolate PolyViteX for *N. gonorrhoeae*; MH + 5% sheep blood for *Campylobacter* spp; MH + 10% defibrinated horse blood for *Helicobacter pylori*; Wilkins-Chalgren + 5% defibrinated blood or Brucella + 1 mg/L vitamin K_1 + 5% blood for anaerobes	ISA + 5% defibrinated horse blood for *Streptococcus pneumoniae*, hemolytic streptococci, *Moraxella catarrhalis*, *Neisseria meningitidis, N. gonorrhoeae*; ISA + 5% defibrinated horse blood + 20 mg/L NAD for *Haemophilus* spp; Columbia + 2% NaCl for staphylococci and for methicillin or oxacillin	None	ISA + 5% defibrinated horse blood + 20 mg/L β-NAD for streptococci, *Haemophilus* spp; *M. catarrhalis, Pasteurella multocida, N. gonorrhoeae*, corynebacteria, anaerobes	Sensitest + 5% defibrinated horse blood for enterococci, *Listeria* spp, streptococci, *M. catarrhalis, N. meningitidis, P. multocida, Campylobacter* spp; HTM for *Haemophilus* spp; chocolate Columbia using 8% defibrinated horse blood for *H. pylori*	HTM for *Haemophilus* spp; GC agar with defined growth supplement (as per NCCLS) for *N. gonorrhoeae*; MH + 5% defibrinated sheep blood for streptococci, *N. meningitidis*; MH + 5% blood unspecified for *M. catarrhalis, Campylobacter* spp; MH + 10% blood unspecified for *H. pylori*
pH	7.2–7.4 at room temperature	7.2–7.4	Not specified in method; manufacturer claims 7.4 ± 0.2	7.2–7.4 at 25°C after sterilization	7.2–7.6 at room temperature	Not specified; manufacturer claims 7.2–7.6	7.2–7.4

(*continued*)

TABLE 2.6 (Continued)

Details of Current Disk Susceptibility Methods

Technical Detail	NCCLS (105)	CA-SFM (94)	BSAC (6,7)	DIN (43,46)	SRGA (132)	CDS (18,19)	Neo-Sensitabs (119)
Divalent cation concentrations	Not specified; performance testing of quality control strains (esp. *Pseudomonas aeruginosa*) recommended (106)	Ca^{++} 50 mg/L, Mg^{++} 25 mg/L	Not specified but 200 mg/L Ca gluconate and 100 mg/L Mg glycerophosphate is in formulation	Not specified	Not specified but 200 mg/L Ca gluconate and 100 mg/L Mg glycerophosphate is in formulation	Not specified	Not specified
Plate diameter	(90 mm), 100 mm, 150 mm	90 mm, 140 mm, or 120 mm square	90 mm	90–100 mm, 140–150 mm, or 120 mm or 210-mm square	90 mm, 140 mm	90 mm	Not specified
Depth of agar	~4 mm = 25–30 mL per 100-mm plate, 60–70 mL per 150-mL plate	~4 mm = 25 mL per 90-mm plate, 60 mL per 140-mm plate, 55 mL per 120-mm square plate	4 mm (25 mL per 90-mm plate)	3–4 mm (20 mL in 90-mm and 48 mL in 140-mm plate = 3.1 mm; 25 mL in 90-mm and 61 mL in 140-mm plate = 3.9 mm; for square 120-mm plate, these volumes are 45 mL and 57 mL, respectively)	4 ± 0.5 mm (25 mL in 90-mm plate, 60 mL in 140-mm plate)	~3 mm (20 mL in 90-mm plate)	4 mm
Storage of plates	Up to 7 d at 2–8°C, with precautions to prevent drying	Up to 3 d at 2–8°C	Up to 1 wk in vented plastic boxes or sealed plastic bags at 8–10°C	Not stated	Refrigerate for up to 1 mo; sealed plastic bags are not necessary	In plastic bags at 4°C for up to 4 wk	Not specified

Disk storage	Refrigerate at −8°C or freeze in non-frost-free freezer at −14°C	Refrigerate at 4–8°C in a tightly closed container	In a sealed container at −20°C ideally or at least <8°C	Refrigerate in a tightly sealed container with desiccant	As per manufacturer's recommendations	Stock disks should be stored at −20°C	Stored at room temperature except cefepime, cefepime + clavulanate, cefpodoxime, temocillin, ticarcillin, ticarcillin + clavulanate (2–8°C)
Disk handling	Remove from fridge or freezer 1–2 h before use, avoiding formation of condensation; store in well-sealed desiccated dispenser, refrigerated between use	Bring to room temperature before opening containers or disk dispensers; once disk container is opened, use within 5 d	Allow disks to warm to room temperature before opening; store disk dispensers in sealed containers with an indicating desiccant at <8°C	Store disk dispensers at 2–8°C; bring to room temperature before use	As per manufacturer's recommendations	Store disk dispensers at 4°C with active desiccant; bring to room temperature before opening	For the stock storage exceptions, store at room temperature; storage up to 2 mo after removal from refrigerator; otherwise disks are stable for 4 yr
Fluid for preparing the inoculum	Growth method, use TS broth; direct method, use 0.9% saline or broth	Direct method, use MH broth or 0.9% saline (M/15 PBS pH7.2 for *Neisseria* spp, Brucella broth or saline for *Campylobacter* spp, Brucella or Schaedler broth for anaerobes); growth method, use MHB (Brucella or Schaedler broth for slow-growing anaerobes)	Iso-Sensitest broth	Phosphate-buffered saline or MH broth	Phosphate-buffered saline	0.9% saline	Growth methods, broth unspecified; direct method, use 0.9% saline

(continued)

TABLE 2.6 (Continued)

Details of Current Disk Susceptibility Methods

Technical Detail	NCCLS (105)	CA-SFM (94)	BSAC (6,7)	DIN (43,46)	SRGA (132)	CDS (18,19)	Neo-Sensitabs (119)
Number of colonies for preparing inoculum	3–5 well-isolated colonies touched with a loop	At least 3	At least 4 morphologically similar colonies	4–5 morphologically uniform colonies	5–10 touched with a sterile loop	1 colony (if visible material on wire), 3–5 colonies (if no visible material)	2–5 depending on method; either ICS (53) or NCCLS method is acceptable
Inoculum preparation	Growth method, in TSB at 35°C for 2–6 h; direct method, into saline or broth (recommended for fastidious organisms)	Most inocula are prepared from subcultures 24 h old; direct method, into saline or broth; growth method, at 37°C for 3–5 h; unstated for slow-growing anaerobes	Growth method, incubate at 35–37°C until visible turbidity; direct method, directly into broth (recommended for fastidious organisms)	From a pure subculture, pick or flush colonies from the plate surface and suspend	Dilute inoculum 1 in 100 in phosphate-buffered saline, except for streptococci (1 in 20) and corynebacteria (1 in 50)	Stab straight wire (must be 0.56 mm in diameter) into colony and then transfer to saline, rotating 10 times and then mixing with repeated pipette action; alternatively pick up material from colony at an angle to get visible material	As per ICS or NCCLS
Inoculum calibration	0.5 $BaSO_4$ McFarland	General, 0.5 McFarland; *N. gonorrhoeae*, 1 McFarland; *H. pylori*, 3 McFarland; anaerobes, 1 McFarland; slow-growing anaerobes, 2 McFarland	0.5 McFarland	0.5 McFarland	0.5 McFarland	Not calibrated routinely	0.5 McFarland (NCCLS method) except *Campylobacter* spp (1.0 McFarland) and *H. pylori* (3–4 McFarland)

Means of applying inoculum	Dip swab into inoculum and press against side of tube before swabbing entire surface of plate in 2 or more directions at 60° angle	Dilute inoculum 1 in 100 (1 in 10 for staphylococci and oxacillin, *Streptococcus* spp, *H. influenzae,* and *N. gonorrhoeae,* neat for *H. pylori* and anaerobes); flood or swab plate	Dilute inoculum 1 in 100 except for staphylococci, *S. pneumoniae, N. meningitidis, M. catarrhalis* (1 in 10), and *N. gonorrhoeae* (neat); dip sterile cotton swab and turn it against the side of the tube to remove excess liquid; swab plate in 3 directions	Dilute inoculum 1 in 100 for Gram-positive bacteria and 1 in 1000 for Enterobacteriaceae	Dip swab into inoculum and roll against side of tube to remove excess; swab surface in at least 2 different directions; it is also acceptable to flood plate, remove excess fluid, and allow plate to dry for 10–15 min	Flood plate, rock it, and remove excess fluid; dry plate by placing it uncovered next to a Bunsen burner for 5–10 min	ICS method, spread inoculum using bent glass rod or Drigalski spatula after applying 1–2 drops (90-mm plate) or 3–4 drops (140-mm plate); for NCCLS method, see NCCLS column
Number and spacing of disks	12 per 150-mm plate, 5 per 100-mm plate; spacing at least 24 mm from center to center	Number not specified but disks must be at least 30 mm apart and at least 10 mm from the plate edge	Not specified (up to 6 allowed per plate)	6 disks per 90- to 100-mm plate, 12 disks per 140- to 150-mm plate	Not specified; disks should be evenly spaced	No more than 6	7–9 per 80- to 100-mm plate, 12 per 140- to 150-mm plate, and 16 per 120-mm square plate, except for *Haemophilus* spp, *Neisseria* spp, streptococci, *Campylobacter* spp, and *H. pylori* (4 per 90-mm to 100-mm plate, 9 per 150-mm plate)
Time between inoculation and disk application	No more than 15 min	No more than 15 min	No more than 15 min	5–15 min	No more than 30 min	No more than 45 min	Not specified

(continued)

TABLE 2.6 (Continued)

Details of Current Disk Susceptibility Methods

Technical Detail	NCCLS (105)	CA-SFM (94)	BSAC (6,7)	DIN (43,46)	SRGA (132)	CDS (18,19)	Neo-Sensitabs (119)
Incubation temperature and time	35°C for 16–18 h, except for *S. maltophilia, B. cepacia, N. gonorrhoeae,* streptococci (35°C for 20–24 h); staphylococci and oxacillin, methicillin, nafcillin, or vancomycin (35°C for 24 h); enterococci and vancomycin (35°C for 24 h)	35–37°C for 18–24 h; 30°C for 24 h for staphylococci and oxacillin; 35–37°C for 72 h for *H. pylori*; 35–37°C for 48 h for anaerobes	35–37°C for 18–20 h; 30°C for 24 h for staphylococci and methicillin or oxacillin	36±1°C for 16–20 h	Allow diffusion of antibiotic for 30–60 min prior to placing in incubator; 35–37°C for 16–20 h	35°C overnight (minimum 16 h), except for *S. pneumoniae, Streptococcus milleri* group, *N. meningitidis, Haemophilus* spp, *Corynebacterium* spp, *M. catarrhalis* (35–37°C); *Campylobacter* spp (42°C); *Yersinia enterocolitica* (30°C); *H. pylori* (35°C for 72 h)	35°C overnight except for *Haemophilus* spp, *Vibrio cholerae* (16–18 h), *N. gonorrhoeae,* streptococci, *Campylobacter* spp (20–24 h); *Steriotrophomonas maltophilia, Burkholderia cepacia* (30°C for 18–24 h); *Acinetobacter* spp (35°C for 18–24 h); *H. pylori* (35–37°C for 48 h)

Atmosphere	Air except *Haemophilus* spp, *N. gonorrhoeae*, streptococci (5% CO_2)	Air except for *Neisseria* spp (5% CO_2); *Campylobacter* spp, and *H. pylori* (microaerophilic atmosphere); anaerobes (anaerobic atmosphere)	Air except for *N. meningitidis, S. pneumoniae, Haemophilus* spp, *N. gonorrhoeae* (4–6% CO_2)	Air	Air except for *Haemophilus* spp, *Neisseria* spp, streptococci (5% CO_2); anaerobic atmosphere for anaerobes	Air except for *S. pneumoniae, S. milleri group, N. meningitidis, Haemophilus* spp, *Corynebacterium* spp, *M. catarrhalis* (5% CO_2); *Campylobacter* spp, *H. pylori* (microaerophilic atmosphere)	Air except for *Haemophilus* spp, *N. gonorrhoeae*, streptococci (5–7% CO_2); *Campylobacter* spp (Campylobacter atmosphere)
Plate stacking	Not addressed	No more than 10 in a stack	No more than 6 in a stack	Not specified	Not specified	Not specified	Not specified
Zone reading	Use ruler or sliding calipers to measure zone to the nearest whole millimeter; hold Petri dish a few inches above a nonreflecting black surface; for opaque media, measure zone from surface; for transparent media, measure zone from the base	From zone edge of complete inhibition, measure with sliding caliper (preferred) or half-millimeter graded ruler	Use ruler, calipers, or automated zone reader and measure to the nearest millimeter; a template can be used	Measure in whole millimeters	Use calipers or another suitable tool; read 80% inhibition for diffuse zone edges	Measure the annular radius with ruler or calipers to the sharpest part of the zone edge	Use sliding calipers, ruler, or template, using back of plate where possible, illuminated with reflected light; measure to the nearest whole millimeter; ignore faint growth of tiny colonies at the edge

(continued)

TABLE 2.6 (Continued)

Details of Current Disk Susceptibility Methods

Technical Detail	NCCLS (105)	CA-SFM (94)	BSAC (6,7)	DIN (43,46)	SRGA (132)	CDS (18,19)	Neo-Sensitabs (119)
Interpretation	Regularly updated tables (106)	Regularly updated tables (94)	Tables supplied (7)	Regularly updated tables (43); if there are more than 3 colonies inside the zone, the result is called resistant (after checking for purity)	Regularly updated tables (134)	Disk content designed so that most zone annular radii are 6 mm for S and <6 mm for R; some exceptions provided in regular updates (19)	Regularly updated tables with zone diameter interpretations for MIC breakpoints from NCCLS, Dutch CRG, SRGA, Norwegian AFA, Denmark Aflæsningsskema, CA-SFM, DIN, BSAC (119)
Interpretative categories	S, I, R	S, I, R	S, R; I used to a very limited extent	S, I, R	S, I, R	S, R	Varies with interpretive guidelines

TABLE 2.7

Features of Disk Susceptibility Test Methods

NCCLS method (105)	
Basic medium	Mueller-Hinton
Additional media	HTM (*Haemophilus* test medium, see agar dilution section for recipe) for *Haemophilus* spp MH + 5% defibrinated sheep blood for *Streptococcus* spp GC agar with 1% defined growth supplement for *Neisseria gonorrhoeae*
pH	7.2–7.4 at room temperature
Divalent cation concentrations	Not specified; performance testing of quality control strains (esp. *Pseudomonas aeruginosa*) recommended (106)
Plate diameters	(90 mm), 100 mm, 150 mm
Depth of agar	~4 mm = 25–30 mL per 100-mm plate, 60–70 mL per 150-mL plate
Storage of plates	Up to 7 days at 2–8°C, with precautions to prevent drying
Disk storage	Refrigerate at −8°C or below or freeze in non-frost-free freezer at −14°C or below
Disk handling	Remove from fridge or freezer 1–2 h before use, avoiding formation of condensation; store in well-sealed desiccated dispenser, refrigerate between use
Fluid for preparing inoculum	Growth method: TSB Direct method: 0.9% saline or broth
Number of colonies for inoculum	3–5 well-isolated colonies touched with a loop
Inoculum preparation	Growth method: in TSB at 35°C for 2–6 h Direct method: into saline or broth (recommended for fastidious organisms)
Inoculum calibration	0.5 $BaSO_4$ McFarland
Application of inoculum	Swab dipped and pressed against side of tube before swabbing entire surface of plate in 2 or more directions at 60° angle
Number and spacing of disks	Spacing at least 24 mm from center to center, i.e. about 12 per 150 mm plate or 5–6 per 100 mm plate. Disks that give large zones should be placed next to those giving smaller zones.
Time between inoculation and disk application	No more than 15 min
Incubation temperature and time	35° for 16–18 h except for *Stenotrophomonas maltophilia, Burkholderia cepacia, N. gonorrhoeae*, streptococci (35°C for 20–24 hours); staphylococci and oxacillin, methicillin, nafcillin, or vancomycin (35°C for 24 h); enterococci and vancomycin (35°C for 24 h)
Atmosphere	Air except *Haemophilus* spp, *N. gonorrhoeae*, streptococci (5% CO_2)
Plate stacking	Not addressed
Zone reading	Use ruler or sliding calipers to measure zone to the nearest whole; hold Petri dish a few inches above a nonreflecting black surface; for opaque media, measure zones from surface; for transparent media, measure zone from the base
Interpretation	Regularly updated tables (106)
Interpretative categories	S, I, R
QC strains	*Enterococcus faecalis* ATCC 29212, *Escherichia coli* ATCC 25922, *E. coli* ATCC 35218, *Haemophilus influenzae* ATCC 49247, *H. influenzae* ATCC 49766, *N. gonorrhoeae* ATCC 49226, *P. aeruginosa* ATCC 27853, *Staphylococcus aureus* ATCC 25923, *Streptococcus pneumoniae* ATCC 49619
CA-SFM method (38,94)	
Basic medium	Mueller-Hinton

(continued)

TABLE 2.7 (Continued)

Features of Disk Susceptibility Test Methods

Additional media	HTM or Chocolate PolyViteX for *Haemophilus* spp Chocolate PolyViteX for *N. gonorrhoeae* MH + 5% sheep blood for *Campylobacter* spp MH + 10% defibrinated horse blood for *Helicobacter pylori* Wilkins-Chalgren + 5% defibrinated blood or Brucella + 1 mg/L vitamin K_1 + 5% blood for anaerobes
pH	7.2–7.4
Divalent cation concentrations	Ca^{++} 50 mg/L, Mg^{++} 25 mg/L
Plate diameters	90 mm, 140 mm, or 120 mm square
Depth of agar	~4 mm = 25 mL per 90-mm plate, 60 mL per 140-mm plate, 55 mL per 120-mm square plate
Storage of plates	Up to 3 days stored at 2–8°C
Disk storage	Refrigerate at 4–8°C in a tightly closed container
Disk handling	Bring to room temperature before opening containers or disk dispensers; once disk container is opened, use within 5 days
Fluid for preparing inoculum	Direct method: MH broth or 0.9% saline (M/15 PBS pH 7.2 for *Neisseria* spp, Brucella broth or saline for *Campylobacter* spp, Brucella, or Schaedler broth for anaerobes) Growth method: MHB (Brucella or Schaedler broth for slow-growing anaerobes)
Number of colonies for inoculum	At least 3
Inoculum preparation	Most inocula are prepared from subcultures 24 h old Direct method: into saline or broth Growth method: at 37°C for 3–5 h; unstated for slow-growing anaerobes
Inoculum calibration	General, 0.5 McFarland; *N. gonorrhoeae,* 1 McFarland; *H. pylori*, 3 McFarland; anaerobes,1 McFarland; slow-growing anaerobes, 2 McFarland
Application of inoculum	Dilute inoculum 1 in 100 (1 in 10 for staphylococci and oxacillin, *Streptococcus* spp, *H. influenzae*, and *N. gonorrhoeae*, neat for *H. pylori* and anaerobes); flood or swab plate
Number and spacing of disks	Number not specified but disks must be at least 30 mm apart and at least 10 mm from the plate edge
Time between inoculation and disk application	No later than 15 min
Incubation temperature and time	35–37°C for 18–24 h; 30°C for 24 h for staphylococci and oxacillin; 35–37°C for 72 h for *H. pylori*; 35–37°C for 48 h for anaerobes
Atmosphere	Air except for *Neisseria* spp (5% CO_2); *Campylobacter* spp and *H. pylori* (microaerophilic atmosphere); anaerobes (anaerobic atmosphere)
Plate stacking	No more than 10 in a stack
Zone reading	From zone edge of complete inhibition, measure with sliding caliper (preferred) or half-millimeter graded ruler
Interpretation	Regularly updated tables (94)
Interpretative categories	S, I, R
QC strains	
BSAC (7)	
Basic medium	Iso-Sensitest

(*continued*)

TABLE 2.7 (Continued)

Features of Disk Susceptibility Test Methods

Additional media	ISA + 5% defibrinated horse blood for *S. pneumoniae*, hemolytic streptococci, *M. catarrhalis, N. meningitidis, N. gonorrhoeae* ISA + 5% defibrinated horse blood + 20 mg/L NAD for *Haemophilus* spp Columbia + 2% NaCl for staphylococci and methicillin or oxacillin
pH	Not specified in method; manufacturer claims 7.4 ± 0.2
Divalent cation concentrations	Not specified but 200 mg/L calcium gluconate and 100 mg/L magnesium glycerophosphate is in formulation
Plate diameter	90 mm
Depth of agar	4 mm (25 mL per 90-mm plate)
Storage of plates	Up to 1 week in vented plastic boxes or sealed plastic bags at 8–10°C
Disk storage	In a sealed container at −20°C ideally or at least <8°C
Disk handling	Allow disks to warm to room temperature before opening; store disk dispensers in sealed containers with an indicating desiccant at <8°C
Fluid for preparing inoculum	Iso-Sensitest broth
Number of colonies for inoculum	At least 4 morphologically similar colonies
Inoculum preparation	Growth method: incubate at 35–37°C until visible turbidity Direct method: direct into broth (recommended for fastidious organisms)
Inoculum calibration	0.5 McFarland
Application of inoculum	Dilute inoculum 1 in 100 except for staphylococci, *S. pneumoniae, N. meningitidis*, and *M. catarrhalis* (1 in 10) and *N. gonorrhoeae* (neat); dip sterile cotton swab and turn it against the side of the tube to remove excess liquid; swab plate in 3 directions
Number and spacing of disks	Not specified (up to 6 allowed per plate)
Time between inoculation and disk application	No more than 15 min
Incubation temperature and time	35–37°C for 18–20 h; 30°C for 24 h for staphylococci and methicillin or oxacillin
Atmosphere	Air except for *N. meningitidis, S. pneumoniae, Haemophilus* spp, *N. gonorrhoeae* (4–6% CO_2)
Plate stacking	No more than 6 plates per stack
Zone reading	Use ruler, calipers, or automated zone reader and measure to the nearest millimeter; a template can be used
Interpretation	Tables supplied (7)
Interpretative categories	S, R; I used to a very limited extent
QC strains	*E. coli* ATCC 12241 (NCTC 12241) or NCTC 10418, *S. aureus* ATCC 25923 (NCTC 12981) or NCTC 6571, *P. aeruginosa* ATCC 27853 (NCTC 12934) or NCTC 10662, *E. faecalis* ATCC 29212 (NCTC 12697), *H. influenzae* ATCC 49247 (NCTC 12699) or NCTC 11931, *S. pneumoniae* ATCC 49619 (NCTC 12977), *N. gonorrhoeae* ATCC 49226 (NCTC 12700)
DIN (46)	
Basic medium	Mueller-Hinton
Additional media	None
pH	7.2–7.4 at 25°C after sterilization
Divalent cation concentrations	Not specified
Plate diameters	90–100 mm, 140–150 mm, or 120 mm or 210 mm square

(continued)

TABLE 2.7 (Continued)

Features of Disk Susceptibility Test Methods

Depth of agar	3–4 mm (20 mL in 90-mm and 48 mL in 140-mm plate = 3.1 mm; 25 mL in 90-mm and 61 mL in 140-mm plate = 3.9 mm; for square 120-mm plate, these volumes are 45 mL and 57 mL, respectively)
Storage of plates	Not stated
Disk storage	Refrigerate in a tightly sealed container with desiccant
Disk handling	Store disk dispensers at 2–8°C; bring to room temperature before use
Fluid for preparing inoculum	Phosphate-buffered saline or MH broth
Number of colonies for inoculum	4–5 morphologically uniform colonies
Inoculum preparation	From a pure subculture, pick or flush colonies from the plate surface and suspend
Inoculum calibration	0.5 McFarland
Application of inoculum	Dilute inoculum 1 in 100 for Gram-positive bacteria and 1 in 1000 for enterobacteriaceae
Number and spacing of disks	6 disks per 70-mm to 100-mm plate, 12 disks per 140-mm to 150-mm plate
Time between inoculation and disk application	5–15 min
Incubation temperature and time	36 ± 1°C for 16–20 h
Atmosphere	Air
Plate stacking	Not specified
Zone reading	Measure in whole millimeters
Interpretation	Regularly updated tables (43); if there are more than 3 colonies inside the zone, the result is called resistant (after a check for purity)
Interpretative categories	S, I, R
QC strains	*S. aureus* ATCC 25923 (DSM 1104), *S. aureus* ATCC 29213 (DSM 2569), *S. aureus* (MRSA) ATCC 43300, *E. faecalis* ATCC 29212 (DSM 2570), *E. coli* ATCC 25922 (DSM 1103), *E. coli* (β-lactamase) ATCC 35218, *Klebsiella pneumoniae* (ESBL) ATCC 700603, *P. aeruginosa* ATCC 27853 (DSM 1117), *H. influenzae* ATCC 49247, *H. influenzae* ATCC 49766, *S. pneumoniae* ATCC 49619, *S. pneumoniae* PEN-R, *M. catarrhalis,* (DSM 11994) *N. gonorrhoeae* ATCC 49226 (DSM 11994)
SRGA (132)	
Basic medium	Iso-Sensitest
Additional media	ISA + 5% defibrinated horse blood + 20 mg/L β-NAD for streptococci, *Haemophilus* spp, *M. catarrhalis, Pasteurella multocida, N. gonorrhoeae*, corynebacteria, anaerobes
pH	7.2–7.6 at room temperature
Divalent cation concentrations	Not specified but 200 mg/L calcium gluconate and 100 mg/L magnesium glycerophosphate is in formulation
Plate diameters	90 mm, 140 mm
Depth of agar	4 ± 0.5 mm (25 mL in 90-mm plate, 60 mL in 140-mm plate)
Storage of plates	Refrigerate for up to 1 month; sealed plastic bags are not necessary
Disk storage	As per manufacturer's recommendations
Disk handling	As per manufacturer's recommendations
Fluid for preparing inoculum	Phosphate-buffered saline
Number of colonies for inoculum	5–10 touched with a sterile loop
Inoculum preparation	Dilute inoculum 1 in 100 in PBS except for streptococci (1 in 20) and corynebacteria (1 in 50)

(*continued*)

TABLE 2.7 (Continued)

Features of Disk Susceptibility Test Methods

Inoculum calibration	0.5 McFarland
Application of inoculum	Dip swab into inoculum and roll against side of tube to remove excess, then swab surface in at least 2 different directions; it is acceptable to flood plate, then remove excess fluid and allow to dry for 10–15 min
Number and spacing of disks	Not specified; disks should be evenly spaced
Time between inoculation and disk application	No more than 30 min
Incubation temperature and time	Allow diffusion of antibiotic for 30–60 min prior to placing in incubator; 35–37°C for 16–20 h
Atmosphere	Air except for *Haemophilus* spp, *Neisseria* spp, streptococci (5% CO_2); anaerobic atmosphere for anaerobes
Plate stacking	Not specified
Zone reading	Use calipers or another suitable tool; read 80% inhibition for diffuse zone edges
Interpretation	Regularly updated tables (134)
Interpretative categories	S, I, R
QC strains	*E. coli* ATCC 25922 (CCUG 17620), *P. aeruginosa* ATCC 27853 (CCUG 17619)
CDS (18,19)	
Basic medium	Sensitest
Additional media	Sensitest + 5% defibrinated horse blood for *Enterococcus* spp, *Listeria* spp, streptococci, *M. catarrhalis, N. meningitidis*, *P. multocida*, *Campylobacter* spp HTM for *Haemophilus* spp Chocolate Columbia with 8% defibrinated horse blood for *H. pylori*
pH	Not specified; manufacturer claims 7.2–7.6
Divalent cation concentrations	Not specified
Plate diameter	90 mm
Depth of agar	~3 mm (20 mL in 90-mm plate)
Storage of plates	In plastic bags at 4°C for up to 4 wk
Disk storage	Stock disks should be stored at −20°C
Disk handling	Disk dispensers stored at 4°C with active desiccant; brought to room temperature before opening
Fluid for preparing inoculum	0.9% saline
Number of colonies for inoculum	1 colony if gives visible material on wire; 3–5 colonies if no visible material
Inoculum preparation	Alternatively pick up material from colony at an angle to get visible material
Inoculum calibration	Not calibrated routinely
Application of inoculum	Flood plate, rock it, and remove excess fluid; dry plate by placing it uncovered next to a Bunsen burner for 5–10 min
Number and spacing of disks	No more than 6
Time between inoculation and disk application	Within 45 min
Incubation temperature and time	35°C overnight (minimum = 16 h) except for *S. pneumoniae*, *Streptococcus milleri* group, *N. meningitidis, Haemophilus* spp, *Corynebacterium* spp, *M. catarrhalis* (35–37°C); *Campylobacter* spp (42°C); *Yersinia enterocolitica* (30°C); *H. pylori* (35°C for 72 h)

(continued)

TABLE 2.7 (Continued)

Features of Disk Susceptibility Test Methods

Atmosphere	Air except for *S. pneumoniae, S. milleri* group, *N. meningitidis, Haemophilus* spp, *Corynebacterium* spp, *M. catarrhalis* (5% CO_2); *Campylobacter* spp, *H. pylori* (microaerophilic atmosphere)
Plate stacking	Not specified
Zone reading	Measure the annular radius with ruler or calipers to the sharpest part of the zone edge
Interpretation	Disk content designed so that most zone annular radii are 6 mm for S and <6 mm for R; exceptions are provided in regular updates (19)
Interpretative categories	S, R
QC strains	*B. fragilis* ATCC 25285 (ACM 5196), *C. jejuni* NCTC 11168 (ACM 5183), *E. faecalis* POW 1994 (ACM 5184), *E. coli* NCTC 10418 (ACM 5185), *E. coli* NCTC 4560 (ACM 5186), *H. influenzae* NCTC 4560 (ACM 5187), *H. influenzae* NCTC 11315 (ACM 5188), *P. aeruginosa* NCTC 10662 (ACM 5189), *S. aureus* NCTC 6571 (ACM 5190), *S. pneumoniae* ARL 10582 (ACM 5191).
Neo-Sensitabs (70)	
Basic medium	Mueller-Hinton (or Iso-Sensitest or Danish Blood Agar)
Additional media	HTM for *Haemophilus* spp GC agar with defined growth supplement (as per NCCLS) for *N. gonorrhoeae* MH + 5% defibrinated sheep blood for streptococci, *N. meningitidis* MH + 5% blood unspecified for *M. catarrhalis, Campylobacter* spp MH + 10% blood unspecified for *H. pylori*
pH	7.2–7.4
Divalent cation concentrations	Not specified
Plate diameter(s)	Not specified
Depth of agar	4 mm
Storage of plates	Not specified
Disk storage	Stored at room temperature except cefepime, cefepime + clavulanate, cefpodoxime, temocillin, ticarcillin, ticarcillin + clavulanate (2–8°C)
Disk handling	For the stock storage exceptions, store dispensers at room temperature; storage up to 2 months after removal from refrigerator; otherwise disks are stable for 4 yr
Fluid for preparing inoculum	Growth methods: broth unspecified Direct method: 0.9% saline
Number of colonies for inoculum	2–5 depending on method; either ICS (53) or NCCLS method is acceptable
Inoculum preparation	As per ICS (53) or NCCLS
Inoculum calibration	0.5 McFarland (NCCLS method) except for *Campylobacter* spp (1.0 McFarland), *H. pylori* (3–4 McFarland)
Application of inoculum	ICS method: spread using bent glass rod or Drigalski spatula after applying 1–2 drops (90-mm plate) or 3–4 drops (140-mm plate) NCCLS method (see NCCLS section)
Number and spacing of disks	7–9 per 80-mm to 90-mm plate; 12 per 140-mm to 150-mm plate; 16 per 120-mm square plate except for *Haemophilus* spp, *Neisseria* spp, streptococci, *Campylobacter* spp, *H. pylori* (4 per 90-mm to 100-mm plate, 9 per 150-mm plate)
Time between inoculation and disk application	Not specified

(*continued*)

TABLE 2.7 (Continued)

Features of Disk Susceptibility Test Methods

Incubation temperature and time	35°C overnight except for *Haemophilus* spp, *V. cholerae* (16–18 h), *N. gonorrhoeae*, streptococci, *Campylobacter* spp (20–24 h); *S. maltophilia, B. cepacia* (30°C for 18–24 h); *Acinetobacter* spp (35°C for 18–24 h); *H. pylori* (35–37°C for 48 h)
Atmosphere	Air except for *Haemophilus* spp, *N. gonorrhoeae*, streptococci (5–7% CO_2); *Campylobacter* spp (campylobacter atmosphere)
Plate stacking	Not specified
Zone reading	Use sliding calipers, ruler, or a template, using back of plate where possible, illuminated with reflected light; measure to the nearest whole millimeter; ignore faint growth of tiny colonies at the edge
Interpretation	Regularly updated tables with zone diameter interpretations for MIC breakpoints from NCCLS, Dutch CRG, SRGA, Norwegian AFA, Denmark Aflæsningsskema, CA-SFM, DIN, BSAC (119)
Interpretative categories	Varies with interpretive guidelines
QC strains	*E. coli* ATCC 25922, *S. aureus* ATCC 25924, *P. aeruginosa* ATCC 27853, *E. faecalis* ATCC 29212

especially the inoculum density. Intrinsically, there is nothing to recommend one method over another, although the NCCLS process of setting MIC breakpoints and zone diameter criteria is based on the most comprehensive data set, which includes pharmacodynamic considerations and a large amount of clinical outcome data (Table 2.8). As most new drug development is based in the United States and driven by FDA criteria for clinical trials, it is likely that the NCCLS disk method will remain the one based on the best available data sets. Efforts toward standardization in Europe and possibly internationally will eventually see all disk methods calibrated against an agreed standard, although this is likely to take a considerable number of years. Because zone diameter interpretive criteria are standardized for each individual method, it is not possible to either deviate from the method or use zone diameter criteria from another method.

Testing of Problematic Species

Anaerobes

With the singular exception of the CA-SFM method (using Wilkins-Chalgren agar), no method has provided fully developed disk susceptibility testing of anaerobes. There have been several significant attempts to develop such methods in the United States (15,70,130), but the results have never been considered sufficiently robust for full development. In part this relates to the prevailing view that routine testing of anaerobic bacteria is not required. Rather it is believed that these bacteria should be tested in specific clinical circumstances or in batches to determine trends in resistance (102). BSAC has recently provided disk susceptibility testing methods for rapidly growing anaerobes on Wilkins-Chalgren agar supplemented with 5% horse blood, including interpretative criteria for a limited number of drugs (81). This effort must be considered tentative.

Campylobacter Species

There have been a small number of pilot studies examining the feasibility of testing *Campylobacter* species by a disk diffusion method (59,73,118). The CA-SFM has introduced a disk diffusion test using Mueller-Hinton supplemented with 5% defibrinated sheep or horse blood (94). There have been other recent studies examining the prevalence of resistance in human or animal isolates using the NCCLS method (83,126), although it is unclear what interpretive criteria were used, as the NCCLS method itself has none. Disk testing on Iso-Sensitest agar supplemented with 5% horse blood has been proposed recently by BSAC (81) and has been employed in epidemiological studies (110). Further multilaboratory studies in this area are awaited, as well as data correlated with clinical outcomes.

Helicobacter Pylori

Some authorities believe that disk susceptibility testing of *H. pylori* is not feasible (81). Their doubts are understandable given the slow-growing nature and special growth requirement of this species. However, CA-SFM

TABLE 2.8

NCCLS Criteria for Tolerable Discrepancy Rates in Setting Zone Diameter Breakpoints

MIC Category	Discrepency Rates (% of MIC category)[a]		
	Very Major	Major	Minor
No intermediate range[b]			
MIC > 1 dilution above resistance breakpoint	<2%	NA	<5%
MIC < 1 dilution below susceptible breakpoint	NA	<2%	<5%
MIC = resistant and susceptible breakpoint	<10%	<10%	<40%
Single or two intermediate dilutions[b]			
MIC > 1 dilution above resistance breakpoint	<2%	NA	<5%
MIC = 1 dilution above resistance breakpoint to 1 dilution below susceptible breakpoint	<10%	<10%	<40%
MIC < 1 dilution below susceptible breakpoint	NA	<40%	<5%

[a] Percentages are the proportion of strains in that particular category, not the whole population.
[b] The resistance breakpoint is the MIC *at or above* which the strain is resistant; the susceptible breakpoint is the MIC *at or below* which the strain is susceptible.

has standardized a disk test on Mueller-Hinton supplemented with 10% defibrinated horse blood and developed interpretive criteria for erythromycin (94). There have also been several preliminary studies looking at the action of macrolides and other agents against this species (63,74,92,96,127,149). There is generally excellent agreement between disk and MIC results in these methods, and testing for resistance to macrolides and metronidazole by disk only requires multilaboratory comparison and quality control development to become a fully validated method, as clinical correlates are well established (92).

Quality Control

The main features of quality control in disk susceptibility testing revolve around the regular testing of quality control strains. Each methodology has a slightly different approach and range of quality control strains. Many advocate the testing of β-lactamase–producing strains of *E. coli* and *H. influenzae* as control organisms for β-lactamase inhibitor combinations. Careful attention must be paid to the storage of quality control strains (see the earlier discussion on agar dilution). Suitable detailed guidance is provided by NCCLS (105). Quality control limits are defined for the common antimicrobials and relevant control strains. Ideally, quality control tests are conducted every time that the susceptibility tests are performed. Some methods allow the shift to weekly testing if daily testing has proven satisfactory. Usually 1 in 20 or 3 in 30 results out of range can be tolerated. Better still is the option of graphing daily results on a Shewhart chart to detect obvious trends (133). If there is no obvious cause for out-of-range testing, the suspect combination should be tested daily for 5 days. If all the results are within the acceptable range, normal quality control procedures can be resumed. Otherwise, a detailed analysis of the source of errors should be undertaken. Sources of error include (a) incorrect measurement or transcription of zone diameters; (b) inadequately mixed, expired, or incorrectly stored turbidity standard; (c) one or more of the materials out of date or incorrectly stored; (d) incorrect incubation temperature or atmosphere; (e) malfunctioning equipment (e.g., pipettors); (f) incorrectly stored disks; (g) altered or contaminated control strain; (h) incorrectly prepared inocula; and (i) inoculum source more than 24 hours old. Judgment is required when deciding whether patient results relevant to the out-of-range quality control tests should be reported.

Reading of Zone Diameters

Manual Methods

Good lighting is essential to proper manual reading of zone diameters. Optimally, the plate is held a few centimeters above a black, nonreflecting background illuminated with reflected light. For transparent media, zones should

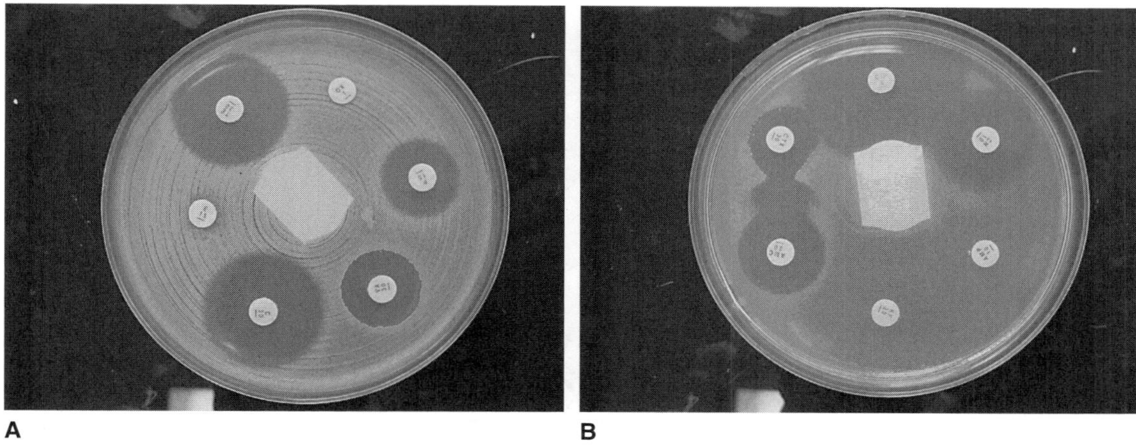

A B

FIGURE 2.3 • Disk diffusion test: NCCLS method on 90-mm plates. (A) *Staphylococcus aureus*. (B) *Escherichia coli*. This strain possesses an extended-spectrum β-lactamase and shows "keyhole" synergy between cefotaxime and amoxycillin-clavulanate.

be measured from the back of the plate; for opaque media such as those containing blood, zones are measured on the upper agar surface in reflected light. Two typical plates are shown in Figure 2.3. All methods normally recommend that zone diameters be measured and recorded. Although measurement is time-consuming, there are long-term advantages, as interpretive criteria can change, and retrospective adjustment of interpretation is possible when breakpoints change (as they do from time to time when new resistance emerges). Measuring and recording zone diameters are probably less frequently practiced (123). Most zone diameters are simple to read. The important exceptions are where the zone edge is not sharp, as noted earlier. Very faint growth inside the zone can be ignored. When there are multiple discrete colonies within the zone, either the strain has resistant mutants (and should be reported as resistant) or the inoculum was mixed. Either way, these colonies should be subcultured and the test repeated from the original plate or inoculum. Care should be taken with hemolytic streptococci not to read the zone of hemolysis rather than the zone edge.

Automated Methods

Significant advances have been made in recent years in imaging and scanning technology. As a result, there are now a small range of commercial systems that can read and interpret zone diameters. These include the Oxoid Aura (Oxoid, Basingstoke, UK), the BioMIC system (Giles Scientific, Santa Barbara, CA), and the Osiris system (Bio-Rad Laboratories, Hercules, CA). These systems have been developed over a long period and have been extensively validated. They have benefited from significant advances in scanning and imaging technology as well as in computer software. Intersubject variability in reading is virtually eliminated, although all systems allow for manual override. Zone diameter breakpoints can be adjusted to whatever method is being used. When interfaced with laboratory information systems, zone-reading systems can save reporting time and reduce transcription errors.

Establishment of Interpretive Criteria

Although formulas have been devised for the relationship between the zone diameter and the MIC of the organism (discussed earlier), in practice it turns out that breakpoint zone diameter criteria cannot really be defined using such formulas. One obstacle is that zone diameters vary continuously and MICs are measured on a discontinuous (grouped) scale of twofold dilutions. An MIC measurement implies that the strain has an MIC within the range of that particular twofold dilution; for example, a measured MIC of 16 mg/L implies that the true MIC is somewhere between 8 mg/L and 16 mg/L. Also, as can be seen from the theoretical example in Fig. 2.4, there is often a broad range (scatter) of zone diameters for strains with the same MIC. Finally, it is common for both zone diameters and MICs to have "off-scale" values (less than or equal to some number or greater than some number).

"Linear" regression is often applied to the paired MIC–zone diameter data. It is linear regression only in the sense that it uses standard linear regression methods on log-transformed MIC versus untransformed zone diameter data. However, it has little value, and its validity can be questioned. First, it is not possible to perform true

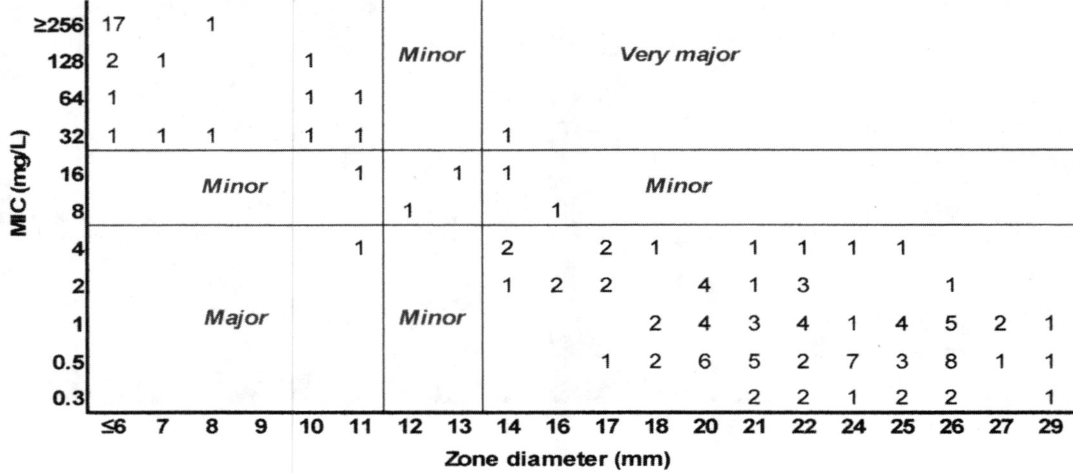

FIGURE 2.4 ● Relationship between zone diameters and MICs.

linear regression if there are off-scale values. Either these data must be assigned some arbitrary value or omitted. Either way, bias is introduced into the regression as a result. Second, as the MIC data are discontinuous, there are unproven assumptions that the true MICs at each point are log-normally distributed. Third, no one has yet defined a satisfactory way of "reading out" the breakpoint zone diameters from linear regression. Instead, alternative statistical methods have been developed (and are evolving) to select zone diameter criteria given previously selected MIC breakpoint criteria.

At present, there are no internationally agreed approaches. The most popular method is that devised by Metzler and DeHaan (95), the so-called error-rate bounded method. This is based on the minimization of "errors" (discrepancies between the zone diameter and MIC) with potential clinical impact. In the modern interpretation of MIC–zone diameter discrepancies, assuming that an intermediate category is desired, there are three types of errors: *minor*, where the MIC is intermediate (I) and the zone diameter is either susceptible (S) or resistant (R) or where the zone diameter is I and the MIC is either S or R; *major*, where the MIC is S and the zone diameter is R (i.e., the zone diameter is falsely resistant), which would deter the prescriber from choosing this drug; and *very major*, where the MIC is R and the zone diameter is S (i.e., the zone diameter is falsely susceptible), which could cause the prescriber to choose the drug though the organism is really resistant. Minor errors will not occur if single MIC and zone diameter breakpoints are selected. Metzler and DeHaan proposed that major errors should account for no more than 5% of the sample and very major errors for no more than 1%. They made no proposal for the percentage of minor errors that could be tolerated, other than to suggest that a large intermediate range of zone diameters is "not useful." The selection of zone diameters was based simply on any one or pair of zone diameters that gave the desired percentages of major and very major errors. Metzler and DeHaan's paper examined single MIC breakpoints and one or two zone diameter breakpoints. Brunden et al. extended the observations to the more common modern situation of having or wishing to have two breakpoint criteria each for MICs and zone diameters (27). They also introduced more sophisticated iterative methods for zone diameter selection and applied a recommendation that the minor errors tolerated should be no more than 5%.

This method has been developed even further by NCCLS, which has codified the error-rate tolerances for setting zone diameter breakpoints depending on the size of the intermediate MIC range (0, 1, or 2 dilutions), compensating for both the inherent error in MIC determinations (±1 dilution) and the number of strains in the different susceptibility categories. Even more sophisticated statistical techniques have been proposed and have been proven to work well on published data, but these have yet to be adopted by any authority (40).

By way of showing how these methods work, the data in Fig. 2.4 would yield the following error rates using the Metzler-DeHaan method: very major, 1/132 (<1%); major, 1/132 (<1%); and minor, 3/132 (2.3%). By the NCCLS method (2 intermediate concentrations), the rates for those with an MIC >1 dilution above the resistance breakpoint are as follows: very major, 0/25 (0%); and minor, 0/25 (0%). The rates for those with an MIC from the resistant to the susceptible breakpoint are as follows: very major, 1/21 (4.8%); major, 1/21 (4.8%); and minor, 1/21 (4.8%). The rates for those with an MIC <1 dilution below the susceptible breakpoint are as follows: major, 0/86 (0%); and minor = 0/86 = 0%.

Rapid Disk Testing

As zone diameters for rapidly growing bacteria become visible after a few hours and after the critical time has passed (see Theoretical Aspects earlier in this chapter), interest has been shown in the possibility of reading disk susceptibility results earlier than the conventional 16 to 20 hours (16,24,82,84,121). High degrees of correlation with standard testing have been shown for reading at 4–5 hours for Enterobacteriaceae (98.9%), Gram-positive cocci (98.7%), and *Pseudomonas* species (97.9%) (2). One quarter of the strains of *P. aeruginosa* will have grown insufficiently at 5 hours and will require longer incubation times (84). In the single study of *Salmonella typhi*, results of reading at 8 hours were 100% concordant with test results after conventional incubation (121).

In order to achieve good correlation with standard disk testing, conditions for the test need to be modified. Plates should be prewarmed to 37°C prior to inoculation, the inoculum should be adjusted to McFarland 1.0 (not 0.5), 5% blood should be added for testing all Gram-positive cocci to maximize growth rates, and strains classified as intermediate but with zones close to the susceptible borderline should be reclassified as susceptible (2).

Rapid reading has not become popular despite its good performance, and it is not currently offered as an alternative by any standard-setting organization. This relates partly to workflow in the laboratory; unless plates can be set up early in the day, it is often not possible to generate the results in sufficient time for the clinician to make use of them on the same day.

Direct Disk Testing

Direct susceptibility testing involves the use of the specimen as the source of the inoculum. Few specimens are suitable for direct testing, because the organism being tested in the specimen may be mixed with other pathogens and contaminants. Considerable error can occur when mixed strains are present in the disk test (124).

Studies on direct testing have been conducted principally on urine and positive blood cultures, although direct testing is feasible on a wider range of specimens, especially those obtained from sterile body sites such as cerebrospinal fluid. A single study on testing wound exudates gave unreliable results (52). The results of all such tests must be considered preliminary, and tests should be repeated by a standardized method once the organism or organisms have been isolated. The benefit of direct testing is that it can generate a preliminary result a day sooner and guide the clinician in choosing an antibiotic earlier in treatment. It is of greatest value when the clinical circumstances are urgent and/or life-threatening. In the one prospective study that compared rapid testing with conventional testing, significant benefits were seen for patient care and outcomes in the group whose results were generated rapidly (49).

Urine

The possibility of direct antimicrobial susceptibility testing of potentially infected urine was recognized many years ago (10). A number of prospective studies have been conducted examining the accuracy of direct disk diffusion testing (23,25,50,51,61,69,75,77,80,99,107, 111,122,147). With few exceptions, direct susceptibility testing shows a high degree of accuracy (94% to 98% agreement with conventional testing), provided strict criteria are followed for the selection of results that can be interpreted. Problems encountered that might prevent interpretation include (a) low bacterial concentrations despite true urinary infection, (b) inaccuracies due to the nonstandardized inoculum, and (c) mixed cultures (77).

The most recent studies in which NCCLS methods were used have provided the best examples of how direct testing of urine should be undertaken (61,77,107). Specimens for direct testing should be selected using microscopy criteria indicating probable urinary tract infection: an elevated white cell count (=8–10 cells per mm^3) and an absence or a paucity of squamous epithelial cells, with or without the visible presence of bacteria. The inoculum is prepared simply by dipping a sterile cotton-tipped swab into the urine specimen, squeezing out the excess fluid against the side of the tube, and streaking a plate of plain Mueller-Hinton agar as in the standardized test. After disk placement, the plates are incubated overnight as normal. The results are interpreted using the standard criteria for those tests where the culture confirms urinary tract infection, there is adequate growth on the medium, the cultures are not mixed (even if they are all pathogens), and the quantitative culture of the original specimen is $=10^4$ CFU/mL. The issue whether to report results as susceptible when they are categorized as intermediate because of high urinary antibiotic concentrations remains unresolved. Doing so increases the "accuracy" of the direct test (107). Intermediate results are sometimes seen when the urine bacterial concentration is higher than the inoculum in the standardized test. Some authors have also noted that the accuracy of direct testing drops when resistance to an antibiotic class is prevalent (77) and have attributed this to the proximity of many zone diameters to breakpoint values when resistance is present. If all the just described criteria are followed, then direct results could be considered valid and should not require repeat testing by the conventional method (77).

Direct susceptibility testing of urine has also been successfully attempted using disk elution (66) and agar dilution breakpoint plates (25).

Blood Cultures

If blood cultures become positive, it is possible to use the blood culture broth to perform direct disk susceptibility testing. This method has been confirmed to perform well in a range of studies (39,55,76,97,148). Rates of overall agreement with standardized testing range from 90% to 95%. One study showed that these rates of agreement could be reached after 6 hours for Gram-positive bacteria, although Gram-negative bacteria required overnight incubation. One advantage of blood culture broth as a source for the inoculum is that the inoculum can be standardized turbidometrically, provided the blood is not lysed (a common problem with *E. coli* and *S. pneumoniae*), although at least one study showed good agreement by using the positive blood culture broth directly (39). There are several options for preparing the inoculum, including direct use of the blood culture broth (39), subculture of a fixed withdrawn volume and further broth incubation to reach McFarland 0.5 (97), and mixing the blood culture broth with broth or distilled water to adjust to the McFarland standard (2). A further advantage of direct blood culture broth use is that knowledge of the Gram-stain characteristics of the isolate can guide the choice of a test medium.

There are some drawbacks to direct testing from blood culture bottles: the presence of high thymidine concentrations in blood culture media will carry over and antagonize the sulfonamides and trimethoprim, and the presence of sodium polyanethol sulfonate (SPS) in older blood culture media to remove antibiotics can antagonize some penicillins, aminoglycosides, and glycopeptides (2). All results generated by direct testing should be confirmed by standardized testing the next day, as bacteremia is a serious condition requiring confident antimicrobial choices.

GRADIENT DIFFUSION SUSCEPTIBILITY TESTING

Gradient diffusion susceptibility testing has been pioneered by a Swedish company, AB Biodisk (Solna, Sweden), under the brand name Etest. The technology exploits the properties of antibiotic diffusion in agar to generate MIC values. It achieves this by applying a gradient of antibiotic along a carrier strip placed on the inoculated surface of an agar plate in the same way that antibiotic disks are placed. The antibiotic gradient is created on the strip by applying different concentrations of antibiotics in repeated arrays of an increasing number of small dots. When applied to the agar surface, the antibiotic diffuses into the surrounding medium in high to low amounts from one end of the strip to the other. The gradient remains stable after diffusion, and the zone of inhibition created takes the form of a pointed ellipse. The MIC is read off the scale printed on the upper side of the strip at the point where the zone edge meets the strip edge (9) (Fig. 2.5).

The first evaluations of this product proved the Etest was comparable to conventional MIC testing (26,79). The

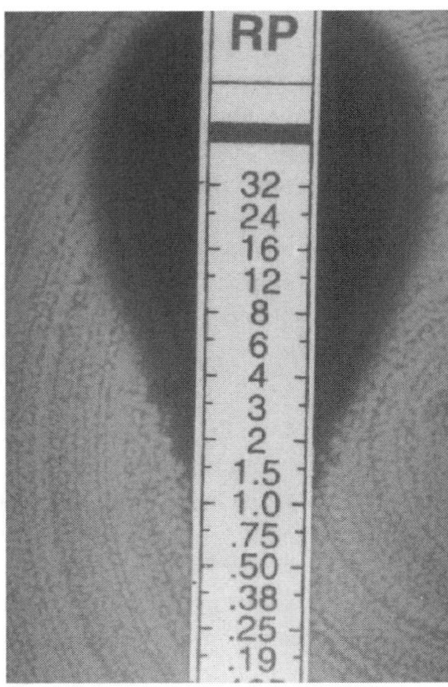

FIGURE 2.5 ● Etest gradient diffusion test for *Streptococcus pneumoniae* and quinupristin/dalfopristin. The MIC is where the growth of the strain meets the strip (1.5 mg/L), ignoring the zone of hemolysis.

Etest has since been evaluated against a very broad range of bacteria, including mycobacteria, as well as yeasts and molds. In general, the Etest produces results similar to those of conventional MIC tests against almost all bacteria. Its attraction is that it is simple to set up (as simple as disk diffusion) and takes less work, time, and materials than any agar or broth dilution method. Difficulties are encountered with some organism-antibiotic combinations, because finding the endpoint (where the zone intersects the strip) suffers from the same problems as zone edge interpretation in disk diffusion. Indeed, the effect is sometimes exaggerated with the Etest. However, as the product has undergone constant reevaluation over the 14 years since its release, the company has provided an excellent range of technical guides, charts, and other visual materials to assist the user in reading and interpreting the results correctly. Problems such as microcolonies at the intersection, swarming, paradoxical effects, hemolysis, resistant subpopulations, endpoints for bacteriostatic drugs, and technical errors are all dealt with and examples provided.

Like all such products, Etest strips must be properly stored and handled. The details of how to store the strips are provided by the manufacturer. Although Etest strips can be readily handled individually by sterile (flamed) forceps, the company also sells two devices, one for handling single strips and one for placing multiple strips on a single plate. The strips are made of plastic and are flexible enough to allow misplacement if forceps are used. As in the case of routine disks, the antibiotic will commence rapid diffusion as soon as the Etest strip is placed. Hence, it is not possible to relocate the strip once it is placed. The length of the strips is such that one fits comfortably on a 90-mm Petri dish. With careful placement, two different antibiotics can be tested on a single 90-mm plate, although this practice is not recommended. If done, the strips must be oriented in opposite directions. Larger plates are recommended if more than one strip is to be used. A normal 150-mm Petri plate will comfortably accommodate six strips provided that the bottoms of the strips are all facing the center of the plate.

Etest strips have the MIC scale printed on the upper side. The scale is often modified from the conventional base 2 logarithmic scale and includes intermediate "dilutions," such as 3 mg/L between the values of 2 and 4 mg/L. These values are not true halfway points on the $\log_2$ scale but rather rounded values, and the lines on the strip at these dilutions are placed accordingly.

The greatest advantage of the Etest is that it provides a laboratory with the ability to conveniently perform an MIC determination on a single strain without the full setup required for a conventional MIC test. If the clinical circumstances demand it, a quantitative susceptibility value can be easily generated. As an example, suppose a serious invasive infection such as meningitis or septicemia has been caused by *Streptococcus pneumoniae* but the categorical susceptibility results (susceptible, intermediate, resistant) provide insufficient information to guide clinical antibiotic decision making. The Etest can also be used to validate unusual resistances generated by conventional testing.

OTHER AGAR-BASED METHODS

Gradient Agar Plates

The concept of creating a single agar plate with a gradient of antibiotic concentration is an old one (72,135). Gradient plates provide a range of concentrations in a single plate and have been used principally to compare the susceptibilities of a range of strains on a single plate, especially when the MIC differences are likely to be small. More recently, gradient plates have also been used to select for resistant variants. When a gradient plate is used for this purpose, the strain being examined must be exposed to subinhibitory concentrations in one part of the plate (29).

In the most common method for preparing a gradient plate, a square Petri plate (100 mm by 100 mm usually) is tilted at a 12° angle while kept precisely level along the perpendicular axis (152). Agar (~25 mL per 100-mm plate) containing the antibiotic of interest at a known concentration is poured into the tilted plate and allowed to set. The plate is then set flat and precisely level, and a second identical volume of agar containing no antibiotic is poured over the top. The plate is ready to use after this second layer has set. Strains under test are usually streaked in a linear fashion starting from the lowest to the highest concentration (from the thin to the thick end of the lower layer).

MUTANT PREVENTION CONCENTRATION

See "Killing Curve" in Chapter 3 for a discussion of the Mutant prevention concentration (MPC).

POPULATION ANALYSIS PROFILING

The emergence of low-level resistance to vancomycin in a number of countries has led to the reintroduction of a research tool now called *population analysis profiling*. The technique was successfully applied to demonstrate the emergence of resistance during treatment of *P. aeruginosa* in an animal model with single agents (60). It was later applied to the characterization of methicillin resistance in *S. aureus* (21). Its application to the study of reduced vancomycin susceptibility in *S. aureus* began with Hiramatsu et al., who successful applied this technique to strains with homogeneous and heterogeneous reduced susceptibility (68). Refinements have been made to the technique in an attempt to minimize false positivity by comparing the area under the curve (AUC) of the population profile (log-transformed CFU/ml) with that of the original heteroresistant strain (Mu3) isolated in Japan (152). AUC ratios of =0.9 comparing the test strain with Mu3 were considered positive for heteroresistance. A ratio of =1.3 was used in a later study to define strains with homogeneous reduced resistance (141). There is ongoing uncertainty about the sensitivity and specificity for detecting hetero- and homogeneous reduced glycopeptide susceptibility in staphylococci using this test. It is very labor-intensive and consumes significant resources and thus is likely to remain a research tool.

CLINICAL VALUE OF *IN VITRO* TESTING

The artificial nature of *in vitro* susceptibility testing frequently raises questions about the interpretation and meaning of results for patient management. Certainly, there are significant differences between the *in vitro* and *in vivo* situations on a range of factors such as (a) fixed versus varying drug concentrations, (b) no protein binding versus protein binding, (c) 16–24 hours of drug exposure versus days for treatment courses, (d) fixed versus variable physiological conditions such as pH and eH, (e) absence versus presence of host immune response, (f) optimum growth conditions versus restricted growth *in vivo*, and (g) low versus high inocula at the start of drug exposure. It is likely, therefore, that the MIC *in vitro* is different from the MIC *in vivo* in some, many, or all situations.

The differences between the morphological and physiological characteristics of bacterial growth *in vitro* and *in vivo* can be stark, suggesting that *in vitro* simulation of conditions might aid in getting *in vitro* responses to better mimic *in vivo* responses to therapy (86,87). Tests on solid surfaces may approximate the state of organisms *in vivo* more closer. Standard laboratory susceptibility tests do not detect the range of antibacterial effects of an antimicrobial, such as sub-MIC effects (85,108), postantibiotic effects (41,89), postantibiotic sub-MIC effects (28), leukocyte enhancement effects (112), and supra-MIC effects.

Yet there is evidence that *in vitro* testing as conducted in the routine laboratory is predictive of response to therapy. Although there are very few studies that have examined test results versus patient outcomes in the routine setting (88), those that have been done, together with clinical experience and the findings of some prospective clinical studies, suggest that there is a high correlation. The question is why such correlation is possible.

The first part of the answer is that although MICs and their susceptibility testing correlates are artificial and indeed somewhat arbitrary, this does not matter. The yard and the meter are also arbitrary units of measurement, yet no one would deny their universal value for making measurements and, more importantly, comparing of measurements. Provided that there are MIC methods that are simple and reproducible and have low degrees of scatter, MICs can be used as a basis for comparing *in vitro* activity with the outcomes of treatment.

Second, if reproducible correlations can be shown between MICs (whatever values are generated) and bacteriological and clinical outcomes, concerns about their poor reflection of *in vivo* activity can be bypassed. In essence, MICs become a convenient "yardstick" for predicting treatment outcomes. Prediction of outcomes has always been the goal of *in vitro* susceptibility testing. It is only then necessary to demonstrate that routine methods themselves correlate with MICs obtained using standardized methods.

Correlations between MICs and outcomes are now being generated through the emergence of the science of antimicrobial pharmacodynamics (42). By the use of *in vitro* and animal models, it has been possible to define the key pharmacodynamic parameters for a broad range of antimicrobial classes, including the β-lactams (42), the aminoglycosides (140), the macrolides (90), the quinolones (4), and the glycopeptides, and to provide guidance on the polymyxins (67), the tetracyclines, the lincosamides, and the oxazolidinones (41). Extrapolation of these findings to human infections has so far not revealed major discrepancies. Extrapolation is frequently necessary, as it is unethical to conduct clinical studies in which some patients must fail therapy in order to confirm pharmacodynamic correlates. Occasionally failure to take into account pharmacodynamics has led to poor outcomes (64,128). Data on pharmacodynamics are now being applied as part of the development of breakpoint values (see Chapter 1).

Third, another goal of susceptibility testing is to detect the presence of resistance, defined microbiologically as the acquisition of a mutation or external genetic material or the induction of natural enzymes with an effect on the phenotype. Resistance will be reflected by an increase in MIC to above normal levels. All susceptibility testing methods include the concept of detecting abnormal phenotypes, although many have set breakpoints that will not detect all abnormal phenotypes. This reflects the tension between microbiological and pharmacodynamic breakpoints discussed in Chapter 1, a tension that is not yet fully resolved. In a range of standardized methods, supplementary tests are recommended to increase the chances of detecting abnormal phenotypes, including β-lactamase detection tests and screening plates. How closely abnormal phenotypes that are below the breakpoints correlate with clinical outcomes is largely unknown, but the conservative position is to interpret them as resistant (or at least intermediate) until it is known that they are susceptible clinically.

REFERENCES

1. Acar JF, Goldstein FW. Disk susceptibility testing. In: Lorian V, ed. *Antibiotics in laboratory medicine,* 3rd ed. Baltimore: Williams & Wilkins, 1991:17–52.
2. Acar JF, Goldstein FW. Disk susceptibility testing. In: Lorian V, ed. *Antibiotics in laboratory medicine,* 4th ed. Baltimore: Williams & Wilkins, 1996:1–51.
3. Acar JF, Goldstein FW, Lagrange P. Human infections caused by thiamine- or menadione-requiring *Staphylococcus aureus. J Clin Microbiol* 1978;8:142–147.
4. Ambrose PG, Bhavnani SM, Owens RC. Clinical pharmacodynamics of quinolones. *Infect Dis N Am* 2003;17:529–543.
5. Andrews JM. Determination of minimum inhibitory concentrations. *J Antimicrob Chemother* 2001;48(Suppl S1): 5–16.
6. Andrews JM. The development of the BSAC standardized method for disc diffusion testing. *J Antimicrob Chemother* 2001;48(Suppl S1):29–42.
7. Andrews JM, for the BSAC Working Party on Susceptibility Testing. BSAC standardized disc susceptibililty testing method. *J Antimicrob Chemother* 2001;48(Suppl S1):43–57.
8. Annear D. Full expression of methicillin resistance in *Staphylococcus aureus. J Antimicrob Chemother* 1985; 15:253–254.
9. Anon. *Etest for MIC determination.* Etest technical guide 3B. Solna, Sweden: Ab Biodisk. Available at: www.abbiodisk.com.
10. Bacteriology Committee of the Association of Clinical Pathologists. Report on antibiotic sensitivity test trial organized by the Bacteriology Committee of the Association of Clinical Pathologists. *J Clin Pathol* 1965;18: 1–5.
11. Baker CN, Huang MB, Tenover FC. Optimizing testing of methicillin-resistant Staphylococcus species. *Diagn Microbiol Infect Dis* 1994;19:167–170.
12. Barry AL. *The antimicrobic susceptibility test: principles and practices.* Philadelphia: Lea and Febiger, 1976.
13. Barry AL. Procedure for testing antibiotics in agar media: theoretical considerations. In: Lorian V, ed. *Antibiotics in laboratory medicine.* Baltimore: Williams & Wilkins, 1980:1–23.
14. Barry AL, Fay GD. The amount of agar in antimicrobic

disk susceptibility test plates. *J Clin Pathol* 1973;59:196–198.

15. Barry AL, Fuchs PC, Gerlach EH, et al. Multilaboratory evaluation of an agar diffusion disk susceptibility test for rapidly growing anaerobic bacteria. *Rev Infect Dis* 1990;12(Suppl 2):S210–S217.
16. Barry AL, Joyce LJ, Adams AP, et al. Rapid determination of antimicrobial susceptibility for urgent clinical situations. *Am J Clin Path* 1973;59:693–699.
17. Bauer AW, Kirby WMM, Sherris JC, et al. Antibiotic sensitivity testing by a standardized single disk method. *Am J Clin Path* 1966;45:493–496.
18. Bell SM. The CDS disc method of antibiotic sensitivity testing (calibrated dichotomous sensitivity test). *Pathology* 1975;7:1–48.
19. Bell SM, Gatus BJ, Pham JN, et al. *Antibiotic susceptibility by the CDS method,* 2nd ed. Available at: www.med.unsw.edu.au/pathology-cds.
20. Bemer-Melchior P, Juvin M-E, Tassin S, et al. In vitro activity of the new ketolide telithromycin compared to those of the macrolides against *Streptococcus pyogenes*: influences of resistance mechanisms and methodological factors. *Antimicrob Agents Chemother* 2000;44:2999–3002.
21. Berge-Bachi B, Strassle A, Kayser FH. Characterization of an isogenic set of methicillin-resistant and susceptible mutants of *Staphylococcus aureus. Eur J Clin Microbiol* 1986;5:697–701.
22. Berkman S, Henry RJ, Housewright RD. Studies on streptomycin, I: Factors influencing the activity of streptomycin. *J Bacteriol* 1947;53:567.
23. Blue AP, Gordon DL. Is primary sensitivity testing on urine samples valid? *Pathology* 1991;23:149–152.
24. Boyle VJ, Faucher ME, Ross RW. Rapid modified Kirby Bauer susceptibility test with single high concentration antimicrobial discs. *Antimicrob Agents Chemother* 1973;3:418–424.
25. Bronnestam R. Direct antimicrobial susceptibility testing in bacteriuria. *APMIS* 1999;107:437–444.
26. Brown DF, Brown L. Evaluation of the Etest, a novel method of quantifying antimicrobial activity. *J Antimicrob Chemother* 1991;27:185–190.
27. Brunden MN, Zurenko GE, Kapik B. Modification of the error-rate bounded classification scheme for use with two MIC break points. *Diagn Microbiol Infect Dis* 1992;15:135–140.
28. Cars O, Odenholt-Tornqvist I. The post-antibiotic sub-MIC effect in vitro and in vivo. *J Antimicrob Chemother* 1993;31(Suppl D):159–166.
29. Carsenti-Etesse H, Roger PM, Dunais B, et al. Gradient plate method to induce *Streptococcus pyogenes* resistance. *J Antimicrob Chemother* 1999;44:439–443.
30. Casals JB, Gylling Pedersen O. Tablet sensitivity testing: a comparison of methods. *Acta Pathol Microbiol Scand* [B] 1972;80:860–816.
31. Cavenaghi LA, Biganzoli E, Danese A, et al. Diffusion of teicoplanin and vancomycin in agar. *Diag Microbiol Infect Dis* 1992;15:253–258.
32. Cooper GL, Louie A, Baltch AL, et al. Influence of zinc on *Pseudomonas aeruginosa* susceptibilities to imipenem. *J Clin Microbiol* 1993;31:2366–2370.
33. Cooper KE. Theory of antibiotic inhibition zones in agar media. *Nature* 1955;176:510–511.
34. Cooper KE, Gillespie WA. The influence of temperature on streptomycin inhibition zones in agar cultures. *J Gen Microbiol* 1952;7:1–7.
35. Cooper KE, Linton AH. The importance of the temperature during the early hours of incubation of agar plates in assays. *J Gen Microbiol* 1952;7:8–17.
36. Cooper KE, Linton AH, Sehgal SN. The effect of inoculum size on inhibition zones in agar media using staphylococci and streptomycin. *J Gen Microbiol* 1958;18:670–687.
37. Cooper KE. The theory of antibiotic inhibition zones. In: Kavanaugh F, ed. *Analytical microbiology.* New York: Academic Press, 1964;1–86.
38. Couvalin P, Soussy J-C, eds. Technical recommendations for in vitro susceptibility testing. 1996 Report of the Comité de l'Antibiogramme de la Société Française de Microbiologie. *Clin Microbiol Infect* 1996;2(Suppl 1):S11–S34.
39. Coyle MB, McGonagle LA, Plorde JJ, et al. Rapid antimicrobial susceptibility testing of isolates from blood cultures by direct inoculation and early reading of disk diffusion tests. *J Clin Microbiol* 1984;20:473–477.
40. Craig BA. Modeling approach to diameter breakpoint determinations. *Diagn Microbiol Infect Dis* 2000;36:193–202.
41. Craig WA. Post-antibiotic effects in experimental animal models: relationship to in-vitro phenomena and the treatment of infections in man. *J Antimicrob Chemother* 1993;31(Suppl D):149–158.
42. Craig WA. Basic pharmacodynamics of antibacterials with clinical applications to the use of β-lactams, glycopeptides and linezolid. *Infect Dis N Am* 2003;17:479–501.
43. D'Amato RF, Thornsberry C, Baker CN, et al. Effect of calcium and magnesium on the susceptibility of *Pseudomonas* species to tetracycline, gentamicin, polymyxin B, and carbenicillin. *Antimicrob Agents Chemother* 1975;7:596–600.
44. Davis WW, Stout TR. Disc plate method of microbiological antibiotic assay, I: Factors influencing variability and error. *Appl Microbiol* 1971;22:659–665.
45. Dibb WL, Digranes A, Bottolfson KL. Effects of carbon dioxide upon the in vitro activity of erythromycin. *Acta Pathol Microbiol Immunol Scand* [B] 1986;94:173–176.
46. DIN 58940–3. *Medical microbiology: susceptibility testing of pathogens to antimicrobial agents,* Part III*: Agar diffusion test.* Berlin: Deutsches Institut für Normung, December 2002.
47. DIN 58940–3. Data for the interpretation of inhibition zone diameters (Suppl 1). *Medical microbiology: susceptibility testing of pathogens to antimicrobial agents,* Part III: *Agar diffusion test.* Berlin: Deutsches Institut für Normung, January 2000.
48. DIN 58940–6. *Medical microbiology: Susceptibility testing of pathogens to antimicrobial agents,* Part VI: *Determination of minimum inhibitory concentration (MIC) with the agar dilution method.* Berlin: Deutsches Institut für Normung, April 2003.
49. Doern GV, Vautour R, Gaudet M, et al. Clinical impact of rapid in vitro susceptibility testing and bacterial identification. *J Clin Microbiol* 1994;32:1757–1762.
50. Dornbusch K, Lindeberg B, Nord C-E, et al. Bacteriuria diagnosis and antibiotic susceptibility testing in a group practice by dip-slide techniques. *Chemotherapy* (Basel) 1979;25:227–232.
51. Dornbusch K, Nord C-E, Olsson B, et al. Antibacterial susceptibility testing by the dip-slide technique: a methodological evaluation. *Chemotherapy* (Basel) 1976;22:190–202.
52. Ellner PD, Johnson E. Unreliability of direct susceptibility testing on wound exudates. *Antimicrob Agents Chemother* 1976;9:355–356.
53. Ericsson HM, Sherris JC. Antibiotic sensitivity testing: report of an international collaborative study. *Acta Pathol Microbiol Scand* 1971;217(Suppl B):1–90.
54. European Committee for Antimicrobial Susceptibility Testing (EUCAST) of the European Society for Clinical Microbiology and Infectious Diseases (ESCMID).

Determination of minimum inhibitory concentrations (MICs) of antibacterial agents by agar dilution. *Clin Microbiol Infect* 2000;6:509–515.
55. Fay D, Oldfather JE. Standardization of direct susceptibility test for blood cultures. *J Clin Microbiol* 1979;9:347–350.
56. Franklin JC. Quality control in agar dilution sensitivity testing by direct assay of the antibiotic in solid medium. *J Clin Path* 1980;33:93–95.
57. Fuchs PC, Barry AL, Brown S. Daptomycin susceptibility tests: interpretive criteria, quality control, and the effect of calcium on in vitro tests. *Diagn Microbiol Infect Dis* 2000;38:51–58.
58. Fuchs PC, Barry AL, Brown SD. Evaluation of daptomycin susceptibility testing by Etest and the effect of different batches of media. *J Antimicrob Chemother* 2001;48:557–561.
59. Gaudreau C, Gilbert H. Comparison of disc diffusion and agar dilution methods for antibiotic susceptibility testing of *Campylobacter jejuni* subsp.jejuni and *Campylobacter coli*. *J Antimicrob Chemother* 1997;39:707–712.
60. Gerber AU, Vastola AP, Brandel J, et al. Selection of aminoglycoside-resistant variants of *Pseudomonas aeruginosa* in an in vivo model. *J Infect Dis* 1982;146:691–697.
61. Gillenwater JY, Clark MM. Tentative direct antimicrobial susceptibility testing in urine. *J Urol* 1996;156:149–153.
62. Goldstein EJC, Sutter VL, Kwok Y-Y, et al. Effect of carbon dioxide on in vitro susceptibility of anaerobic bacteria to erythromycin. *Antimicrob Agents Chemother* 1981;20:705–708.
63. Hachem CY, Clarridge JE, Reddy R, et al. Antimicrobial susceptibility testing of *Helicobacter pylori*. *Diagn Microbiol Infect Dis* 1996;24:37–41.
64. Harding I, MacGowan AP, White LO, et al. Teicoplanin therapy for *Staphylococcus aureus* septicaemia: relationship between pre-dose serum concentrations and outcome. *J Antimicrob Chemother* 2000;45:835–841.
65. Hecht DW, Lederer L. Effect of the choice of medium on the results of in vitro susceptibility testing of eight antimicrobials against the *Bacteroides fragilis* group. *Clin Infect Dis* 1995;20(Suppl 2):S346–S349.
66. Heinze PA, Thrupp LD, Anselmo CR. A rapid (4–6 hour) urine-culture system for direct identification and direct antimicrobial susceptibility testing. *Am J Clin Pathol* 1979;71:177–183.
67. Hermsen ED, Sullivan CJ, Rotschafer JC. Polymyxins: pharmacology, pharmacokinetics, pharmacodynamics and clinical applications. *Infect Dis N Am* 2003;17:545–562.
68. Hiramatsu K, Arikata N, Hanaki H, et al. Dissemination in Japanese hospitals of strains of *Staphylococcus aureus* heterogeneously resistant to vancomycin. *Lancet* 1997;350:1670–1673.
69. Hollick GE, Washington JA. Comparison of direct and standardized disk diffusion susceptibility testing of urine cultures. *Antimicrob Agents Chemother* 1976;9:804–809.
70. Horn R, Bourgault A-M, Lamothe F. Disk diffusion susceptibility testing of the *Bacteroides fragilis* group. *Antimicrob Agents Chemother* 1987;31:1596–1599.
71. Humphrey JH, Lightbown J. A general theory for plate assay of antibiotics with some practical applications. *J Gen Microbiol* 1952;7:129–143.
72. Hunt DE, Sandham HJ. Improved agar gradient-plate technique. *Appl Microbiol* 1969;17:329–330.
73. Huysmans M, Turnidge J. Disc susceptibility testing for thermophilic campylobacters. *Pathology* 1997;29:209–216.
74. Iovene MR, Romano M, Pilloni AP, et al. Prevalence of antimicrobial resistance in eighty clinical isolates of *Helicobacter pylori*. *Chemotherapy* 1999;45:8–14.
75. Jenschke WJ, Trevino E, Vaqnce PH, et al. Comparison of direct urine and standard Kirby-Bauer sensitivities. In: Abstracts of the 93rd General Meeting of the American Society for Microbiology 1993; American Society for Microbiology, Washington, DC. Abstract C-190.
76. Johnson JE, Washingon JA. Comparison of direct and standardized antimicrobial susceptibility testing of positive blood cultures. *Antimicrob Agents Chemother* 1976;10:211–214.
77. Johnson JR, Tiu FS, Stamm WE. Direct antimicrobial susceptibility testing for acute urinary tract infection in women. *J Clin Microbiol* 1995;33:2316–2323.
78. Johnson MM, Hill SL, Piddock LJV. Effect of carbon dioxide on testing of susceptibilities of respiratory tract pathogens to macrolides and azalide antimicrobial agents. *Antimicrob Agents Chemother* 1999;43:1862–1865.
79. Jorgensen JH, Howell AW, Maher LA. Quantitative antimicrobial susceptibility testing of *Haemophilus influenzae* and *Streptococcus pneumoniae* by using the E-test. *J Clin Microbiol* 1991;29:109–114.
80. Källenius G, Dornbusch K, Hallander HO, et al. Comparison of direct and standardized antibiotic susceptibility testing in bacteriuria. *Chemotherapy* (Basel) 1981;27:99–105.
81. King A. Recommendations for susceptibility tests on fastidious organisms and those requiring special handling. *J Antimicrob Chemother* 2001;48(Suppl S):77–80.
82. Kluge RM. Accuracy of Kirby-Bauer susceptibility tests read at 4, 8 and 12 hours of incubation: comparison with reading at 18 to 20 hours. *Antimicrob Agents Chemother* 1975;8:139–145.
83. Ledergerber U, Regula G, Stephen R, et al. Risk factors for antibiotic resistance in *Campylobacter* species isolated from raw poultry meat in Switzerland. *BMC Public Health* 2003;3:39–47.
84. Lorian V. A five hour disc antibiotic susceptibility test. In: Lorian V, ed. *Significance of medical microbiology in the care of patients*. Baltimore: Williams & Wilkins, 1977:203–212.
85. Lorian V. Low concentrations of antibiotics. *J Antimicrob Chemother* 1985;15(Suppl A):15–26.
86. Lorian, V. Differences between in vitro and in vivo studies. *Antimicrob Agents Chemother.* 1988;32:1600–1601.
87. Lorian V. In vitro simulation of in vivo conditions: physical state of the medium. *J Clin Microbiol* 1989;27:2403–2406.
88. Lorian V, Burns L. Predictive value of susceptibility tests for the outcome of antibacterial therapy. *J Antimicrob Chemother* 1990;25:175–81.
89. MacKenzie FM, Gould IM. The post-antibiotic effect. *J Antimicrob Chemother* 1993;31(Suppl D):519–537.
90. Maglio D, Nicolau DP, Nightingale CH. Impact of pharmacodynamics on dosing of macrolides, azalides and ketolides. *Infect Dis N Am* 2003;17:563–577.
91. McDermott SN, Hartley TF. New datum handling methods for the quality control of antibiotic solutions and plates used in the antimicrobial susceptibility test. *J Clin Microbiol* 1989;27:1814–1825.
92. McNulty C, and the PHLS Helicobacter Working Group. *Helicobacter pylori* susceptibility testing by disc diffusion. *J Antimicrob Chemother* 2002;49:601–609.
93. Medeiros AA, O'Brien TF, Wacker WEC, et al. Effect of salt concentration on the apparent in vitro susceptibility of Pseudomonas and other Gram-negative bacilli to gentamicin. *J Infect Dis* 1971;124(Suppl):S59–S66.
94. Members of the SFM Antibiogram Committee. Comité de l'Antibiogramme de la Société Française de Microbiologie Report 2003. *Int J Antimicrob Agents* 2003;21:364–391.

95. Metzler CM, DeHaan RM. Susceptibility tests of anaerobic bacteria: statistical and clinical considerations. *J Infect Dis* 1974;130:588–594.
96. Midolo PD, Bell JM, Lambert JR, et al. Antimicrobial resistance testing of *Helicobacter pylori*: a comparison of Etest and disk diffusion methods. *Pathology* 1997;29:411–414.
97. Mirrett S, Reller LB. Comparison of direct and standard antimicrobial disk susceptibility testing for bacteria isolated from blood. *J Clin Microbiol* 1979;10:482–487.
98. Moosdeen F, Williams JD, Secker A. Standardisation of inoculum size for disc susceptibility testing: a preliminary report of a spectrophotometric method. *J Antimicrob Chemother* 1988;21:439–443.
99. Mukerjee C, Reiss-Levy E. Evaluation of direct disc diffusion susceptibility testing for bacteriuria using diluted urine against the standard CDS method. *Pathology* 1994;26:201–207.
100. Murray CK, Walter EA, Crawford S, et al. Abiotrophia bacteremia in a patient with neutropenic fever and antimicrobial susceptibility testing of Abiotrophia isolates. *Clin Infect Dis* 2001;32:e140–e142.
101. National Committee for Clinical Laboratory Standards. *Protocols for evaluating dehydrated Mueller-Hinton agar: approved standard.* Wayne, PA: National Committee for Clinical Laboratory Standards, 1996. NCCLS document M6-A.
102. National Committee for Clinical Laboratory Standards. *Methods for antimicrobial susceptibility testing of anaerobic bacteria: approved standard–fifth edition.* Wayne, PA: National Committee for Clinical Laboratory Standards, 2003. NCCLS document M11-A6.
103. National Committee for Clinical Laboratory Standards. *Methods for dilution antimicrobial susceptibility tests for bacteria that grow aerobically: approved standard–sixth edition.* Wayne, PA: National Committee for Clinical Laboratory Standards, 2003. NCCLS document M7-A6.
104. National Committee for Clinical Laboratory Standards. *Quality control for commercially prepared microbiological culture media: approved standard–second edition.* Wayne, PA: National Committee for Clinical Laboratory Standards, 2003. NCCLS document M22-A2.
105. National Committee for Clinical Laboratory Standards. *Performance standards for antimicrobial disk susceptibility tests: approved standards–seventh edition.* Wayne, PA: National Committee for Clinical Laboratory Standards, 2003. NCCLS document M2-A8.
106. National Committee for Clinical Laboratory Standards. *Performance standards for antimicrobial susceptibility testing: fourteenth informational supplement.* Wayne PA: National Committee for Clinical Laboratory Standards, 2004. NCCLS document M100-S14.
107. Oakes AR, Badger R, Grove DI. Comparison of direct and standardized testing of infected urine for antimicrobial susceptibilities by disk diffusion. *J Clin Microbiol* 1994;32:40–45.
108. Odenholt I. Pharmacodynamic effects of subinhibitory antibiotic concentrations. *Int J Antimicrob Agents* 2001; 17:1–8.
109. The Oxoid manual, 8th Edition, 1998. Ed. Bridson EY. Oxoid Limited, Basing stoke, UK.
110. Oza AN, McKenna JP, McDowell SWJ, et al. Antimicrobial susceptibility of *Campylobacter* spp. isolated from broiler chickens in Northern Ireland. *J Antimicrob Chemother* 2003;52:220–223.
111. Perez JR, Gillenwater JY. Clinical evaluation of testing immediate antibiotic disk sensitivities in bacteriuria. *J Urol* 1973;110:452–456.
112. Pruul H, McDonald PJ. Damage to bacteria by antibiotics in vitro and its relevance to antimicrobial chemotherapy. *J Antimicrob Chemother* 1988;21:695–698.
113. Reller LB, Schoenknecht FD, Kenny MA, et al. Antibiotic susceptibility testing of *Pseudomonas aeruginosa:* selection of a control strain and criteria for magnesium and calcium content of media. *J Infect Dis* 1974;130:454–463.
114. Retsema JA, Brennan LA, Girard AE. Effects of environmental factors on the in vitro potency of azithromycin. *Eur J Clin Microbiol Infect Dis* 1991;10:834–842.
115. Reynolds AV, Hamilton-Miller JM, Brumfitt W. Diminished activity of gentamicin under anaerobic or hypercapnic conditions. *Lancet* 1976;1(7957):447–449.
116. Roe DE, Hecht DW, Finegold SM, et al. Multilaboratory comparison of anaerobe susceptibility results using three different agar media. *Clin Infect Dis* 2001;35(Suppl 1): S40–S46.
117. Roe DE, Hecht DW, Finegold SM, et al. Multilaboratory comparison of growth characteristics for anaerobes using five different media. *Clin Infect Dis* 2001;35(Suppl 1): S36–S45.
118. Rogol M, Michel J. Detection of resistant isolates of *Campylobacter jejuni* by the disc susceptibility method. *Eur J Clin Microbiol* 1984;3:40–42.
119. Rosco Diagnostica A/S. Users guide: Neo-Sensitabs™ susceptibility testing, 16th ed. 2003. Available at: www.rosco.dk/Default.asp?ID=198.
120. Rosenblatt JE, Schoenknecht F. Effect of several components of anaerobic incubation on antibiotic susceptibility results. *Antimicrob Agents Chemother* 1972;1:433–440.
121. Saha SK, Darmstadt GL, Baqui AH, et al. Rapid identification and antibiotic susceptibility testing of *Salmonella enterica* serovar *typhi* isolated from blood: implications for therapy. *J Clin Microbiol* 2001;39:3583–3585.
122. Scully PG, O'Shea B, Flanagan KP, et al. Urinary tract infection in general practice: direct antibiotic sensitivity testing as a potential diagnostic method. *Irish J Med Sci* 1990;159:98–100.
123. Shah PM. Recording zone diameters—a rare phenomenon in microbiology laboratories? [letter]. *Int J Antimicrob Agents* 2004;23:208.
124. Shahidi M, Ellner PD. Effect of mixed cultures on antibiotic susceptibility testing. *Appl Microbiol* 1969;18:766–770.
125. Shungu D. Chemical and physical properties of antibiotics: preparation and control of antibiotic susceptibility disks and other devices containing antibiotics. In: Lorian V, ed. *Antibiotics in laboratory medicine,* 4th ed. Baltimore: Williams & Wilkins.
126. Sjögren E, Lindblom G-B, Kaijser B. Norfloxacin resistance in *Campylobacter jejuni* and *Campylobacter coli* isolates from Swedish patients. *J Antimicrob Chemother* 1997;40:257–261.
127. Smith C, Perkins J, Tompkins D. Conparison of Etest and disc diffusion for detection of antibiotic resistance in *Helicobacter pylori. Microbiol Digest* 1997;14:21–23.
128. Snydman DR, Cucheral GJ Jr, McDermott L, et al. Correlation of various in vitro testing methods with clinical outcomes in patients with *Bacteroides fragilis* group infections treated with cefoxitin: a retrospective analysis. *Antimicrob Agents Chemother* 1992;36:540–544.
129. Spangler SK, Jacobs MR, Appelbaum PC. Effect of CO_2 on susceptibilities of anaerobes to erythromycin, azithromycin, clarithromycin, and roxithromycin. *Antimicrob Agents Chemother* 1994;38:211–216.
130. Sutter VL, Kwok YY, Finegold SM. Standardized antimicrobial disc testing of anaerobic bacteria, I: Susceptibility of *Bacteroides fragilis* to tetracycline. *Appl Microbiol* 1973;3:188–193.

131. Swedish Reference Group on Antibiotics. Dilution methods. Available at: www.srga.org/RAFMETOD/Basmet2.htm.
132. Swedish Reference Group on Antibiotics. Disk diffusion. Available at: www.srga.org/RAFMETOD/rafmet.htm.
133. Swedish Reference Group on Antibiotics. Validation and internal quality control of antibiotic susceptibility testing. Available at: www.srga.org/RAFMETOD/qcmet.htm.
134. Swedish Reference Group on Antibiotics. Zone breakpoints from SRGA and SRGA-M. Available at: www.srga.org/RAFMETOD/Zontab.htm.
135. Szybalski W. Microbial selection, I: Gradient plate technique for study of bacterial resistance. *Science* 1952;116:46–48.
136. Tapsall JW, Wilson E, Harper J. Thymine dependent strains of Escherichia coli selected by trimethoprim-suphamethoxazole during therapy. *Pathology* 1974;6:161–167.
137. Toohey M, Francis G, Stingemore N. Variation in Iso-Sensitest agar affecting β-lactam testing. *ASIGnation* (newsletter of the Antimicrobial Special Interest Group of the Australian Society for Microbiology) 1990;1(6):5–8.
138. Touhy MJ, Procop GW, Washington JA. Antimicrobial susceptibility of *Abiotrophia adiacens* and *Abiotrophia defectiva*. *Diagn Microbiol Infect Dis* 2000;38:189–191.
139. Traub WH, Leonhard B. Antibiotic susceptibility tests with fastidious and nonfastidious bacteria reference strains: effects of aerobic versus hypercapnic incubation. *Chemotherapy* 1995;41:18–33.
140. Turnidge JD. Pharmacodynamics and dosing of aminoglycosides. *Infect Dis N Am* 2003;17:503–528.
141. Walsh TR, Bolmström A, Qwärnström A, et al. Evaluation of current methods for detection of staphylococci with reduced susceptibility to glycopeptides. *J Clin Microbiol* 2001;39:2439–2444.
142. Ward PB, Palladino S, Looker JC, et al. P-nitrophenylglycerol in susceptibility testing media alters the MICs of antimicrobials for *Pseudomonas aeruginosa*. *J Antimicrob Chemother* 1993;31:489–496.
143. Ward PB, Palladino S, Looker JC. P-nitrophenylglycerol in susceptibility testing media alters the MICs of antimicrobials for aerobic Gram-negative bacilli. *J Antimicrob Chemother* 1993;31:803–805.
144. Washington JA, Snyder RJ, Kohner PC, et al. Effect of cation content of agar on the activity of gentamicin, tobramycin and amikacin against *Pseudomonas aeruginosa*. *J Infect Dis* 1978;137:103–111.
145. Waterworth PM. Sulphonamides and trimethoprim. In: Reeves DS, Phillips I, Williams JD, et al., eds. *Laboratory methods in antimicrobial chemotherapy*. Edinburgh: Churchill Livingstone, 1978:82–84.
146. Waterworth PM. The aminoglycosides. In: Reeves DS, Phillips I, Williams JD, et al., eds. *Laboratory methods in antimicrobial chemotherapy*. Edinburgh: Churchill Livingstone, 1978:85–87.
147. Waterworth PM, Del Piano MD. Dependability of sensitivity tests in primary culture. *J Clin Pathol* 1976;29:179–184.
148. Wegner DL, Mathis CR, Neblett TR. Direct method to determine the antibiotic susceptibility of rapidly growing blood pathogens. *Antimicrob Agents Chemother* 1976;9:861–862.
149. Weiss K, Laverdiere M, Restieri C. Comparison of 10 antibiotics against clinical strains of *Helicobacter pylori* by three different techniques. *Can J Gastroenterol* 1998;12:181–185.
150. Winstanley T, Edwards C, Limb D, et al. Evaluation of a surfactant, Dispersol LN, as an anti-swarming agent in agar dilution susceptibility testing. *J Antimicrob Chemother* 1994;33:353–356.
151. Wise R, Phillips I. Towards a common susceptibility testing method? *J Antimicrob Chemother* 2000;45:919–920.
152. Wootton M, Howe RA, Hillman R, et al. A modified population analysis profile (PAP) method to detect hetero-resistance to vancomycin in *Staphylococcus aureus* in a UK hospital. *J Antimicrob Chemother* 2001;47:399–403.
153. Working Party on Antibiotic Sensitivity Testing of the British Society for Antimicrobial Chemotherapy. A guide to sensitivity testing. *J Antimicrob Chemother* 1991;27(Suppl D):1–50.

CHAPTER 3

Susceptibility Testing of Antimicrobials in Liquid Media

Daniel Amsterdam

Fleming's serendipitous observation of the action of *Penicillium notatum* against several species of bacteria initiated what was to become known as the chemotherapy era. From that discovery, Fleming developed two approaches for assessing antimicrobial activity that are currently used. The initial discovery was determined by an agar diffusion methodology. Subsequent experiments that attempted to characterize this newly found antibacterial substance can be recognized as exemplifying the broth dilution method for susceptibility testing (80). One method Fleming used to obtain quantitative assessments of the degree of activity of an antimicrobial agent was to inoculate a suspension of the organism into a liquid growth medium that incorporated serial twofold dilutions of the agent. This we recognize as the broth macrodilution method. Obviously, it is not the broth that is diluted. The potentially active compound is the component that is diluted. As penicillin became available for therapeutic use, other medical microbiologists quickly adopted this procedure in order to guide therapy (182). No doubt another impetus for antimicrobial susceptibility testing became manifest as a result of financial considerations. Before World War II, the production of penicillin was limited and extremely expensive. Thus, it was evident that a procedure capable of predicting when the use of penicillin would be effective in a particular infectious disease needed to be developed. In the 1940s, several antibiotics were discovered. Although the broth susceptibility method was the first procedure developed for assessing the *in vitro* efficacy of antimicrobial agents (and it still serves today as a reference method), it was replaced by methods using antibiotic-impregnated filter paper strips (82) and later disks (245).

Toward the end of the 1950s, the status of antimicrobial susceptibility testing was in disarray as a result of the lack of acceptable standard procedures. To remedy this situation, an international group of experts was convened. They outlined general guidelines and reported on the need for standards (261). After the World Health Organization report, an international collaborative group was formed to address the problems of standardization. The report by this group (74) was later followed by adoption of the procedures of Bauer et al. (25) in the *Federal Register* (76,77), which in large part was directed toward agar disk diffusion susceptibility testing. The International Collaborative Study (ICS) report (74) was the springboard for establishing a database and objectives of standardization for current methods (77,167,168).

As it evolved from Fleming's pioneering studies, the technique of using serial twofold dilutions in a liquid medium for studying the antimicrobial action of therapeutic agents is referred to as the broth dilution method, although the component diluted is clearly the antimicrobial agent. Initially, this technique was performed in test tubes in a final volume of 1–2 mL, and most laboratories followed the procedure detailed by the ICS (74). As the number of antimicrobial agents for testing increased, a more manipulative assay was automated and became popular. This procedure, referred to as the microdilution technique because the final volume was only 50 μL, has gained much wider acceptance than the earlier dilution methodology, known as the macrobroth or macrodilution technique.

Commercial development and application of the miniaturized technique has made it accessible to all laboratories. Thus, minimal inhibitory concentrations (MICs) can be provided by any laboratory regardless of its technical resources. Microdilution test results have been nearly equivalent to those obtained with the conventional macrodilution method, with little exception. For Gram-negative microorganisms, the microdilution procedure yields MICs approximately one dilution lower than does the macrodilution method (see "Standard Broth Dilution Procedures").

The focus of this chapter is on selected elements in the design and performance of standard methods and new rapid, automated, and instrumental approaches to antimicrobial susceptibility testing in liquid media. Although reference is made to a variety of fastidious microorganisms, anaerobes and mycobacteria are not discussed (see Chapters 4 and 5).

GENERAL CONSIDERATIONS

Test Procedure

In selecting a procedure to determine the outcome of the interaction of microbe and antimicrobial compound, the laboratory must first determine whether qualitative or quantitative information is desired or required. Although, as stated, the central focus of this discussion is on the interaction of bug and drug in a liquid (broth) environment, a comparison of broth and agar diffusion methodologies is warranted (Table 3.1).

TABLE 3.1

Comparative Feature of Disk Diffusion and Dilution Methods

Feature	Disk Diffusion	Agar Dilution	Broth Dilution[a]
Contamination readily observed	Yes	Yes	No[b]
Test for most resistant members of inoculum	No	No	Yes
Inoculum effect	No[c]	No	Yes[c]
Quantitative result	No[d]	Yes	Yes
MBC result	No	No	Yes
Direct test from clinical material	Yes	?	No
Applicable for slow-growing and fastidious organisms	No[e]	Yes	Yes
Readily amenable to automation	No	?	Yes

[a] Micro (0.1 mL) or macro (1.0 to 2.0 mL).
[b] Contaminants can be detected on subculture to appropriate medium.
[c] Slow-growing subpopulations (e.g., methicillin-resistant *S. aureus*, MRSA; methicillin-resistant *S. epidermidis*, MRSE) require additional incubation interval and/or medium advantage.
[d] Zone diameters are inversely related to MIC and require regression analysis for development of interpretive guidelines (*S*, susceptible: *I*, intermediate or indeterminate: *R*, resistant).
[e] Current standards apply to aerobic organisms.

It is evident that a distinct advantage of broth methods is that they permit the determination of a minimal bactericidal concentration (MBC) endpoint. For those laboratories involved in special clinical pharmacologic studies, the assessment of the clinical efficacy of antimicrobial compounds (older or newly formulated), detailed assays of drug levels, distribution, and toxicity, and fully quantifiable results determined by MIC endpoints derived from broth dilution studies are required. The MIC can in turn be used to calculate therapeutic ratios, that is, the ratio of serum (or tissue) fluid concentration to MIC. The MIC can be determined from standard quantitative broth (or agar) dilution methods and derived from regression analysis of the diameter of zone inhibition (48,145) (Table 3.1). If the laboratory has established a database and has experience with one methodology, changing procedures for an alternative method can create new problems.

The advantages of one approach over another are summarized in Table 3.1. In certain clinical therapeutic situations (e.g., in cases of endocarditis or osteomyelitis), MICs may be indicated. When MICs are obtained, they can be used to calculate therapeutic regimens to minimize the adverse effects of potentially toxic drugs, giving added confidence in the selected therapeutic regimen. If broth is used, the simultaneous or sequential determination of MIC and MBC values can be achieved or the killing rate determined (6). Furthermore, the quantitative assay of drug combinations to detect synergy is more readily achievable in liquid systems and may be required in certain clinical situations (e.g., in cases of infection with *Enterococcus*).

For clinical laboratories, combining two approaches could prove to be more useful and cost-effective. For example, antimicrobial susceptibility testing of urine samples could be done by agar disk diffusion, and broth dilution could be reserved for isolates recovered from putatively sterile compartments (blood, spinal fluid, synovial fluid, etc.). With this strategy, isolates recovered from nonsterile compartments would not require quantitative studies.

Results obtained from broth dilution susceptibility testing may be less than optimal with certain antimicrobial-microorganism combinations. The bacteria that have produced difficulties in the past decade are *Enterococcus*, methicillin-resistant *Staphylococcus aureus* (MRSA), *Pseudomonas aeruginosa*, *Haemophilus influenzae*, and *Neisseria gonorrhoeae*. Antimicrobials that delivered unreliable data included the sulfonamides, trimethoprim, nitrofurantoin, and newer combination drugs as the β-lactam–β-lactamase inhibitors. These problems were attributable to lack of appropriate standardization of inoculum and medium and have been resolved.

Several variables must be controlled to obtain accurate reproducible results. As with any assay system, deviation from a standard procedure modifies the results obtained.

TABLE 3.2

Factors That Modify the Results of Broth Dilution Tests

Dilution schedule
Serial twofold vs arithmetic intervals
Medium composition
pH
Cation concentration
Osmolarity
Supplements
Volume
Inoculum size and growth phase
Temperature of incubation
Duration of incubation
Varying quality control and standardization procedures

Table 3.2 outlines some elements of the broth dilution test that have produced variable results. These are discussed in the pages that follow.

Limitations

One must recognize that the laboratory brings together in an artificial way (*in vitro*) the bug and drug in a setting outside of the host environment. Whether liquid (broth) or semisolid (agar) environments more truly represent the living human milieu is a subject of ongoing discussion and controversy (133). More pointedly, is the microorganism selected for study representative of the infectious agent offending the host? Because nosocomial infections predominate in hospital settings, a key question is whether the microorganisms recovered from patient specimens are representative of infection or colonization. Usually this question cannot be answered, but it is clear that the most likely pathogen from a specific specimen should be tested and that routine testing of mixed flora should not be done. The identity of the isolate to be tested frequently dictates or influences the methodology. For certain microorganisms, such as, *Streptococcus pyogenes* and *Neisseria meningitidis*, testing may not be necessary because the outcome can be readily assured using certain antimicrobial agents (see Chapter 17) or the method and interpretative standard are not yet fully established for the species. For certain rare pathogens or microorganisms with slow growth potential, clearer endpoints may be obtainable in broth as compared with agar.

In the final analysis, it is necessary to realize that in the laboratory setting there is a continuous exposure of 10^5 to 10^6 colony-forming units (CFU) of microorganism per milliliter to a static (albeit minimally varying) drug concentration during the entire incubation period. These conditions do not prevail *in vivo*, where larger (or smaller) numbers of bacteria at the infected site are exposed to fluctuating drug concentration gradients.

ANTIMICROBIAL AGENTS

Selection of Antimicrobial Compounds for Evaluation

As the number of approved compounds continues to increase (although now at a limited rate), the challenge for the laboratory is to select rationally a limited number of antimicrobial agents for testing. To test all licensed drugs would be impractical and, in this era of constrained laboratory budgets, uneconomical. In the past, the selection of agents for testing was aided in part by the US Food and Drug Administration (FDA) as it recognized class compounds or, as they apply to agar disk diffusion testing, class disks. However, as the number of chemical classes and congeners within each class increases, the unique pharmacokinetic properties frequently dictate separate disks for each newly approved compound. With the current proliferation of newer β-lactam agents and quinolones, the class idea of drug selection has become even more important for achieving economy of testing, especially given the availability of the several commercial systems.

Each laboratory and clinical setting should develop a strategy for testing compounds based on previously accrued information on resistance patterns of class agents. Patient demographics as well as patterns of antibiotic use (and abuse) will assist in this selection process. Guidelines to assist laboratories in this process have been proposed by the National Committee for Clinical Laboratory Standards (NCCLS) (167,168) and are included here for convenience (Table 3.3)

It should be noted that the represented groups of organisms are those for which it is most difficult to predict, with any degree of certainty, a susceptibility result based on prior experimental data. The agents in the primary and secondary groups achieve peak levels in serum, whereas those noted in the urine group attain maximum concentrations in that compartment. Final drug selection should represent a consensus opinion at each site or medical center and should include input from the clinical microbiologist, infectious disease specialist, and clinical pharmacist. As noted, these decisions require information about the antimicrobial nature (toxicity and pharmacokinetics) and the probability of resistance for each drug-bug pair previously tested. Acquisition and use costs also need to be considered. Frequently, these data are incorporated into a quarterly or annual summary report distributed by the institution.

(*text continues on page 67*)

TABLE 3.3

Antimicrobial Agents That Should Be Considered for Standard Antibiotic Susceptibility Testing and Reporting by the Clinical Microbiology Laboratory[a]

	Gram-Negative Organisms		
Enterobacteriaceae[b]	*Pseudomonas aeruginosa* Non-Enterobacteriaceae	*Haemophilus*[p]	*Neisseria gonorrhoeae*[q]
Primary agents	*Primary agents*	*Primary agents*	*Supplemental agents*
Amikacin	Amikacin	Amoxicillin/clavulanic acid or	Penicillin
Amoxicillin/clavulanic acid	Aztreonam	ampicillin/sulbactam	Cefixime or cefotaxime
or ampicillin/sulbactam	Cefepime	Ampicillin	or cefpodoxime or ceftizoxime
Ampicillin[d]	Cefoperazone	Azithromycin or clarithromycin	or ceftriaxone
Cefepime	Cefotaxime or ceftriaxone	Cefaclor or cefprozil or loracarbef	Cefmetazole
Cefmetazole	Ceftazidime	Cefaclor or clarithromycin	Cefotetan
Cefoperazone	Ciprofloxacin	Cefixime or cefpodoxime	Cefoxitin
Cefotaxime[h] or ceftizoxime	Clavulanate	Ceftriaxone or cefotaxime	Ciprofloxacin or gatifloxacin
or ceftriaxone	Gentamicin	or ceftizoxime or ceftazidime	or ofloxacin
Cefoxitin/cefotetan	Imipenem	Cefuroxime	Spectinomycin
Cefoperazone	Levofloxacin	Chloramphenicol	Tetracycline[g]
Cephalothin[e]	Meropenem	Meropenem	
Chloramphenicol	Mezlocillin or ticarcillin	Trimethoprim/sulfamethoxazole[f]	
Ciprofloxacin or levofloxacin	Norfloxacin[j,k]	*Supplemental panel*[c]	
Entapenem, imipenem, or meropenem	Piperacillin	Amoxicillin/clavulanic acid	
Gentamicin	Sulfisoxazole[j,k]	Azithromycin or clarithromycin	
Mezlocillin or piperacillin	Tetracycline[j,k]	Aztreonam	
Piperacillin-tazobactam	Tircarcillin/clavulanic acid	Cefonicid	
Ticarcillin	Tobramycin	Ciprofloxacin or gemifloxacin or	
Ticarcillin/clavulanic acid	Trimethoprim/sulfamethoxazole	gatifloxacin or levofloxacin	
Trimethoprim/sulfamethoxazole	*Supplemental panel*[c]	or lomefloxacin or moxifloxacin	
Supplemental panel[c]	Carbenicillin	or ofloxacin or sparfloxacin	
Aztreonam	Cefotaxime or ceftriaxone	Ertapenem or imipenem	
Carbenicllin	Ceftizoxime[l]	Rifampin	
Ceftazidime	Chloramphenicol[l]	Tetracycline	

Gatifloxacin	Lomefloxacin or norfloxacin or ofloxacin		
Lomefloxacin,[j] or norfloxacin or ofloxacin	Tetracycline[g,j]		
Nitrofurantoin[j]			
Tetracycline[g]			
Tobramycin			
Gram-Positive Cocci			
Staphylococcus	*Enterococcus*	*Stretococcus pneumoniae*	*Streptococcus*
Primary agents	*Primary agents*	*Primary agents*	*Primary agents*
Amikacin	Gentamicin (high level)	Cefepime	Chloramphenicol
Amoxicillin/clavulanic acid	Linezolid	Cefotaxime or ceftriaxone	Clindamycin
or ampicillin/sulbactam	Penicillin or ampicillin	Chloramphenicol	Erythromycin
Cephalothin	Quinupristin-dalfopristin	Clindamycin	Penicillin or ampicillin
Chloramphenicol	Streptomycin (high level)	Erythromycin	Vancomycin
Clindamycin	Vancomycin	Gatifloxacin or gemifloxacin or	*Supplemental panel*[c]
Erythromycin or azithromycin	*Supplemental panel*[c]	levofloxacin or ofloxacin	Cefepime or
or clarithromycin	Chloramphenicol	or moxifloxacin or sparfloxacin	cefotaxime or ceftriaxone
Gentamicin	Ciprofloxacin	Meropenem	Levofloxacin or ofloxacin
Linezolid	Erythromycin	Penicillin	Linezolid
Oxacillin[n] or methicillin	Levofloxacin	Tetracycline	Quinupristin-dalfopristin
Penicillin[m]	Nitrofurantoin[j]	Trimethoprim/sulfamethoxazole	
Trimethoprim/sulfamethoxazole	Norfloxacin[j]	Vancomycin	
Vancomycin	Rifampin	*Supplemental panel*	
Supplemental panel[c]	Tetracycline[g]	Amoxicillin or	
Cefotaxime or ceftriaxone		amoxicillin/clavulanic acid	
Chloramphenicol		Chloramphenicol	
Ciprofloxacin or gatifloxacin		Ertapenem or imipenem	
or levofloxacin or ofloxacin		Linezolid	
Gentamicin		Rifampin	
Lomefloxacin or norfloxacin[j]			
Nitrofurantoin[j]			
Quinopristin-dalfopristin			
Rifampin			
Tetracycline[g]			

TABLE 3.3 (Continued)

Antimicrobial Agents That Should Be Considered for Standard Antibiotic Susceptibility Testing and Reporting by the Clinical Microbiology Laboratory[a]

[a] Final selection of appropriate antimicrobials for regular reporting must be made by each laboratory in consultation with infectious disease specialists and pharmacy staff. Susceptibility patterns of nosocomial pathogens in each hospital should be considered. "Primary" and "supplemental panels" are designed for specificity in utilization of newer expensive agents and thereby minimize costs and selection of multiresistant strains.

[b] Also applied to other Gram-negative species which are not apparent on primary isolation plates (e.g., *Acinetobacter*, *Aeromonas*, and nonpigmented *Pseudomonas* species).

[c] Supplemental panels comprise alternative drugs to be tested (1) against strains that are resistant to multiple primary agents, especially to primary drugs in a given family (e.g., β-lactams or aminoglycosides) by initial disk diffusion or primary set of dilution tests; (2) in some institutions known to harbor multiple resistant strains, where selected secondary agents, e.g., cefoxitin or amikacin, may warrant testing with the primary set; (3) for epidemiologic purposes; or (4) as alternate treatment for patients allergic to penicillin or other primary drugs.

[d] Results generally equivalent for amoxicillin, bacampicillin, and mecillinam.

[e] Generally representative of first-generation cephalosporins such as cephapirin, cephradine, cephalexin, ceforanide, and cefazolin. Note: Occasional strains of Enterobacteriaceae, particularly some *Escherichia coli*, may be more susceptible to cefazolin or to ceforanide than to cephalothin or other first-generation cephalosporins. Thus, while cephalothin can be utilized reliably to predict susceptibility to cefazolin and ceforanide, the reverse is not necessarily true, e.g., cefazolin-susceptible enterics may occasionally be resistant to cephalothin.

[f] Usually representative also of additional second-generation cephalosporin agents such as cefamandole, cefonicid, or ceftriaxone. Generally, one agent from the group can be tested.

[g] Generally representative of the tetracycline group, although doxycycline or minocycline may be more active for selected nonfermenting Gram-negative bacilli or occasional staphylococci.

[h] Usually representative also of additional third-generation cephalosporin agents such as moxalactam, ceftazidime, ceftizoxime, or cefotetan. Generally, one agent from the group can be tested.

[j] Tested only for pathogens recovered from urinary tract infections.

[k] May be useful against selected nonfermenters and *Pseudomonas* spp other than *P. aeruginosa.*

[l] Other drugs absent from this column such as cephalosporins, clindamycin, or the aminoglycosides (low level concentrations) should not be tested against enterococci because of the prevalence of high-level resistance indicating resistance to synergy (see text and Chapter 10).

[m] Results against staphylococci are equivalent for ampicillin (see text).

[n] Representative of the semisynthetic β-lactamase–resistant penicillins. Oxacillin or nafcillin may be preferable to methicillin because of better stability characteristics.

[o] Penicillin is representative of ampicillin, ampicillin cogeners, amoxicillin, acylamino penicillins, etc. It may be used to predict susceptibility to ampicillin, amoxicillin, ampicillin-sulbactam, amoxicillin-clavulanic acid, piperacillin, and piperacillin-tazobactam for non-β-lactamase–producing enterococci.

[p] For isolates recovered from blood and cerebrospinal fluid, only results of testing with ampicillin, chloramphenicol, and a third-generation cephalosporin should be reported. Results of tests with oral agents should be reported only against isolates recovered from localized uncomplicated infection (e.g., otitis media, sinusitis).

[q] A β-lactamase test should be used to detect the most common form of penicillin resistance. It will also provide useful epidemiological information.

Although costs and test constraints may limit the number of agents tested (usually 8–12), hospital and/or laboratory information systems can specify the distribution of reports of susceptibility test results to the patient's chart. In a sense, the problem of selecting agents for testing prompts the following question: what information about which agent should be routinely reported? Compounds that are on restricted or limited formulary status need not be routinely reported, but the data can be stored for consultation and future consideration of routine testing and reporting. The laboratory may also wish to consider testing those agents that are soon to be approved by the FDA, in anticipation of acquiring a database for setting new priorities.

In the performance of any susceptibility assay, the laboratory needs to define its objectives clearly. These should include the following:

1. To test organisms recovered from significant sites (e.g., blood or cerebrospinal fluid) to provide a guide for rational therapy.
2. To evaluate the susceptibility of selected nosocomial agents to determine variations in resistance patterns.
3. To determine and monitor antibiotic susceptibility (resistance) patterns as epidemiological markers and thus as evidence of the effective use of antibiotics for coverage.
4. To study the activity of recently approved and introduced agents as well as experimental agents.

For routine clinical laboratories, an integrated approach is prudent. This approach serves to discourage the potential abuse of newer agents and thus can help minimize the selective pressure on nosocomial isolates, limiting their potential for developing resistance (Table 3.3).

Several caveats need to be mentioned in regard to Table 3.3, which represents a guide for general test selection of antimicrobial agents against selected bacterial genera.

- For bacteria recovered from cerebrospinal fluid, cefotaxime and ceftriaxone should be tested and reported. Several antimicrobial agents and types may not be effective for treatment. These include:
  - Agents administered orally.
  - First- and second-generation cephalosporins (except cefuroxime).
  - Clindamycin.
  - Macrolides.
  - Tetracyclines.
  - Fluoroquinolones.
- Rifampin should not be used as the sole antimicrobial agent.
- The macrolides and clindamycin should not be routinely reported for microorganisms recovered from the urinary tract.

Concentration Range for Testing

When susceptibility plates are prepared in-house or ordered from a commercial supplier, specific concentrations must be selected that conform to the microtiter configuration (conventionally, 8 × 12 wells) or the containers being used. The concentrations selected must satisfy several criteria.

1. The concentrations should extend over the endpoints of a large series of isolates, taking into consideration whether the distribution of endpoints is dichotomous, unimodal, or bimodal. For example, *Streptococcus pneumoniae* and other streptococci (e.g., *Streptococcus viridans*) are exquisitely susceptible to penicillin. For these organisms, limiting the lower end of the concentration range to 0.5 or 0.1 μg/mL may fail to detect minor but significant variations in the susceptibility pattern. Although such shifts may be minor, they provide a way of tracking emerging resistance. The development of emerging resistance of *S. pneumoniae* to penicillin has been documented (8,122), but has limited clinical relevance, since the large doses of penicillin that can be administered to patients will kill pneumococci with an MIC 10 times higher than the normal.
2. The concentrations tested should include and exceed (by at least one dilution step) the highest concentration found in biologic fluids. For those compounds that are concentrated in the urine in their active form, such levels can be quite high. Pharmacokinetic data for compartmentalized antimicrobics in specific compartments must be reviewed when making these selections. Similarly, for potentially toxic agents, such as the aminoglycosides, it is pointless to test expanded upper ranges of concentrations beyond one or two dilutions above the pharmacologically toxic level. Here is one example of the failure of the twofold serial dilution schedule. Because of the narrow safety margin (therapeutic index) of aminoglycosides, rather than increasing the range above (in this case) the urinary level and taking the drug outside the therapeutic index range, it would be more prudent to prepare small arithmetic incremental dilutions for gentamicin (as well as tobramycin) in the 6–12 μg/mL range (259), as follows: 0.5, 1.0, 2.0, 4.0, 6.0, 8.0, 10.0, 12.0, and perhaps 16.0 μg/mL. For amikacin, a similar stepping range from 1.0 to 32 μg/mL is appropriate. Table 3.4 fails to note these figures, because the panels are not commercially available and are difficult to prepare. However, they are presented here for the reader's consideration.
3. The range of concentrations included in the panel should permit the endpoint detection of quality control (QC) strains (see "Quality Control"). Although routine plates and tubes cannot be prepared in anticipation of predicting synergy-checkerboard patterns

(*text continues on page 71*)

TABLE 3.4

Standard Dilution Ranges of Antimicrobial Agents for Antimicrobial Testing in the Clinical Laboratory[a]

Antimicrobial Agent	Concentration (μg/mL) 0.015	0.03	0.06	0.12	0.25	0.5	1.0	2.0	4.0	8.0	16	32	64	128
β-Lactam penicillins														
Ampicillin[b]														
Gram-positive[c]	+	+	x	x	x	x	x	x	x	x	+	+		
Ampicillin														
Gram-negative[d]				+	+	x	x	x	x	x	x	x	x	+
Carbenicillin														
Gram-negative							x	x	x	x	x	x	x	x
Carbenicillin														
Pseudomonas[e]							x	x	x	x	x	x	x	x
Extended spectrum penicillins[f]							(8)	(16)	(32)	(64)	(128)	(256)	(512)	
Gram-negative				+	x	x	x	x	x	x	x	x	+	+
Pseudomonas				+	+	+	x	x	x	x	x	x	x	x
Oxacillin[g] or nafcillin or		+	+	x	x	x	x	x	x	x	x	+	+	
methicillin		+	+	x	x	x	x	x	x	x	x	+	+	
Penicillin	+	+	x	x	x	x	x	x	x	x	+	+		
β-lactam/β-lactamase inhibitor combination														
Amoxicillin/clavulanic acid or empicillin/sulbactam			+	+	x	x	x	x	x	x	x	x		
Piperacillin/tazobactam or ticarcillin/clavulanic acid					+	x	x	x	x	x	x	x	+	+(256)
Cephalosporins and cephems														
Cephalosporin 1°[h,i]														
Gram-positive	+	+	x	x	x	x	x	x	x	x	+	+		
Gram-negative[d]				+	+	x	x	x	x	x	x	x	x	+

Cephalosporin 2°,[j] and 3°,[k]														
Gram-negative		+	+		x	x	x	x	x	x	x	+	+	
Cephalosporin 3°,[k]														
Pseudomonas				+	+	x	x	x	x	x	x	x	x	+
Cephalosporin 4°														
Cefepime				+	+	x	x	x	x	x	x	x	x	+
Carbenems/monobactams														
Aztreonam							x	x	x	x	x	x	x	x
Imipenem						x	x	x	x	x	x	x	x	
Ertapenem						x	x	x	x	x	x	x	x	
Meropenem						x	x	x	x	x	x	x	x	
Glycopeptides														
Teicoplanin	+	+	x	x	x	x	x	x	x	x	+	+		
Vancomycin	+	+	x	x	x	x	x	x	x	x	+	+		
Aminoglycosides[j]														
Amikacin[m] or kanamycin			+	+	x	x	x	x	x	x	x	x	x	+
Gentamicin or tobramycin[m]		+	+	x	x	x	x	x	x	x	x	x	x	
Macrolides														
Azithromycin or clarithromycin, or dirithromycin				x	x	x	x	x	x	x	x			
Erythromycin		+	+	x	x	x	x	x	x	x	x	+		
Telithromycin			+	x	x	x	x	x	x	x	x	+		
Tetracycline[n]			+	+	x	x	x	x	x	x	x	x	+	
Quinolones[o]	+	+	+	x	x	x	x	x	x	x	x	+		
Others														
Chloramphenicol			+	+	x	x	x	x	x	x	x	x	+	+
Clindamycin	+	+	x	x	x	x	x	x	x	x	+	+		
Linezolid						x	x	x	x	x	x	x	x	
Nitrofurantoin[p]							x	x	x	x	x	x	x	x
Quinupristin-dalfopristin				x	x	x	x	x	x	x	x			
Rifampin	+	+	x	x	x	x	x	x	x	x	+	+		
Trimethoprim/ sulfamethoxazole		+ (0.6)	+ (1.2)	+ (2.4)	x (4.8)	x (9.5)	x (19)	x (38)	x (76)	x (152)	x (304)	x (608)	x (1216)	

TABLE 3.4 (Continued)

Standard Dilution Ranges of Antimicrobial Agents for Antimicrobial Testing in the Clinical Laboratory[a]

[a] x = concentrations designed for a basic 8-dilution series, such as for an 8-well or tube tray (see text).
+ = added dilutions designed for comprehensive 12-dilution series, such as for a 12-well or tube tray (see text).

[b] Also applicable to amoxicillin and bacampicillin.

[c] Gram-positive and "sensitive" Gram-negative organisms, e.g., *Staphylococcus* spp, *Streptococcus* spp, including *Streptococcus pneumoniae*, *Neisseria* spp, and *Haemophilus* spp (ampicillin only).

[d] Gram-negative bacilli (e.g., Enterobacteriaceae and miscellaneous nonfermentative Gram-negative bacilli).

[e] If special panel is used for *Pseudomonas aeruginosa*.

[f] Applicable to ticarcillin, mezlocillin, piperacillin, and azlocillin.

[g] Interpretive results representative of penicillinase-resistant penicillin group such as nafcillin, oxacillin, cloxacillin, and dicloxacillin.

[h] Dilution ranges usually apply to all cephalosporins and monobactams. (See text and Table 3.1 for discussion of interpretive standards and of selection of representative first-, second-, and third-generation cephalosporins and analogs for testing in usual clinical microbiology procedures.)

[i] Applicable for cephalothin, cephapirin, cefazolin, cephradine, cephalexin, ceforamide, and cefadroxil.

[j] Applicable for cefamandole, cefuroxime, cefotixin, and cefonicid.

[k] Applicable for cefotaxime, moxalactam, cefoperazone, ceftazidime, ceftizoxime, and cefsulodin.

[l] Concentrations listed are for standard $\log_2$ dilutions. Some authors suggest added precision is warranted for aminoglycosides by adding "half" dilutions such as 6 (and 12) for gentamicin and tobramycin and 12 (and 24) for kanamycin and amikacin.

[m] May be reserved for secondary testing or reporting of strains resistant to gentamicin or to multiple other agents on primary tests (see text).

[n] Dilutions and interpretive results representative of tetracycline group.

[o] Applicable to ciprofloxacin, norfloxacin (see note p) and ofloxacin gatifloxacin, gemifloxacin, levofloxacin, moxifloxacin, and sparfloxacin.

[p] To be tested only against Gram-negative pathogens from urinary tract infections.

(see Chapter 9), it is worth noting that certain species, such as those in the genus *Enterococcus,* can be readily treated with a combination of penicillin G or ampicillin and an aminoglycoside, usually gentamicin, to produce synergistic bactericidal activity. Testing for synergistic and bactericidal activity is discussed elsewhere in this volume. Although dilution and synergy or killing curves in broth underscore a conventional basis for quantitative methods of testing synergy, such tests represent a special objective outside the scope of standard broth dilution procedures for routine susceptibility tests. However, the enterococci can be challenged with a single aminoglycoside concentration to determine whether the organisms demonstrate high-level resistance and would be susceptible to the synergistic action of a β-lactam and an aminoglycoside (156). Such high-level resistance can be determined with a single concentration outside of the clinically useful range included in Table 3.4. A 500- to 2000-μg/mL concentration of aminoglycoside (usually gentamicin) could be included to screen for this type of resistance to synergy in the *enterococci,* as is common in some commercial systems. It is wise to consider whether this single high-level dilution should be added to the standard series or whether it should be part of a separate screening process for all Gram-negative bacilli.

It is difficult to arrange a series of concentrations that satisfy all of the criteria noted earlier and that are applicable in the clinical laboratory setting. However, Table 3.4 presents a suggested outline of concentration ranges designed to approach the goals. Two series ranges are indicated in the table. The first (denoted by "X") represents a basic set of eight dilutions that cover minimum concentrations. These usually include MIC breakpoints suggested for assigning a general interpretive result to three or four categories, regardless of the terminology used to define the interpretive scheme. The use of widely spaced, selected, screening dilution steps frequently employed for certain drugs in commercial microdilution trays should be avoided. The use of widely spaced (skip-step) dilutions results in a less accurate quantitative assay than does a continuum of concentrations (see "Standard Interpretive Guidelines") and fails to detect upward trending of resistance. Also noted in Table 3.4 are extended concentrations (denoted by "+") for expanding the basic dilution series to provide additional relevant concentrations. These additional concentrations are added to either the upper or lower end of the range to permit better estimation of possible clinical utility against partially resistant strains in uncomplicated urinary tract infections, where high levels of drugs may be achieved in the urine (34). The addition of the end dilutions (concentrations) allows detection of modest changes in the susceptibility patterns frequently seen with highly susceptible isolates (as mentioned in the preceding section) for organisms such as *S. pneumoniae* or *N. gonorrhoeae* or occasional Gram-negative bacilli that might be especially susceptible to newer agents. If the laboratory determines that the scheme outlined in Table 3.4 is unacceptable and represents a far too customized situation, a compromise standard series of dilutions can be prepared, as outlined by the ICS (74). Table 3.5 lists dilution concentrations recommended for preparation of standard twofold dilutions in 13 × 100-mm tubes. The scheme represented in Table 3.5 can be extended to include as many endpoints as desired. As indicated, 14 dilution steps are included, making the scheme broad enough to address most of the problems noted earlier, but it may not be practical or necessary for the average clinical laboratory. For larger volumes of work, when more tubes are necessary, the scheme outlined in Table 3.6 is recommended (74). Here again, although the series may be customized for specific bacterial agents, employing the same standard dilution for all drugs has the advantage of simplicity and utility for routine use.

Preparation and Storage of Stock Solutions

The decision to purchase commercial test systems or to prepare in-house panels depends on the laboratory type (clinical, developmental, etc.) and the objectives. Prior to the development of commercial antimicrobial susceptibility test systems, there was little choice, except for deciding whether agar or broth dilution would be used. In either case, rigorous standards have to be followed for controlling the preparation and maintenance of stock solutions of antimicrobial agents.

Reagent-quality antimicrobial powders can be obtained from the pharmaceutical manufacturer, the FDA, or the US Pharmacopeia (Rockville, MD). Drug preparations stocked by pharmacies for clinical administration should not be used in the laboratory because they may contain preservatives and may not be standardized as carefully as assay-quality powders. Additionally, some clinical preparations (e.g., chloramphenicol sodium succinate) require hydrolysis *in vivo* to be in the active form.

Laboratories need to maintain a detailed registry of the antibiotic powders requested that indicates the date of receipt, supplier, lot number, assay potency, outdate, and storage conditions and incorporates information supplied by the manufacturer. Frequently, along with the powder the supplier sends a material safety data sheet (MSDS) detailing the method of disposal and other pertinent information on the use of the powder and its potential danger to the user.

Once opened, sealed vials must be stored in a dessicator; some require refrigerated storage in a dessicator. Antimicrobials vary in their storage requirements. Aminoglycosides are stable at room temperature (in a dessicator), whereas β-lactams need to be kept at 20°C or lower. A general rule to heed is that the lower temperatures add to

TABLE 3.5

System for Preparing Dilutions for the Broth Dilution Method[a]

Directions for Preparing Dilutions			Final IU or μg per mL[b]	Log2 IU/μg per mL
2 mL	2,000 IU/μg per mL stock + 13.62 mL	broth = 256 μg or IU per mL	128	7
2 vols	256 IU/μg per mL (above) + 2 vols	broth = 128 μg or IU per mL	64	6
1 vol	256 IU/μg per mL (above) + 3 vols	broth = 64 μg or IU per mL	32	5
1 vol	256 IU/μg per mL (above) + 7 vols	broth = 32 μg or IU per mL	16	4
2 vols	32 IU/μg per mL (above) + 2 vols	broth = 16 μg or IU per mL	8	3
1 vol	32 IU/μg per mL (above) + 3 vols	broth = 8 μg or IU per mL	4	2
1 vol	32 IU/μg per mL (above) + 7 vols	broth = 4 μg or IU per mL	2	1
2 vols	4 IU/μg per mL (above) + 2 vols	broth = 2 μg or IU per mL	1	0
1 vol	4 IU/μg per mL (above) + 3 vols	broth = 1 μg or IU per mL	0.5	−1
1 vol	4 IU/μg per mL (above) + 7 vols	broth = 0.5 μg or IU per mL	0.25	−2
2 vols	0.5 IU/μg per mL (above) + 2 vols	broth = 0.25 μg or IU per mL	0.125	−3
1 vol	0.5 IU/μg per mL (above) + 3 vols	broth = 0.125 μg or IU per mL	0.063	−4
1 vol	0.5 IU/μg per mL (above) + 7 vols	broth = 0.063 μg or IU per mL	0.031	−5
2 vols	0.063 IU/μg per mL (above) + 2 vols	broth = 0.031 μg or IU per mL	0.016	−6
etc.			etc.	etc.

[a] Reproduced with permission from Ericsson and Sherris (74).
[b] The final concentration is obtained in the test tubes after 1 mL of the concentration given in the first column is diluted with 1 mL of inoculum.
Note: Any multiple of the volumes in the table may be used, according to the number of tests to be made, i.e., 0.5 mL vols suffice for two tests and 4 mL vols for eight tests.

TABLE 3.6

Alternative Dilution System for Large Numbers of Broth Dilution Tests[a]

Initial Concentration Required (μg or U per mL)	Amount of Antibiotic for 50 mL	Concentration of Stock Solution (μg or U per mL)	Stock Solution (mL)	Broth or Other Diluent (mL)	Concentration after Adding Inoculum (μg or U per mL)	Log2
256	12,800	1,280	10	40	128	64
128	6,400	1,280	5	45	64	32
64	3,200	1,280	2.5	47.5	32	16
32	1,600	1,280	1.25	48.75	16	8
16	800	80 (1:16 of 1,280)	10	40	8	4
8	400	80 (1:16 of 1,280)	5	45	4	2
4	200	80 (1:16 of 1,280)	2.5	47.5	2	1
2	100	80 (1:16 of 1,280)	1.25	48.75	1	0
1	50	5 (1:16 of 80)	10	40	0.5	−1
0.5	25	5 (1:16 of 80)	5	45	0.25	−2
etc.	etc.					

[a] Reproduced with permission from Ericsson and Sherris (74). The example is for 50 tests. Diluent may be dispensed with a sterile automatic buret and volumes distributed with automatic pipettes.

TABLE 3.7

Storage of Primary Concentrated Reconstituted Therapeutic Solutions[a]

Drug	Essentially Complete Stability (or Approximate Percent Original Activity) for Storage Time at Temperature			pH of Primary Compound
	−15 to −20°C	4 to 5°C	23 to 25°C	
Amikacin sulfate	>36 mo	>36 mo	36 mo	3.5–5.5
Ampicillin sodium (20 mg/mL in 0.9% NaCl)	92–96%/24 h	97%/24 h	85–92%/24 h	8–10
Carbenicillin sodium	<1 mo	6 d	80%/3 d	6–8
Cefazolin sodium	<3 mo	14 d	90–92%/4 d	4.2–7.0
Cefotaxime	>3 mo	10 d	24 h	
Cefoxitin sodium	<8 mo	26 d	33–44 h	4.2–7.0
Cephalothin sodium	<6 wk	4 d	12 h	6.0–8.5
Cephapirin sodium	<2 mo	10 d	12 h	6.5–8.5
Clindamycin phosphate	>1 mo	32 d	16 d	5.5–7.0
Gentamicin sulfate			2 yr	3.5–5.5
Methicillin sodium	1 mo	4–24 d	24 h	6.0–8.5
Nafcillin sodium	3–9 mo	7 d	3 d	5–8
Oxacillin sodium	3 mo	7 d	3 d	8
Penicillin G potassium	3 mo	7 d		6–7
Tetracycline HCl	>1 mo		12–24 h	2–3
Ticarcillin disodium	>1 mo	91%/7 d	93%/24 h 63%/3 d	6–8
Tobramycin sulfate	>3 mo	4 d	24 h	6–8

[a] From Trissel (239), primarily reconstituted concentration solutions of therapeutic products. Most diluents sterile distilled H_2O. Drug concentration varied in different studies cited, but most ranged from 10 to 300 mg/mL.

the risk of water condensation and the associated problems of ensuring adequate dessication. When preparing to open a sealed dessicator unit, it is necessary to hold the unit and its contents at room temperature and permit both to equilibrate. Before being returned to the freezer or refrigerator, the dessicator should be resealed and the accumulated moisture dessicated. Because of their instability, some β-lactams (ampicillin, amoxicillin, and methicillin) should not be stored for longer than 6 weeks. Although there is a paucity of data on the stability of laboratory stock standards, Table 3.7 provides some relevant information (239).

When antibiotic stock solutions are being prepared, powdered (lyophilized) material must be completely dissolved. Because all antimicrobials are not soluble in water, Table 3.8 indicates the nonaqueous solvents that are usually used. Some solvents, such as dimethylformamide (DMF), are intrinsically antibacterial. Barry and Lasner (21) found that use of DMF as a solvent for nitrofurantoin introduced errors in nitrofurantoin diluted 1:50. However, if DMF was diluted in Mueller-Hinton broth (MHB) at 1:100 to 1:200 (i.e., 0.1 to 0.2 mL of DMF), there was no detectable inhibition or antagonism associated with the residual DMF concentration when tested against *S. aureus* or *Escherichia coli* (Fig. 3.1).

When stock solutions are prepared, they frequently need to be sterilized by filtration. At the level of concentrated stock solutions, it may not be necessary to filter-sterilize, because these highly active solutions may be self-sterilizing. Aseptic precautions should be followed when further dilutions are warranted. When filtration through a matrix is needed, care should be taken to avoid the use of fiber pads owing to their absorbent nature, especially with antimicrobial agents of protein structure. The characteristics of four filter types in the retention of

TABLE 3.8

Solvents and Diluents for Preparation of Stock Solutions of Antimicrobial Agents Requiring Solvents Other Than Water[a,b]

Antimicrobial Agent[c]	Solvent[d]	Diluent
Amoxicillin, ticarcillin, clavulanic acid, and sulbactam	Phosphate buffer, pH 6.0, 0.1 M	Phosphate buffer, pH 6.0, 0.1 M
Ampicillin	Phosphate buffer, pH 8.0, 0.1 M	Phosphate buffer, pH 6.0, 0.1 M
Azithromycin and erythromycin	95% ethanol	Broth medium
Aztreonam	Saturated solution sodium bicarbonate	Water
Cefepime, cefadroxil, cefazolin, cefdinir, cefditoren, cefetamet, cefuroxime	Phosphate buffer, pH 6.0, 0.1 M	Phosphate buffer, pH 6.0, 0.1 M
Cefixime	Phosphate buffer, pH 7.0, 0.1 M	Phosphate buffer, pH 7.0, 0.1 M
Ceftibuten	1/10 vol DMSO	Water
Cefotetan	DMSO	Water
Cefpodoxime	0.10% aqueous sodium bicarbonate	Water
Ceftazidime[e]	sodium bicarbonate[e]	Water
Cephalothin	Phosphate buffer, pH 6.0, 0.1 M	Water
Chloramphenicol	95% ethanol	Water
Cinoxacin and nalidixic acid	½ volume of water, then add 0.1 N NaOH dropwise to dissolve	Water
Clarithromycin	Methanol or glacial acetic acid	Phosphate buffer, pH 6.5, 0.1 M
Clavulanic acid	Phosphate buffer, pH 6.0, 0.1 M	Phosphate buffer, pH 6.0, 0.1 M
Dirithromycin	Glacial acetic acid	Water
Enoxacin, fleroxacin, norfloxacin, and ofloxacin	½ volume of water, then 0.1 N NaOH dropwise	Water
Ertapenem	Phosphate buffer, pH 7.2, 0.01 M	Phosphate buffer, pH 7.2, 0.01 M
Erythromycin	95% ethanol or glacial acetic acid	Water
Enoxacin, fleroxacin, norfloxacin, and ofloxacin	½ volume of water, then 0.1 M NaOH dropwise to dissolve	Water
Imipenem	Phosphate buffer, pH 7.2, 0.01 M	Phosphate buffer, pH 7.0, 0.1 M
Levofloxacin	½ volume of water, then 0.1 M NaOH dropwise to dissolve	Water
Metronidazole	DMSO	Water
Moxalactam[f] (diammonium salt)	0.04 N HCl (let sit for 1.5 to 2 h)[g]	Phosphate buffer, pH 7.0, 0.1 M
Nitrofurantoin[h]	Phosphate buffer, pH 8.0, 0.1 M	Phosphate buffer, pH 8.0, 0.1 M
Rifampin	Methanol	Water (with stirring)
Sulfonamides	½ volume of hot water and minimal amount of 2.5 M NaOH to dissolve	Water
Telithromycin	Glacial acetic acid	Water
Trimethoprim	0.05 N lactic or hydrochloric acid, 10% of final volume	Water (may require heat)

[a] Adapted from Baker et al. (13) and NCCLS (167). See Shungu (205).

[b] The agents known to be suitable for water solvents and diluents are amikacin, azlocillin, carbenicillin, cefaclor, cefamandole, cefmetazole, cefonicid, cefotaxime, cefoperazone, cefoxitin, cefprozil, ceftizoxime, ceftriaxone, ciprofloxacin, clinafloxacin, clindamycin, garenoxacin, gatifloxacin, gemifloxacin, gentamicin, kanamycin, linezolid, loracarbef, mecillinam, meropenem, methicillin, mezlocillin, moxifloxacin, nafcillin, netilmicin, oxacillin, penicillin G, piperacillin, quinupristin-dalfopristin, sparfloxacin, spectinomycin, streptomycin, sulbactam, tetracyclines, tobramycin, trimethoprim (lactate), and vancomycin.

TABLE 3.8 (Continued)

Solvents and Diluents for Preparation of Stock Solutions of Antimicrobial Agents Requiring Solvents Other Than Water[a,b]

[c] Some agents are included for completeness but are not listed in Table 3.4.
[d] Some of these solvents are potentially toxic; consult manufacturer's material data safety sheet (MDS). These solvents and diluents are for making stock solutions of antimicrobial agents requiring solvents other than water. They can be further diluted as necessary with water or broth.
[e] Use anhydrous sodium carbonate at a weight exactly 10% of the ceftazidime to be used. Put the soldium carbonate in solution in most of required water. Dissolve the antibiotic in this sodium carbonate solution and add water to the desired volume. Use the solution as soon as possible, but it can be stored up to 6 h at no more than 25°C.
[f] The diammonium salt of moxalactam is very stable but is almost pure R isomer. Moxalactam clinical is a 1:1 mixture of R and S isomers. Therefore, dissolve the salt in 0.04 N HCl and allow it to react for 1.5 to 2.0 h to convert to equal parts of both isomers.
[g] Solubilize other cephalosporins and cephamycins (unless manufacturer indicates otherwise) in phosphate buffer, pH 6.0, 0.1M, and further dilute in sterile distilled water. These include cephalothin, cefazolin, and cefuroxime.
[h] Alternatively, dissolve nitrofurantoin in dimethyl sulfoxide (DMSO).

antimicrobial activity were studied by Murray and Niles (160) and are listed in Table 3.9.

FACTORS THAT MODIFY THE RESULTS AND REPRODUCIBILITY OF THE BROTH DILUTION TEST

Several factors influence the outcome and reproducibility of broth susceptibility results. First, the microorganism manifests its own genetic background, structure, and metabolic behavior, which strongly influence the development of resistance and disease-producing potential. Second, the antimicrobial agent possesses characteristics that affect solubility, protein binding, distribution, absorption, stability, and metabolic modification. The third factor is the milieu in which these interactions are tested and evaluated. These variables are noted in Table 3.2 and are discussed in the following pages. The problems associated with dilution schedules are discussed in "Concentration Range for Testing."

Media

Ideally, the medium in which the microorganism and antimicrobial agent interact should mimic the serum or interstitial fluid of the patient. The problem of medium influencing the results and reproducibility of susceptibility tests has long been recognized. Liquid (and agar) media

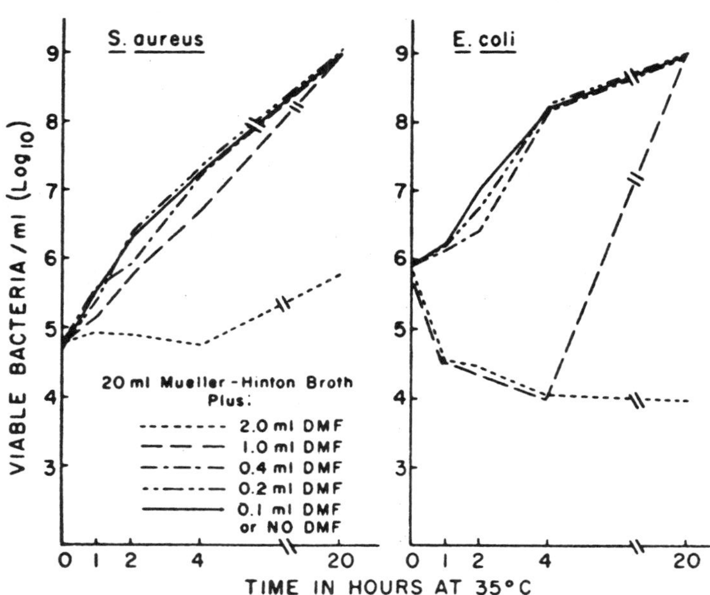

FIGURE 3.1 • Inhibition of baterial growth by DMF. Growth curves obtained in MHB with 0.1 mL of DMF are superimposed on those obtained in control broth with no DMF. (Reproduced with permission from Barry and Lasner [21].)

TABLE 3.9

Effect of Filtration on 20 Antimicrobial Agents[a]

Antimicrobial Agent[b]	Percent Antimicrobial Activity Recovered after Filtration Through			
	Glass Fiber	Cellulose Triacetate	Mixed Esters	Polycarbonate
Amikacin	100	100	96	102
Ampicillin	99	102	97	97
Carbenicillin	99	99	97	97
Cefoxitin	96	107	96	96
Cephalothin	95	102	102	94
Clindamycin	100	101	101	102
Erythromycin	102	103	101	100
Gentamicin	97	98	100	100
Kanamycin	102	98	95	98
Methicillin	100	98	101	98
Nafcillin	98	100	99	98
Nalidixic acid	97	99	102	98
Nitrofurantoin	101	100	100	100
Oxacillin	101	102	98	98
Penicillin G	101	101	103	101
Rifampin	96	96	94	98
Sulfadiazine	104	101	101	100
Tetracycline	101	102	98	102
Tobramycin	102	102	98	100
Vancomycin	101	101	103	101

[a] From Murray and Niles (160).
[b] Initial concentration, 100 μg/mL.

suffers from variations in the lots produced by the manufacturer, in part because of the variability of raw materials and the intrinsically undefined nature of the formulations. It is clear that no single medium could ever completely satisfy the goals of providing relevant reproducible endpoints for all antimicrobial agents tested against all potential pathogens. The requirements for an ideal medium (liquid or solid) have been summarized by Barry (17) as follows:

1. The medium should support the growth of a variety of pathogens for which susceptibility tests are required, without the need for special supplements or enrichments.
2. Medium contents should be defined, at least to the point of specific production details for crude components such as peptone and agar.
3. Different batches of the medium prepared by different manufacturers should yield reproducible results.
4. The medium should be free of components that are known to interact with antimicrobial agents that will be tested.
5. The medium should be capable of controlling pH (especially on the acid side) during the growth of common pathogens.
6. The broth and agar versions of the medium should have the same formulation, except for the solidifying agent.
7. The medium should be approximately isotonic for bacteria, and the agar version should be able to accept the addition of blood when required for the growth of fastidious microorganisms.

Over the years, several different media representing compromises from the ideal have been used. In a coordinated effort, the ICS (74) directed a study to determine the effects of variations in medium constituents. When two media, namely Grove and Randall no. 9 medium (96) and Mueller-Hinton medium (26,27), were compared (80), it

TABLE 3.10

Effect of Growth Media on MIC (*Escherichia coli*)[a]

Antibiotic	*E. coli* Control Organism	Significant Difference	Media[b]			
			OST	BHI	TS	MH
Ampicillin	WHO-5	$P<0.001$	8.69	9.33	9.80	8.69
Cephalothin	WHO-5	N.S.	10.20	10.50	10.50	10.44
Chloramphenicol	WHO-5	$P<0.001$	7.82	8.90	9.40	8.44
Kanamycin	WHO-5	$P<0.02$	8.81	9.90	10.00	9.33
Tetracycline	WHO-16	$P<0.001$	7.11	7.99	8.56	7.61
Gentamicin	4883	N.S.	7.94	7.99	9.10	8.19
Colistin	WHO-5	$P<0.001$	7.62	7.34	8.56	8.61

[a] From Tilton et al. (231). Results expressed as $\log_2 \bar{\chi}$ MIC + 9.
[b] OST, Oxoid sensitivity test; BHI, brain heart infusion; TS, trypticase soy; MH, Mueller-Hinton.

was found by the ICS that Mueller-Hinton was more suitable for supporting the rapid growth of enteric Gram-negative bacilli and group A streptococci, whereas Grove and Randall no. 9 produced better growth of these Gram-positive organisms: *S. aureus,* the enterococci, and the *S. viridans* streptococci. When two commercial sources of Mueller-Hinton were evaluated, notable differences were found only for the aminoglycosides (at that time, streptomycin and kanamycin). It is likely that varying cation content accounted for these differences (discussed later).

MHB is probably the most widely recommended liquid medium for broth dilution tests (19,74,87,89, 142,247). However, this medium was originally intended not for susceptibility testing but for the isolation of pathogenic *Neisseria* species (159). Because MHB contained low levels of paraaminobenzoic acid (*p*-ABA), it was used in agar form to determine the susceptibility of microorganisms to sulfonamide (39). The beef extract and casein hydrolysate in MHB are poor credentials for a reference medium. The former is difficult to standardize, and the high salt content of the latter needs to be compensated for. In spite of these deficiencies, the ICS group decided to use MHB in several studies because of the relatively good reproducibility and simplicity. An added feature was the low content of *p*-ABA, which made the medium suitable for testing sulfonamides. When MHB, brain-heart infusion (BHI), trypticase soy (TS), and Oxoid media were used in comparing tube (macrodilution) and broth microdilution results, MHB fared extremely well (232). In a replicate test series with *S. aureus,* none of the means of MICs varied by more than one dilution. For Gram-negative organisms, the MICs were generally lower for MHB than for the other media tested. The greatest variation was with the Oxoid medium, which produced differences of as much as three dilutions between the macrodilution and microdilution methods. In another study in which the same four media were evaluated, Tilton et al. (231) found significant differences among the media when tested against reference strains of *E. coli* (Table 3.10), *S. aureus,* and *Pseudomonas* spp. The highest MICs were obtained in TS broth for the Gram-negative strains. Differences between the media rarely exceeded 1.5 dilution steps, and the authors concluded that MHB, at cation-adjusted concentrations, was an acceptable medium. Other researchers have reached the same conclusion (173).

The issue of Mueller-Hinton being designated as a reference medium, even though its deficiencies have been recognized, has become moot. The medium has been used extensively, and there appear to be no proposals or contenders to replace it. NCCLS has established a reference lot for Mueller-Hinton agar (163). Cation-adjusted MHB (CAMHB), once recommended by NCCLS for routine testing of commonly encountered microorganisms, is now recommended when testing all species and antimicrobial agents. CAMHB is available from commercial manufacturers with Ca^{2+} (20–25 mg/L) and Mg^{2+} (10–12.5 mg/L) supplemented for convenience and uniformity. It is necessary to use CAMHB when aminoglycosides are tested against *P. aeruginosa* and when tetracycline is tested against other bacteria.

pH, Buffer, and Incubation

The mechanisms of the effect of antimicrobial pH is not precisely understood and is not consistent from drug to drug. In addition, the pH of the medium affects the activity of certain antibiotics. For some drugs, the pH variation

TABLE 3.11

Examples of General Optimum pH for Activity of Groups of Antimicrobial Agents[a]

Drug Group	Optimum pH
Tetracycline	6.6
Penicillin and cephalosporins	6.8
Trimethoprim and sulfonamides	7.3
Erythromycin and clindamycin	7.8
Aminoglycosides	7.8
Vancomycin	7.8

[a] Adapted from Garrod and Waterworth (85).

TABLE 3.12

Fold Increase (+) or Decrease (−) in the MIC of Different Aminoglycosides for *Staphylococcus aureus* in Broth at Different pH[a]

Drug	pH 5.5	pH 6.5	pH 7.5	pH 8.5
Streptomycin	+64	+16	1	−8
Gentamicin	+16	+4	1	−2
Tobramycin	+16	+8	1	−2
Kanamycin	+16	+4	1	1
Amikacin	+32	+4	1	−2
Sisomicin	+16	+4	1	−2

[a] From Waterworth (250).

is minor. For example, the non-ionized side chain of penicillin G is slightly more active in acidic medium, but the effect is inconsequential, in that it can be demonstrated only by utilizing special experiments. The effect of the pH of the medium on the activity of six classes of antimicrobial agents is indicated in Table 3.11.

Penicillins that are non-ionized or weak acids demonstrated minor variations according to the broth medium used, even when the pH was adjusted to approximately 7.0, and the MICs observed were generally within experimental error (one or two dilutions) for five different broths (180). This situation is in contrast to that of the aminoglycosides. Streptomycin is 500 times more active in alkaline medium than in acidic medium (60). Other aminoglycosides show similar but less drastic shifts in activity with changes in pH (Table 3.12).

The buffering capacity inherent in the formulation of a medium contributes to the stability of the pH during incubation; the inclusion of glucose in the medium results in some lowering of pH during the growth of strains that can ferment the substrate. These differences were observed in medium with and without glucose when *E. coli* was used as the test organism (17). The effect of adding specific buffers to stabilize a defined synthetic amino acid medium (SAAM) (101) has also been demonstrated.

Does the pH of the medium modulate the outcome of susceptibility results to the extent that the interpretation of the test and, its clinical relevance would be altered? Can the pH environment of the patient be clinically manipulated significantly for therapeutic purposes? The answer to both questions is in the affirmative. Such examples probably occur more readily with the macrolide and aminoglycoside groups, which are more active in slightly basic media, and the tetracyclines, which are more active in acidic environments. Definitive changes in interpretive results have occurred with gentamicin, kanamycin, erythromycin, novobiocin, and tetracycline (33) (Table 3.13).

The marked pH effect on the aminoglycosides may be explained by the degree of ionization of these compounds. However, this explanation is not plausible for changes with the prototypic penicillin G, which is intrinsically slightly acidic but allows for minimal changes of antibacterial activity in the range pH 6–8. Another mechanism proposed for non-ionized erythromycin may be directly responsible for antimicrobial activity (188). The antimicrobial activity of this macrolide is enhanced vividly as the pH approaches a pK_a of 8.6 (Fig. 3.2). This enhanced activity of erythromycin at alkaline pH extends the spectrum of activity of this compound to include Gram-negative organisms, particularly *E. coli* (135). These observations have been used in the clinical treatment of urinary tract infections. It has been shown that alkalinization of the urine is sufficient to activate erythromycin and produces successful clinical treatment (188). Theoretically, laboratories should set up an environment that mimics this pH difference, but rarely is this needed or accomplished.

Another example of the effect of pH on the outcome of susceptibility test results and treatment can be found in studies with *Campylobacter* species. During the past several years, *Campylobacter*-like organisms have been implicated in a wide variety of conditions involving the stomach and duodenum, from gastritis to dyspepsia, as well as potentially gastric carcinoma (23). *Campylobacter pylori* (now *Helicobacter pylori*) is generally regarded as the agent associated with or implicated in these conditions. *H. pylori* is susceptible to a wide variety of antimicrobial agents, including penicillins, cephalosporins,

TABLE 3.13

Effect of pH on Antimicrobial Activity[a]

Increased			
Acidic	Alkaline	Decreased Acidic	Variable to Little
Amoxicillin	Amikacin	Azithromycin	Aztreonam
Ampicillin	Azlocillin	Clarithromycin	Cefamandole
Carbenicillin	Clarithromycin	Clindamycin	Cefoperazone
Cloxacillin	Erythromycin	Metronidazole	Ceftazidime
Doxycycline	Mezlocillin	Trospectomycin	Ceftriaxone
Minocycline	Nalidixic acid		Cephalexin
Nitrofurantoin	Netilmicin		Cephalothin[b]
Piperacillin	Quinolones		Chloramphenicol
Tetracyclines	Streptomycin		Moxalactam
	Tobramycin		Nafcillin
			Penicillin[b]
			Polymixin B
			Sulfonamide[b]
			Trimethoprim

[a] Adapted from Nicolle LE, 174a.
[b] Variable effect.

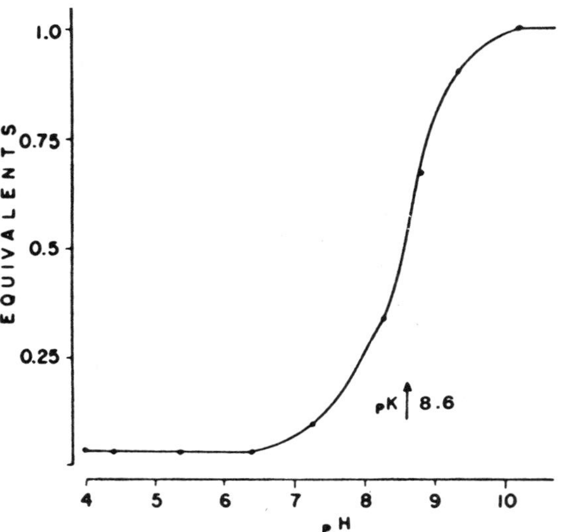

FIGURE 3.2 • Ionization of erythromycin. (Reproduced with permission from Sabath et al. [188].)

macrolides, nitrofurantoins, and quinolones (23,150). The relative efficacy of these treatments is unknown, and many patients have gastric intolerance as a side effect (23). It is uncertain at which pH antimicrobial agents demonstrate maximum effectiveness *in vivo*. Similarly, it is questionable at what pH antimicrobial susceptibility testing should be executed. Recently, Grayson et al. (94) tested the susceptibility of 22 isolates of *H. pylori*, (obtained from gastric mucosal biopsies) against eight antimicrobial agents. Antimicrobial susceptibility studies utilized the agar dilution methodology with an inoculum of 5×10^5 CFUs/spot. The comparative efficacies of the agents are shown in Table 3.14. The macrolides, quinolones, and clindamycin demonstrated diminished activity at acidic pH, compared with their activity at pH 7.4. In the alkaline pH range, MIC_{90} values were moderately but uniformly decreased (increased potency) for these same drugs. The MICs for ampicillin and metronidazole were essentially constant and within clinically achievable levels in the three pH ranges tested. The authors concluded, based on the results of their study, that if the pH of a human gastric environment was only slightly below pH 7.4, a significant loss of antimicrobial activity could result. They suggested that

TABLE 3.14

Comparative Activity (MIC_{90}) of Eight Antimicrobial Agents against *Campylobacter pylori* at Three pH Ranges[a]

Antimicrobial Agents	MIC_{90} at		
	pH 7.4	pH 5.7–6.0	pH 7.8–8.0
Ampicillin	0.5	2.0	0.25
Erythromycin	0.25	>4.0	0.125
Dirythromycin	1.0	>4.0	1.0
Ciprofloxacin	0.5	4.0	0.5
Ofloxacin	1.0	2.0	0.5
Metronidazole	4.0	4.0	4.0
Doxycycline	2.0	2.0	4.0
Clindamycin	2.0	8.0	1.0

[a] Adapted from Grayson et al. (94).

the modulating effect of pH on antimicrobial activity may explain the apparent discrepancy between *in vitro* susceptibility results and observed therapeutic failures and that clinicians need to consider the effect of pH when selecting an agent for the treatment of *H. pylori*. Added data from a study of 30 clinical isolates of *H. pylori* with trospectomycin, ampicillin, metronidazole, clarithromycin, azithromycin, and clindamycin under varying pH conditions showed that an acidic environment unfavorably affected the activity of all of the agents tested (50).

The gaseous environment is important in stabilizing the pH of media, particularly solid media; it can also affect broth. The presence of CO_2 in the incubation atmosphere, for example, may produce acidic changes, at least early in the course of incubation. Standardized susceptibility testing should not be performed in a CO_2 environment. If capnophilic organisms are being tested, their growth would be scanty in an aerobic atmosphere, and so they can be incubated in CO_2, but interpretation of the results is not considered routine. When susceptibility results obtained in an aerobic environment and a 10% CO_2 incubator were compared, the MICs of aminoglycosides and erythromycins were higher (i.e., the antimicrobials were less active) and tetracyclines, methicillin, and novobiocin were more active in the CO_2 environment (74). These studies pertained to diffusion tests; however, the net effect of the 10% CO_2 environment was a lowering of pH.

Although one would expect that the target temperature for incubation of antimicrobial susceptibility tests would be between 35°C and 37°C, the temperature of incubation has been studied, particularly in regard to the detection of MRSA. Because MRSA strains are known to grow at reduced rates, it would be anticipated that these would be favored at lower incubation temperatures, compared with their more rapidly growing susceptible counterparts. In a study by Mackowiak (141), incubation at 35°C proved satisfactory for routine growth of MRSA strains as well as for all susceptibility tests. However, the heteroresistance of MRSA may be missed at 37°C. At elevated temperatures (from 35°C to 41.5°C), incubation of routine susceptibility tests (microtiter and serum bactericidal tests) indicated that more than 20% of the MIC values were lowered significantly (Fig. 3.3), and serum activity was enhanced at the higher temperatures.

The molarity (i.e., the strength) of a buffer used in the formulation of a medium can also affect the antimicrobial activity of certain compounds. In tobramycin assay systems, it was shown that the activity of the drug was generally increased with decreasing molarity, and the effect was dependent on the type of assay system used (123). For gentamicin, increasing concentrations of phosphate buffer in concert with shifts in pH produced a greater degree of error.

The extent of incubation has been studied in relationship to its effect on MIC. As incubation was prolonged, increasing MICs of cephalothin were observed beyond 12 hours (254). Such effects may be partly due to progressive antibiotic inactivation with increasing incubation interval and are more likely to be encountered with the relatively unstable penicillins and cephalosporins (201,253). Broth and agar dilution methods were compared (204) in

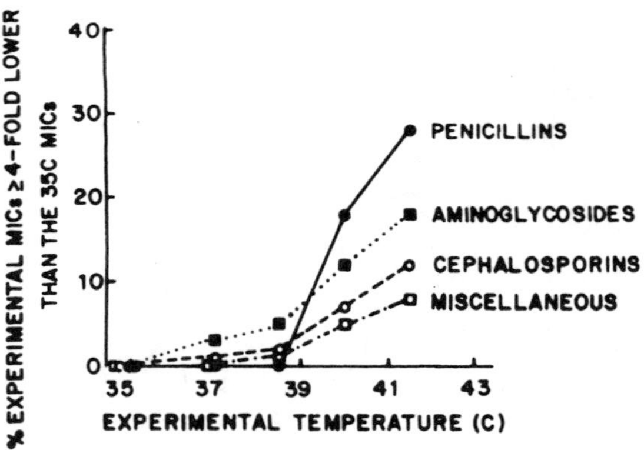

FIGURE 3.3 ● Effect of temperature on the antimicrobial susceptibility of 432 bacterial strains to classes of antimicrobial agents. Data are the percentages of experimental MICs (determined at the indicated temperatures) that were four or more times lower than standard MICs (determined at 35°C). Comparison of the results at 40°C and 41.5°C with those at 35°C by Fisher's one-tailed exact test showed statistically significant differences for all antibiotic classes ($p < 05$). (Reproduced from Mackowiak et al. [141].)

TABLE 3.15

Increase of Ampicillin and Cephalothin MIC for 18 Bacterial Strains between 12 and 24 Hours of Incubation[a]

		Fold Increase in MIC		
Antibiotic	**Test Method**	0	2	4
Ampicillin	Broth[b] dilution	5[c]	9	4
	Agar[b] dilution	13	5	0
Cephalothin	Broth dilution	8	9	1
	Agar dilution	14	4	0

[a] From Sherris et al. (204). Strains tested were 8 *Staphylococcus aureus*, 4 enterococci, 4 *Escherichia coli*, and 2 *Aerobacter-Klebsiella*.
[b] Mueller-Hinton broth and agar (Difco).
[c] Number of strains.

relationship to the duration of incubation (12 and 24 hours) (Table 3.15).

For the broth dilution techniques, the MICs increased at least twofold more than twice as often with prolonged incubation, compared with the changes that occurred between 12 and 24 with agar dilutions. This effect can be observed for ampicillin and cephalothin as well as newer broad-spectrum β-lactams. In broth dilution systems, the best reproducibility and minimal alteration in MICs from the late growth of residual persister cells can be seen if a routine is followed of reading broth dilution endpoints after overnight incubation (usually 18 hours). (See "Automated, Rapid, and Instrument-associated Methods" for the adverse effects of short-term incubation.)

When microorganisms are exposed in broth to antibiotic concentrations for short durations and then the antibiotic is removed or inactivated, the resultant effect has been termed the postantibiotic effect, defined by Craig and Gudmundsson (46). This phenomenon may be relevant to clinical responses to therapy and can be used to establish dosage schedules (66,146). Extended incubation over a number of hours in antibiotic-deficient medium must be used to determine the residual effect of brief exposure (0.5 to 4 hours) to the antimicrobial agent, so this type of assay cannot be considered a routine or rapid test.

Cation Concentration and Osmolality

The divalent cations calcium and magnesium have a profound modulating impact on the effects of the aminoglycosides, especially gentamicin. For example, the general results of broth dilution tests with gentamicin show MICs one $\log_2$ unit higher than the results for agar medium, probably reflecting variations in cation concentrations. Other aminoglycosides, as well as tetracycline, are also affected. Varying cation content has posed significant problems in agar medium (118). However, different concentrations of magnesium in broth medium have also been responsible for marked MIC variations in the activity of gentamicin against many *Pseudomonas* strains (85). Falsely low MICs are observed with media not supplemented with calcium and magnesium. A similar but less pronounced effect can be seen against other Gram-negative organisms in unsupplemented media (75,85). The data in Table 3.16 indicate results obtained by varying the concentrations of magnesium, calcium, and sodium salts in nutrient broth for susceptibility studies of *Pseudomonas* with gentamicin. After extensive surveys (185), it was suggested that final concentrations of magnesium of 20–35 mg/L and concentrations of calcium of 50–100 mg/L should supplement broth. These concentrations modify the medium and bring it into the physiologic concentration range found in serum (Table 3.17). In commercial microdilution systems, the medium is cation-supplemented.

In studies with the tetracyclines, different MICs were obtained in TS broth compared with MHB (107). These differences were attributed to variations in cation concentrations. MHB produced eightfold lower MICs against *S. aureus, E. coli,* and *Klebsiella* species, but the antibiotic inhibitory effect of the TS broth was reversed by the apparent chelating effects of phosphate, oxalate, or citrate. The opposite effects (increased MICs) on tetracycline in MHB were produced by adding the cations magnesium, calcium, or iron (107,252).

Sodium chloride concentrations change the osmolarity of medium and have a marked effect on the activity of the aminoglycosides gentamicin (151) and tobramycin (123). A sixfold decrease in activity and increase in MIC was

TABLE 3.16

Growth of *Pseudomonas aeruginosa* 41501 in Nutrient Broth Containing Serial Dilutions of Gentamicin and Various Concentrations of Salts[a]

Salt	Concentration of Salt (mM)	Conductivity ($m\Omega^{-1}$) at 0°C	Gentamicin (μg/mL)											
			31.3	15.6	7.8	3.9	2.0	1.0	0.5	0.25	0.13	0.06	0.03	0.015
NaCl	174	8.1	0	0	0	0	0	0	+	+	+	+	+	+
	87		0	0	0	0	0	0	0	0	+	+	+	+
	44		0	0	0	0	0	0	0	0	0	+	+	+
	22		0	0	0	0	0	0	0	0	0	0	0	+
	11		0	0	0	0	0	0	0	0	0	0	0	+
	5.4		0	0	0	0	0	0	0	0	0	0	0	+
	2.7		0	0	0	0	0	0	0	0	0	0	0	+
$MgCl_2$	29.5	3.4	0	0	+	+	+	+	+	+	+	+	+	+
	14.8		0	0	0	0	+	+	+	+	+	+	+	+
	7.4	1.6	0	0	0	0	0	0	+	+	+	+	+	+
	3.7		0	0	0	0	0	0	0	+	+	+	+	+
	1.8		0	0	0	0	0	0	0	0	+	+	+	+
	0.9		0	0	0	0	0	0	0	0	0	+	+	+
	0.5		0	0	0	0	0	0	0	0	0	0	+	+
$MgSO_4$	29.5		0	0	+	+	+	+	+	+	+	+	+	+
	14.8		0	0	0	0	+	+	+	+	+	+	+	+
	7.4		0	0	0	0	0	0	+	+	+	+	+	+
	3.7		0	0	0	0	0	0	0	+	+	+	+	+
	1.8		0	0	0	0	0	0	0	0	+	+	+	+
	0.9		0	0	0	0	0	0	0	0	0	+	+	+
	0.5		0	0	0	0	0	0	0	0	0	0	+	+
$CaCl_2$	2.95		0	0	0	0	0	+	+	+	+	+	+	+
	1.5		0	0	0	0	0	0	0	+	+	+	+	+
	0.8		0	0	0	0	0	0	0	0	+	+	+	+
	0.4		0	0	0	0	0	0	0	0	0	+	+	+
	0.2		0	0	0	0	0	0	0	0	0	0	+	+
	0.1		0	0	0	0	0	0	0	0	0	0	+	+
	0.05		0	0	0	0	0	0	0	0	0	0	+	+
None		0.8	0	0	0	0	0	0	0	0	0	0	0	+

[a] Reproduced with permission from Medairos et al. (151).

noted by changing (increasing) the NaCl concentration from 22 to 174 mmol/L.

β-Lactams that bind to varying penicillin-binding proteins (PBPs) may be uniquely affected by the osmolarity and, in turn, the conductivity of the test medium. This effect of osmolarity varies from strain to strain of bacterium. For some strains of *Proteus* or *Klebsiella* tested against mecillinam, a 500-fold increase in MIC as a result of increasing molarity from 185 to 402 mOsmol/L was observed. In contrast, a strain of *Enterobacter cloacae* showed no change in the MIC for mecillinam between the same osmolarity levels in the same broth (NIH medium) (170).

Supplements and Other Additives

Recently, MHB has been shown to be acceptable for a wide variety of antimicrobial susceptibility tests and to be well suited for standard, rapidly growing pathogens such as enteric Gram-negative bacilli, *Pseudomonas* spp, staphylococci, and *Enterococcus* spp. For organisms that grow rapidly and have been studied adequately, there are

TABLE 3.17

Total Concentrations of Magnesium and Calcium in Normal Serum and Commercial Batches of Mueller-Hinton (MH) Media[a]

Medium (No. Batches Tested)[b]	Concentration (mg/L)[c]	
	Mg^{2+}	Ca^{2+}
MH broth		
BBL (5)	3.0 ± 0.8 (2.0–4.7)	10.8 ± 10.4 (4.1–31.6)
Difco (5)	4.2 ± 1.0 (2.9–5.6)	15.0 ± 10.5 (8.0–35.8)
Human serum[d] (60)	21.7 ± 1.2	98.0 ± 2.5

[a] Adapted from Reller et al. (185).
[b] BBL, Baltimore Biological Laboratories; Difco, Difco Laboratories.
[c] Mean ± S.D. (range).
[d] Adapted from Pybus, cited by Reller et al. (185).

well-standardized interpretive guidelines and QC standards (167,168). For bacteria that do not grow readily on this medium, other supplements or alternative media may be required. The addition of blood or hemoglobin or of special additives such as IsoVitaleX (Baltimore Biological Laboratories) has been proposed to enhance the growth of many fastidious organisms that may frequently require susceptibility testing (see "Fastidious and Unusual Pathogens"). Because some of the supplements produce an opacity that cannot be readily used in standard macrodilution or microdilution broth systems, they are more suitable to solid agar medium. The susceptibility testing of *H. influenzae* has long been a problem in this regard. Only recently, Jorgensen et al. (116) studied the problem and developed a special test medium, *Haemophilus* test medium (HTM), that has become commercially available and provides a solution to this problem.

The addition of various supplements of unknown chemical composition may in some instances alter antibiotic activity. However, if adequate controls are incorporated, standards are developed for appropriate interpretation, and additional control strains are utilized in the testing protocol, media supplemented with various components may be used successfully for broth dilution susceptibility tests.

Supplementation of test media with previously used (but undefined) components can result in unusual effects. Eliopoulos et al. (69) reported on the effect of 5% sheep blood added to Mueller-Hinton agar on the activity of cefotaxime and other cephalosporins against *Enterococcus faecalis*. They determined that the activities of cefotaxime and other aminothiazoyl oxime cephalosporins (e.g., cefpirome, ceftazidime, cefmenoxime, ceftriaxone, and ceftizoxime) against *E. faecalis* were enhanced by the addition of 5% sheep blood. This effect was not documented for aztreonam (a nonoxime aminothiazoyl), cefotiam, or other cephalosporins and was specific to the *syn*-configuration of the oxime moiety. Enhancement of cefotaxime activity was shown against 50% of 85 clinical isolates and could be demonstrated only with low bacterial inocula. The α-globulin fraction of serum mimicked this enhancing activity, whereas α_1-, β-, and γ-globulin fractions and albumin frequently antagonized or did not significantly affect the antimicrobial activity. Although these observations may not have direct clinical relevance, they present a possible explanation for the relatively infrequent occurrence of enterococcal superinfection in patients treated with cefotaxime, which demonstrates poor *in vitro* activity.

When 5% sheep blood or 10% fetal calf serum was added to liquid media for testing *H. pylori* susceptibility (45), sheep blood inhibited growth. When the effect of bismuth was evaluated, it was found that the compound inhibited growth in medium containing starch but that the inhibition was neutralized in medium containing serum (Fig. 3.4).

Prior to the development of HTM, broth dilution tests were satisfactorily done using MHB (171). Today, susceptibility testing of sulfonamides does not pose a serious, relevant clinical problem. Sulfonamides are rarely used in treatment, and their testing is not usually required. Media enriched with various digests or supplements may contain *p*-ABA, thus obviating sulfonamide inhibition and rendering the tests inaccurate or useless. Testing of trimethoprim or a combination of trimethoprim and sulfamethoxazole presents similar problems, in that the activity of trimethoprim or sulfamethoxazole is antagonized by the high thymidine content of enriched media. This problem exists *in vitro* although apparently not *in vivo*, because thymidine and thymine both seem to be present in sufficiently low levels in blood and urine so as not to interfere with *in vivo* bacteriostatic and bactericidal activity during treatment (244,250). Thus, media have to be adjusted so that the thymidine content is diminished or absent. A suitable formulation was designated SF medium base (225). Dramatic differences between a standard broth medium and one enriched with 5% lysed horse blood can be seen in Fig. 3.5. The supplement of 5% lysed horse blood contains sufficient thymidine phosphorylase to inactivate thymidine in various media (78,225). In the United States, most commercial lots of Mueller-Hinton medium have proven satisfactory for overnight incubation as a result of careful QC measures by the manufacturers. Other technical problems encountered with broth dilution methods when testing sulfonamides and trimethoprim result in hazy endpoints. These problems have been resolved by manipulation of the medium and the use of small inocula (78).

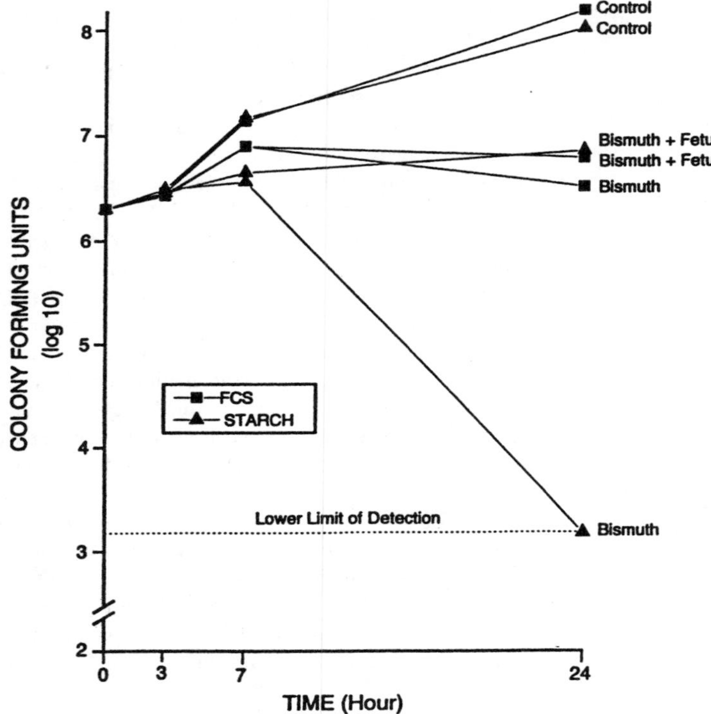

FIGURE 3.4 ● Effect of broth components, fetal calf serum (*FCS*) (10%), starch (0.5%), and fetuin (1.2 mg/mL) on the bactericidal activity of bismuth (32 g/mL). (Reproduced from Coudron and Stratton [141].)

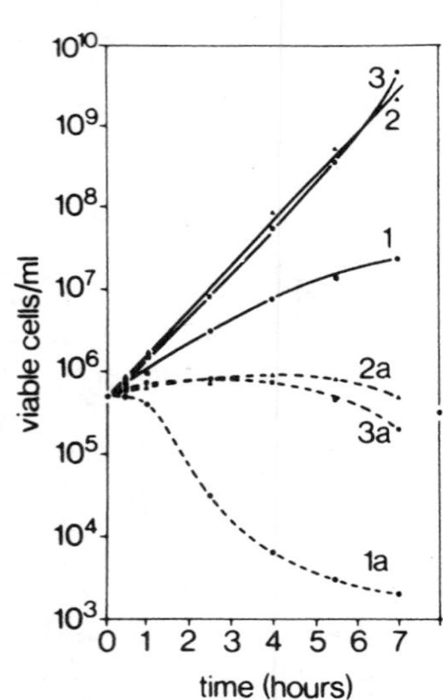

FIGURE 3.5 ● Influence of 5% lysed horse blood on the effect of trimethoprim (2 g/mL) on growth of *E. coli* B in different media. The blood-containing media were heated for 30 minutes to 56°C before inoculation. Media: *1*, sensitivity test broth (Oxoid); *1a*, medium 1 plus 5% lysed horse blood; *2*, nutrient broth no. 2 (Oxoid); *2a*, medium 2 plus 5% lysed horse blood; *3*, BHI (Difco); *3a*, medium 3 plus 5% lysed horse blood. (Adapted from Then [225].)

Other Media

It appears that MHB and CAMHB have established a foothold in the antimicrobial susceptibility literature. Presently, no other medium has been studied sufficiently to replace them. There have been investigations into one defined medium, namely, SAAM (101). Although this medium proved comparable in growth support and antagonism of sulfatrimethoprim, it has not gained acceptance for routine use. Similarly, another defined medium free of purines or pyrimidines (59) has been studied. However, a large proportion of *Streptococcus* and *Staphylococcus* strains failed to grow on this medium; thus, it is unsuitable for use in routine clinical laboratories. There has been little investigation into other media that would meet the ideal criteria defined by Barry. It is more likely that, with the aid of organizations like NCCLS, reference lot media may be designed and accepted. As noted, a reference lot has been defined for Mueller-Hinton agar with regard to susceptibility testing of *H. influenzae* on agar surfaces. MHB has yet to be defined.

INOCULUM SIZE, EFFECTS, AND STANDARDIZATION

The density of inoculum in an antimicrobial susceptibility assay is critical for the generation of reliable and reproducible susceptibility test results. The adjustment of inoculum density is more important for broth dilution tests than for disk diffusion and agar dilution methods. The reason is that, with agar methods, visual (macroscopic) inspection of growth permits semiquantitative evaluation of inoculum density. In contrast, it is difficult to estimate the growth density in the growth control tubes (Table 3.1).

Susceptibility test results differ according to the species, strain, and antimicrobial agent tested (32,44,204,231). During growth of a particular bacterial strain, it can be assumed that homogeneous progeny develop. However, some degree of inoculum size effect may result from the MICs of individual bacterial cells that follow a normal distribution. Thus, with larger inocula, there is a greater probability that there will be some cells or variants from the more resistant end of the distribution curve. In broth, the cells from this extreme of the normal distribution are more likely to survive and grow.

As mentioned, large bacterial populations are less promptly and completely inhibited than smaller ones. Also, the likelihood of the emergence of resistant mutants is greater in a large population of bacterial cells. This is exemplified by the emergence and recognition of MRSA and methicillin-resistant *Staphylococcus epidermidis* (199). To detect and define these particular populations more accurately, it is necessary to depress the growth of the more rapidly growing, susceptible population and to extend the incubation interval beyond the usual 18–24 h so as to readily detect the presence of the more slowly growing, resistant population (226). There is less chance of observing the resistant population if the critical inoculum is small. According to Sanders et al. (154,192,193), low-frequency mutant subpopulations of antimicrobial-resistant organisms are best detected by broth dilution systems at an inoculum concentration of more than 10^5 CFU/mL.

The inoculum effect, first reported in 1940 for the interaction of *Streptococcus haemolyticus* and a sulfa compound (258), was later described for penicillin and *S. aureus* (104a). The effect has been found in several bacterial species and is particularly widespread among the β-lactam antimicrobial agents when their activity is directed against β-lactamase–producing bacteria. Although the inoculum effect has been most widely studied in the staphylococci, it has been shown to be associated with a variety of bacterial species and almost every class of antimicrobial agent. Table 3.18 outlines the antibiotic-organism pairs that generally exhibit an inoculum effect. This effect is generally attributed to the inactivation of the antimicrobial agent by β-lactamase (37). However, it is known to occur with antimicrobial agents lacking the β-lactam ring. Other possible causes of the inoculum effect include the selection of resistant mutants and drug breakdown by other drug-targeted inactivating enzymes. The inoculum effect can be defined as a significant increase in MIC (plus two dilutions) when the inoculum size is increased (at least by 0.5 log unit). In some studies, the effect was noted when the inoculum was varied by four orders of magnitude. Early studies investigating this phenomenon need to be considered in light of the standardized elements of testing recommended by NCCLS (167). Additionally, studies elucidating the inoculum phenomenon have not been well standardized; they vary in incubation interval, reagent volume, and size of the test vessel.

The clinical implications of the inoculum effect are uncertain. Clearly, the inoculum standard established by

TABLE 3.18

Evidence of Occurrence of an Inoculum Effect[a]

Antimicrobial Agent	*S. aureus*	Enterobacteriaceae	*Pseudomonas*	*H. influenzae*	*N. gonorrhoeae*	*Branharmella catarrhalis*
Penicillins	+	+	+	+	+	+
1° Cephalosporin	+	V	V	+	+	+
2° Cephalosporin	+	V	V	+	+	+
3° Cephalosporin	–	+	+	+	+	+
Aminoglycoside	+	0	0	U	U	U
Chloramphenicol	–	0	0	+	U	U
Quinolones	V	0	0	U	U	U
Imipenem	V	U	U	+	U	U

[a] Data derived from Bartlett (23).
Symbols: +, effect observed; 0, effect not observed; V, variable response; U, undetermined.

NCCLS (5×10^5 CFU/mL final concentration for broth dilution and 10^4 CFU/spot) is not applicable to all clinical situations. At best, it represents a compromise between various clinical infections and the procedural manipulation for eliminating the potential for trailing endpoints. This methodologic result occurs when the inoculum exceeds a final concentration of 10^7CFU/mL. With several of the antibiotic-organism pairs that have exhibited the inoculum effect (Table 3.18), the final MIC result, although elevated compared with the result obtained with a smaller inoculum size, would still have yielded an interpretation of susceptible based on the MIC:level ratio.

Of the several factors that can modulate the outcome of antimicrobial susceptibility tests, the inoculum size, besides being relatively easy to measure, should be among the easiest to standardize. The role of inoculum size was shown in studies of penicillin-sensitive and penicillin-resistant strains of *S. aureus* treated with cephalexin (40,119). Marked changes in MICs and MBCs were observed for 100-fold changes in inoculum density (Fig. 3.6). The effects of 10-fold dilutions of inoculum, from 10^3 to 10^7 CFU/mL, can be seen for several antibiotic groups used against *E. coli* (Table 3.19), Gram-positive and -negative organisms (Table 3.20), and *Pseudomonas* spp (Tables 3.21 and 3.22). Against *E. coli*, tetracycline was found to be the most refractory to inoculum effects, whereas significant changes were recorded with the other antimicrobial agents, especially at the high end of the inoculum range (Table 3.10). For *P. aeruginosa*, the effect of varying inoculum size on the activity of the antimicrobials tested was related to the agent tested (44). When the inoculum was increased to 5×10^5 CFU/mL, the MIC_{90} values for all drugs tested were increased (Table 3.21). When the inoculum was increased further to 5×10^7 CFU/mL, the MIC_{90} values could be determined only for gentamicin and thienamycin. The MBC_{90} values at an inoculum of 5×10^5 CFU/mL ranged from 8 μg/mL for gentamicin and thienamycin to 128 μg/mL for cefotaxime (Table 3.21). With the largest inoculum, the MBC_{90} values for gentamicin and thienamycin remained constant, but the MBC_{90} values for the other drugs tested were less than 128 μg/mL. The susceptibility results for *H. influenzae* are seriously influenced by the size of the inoculum (67,72,220). The effect is more pronounced for ampicillin-resistant isolates (β-lactamase producers?) and penicillin than for cephalosporins. Now that inoculum size and medium have been defined for *H. influenzae* susceptibility testing, variation in susceptibility test results is anticipated to diminish.

The effect of inoculum density variation on various antimicrobial agents tested against several species must be considered in any recommendation for a standard or reference method. Most investigations support the earlier work of the ICS (74), which suggested that an inoculum of 10^5–10^6 CFU/mL would yield acceptable results in a macrobroth dilution test. Some workers adjust the inoculum closer to the range of 1 to 5×10^5 CFU/mL. For microdilution, the average recommended inoculum is 1×10^6 CFUs (89).

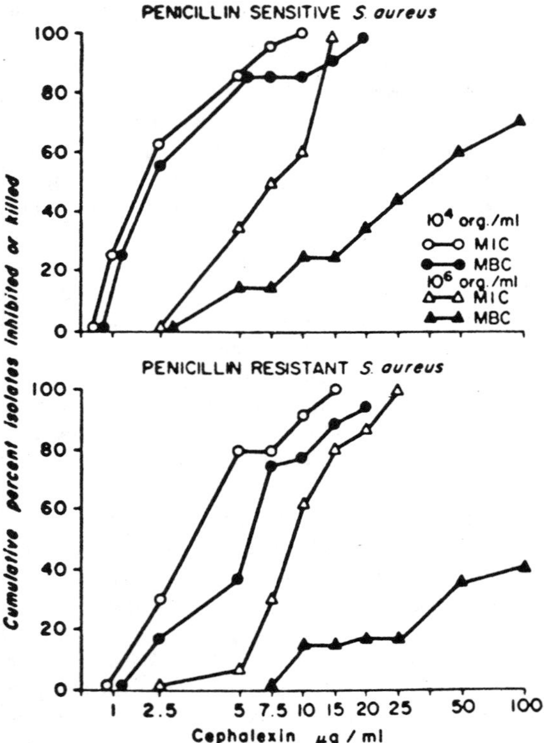

FIGURE 3.6 ● Cumulative percentages of 16 isolates of penicillin-susceptible *S. aureus* and 13 isolates of penicillin-resistant *S. aureus* inhibited (MIC) or killed (MBC) by increasing concentrations of cephalexin, tested in nutrient broth medium with bacterial inocula of two different sizes. (Reproduced with permission from Clark and Turck [40].)

Methodology for Standardizing Inocula

For the reasons mentioned earlier, it is imperative that each culture inoculum be individually standardized. The procedures frequently used for both the macrodilution and microdilution systems involve either adjustment of a logarithmic-phase broth culture to a McFarland 0.5 turbidity standard (25,167) or defined direct dilutions from 0.5-mL volumes of stationary-phase broth cultures (167). Several discrete colonies, usually three to seven, are subcultured to the inoculum growth broth, to avoid single-colony variance. The inoculum is usually cultured in the

TABLE 3.19

Effect of the Inoculum Concentration *Escherichia coli* on MIC[a]

Antibiotic	*E. coli* Control Organism	Significant Difference	Inoculum Concentration (CFU)			
			10^4	10^5	10^6	10^7
Ampicillin	WHO-5	$P<0.05$	8.71	8.57	8.71	10.00
Cephalothin	WHO-5	$P<0.01$	10.28	10.28	11.00	12.00
Chloramphenicol	WHO-5	$P<0.05$	8.76	8.58	8.91	9.54
Kanamycin	WHO-5	$P<0.01$	8.77	9.25	10.08	10.77
Tetracycline	WHO-16	N.S.	7.40	7.50	7.29	7.86
Gentamicin	4883	$P<0.001$	6.50	7.67	8.75	10.00
Colistin	WHO-5	$P<0.001$	6.00	8.50	9.00	9.75

[a] Adapted from Tilton et al. (231). Results expressed as $\log_2 \bar{\chi}$ MIC + 9.

same broth medium used for the test, such as MHB or CAMHB (richer media such as TS broth and BHI can also be used satisfactorily). For rapidly growing pathogens, overnight broth cultures (4–8 mL) grow to approximately 10^9 CFU/mL. A 1:1000 or 1:2000 dilution of this growth brings the inoculum density to the range of 5×10^5 to 5×10^6 CFU/mL. Results have generally been satisfactory with such methods, because most rapidly growing pathogens achieve stationary-phase growth at density levels that fall within a reasonable range. Alternatively, one can adjust the turbidity of a 4- to 8-mL overnight culture or a 4- to 6-hour broth culture (both are considered to be in the stationary phase) to a standardized density. This can be accomplished nephelometrically with instruments frequently provided with automated units for determining susceptibility or manually by dilution to match the visual turbidity of the McFarland 0.5 $BaSO_4$ standard, which approximates 10^5 CFU/mL. The 4- to 6-hour broth culture offers a significant time advantage compared with the overnight incubation. However, for some more slowly growing, more fastidious strains, such as *Haemophilus* or *Neisseria* strains, overnight growth may be required. Satisfactory results have been obtained by emulsifying colony plate growth to match either nephelometric or McFarland turbidity standards. Then, appropriate dilutions (e.g., 1:2000) are made for the final inoculum.

It has been shown that turbidity-adjusted direct suspensions can also yield reproducible and accurate results for commonly encountered Gram-negative or Gram-positive, rapidly growing microorganisms (23). When the growth phase of the inoculum was studied systematically by Barry et al. (20), they found that generally satisfactory reproducibility with control strains was dependent on whether the inoculum standard utilized required harvesting direct suspensions from overnight colonies or from logarithmic-phase (2- to 4-hour) or stationary-phase (5- to 6-hour) broth cultures.

After an inoculum has been prepared, variability has been observed in the delivery of the inoculum to the test system. In some systems, this was more dependent

TABLE 3.20

Effect of Increasing Inoculum Concentrations of Gram-positive and Gram-negative Bacteria[a] on the MICs of Cefuroxime and Four Other Cephalosporins[b]

Cephalosporins	MIC_{50} at Inoculum Concentrations (CFU/mL)		
	10^3	10^5	10^7
Cefuroxime	2	4	>32
Cefamandole	0.5	1	>32
Cefoxitin	4	4	16
Cephalothin	4	8	>32
Cefazolin	2	4	>32

[a] Includes the following species (number of strains): *Escherichia coli* (22), *Klebsiella* spp. (20), *Enterobacter* spp. (20), *Proteus mirabilis* (19), *Proteus* spp. (20), *Pseudomonas capacia* (3), *Pseudomonas maitophilla* (5), *Aeromonas hydrophila* (4), and *Staphylococcus aureus* (26).

[b] From Barry et al. (22).

TABLE 3.21

Influence of Inoculum Size on Concentrations of Gentamicin, *N*-formimidoyl Thienamycin, Moxalactam, Cefotaxime, and Piperacillin Required to Inhibit the Growth of 40 Isolates of *Pseudomonas aeruginosa* by a Broth Microtiter System[a]

	MIC (μg/mL of Medium)								
				For % of Isolates					
	Range			50			90		
Compound	5×10^3	5×10^5	5×10^7	5×10^3	5×10^5	6×10^7	5×10^3	5×10^5	5×10^7
Gentamicin[b]	0.06–64	0.125–64	0.5–128	0.25	0.5	1	1	2	4
N-formimidoyl thienamycin	0.06–8	0.25–16	0.5–16	0.5	1	4	2	8	8
Moxalactam	0.5–32	0.5–64	16–>128	4	8	128	16	32	>128
Cefotaxime	1–64	4–128	16–>128	4	8	>128	16	32	>128
Cefoperazone	0.5–16	1–32	16–>128	2	4	>128	4	8	>128
Piperacillin	0.5–16	2–64	32–>128	2	4	>128	8	16	>128

[a] From Corrado et al. (44).

TABLE 3.22

Influence of Inoculum Size on Concentrations of Gentamicin, *N*-formimidoyl Thienamycin, Moxalactam, Cefotaxime, Cefoperazone, and Piperacillin Required for Bactericidal Activity for 40 Isolates of *Pseudomonas aeruginosa* by a Broth Microtiter System[a]

	MBC (μg/mL of Medium)								
				For % of Isolates					
	Range			50			90		
Compound	5×10^3	5×10^5	5×10^7	5×10^3	5×10^5	5×10^7	5×10^3	5×10^5	5×10^7
Gentamicin[b]	0.06–128	0.25–128	0.5–128	0.5	1	2	1	8	8
N-formimidoyl thienamycin	0.25–8	0.5–16	1.0–16	1	2	4	4	8	8
Moxalactam	0.5–64	4–64	16–>128	8	16	>128	32	32	>128
Cefotaxime	1–128	8–>128	64–>128	8	16	>128	32	128	>128
Cefoperazone	0.5–32	1–>128	32–>128	2	4	>128	8	64	>128
Piperacillin	1–16	2–>128	64–>128	2	4	>128	16	32	>128

[a] From Corrado et al. (44).

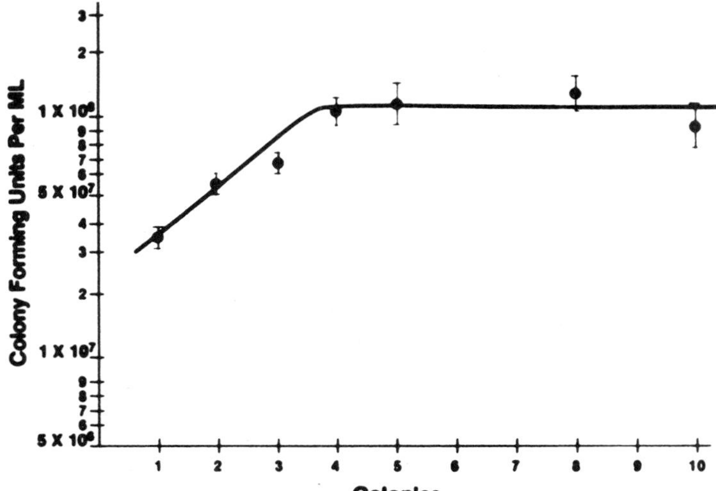

FIGURE 3.7 ● Inoculum standardization with RISS. The range and mean of viable *E. coli* ATCC strain 25922 obtained with the inoculation rod versus the number of colonies picked are shown. (Reproduced from Wicks et al. [255].)

on a mechanical inoculum preparation and transfer system and independent of the growth phase of the organism. Inocula prepared with *Pseudomonas* strains demonstrated lower counts, perhaps due to clumping, than did those prepared with other organisms (18). Final MIC results were generally reproducible and consistent regardless of the method of inoculum preparation and despite the system-dependent inoculum variations from 2×10^4 to 1×10^6 CFU/mL (23). Table 3.19 indicates that, with some drug-organism combinations (10%), statistically significant differences in geometric mean MICs resulted from different growth or inoculum preparation methods tested in two different microdilution systems (18).

Numerous techniques have been developed for inoculum preparation, standardization, and transfer and been incorporated into the expanding range of commercial microdilution test systems (see "Standard Broth Dilution Procedures"). Several systems adjust turbidity suspensions instrumentally. However, most recommend the use of a mechanical device that involves touching five colonies directly with a wand containing grooves at its bottom crosshatch, followed by emulsification in an appropriate volume of saline. This system, referred to as RISS and marketed as PROMPT, eliminates prior broth incubation and turbidity adjustment (1,216). Figure 3.7 illustrates how the CFU/mL values in the inoculum are affected by increasing the number of colonies touched; a maximum colony count is achieved after selecting four colonies.

STANDARD BROTH DILUTION PROCEDURES

The focus of this chapter is on broth dilution procedures. However, it is worthwhile to note that comparisons of results of broth and agar dilution methodologies have shown them to be similar (143). In some instances, as noted by Lorian (130), the differences for quinolones have been significant. There has been a considerable range of variability in studies, depending on the method used, the antimicrobial agent studied, and the organisms tested. A number of investigations have also compared microdilution and macrotube dilution techniques (91,92,173). Tables 3.23 and 3.24 present some of the results. Clearly, for the majority of agents tested, there were few strains that varied by more than plus or minus one dilution.

Comparative evaluations of the microdilution and macrodilution broth procedures are noted here to provide a historical perspective. Since the 1980s, there have been no evaluations of these two broth methodologies, owing in part to the popularity of the microdilution procedure. Furthermore, commercial applications of the miniaturized technique that began in the mid-1970s have made it practical for laboratories to provide MICs for all isolates, or at least for all those they wish to report on. In general, microdilution test results are essentially equivalent to those obtained with the standardized macrobroth dilution procedure. For certain organisms, such as Gram-negative bacilli, the microdilution results are approximately one dilution step lower than those obtained with the macrodilution broth technique. This seems to be a general feature of the microdilution technique and may be partially due to the way endpoints are read. Minimal turbidity, which is visible in a test tube, may not be readily observed in a microtiter well. Another possible explanation may involve the inoculum. Although in their final concentrations the inocula in the two systems contain approximately 5×10^5 organisms and are comparable, the absolute number of viable cells delivered into the microtiter well is one log unit less than that inoculated into the test tube.

TABLE 3.23

Comparison of Microdilution[a] and Macrodilution[b] Results: Frequency of Agreement and Variation of Microdilution MICs When Compared with Macrodilution MICs as the Reference Standard[c]

Antibiotic	Microdilution		>Macrodilution			Microdilution and Macrodilution Identical	Microdilution		<Macrodilution			Totals
	>4	4	3	2	1		1	2	3	4	>4	
Penicillin G					4	14	7					25
Methicillin					4	18	3					25
Ampicillin					5	14	5	1				25
Cephalothin				2	12	11						25
Erythromycin					2	18	5					25
Tetracycline-HCl					3	17	3	1		1		25
Kanamycin					7	14	4					25
Gentamicin					7	4	7	6	1			25
Colistin				2	2	10	5	5	1	1		25
Total no.	0	0	0	4	45	120	39	13	2	1	0	225
(% distribution)				(2)	(20)	(54)	(17)	(6)	(1)	(0.5)		(100)

[a] Automated dilutions in Mueller-Hinton broth using microtiter trays and the Canalco Autotiter apparatus.
[b] Manual macrotube dilutions in Mueller-Hinton broth according to Ericsson and Sherris (74).
[c] Adapted from Geriach (91). Twenty-five strains were tested by both methods with each antibiotic.

TABLE 3.24

Occurrence of Discrepant Test Results against *Pseudomonas* Strains, Based on the Susceptibility Test Method Used[a]

Drug	Microdilution MIC > Tube MIC		Microdilution MIC = Tube MIC	Microdilution MIC < Tube MIC	
	Two Dilutions	One Dilution		One Dilution	Two Dilutions
Gentamicin	0	5	24	70	1
Tobramycin	0	34	51	15	0
Amikacin	1	19	61	19	0
Carbenicillin	0	13	61	26	0

[a] From Jorgensen et al. (115).

Standard Microdilution Broth Procedure

The performance of microdilution tests has been described by a number of authors using in-house panels prepared by mechanical semiautomated or automated equipment (87,88,91,110,112,149,249,260) or commercial test panels routinely prepared or customized for the user. Commercially prepared test panel systems employ either frozen antimicrobial solutions in medium or dried preparations that need to be rehydrated by adding diluent and inoculum to each well. The test panel state of some commercial preparations and their method of inoculation are noted in Table 3.25.

For preparation of standard microdilution panels in the laboratory, the following general recommendations and directions can be followed (87,228). The antimicrobial agent stock solutions are prepared and stored as noted in Tables 3.4 and 3.7 and as found in NCCLS standard M7-A6 (167). The recommended dilutions have been included in Table 3.4, and the flexibility dilution schedule need not be limited to serial twofold increments.

The recommended broth for testing is MH supplemented with 50 mg/L Ca^{2+} and 25 mg/L Mg^{2+}. These concentrations are achieved by the addition of the appropriate amounts of filter-sterilized $CaCl_2$ and $MgCl_2$ stock solutions to cold sterile broth. Ideally, microdilution trays should be prepared each day they are used. However, with the availability of semiautomated dispensing devices for preparing dilutions and dispensing prediluted agent, it is possible to prepare large numbers of trays at one time and store them frozen until required. As trays are filled, they are stacked in groups of five to ten and are either covered with an empty tray on top or placed and sealed in plastic bags and frozen at 20°C or 70°C. Household freezers are satisfactory, but they should not contain self-defrosting units, because fluctuations in temperature during the defrost cycle thaw and refreeze the antimicrobial agents and thus contribute to their deterioration. Trays quick-frozen at 70°C and stored at 20°C have a useful shelf-life of about 6 weeks. Storage at 70°C significantly increases the shelf-life to approximately 3 months. Once a group of trays is removed from the freezer, they should be allowed to warm at room temperature prior to use. Unused thawed trays should be discarded and never refrozen.

Actively growing broth cultures are diluted to a McFarland value of 0.5 (as described earlier). Multipoint plastic or metal replicators (inoculators) are used in several commercial and semiautomated systems. After inoculation, each well should contain approximately 5×10^5 CFU/mL (5×10^4 CFU/well).

After inoculation of microdilution trays, they should be covered with sealing tape to minimize evaporation. Alternatively, large numbers of trays can be stacked and covered with an empty tray. After 16–20 hours of incubation, trays may be examined from below with a reflective viewer and MICs determined. The trays can also be read visually from the top. The endpoint MIC is the lowest concentration of drug at which the microorganism tested does not demonstrate visible growth. In judging the endpoint, it is necessary to compare the growth (or absence of growth) in the test wells with the growth (or absence of growth) in the well without the antimicrobial agent. Endpoints are easily read as turbid wells or clear wells. For some antimicrobials, such as the sulfonamides and trimethoprim, endpoints may trail. The endpoint for these drugs should be read as an 80% to 90% decrease in growth compared with growth in the control well.

Standard Macrodilution Broth Procedure

The variables that affect the outcome of dilution tests were outlined earlier and were reviewed in the preceding section. The procedures for performing the macrodilution

TABLE 3.25

Historical Overview of Automated and Instrument-associated Antimicrobial Susceptibility Test Systems[a]

System (Manufacturer)	Antimicrobial State	Inoculation	Instrument	Incubation Interval (Hours)
Autobac (Organon Teknika)[b]	Disk	Channel distribution	Light scatter at 665 nm, 35°/log index	3–5
Advantage (Abbott)[b]	Disk	Channel distribution	Absorbance at 665 nm/algorithm	3–6
AMS-Vitek (McDonnell Douglas)[c]	Card	Channel distribution	Absorbance at 665 nm/algorithm	6–10
Sceptor (BBL)	Dry	Multitip pipet	Visual turbidity	16–18
Sensititre (Radiometer)	Dry	Sequential auto-inoculation	Fluorometer/algorithm	5–18
Uniscept (API)[b]	Dry	Sequential auto-inoculation	Absorbance/AC[d]	16–24
MicroScan (Baxter)[e]	Frozen	Multiprong	Absorbance/AC	16–24 or 4–89[f]
Microcoder II (Beckman)[b]	Frozen	Multiprong	Visual AC	16–24
Precept (Austin Biological)[b]	Dry	Multiprong	Visual growth/no growth, light pen	16–24
MIC BioPlate (Plasco/Difco)[b]	Frozen	Multiprong	Visual turbidity, light pen	16–24
Repliscan (Cathra)	In medium	Multiprong	Visual growth/no growth, light pen	16–24

[a] Adapted from Amsterdam (5).
[b] These systems are no longer commercially available. See Table 3.29.
[c] Vitek bioMerieux. See Table 3.29.
[d] AC, analog conversion.
[e] New corporate sponsor. See Table 3.29.
[f] Fluorogenic substrates permit rapid readings.

broth test have been described by several authors (17,74,86,96,104,246–248). Errors and statistical variability of dilution procedures have been reviewed (89). The basic methodology described in the ICS report (74) has proven satisfactory for many laboratories, and Table 3.5 presents a scheme recommended in the ICS report for the preparation of antibiotic dilutions. An alternative dilution schedule for preparing a larger number of tubes is shown in Table 3.6. Because the dilutions are pipetted directly into blocks of three dilution tubes with one pipette, the chance of error is significantly reduced. A sequential twofold dilution method is summarized from the work of Jones et al. (109) as follows. The working antimicrobial solution is prepared by diluting the drug and MHB to the highest final concentration desired. The test is performed in thirteen 100-mm screw-capped (or cotton-plugged, etc.) test tubes. For a limited number of tests, twofold dilutions are prepared directly in test tubes, as follows: 2.0 mL of the working solution of the drug is added to test tube 1 of the dilution series. To each remaining tube, 1.0 mL of MHB is added. With a sterile pipette, 1.0 mL is transferred from tube 1 to tube 2. After thorough mixing, 1.0 mL is transferred (using a separate pipette for this and each succeeding transfer) to tube 3. This process is continued to the next to last tube, from which 1.0 mL is removed and discarded. The last tube receives no antimicrobial agent and serves as a growth control. The final concentrations of antimicrobial agents in this test are half those of the initial dilution series because of the addition of an equal volume of inoculum in broth. The inoculum is prepared and adjusted, as noted above, to contain 10^5 to 10^6 CFU/mL, by adjusting the turbidity of the broth culture to match the McFarland 0.5 standard. It is then further diluted 1:200 in broth, and 1.0 mL of the adjusted inoculum is added to each test tube. Tubes are incubated at 35°C for 16–20 hours. The lowest concentration of antimicrobial agent that results in complete inhibition of visible growth represents the MIC. A very faint haziness or a small button is usually disregarded.

Quality Control

For *in vitro* susceptibility test results to be meaningful for selecting appropriate antimicrobial agents and monitoring their use for the treatment of infection, they need to be accurate and reproducible. Because of the potential for variation, emphasis has been focused on strict adherence to methods and reference procedures (167,168). The development of QC parameters has played a significant role in the high level of performance obtained by most laboratories. Keys to this performance are the application of standard reference strains with known reactivity and the assessment of qualitative and quantitative endpoints.

The ideal reference strain for QC of dilution susceptibility methods should have MIC endpoints near the middle of the range of concentrations being tested for a given drug, or at least no closer than two dilutions from the extremes of the test range included (228). Thus, in QC for dilution testing, it has been necessary to deviate from established QC strains that have been used for disk diffusion testing. For example, *S. aureus* American Type Culture Collection (ATCC) strain 29213, a weak β-lactamase producer, is recommended instead of ATCC strain 25923. Additionally, *S. faecalis* ATCC strain 29212 and *E. coli* ATCC strain 35218 have been recommended as controls for β-lactamase inhibitors such as clavulanic acid and sulbactam. A sixth control strain, *H. influenzae* ATCC strain 49247, has recently been proposed (by NCCLS) for testing drugs against *H. influenzae* (167).

Studies of the precision and accuracy of macrodilution and microdilution MIC endpoints with the older established QC strains have shown that reproducibility should be within plus or minus one $\log_2$ dilution interval for 95% of the replicates (86,247) and that most tests should fall at the modes. The ranges of MICs expected for several contemporary antimicrobial agents against the reference strains are indicated in Table 3.26.

Control reference strains should remain genetically and phenotypically stable over many replications and long-term storage. Control strains must be stored using procedures designed to minimize chances of mutation or variant selection (247). It is suggested that, for long-term storage, QC strains be lyophilized or frozen in a stabilizing medium such as whole sheep blood or 15% glycerol in an enriched broth such as BHI or 50% serum in broth. Freezing at 60°C (or below) is preferable to storing in conventional freezers (20°C). Strains can be maintained for short-term storage at 4°C for approximately 2 weeks on agar (soybean digest casein).

When new batches or lots of microdilution trays are received from a commercial source or prepared, they should be tested with reference strains to determine their acceptability. The MICs resulting from QC testing should be no more than one dilution interval above or below the anticipated MIC. If the difference is greater, either the batch is rejected or the results with the affected antimicrobial agent are not recorded or reported. Additionally, representative uninoculated trays should be tested for sterility of the medium. QC should be done on a periodic basis after reproducibility and accuracy have been documented by daily QC practice (153,167). These QC procedures provide a review of variables such as antimicrobial potency and stability, instrument function, and technical proficiency. The MICs obtained with each reference strain should be maintained in a record book for ongoing review.

Some additional QC procedures are necessary for broth dilution tests but are less critical for agar or disk diffusion tests. A purity control plate for each isolate tested is subcultured, for isolation on an appropriate agar medium, directly from the final inoculum suspension to detect potential contamination or mixed cultures. A growth control tube (or well) free of antimicrobial agents is included within each panel set to ensure adequate growth. This also serves as a turbidity control (a comparative aid) when reading endpoints. The inoculum should be measured periodically by a direct dilution plate count of the time 0 inoculum from the growth tube or well. Finally, the proficiency of the observers determining endpoints should be monitored periodically by comparing their results with those from a standard reader to ensure uniformity between different observers reading the same plate.

There are several types of susceptibility test results that, when obtained, require further confirmation or investigation. Forty-five nonsusceptible phenotypes are listed in Table 3.27, and these may be associated with pre- or postanalytical (test) errors. In any event, these phenotypes warrant follow-up study.

FASTIDIOUS AND UNUSUAL PATHOGENS

The standard broth procedures described thus far are applicable to routine antimicrobial susceptibility testing. The term "routine" reflects the fact that the testing is of rapidly growing, nonfastidious pathogens frequently encountered in the clinical setting. Routine susceptibility procedures, however, may not be applicable to predictably slow growing microorganisms with prolonged lag times and/or slow generation times (125). Some clinically significant bacteria have characteristics that preclude their being tested by standard methods. They may grow too slowly, may require special nutrients or atmospheres, or simply may not have been tested enough to demonstrate that they can be tested accurately and reproducibly by the standard methods. These microorganisms have been termed "fastidious" and/or "unusual." Specifically, fastidious organisms do not readily grow on Mueller-Hinton medium without supplementation. Unusual organisms may grow well on Mueller-Hinton medium, but studies have not been completed to demonstrate that they can be tested reliably by standard methods. Testing the

TABLE 3.26

Acceptable Quality Control Ranges (NCCLS)[a] of MICs (μg/mL)[b] for Reference Strains

Antimicrobial Agent	*Staphylococcus aureus* ATCC 29213[a]	*Enterococcus faecalis* ATCC 29212	*Escherichia coli* ATCC 25922	*Pseudomonas aeruginosa* ATCC 27853	*Escherichia coli* ATCC 35218[b]
Amikacin	1–4	64–256	0.5–4	1–4	
Amoxicillin-clavulanic acid	0.12/0.06–0.5/0.25	0.25/0.12–1.0/0.5	2/1–8/4		4/2–16/8
Ampicillin	0.5–2	0.5–2	2–8		
Ampicillin-sulbactam			2/1–8/4		8/4–32/16
Aziocillin	2–8	1–4	8–32	2–8	
Azithromycin	0.5–2				
Aztreonam			0.06–0.25	2–8	
Carbenicillin	2–8	16–64	4–16	16–64	
Cefaclor	1–4		1–4		
Cefamandole	0.25–1		0.25–1		
Cefazolin	0.25–1		1–4		
Cefdinir	0.12–0.5		0.12–0.5		
Cefditoren	0.25–2		0.12–1		
Cefepime	1–4		0.016–0.12	1–8	
Cefetamet			0.25–1		
Cefixime	8–32		0.25–1		
Cefmetazole	0.5–2		0.25–1	>32	
Cefonicid	1–4		0.25–1		
Cefoperazone	1–4		0.12–0.5	2–8	
Cefotaxime	1–4		0.03–0.12	8–32	
Cefotetan	4–16		0.06–0.25		
Cefoxitin	1–4		2–8		
Cefpodoxime	1–8		0.25–1		
Cefprozil	0.25–1		1–4		
Ceftazidime	4–16		0.06–0.5	1–4	
Ceftibuten			0.12–0.5		
Ceftizoxime	2–8		0.03–0.12	16–64	
Ceftriaxone	1–8		0.03–0.12	8–64	
Cefuroxime	0.5–2		2–8		
Cephalothin	0.12–0.5		4–16		
Chloramphenicol	2–8	4–16	2–8		
Cinoxacin			2–8		
Ciprofloxacin	0.12–0.5	0.25–2	0.004–0.016	0.25–1	
Clarithromycin	0.12–0.5				
Clinafloxacin	0.008–0.06	0.03–0.25	0.002–0.016	0.06–0.5	
Clindamycin	0.06–0.25	4–16			
Daptomycin[c]	0.25–1	1–8			
Dirithromycin	1–4				
Doxycycline			0.5–2		
Enoxacin	0.5–2	2–16	0.06–0.25	2–8	

(continued)

TABLE 3.26 (Continued)

Acceptable Quality Control Ranges (NCCLS)[a] of MICs (μg/mL)[b] for Reference Strains

Antimicrobial Agent	*Staphylococcus aureus* ATCC 29213[a]	*Enterococcus faecalis* ATCC 29212	*Escherichia coli* ATCC 25922	*Pseudomonas aeruginosa* ATCC 27853	*Escherichia coli* ATCC 35218[b]
Ertapenem	0.06–0.25	4–16	0.004–0.016	2–8	
Erythromycin	0.25–1	1–4			
Fleroxacin	0.25–1	2–8	0.03–0.12	1–4	
Fostomycin	0.5–4	32–128	0.5–2	2–8	
Garenoxacin	0.004–0.03	0.03–0.25	0.004–0.03	0.5–2	
Gatifloxacin	0.03–0.12	0.12–1.0	0.008–0.03	0.5–2	
Gemifloxacin	0.008–0.03	0.016–0.12	0.004–0.016	0.25–1	
Gentamicin	0.12–1	4–16	0.25–1	0.5–2	
Grepafloxacin	0.03–0.12	0.12–0.5	0.004–0.03	0.25–2.0	
Imipenem	0.016–0.06	0.5–2	0.06–0.25	1–4	
Kanamycin	1–4	16–64	1–4		
Levofloxacin	0.06–0.5	0.25–2	0.008–0.06	0.5–4	
Linezolid	1–4	1–4			
Lomefloxacin	0.25–2	2–8	0.03–0.12	1–4	
Loracarbef	0.5–2		0.5–2	>8	
Mecillinam			0.03–0.25		
Meropenem	0.03–0.12	2–8	0.008–0.06	0.25–1	
Methicillin	0.5–2	>16			
Meziocillin	1–4	1–4	2–8	8–32	
Minocycline	0.06–0.5	1–4	0.25–1		
Moxalactam	4–16		0.12–0.5	8–32	
Moxifloxacin	0.016–0.12	0.06–0.5	0.008–0.06	1–8	
Nafcillin	0.12–0.5	2–8			
Nalidixic acid			1–4		
Netilmicin	≤0.25	4–16	≤0.5–1	0.5–8	
Nitrofurantoin	8–32	4–16	4–16		
Norfloxacin	0.5–2	2–8	0.03–0.12	1–4	
Ofloxacin	0.12–1	1–4	0.015–0.12	1–8	
Oritavancin	0.5–2	0.12–1			
Oxacillin	0.12–0.5	8–32			
Penicillin	0.25–2	1–4			
Piperacillin	1–4	1–4	1–4	1–8	
Piperacillin-tazobactam	0.25/4–2/4	1/4–4/4	1/4–4/4	1/4–8/4	0.5/4–2/4
Quinupristin-dalfopristin	0.25–1	2–8			
Rifampin	0.004–0.016	0.5–4	4–16	16–64	
Sparfloxacin	0.03–0.12	0.12–0.5	0.004–0.016	0.5–2	
Sulfisoxazole	32–128	32–128	8–32		
Teicoplanin	0.25–1	0.06–0.25			
Telithromycin	0.06–0.25	0.016–0.12			
Tetracycline	0.12–1	8–32	0.5–2	8–32	

(continued)

TABLE 3.26 (Continued)

Acceptable Quality Control Ranges (NCCLS)[a] of MICs (μg/mL)[b] for Reference Strains

Antimicrobial Agent	*Staphylococcus aureus* ATCC 29213[a]	*Enterococcus faecalis* ATCC 29212	*Escherichia coli* ATCC 25922	*Pseudomonas aeruginosa* ATCC 27853	*Escherichia coli* ATCC 35218[b]
Ticarcillin	2–8	16–64	4–16	8–32	
Ticarcillin-clavulanic acid	0.5/2–2/2	16/2–64/2	4/2–16/2	8/2–32/2	8/2–32/2
Tobramycin	0.12–1	8–32	0.25–1	0.25–1	
Trimethoprim[g]	1–4	≤1	0.5–2	>64	
Trimethoprim-sulfamethoxazole	≤0.5/9.5	≤0.5/9.5	≤0.5/9.5	8/152–32/608	
Trospectomycin	2–16	2–8	8–32		
Trovafloxacin	0.008–0.03	0.06–0.25	0.004–0.016	0.25–2	
Vancomycin[f]	0.5–2	1–4			

[a] Adapted from NCCLS document M100–S14 (M7–A6) (167).
[b] MICs were obtained from several reference laboratories by broth microdilution with CAMHB.

TABLE 3.27

Antimicrobial Test Results That Require Confirmation and/or Investigation[a]

Microorganism[b]	Nonsusceptible Phenotypes[c]
Gram-negative	
Enterobacteriaceae	Amikacin, carbapenems,[d] fluoroquinolones
Pseudomonas aeruginosa	Aminoglycosides (multiple)
Stenotrophomonas maltophilia	Trimethoprim-sulfamethoxazole
Hemophilus influenzae	Ampicillin, amoxicillin-clavulanic acid,[e] aztreonam, carbapenem, 3rd-generation cephalosporins, fluoroquinolones
Neisseria gonorrhoeae	3rd-generation cephalosporins, fluoroquinolones
Neisseria meningitidis	Penicillin, ciprofloxacin
Gram-positive	
Enterococcus faecalis	Ampicillin or penicillin, linezolid, high-level aminoglycosides, quinupristin-dalfopristin
Enterococcus faecium	High-level aminoglycoside, linezolid, quinupristin-dalfopristin
Staphylococcus aureus	Linezolid, oxacillin, quinupristin-dalfopristin, vancomycin
Staphylococcus, coagulase-negative	Linezolid, vancomycin
Streptococcus pneumoniae	Fluoroquinolones, linezolid, meropenem, 3rd-generation cephalosporins, penicillin, vancomycin
Streptococcus, beta	Ampicillin or penicillin, 3rd-generation cephalosporins, linezolid, vancomycin
Streptococcus viridans	Penicillin, linezolid, vancomycin

[a] See Livermore (128) and NCCLS (168).
[b] Any microorganism that is resistant to all agents tested warrants review and investigation.
[c] Microorganisms that fail to meet the interpretive criteria for S (susceptible); they may be I or R.
[d] *Proteus* spp are an exception for imipenem.
[e] β-Lactamase negative.

susceptibility of unusual organisms to antimicrobial agents may also present special problems.

In the past, many of these organisms did not require susceptibility tests because they were known to be universally susceptible to an appropriate antimicrobial agent that was not toxic and could reach sufficient levels to effect a clinical cure. Resistant strains have emerged, however. Resistance to β-lactams is most often due to production of β-lactamase, which may be constitutive or inducible and may be mediated by either chromosomal or plasmid genes (187,193). In some species, such as *H. influenzae* and *N. gonorrhoeae,* penicillin and ampicillin resistance has been typically caused by the acquisition of plasmids that mediate constitutive β-lactamase production by the organisms (70,71). In other species, such as *S. pneumoniae,* penicillin resistance is not due to β-lactamase production caused by plasmids but is chromosomally mediated and is due to the alteration of penicillin-binding proteins (PBPs) (268).

These developments have produced challenges for clinicians because previously employed empirical therapies associated with these fastidious or unusual organisms may not be adequate. Additional laboratory testing is sometimes required to support a prediction of therapic success.

For some organisms, such as group A streptococci, susceptibility tests are not necessary because these organisms have maintained (with some exceptions) universal susceptibility to penicillin, the drug of choice. However, for *S. pneumoniae,* especially if it was isolated from a putatively sterile site, a test to determine susceptibility to penicillin is indicated, because some of the strains may be relatively or completely resistant to penicillin. If it becomes necessary to perform susceptibility tests on clinical isolates for which no standard method has been described, it is usually best to determine the MIC using the general broth dilution method described earlier and in NCCLS standard M7-A6. Table 3.28 details the antimicrobial susceptibility methods that can be used for these fastidious or unusual organisms. It is obvious that certain microorganisms have been omitted, notably anaerobes, *Mycobacterium tuberculosis, Chlamydia* spp, *Mycoplasma* spp, and spirochetes. For these groups, readers can refer to appropriate chapters in this volume.

Haemophilus Influenzae

H. influenzae and other *Haemophilus* species are examples of common clinical pathogens with special growth requirements. The widespread emergence of β-lactamase–producing strains has made rapid detection of β-lactamase production and, in turn, detection of ampicillin resistance in this organism important objectives (13,169,227,228).

Antimicrobial resistance among clinical isolates of *H. influenzae* has been monitored in the United States, Canada, and Europe. In a comprehensive study (54) involving isolates in the United States, 20% of all *H. influenzae* isolates were ampicillin-resistant by virtue of β-lactamase production. Enzyme-mediated resistance to ampicillin is approximately twice as common in serotype B strains (31.7%) as in non-B strains (15.6%). As a result of the production of the inactivating enzyme chloramphenicol acetyltransferase (9), occasional resistance has been noted with chloramphenicol, as well as resistance to tetracycline, trimethoprim/sulfamethoxazole, rifampin, and first-generation cephalosporins.

Because of the worldwide prevalence of β-lactamase–producing strains of *H. influenzae,* it is imperative that clinical laboratories routinely perform β-lactamase studies on all clinically significant isolates. Several media formulations have been employed for dilution or diffusion susceptibility testing with *H. influenzae* (114,116). Although individual methods may have been useful in individual laboratories, a common problem with these media formulations has been the complexity of their preparation and their opaque nature. Recently, a new simplified medium, HTM, has been developed; it avoids many of these problems (116). HTM is optically clear, stable, and reproducible from lot to lot and is currently available commercially from several manufacturers. The use of HTM has been advocated by NCCLS for both dilution and diffusion tests with *H. influenzae* (167). Guidelines for the interpretation of MIC and QC results with a *H. influenzae* reference strain are included in this chapter and are contained in Tables 3.28 and 3.30.

In addition to *H. influenzae,* other problem organisms have been tested, as indicated in Table 3.28. Following is a discussion of current approaches to the testing of MRSA, *N. gonorrhoeae, S. pneumoniae, S. viridans, Listeria monocytogenes, Eikenella corrodens,* and *Chlamydia* spp, along with appropriate references. In general, the use of a full incubation interval of 24 hours and the addition of 2% sodium chloride to cation-supplemented MHB have facilitated the testing of MRSA and have greatly enhanced the reliability of standard microdilution tests in detecting such organisms (53,147,229). Variable results have been obtained with different dilution methods for testing MRSA strains with cephalosporins, and many strains appear fully susceptible to cephalosporins, which is inconsistent with treatment results. This has led to the standard recommendation that cephalosporin tests not be reported for MRSA and methicillin-resistant *S. epidermidis* (168).

Neisseria Gonorrhoeae

The changing antimicrobial susceptibility of *N. gonorrhoeae* is an example of how clinical laboratories have had to modify their approaches and strategies in susceptibility testing. *N. gonorrhoeae* has developed resistance to all of the agents that have been recommended for gonorrhea therapy. When penicillin was the recommended

(*text continues on page 103*)

TABLE 3.28

Susceptibility Testing of Fastidious and Unusual Pathogens[a]

Organism	Method	Medium	Incubation/Environment	Comments
Campylobacter spp	Broth microdilution (166) Agar dilution	CAMHB + 5% LHB[c] MHA + 5% blood	35°C, 18–24 h in 85% N_2 10% CO_2 5% O_2	Some strains may require 48 h for adequate growth. Does not require routine testing, as many cases of gastrointestinal disease are self-limiting. Empirical treatment with a macrolide is usually successful.
Corynebacterium spp	Broth microdilution (166) Agar dilution	CAMHB MHA	35°C, 18–24 h	Some strains may require a more nutritive medium, e.g., blood or serum additives. Test JK against vancomycin and rifampin.
Haemophilus spp	Broth microdilution (116, 166, 227, 228) QC: *H. influenzae* ATCC 49247 & 49766	HTM[d] (inoculum from choc)	35°C, 20–24 h	See the most recent NCCLS dilution standard for recommendations on drugs and breakpoints.
	β-lactamase (228)		Room temperature up to 1 h	Do not need induction. Any β-lactamase method can be used. Some strains may be ampicillin-resistant but β-lactamase–negative.
Helicobacter pylori	Agar dilution (NCCLS) QC: *H. pylori* ATCC 43504	MHA	35°C, 3 d in special *Campylobacter* gas systems	Interpretive criteria only for clarithromycin.
Legionella spp	Do not test routinely (230)			Therapy can be empirical (macrolide and/or rifampin). Susceptibility testing should be done only in reference laboratories.
Listeria monocytogenes	Broth microdilution (166) Agar dilution QC: *Streptococcus pneumoniae* ATCC 49619	CAMHB + 5% LHB MHA + 5% sheep blood	35°C, 16–20 h	*L. monocytogenes* may be susceptible to cephalosporins *in vitro* but they are not effective clinically. Drugs of choice are ampicillin and TMP-SMX. Ampicillin MICs are usually 0.5–1.0 μg/mL. Ampicillin is usually the drug of choice in meningitis.

Moraxella catarrhalis	Broth microdilution (166) Agar dilution β-lactamase (228, 230)	CAMHB[b] MHA[b]	35°C, 18–24 hr Room temp. up to 1 h	Some strains may require a more nutritive medium. Use only the nitrocefin method. Other methods must be proven to be equivalent. 80% or more of strains are β-lactamase–positive. The β-lactamase is not the TEM type but is inhibited by clavulanic acid and sulbactam.
Mycobacterium fortuitum and *Mycobacterium chelonae*	Broth microdilution; inoculum is prepared from overnight growth in MHB + 0.02% Tween 80 (230)	CAMHB	35°C, 72 h	Avoid creating aerosols. Test aminoglycosides, doxycycline, cefoxitin, crythromycin, and sulfonamides. Ciprofloxacin also has activity against *M. fortuitum*. Other *Mycobacterium* spp are not tested by this method.
Neisseria meningitidis	Broth microdilution (166)	CAMHB+ 2–5% LHB	35°C, 24 h in CO_2	Test penicillin, rifampin, and sulfonamide. Organisms in broth may lyse after 24 h. Rifampin and sulfa data are for decisions on prophylaxis and not therapy (230).
	Agar dilution (166)	MHA	35°C, 18–24 h in CO_2	
Neisseria gonorrhoeae	Agar dilution or disk diffusion (See text and Jones et al. [111])	GC agar base with "XV" supplement	35°C, 24 h in CO_2	Ideally, test for penicillin, tetracycline, spectinomycin, and ceftriaxone.
	β-lactamase (228)	From isolation media	Room temp. up to 1 h	Occasional strains may be resistant to penicillin but β-lactamase–negative. Induction not required: any β-lactamase method can be used.
Nocardia spp	Broth microdilution (166)	CAMHB	35°C, 48 h	*N. asteroides* has four or five different susceptibility patterns; *N. brasiliensis* has one. Sulfas are generally drugs of choice, but intolerance or allergy is fairly common. Test a variety of antimicrobials including third-generation cephalosporins and β-lactam–β-lactamase inhibitor combinations (personal communication from Dr. Richard Wallace, University of Texas Health Science Center, Tyler, TX).

(*continued*)

TABLE 3.28 (Continued)

Susceptibility Testing of Fastidious and Unusual Pathogens[a]

Organism	Method	Medium	Incubation/Environment	Comments
Nonfermentative bacteria (other than *Acinetobacter* spp)	Broth microdilution (166)	CAMHB or CSMHB + supplements if needed	35°C, 18–24 h or longer; use CO_2 if necessary	Some of these isolates may require a more enriched medium.
	Agar dilution (166)	MHA + supplements if needed		
"Organisms causing endocarditis:" nonenterococcal streptococci	See *Streptococcus* spp section for MIC methods			If penicillin MIC >0.1 μg/mL, β-lactam plus aminoglycoside (streptomycin or gentamicin) therapy should be considered.
Enterococcus spp	See *Streptococcus* spp section for MIC methods			Use β-lactam and aminoglycoside (streptomycin or gentamicin) for therapy. Some strains will not respond synergistically to the combination (see below).
	High-level aminoglycosides test for synergy *E. faecalis* ATCC 29212 (S) ATCC 51299 (R)	BHI broth	35°C, 24 h; additional 24 h if necessary	Test streptomycin at 1000 μg/mL and gentamicin at 500 μg/mL. If there is no growth, synergy between the β-lactam and the aminoglycoside is likely to occur; if there is growth, synergy is unlikely. Blood may influence susceptibility tests with aminoglycosides and cephalosporins and some enterococci (47). It is assumed that most oxacillin-resistant staphylococci can be detected by agar dilution, although there are no data or recommendations for adding NaCl (169).
S. pneumoniae	Broth microdilution (166, 230) QC: *S. pneumoniae* ATCC 49619	CAMHB + 5% LHB	35°C, 18–24 h	MIC breakpoints for penicillin are: susceptible, ≤0.06; intermediate, 0.12–1.0; and oxacillin disk diffusion zone diameter of ≥20 MICs indicate susceptibility.

Streptococcus spp	Broth microdilution (166) QC: *S. pneumoniae* ATCC 49619	CAMHB + 5% LHB	35°C, 18–24 h in CO_2 if necessary	Nonenterococcal streptococci that grow well in this medium (and may require CO_2) may also be tested by the standard NCCLS disk diffusion methods (123). The oxacillin screen test as used for pneumococci (i.e., to indicate penicillin resistance) does not work for these organisms. Penicillin resistance occurs most often in *S. mitis* but does occur in other species. For group A streptococci, erythromycin resistance occurs; zones of ≥18 mm correlate well with MICs of ≤0.12 μg/mL, and zones of <18 mm with MICs of ≥2 μg/mL (169).
Streptococci, pyridoxal-dependent	Broth microdilution (43, 166)	CAMHB + 5% LHB + 0.001% pyridoxal HCl	35°C, 18–24 h in CO_2 if necessary	Grow organisms on agar containing 0.001% pyridoxal HCl. Alternatively 1% pyridoxal HCl can be swabbed onto the surface of a blood agar plate prior to inoculation. Prepare inoculum suspension from growth on plate.
Fastidious or unusual organisms not mentioned previously	Broth dilution (166) Agar dilution (166)	Use CAMHB/A plus supplements as necessary. Trial and error may be necessary to determine needs	35°C, 18–24 h or longer. Use required atmosphere. Trial and error may be necessary to determine needs	If unusual supplements or atmosphere is necessary, report MIC as not done with a standardized test.
Staphylococcus[e,f] *aureus* Oxacillin-resistant (methicillin-resistant)	Agar screen (226,229) *S. aureus* 29213 (OS) *S. aureus* ATCC 433000 (OR)	MHA + 4% NaCl and 6 μg/mL oxacillin or 10 μg/mL methicillin	35°C, full 24 h but no longer	Use as a screening test for methicillin, oxacillin, nafcillin, or cloxacillin resistance. Oxacillin is the preferred test agent in most institutions. Inoculate plate by "pie-plating" or by "spot" inoculation with swab. Growth indicates chromosomal intrinsic resistance. Use as a second test in addition to the broth microdilution or disk diffusion test. Note: this method not reliable for detecting oxacillin resistance coagulase-negative staphylococci.
	Broth microdilution—for methicillin and oxacillin and methicillin and oxacillin only (cephalothin or other β-lactams, excluding cefamandole, if desired) (166,226,229)	CAMHB +2% NaCl	35°C, full 24 h but no longer	For *S. aureus*, S ≤ 2 and R ≥ 4. For coagulase-negative staphylococci, S ≤ 0.25 and R ≥ 0.5. The above breakpoints are to be used only with this MIC method. Oxacillin is the preferred test agent. To prepare inoculum, suspend colonies from an overnight agar plate into broth or saline to equal the turbidity of a 0.5 McFarland standard (1,20). Final inoculum should be 3–5 × 10^5 CFU/mL. Some strains are hyperproducers of β-lactamase and yield resistant or borderline MICs to oxacillin and methicillin but will not be intrinsically resistant. These strains are not usually multiresistant to drugs other than β-lactams. These strains are usually susceptible to amoxicillin-clavulanic acid (intrinsically oxacillin-resistant strains are not).

(*continued*)

TABLE 3.28 (Continued)

Susceptibility Testing of Fastidious and Unusual Pathogens[a]

Organism	Method	Medium	Incubation/Environment	Comments
				Clues (flags) indicating resistance to methicillin, oxacillin, or nafcillin: 1. Multiple resistance to any or all of the following: • erythromycin • aminoglycosides • chloramphenicol • tetracycline • clindamycin 2. Intermediate MIC to methicillin or oxacillin. 3. Failure to show cross-resistance between methiciilin, nafcillin, and oxacillin.

[a] In general, the inoculum for most of these tests is preferably prepared directly from growth off of agar plates (11). It is best to use a fresh plate, but some organisms may require 48 h for adequate growth. Suspend the growth into a clear broth and standardize the suspension to match a 0.5 McFarland standard. Then make appropriate dilutions depending on type of system or method being used (see directions for specific organisms). Inoculum for broth microdilution should be 10^5 to 5×10^5 CFU/mL and for agar. 10^4 to 5×10^4 CFU/spot.

[b] Abbreviations for media or reagents: MHA, Mueller-Hinton agar; CAMHB, cation-adjusted Mueller-Hinton broth (26); BHI, brain heart infusion broth; NAD, nicotinamide adenine dinucleotide; SXT, sulfamethoxazole-trimethoprim.

[c] The lysed blood used in these tests is lysed by freezing, thawing at least 6 times, and then adding an equal volume of sterile distilled water. The solution is clarified by centrifugation (10,000 $\times$ g) for 20 min and subsequent decantation of the supernate (not necessary if it is to be added to agar). Sheep blood is not recommended for tests with *Haemophilus* spp or with sulfonamides.

[d] To make *Haemophilus* test medium (HTM), first prepare a fresh hematin stock solution by dissolving 50 mg of powder in 100 mL of 0.01 N NaPH with heat and stirring until the powder is thoroughly dissolved. Add 30 mL of the hematin stock. After autoclaving and cooling, cations are added aseptically, if needed as in CAMHB, and 3 mL of a NAD stock solution (50 mg of NAD dissolved in 10 mL of filter distilled water) also aseptically added. If sulfonamides or trimethoprim are to be tested, 0.2 IU/mL thymidine phosphorylase should also be aseptically added to the medium.

[e] *S. aureus* exhibiting resistance to one of the penicillinase-resistant penicillins (MRSA) must be reported as resistant to cephalosporin-like antimicrobial agents, regardless of *in vitro* dilution test results, because in most cases of documented MRSA infections, patients have responded poorly to cephalosporin chemotherapy. Methicillin-resistant, coagulase-negative *Staphylococcus* spp also appear not to respond well to cephalosporin treatment, but the data are less clear than with *S. aureus*.

[f] Also applies to other *Staphylococcus* spp.

therapy for *N. gonorrhoeae* infection, most isolates were initially susceptible. From the mid-1940s to the 1970s, there was a 24-fold increase in the dosage of procaine penicillin (2×10^5 units to 4.8×10^6 units). Penicillin is no longer the recommended therapy.

The resistance of *N. gonorrhoeae* to antibacterials is due either to multiple chromosomal mutations or to R factor plasmids. In 1987, the increasing prevalence of strains with β-lactamase plasmids prompted discontinuation of the use of penicillin as a single-dose therapy. Determining resistance, which is primarily a laboratory responsibility, affects epidemiological surveillance and patient care.

A standardized laboratory method for monitoring the susceptibilities of gonococcal isolates was formulated and has been recommended by NCCLS based on a multicenter laboratory study whose purpose was to standardize disk diffusion and agar susceptibility tests (111). The recommended test medium is GC agar base with a defined XV-like supplement. Three QC organisms are required: *N. gonorrhoeae* ATCC strain 49226 (CDC F-18), *N. gonorrhoeae* World Health Organization (WHO) strain V, and *S. aureus* ATCC strain 25923.

The publication of the multicenter guidelines does not alter the need or methodology for detecting penicillinase-producing *N. gonorrhoeae*. Penicillinase-producing *N. gonorrhoeae* strains may be identified by detection of β-lactamase with a nitrocefin substrate (Table 3.28). Strains of *N. gonorrhoeae* that have chromosomally mediated resistance to antimicrobial agents or plasmid-mediated resistance to penicillin and/or tetracycline may be detected by measuring their susceptibilities by disk diffusion (111) and are not discussed here. Agar dilution methodology is preferred to broth dilution, as *N. gonorrhoeae* is known to autolyze in liquid media.

Streptococcus Pneumoniae

Throughout the world, there have been increasing reports of the relative resistance of *S. pneumoniae* to penicillin as well as to other drugs such as tetracycline, erythromycin, clindamycin, and chloramphenicol (8,122). Nonsusceptible strains have been isolated in the United States with increasing frequency; thus, routine testing of isolates of *S. pneumoniae* is probably warranted. Satisfactory broth dilution tests can be performed with *S. pneumoniae*, provided that the broth medium is appropriately supplemented by adding 5% defibrinated sheep blood to freshly thawed MHB in microdilution trays that have been stored for no more than 2 months at 20°C. Commercially prepared test systems are available but have limitations and need to be verified and validated (223). Tests for other streptococci are indicated in Table 3.28.

Special studies related to susceptibility testing of several other species have been performed and are noted here. MICs, MBCs, and killing curves have been studied for *L. monocytogenes* using TS broth (43,257). *Pasteurella multocida* was tested in microtiter panels using MHB supplemented with 10% horse serum (214). Vanhoof et al. (243) evaluated inhibition and killing of *Campylobacter jejuni* in MHB. *Eikenella corrodens* susceptibility testing has been accomplished using MHB supplemented with 0.5% lysed sheep blood (93). *Mycoplasma* spp have also been studied (106) in macrotube systems and by microdilution susceptibility testing (207, 209). Unlike conventional bacteria, which can grow in artificial media, *Chlamydia trachomatis* has been tested against a variety of antimicrobial agents by incorporating antibiotic dilutions in cycloheximide-treated McCoy cell cultures (31,98). Utilizing this approach, MICs and MBCs can be determined (see Chapter 7).

AUTOMATED, RAPID, AND INSTRUMENT-ASSOCIATED METHODS

Direct Microscopy and Observation of Bacterial Morphology

Early in the use of penicillin, it was noted that cultures of either spinal fluid or blood taken from individuals who had been treated with penicillin demonstrated aberrant forms in these clinical specimens. Observations of morphological alterations in bacteria produced during early exposure to various antimicrobial agents were recorded by several investigators (65,83). Growth can be observed by a variety of means, including light, phase-contrast, and electron microscopy, with different changes being produced by an antibiotic, depending on the bacterial species and the mode of action and concentration of the agent. Antibiotics, especially those of the β-lactam class, which interfere with cell wall synthesis and bind to the lytic PBPs (see "Minimal Bactericidal Concentration"), can produce various filamentous forms or protoplasmic enlargements (95). Similar morphological alterations can be seen in inocula exposed to concentrations that are below the MIC but that nonetheless modify the characteristics of the affected bacterial population (131).

The minimum amount of antimicrobial agent necessary to induce such alterations has been termed the minimal antibacterial concentration (MAC) (131,132). When visualized by light microscopy, this approach represents a rapid method, because the changes may occur rapidly, occasionally within minutes. However, these observations are qualitative, the methods are not standardized, and the observations are labor-intensive.

Clinical data demonstrating the relevance of a given alternative antibiotic susceptibility test method in the care and management of infectious disease are based primarily on the MIC of the agent against the infecting organism. Additional investigation is needed to establish the interpretive significance of a standard derived from the new approach. Thus, in the MAC approach, one would have

TABLE 3.29

Comparison of Overnight MIC Readings with Inocula of 10^5/mL[a] to 3-Hour Readings with Inocula of 10^7/mL[b]

Determinants	Ratio of 18- to 3-Hour Readings								Total Strains
	0.03	0.125	0.25	0.5	1	2	4	8	
3- and 18-hour MICs within range tested		2	5	20	32	9	2	1	71
One of the two MICs above the range tested[c]	1	1	2	6	—[d]		1		11[d]
One of the two MICs below the range tested[c]				4					4
Subtotals	1	3	7	30	32[d]	9	3	1	
Total		11			71[d]		4		86[d]

[a] ICS broth tube dilution method (74).
[b] Adapted from Lampe et al. (124).
[c] Ratios calculated by considering MIC readings of, e.g., >128 as 256 and <0.25 as 0.125.
[d] In 22 cases, both MICs were above the range tested and were excluded.

to study the MAC/MIC ratios (131,267) to determine the MAC's clinical utility.

Early Reading of Conventional Tests

Like in the early reading of disk diffusion tests, where the kinetics of growth and zone formation are fairly well stabilized for many drug-bug interactions within 8 hours of incubation and frequently within 5 hours (136) or 6 hours (20), results of rapid or early reading can be estimated in liquid media. It is suggested, however, that early estimated results be confirmed by a later reading or by retesting with conventional incubation intervals. Lampe et al. (124) determined the accuracy of early reading compared with standard ICS macrotube dilution (i.e., 3 hour in comparison with the conventional 18-hour incubation time). Values from the conventional incubation were at least 4 times higher than those from the early 3-hour reading for 43% of the strains tested. Agreement was improved with the 8-hour incubation period. When procedural modifications were initiated for the purpose of producing rapid results that would conform to conventional endpoints, comparisons of different media, shaking versus static cultures, and reading by particle count versus visually did not eliminate the discrepancies (124). However, increasing the inoculum size to possibly 10^7 CFU/mL produced better agreement, with 14% of the test isolates demonstrating fourfold dilution errors (Table 3.29). Because this approach is not applicable to all species, especially in view of variable mechanisms of resistance, additional clinical investigations of these interpretations are warranted. Until such investigations for establishing clinical guidance in earlier time frames are completed, the focus will be on the reference overnight method.

There have been attempts over the years to develop methods that could enhance the apparent growth of bacteria and thereby reduce the conventional overnight incubation required to determine an MIC. Investigators have used colorimetric indicators and leuco dyes to amplify the macroscopic observation of turbidity. In macrodilution assays, phenol red was added to assay tubes containing glucose and yeast extract to enhance growth. If the test organism grew utilizing the glucose, tubes would turn yellow as a result of the pH change. If the antimicrobial agent inhibited the organism, the indicator would remain red. Nonfermenter organisms could be detected by an orange-red color if they grew in the antibiotic-free tubes.

Redox indicators such as resazurin, triphenyltetrazolium chloride, and methylene blue have been used as indicators of growth (208). Because these dyes may be antibacterial, the strategy was to add them to the control tube after a brief (3- to 5-hour) incubation period. If sufficient growth was then detectable, the indicator would be added to all assay tubes. Bartlett and Mazens (24)

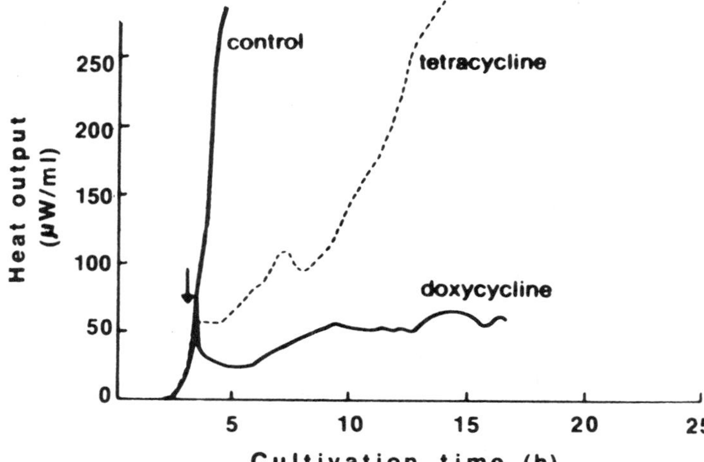

FIGURE 3.8 ● Microcalorimetric response of logarithmic-phase cells of *E. coli* toward two antibiotics. *Arrow*, time of addition of drugs. (Reproduced from Mardh et al. [144].)

enhanced the sensitivity of triphenyltetrazolium chloride by the addition of phenazine methosulfate, which accelerated formation of the red formazan precipitate resulting from growth of the bacteria. The indophenol reagent dichlorophenolindophenol is another redox dye that has been tested (130). A proprietary tetrazolium-type reagent (Alamar blue) incorporated into commercially prepared antibiotic-containing testing panels has received some attention (10).

In a unique approach, bacterial respiration was detected utilizing the respiration of hemoglobin as an indicator. A 3% suspension of red blood cells (outdated human or animal) served as the indicator (200).

The rapid approaches described in these early reports have not been accepted by and are not applied in clinical or reference laboratories. Had they received some commercial impetus and if ample reference and QC measures had been developed to ensure reliability, they might have achieved acceptance.

Alternative Rapid Instrumental Methods

Detection of Bacteria and Bacterial Products

In the search for rapid methods for determining the interaction of antimicrobial agents and organisms, microbiologists have examined the products of bacterial metabolism (intermediate and end products) as well as the interaction of the organism with various energy sources. In addition to the more complex products of bacterial metabolism detectable by gas chromatographic methods (155), there are the more immediate endproducts of glucose degradation (i.e., carbon dioxide, water, energy, ATP, and heat). Thus, if glucose is tagged with radioactive carbon or some other substrate is similarly tagged, then the CO_2 released via bacterial metabolism is radioactive and can be detected by radiometry (51,52,126,127). Alternatively, the CO_2 produced can be monitored by infrared spectroscopy to detect growth. Also, the ATP produced by metabolism can be measured by the luciferin-luciferase reaction, and the energy quanta derived from this interaction can be measured with an ATP luminometer (38). Similarly, heat in the form of nonutilizable energy derived from the enzymatic degradation of glucose can be detected (Fig. 3.8) and measured by microcalorimetry (27). As bacteria replicate in the growth medium, they decrease the measured electrical resistance (impedance in alternating-current circuits) in the medium (Fig. 3.9). Impedance has been measured in bacterial cultures by passing a high-voltage, alternating-current signal through the medium and monitoring its effect (35,36,242). All of these approaches are bacteriologically sound, in that any method used to detect bacterial growth can be applied to the measurement of the interaction of antimicrobial and bacterium and thus to the testing of susceptibility (27,42).

Of the several methods noted here, two persist in commercial instrumentation suitable for clinical laboratories: radiometry and ATP luminometry. Only the former is currently applied to antimicrobial susceptibility testing, specifically with mycobacteria (102,108).

Another approach to the detection of bacteria and, in turn, the determination of susceptibility involves measuring bacteria interacting with some component of the electromagnetic spectrum. Theoretically, one can measure single particles (individual bacteria) or, for better accuracy, a population of particles (bacteria). The origin of using densitometry (turbidity and visual turbidity) (Fig. 3.10) can be traced to the hallmark works of McFarland (148) and Longsworth (129). Specialized light-scattering methods (Fig. 3.11) using coherent light emanating from a

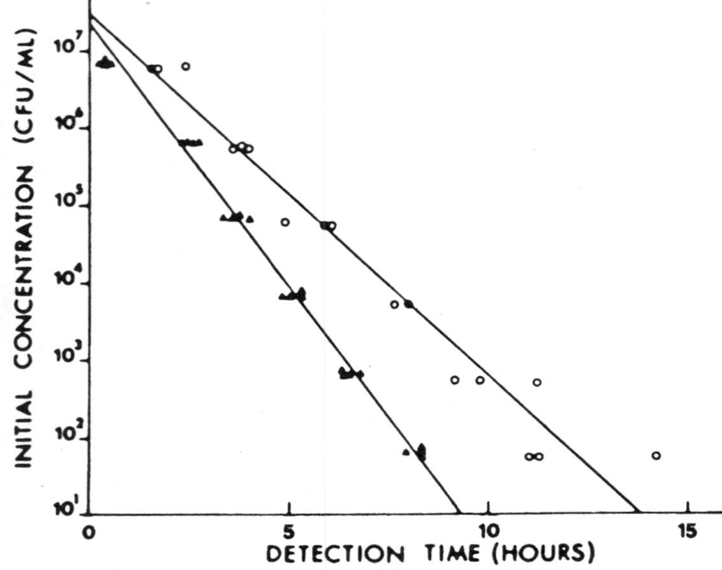

FIGURE 3.9 ● Detection times by electrical impedance monitoring graphed against initial concentrations of microorganisms for *E. coli* (▲) and *S. aureus* (○), both growing in TS broth at 35°C. The *solid lines* represent least-squares linear fits to the data points for each organism. The slopes of the lines reflect the organisms generation times (26 minutes for *E. coli* and 38 minutes for *S. aureus*). The correlation between log initial concentration and detection time was 0.95 for *E. coli* and 0.94 for *S. aureus*. (Reproduced with permission from Cady et al. [36].)

laser have also been applied (262, 263). Infrared light (43) and ultraviolet light have been used as energy sources to detect bacteria. Radiation of the latter type interacts with nucleic acids at 260 nm. The uptake of thymidine, a DNA precursor, by microorganisms in the presence and absence of antimicrobial agents has been assessed by Amaral et al. (3). In this assay, labeled thymidine (with either tritium or carbon as the label) is used to determine susceptibility profiles directly from a patient's specimen, thereby obviating the need for a primary culture and the time delay associated with the initial culture. The assay determines the amount radioactive thymidine incorporated into DNA compared with control and antibiotic-containing cultures. Clear drawbacks of this approach include the potential

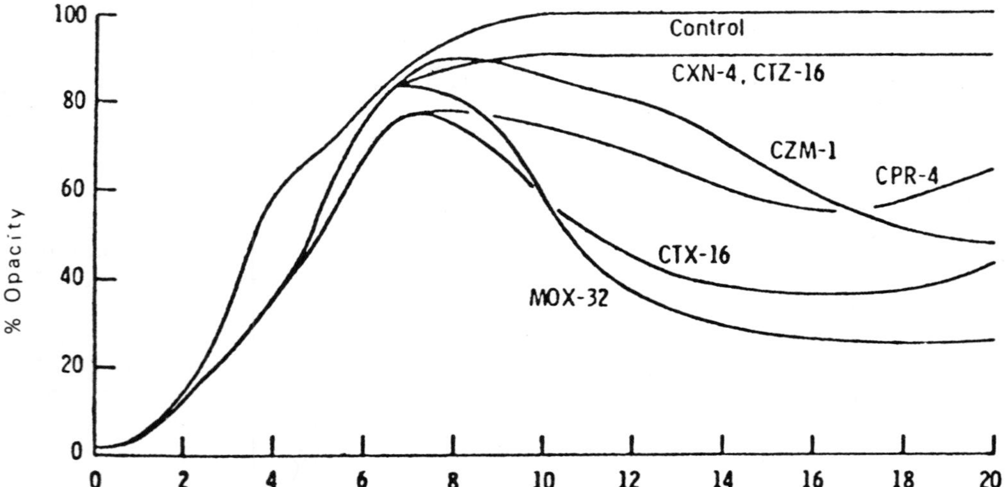

FIGURE 3.10 ● Growth response, as measured by turbidity (opacity) of *P. aeruginosa* toward several β-lactam antibiotics. The drop in turbidity due to lysis varied depending on the antibiotic. Regrowth was observed with cefoperazone at 4 μg/mL and cefotaxime at 16 μg/mL. The initial population at time 0 was about 10^6 cells/mL, at which time drugs were added. MOX, moxalactam; CTX, cefotaxime; CPR, cefoperazone; CZM, ceftazidime; CXN, ceftriaxone; CTZ, ceftizoxime. Numerals refer to concentrations in μg/mL, which were equivalent to twice the MIC for each of the drugs. (Reproduced from Greenwood and Eley [95].)

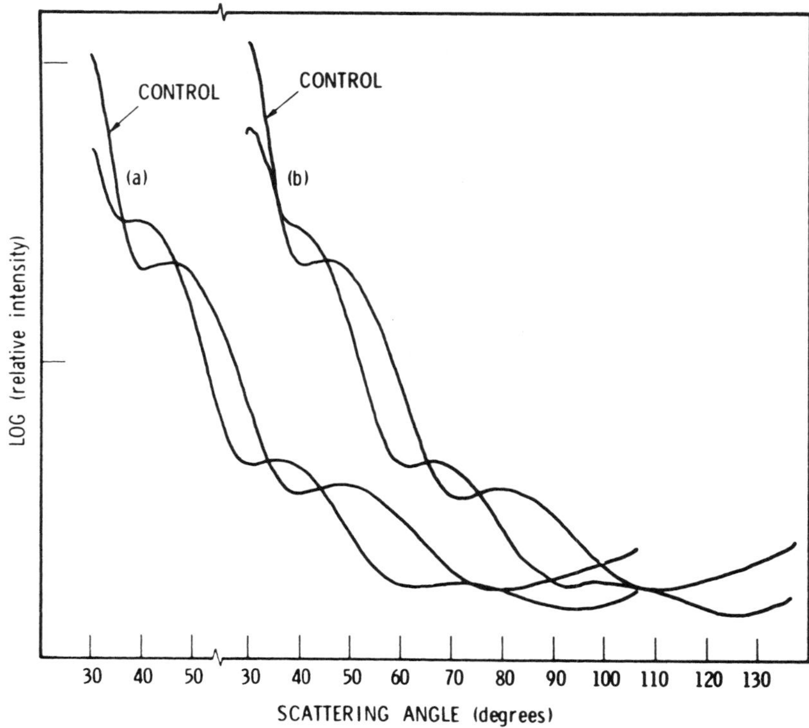

FIGURE 3.11 • Effects of (a) ampicillin (0.20 μg/mL) and (b) penicillin (0.14μg/mL) on the light-scattering patterns from a suspension of susceptible *S. aureus*. (Reprinted with permission from Wyatt [263].)

contamination of the workplace and technical staff and the costs associated with the necessity to routinely monitor the environment and personnel and dispose of materials.

Flow Cytometry

A recent significant development in antimicrobial susceptibility testing is the application of flow cytometry (176). The technology of flow cytometry encompasses aspects of immunology, biochemistry, molecular biology, and histology. Any cellular analyte or metabolic event that can be tagged with a fluorescent dye is a potential candidate for analysis by flow cytometry. Flow cytometers are complex instruments linked to powerful computers still largely dependent on manual procedures. The essence of current multiparameter flow cytometry resides in the capability of the instrument to analyze individual cells (and cell types) of a subpopulation within a larger heterogeneous population without the need for separating or isolating the subpopulation. During flow cytometric analyses, cells in suspension are pushed (flow) single file through a flow cell (Figs. 3.12 and 3.13), where the cells are exposed to monochromatic light emanating from a laser beam, usually of the argon-ion type (162,202). Two cellular parameters derived from the scatter of the laser light are measured: size (forward light scatter) and internal complexity or surface irregularity (right-angle scatter). Detectors in the flow cytometers are sensitive to the colors emitted by fluorochrome-tagged antibodies or fluorescent tracers after excitation by the laser beam.

The technique, as applied to antimicrobial susceptibility testing of microbes, exposes the organism to an antimicrobial agent for 2–6 hours at an appropriate incubation temperature. After exposure, organisms are stained with a fluorescent stain like ethidium bromide, which results in increased fluorescence due to breakdown of the cells. The increased fluorescence is then interpreted as death and could be used to determine the MIC. This approach has been applied to *M. tuberculosis* (174). There is no commercial instrument exclusively for this specific application. The current drawbacks of using flow cytometry for bacterial susceptibility testing are the cost of the system and the limited data accumulated for bacteria.

Automated Antimicrobial Susceptibility Test Systems

During the 1980s, clinical microbiology laboratories increased their use of commercial instrument-associated antimicrobial susceptibility testing methods. The growing

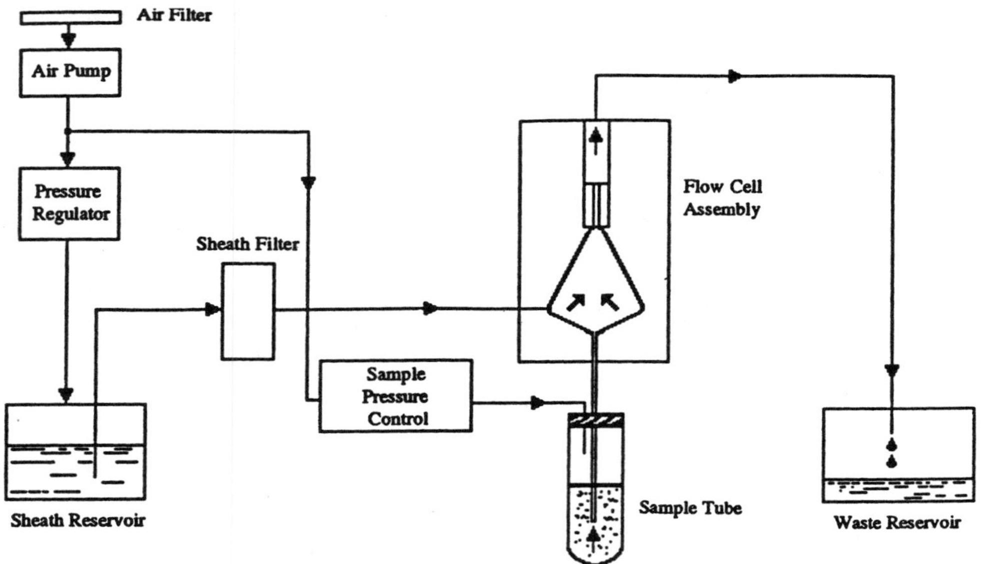

FIGURE 3.12 ● Simplified fluidics system of a flow cytometer concerned with moving the cells. The sample moves in a uniform stream across the laser intersection. (Reproduced from the National Center for Infectious Diseases [162].)

acceptance of these commercial instruments by laboratories parallels progress in electronics, robotics, and microcomputers—progress that permitted manufacturers to develop instrumentation able to identify routine Gram-negative and Gram-positive bacteria of medical importance, determine the associated antimicrobial susceptibility, and combine the results into a single report. The broth microdilution susceptibility tests and associated identification component have become the most popular of the systems currently available to clinical microbiology laboratories in the United States (41).

Background, Development, and Description of Automated Susceptibility Test Systems

The earliest automated and probably rapid susceptibility test system was the TAAS (Technicon Automated Antimicrobial Susceptibility) system. It was developed in the early 1970s by Technicon Instrument Corporation (Tarrytown, NY). It was never marketed. In this system, an antimicrobial agent was delivered by dropping antibiotic-impregnated disks into broth. Through the process of elution, the antimicrobial agent was free to act in a short

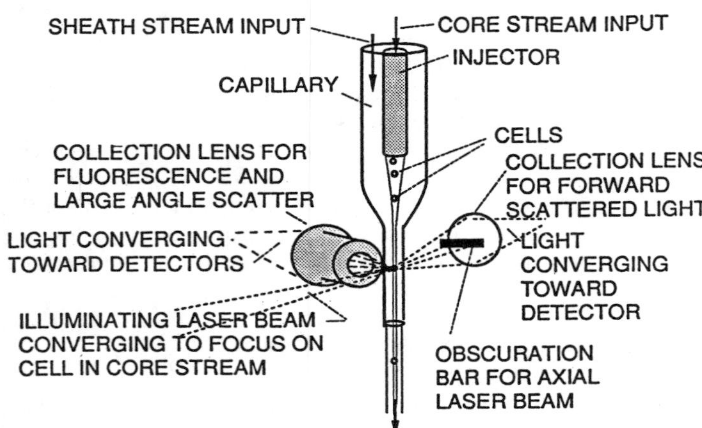

FIGURE 3.13 ● Schematic diagram of a typical flow cytometer. (Reproduced from Shapiro [202].)

period of time. After bacterial inoculation and growth for 3 hours in the presence of the single antimicrobial concentration, growth was compared with a control broth without antibiotic. A growth index was calculated based on the ratio of the growth in the presence and absence of the antimicrobial agent. From this index, an evaluation was made as to whether the bacterial population was susceptible (or resistant) to the antimicrobial agent. Instruments that immediately followed, such as the Autobac system (developed and marketed by Pfizer Diagnostics), also used antibiotic elution from paper disks as a means to initiate antimicrobial activity.

Subsequent systems utilized the microtiter 12 × 8 (96-well) format, in which antibiotic was prepared and frozen until used. In some cases a lyophilized dry powder was used. Clearly, there are advantages associated with dry powders, such as increased shelf life and storage flexibility. Systems utilizing microtiter formats became increasingly automated, to such an extent that the inoculation, incubation, and readout could be handled without human intervention. Once microcomputers with expanded memory became available, along with the capability of printing susceptibility results with bacterial identification and associated patient demographics, data management systems that could be used for the generation of cumulative susceptibility profiles were developed.

An abbreviated list of automated susceptibility systems available during the past two decades is presented in Table 3.25. As noted, most systems are no longer manufactured, and the commercial sponsors of the viable systems have changed.

Of the several antimicrobial susceptibility testing systems listed in Table 3.25, all but one use visible light as a measuring parameter (5). The Sensititre system uses fluorometric monitoring for determining the interaction of antimicrobial agent and bacterium (213). The systems that detect early growth with limited incubation (less than 6 hours) are the Autobac, the Advantage, and the ASM Vitek and Sensititre systems. If one considers the operational definition of rapid as 4 to 6 hours, then only the Autobac and Advantage systems fall into this category. All of the other systems require 6 hours or overnight incubation. However, the effects of limited incubation intervals, especially with β-lactam drugs, warrant serious evaluation (73). The accuracy of these systems (plus or minus one dilution) ranges from 87.6% to 98.3% (111).

It is not productive to describe in detail the varied commercial systems that were available, because frequent changes and corporate direction have modified the design and features of these instruments. Table 3.30 outlines contemporary instruments currently available and widely used. The descriptions of the two systems that follow—the MicroScan system, originally developed by Baxter, and the system from Vitek/McDonnell Douglas, now Vitek bioMerieux (Hazelwood, MO)—represent different approaches to automated susceptibility testing.

The MicroScan system developed in the 1980s uses the conventional 96-well format or an extended design coupled with fluorogenic or standard substrates to detect bacterial growth. The system includes a large computer-controlled microprocessor that incubates standard microdilution trays and interprets biochemical and/or susceptibility results with either a fluorometer for fluorogenic substrates or a conventional photometer for standard plates. (Panels with fluorogenic substrates have been discontinued.) The WalkAway model is available in two sizes, with a 40- or 96-test panel capacity. It consists of a large, self-contained incubator-reader with humidifier, a carousel that rotates towers containing the panels, a bar code scanner, photometers (spectrophotometer/fluorometer), and associated robotic mechanisms to move panels and perform designated computer-controlled robotic steps to access and position trays, add reagents, and position trays for reading. The instrument is associated with a microcomputer, a video display terminal, and a printer. The database management system is capable of producing a patient report and storing that information to subsequently reproduce cumulative reports, epidemiological reports, and antibiograms. Although the instrument discussed is automated, preparation of the inoculum is done individually and manually using a seed trough, which is transferred to the test panel with a rehydrator/inoculator (RENOK). This approach is more conventional, using the microtiter format with multiple antibiotic concentrations directed by microcomputer-controlled robotics (except for inoculum preparation) to achieve a final MIC result.

In contrast to the microtiter panel approach platform is the specialized design and concept of the Vitek system. The essence of this system is the reagent card, a small thin plastic unit that contains 30 wells or microcuvettes in the Legacy version and 45 wells in the Vitek 2 version. The wells are connected by capillaries in which bacterial test suspension passes for rehydration and inoculation. The cards are available with a variety of predetermined configurations of antimicrobial agents and reagents to identify Gram-positive or Gram-negative organisms. The MIC endpoint is determined by an algorithm from results of testing one to five antimicrobial concentrations. Cards are stored at 4°C, with a shelf life of approximately 12 months. The system includes integrated hardware consisting of a filler/sealer that serves as the inoculator and sealer for up to 10 cards, a reader/incubator that contains the robotic system to move the cards on a timely basis from a carousel to a position in the instrument where optical density or biochemical reactions are determined by a photometer, and a computer module that contains software, a video display terminal, a and printer. Systems are available in different capacities and can hold from

TABLE 3.30

Contemporary Automated Susceptibility Test Systems

System (Manufacturer)	Test Panel	Inoculation	Readout	System Components	Expert System
MicroScan WalkAway (Dade Behring, Inc.)	Conventional 8 × 12 microdilution trays; 40/96 panel capacity	Multiprong manual device	Turbidometric direct MIC or breakpoint	Incubator/reader, PC with video monitor and printer; data management system	Yes
Phoenix (Becton Dickinson)	Proprietary test panel with 136 wells; 100 panel capacity	Manual by self-filling transfer device into opening of test panel	Turbidometric with redox indicator system for direct MIC	Incubator/reader with integrated PC/monitor	EpiCenter software package available separately
Sensititre ARIS (Trek Diagnostics)	Conventional 8 × 12 microdilution trays; 64 panel capacity	Autoinoculator	Fluorometric direct MIC or breakpoint	Incubator/reader PC with video monitor and printer; autoinoculator	
Vitek Legacy (bioMerieux)	Proprietary plastic reagent cards with microchannels to 30/45 wells; 120 card capacity	Manual inoculum prep, filler-seal module, density verification	Turbidometric kinetic measurements of growth perform linear regression plots and derive MICs algorithmically	Incubator/reader; PC with video monitor and printer	Yes
Vitek 2 (bioMerieux)	Proprietary plastic reagent cards with microchannels to 64 wells; 60/120 card capacity	Automated inoculum dilution, density verification, card filling and sealing	As for legacy, some agents are direct MICs	Incubator/reader; filler-sealer; PC with video monitor and printer; data management system	Yes

30 to 240 cards. Growth is determined turbidometrically at hourly intervals for up to 15 hours, and is compared to the baseline and expressed as a ratio. Normalized linear regression of the growth is used to calculate a best fit to determine the MIC. The user can opt to print susceptibility results as discrete MICs or qualitative breakpoint results (susceptible to resistant).

Each of the systems described here can be linked to the main laboratory information system through a standard RS232 interface. The data management system is designed for storing and retrieving data for laboratory pharmacy and infection control purposes as well as printing chartable patient reports.

In addition to the instruments listed in Table 3.30, there are available several semiautomated devices that only turbidometrically or fluorometrically read/scan test panels inoculated manually and incubated overnight (18–24 hours). These include the AutoScaptor (Becton Dickinson), MicroScan autoSSCAN-4 (Dade Behring), mini API (bioMerieux), and Sensititre AutoReader (Trek Diagnostic). Also not included in Table 3.30 are the several computer-assisted semiautomated devices that measure disk diffusion zone diameters by image analysis (see Chapter 2). This latter group of instruments interpret zone diameter readings according to a user-selected database for reporting S, I, or R categories. One system, BIOMIC (Giles Scientific), determines MICs by regression analysis of measured zone diameters. Clear advantages of this instrument group are that they generally provide results that are more reproducible than those achieved by manual observation, measurement, and recording and that they can be interfaced to laboratory information systems, thereby reducing the potential for transcription errors in patient reports.

Advantages of Automated Systems

A perceived advantage of the automated approach to antimicrobial susceptibility testing is the apparently more efficient use of robotics, rather than humans, in executing these tests. However, the gain in labor savings is not extensive. Perhaps a more meaningful advantage is the reproducibility of results obtained by using this type of instrumentation. Because procedures for inoculum preparation, the specified duration of incubation, and the assessment of growth are standardized in these systems, subjective components are removed, and intralaboratory and interlaboratory standardization is readily achieved. For high-volume laboratories that demand high throughput, the time required for reading and interpreting routine susceptibility tests is diminished. The associated capability of performing identifications is an additional advantage. Considerable labor savings are also derived from the potential to establish a link between the computer and the laboratory information system. This capability precludes technologist error in transcribing, sorting, and entering results in individual reports.

Limitations and Problems of Automated Systems

Systems that mimic and merely robotize a multiwell approach to performing conventional MICs seem to have only minor disadvantages. However, when the systems associated with these instruments offer limited testing panel capacity, are not applicable to all groups of bacteria, and fail to incorporate QC endpoints that are on scale (i.e., within the MIC range of the test panel), their flexibility and precision are questionable. Furthermore, the capital outlay required for purchase and the high cost per test for reagent rental acquisition need to be assessed and compared with the expense of manual test methods. If the clinical impact significantly improves the quality of patient care and reduces hospital costs overall, then the financial costs of the testing itself become irrelevant.

The design of automated instruments that utilize extremely small volumes, modify the inoculum, and reduce the incubation interval has created several problems in the detection of resistance. The detection of type 1 inducible β-lactamase resistance associated with *Citrobacter, Enterobacter, Serratia, Providencia, Pseudomonas,* and indole-positive *Proteus* strains is hampered by short detection (incubation) intervals. Owing to their inherent nature, inducible-type resistors are missed because a longer incubation is required for induction and expression and subsequent detection of spontaneous mutants.

Because of the failure to detect emerging vancomycin resistance in *enterococci,* the FDA had imposed prohibitions for automated testing of *enterococci* with vancomycin. Similarly, these restrictions have been applied to *S. pneumoniae* susceptibility testing. As noted earlier, the limitations associated with short incubation times contribute to these problems.

Other specific problems related to automated susceptibility systems have been encountered. These include false resistance to aztreonam, especially for *Proteus* and *Morganella* spp, and false resistance to imipenem associated with *Pseudomonas* spp.

A serious limitation of contemporary instrumentation concerns the newly recognized need to verify methicillin resistance. This is especially pertinent when testing coagulase-negative staphylococci. Verification can be accomplished by molecular detecting of *mecA* or its surrogate-encoded protein product, PBP-2A, by latex agglutination. *mecA* detection is the gold standard. Alternatively, NCCLS has recently recommended a cefoxitin agar diffusion methodology (168).

During the development and evaluation of each commercial automated systems, reports have cited problems. As problems are identified, the manufacturer has attempted to address then by modifying the system by adjusting the growth support and cation content of the growth medium, modifying the reagents, and revising the software and/or algorithms associated with the optical reading device. Due to ongoing modifications, it is difficult to compare and evaluate the accuracy of the systems. As clinical microbiology laboratories come to understand the limitations of these systems, they may rethink the apparent benefit of automation and return to classical approaches, which are more flexible, less fraught with resistance problems, and less costly.

Verification of Antimicrobial Susceptibility Test Systems

When the laboratory considers endorsing a newly acquired automated test system or transitions from an extant system or conventional microdilution method to a new system, it is critical that the test performance of the new system is verified. Verification is accomplished by using the new or revised test method in parallel with a reference method with a known and satisfactory level of performance. The evaluation of susceptibility test methods should be done using a distribution of organisms typically encountered at the institution, ideally including susceptible and resistant strains for each antimicrobial agent. Guidelines are available, but generally the evaluation should be designed to include at least 100 strains and detect three types of errors categorized as *very major* (reference method R; new system S), *major* (reference method S, new system R), and *minor* (reference method R or S, new system I). Very major errors should be $\leq$3% and major and minor errors should be $\leq$7% (68).

Clinical Impact of Automated or Rapid Testing

Early evaluations of automated systems now more than 20 years old have failed to show that rapid susceptibility tests produce a sustained significant positive impact on patient care. In studies of patients with bacteremia, Doern et al. (55) found that, among 173 patients who were receiving antibiotics, rapid susceptibility testing indicated a change in therapy for 48 of these patients. For 32 of the 48 patients, the change in therapy was made 24 hours earlier as the result of 1-day earlier testing. Trenholme et al. (238) found that, for 226 bacteremic patients, rapid automated susceptibility results were associated with a greater likelihood of administration of appropriate antimicrobial therapy, a change to more effective therapy, and/or use of less costly therapy. These studies failed to find a change in patient outcome.

In a follow-up study, Doern et al. (56) evaluated two controlled patient groups in a tertiary care institution. One group was tested with conventional overnight microbiological procedures for identification and susceptibility testing. The other group had the benefit of rapid, same-day procedures. The investigators found that, with regard to mortality rates, the patients receiving the advantage of rapid, same-day testing experienced a lower mortality rate (8.8% versus 15.3% in the conventional testing group). Other advantages associated with rapid testing were fewer laboratory studies, fewer days of incubation, fewer days in critical care units, and shortened times prior to modifications in antimicrobial therapy. In a more recent study, Barenfanger et al. (14) documented clinical and financial benefits (reduced length of stay) of rapid identification and antimicrobial susceptibility testing.

Schifman et al. (195) determined that a significant issue impacting patient outcome was the slow reporting of and response to results in the postanalytical phase of testing. These authors found that the value of susceptibility test results in initiating or modifying therapy was reduced by inefficient reporting practices. In many institutions, getting clinicians to respond promptly to actionable health care information is an ongoing quality improvement concern.

Rapid methods to determine susceptibility (actually resistance) have been used and no doubt will continue to be used as an adjunct to conventional susceptibility testing. Mention has been made of the use of β-lactamase testing using nitrocefin disks and the detection of chloramphenicol resistance by chloramphenicol acetyltransferase assay (9,49). Tests modeled on this strategy have been designed using the breakthroughs in recombinant nucleic acid technology to promptly assess resistant mechanisms (222) (see Chapter 11). For example, by testing for the presence of a plasmid product (an enzyme) or the nucleotide sequence that directs the synthesis of the product, a laboratory can report results within hours. Several nucleic acid probes for detecting and identifying specific infectious agents are already FDA-approved, and they are useful in the clinical laboratory. At recent count, 106 plasmids have been identified, and the gene products probed can be used to detect resistance for 16 classes of antimicrobial agents (183,224). Recently, York et al. (265) evaluated the molecular detection of *mecA* by polymerase chain reaction and the standard method for determining methicillin resistance in coagulase-negative staphylococci. Since *mecA* encodes for a low-affinity penicillin-binding protein, PBP-2a, one could alternatively detect this protein product using a commercially available latex agglutination kit. It can be anticipated that commercial probes for resistance markers may be available in the near future. This approach to susceptibility testing (actually determining resistance) can be extremely useful, especially in therapeutic situations in which meningitis is present. A note of caution: the presence of a particular nucleotide sequence that indicates the potential for producing the plasmid-mediated resistance product does not always mean that the product is expressed by the bacterium.

Indirect guides to determine the susceptibility of *S. viridans* group streptococci associated with endocarditis have been proposed (47). Studies have shown that the quantity of glycocalyx produced by these organisms is correlated with the size of infected cardiac vegetations and resistance to antimicrobial therapy (174). Other approaches to screening resistance of selected pathogens using antimicrobial agents incorporated into agar have been used successfully (219).

INTERPRETIVE GUIDELINES FOR SUSCEPTIBILITY OR RESISTANCE

It is clear that in contemporary medical practice antimicrobial susceptibility testing is necessary component for the delivery of effective, cost-efficient medical care. The MIC is of major import in the comparative evaluation of antimicrobial agents and in the ability to predict their clinical effectiveness by gauging bacteriologic outcome. Ever since Fleming's discovery of the activity of penicillin and the subsequent development of antimicrobial agents, methods have been evaluated to measure and define the true value and meaning of this interaction—the MIC. The testing of the interaction between microorganism and antimicrobial agent is clinically applicable when it defines a breakpoint that parts the susceptible from the resistant. Test conditions and parameters can indeed modulate the outcome of test results, as discussed. In basic microbiology research laboratories, the endpoint of a standardized test, with the resultant MIC, yields an operational definition that identifies the organism tested as susceptible to the lowest concentration in the series. This does not require further clarification. However, in clinical microbiology laboratories, the medical relevance of that susceptibility test result is paramount. The variables and considerations that form the basis of the recommendations for the development of susceptibility testing interpretive guidelines were discussed in a landmark report by Ericsson and Sherris (74) and formed the basis for the interpretive categories recommended by Bauer et al. (25) and the NCCLS documents on dilution susceptibility testing (167). A commonly held misconception is that the MIC and its interpretation are based solely on the ratio of the MIC and the peak achievable serum level. This is incorrect. In fact, the interpretive guidelines, as evaluated by NCCLS (Table 3.31), are based on a tripartite set of databases, as originally recommended by Ericsson and Sherris (74), Bauer et al. (25), and NCCLS. The database for evaluating interpretive standards is dependent on the susceptibility of isolates in a large population distribution, the clinical pharmacology of the drug, and the drug's clinical efficacy. When examining the MIC of new drugs for isolates or reviewing the efficacy of older drugs, the results are compared with the mode (or modes), range, and character (i.e., unimodal, bimodal, or skewed) of the distribution of MICs for populations of strains of the same species being tested. These ranges are then compared with the distribution of MICs of other species within the same group for the same drug and other agents of the same class.

In evaluating the clinical pharmacology of the drug, one includes the range, peak, mean, and trough serum levels expected from the variety of dosage schedules and also considers other pharmacokinetic parameters such as protein binding, volume of distribution, tissue level, and level of the active drug in urine. The range of mean serum levels rather than peak values more appropriately reflects overall tissue levels and avoids inappropriately amplified therapeutic ratios that result from comparing transient, maximally achievable peak serum levels with the MIC of the organism. Lastly, data are collected and evaluated from prospective clinical investigations that reflect the *in vivo* response to treatment of patients with specific infections caused by various strains of species with known MICs. Guidelines for performing these types of experiments have been included in a new NCCLS document (161).

The problems of developing the interpretive breakpoints are usually more difficult for disk diffusion assays, where one has to establish the appropriate disk mass to produce zones of inhibition of a range usable in clinical microbiology laboratories. This is often done initially with customized or handmade disks and then confirmed later with commercially prepared formulations. The usual practice is to construct regression lines of a zone of inhibition versus MIC for about 500 separate isolates covering the spectrum of the new antimicrobial agent. These studies often include one or more comparative agents of the same class as the test agent. The bacterial strains used are obtained from geographic areas within the United States and represent the major routine isolates that would be expected to be treated with the agent under development. Breakpoints are selected based on the pharmacokinetics of the agent in humans, the ability to separate resistant and susceptible bacterial species, and the minimization of major errors of interpretation (false-susceptible or false-resistant). Additionally, for disk development, the paper containing the antimicrobial reagent has to be evaluated for content and stability over time and under storage conditions.

Over time, the criteria that have been used to establish breakpoints have changed, and various countries and organizations have adapted differing criteria (see Chapter 1). Early in antimicrobial susceptibility studies, it was observed that all strains of a bacterial species do not demonstrate the same degree of susceptibility and that the susceptibilities (i.e., MICs) for a population of strains are distributed according to a bimodal or normal distribution. Eventually, national committees and organizations such as NCCLS came to conclude that in the derivation of a breakpoint the pharmacokinetic (PK) properties (e.g., drug distribution in the host) and pharmacodynamic (PD) properties (e.g., activity against the infecting agent) of the antimicrobial compound indicated that the MIC (interpreted as "susceptible") would suggest the possibility—perhaps the probability (not quantitatively defined)—of antimicrobial therapy success and "resistant" would connote failure. It is of interest to note the differing approaches used in various countries by the empowered organized committees that oversee or regulate antimicrobial susceptibility

(*text continues on page 120*)

TABLE 3.31

MIC Interpretive Standards for Two Categories of Susceptibility[a]

Antimicrobial Agents	MIC Standards (μg/mL)	
	Susceptible	Resistant
β-Lactam penicillins		
Ampicillin[b]		
When testing Enterobacteriaceae	≤8	≥32
When testing *Vibrio cholerae*	≤8	≥32
When testing *staphylococci*[c] and *Moraxella catarrhalis*[d]	≤0.25	≥0.5
When testing *Listeria monocytogenes*	≤2	≥4
When testing enterococci	≤8	≥16
When testing streptococci and other Gram-positive organisms	≤0.12	≥4
When testing *Haemophilus* spp	≤1	≥4
When testing *Streptococcus pneumoniae*[e]	≤0.06	≥4
When testing other *Streptococcus* spp β-hemolytic group	≤0.25	
Azlocillin, when testing *Pseudomonas aeruginosa*[f]	≤128	≥128
Carbenicillin		
When testing *P. aeruginosa*	≤128	≥512
When testing other Gram-negative organisms	≤16	≥64
Methicillin, when testing staphylococci[g]	≤8	≥16
Mezlocillin		
When testing *P. aeruginosa*	≤64	≥128
When testing other Gram-negative organisms	≤16	≥128
Nafcillin, when testing staphylococci[e]	≤2	≥4
Oxacillin, when testing staphylococci[e]	≤2	≥4
Penicillin		
When testing staphylococci[c] and *M. catarrhalis*[d]	≤0.12	≥0.25
When testing *L. monocytogenes*	≤2	≥4
When testing enterococci	≤8	≥16
When testing streptococci	≤0.12	≥4
When testing *S. pneumoniae* and *N. gonorrhoeae*	≤0.06	≥2
Piperacillin		
When testing *P. aeruginosa*	≤64	≥128
When testing other Gram-negative organisms	≤16	≥128
Ticarcillin		
When testing *P. aeruginosa*	≤64	≥128
When testing other Gram-negative organisms	≤16	≥128
β-Lactam–β-lactamase inhibitor combinations		
Amoxicillin–clavulanic acid[f]		
When testing *staphylococci*[c]	≤4/2	≥8/4
When testing *Haemophilus* spp	≤4/2	≥8/4
When testing other organisms	≤8/4	≥32/16

(continued)

TABLE 3.31 (Continued)

MIC Interpretive Standards for Two Categories of Susceptibility[a]

Antimicrobial Agents	MIC Standards (μg/mL)	
	Susceptible	Resistant
Ampicillin-sulbactam[f]		
When testing Gram-negative enteries and staphylococci[c]	≤8/4	≥32/16
When testing *Haemophilus* spp	≤2/1	≥412
Piperacillin-tazobactam		
When testing *P. aeruginosa*	≤64/4	≥128/4
When testing other Gram-negative organisms	≤16/4	≥128/4
When testing *staphylococci*[c]	≤8/4	≥16/4
When testing *Haemophilus* spp	≤2/1	≥2/4
Ticarcillin-clavulanic acid		
When testing *P. aeruginosa*	≤64/2	≥128/2
When testing other Gram-negative organisms	≤16/2	≥128/2
When testing *staphylococci*[c]	≤8/2	≥16/2
Cephalosporins and other cephems		
Cefaclor, when testing *Haemophilus* spp	≤8	≥32
Cefazolin	≤8	≥32
Cefapime		
When testing *S. pneumoniae*	≤0.5	≥2
When testing *Haemophilus* spp	≤2	
When testing *N. gonorrhoeae*	≤0.5	≥2
When testing other organisms	≤8	≥32
Cefetamet		
When testing *Haemophilus* spp	≤4	≥16
When testing *N. gonorrhoeae*	≤0.5	
When testing other organisms	≤4	≥16
Cefixime		
When testing *Haemophilus* spp	≤1	
When testing *N. gonorrhoeae*	≤0.25	
When testing other organisms	≤1	≥4
Cefmetazole		
When testing *N. gonorrhoeae*	≤2	≥8
When testing other organisms	≤16	≥64
Cefonicid		
When testing *Haemophilus* spp	≤4	≥16
When testing other organisms	≤8	
Cefoperazone	≤16	≥64
Cefotaxime		
When testing *S. pneumoniae*	≤0.5	≥64
When testing *Haemophilus* spp	≤2	
When testing *N. gonorrhoeae*	≤0.5	
When testing other organisms	≤8	≥64

(continued)

TABLE 3.31 (Continued)

MIC Interpretive Standards for Two Categories of Susceptibility[a]

Antimicrobial Agents	MIC Standards (μg/mL)	
	Susceptible	Resistant
Cefotetan		
When testing *N. gonorrhoeae*	≤2	≥64
When testing other organisms	≤16	≥64
Cefoxitin		
When testing *N. gonorrhoeae*	≤2	≥8
When testing other organisms	≤8	32
Cefpodoxime		
When testing *Haemophilus* spp	≤2	
When testing *N. gonorrhoeae*	≤0.5	
When testing other organisms	≤2	≥8
Cefprozil		
When testing *Haemophilus* spp	≤8	≥32
When testing other organisms	≤8	≥32
Ceftazidime		
When testing *Haemophilus* spp	≤2	
When testing *N. gonorrhoeae*	≤0.5	
When testing other organisms	≤8	≥32
Ceftibuten[g]		
When testing *Haemophilus* spp	≤2	
When testing other organisms	≤8	≥32
Ceftizoxime		
When testing *Haemophilus* spp	≤2	
When testing *N. gonorrhoeae*	≤0.5	
When testing other organisms	≤8	
Ceftriaxone		
When testing *S. pneumoniae*	≤0.5	≥2
When testing *Haemophilus* spp	≤2	
When testing *N. gonorrhoeae*	≤0.25	
When testing other organisms		≥64
Cefuroxime		
When testing *S. pneumoniae*	≤0.5	≥2
When testing *Haemophilus* spp	≤4	≥16
When testing *N. gonorrhoeae*	≤1	≥4
When testing other organisms	≤4–8	≥32
Cephalothin[h]	≤8	≥32
Loracarbef,[c] when testing *Haemophilus* spp	≤8	≥32
Moxalactam	≤8	≥64

(continued)

TABLE 3.31 (Continued)

MIC Interpretive Standards for Two Categories of Susceptibility[a]

Antimicrobial Agents	MIC Standards (μg/mL)	
	Susceptible	Resistant
Carbapenems[c]		
Ertapenam		
When testing *S. pneumoniae*	≤1	≥4
When testing *Haemophilus* spp	≤0.5	
When testing other organisms	≤2	≥8
Imipenem		
When testing *S. pneumoniae*	≤0.12	≥1
When testing *Haemophilus* spp	≤0.5	
When testing other organisms	≤4	≥16
Meropenem		
When testing *S. pneumoniae*	≤0.25	≥1
When testing *Haemophilus* spp	≤0.5	
When testing other organisms	≤4	≥16
Monobactams		
Aztreonam		
When testing *Haemophilus* spp	≤2	
When testing other organisms	≤8	≥32
Glycopeptides		
Teicoplanin	≤8	≥32
Vancomycin		
When testing *S. pneumoniae*	≤1	≥32
When testing *Streptococcus* spp	≤1	
When testing other organisms	≤4	≥32
Aminoglycosides		
Amikacin[i]	≤16	≥64
Gentamicin		
When testing enterococci	≤500	≥500
When testing other organisms	≤4	≥16
Kanamycin[i]	≤16	≥64
Netilmicin[i]	≤8	≥32
Streptomycin		
When testing enterococci by broth microdilution screen test	<1000	>1000
When testing enterococci by agar screen test	≤2000	>2000
Tobramycin[i]		
Macrolides	≤4	≥16
Azithromycin		
When testing *S. pneumoniae*	≤0.5	≥2
When testing *Haemophilus* spp	≤4	
When testing other organisms	≤2	≥8

(continued)

TABLE 3.31 (Continued)

MIC Interpretive Standards for Two Categories of Susceptibility[a]

Antimicrobial Agents	MIC Standards (μg/mL)	
	Susceptible	Resistant
Clarithromycin		
When testing *S. pneumoniae*	≤0.5	≥2
When testing *Haemophilus* spp	≤4	
When testing *H. pylori*	≤0.25	≥1
When testing other organisms	≤2	≥8
Erythromycin when testing *S. pneumoniae*	≤0.5	≥8
	≤0.5	≥4
Tetracyclines[j]		
Tetracycline		
When testing *S. pneumoniae*	≤2	≥8
When testing *V. cholerae*	≤4	≥16
When testing *Streptococcus* spp	≤2	≥8
When testing other organisms	≤4	≥16
Quinolones		
Cinoxacin[g]	≤16	≥64
Ciprofloxacin		
When testing *Haemophilus* spp	≤1	
When testing *N. gonorrhoeae*	≤0.06	
When testing other organisms	≤1	≥4
Enoxacin, when testing *N. gonorrhoeae*	≤2	≥8
	≤0.5	
Fleroxacin		
When testing *Haemophilus* spp	≤2	
When testing *N. gonorrhoeae*	≤0.25	≥1
When testing other organisms	≤2	≥8
Gemifloxacin		
When testing *S. pneumoniae*	≤0.12	≥0.5
When testing *Klebsiella pneumoniae*	≤0.25	≥1
When testing *Haemophilus* spp	≤0.12	
Gatifloxacin		
When testing *S. pneumoniae*	≤1	≥4
When testing *Haemophilus* spp	≤1	
When testing *N. gonorrhoeae*	≤0.25	≥2
When testing other organisms	≤2	≥8
Grepafloxacin		
When testing *S. pneumoniae*	≤0.5	≥2
When testing *Haemophilus* spp	≤0.5	
When testing *N. gonorrhoeae*	≤0.06	≥1
When testing other organisms	≤1	≥4

(continued)

TABLE 3.31 (Continued)

MIC Interpretive Standards for Two Categories of Susceptibility[a]

Antimicrobial Agents	MIC Standards (μg/mL)	
	Susceptible	Resistant
Levofloxacin		
When testing *S. pneumoniae*	≤2	≥8
Lomeflaxicin		
When testing *Haemophilus* spp	≤2	
When testing *N. gonorrhoeae*	≤0.12	
When testing other organisms	≤2	
Moxifloxacin		
When testing *S. pneumoniae*	<1	≥4
Nalidixic acid[g]	≤16	≥32
Norfloxacin,[g] when testing other organisms	≤4	≥16
Ofloxacin[g]		
When testing *S. pneumoniae*	≤2	≥8
When testing *Haemophilus* spp	≤2	
When testing *N. gonorrhoeae*	≤0.25	
When testing other organisms	≤2	≥8
Sparfloxacin		
When testing *S. pneumoniae*	≤0.5	≥2
Trovofloxacin		
When testing *S. pneumoniae*	≤1	≥4
Others		
Chloramphenicol		
When testing *S. pneumoniae*	≤4	≥8
When testing *V. cholerae*	≤8	≥32
When testing other *Streptococcus* spp	≤4	≥16
When testing other organisms	≤8	≥32
Clindamycin		
When testing *S. pneumoniae*	≤0.25	≥1
When testing *Streptococcus* spp	≤0.25	≥1
When testing other organisms	≤0.5	≥4
Linezolid		
When testing staphylococci	≤4	
When testing enterococci	≤2	≥8
Nitrofurantoin[g]	≤32	≥128
Quinupristin-dalfopristin		
When testing *S. pneumoniae*	≤1	≥4
When testing staphylococci	≤1	≥4
When testing enterococci	≤1	≥4
Rifampin		
When testing *S. pneumoniae*	≤1	≥4
When testing other organisms	≤1	≥4

(continued)

TABLE 3.31 (Continued)

MIC Interpretive Standards for Two Categories of Susceptibility[a]

Antimicrobial Agents	MIC Standards (μg/mL) Susceptible	Resistant
Spectinomycin, when testing *N. gonorrhoeae*	≤32	≥128
Sulfonamides[g,i]	≤256	≥512
Telithromycin		
When testing *S. pneumoniae*	≤1	≥4
When testing *Haemophilus* spp	≤4	≥16
When testing staphylococci	≤1	≥4
Trimethoprim[g]	≤8	≥16
Trimethoprim/sulfamethoxazole		
When testing *S. pneumoniae*	≤0.5/9.5	≥4/76
When testing *Haemophilus* spp	≤0.5/9.5	≥4/76
When testing *V. cholerae*	≤2/38	≥32
When testing other organisms	≤2/38	≥4/76

[a] Adapted from NCCLS M100-S14 (M7-A6) (167).
[b] Class representative for ampicillin, amoxicillin, bacampicillin, cyclacillin, and hetacillin.
[c] Penicillin should be used to test the susceptibility of all staphylococci to all penicillinase-sensitive penicillins, such as ampicillin, amoxicillin, azlocillin, bacampicillin, hetacillin, carbenicillin, mezlocillin, piperacillin, and ticarcillin. Staphylococci exhibiting resistance to methicillin, oxacillin, or nafcillin should be reported as also resistant to other penicillins, cephalosporins, carbacephems, carbapenems, and inhibitor combinations despite apparent *in vitro* susceptibility of some strains to the latter agents. This is because infections with methicillin-resistant staphylococci have not responded favorably to therapy with antibiotics.
[d] Testing the clinical utility of penicillin, ampicillin, and amoxicillin for treatment of *M. catarrhalis* infections is best done with a nitrocefin-based β-lactamase assay. Usually, dilution tests with these agents are unnecessary.
[e] Interpretive guideines imply the use of CAMHB or MHA containing 2% (w/v) NaCl. Of the antistaphylococcal, β-lactamase–resistant penicillins, either oxacillin or methicillin may be tested, and results can be applied to other penicillinase-resistant penicillins, nafcillin, cloxacillin, and discloxacillin. Oxacillin is preferred because it has more resistance to degradation in storage and because it is more likely to detect heteroresistant strains. Nafcillin is not used with blood-containing media. Cloxacillin should not be used because it may not detect methicillin-resistant *S. aureus* strains.
[f] Ampicillin test results may be used to determine susceptibility to amoxicillin–clavulanic acid and ampicillin-sulbactam among streptococci and non-β-lactamase-producing enterococci.
[g] Susceptibility data for ceftibuten, cinoxacin, nalidixic acid, nitrofurantoin, norfloxacin, sulfonamides, and trimethoprim apply only to organisms isolated from urinary tract infections.
[h] Cephalothin can be used to represent cephalothin, cephapirin, cephradine, cephalexin, cefaclor, cefadroxil, cefazolin (except against *Enterobacteriaceae*), cefuroxime, cefpodoxime, cefprozil, and loracarbef (except against *Enterobacteriaceae*). Cephalosporins (with exceptions in parentheses) may be tested individually against *Enterobacteriaceae* because they may be active when cephalothin is not.
[i] Sulfisoxazole can be used to represent any of the currently avalable sulfonamide preparations. Blood-containing media (except for lysed horse blood) are generally not suitable for testing sulfonamides. Mueller-Hinton broth or agar should be checked for excessive levels of thymidine as described in Table 3.3.
[j] Tetracycline is the representative for all tetracyclines, and the results can be applied to chlortetracycline, demeclocycline, doxycycline, methacycline, minocycline, and oxytetracycline. Certain organisms, however, may be more susceptible to minocycline and doxycycline than to tetracycline (e.g., some staphylococci and *Acinetobacter* spp).

testing. The Dutch committee for regulating antimicrobial susceptibility testing, the CRG, states, "Micro-organisms are categorized susceptible (S), as opposed to resistant (R) to an antimicrobial agent; if concentrations of the non-protein bound fraction in vivo, based on the dosing regimen proposed, are above the MIC of a microorganism for a sufficient time period in order to eradicate the microorganism, and thereby cure of the patient can be reasonably expected." In contrast, the British Society for Antimicrobial Chemotherapy uses this formula; breakpoint concentration = $C_{max} \cdot csf$ (e.t), where C_{max} is the maximum serum concentration following a stated dose at steady state, e is the factor by which the C_{max} should exceed the MIC, f is a protein-binding factor, s is a reproducibility factor, and t represents the serum half-life. Clearly, organized groups have used varied data and criteria in

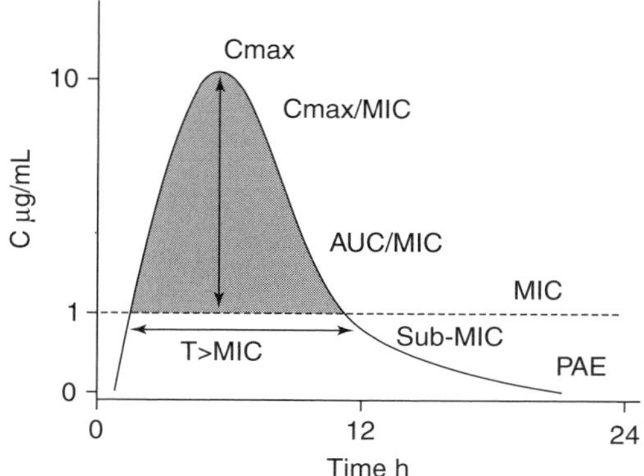

FIGURE 3.14 • Relationship of pharmacokinetic and pharmacodynamic properties of antimicrobial agents: Cmax, peak concentration; MIC, minimum inhibitory concentration; AUC, area under the curve; T> MIC, time over the MIC; PAE, postantibiotic effect.

establishing breakpoints, although the trend is toward the inclusion of PK and PD information.

In the United States, the FDA and the NCCLS Subcommittee on Antimicrobial Susceptibility Testing have the responsibility for the development of standards that promote accurate and reproducible antimicrobial susceptibility testing and appropriate reporting. Data reviewed for establishing susceptibility breakpoints include *in vitro* drug characteristics, necessary distributions of microorganisms, PK/PD parameters, and the correlation of test results with outcome statistics.

As suggested, organizing committees in several countries are now using PK/PD relationships in their breakpoint estimations. For many drugs, data were accumulated documenting the relationship between drug concentration and effect. Three major characteristics of the concentration-time curve of a drug have been delineated: concentration (C_{max}), area under the concentration-time curve (AUC), and the time the concentration remains above the MIC (T>MIC) (Fig. 3.14). From these are derived PK/PD indices by relating the drug parameter to the MIC: AUC/MIC, C_{max}/MIC, and T>MIC. Studies of animal models of infection show an evident relationship between the PK/PD indices and efficacy. The setting of these breakpoints is derived from highest generally achieved indices: 100–125 for the AUC/MIC and 8–12 for the C_{max}/MIC (156). Examples of PK/PD relationships and breakpoints are shown in Table 3.32.

Although it was generally considered instructive and meaningful to classify antimicrobial agents as bacteriostatic or bactericidal (all antibiotics are bacteriostatic but not necessarily bactericidal), contemporary interpretation identifies two patterns of bacterial killing: time-dependent killing or concentration-dependent killing. Time-dependent killing agents are characterized by the PD parameter T>MIC whereas concentration-dependent killing agents are characterized by C_{max}/MIC or AUC/MIC. Several antimicrobial classes classified by these PD parameters are listed in Table 3.33.

Although the MIC of a particular strain of microorganism recovered from a patient can be considered constant and reproducible (it may differ from other strains of the same species), it is known that the PK parameters of absorption rate, volume of distribution, and clearance can differ among individuals. Drusano and colleagues acknowledged these variations and presented an integrated approach to population pharmacokinetics and microbiological susceptibility information. Statistical simulation Monte Carlo using (a computer-generated program that integrates variously attainable PK/PD indices and MICs) can provide insight into the proportion of the population who can achieve an effective AUC/MIC and for whom clinical success can be quantitative by predicted (4,61,62). Monte Carlo simulation incorporates a probability function to generate random AUC and MIC values from a sampling distribution. Thousands of single-point estimates are made and their probabilities plotted (Figure 3.15). Whereas single-point AUC/MIC estimates provide information on what is possible, Monte Carlo simulations can determine probability. Thus, one could predict the probability of achieving a targeted AUC/MIC ratio at different MIC breakpoints (Fig. 3.16).

Monte Carlo simulations and other statistical approaches, such as analysis using CART (Classification and Regression Tree Analysis, a statistical computer program for predicting the probability of a clinical response to infection by a microorganism as a function of the peak-C_{max}/MIC ratio) (158), are and will be useful in developing more meaningful clinically applicable breakpoints. They do not enhance the value of the clinical laboratory providing comparative MICs for an infective organism with only an S, I, or R interpretation. What would prove applicable in light of this discussion is to provide the clinician with the number of $\log_2$ concentrations below the S breakpoint concentration that was achieved; indirectly this would be relative to AUC/MIC and C_{max}/MIC.

These considerations have led, at least in the United States, to the separation of data into three (or possibly four) interpretive categories: "susceptible," "intermediate" (or "moderately susceptible"), and "resistant." Susceptible organisms attain MICs that fall into the susceptible range of MICs and would generally be below serum or tissue levels of the drug achievable with usual dosage regimens; the implication is that infections attributable to such organisms may be appropriately treated with that drug. Strains classified as resistant would not be inhibited by typically achievable systemic concentrations.

"Intermediate" refers to organisms with MICs in the middle of the overall range of distribution of MICs. In some population distributions, there may be isolates that

TABLE 3.32

PK/PD Parameters of Seven Fluoroquinolones with Derived Breakpoints[a]

Fluoroquinolone[b]	Dosing Regimen	C_{max} μg/mL	AUC μg h/mL	Protein Binding %	S-Breakpoint[d] μg/mL	
					Pd[d]	NCCLS
Ciprofloxacin	500 mg/12 h	2.6	22.2	22	0.25	1.0
Sparfloxacin[c]	200 mg/24 h	0.6	16.4	45	0.125	0.5
Levofloxacin	500 mg/24 h	5.2	61.1	30	0.5	2.0
Ofloxacin	200 mg/12 h	2.2	29.2	30	0.25	2.0
Grepafloxacin[c]	400 mg/24 h	0.9	11.4	50	0.125	0.5
Trovofloxacin[c]	200 mg/24 h	2.2	30.4	70	0.125	1.0
Moxifloxacin	400 mg/24 h	4.5	48.0	40	0.5	1.0

[a] Adapted from Mouton (158).
[b] Does not include recently FDA-approved gemifloxacin.
[c] Discontinued in the United States.
[d] Based on AUC/MIC of 100–125 h and a C_{max}/MIC of 8–12.

TABLE 3.33

Pharmacodynamic (PD) Indices as Surrogate Markers of Time-dependent and Concentration-dependent Antimicrobial Agents

Antibiotic Class	PD Index
Time-dependent	
β-Lactams	T>MIC
Penicillins	
Cephalosporins	
Monobactams	
Carbapenem	
Glycopeptides	T>MIC C_{max}-free/MIC
Concentration-dependent	
Aminoglycosides	C_{max}/MIC AUC/MIC
Fluoroquinolones	C_{max}/MIC AUC/MIC
Macrolides	C_{max}/MIC
Azithromycin	AUC/MIC
Clarithromycin	
Crythromycin	
Ketolides	C_{max}/MIC
Telithromycin	AUC/MIC

Adapted from Chung E et al (39a).

have no strains with fully susceptible MICs. For example, the action of penicillin or ampicillin against *Enterococcus* strains is such that serious infections with such strains would have to be treated synergistically with penicillin or ampicillin combined with an aminoglycoside, as already noted. For some organism-drug pairs, the "moderately susceptible" category represents a narrow range that is really intermediate or equivocal and cannot defined clearly. This range is a buffer zone and allows for technical or biological (plus or minus one dilution) variation in MIC reproducibility.

The "resistant" category encompasses organisms whose MICs indicate they are not readily amenable to treatment with that drug although the tissue or drug concentration is readily attainable. It provides the most relevant clinical guidance of any of the interpretive categories and implies with reasonable assurance that normally a serious infection would not respond to treatment. However, it should be noted that, for the typical MICs interpreted as resistant, subinhibitory concentrations may produce a potentially beneficial clinical effect on some strains by modifying some pathogenicity traits, such as rate of growth, ability to adhere, toxin production, or susceptibility to phagocytic action.

In the past, for selected multiresistant strains producing urinary tract infections, NCCLS documents defined a fourth category, "conditionally susceptible." This category was utilized because of the high levels achieved by certain drugs and the occasional value of utilizing these drugs in uncomplicated urinary tract infections associated with multiresistant enteric bacteria with high MICs. This interpretive category is absent from current documents, and the "Intermediate" category now encompasses this group.

A new term has emerged, "nonsusceptible," which has two different interpretations. NCCLS uses this term

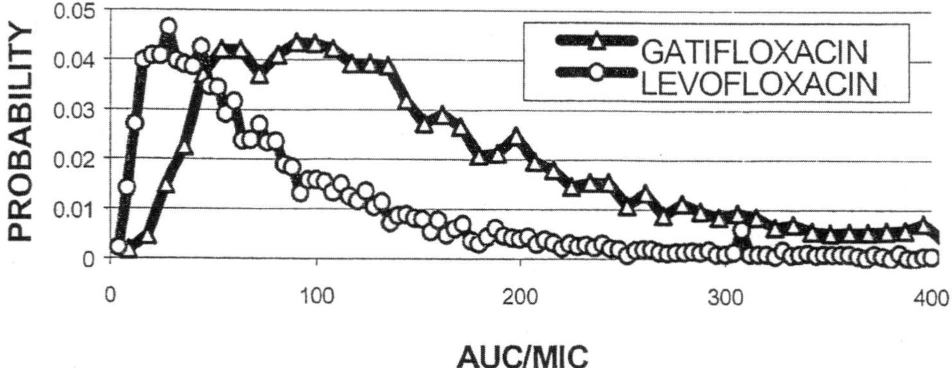

FIGURE 3.15 • Probability distribution curves for two quinolones, gatifloxacin and levofloxacin, depicting AUC/MIC ratios against *S. pneumoniae*. Distributions integrate AUC and MIC. If an AUC/MIC of 120 (or less) is associated with a positive clinical outcome, then gatifloxacin has a greater probability of achieving that ratio (4).

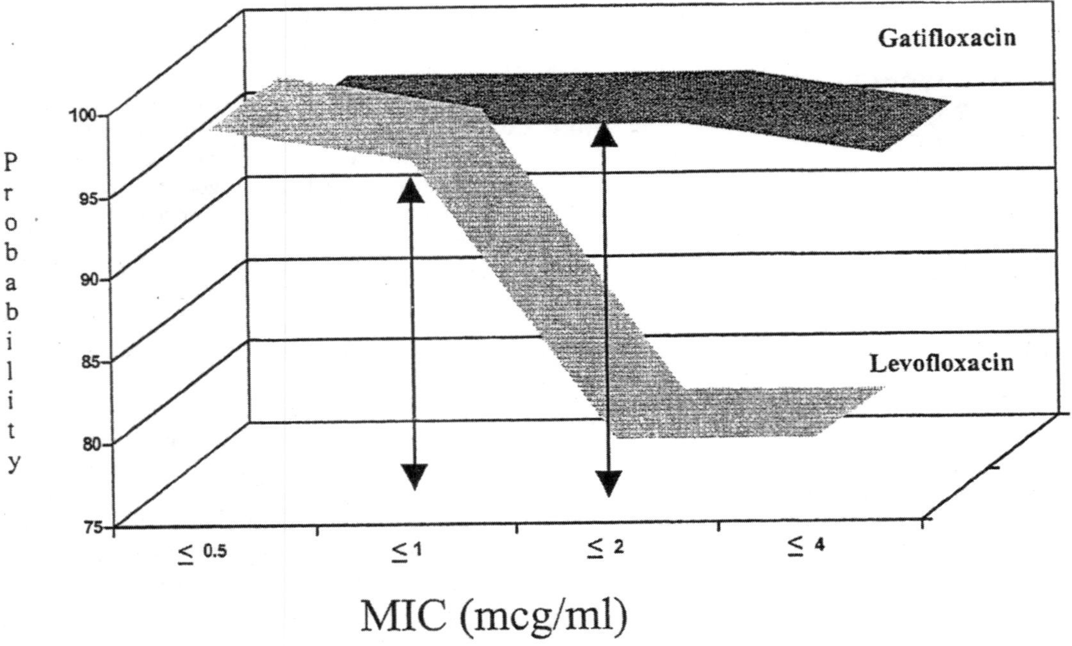

FIGURE 3.16 ● Probability of achieving an AUC/MIC ratio of 30 at differing MICs for two quinolones, gatifloxacin and levofloxacin. Note gatifloxacin maintains a near 90% probability from =0.5–3.0 μg/mL, whereas levofloxacin declines abruptly at 0.75 μg/mL (4).

for characterizing some organism-antimicrobial combinations where there are no or very few resistant strains to define a resistant category (see Table 3.31). "Clinically nonsusceptible" refers to that population of microorganisms that qualify as either "intermediate" or "resistant."

Because the interpretation of these guidelines cannot be arithmetically quantified and cannot be agreed upon with a great deal of reliability, this author has taken the view that the interpretive guidelines should clearly represent the extremes of the susceptibility spectrum (i.e., susceptible and resistant). These guidelines are presented in Table 3.31 for reference. Additionally, it should be recognized that the extreme categoric interpretations are relatively constant. The "intermediate" (or "moderately susceptible") category is subject to greater fluctuations, due to periodic reevaluation. Interpretive standards for phenotypic screening and confirmation of extended-spectrum β-lactamase (ESBL) in *Enterobacteriaceae* (specifically *E. coli, Klebsiella pneumoniae,* and *Klebsiella oxytoca*) are presented in Table 3.34.

It must be emphasized that the breakpoints presented in Table 3.31 and supported by NCCLS are not necessarily the values used in all countries. Examples of breakpoints used in various countries are shown in Table 3.35 (194). In addition to NCCLS, there are working committees in other countries, notably France and Great Britain, that have been active in developing breakpoints based on experiences in their particular geographic regions (194).

At many institutions, considerable efforts have been made to educate physicians not trained as infectious disease specialists in the utilization of MICs. However, one frequently sees that in daily practice MICs are poorly understood and interpreted. One type of error involves the choice of the wrong class of drug. For instance, an aminoglycoside might unnecessarily be used to treat a relatively benign infection with *E. coli* that is susceptible to multiple drugs merely because an MIC of 1 for amikacin appears to indicate greater susceptibility than the MIC of 2 for tetracycline or the MIC of 4 for ampicillin. Another type of error leads to a false categorical interpretation of the wrong drug within a class when the absolute values of the MICs are seemingly different. For these reasons, it is recommended that the appropriate interpretative category always be reported along with the numerical value of the MIC. In some clinical settings, there has been a tendency to report the ratio of the MIC to theoretical peak serum (or urine) levels for various dosages. The reports are sometimes computerized and are semiquantitated by a single plus sign or several plus signs, indicating the degree of susceptibility (or resistance). Such reports really are somewhat arbitrary and falsely quantitative. Although theoretically such calculations are possible, they omit other PK parameters such as the possibility of protein binding (should it be subtracted?), the use of peak or mean levels, and the use of trough levels in the numerator. What about renal or liver function tests, and in whom have the

TABLE 3.34

Screening and Confirmatory Tests[a] for ESBLs[b]

Initial/Screen		Confirmatory	
Antimicrobial Agent[c]	MIC	Antimicrobial Agent[d]	MIC
Aztreonam	≥2	Cefotaxime	>8 or
Cefotaxime	≥2	Cefotaxime-clavulanic acid (4 μg/mL)	≥3 twofold decrease
Cefpodoxime	≥8	AND	
Ceftazidime	≥2	Ceftazidime	>8 or
Ceftriaxone	≥2	Ceftazidime-clavulanic acid (4 μg/mL)	≥3 twofold decrease

[a] Standard broth dilution with CAMB. For QC: *E. coli* ATCC 25922 for screening and *Klebsiella pneumoniae* ATCC 700603 for confirmatory testing.
[b] Although several species of Enterobacteriaceae produce ESBLs, these interpretations are for *Klebsiella pneumoniae, Klebsiella oxytoca,* and *E. coli.*
[c] The use of multiple antimicrobial agents will improve detection.
[d] Confirmatory testing requires the use of cefotaxime and ceftazidime alone *and* in combination with clavulanic acid.

levels been determined? The patient under consideration has a specific disease and may not be compartmentalizing the drug in the typical way that the manufacturer's product insert indicates for that antibiotic. Such specific pseudoquantitative reporting systems are based on oversimplified pharmacological assumptions and may be misleading.

The general concept of therapeutic ratios is useful in teaching antimicrobial management. Thus, it may be appropriate and informative for laboratories to include, in their quarterly or annual reports, tables summarizing the standard interpretive breakpoints (as noted in Table 3.31) and the ranges of mean serum levels. Additionally, this information can be placed at the back of a patient's report. Lastly, since the bottom line is always cost, it is often necessary in many clinical settings for the laboratory, through the pharmacy and therapeutics committee, to supply clinicians with the average daily cost of an antibiotic, as determined at that institution, for treatment of severe to moderate infections. The clinicians can then use the laboratory susceptibility data along with the cost data to determine the most clinically efficacious and least expensive therapy.

MICs: Predictive Value of Clinical Outcome

Earlier, reference was made to the inoculum concentration, rate of replication, and phase as modifying factors in obtaining accurate, reproducible MIC results. Recently, it has been learned that microbial interactions in biofilms can confound the interpretation and predictive value of *in vitro* systems using homogeneous bacterial populations. The model of the way bacteria reproduce and grow as free-swimming planktonic cells is not truly realized in nature. Planktonic cells attach to inanimate surfaces (e.g., plastic catheters or sand) or to the epithelial cells of an airway system. Their ability to detach or remain attached is dependent on several characteristics of the host system. Typically, the ability of clusters of bacteria to remain attached and form biofilms relates to availability of a foreign object (catheter) or dead tissue and to protection from host defenses and antibodies. Microbial biofilms are slow to develop, cause collateral damage to tissues, and are persistent. They are regarded as communities of bacteria that grow on surfaces, as opposed to microorganisms that are dispersed or free floating, and they complicate several medical problems, namely, periodontitis, osteomyelitis, infected catheters (pacemaker leads and urinary catheters), and cystic fibrosis.

It is expected that within communities the bacteria communicate. In the 1960s, marine microbiologists discovered that for *Vibrio fischeri* the ability to produce light (bioluminescence) is dependent on a critical population size. The signal that turned on the light was genetically controlled by an autoinducer (AI). Infectious disease specialists and microbiologists who study pathogenic mechanisms and virulence have learned that the changes in gene expression patterns in response to the host environment are a prerequisite for bacterial infection, and autoinducers and associated genes have been found in Gram-positive and Gram-negative bacteria. In studies of *Pseudomonas aeruginosa* in cystic fibrosis patients, it was found that the prophylactic administration of macrolides that do not kill *P. aeruginosa* (e.g., azithromycin) can bring about clinical relief. This might be attributable to the activity

TABLE 3.35

Examples of Breakpoints Used in Various Countries Compared with Breakpoints Determined by the Proposed Method for the Species *Yersinia enterocolitica*[a]

	CAR[b]		MEZ		CXT	
	≤	≥[c]	≤	≥	≤	≥
US[d]	32.16		16.64		8.8	
France	128		8	21	8	
FRG	32		4	22	1	
Great Britain	32		16			
Sweden	16	24			4	25
Netherlands	16	22	8	23	4	25
Proposed method	8	24	4	30[e]	4	29

[a] The breakpoints shown separate the sensitive strains from the others. These data were published in the papers cited in references (Swedish reference group 1981, US national committee 1983 and 1984, European committee 1985, British society 1985, Comité de l'antibiogramme 1985).
[b] Abbreviations: CAR, carbenicillin: MEZ, meziocillin; CXT, cefoxitin; MIC, minimum inhibitory concentration.
[c] Symbols: ≤, a strain is sensitive when its MIC expressed in μg/mL is inferior or equal to the breakpoint concentration; ≥, a strain is sensitive when its diameter expressed in mm is superior or equal to the breakpoint diameter. This is indicated only when the same breakpoint concentration and the same ICS diffusion technique (52) are used.
[d] In the United States, the interpretive standards proposed for dilution tests (first number) should not be confused with the values of approximate MIC correlates obtained from diffusion tests (second number).
[e] This value is proposed in the meantime, until new cluster(s) eventually appear.

of the drug on the normal oropharyngeal flora, thus minimizing the release of autoinducer-2 (AI-2) of *P. aeruginosa*. AI-2 is responsible for the induction of virulence genes for exotoxin and elastase (63). For glycopeptide intermediate-level resistant *S. aureus* (GISA), the majority of infections originate on biomedical devices. The loss of accessory gene regulator *(agr)*, a gene cluster comprising five different genes, involved in quorum sensing (the mechanism bacteria use to communicate with each other) has been suggested as contributing to their ability to produce biofilms. All VISA/GISA strains tested belong to *agr* group II and have defective *agr* function (190). In *Enterococcus faecalis*, the gene locus *fsr* has been identified as present in 70% of clinical isolates. It appears responsible for regulation of two virulence genes, genes-gelatinase and a gelatinase and a serine protease (175). Homology between *fsr* and the *agr* gene of *Staphylococcus* has been noted (181).

The role of these virulence genes in diverse bacterial groups interacting with normal or commensal microflora and/or growing as biofilms poses challenging questions for medical microbiologists. What is the value of isolating a single offending species and determining the MICs of a variety of antimicrobial agents when in situ its role may be regulated by other bacterial populations within the community it resides in?

Given this background, what is the reliability of an MIC and its S/R interpretation in predicting the clinical outcome of antimicrobial therapy? Apart from pharmaceutical-sponsored studies of directed single agent activity against a particular bacterial target or group, there is a paucity of reports on the relevance of *in vitro* bacterial susceptibility to the outcome of antimicrobial therapy.

In a retrospective study (134) of 510 patients who received antimicrobial therapy, 382 (75%) had susceptibility tests performed on at least one culture prior to the administration of antimicrobial therapy. Eighteen bacterial species (~75% due to Gram-negative rods) were recovered from 298 patients, and of these patients, 271 (91%) received antimicrobial therapy to which the organisms were susceptible and 219 (81%) improved. Of the 271 patients who received therapy to which the bacteria were resistant, 3% demonstrated improvement and 82% did not improve. This study clearly shows the value of selecting therapy according to *in vitro* susceptibility test results. Similarly, a prospective observational study of 2,634 septic patients showed that "adequate antibiotic treatment" defined on the basis of *in vitro* susceptibility of an isolated microorganism (at least five species were identified) and/or initiation of antibiotic treatment between 24 hours before and 72 hours after study enrollment resulted in a 10% decrease (33% vs. 43%) in mortality (140). In contrast, an international prospective observational study (266) of 844 hospitalized patients with blood cultures positive for *S. pneumoniae* reported that "discordant therapy" (inactive *in vitro* susceptibility with penicillins, cefotaxime, and ceftriaxone but not cefuroxime), as compared with "concordant antibiotic therapy" (i.e., receipt of a single antibiotic with *in vitro* activity against *S. pneumoniae*), did not result in a higher mortality rate. Similarly, the time required for defervescence and the frequency of suppurative complication did not result in a higher mortality rate. The conclusion from these data is that β-lactam antibiotics could prove useful for pneumococcal bacteremia regardless of *in vitro* susceptibility as defined by NCCLS breakpoints.

Research on acute exacerbation of chronic bronchitis (AECB), includes several studies that compared the activity of quinolones and macrolides against *H. influenzae*. There are differences in the impact of compounds of these two types. Apart from the direct antibacterial-PD properties of these agents, the macrolides appear to possess an immunomodulatory effect that prevents recurrence of infection. A conclusion of Martinez in cases of AECB is that *in vitro* antimicrobial resistance is of unclear significance (79,139).

Against nosocomial pneumonia, antimicrobial agents are the mainstay of pharmacologic measures. It is worth noting that in these studies Gram-negative bacteria were the most frequently isolated microorganisms. Several studies examined the mortality rate in association with inadequate antimicrobial therapy. When antibiotic therapy was "appropriate" (i.e., the infective organisms were susceptible), there was a 60% decrease in mortality from 90% (inappropriate) therapy to 30% (appropriate) (2,120,137).

Prior to the publication of the Yu et al. study cited earlier, Rex and Pfaller (186) reviewed multiple reports examining the correlation of therapeutic outcome with *in vitro* susceptibility. They proposed the "90–60 rule," which states that infections that are due to susceptible isolates respond to appropriate therapy about 90% of the time whereas infections that are due to resistant isolates or are treated inappropriately respond to therapy about 60% of the time.

ASSAY OF BACTERICIDAL ACTIVITY

MIC values estimate the bacteriostatic or inhibitory activity of antimicrobial agents. An MIC, when determined according to the standards and references detailed, is a reproducible parameter for a given antimicrobial agent against a variety of rapidly growing pathogens. In clinical practice, the MIC usually suffices for guiding chemotherapy. The success of *in vivo* antimicrobial action depends to a large extent on the host's defense mechanisms, which ultimately sequester and kill the microorganisms that have been reduced by the bacteriostatic action of the chemotherapeutic agent. The main body of medical microbiology, clinical pharmacology, and infectious disease literature utilizes MIC data in studying the effects of antimicrobials and in establishing criteria for application in therapy.

For antimicrobial agents that possess bactericidal action (mainly aminoglycosides and β-lactams), it is sometimes necessary to perform additional quantitative assessments of the killing effect on a given offending microorganism. The parameter known as the MBC can be determined in several ways:

1. By estimating the MBC as a result of the MIC for an infecting organism.
2. By estimating the titer of serum of a patient receiving antimicrobial therapy that kills the infecting organism after fences (i.e., the serum bactericidal titer or test [SBT]).
3. By determining the number of surviving bacteria in a fixed concentration of the drug using the average obtainable blood level at defined time intervals (i.e., the killing curve).

The assessment of bactericidal activity, although methodologically feasible, is fraught with microbiological phenomena and technical problems requiring consummate understanding on the part of those who consider their application and those who execute the assays.

Microbiologic Factors

Since the interactions of bacteria and antimicrobial agents began to be gauged, investigators have observed unusual and complex phenomena that remain incompletely understood in the modern molecular era. One such phenomenon is known as the paradoxical effect (or the Eagle phenomenon) (66). Discovered in the early days of penicillin therapy, the paradoxical effect manifests as the puzzling appearance of increasing numbers of bacterial survivors at concentrations higher than the MBC. Since its discovery, it has been observed for several species of bacteria and for antimicrobial agents other than the β-lactam group and is believed to be the result of interference with protein synthesis of the organism by higher concentrations of the β-lactam. The paradox occurs when the proportion of surviving cells increases significantly even as the concentration of antimicrobial agent increases beyond the MBC. It has been theorized that the high concentration of antimicrobial agent inhibits protein synthesis to a degree that prevents the growth necessary for expression of the lethal effect of the drug. No therapeutic implications appear associated with this effect.

A second complexity involving incomplete killing has been referred to as the persistence phenomenon and relates to the small proportion (usually less than 0.1%) of the inoculum cells that persist (survive) despite the lethal activity of antimicrobial agents. Again, this is especially common with β-lactam agents. If the persisters are subcultured and retested, they appear as susceptible to the effects of the antimicrobial agent as the original isolate, and no greater proportion of cells persist. Persisters have been considered to be metabolically inactive forms that were not actively growing at the time of the interaction of the drug with the inoculum and consequently were not killed by the β-lactam compound.

Of the several mechanisms by which bacteria seemingly evade the killing effect of antimicrobial agents, perhaps the least understood is that of tolerance. The term was coined in 1970 by Tomasz et al. (237) to describe the atypical *in vitro* response of pneumococcal strains to penicillin. This response was later recognized as genotypic tolerance. The more common and perhaps more clinically relevant type of tolerance, phenotypic tolerance, was described earlier, in 1942, by Hobby et al. (100).

Reports related to the phenomenon of tolerance have accumulated rapidly over the past few years, and several reviews deal with it (99,203,240,241). Operationally, tolerance can be defined as the ability of bacteria to grow in the presence of high concentrations of antimicrobials, so that the killing action of the drug is avoided but the MIC remains the same. In Tomasz's original observation, typical pneumococcal isolates were quickly lysed and lost viability at penicillin concentrations greater than the MIC. However, the selected tolerant strain was not lysed and lost viability at a significantly reduced rate. Recently, it has been suggested that four different mechanisms may contribute to the ability of organisms to survive (or survive at a higher rate) during treatment with penicillin or other cell wall–directed compounds. Tuomanen et al. (241) proposed the term *survivor mutation* and attributed the mechanism of survival to ancillary bactericidal and lytic processes. Moreover, they cautioned against using the term *tolerant* to describe all of these isolates. The relationship between the killing rates in different bacterial populations and the MBC is depicted in Figure 3.17.

Tolerance in the main has been associated with -lactam agents and has been reported for a number of genera, including *Streptococcus, Staphylococcus, Listeria, Lactobacillus,* and *Clostridium.* A growing debate revolves around the criteria used to define tolerance. The generally acceptable definition has been a ratio of the MBC to the MIC of more than 32, as originally defined by Sabath et al. (189). However, differences among investigators have led to an assortment of values ranging from 8 to 32 to 100 (203). A more precise approach for detecting tolerant strains is to use quantitative killing curve methods. More than 20 bacterial species recovered from clinical material have been implicated as tolerant strains. However, because of a lack of consensus, the true incidence of tolerance among clinical isolates remains to be determined. The problem is muddied by the variable application of adequate bacteriological techniques, the variable definition of tolerance, and the lack of suitable reference strains.

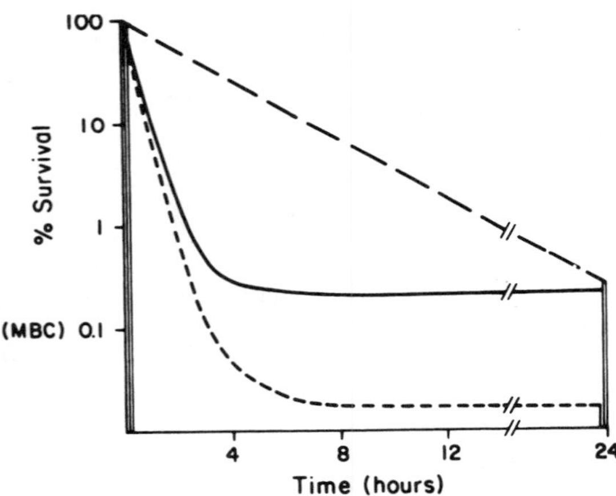

FIGURE 3.17 ● Relationship between killing rates and MBC values. Curves show three possible types of kinetics for the loss of viability during treatment with penicillin at a concentration of one time the MIC value. The *vertical bar* at 0 minutes indicates the inoculum; the *bars* at 24 hours represent percent survival, as determined by the MBC value. The *lower bar* represents less than 0.1% survival reached along the rapidly declining killing curve of the nontolerant bacterium (- - -). The *higher bars* indicate survival of more than 0.1% of the cells, which indicates tolerance by the MBC test. However, rates (and mechanisms) of killing in the two tolerant cultures are different. The truly tolerant mutant undergoes slow loss of viability (- - -), whereas the other culture (—) has an initially rapid rate of killing typical of nontolerant cells but a higher survival rate, which may be due to a physiologically heterogeneous inoculum (e.g., higher percentage of dormant cells that are phenotypically tolerant). Alternatively, these cells may represent increased persisters or a subpopulation of resistant cells. (Reprinted with permission from Handwerger and Tomasz [99].)

To study the effects of antimicrobials on bacteria with decreased or arrested division rates, two new parameters have been suggested for assessing the efficacy of killing. One of them, the MnBC, is analogous to the MBC but applicable to conditions (phenotypic) of slower growth; it is defined as the concentration of drug that achieves a one-log killing in 24 hours of cells starved for 10 m before the addition of antibiotic (241).

Whatever the terms and categories used to describe these events, it is necessary to recognize that the organisms involved may be present in various clinical situations. Although it is generally accepted that rapidly growing and dividing organisms are more susceptible to the inhibiting effects of cell wall–directed antimicrobial agents, it is recognized that rapidly growing bacteria flourish under broth-related clinical conditions like bacteremia. In other clinical conditions, specifically osteomyelitis, it has been demonstrated that microorganisms divide at a much reduced rate and thus would be less susceptible to the effects of antimicrobial agents. A perceived problem in dealing with this clinical dilemma is how to select antimicrobial agents that would be well targeted in arrested growth situations (240). It is of utmost interest and importance to determine whether these isolates are the result of technical manipulation in the laboratory or are indicative of a real clinical phenomenon (Fig. 3.18).

The concept of tolerance is derived from the bactericidal mode of action of β-lactam antibiotics. β-Lactam compounds are bactericidal because they inhibit bacterial cell wall synthesis. Basically, their mode of action is to interfere with the transpeptidation process that links the individual peptidoglycan components of the bacterial cell wall to each other (171,232,233,235,264). β-Lactams bind to and inactivate specific targets on the inner surface of the bacterial cell membranes. These targets are referred to as the PBPs (30,210,212,235,264). The PBPs are enzymes—transpeptidases, carboxypeptidases, and endopeptidases—involved in the terminal stages of assembling the bacterial cell wall and maintaining the structure of the cell wall during growth and division (234).

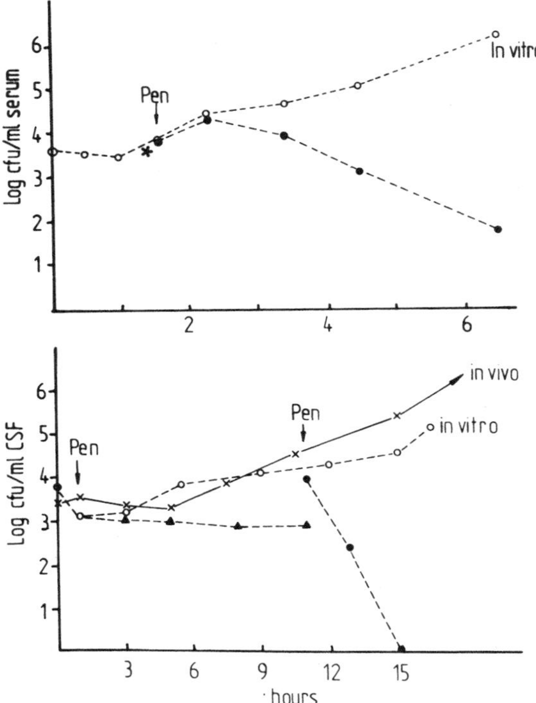

FIGURE 3.18 ● Phenotypic tolerance of nongrowing *S. pneumoniae* upon their transfer from serum to cerebrospinal fluid (CSF). *Top*, *S. pneumoniae* strain S_{111} was grown in a chemically defined medium (38), filtered, and resuspended in heat-treated rabbit serum. During growth (*) the culture was divided into six aliquots. One aliquot was maintained as a control (○), and one was exposed to penicillin at 20 times the MIC (●). Viability was determined over 6 hours. The remaining aliquots were filtered, resuspended in saline, and used in the experiment, whose results are shown in the bottom panel. *Bottom*, pneumococci were either injected into the subarachnoid space of rabbits, as described (182) (×), or suspended in normal CSF *in vitro* (○). Viability was determined over 17 hours. Benzylpenicillin (*Pen*), at 20 times the MIC, was added at two time points (*arrows*) to the *ex vivo* culture aliquots: at 1 hour of the initial 5-hour lag phase (▲) or at 10 hours during the growth phase in CSF (●). *In vivo* and *in vitro* growth rates in the CSF were comparable. Transfer of growing pneumococci from the serum to the CSF resulted in a temporary halt in bacterial growth. Benzylpenicillin was not able to kill the nongrowing, phenotypically tolerant pneumococci. Bacteria actively growing in serum or CSF were killed rapidly. (Reproduced with permission from Tuomanen [240].)

β-Lactam compounds have different attachment sites and binding capacities for the various PBPs and, depending on the specific PBP bound, have different effects on bacteria (90,172,211). The inactivation of some PBPs (PBPs 1A, 1BS, 2, and 3) contributes to bacterial death. In contrast, other PBPs (PBPs 4, 5, and 6) are not essential for bacterial viability, and their inactivation by β-lactam molecules is not lethal for the bacteria (151,236). Currently, it is theorized that β-lactams binding to PBPs inactivate endogenous inhibitors of bacterial autolysins. The autolysins can then disrupt covalent bonds in the bacterial cell wall and cause bacteriolysis. The growth of certain organisms that lack autolysins can be inhibited by β-lactam antibiotics, but such organisms are not killed, thus leading to the phenomenon of bacterial tolerance (237).

Clinical Relevance and Applications

In some clinical situations, both microbiological and clinical data have been accumulated that suggest that MBC determinations or other bactericidal assays may be interpretable and relevant. These have been referred to earlier and include directed activity against *Enterococcus* strains associated with endocarditis (256) and occasional cases of bacterial endocarditis (58) caused by other organisms that may not be fully susceptible, particularly *Pseudomonas* species, MRSA, various species of coagulase-negative *Staphylococcus,* and *S. aureus.* The MBC may also be of value in the management of osteomyelitis (215) and bacteremic infections in granulocytopenic patients (198).

Technical Factors

The application of the MBC (which is founded on the MIC and its derivative, the MBC/MIC ratio) to determine the microbicidal activity of antimicrobial agents has been questioned because the endpoints are based on arbitrary definitions and are often poorly reproducible. Even within a particular methodology, such as macrodilution versus microdilution procedures (184), there is great biologic variability, and different endpoints may be obtained (Table 3.36).

Dilution methods suffer from several technical problems, such as antibiotic carryover, bacteria adhering to the surface of the test vessel, and variations in the medium and growth phase of the inoculum, all of which affect the CFU recovered from subculture plates (152, 197) (see "MBC Procedure"). One step in performing the assay is critical because of an unusual condition that occurs at the surface (meniscus) of the assay container. At the medium interface, viable organisms flourish, perhaps to escape the potential lethal action of the antimicrobial agent. This potential for error is diminished by mixing and reincubating (see "MBC Procedure," steps 13 and 14).

As for MIC assays, the recommended broth is MHB supplemented with Ca^{2+} and Mg^{2+} for testing *P. aeruginosa.* Sodium chloride (2% final concentration) should be added for testing *S. aureus.* MHB can be used with human serum (HS) in a 1:1 ratio. The use of HS depends on the antimicrobial agent to be tested (and its potential for protein binding), the organism, and the bactericidal test executed. The selection of medium may be altered for

TABLE 3.36

Technical Factors Influencing MBC Tests[a]

Variable Factor	Effect
Phase of growth	Increases survivors in stationary phase; paradoxical (Eagle) effect exaggerated in late logarithmic phase
Type of tube or glassware	Adhesion to inside of test vessel varies with material and may elevate counts of survivors, leading to false results
Mode of inoculation	Eliminates adhesion above meniscus by using a small-volume inoculum below the meniscus and avoid shaking
Mixing at 20 h	Vortexing is needed to resuspend all cells
Reincubation for 4 h and vortex again	Allows all cells resuspended at 20 h from above meniscus to be killed before sampling
Antibiotic carryover	Gives falsely low counts of survivors at higher antibiotic concentrations
Reincubation of recovery media	Total of 48 h for staphylococci (72 h for fastidious organisms) may be necessary for final results

[a] Adapted from Schoenknecht et al. (197).

research needs in order to grow fastidious microorganisms. For the serum bacterial titer, a 1:1 combination of MHB and HS is the recommended medium (165).

Adherence to the details outlined in the preceding sections with respect to inoculum size, strain storage, growth phase, assay medium, cation content, and incubation duration and temperature must be strict.

Whereas it is anticipated that for bactericidal drugs the MIC and MBC would be similar, it is accepted that for bacteriostatic drugs the MBC could be several dilutions greater. A procedural problem related to the MBC is the definition of the endpoint as it relates to the number of survivors that remain in the population, because 100% elimination is an impossible goal to achieve (7,197). Several investigators have utilized the definition of a reduction of the number of bacteria present in the inoculum to 99.99% of the original population. This represents a 10^{-3} ($-\log 10^3$) reduction and is somewhat arbitrary, since there is no convincing evidence that a 99.0% or 98.0% reduction actually portrays the outcome and is more clinically relevant. In the United States, NCCLS (162) has written a proposed standard for these tests in which a 1000-fold reduction of the original inoculum is used as a conventional standard. When the ratio of MBC to MIC is 32 or greater for a given bacterium-antimicrobial combination, the organism is said to be tolerant to the action of the antimicrobial, and it is questionable whether a favorable clinical response or outcome can be achieved. The popular definition of tolerance (MBC/MIC greater than 32) has little scientific basis and results in organisms whose response to penicillin is close to the 99.9% definition of kill being artificially divided into susceptible and tolerant categories (152) (Fig. 3.19). In view of the lack of

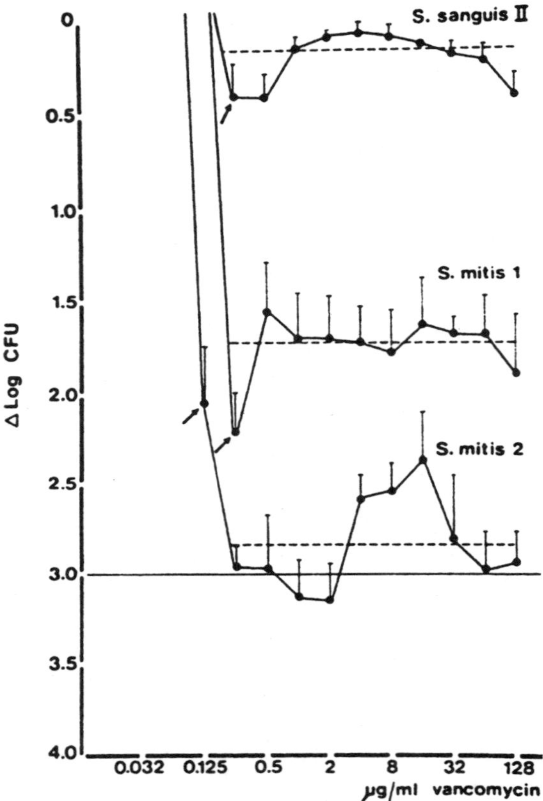

FIGURE 3.19 ● Actual reduction of the viable counts for three representative strains after standard broth dilution testing with vancomycin. *Arrows*, MIC. The *solid line* at 3 $\log_{10}$ represents the cutoff value of 99.9% killing defining the MBC. The *dashed lines* for each strain represent the mean Δlog CFU. The mean Δlog CFU values for *Streptococcus sanguis* II, *Streptococcus mitis* 1, and *S. mitis* 2 were 0.1 (MBC, more than 128 µg/mL), 1.72 (MBC, more than 128 µg/mL), and 2.84, respectively. The MBC for *S. mitis* 2 was difficult to define because of more than 99.9% killing with 1 and 2 µg/mL vancomycin but not above 4 µg/mL vancomycin. (Reproduced with permission from Meylan et al. [152].)

reproducibility of conventional MBC methods, the definition should be treated with caution.

Minimal Bactericidal Concentration

The important studies by Taylor et al. (221) on the MBC determination for staphylococci have shown that much of the variability in the assay results is due to procedural details. In the United States, most of the contention regarding the assay revolves around the issue of whether to use the macrodilution or microdilution method. In an extensive investigation, James (105) compared four methods for determining the MIC and MBC of penicillin against *S. viridans*. In his studies, the macrodilution and microdilution methods were compared, along with the membrane and gradient plate methods. The author studied 28 strains of *S. viridans* streptococci by these methods and determined the MICs and MBCs. From these data, he calculated the mean error span shown in Table 3.37. Note that conventional MIC methods are expected to yield reproducibility between tests within one doubling dilution, which equates to a mean error span of less than 0.5 tube errors. If this criterion is applied, then the macrodilution, membrane, and gradient methods gave acceptable reproducibility, whereas the microdilution method did not and therefore should not be used for the determination of the MIC, at least with *S. viridans* streptococci. When one applies the same criterion to MBC determinations, only the gradient method gave acceptable reproducibility, and it was the most reliable method for predicting penicillin tolerance. James concluded from his studies that the mean error spans for all methods were acceptable, except for the microdilution technique. However, correct and reproducible results were obtained for all control organisms by the gradient method and, to a lesser extent, the membrane method. His study clearly indicated that the microdilution results were unacceptable.

In deciding on a method to adopt for determining the MBC, it is thus best, as shown by the work of James (105), to avoid the microdilution method. Because many reference and clinical laboratories may not have accumulated experience with the gradient or membrane methods, the macrodilution method is the logical choice. It is described here in detail, as adapted from Schoenknecht et al. (195).

TABLE 3.37

Test Variation for 23 Strains of Viridans Streptococci Tested for MIC and MBC by Four methods[a,b]

Method	No. Stains Tolerant[c,d]	MIC Tube Error (range)	MBC Tube Error (range)
Microdilution	13	±1.56 (0–9)	±4.24 (0–18)
Macrodilution	11	±0.48 (0–6)	±3.47 (0–23)
Membrane	12	±0.50 (0–4)	±2.50 (0–20)
Gradient	12	±0.23 (0–1)	±0.22 (0–3)

[a] Adapted from James (105).
[b] Mean error span for each method (±2 SD) expressed as the number of twofold dilutions.
[c] On the basis of mean MBC/MIC >32, 6 strains were tolerant by all methods.
[d] No single organism was responsible for major discrepancies in all methods.

MBC Procedure

MIC

1. Subculture organisms onto appropriate medium (usually a blood agar plate) and incubate overnight at 35°C.
2. Inoculate a tube containing 3 mL of saline or MHB with five or more colonies from the overnight plate to achieve a turbidity equivalent to a no. 1 McFarland standard (approximately 10^8 organisms/mL).
3. Transfer 0.1 mL of turbid inoculum (patient's pathogen) into 10 mL of MHB or other appropriate broth. Incubate in a shaking water-bath or equivalent at 35°C until turbid. This corresponds to an endpoint between a no. 1 McFarland standard and an overnight suspension and requires 5 to 6 hours for rapid growers.
4. Inoculate the standard control organism (*E. coli, S. aureus*, etc.) into 3 mL of broth and incubate (without shaking) at 35°C until turbid.
5. Prepare twofold serial dilutions of the antibiotic in 2 mL of MHB (total volume per acid-washed borosilicate glass tube); 16 × 100-mm glass tubes with loose-fitting metal caps are preferred.
6. Standardize the inocula (patient's organism and control organism) to equal a 0.5 McFarland turbidity standard (approximately 5×10^7 organisms/mL) in 3 mL of saline or broth.
7. Dilute adjusted inocula 1:10 (0.2 mL in 1.8 mL of MHB or appropriate substitute). This equals about 5×10^6 organisms/mL.
8. Dispense, using an Eppendorf or equivalent pipette, 100 μL of diluted inoculum into tubes containing serial dilutions of the antibiotic. To inoculate, insert the pipette tip well under the surface of the antibiotic-containing broth. Avoid any contact between the tip and the walls of the tube. Rinse the tip five times in solution. The same tip may be used throughout the test

if inoculating from lowest to highest concentration of antibiotic. The final inoculum size is approximately 2.5×10^5 organisms/mL.

9. Incubate for 20 hours at 35°C.
10. From the 1:10 dilution of the 0.5 McFarland-adjusted inoculum, which should be about 5×10^6 organisms/mL (step 7), dilute serially 1:10 in MHB four times to achieve a final inoculum of 5×10^2 organisms/mL, as follows: 0.2 mL (5×10^6 CFU/mL) + 1.8 mL MHB; 0.2 mL (5×10^6 CFU/mL) + 1.8 mL MHB 5×10^5 CFU/mL; 0.2 mL (5×10^6 CFU/mL) + 1.8 mL MHB 5×10^4 CFU/mL; 0.2 mL (5×10^4 CFU/mL) + 1.8 mL MHB 5×10^3 CFU/mL; 0.2 mL (5×10^3 CFU/mL) + 1.8 mL MHB 5×10^2 CFU/mL.
11. Aliquot 0.1 mL of this suspension, dispense either into a tube of melted agar for the preparation of pour plates or onto an appropriate agar plate (e.g., blood agar) and distribute evenly using sterile bent glass rods. This procedure should be done in duplicate. Incubate overnight at 35°C.
12. Observe and record MIC of control organisms.
13. For patient's sample only, vigorously vortex-mix tubes without visible growth for 15 seconds and reincubate for an additional 4 hours.
14. Vortex-mix again and sample tubes for MBC determination; spread 100-μL samples across the surface of dried TS agar plates with sterile bent glass rods.
15. Record patient's MIC.

MBC

16. Incubate plates overnight at 35°C for the MBC test.
17. After 1 day (or 2 days), count the number of colonies per plate from the original inoculum plates or pour plates and average. Determine a colony count that represents 0.1% of the original inoculum (i.e., 99.9% reduction).
18. Count colonies from MBC plates. Any number equal to or less than the determined colony count from step 17 is considered as a 99.9% kill or bactericidal result.

When counting the number of colonies to determine the plate average, the mean is referred to as N. Apply the formula $N/2 + 2(\sqrt{N}/2)$ to determine the upper limit of a colony count that represents 0.1% of the original inoculum (approximately 95% confidence limits). Therefore, any colony counts from MBC plates equal to or less than the determined inoculum colony count upper limit are considered 99.9% kill or bactericidal results.

Alternatively, rejection values can be determined from a chart that takes into account the final inoculum size, dual sampling, pipetting error, and the Poisson distribution of sample responses (Table 3.38).

Hacek et al. (97), recognizing the potential variability and complexity imposed by this assay, proposed a modified scheme. Their modified bactericidal testing protocol includes omitting serum supplementation, incubation without agitation, running tests in duplicate with a reduced number of dilutions (six instead of nine), extending the incubation interval for 24 hours to resolve discrepancies, using single 0.1-mL aliquots, and adopting an alternate endpoint calculation. The authors found a 91% agreement between the standard and their modified protocol and suggest the alternative procedure is practical for the clinical laboratory.

TABLE 3.38

Rejection Value (Number of Colonies) and Calculated Sensitivity and Specificity for Each Initial Inoculum Concentration on the Basis of Duplicate 0.01-mL Samples[a,b]

Final Inoculum (CFU/mL)	Rejection Value[c]	Sensitivity[d] (%)	Specificity[d] (%)
1×10^5	4	77	97
2×10^5	8	89	99
3×10^5	15	99	99
4×10^5	20	99	99
5×10^5	25	99	99
6×10^5	29	99	99
7×10^5	33	99	99
8×10^5	38	99	99
9×10^5	42	99	99
1×10^6	47	99	99
2×10^6	91	99	99
3×10^6	136	99	99
4×10^6	182	99	99
5×10^6	227	99	99
6×10^6	273	99	99
7×10^6	318	99	99
8×10^6	364	99	99
9×10^6	409	99	99
1×10^7	455	99	99

[a] Adapted from NCCLS (165).
[b] A 5% error (pipette plus full sampling) is considered for determination of final inoculum based on *duplicate* sampling of final inoculum size.
[c] Number of colonies. When the sum of colonies from duplicate samples is equal to or less than the rejection value, the antibiotic is determined to be lethal (a 0.999 or greater reduction in the final inoculum).
[d] Sensitivity and specificity calculated for each specific final inoculum concentration and rejection value.

Serum Bactericidal Titer/Test

Clinical Relevance and Applications

The seminal work on and application of this test were done by Schlichter and MacLean (196). In its original form, the test determined bacteriostatic activity; it was later modified to include bactericidal activity. However, in the nearly 50 years that the test has been available and used, there has been no clear, universally accepted criteria for its application. Critical reviews of the SBT have not found the test clinical useful and have stressed the need for standardization of the methodology (215, 217). NCCLS has developed a proposed guideline (164), and in a thoughtful review Stratton (216) addressed the specific application and clinical relevance of the test.

Assessing the antimicrobial activity in a patient's serum during treatment by using the offending organisms isolated from the patient as the test strain would appear to be the most logical approach to evaluating and monitoring chemotherapy. The SBT measures the combined effects of absorption and elimination of the antimicrobial agent, its potential binding to serum proteins, the effect of metabolic congeners of the parent compound against the microorganisms, and, if dual antimicrobial therapy is administered, the effects of drug interactions, including synergistic, additive, and antagonistic effects.

As with the determination as MBC, the SBT can be helpful in monitoring the treatment of bacterial endocarditis (58,256), bacteremia in patients with cancer (65), osteomyelitis or septic arthritis (178,215), and bacterial meningitis (191).

As an experimental tool, the SBT has been used in evaluating new drugs and drug combinations and detecting antimicrobial potency in infected body fluids other than blood. When the SBT has been used for drug evaluation (in humans or animals), analysis of the results can be aided by using the titer to measure the area under the bactericidal curve (AUBC) (16).

Although the SBT approach seems to be a logical integration of physiological (PK) and *in vitro* susceptibility, this test, as well as other bacterium-antimicrobial assays, fails to evaluate the cellular and humoral defenses of the host, the site and severity of the infection, the quantity of bacteria present and their virulence, and the continually changing concentration of the antimicrobial agent in the host.

SBT Methodology

As with the MBC procedures, many variations of this test exist. The same care and attention to details and materials used in executing the MBC procedures should be used here. The method that follows is adapted from several sources (7,164,197).

Collection of Patient Serum

Inherent in this procedure is the use of the patient's serum to represent the physiological concentration of the antimicrobial agent. For this purpose, a peak level and a trough level are generally obtained. The peak level is considered the level obtained 30–45 minutes after an intravenous infusion, 60 minutes after an intramuscular infusion, or 90 minutes after an oral dose. The peak level is obtained 30–60 minutes after the drug is absorbed and distributed. The trough level is the level that is considered to occur 30 minutes prior to the following dose.

After the specimen has been collected, it should be transported to the laboratory properly and promptly, to separate the blood and serum. Serum collected from the specimen should be frozen if a delay of more than 2 hours in performing the SBT is anticipated. Ideally, trough and peak serum specimens should be pair-matched rather than collected on different days of therapy.

Patient Organism

The SBT must be anticipated so that the patient's clinical isolate can be saved. Because it is the practice of many clinical laboratories to save bacteremic isolates as well as isolates from spinal and other body fluids, these can be retrieved early. On the other hand, if it is anticipated that the isolate will be needed, this should be kept frozen at 70°C in a TS broth or in a cryoprotectant medium (e.g., glycerol).

SBT Procedure

1. Serially dilute the patient's serum twofold at least 1:64, using MHB as diluent. The final volume per tube should be 1 mL.
2. Add the patient's organism to a 0.1-mL volume of a carefully prepared inoculum (see steps 10 and 11 of the MBC procedure).
3. Prepare pour plates for establishing original inoculum CFU counts (see steps 7 through 11 of the MBC procedure).
4. Include a growth control tube containing MHB and inoculum but no serum.
5. Incubate for 18 to 24 hours.
6. Subculture for the 99.9% bactericidal endpoint, as described for the MBC procedure.

Interpretation

The interpretation of endpoints is controversial. The NCCLS guidelines (164) offer the following: peak titer of 1:2 and trough titer of 1:2, interpretation of inadequate; peak titer of 1:4 to 1:16 and trough titer of 1:4, interpretation of intermediate; peak titer of 1:32 and trough titer of 1:8, interpretation of adequate. According to Stratton (215), in orthopedic infections a titer of 1:8 is prognostic of cure, although higher titers do not necessarily preclude positive outcomes.

Killing Curve

The killing curve or killing rate is represented by a plot of the number of survivors in the host after administration of a typical therapeutic regimen. It has been used to evaluate and compare new drugs and to study differences and changes in the antimicrobial susceptibility of clinically important bacterial isolates. These determinations are rarely used for guiding chemotherapy; they are mainly applied in experimental situations to animal models and are generally used to assess classes of drugs. One concentration of antibiotic is tested, usually that which is representative of an average level obtainable during therapy. At periodic intervals, usually at 0, 4, 12, and 24 hours of incubation, colony counts are performed and charted on semilogarithmic paper, with the survivor colony count on the ordinate (logarithmic scale) and time on the abscissa (arithmetic scale) (Fig. 3.20). For example, when one compares the β-lactam antimicrobial agents with the aminoglycosides, the former are characterized by slower, dose-dependent initial bactericidal activity. The extent of the bactericidal action is related to the time during which the serum level exceeds the MIC. If this level falls below the MIC, there is immediate regrowth of the microorganisms. In contrast, aminoglycosides demonstrate rapid, dose-dependent initial bactericidal activity, followed by a bacteriostatic phase that can last several hours after the serum concentration falls below the MIC.

The kinetics of antimicrobial activity, as described, provide a theoretical basis for dosing frequency and depend on the pathogen and the antibiotic used. Only one antibiotic concentration, representing the average obtainable blood level, or a limited number of concentrations, representing multiples or fractions of the blood level, are used. In the plot in Figure 3.20, the aminoglycoside is shown to be a drug with concentration-dependent bactericidal activity. At increasing drug concentrations, there is an increase in the magnitude and rate of killing. β-Lactam compounds (penicillin in Fig. 3.20) demonstrate little concentration-dependent bactericidal activity. At least for two antimicrobial agents, ampicillin and ciprofloxacin, their activities (expressed as killing rates) were similar in MHB and human urine, as judged by an *in vitro* PD model (60).

Although the protocol outlined below relates to evaluating the lethal activity of individual antimicrobial agents, agents combined for their potential synergistism can also be tested (see Chapter 10).

More recently, modified killing curve investigations have been used to elucidate anticipated multiple resistance mechanisms expressed by *S. pneumoniae* and *Mycobacteria* species against fluoroquinolone compounds (29,57). In this variation of the killing curve procedure, large numbers of microorganisms (10^8 to 10^{10}) are plated on increasing concentrations of antibiotic—in this case fluoroquinolones—and the fraction of cells that can be recovered are then treated as CFUs. The fraction that survive or grow are plotted against the concentration (i.e., the MIC). As can be seen in Fig. 3.21, the first dip in the plot occurs at the MIC; a second inflection point in mutant recovery occurs at a concentration the authors refer to as the MPC (**mutant prevention concentration**), the concentration required to block first-step mutants. This approach has proved valuable in studying the design of the fluoroquinolones in order to anticipate the possible development of stepwise mutants.

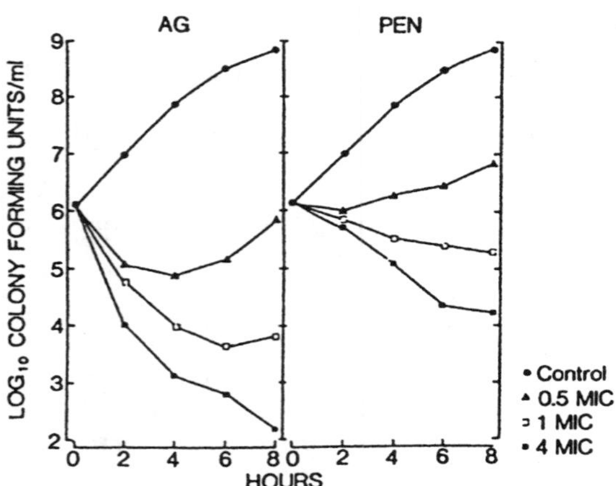

FIGURE 3.20 ● Killing curves. At periodic intervals, usually at 0, 4, 12, and 24 hours of incubation, colony counts are performed and charted on semilogarithmic paper, with the survivor colony count on the ordinate (logarithmic scale) and time on the abscissa (arithmetic scale). *AG*, aminoglycoside; *PEN*, penicillin.

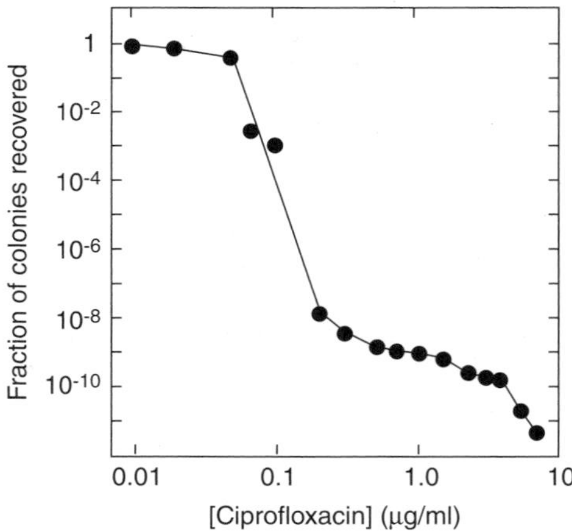

FIGURE 3.21 ● Effect of increasing concentrations of a quinolone (e.g., ciprofloxacin) on selection of resistant mutants. As drug concentration increases, note two inflections in the number of colonies recovered. The first drop equals the MIC. The second drop in mutant recovery occurs at the concentration required to block the growth of first-step mutants—the MPC (29,57).

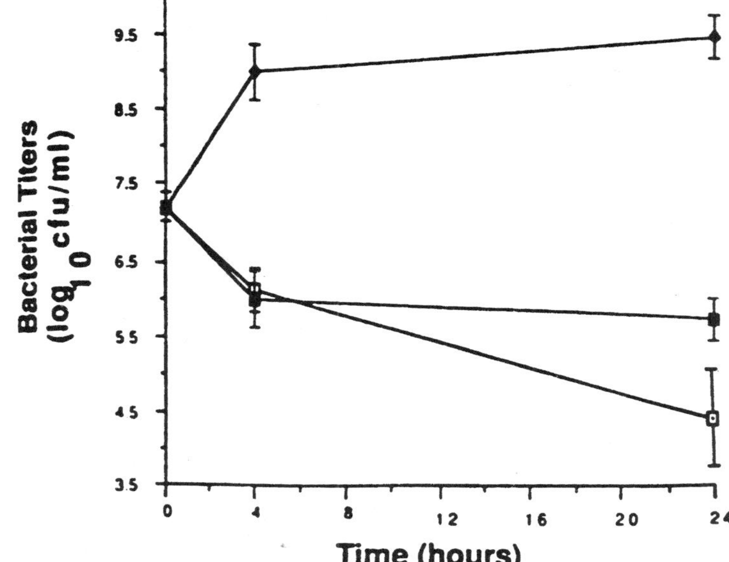

FIGURE 3.22 ● Time-kill curves for nafcillin (□) and vancomycin (■) at a concentration of four times the MIC for 10 clinical isolates of *S. aureus*. ♦, Control. (Reproduced from Small and Chambers [204].)

Killing Curve Procedure

1. Prepare inoculum of approximately 5×10^7 CFU/mL, as in steps 1 through 3 and 5 and 6 of the MBC procedure.
2. Inoculate according to step 8 of the MBC procedure. The final concentration should be 5×10^5 CFU/mL for each tube.
3. Immediately vortex-mix for 15 seconds the zero growth tube and dispense 0.1 mL into a tube of melted agar for the preparation of agar pour plates. Incubate at 35°C for 18 to 24 hours.
4. Similarly, for each subsequent time interval, prepare pour plates.
5. For testing at 24 hours, vortex-mix the last tube at 20 hours and reincubate for an additional 4 hours.
6. At 24 hours, vortex-mix again and prepare pour plates.

Serum Bactericidal Rate

The time-kill curve evaluates the rate at which single or multiple drugs kill bacteria. The serum bactericidal rate represents the rate of serum killing; the method used integrates *in vitro* activity and the *in vivo* pharmacokinetics of antimicrobial drugs and therefore reflects very accurately what happens in the host.

In a novel approach to the application of the serum bactericidal rate, Barriere et al. (16) measured the AUBC to determine the total synergistic bactericidal activity. When the calculated value of the AUBC for a combination was greater than the sum of the values for the individual drugs, the combination was judged to be synergistic.

A therapeutic role for the use of killing curves was shown by Small and Chambers (206). They studied the clinical failure of vancomycin when treating intravenous drug users with *S. aureus* endocarditis. *In vitro* studies with 10 strains of *S. aureus* recovered from this patient group demonstrated that, at 4 times the MIC, vancomycin was less rapidly bactericidal than nafcillin (Fig. 3.22). At 4 hours after incubation, the mean decreases in bacterial counts for vancomycin and the β-lactam were similar. However, after 24 hour the mean count for vancomycin had not significantly changed from the 4-hour titration, though there was a significant reduction (2.8 $\log_{10}$ CFU/mL) for nafcillin. It was on this basis that the authors explained relapses and persistent bacteremia in the vancomycin-treated group and concluded that vancomycin was less effective than nafcillin for treating this infection.

CYTOKINES AND CYTOKINE ACTIVITY

Cytokines represent a broad group of soluble mediators of cell-to-cell communication; the group includes interleukins, interferons, and colony-stimulating factors (102). Cytokine molecules are mediators of specific and nonspecific host defense responses. As such, they play a critical role in effector mechanisms that eliminate foreign antigens such as microorganisms. Advances in our understanding of cytokines have focused on two primary biologic activities: the regulation of inflammation with effective immune responses to pathogen invasions and a wide array of hemopoietic activities that serve to modulate the growth of immune cells. Table 3.39 lists some cytokines and their biologic effects. It is with the understanding that cytokines may play a supportive or synergistic role in conjuction with antimicrobial agents that they are

TABLE 3.39

Selected Cytokines: Sources and Biologic Effects[a]

Cytokine	Cellular Source	Biological Effects
IFN-α, -β (interferon)	Phagocytes	Antivival, pyrogenic
IFN-γ	T cells	Activates mononuclear phagocytes
IL-1 (interleukin-1)[b]	Monocytes, macrophages	Cell activation, fever, cachexia
IL-1 ra	T cells (Th-1)	Blocks IL-1 receptor
IL-2[c]	T cells	T cell proliferation, stimulates B cell proliferation
IL-4	T cells, macrophages, B cells	Isotype (class) switching to IgE
IL-10	T cells, macrophages	Suppresses inflammatory cytokines, enhances B cell proliferation
IL-12	Macrophages, B cells	Stimulates differentiation of Th 1 Cells
TNF-α (tumor necrosis factor)	Numerous cell types	Wide range of inflammatory and immune responses

[a] Compiled from various sources (e.g., Howard, Miyajima, and Coffman [102]).
[b] Lymphocyte activating factor.
[c] T cell growth factor.

included and discussed here. The interferons have demonstrated significant activity in different types of infectious disease, which has resulted in several FDA-approved indications (15). Interferon-α has shown antiviral activity, and some interleukins are known to demonstrate protection against intracellular pathogens (121). Interleukin-1 receptor antagonist serves as an active mediator during severe bacterial infection or septic shock. As recombinant forms of these compounds become available, no doubt clinical trials will be attempted to determine effectiveness.

The cytokines can be readily assayed in human biological fluids by an enzyme-linked immunosorbent assay-type sandwich immunoassay that recognizes both natural human and *E. coli*–derived human cytokines. A typical standard curve from a commercial kit assay is shown in Figure 3.23.

FUTURE CONSIDERATIONS

Laboratory assessments of antimicrobial activity will no doubt attempt to more broadly incroporate microbiological and pharmacological attributes of antibiotics. Advances in PK/PD modeling have made significant contributions to establishing breakpoint determinations that are more clinically relevant. However, the application to direct patient care in real time is not yet fully realized. As currently conceived, some of the approaches that use computer-simulated models are too tedious to execute as part of actionable health care. Aspects of these kinetic

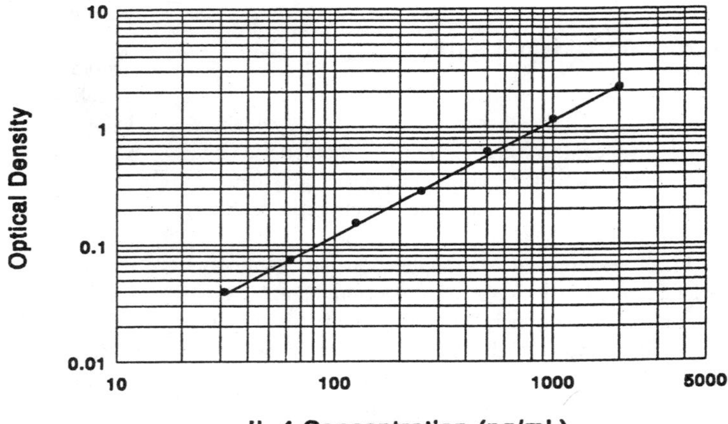

FIGURE 3.23 ● Typical sandwich enzyme-linked immunosorbent assay standard curve obtainable with a commercial kit that recognizes natural human and *E. coli*–derived recombinant interleukin-4 (IL-4).

models have been recently incorporated into programs made available on personal digital assistants (PDAs) at the patient's bedside to help in the delivery of rational, safe, and effective therapy (157). As new pathogens emerge, some associated with resistance mechanisms that threaten to limit the effective therapeutic use of antimicrobial agents, laboratories will be called upon to move rapidly and accurately to screen for the presence of resistant members. Toward this end, screening methods for genetic markers of resistance such as those discussed in this chapter will be used. Additionally, the use of multiple probes directed toward more than one gene target (multiplexing) will no doubt be attempted. Lastly, as the pipeline for the development of new antimicrobial compounds continues to dwindle, pharmaceutical companies may consider developing additional antiinflammatory, antisepsis medicines. In that event, clinical laboratories will have the need to titrate inflammatory cytokines and their immunotherapeutic targets.

REFERENCES

1. Aldridge KE, Janney A, Sanders CV, et al. Interlaboratory variation of antibiograms of methicillin-resistant and methicillin-susceptible *Staphylococcus aureus* strains with conventional and commercial testing systems. *J Clin Microbiol* 1983;18:142–147.
2. Alvarez-Lerma F. Modification of empiric antibiotic treatment in patients with pneumonia acquired in the intensive care unit. ICU-Acquired Pneumonia Study Group. *Intensive Care Med* 1996;22:387–394.
3. Amaral L, Trigenis B, Atkinson BA. The radioactive thymidine incorporation method for the determination of antibiotic susceptibility of Gram-negative bacilli. *Eur J Clin Microbiol* 1982;1:149–154.
4. Ambrose PG, Grasela DM. The use of Monte Carlo simulation to examine pharmacodynamic variance of drugs: fluoroquinolone pharmacodynamics against *Streptococcus pneumoniae*. *Diagn Microbiol Infect Dis* 2000;38:151–157.
5. Amsterdam D. Instrumentation for antimicrobic susceptibility testing: yesterday, today, and tomorrow. *Diagn Microbiol Infect Dis* 1988;9:167–178.
6. Amsterdam D. Principles of antibiotic testing in the laboratory. In: Balows A, Hausler WJ Jr, Lennette EH, eds. *Laboratory diagnosis of infectious disease: principles and practice*. Vol. 1. New York: Springer-Verlag, 1988:22–38.
7. Anhalt JP, Washington JW II. Bactericidal tests. In: Washington JA, ed. *Laboratory procedures in clinical microbiology*. 2nd ed. New York: Springer-Verlag, 1985:431–745.
8. Appelbaum PC. Worldwide development of antibiotic resistance in pneumococci. *Eur J Clin Microbiol* 1987;6:367–377.
9. Azemun P, Stall T, Roberts M, et al. Rapid detection of chloramphenicol resistance in *Haemophilus influenzae*. *Antimicrob Agents Chemother* 1981;20:168–170.
10. Baker CN, Banerjee SH, Tenover FC. Evaluation of Alamar colorimetric MIC method for antimicrobial susceptibility testing Gram-negative bacteria. *J Clin Microbiol* 1994;32:1261–1267.
11. Baker CN, Hollis G, Thornsberry C. Antimicrobial susceptibility testing of *Francisella tularensis* with a modified Mueller-Hinton broth. *J Clin Microbiol* 1988;22:212–215.
12. Baker CN, Thornsberry C, Hawkinson RW. Inoculum standardization in antimicrobial susceptibility testing: evaluation of overnight agar cultures and the Rapid Inoculum Standardization System. *J Clin Microbiol* 1983;17:450–457.
13. Baker CN, Thornsberry C, Jones RN. In vitro antimicrobial activity of cefoperazone, cefotaxime, moxalactam (LY 127935), azlocillin, mezlocillin, and other β-lactam antibiotics against *Neisseria gonorrhoeae* and *Haemophilus influenzae*, including β-lactamase–producing strains. *Antimicrob Agents Chemother* 1980;17:757–761.
14. Barenfanger J, Drake C, Kacich G. Clinical and financial benefits of rapid identification and antimicrobial susceptibility testing. *J Clin Microbiol* 1999;37:1415–1418.
15. Baron S, Tyring SK, Fleischman R, et al. The interferons: mechanisms of action and clinical applications. *JAMA* 1991;266:1375–1383.
16. Barriere SL, Ely E, Kapusnik JE, et al. Analysis of a new method for assessing activity of combinations of antimicrobials: area under the bactericidal curve. *J Antimicrob Chemother* 1985;16:49–59.
17. Barry AL. *The antimicrobic susceptibility test: principles and practices*. Philadelphia: Lea & Febiger, 1976.
18. Barry AL, Badal RE, Hawkinson RW. Influence of inoculum growth phase on microdilution susceptibility tests. *J Clin Microbiol* 1983;18:645–651.
19. Barry AL, Jones RN, Gavan TL. Evaluation of the micromedia system for quantitative antimicrobial drug susceptibility testing: a collaborative study. *Antimicrob Agents Chemother* 1978;13:61–69.
20. Barry AL, Joyce LJ, Adams AP, et al. Rapid determination of antimicrobial susceptibility for urgent clinical situations. *Am J Clin Pathol* 1973;59:693–699.
21. Barry AL, Lasner RA. Inhibition of bacterial growth by the nitrofurantoin solvent dimethylformamide. *Antimicrob Agents Chemother* 1976;9:549–550.
22. Barry AL, Thornsberry C, Jones RN, et al. Cefuroxime, an in vitro comparison with six other cephalosporins. *Proc R Soc Med* 1977;70(Suppl 9):63–71.
23. Bartlett JG. *Campylobacter pylori*: fact or fancy. *Gastroenterology* 1988;94:229–232.
24. Bartlett RC, Mazens MF. Rapid antimicrobial susceptibility test using tetrazolium reduction. *Antimicrob Agents Chemother* 1979;15:769–774.
25. Bauer AW, Kirby WMM, Sherris JC, et al. Antibiotic susceptibility testing by a standardized single disk method. *Am J Clin Pathol* 1966;45:493–496.
26. Bauer AW, Sherris JC. The determination of sulfonamide susceptibility of bacteria. *Chemotherapia* 1964;9:1–19.
27. Binford JS Jr, Binford LF, Adler P. A semiautomated microcalorimetric method of antibiotic sensitivity testing. *Am J Clin Pathol* 1973;59:86–94.
28. Blaser J, Staone BB, Groner MC, et al. Comparative study with enoxacin and netilmicin in a pharmacodynamic model to determine importance of ratio of antibiotic peak concentration to MCI for bactericidal activity and emergence of resistance. *Antimicrob Agents Chemother* 1987;31:1054–1060.
29. Blondeau JM, Zhao X, Hansen G, et al. Mutant prevention concentrations of fluoroquinolones for clinical isolates of *Streptococcus pneumoniae*. *Antimicrob Agents Chemother* 2001;45:433–438.
30. Blumberg PM, Strominger JL. Interaction of penicillin with the bacterial cell: penicillin-binding proteins and penicillin-sensitive enzymes. *Bacteriol Rev* 1974;38:291–335.
31. Bowie WR. Lack of in vitro activity of cefoxitin,

cefamandole, cefuroxime, and piperacillin against *Chlamydia trachomatis. Antimicrob Agents Chemother* 1982;21:339–340.

32. Brook I. Inoculum effect. *Rev Infect Dis* 1989;11:361–368.
33. Brown WJ, Sautter RC. Five-hr minimal inhibitory concentration test of four antimicrobial agents for *Pseudomonas aeruginosa. Antimicrob Agents Chemother* 1977;11:1064–1066.
34. Brumfitt W, Percival A. Laboratory control of antibiotic therapy in urinary tract infection. *Ann NY Acad Sci* 1967;145:329–343.
35. Cady P. Progress in impedance measurements in microbiology. In: Sharpe AN, Clarke DS, eds. *Mechanizing microbiology.* Springfield, IL: Charles C Thomas, 1978:199–239.
36. Cady PS, Dufour W, Draeger SJ. Electrical impedance measurements: rapid method for detecting and monitoring microorganisms. *J Clin Microbiol* 1978;7:265–272.
37. Chapman SW, Steigbigel RT. Staphylococcal β-lactamase and efficacy of β-lactam antibiotics: in vitro and in vivo evaluation. *J Infect Dis* 1983;143:1078–1089.
38. Chappelle EW, Levin GV. Use of firefly bioluminescent reaction for rapid detection and counting of bacteria. *Biochem Med* 1968;2:41–52.
39. Chow BF, McKee CM. Interaction between crystalline penicillin and human plasma proteins. *Science* 1945;101:67–68.

39a. Chung E, Amsden GW, Nafzinger AN, Bertino Jr JS. The application of pharmacodynamics in the optimization of antibiotic therapy. Formulary 2003;38:294–319.

40. Clark H, Turck M. In vitro and in vivo evaluation of cephalexin. *Antimicrob Agents Chemother* 1969;8:296–301.
41. College of American Pathologists. *Proficiency survey program: College of American Pathologists surveys final critique for set D-A 199.* Northfield, IL: College of American Pathologists, 1991.
42. Colvin HJ, Sherris JC. Electrical impedance measurements in the reading and monitoring of broth dilution susceptibility tests. *Antimicrob Agents Chemother* 1977;2:61–66.
43. Cooksey RC, Swenson JM. In vitro antimicrobial inhibition patterns of nutritionally variant streptococci. *Antimicrob Agents Chemother* 1979;16:514–518.
44. Corrado ML, Landesman SH, Cherubin CE. Influence of inoculum size on activity of cefoperazone, cefotaxime, moxalactam, piperacillin, and N-formimidoyl thienamycin (MK 0787) against *Pseudomonas aeruginosa. Antimicrob Agents Chemother* 1980;18:893–896.
45. Coudron PE, Stratton CW. Factors affecting growth and susceptibility testing of *Helicobacter pylori* in liquid media. *J Clin Microbiol* 1995;33:1028–1030.
46. Craig WA, Gudmundsson S. The postantibiotic effect. In: Lorian V, ed. *Antibiotics in laboratory medicine.* 2nd ed. Baltimore: Williams & Wilkins, 1985:515–536.
47. Dall LR, Herndon BL. Association of cell-adherent glycocalyx and endocarditis production by viridans group streptococci. *J Clin Microbiol* 1990;28:1698–1700.
48. D'Amatò RF, Hochstein L, Vernaleg JR, et al. Evaluation of the BIOGRAM antimicrobial susceptibility test system. *J Clin Microbiol* 1985;22:793–798.
49. de la Maza K, Miller ST, Ferraro MJ. Use of commercially available rapid chloramphenicol acetyltransferase test to detect resistance in *Salmonella* species. *J Clin Microbiol* 1990;28:1867–1869.
50. Debets-Ossenkopp YJ, Namarar F, MacLaren DM. Effect of an acidic environment on the susceptibility of *Helicobacter pylori* to trospectomycin and other antimicrobial agents. *Eur J Clin Microbiol Infect Dis* 1995;14:353–355.
51. DeLand FH, Wagner HN Jr. Early detection of bacterial growth with carbon 14-labeled glucose. *Radiology* 1969;92:154–155.
52. DeLand F, Wagner HN Jr. Automated radiometric detection of bacterial growth in blood culture. *J Lab Clin Med* 1970;75:529–534.
53. Dillon LK, Howe SE. Early detection of oxacillin-resistant staphylococcal strains with hypertonic broth diluent for microdilution panels. *J Clin Microbiol* 1984;19:473–476.
54. Doern GV, Jorgensen JH, Thornsberry C, et al. National collaborative study of the prevalence of antimicrobial resistance among clinical isolates of *Haemophilus influenzae. Antimicrob Agents Chemother* 1988;32:180–185.
55. Doern GV, Scott DR, Rashad AL. Clinical impact of rapid antimicrobial susceptibility testing of blood culture isolates. *Antimicrob Agents Chemother* 1982;21:1023–1024.
56. Doern GV, Vaator R, Gaudet M, et al. Clinical impact of rapid in vitro susceptibility testing and bacterial identification. *J Clin Microbiol* 1994;32:1757–1762.
57. Dong Y, Zhao X, Kreisworth BN, et al. Mutant prevention concentration as a measure of antibiotic potency: Studies with clinical isolates of *Mycobacterium tuberculosis. Antimicrob Agents Chemother* 2000;44:2581–2584.
58. Dormer AE. The treatment of bacterial endocarditis. *Br Med Bull* 1960;16:61–66.
59. Dougherty PF, Yotter DW, Matthews TR. Chemically defined medium for susceptibility testing of antimicrobial agents. *Antimicrob Agents Chemother* 1976;10:923–925.
60. Drobot GR, Karlowsky JA, Hoban DJ, et al. Antibiotic activity in microbiological media versus that in human urine: comparison of ampicillin, ciprofloxacin, and trimethoprim-sulfamethoxazole. *Antimicrob Agents Chemother* 1996;40:237–240.
61. Drusano GL, Johnson DE, Rosen M, et al. Pharmacodynamics of a fluoroquinolone antimicrobial agent in a neutropenic rat model of *Pseudomonas sepsis. Antimicrob Agents Chemother* 1993;37:483–90.
62. Drusano GL, Preston SL, Hardalo C, et al. Use of preclinical data for selection of a phase II/III dose for evernimicin and identification of a preclinical MIC breakpoint. *Antimicrob Agents Chemother* 2001;45:13–22.
63. Duan K, Dammel C, Stein J, et al. Modulation of *Pseudomonas aeruginosa* gene expression by host microflora through interspecies communication. *Molec Microbiol* 2003;50:1477–1491.
64. Dugan DL, Wright DN. Quantitative infrared photoanalysis of selected bacteria. *Appl Microbiol* 1974;28:205–211.
65. Duguid JP. The sensitivity of bacteria to the action of penicillin. *Edinb Med J* 1946;53:401–412.
66. Eagle H, Musselman A. The rate of bactericidal action of penicillin in vitro as a function of its concentration, and its paradoxically reduced activity at high concentrations against certain organisms. *J Exp Med* 1948;88:99–131.
67. Eickhoff TC, Ehret JM. In vitro comparison of cefoxitin, cefamandole, cephalexin, and cephalothin. *Antimicrob Agents Chemother* 1976;9:994–999.
68. Elder LB, Hansen SA, Kellogg JA, et al. *Verification and validation of procedures in the clinical microbiology laboratory Cumitech 31.* Washington, DC: ASM Press, 1997.
69. Eliopoulos GM, Reiszner E, Willey S, et al. Effect of blood product medium supplements on the activity of cefotaxime and other cephalosporins against *Enterococcus faecalis. Diagn Microbiol Infect Dis* 1989;12:149–156.
70. Elwell LP, DeGraff J, Seibert D, et al. Plasmid-linked ampicillin resistance in *Haemophilus influenzae* type b. *Infect Immun* 1975;12:404–410.
71. Elwell LP, Roberts M, Mayer L, et al. Plasmid-mediated β-lactamase production in *Neisseria gonorrhoeae. Antimicrob Agents Chemother* 1977;11:533–538.
72. Emerson BB, Smith AL, Harding AL, et al. *Haemophilus*

influenzae type B susceptibility of seventeen antibiotics. *Pediatrics* 1975;86:617–620.

73. Eng RHK, Cherubin CM, Smith SM, et al. Inoculum effect of β-lactam antibiotics on Enterobacteriaceae. *Antimicrob Agents Chemother* 1985;28:601–606.
74. Ericsson HM, Sherris JC. Antibiotic sensitivity testing: report of an international collaborative study. *Acta Pathol Microbiol Scand* 1971;217(suppl B):390.
75. Fass RJ, Barnishan J. Effect of divalent cation concentrations on the antibiotic susceptibilities of nonfermenters other than *Pseudomonas aeruginosa*. *Antimicrob Agents Chemother* 1979;16:434–438.
76. *Federal Register*. Rules and regulations: antibiotic susceptibility disks: correction. *Fed Reg* 1973;38:2576.
77. *Federal Register*. Rules and regulations: antibiotic susceptibility discs. *Fed Reg* 1972;37:20525–20529.
78. Ferone RS, Bushby RM, Burchall JJ, et al. Identification of Harper-Cawston factor as thymidine phosphorylase and removal from media of substances interfering with susceptibility testing to sulfonamides and diaminopyrimidines. *Antimicrob Agents Chemother* 1975;7:91–98.
79. Flaherty KR, Saint S, Fendrick AM, et al. The spectrum of acute bronchitis. *Postgrad Med* 2001;109:39–47.
80. Fleming A. On the antibacterial action of cultures of a penicillium with special reference to their use in the isolation of *B. influenzae*. *Br J Exp Pathol* 1929;10:226–236.
81. Forrest A, Nix DE, Ballow CH, et al. Pharmacodynamics of intravenous ciprofloxacin in seriously ill patients. *Antimicrob Agents Chemother* 1993;37:1073–1081.
82. Foster JW, Woodruff HB. Microbiological aspects of penicillin. *J Bacteriol* 1943;46:187–202.
83. Gardner AD. Morphological effects of penicillin on bacteria. *Nature* 1940;146:837–838.
84. Garrod LP, Lambert HP, O'Grady R, eds. *Antibiotics and chemotherapy*. Edinburgh: Churchill Livingstone, 1973:490–531.
85. Garrod LP, Waterworth PM. Effect of medium composition on the apparent sensitivity of *Pseudomonas aeruginosa* to gentamicin. *J Clin Pathol* 1969;22:534–538.
86. Gavan TL. Broth dilution methods. In: Gavan TL, Cheatle EL, McFadden HW, eds. *Antimicrobial susceptibility testing*. Chicago: American Society of Clinical Pathology, 1971:105–124.
87. Gavan TL, Barry AL. Microdilution test procedures. In: Lennette EH, Spaulding EH, Truant JP, eds. *Manual of clinical microbiology,* 3rd ed. Washington, DC: American Society for Microbiology, 1980:359–362.
88. Gavan TL, Butler D. An automated microdilution method for antimicrobial susceptibility testing. In: Balows A, ed. *Current techniques for antibiotic susceptibility testing*. Springfield, IL: Charles C Thomas, 1973:88–93.
89. Gavan TL, Jones RN, Barry AL. Evaluation of the Sensititre system for quantitative antimicrobial drug susceptibility testing: a collaborative study. *Antimicrob Agents Chemother* 1980;17:464–469.
90. Georgopapadakou NH, Liu FY. Binding of β-lactam antibiotics to penicillin-binding proteins of *Staphylococcus aureus* and *Streptococcus faecalis*: relation to antibacterial activity. *Antimicrob Agents Chemother* 1980;18:834–836.
91. Gerlach EH. Microdilution, I: A comparative study. In: Balows A, ed. *Current techniques for antibiotic susceptibility testing*. Springfield, IL: Charles C Thomas, 1973: 63–76.
92. Gerlach EH. Dilution test procedures for susceptibility testing. In: Bondi A, Bartola JT, Prier JD, eds. *The clinical laboratory as an aid in chemotherapy of infectious disease*. Baltimore: University Park Press, 1977:45–50.
93. Goldstein EJC, Cherubin CE, Shulman M. Comparison of microtiter broth dilution and agar dilution methods for susceptibility testing of *Eikenella corrodens*. *Antimicrob Agents Chemother* 1983;23:42–45.
94. Grayson ML, Eliopoulos GM, Ferraro MJ, et al. Effect of varying pH on the susceptibility of *Campylobacter pylori* to antimicrobial agents. *Eur J Clin Microbiol Infect Dis* 1989;8:888–889.
95. Greenwood D, Eley A. A turbidimetric study of the responses of selected strains of *Pseudomonas aeruginosa* to eight antipseudomonal β-lactam antibiotics. *J Infect Dis* 1982;145:110–117.
96. Grove DC, Randall WA. *Assay methods of antibiotics: methods for the determination of bacterial susceptibility to antibiotics*. New York: Medical Encyclopedia, 1955.
97. Hacek DM, Dressel DC, Peterson LR. Highly reproducible bactericidal activity test results by using a modified rational committee for clinical laboratory standards broth microdilution technique. *J Clin Microbiol* 1999;37:1881–1884.
98. Hammerschlag M, Gleyzer A. In vitro activity of a group of broad-spectrum cephalosporins and other β-lactam antibiotics against *Chlamydia trachomatis*. *Antimicrob Agents Chemother* 1983;23:493–494.
99. Handwerger S, Tomasz A. Antibiotic tolerance among clinical isolates of bacteria. *Rev Infect Dis* 1985;7:368–386.
100. Hobby GL, Meyer K, Chaffee E. Observations on the mechanism of action of penicillin. *Proc Soc Exp Biol Med* 1942;50:281–285.
101. Hoeprich PD, Barry AL, Fay GD. Synthetic medium for susceptibility testing. *Antimicrob Agents Chemother* 1970;1969:494–497.
102. Howard MC, Miyajima A, Coffman R. T-cell derived cytokines and their receptors. In: Paul WE, ed. *Fundamental immunology,* 3rd ed. New York: Raven Press, 1993:763–800.
103. Inderlied CB, Young LS. Radiometric in vitro susceptibility testing of *Mycobacterium tuberculosis*. *Antimicrob Newslett* 1986;3:55–60.
104. Jackson GG, Finland M. Comparison of methods for determining sensitivity of bacteria to antibiotics in vitro. *Arch Intern Med* 1951;88:446–460.
105. James PA. Comparison of four methods for the determination of MIC and MBC of penicillin for viridans streptococci and the implications for penicillin tolerance. *J Antimicrob Chemother* 1990;25:209–216.
106. Jao RL, Finland M. Susceptibility of *Mycoplasma pneumoniae* to 21 antibiotics in vitro. *Am J Med Sci* 1967;253:639–650.
107. Jay VA, Sherris JC. In: Ericcson H, Sherris J, eds. 1965.
108. Johnston Laboratories. Drug susceptibility of *M. tuberculosis* cultures by the Bactec system: Bactec data JL1—664. In: *Bactec news*. Cockeysville, MD: Johnston Laboratories, 1979.
109. Jones RN, Barry AL, Gavan TL, et al. Susceptibility tests: microdilution and macrodilution broth procedures. In: Lennette EH, Balows A, Hausler WJ Jr, et al., eds. *Manual of clinical microbiology,* 4th ed. Washington, DC: American Society for Microbiology, 1985.
110. Jones RN, Gavan TL, Barry AL. Evaluation of the Sensititre microdilution antibiotic susceptibility system against recent clinical isolates: three-laboratory collaborative study. *J Clin Microbiol* 1980;11:426–429.
111. Jones RN, Gavan TL, Thornsberry C, et al. Standardization of disk diffusion and agar dilution susceptibility tests for *Neiserria gonorrhoeae*: interpretive criteria and quality control guidelines for ceftriaxone, penicillin, spectinomycin, and tetracycline. *J Clin Microbiol* 1989;27:2758–2766.
112. Jones RN, Thornsberry C, Barry AL, et al. Evaluation of the Sceptor microdilution investigation. *J Clin Microbiol* 1981;13:184–194.

113. Jorgensen JH. Antimicrobial susceptibility testing of *Haemophilus influenzae*: an update. *Antimicrob Newslett* 1989;6:65–68.
114. Jorgensen JH, Doern GV, Thornsberry C, et al. Susceptibility of mutliple-resistant *Haemophilus influenzae* to newer antimicrobial agents. *Diagn Microbiol Infect Dis* 1988;9:27–32.
115. Jorgensen JH, Lee JC, Jones PM. Chemically defined antimicrobial susceptibility test medium for *Pseudomonas aeruginosa*. *Antimicrob Agents Chemother* 1977;11:415–419.
116. Jorgensen JH, Redding JS, Maher LA, et al. Improved medium for antimicrobial susceptibility testing of *Haemophilus influenzae*. *J Clin Microbiol* 1987;25:2105–2113.
117. Kavanagh F. *Analytical microbiology*. New York: Academic Press, 1963.
118. Kenny MA, Pollock HM, Minshew BH, et al. Cation components of Mueller-Hinton agar affecting testing of *Pseudomonas aeruginosa* susceptibility to gentamicin. *Antimicrob Agents Chemother* 1980;17:55–62.
119. Kind AC, Kestle DG, Standiford HC, et al. Laboratory and clinical experience with cephalexin. *Antimicrob Agents Chemother* 1969;8:361–365.
120. Kollef MH, Sherman G, Ward S, et al. Inadequate antimicrobial treatment of infections: a risk factor for hospital mortality among critically ill patients. *Chest* 1999;115:462–474.
121. Kushner I. Regulation of the acute phase response by cytokines. In: Oppenheim JJ, Rossio JL, Geaniny AH, eds. *Clinical application of cytokines*. New York: Oxford University Press, 1993:27–34.
122. LaForce FM. Pneumonia3—41987: new developments. *Eur J Clin Microbiol* 1987;6:613–617.
123. Lamb JW, Mann JM, Simmons RJ. Factors influencing the microbiological assay of tobramycin. *Antimicrob Agents Chemother* 1972;1:323–328.
124. Lampe MR, Aitken CL, Dennis PG, et al. Relationship of early readings of minimal inhibitory concentrations to the results of overnight tests. *Antimicrob Agents Chemother* 1975;8:429–433.
125. Lebek G, Zund P. R-factors affecting host generation time: their influence on sensitivity testing. *Infection* 1981;9:76.
126. Levin GV. Rapid microbiological determinations with radioisotopes. *Adv Appl Microbiol* 1963;5:95–133.
127. Levin GV, Hein AH, Clendenning JR, et al. Gulliver: a quest for life on Mars. *Science* 1962;138:114–121.
128. Livermore DM, Winstanley TG, Shannon KP. Interpretative reading: recognizing the unusual and inferring resistance mechanisms from resistant phenotypes. *J Antimicrobial Chemother* 2001;48(Suppl 1):87–102.
129. Longsworth LG. The estimation of bacterial populations with the aid of a photoelectric densitometer. *J Bacteriol* 1936;32:307–328.
130. Lorian V. *Antibiotics and chemotherapeutic agents in clinical and laboratory practice*. Springfield, IL: Charles C Thomas, 1966.
131. Lorian V. Some effects on subinhibitory concentrations of antibiotics on bacteria. *Bull NY Acad Med* 1975;51:1046–1055.
132. Lorian V. Effect of low antibiotic concentrations on bacteria. In: Lorian V, ed. *Antibiotics in laboratory medicine*, 2nd ed. Baltimore: Williams & Wilkins, 1986:596–668.
133. Lorian V. *In vitro* simulation of in vivo conditions: physical state of the culture medium. *J Clin Microbiol* 1989;27:2403–2406.
134. Lorian V, Burns L. Predictive value of susceptibility tests for the outcome of antibacterial therapy. *J Antimicrob Chemother* 1990;25:175–181.
135. Lorian V, Sabath LD. Effect of pH on the activity of erythromycin against 500 isolates of Gram-negative bacilli. *Appl Microbiol* 1970;20:754–756.
136. Lorian V, Waluschka A, Carruth C, et al. A five-hour disc susceptibility test. In: Lorian V, ed. *The significance of medical microbiology in the care of patients*. Baltimore: Williams & Wilkins, 1982.
137. Luna CM, Vujacich P, Niederman MS, et al. Impact of BAL data on the therapy and outcome of ventilator-associated pneumonia. *Chest* 1997;111:676–685.
138. Luria SE. A test for penicillin sensitivity and resistance in *Staphylococcus*. *Proc Soc Exp Biol Med* 1946;61:46–51.
139. Lynch JP III, Fernandez JM. Clinical relevance of macrolide-resistant *Streptococcus pneumoniae* for community-acquired pneumonia. *Clin Infect Dis* 2002; 34(Suppl 1):S27–S46.
140. MacArthur RD, Miller M, Albertson T, et al. Adequacy of early antimicrobic antibiotic treatment and survival in severe sepsis: experience from the MONARCS trial. 2004;38:284–288.
141. Mackowiak RA, Marling-Cason M, Cohen RL. Effects of temperature on antimicrobial susceptibility of bacteria. *J Infect Dis* 1982;145:550–555.
142. MacLowry JD, Jaqua MJ, Selepak ST. Detailed methodology and implementation of a semi-automated serial dilution microtechnique for antimicrobial susceptibility testing. *Appl Microbiol* 1970;20:46–53.
143. MacLowry JD, Young MJ, Selepak ST, et al. A semiautomated microtechnique for serial dilution antimicrobial sensitivity testing in the clinical laboratory. *Int J Clin Pharmacol* 1970;3:70–72.
144. Mardh PA, Anderson KE, Wadso I. Kinetics of the actions of tetracyclines on *Escherichia coli* as studied by microcalorimetry. *Antimicrob Agents Chemother* 1976;10:604–609.
145. Matsen J, Koepcke M, Quie P. Evaluation of the Bauer-Kirby-Sherris-Turck and single-disk diffusion methods of antibiotic susceptibility testing. *Antimicrob Agents Chemother* 1970;9:445–453.
146. McDonald PJ, Craig WA, Kunin CM. Brief antibiotic exposure and effect on bacterial growth. In: Williams JD, Geddes AM, eds. *Chemotherapy*, Vol. 2. New York: Plenum Press, 1976:95–102.
147. McDougal LK, Thornsberry C. The role of β-lactamase in staphylococcal resistance to penicillinase-resistant penicillins and cephalosporins. *J Clin Microbiol* 1986;23:832–839.
148. McFarland J. The nephelometer: an instrument for estimating the numbers of bacteria in suspensions used for calculating the opsonic index and for vaccines. *JAMA* 1907;49:1176–1178.
149. McMaster PRB, Robertson E, Witebsky F, et al. Evaluation of a dispensing instrument (Dynatech MIC-2000) for preparing microtiter antibiotic plates and testing potency during storage. *Antimicrob Agents Chemother* 1978;13:842–844.
150. McNulty CAM, Dent J, Wise R. Susceptibility of clinical isolates of *Campylobacter pyloridis* to 11 antimicrobial agents. *Antimicrob Agents Chemother* 1985;28:837–838.
151. Medeiros AA, O'Brien T, Wacker WEC, et al. Effect of salt concentration on the apparent in vitro susceptibility of *Pseudomonas* and other Gram-negative bacilli to gentamicin. *J Infect Dis* 1971;124(Suppl):S59–S64.
152. Meylan PR, Francioli P, Glauser MP. Discrepancies between MBC and actual killing of viridans group streptococci by cell-wall-active antibiotics. *Antimicrob Agents Chemother* 1986;29:418–423.
153. Miller JM, Andersen BV, Caudill SP. New quality control frequency guidelines for antimicrobic susceptibility testing. *Antimicrob Newslett* 1986;3:77–79.

154. Minami S, Yotsuji A, Inoue M, et al. Induction of β-lactamase by various β-lactam antibiotics in *Enterobacter cloacae*. *Antimicrob Agents Chemother* 1980;18:382–385.
155. Mitruka BM. *Gas chromatographic applications in microbiology and medicine*. New York: John Wiley and Sons, 1975.
156. Moellering RC, Wennersten C, Medrek T, et al. Prevalence of high level resistance to aminoglycosides in clinical isolates of enterococci. *Antimicrob Agents Chemother* 1970;10:335–340.
157. Mohr JF, Wanger A, Rex JH. Pharmacokinetic/pharmacodynamic modeling can help guide targeted antimicrobial therapy for nosocomial Gram-negative infections in critically ill patients. *Diag Microbiol Infect Dis* 2004;48:125–130.
158. Mouton JW. Breakpoints: current practice and future perspectives. *Int J Antimicrobial Agents* 2002;19:323–331.
159. Mueller JH, Hinton J. A protein-free medium for the primary isolation of the gonococcus and meningococcus. *Proc Soc Exp Biol Med* 1941;48:330–333.
160. Murray PR, Niles AC. Effect of filtration on antimicrobial solutions. *Antimicrob Agents Chemother* 1981;20:686–687.
161. National Committee for Clinical Laboratory Standards. *Proposed guidelines for pharmaceutical and susceptibility test reagent manufacturers*. Villanova, PA: National Committee for Clinical Laboratory Standards, 1986.NCCLS document M23-P.
162. National Center for Infectious Diseases. *Flow cytometric immunophenotyping procedure manual*. Atlanta: US Department of Health and Human Services, 1993.
163. National Committee for Clinical Laboratory Standards. *Protocols for evaluating dehydrated Mueller-Hinton agar.* Villanova, PA: National Committee for Clinical Laboratory Standards, 1996. NCCLS document M6-A.
164. National Committee for Clinical Laboratory Standards. *Methodology for the serum bactericidal test*. Wayne, PA: National Committee for Clinical Laboratory Standards, 1999. NCCLS document M21-A.
165. National Committee for Clinical Laboratory Standards. *Methods for determining bactericidal activity of antimicrobial agents*. Wayne, PA: National Committee for Clinical Laboratory Standards, 1999. NCCLS document M26-A.
166. National Committee for Clinical Laboratory Standards. *Evaluation of lots of Mueller-Hinton broth for antimicrobial susceptibility testing: proposed guideline*. Wayne, PA: National Committee for Clinical Laboratory Standards, 2001. NCCLS document M32-P.
167. National Committee for Clinical Laboratory Standards. *Methods for dilution antimicrobial susceptibility tests for bacteria that grow aerobically: approved standard*. 6th ed. Wayne, PA: National Committee for Clinical Laboratory Standards. 2003. NCCLS document M7-A6
168. National Committee for Clinical Laboratory Standards. *Performance standards for antimicrobial disk susceptibility tests: approved standard*. 8th ed. Wayne, PA: National Committee for Clinical Laboratory Standards, 2003. NCCLS document M2-A8.
169. Needham CA. *Haemophilus influenzae*: antibiotic susceptibility. *Clin Microbiol Rev* 1988;1:218–227.
170. Neu H. Mecillinam, a novel penicillanic acid derivative with unusual activity against Gram-negative bacteria. *Antimicrob Agents Chemother* 1976;9:973–999.
171. Neu HC. Penicillins: new insights into their mechanisms of activity and clinical use. *Bull NY Acad Med* 1982;58:681–695.
172. Neu HC. Penicillin-binding proteins and role of amdinocillin in causing bacterial cell death. *Am J Med* 1983; 75(Suppl 2A):9–20.
173. Neussel H. Problems of standardization of media. In: Williams JD, Geddes AM, eds. *Chemotherapy*. New York: Plenum Press, 1976:2.
174. Nicolle Norden MA, Kurzyski TA, Bounds SE, et al. Rapid susceptibility testing of *Mycobacterium tuberculosis* (H37Ra) by flow cytometry. *J Clin Microbiol* 1995;33:1231–1237.

174a. Nicolle LE. Measurement and significance of antibiotic activity in the urine. In: Lorian V, ed. Antibiotics in laboratory medicine 4th ed. Baltimore: Williams & Wilkins 1986:793–812.

175. Pillai SK, Sakoulas G, Gold HS, et al. Prevalence of the fsr locus in *Enterococcus faecalis* infections. *J Clin Microbiol* 2002;40:2651–2652.
176. Pore RS. Antibiotic susceptibility testing by flow cytometry. *J Antimicrob Chemother* 1994;34:613–627.
177. Preston SL, Drusano GL, Berman AL, et al. Pharmacodynamics of levofloxacin: a new paradigm for early clinical trials. *JAMA* 1998;279:125–129.
178. Prober CG, Yeager AS. Use of the serum bactericidal titer to assess the adequacy of oral antibiotic therapy in the treatment of acute hematogenous osteomyelitis. *J Pediatr* 1979;95:131–135.
179. Pulliam L, Dall L, Inokuchi S, et al. Effects of exopolysaccharide production by viridans streptococci on penicillin therapy of experimental endocarditis. *J Infect Dis* 1985;151:153–156.
180. Pursiano TA, Misiek M, Leitner F, et al. Effect of assay medium on the antibacterial activity of certain penicillins and cephalosporins. *Antimicrob Agents Chemother* 1973;3:33–39.
181. Qin X, Singh KV, Weinstock GM, et al. Effects of *Enterococcus faecalis fsr* genes on production of gelatinase and a serine protease and virulence. *Infect Immun* 200;68:2579–2586.
182. Rammelkamp CH, Maxon T. Resistance of *Staphylococcus aureus* to the action of penicillin. *Proc Soc Exp Biol Med* 1942;51:386–389.
183. Rasheed JK, Tenover FC. Detection and characterization of antimicrobial resistance genes in bacteria. In: Murray PR, Baron EJ, Pfaller MA, et al. eds. *Manual of clinical microbiology,* 8th ed. Washington, DC: ASM Press, 2003:1196–1212.
184. Reimer LG, Stratton C, Reller LB. Minimum inhibitory and bactericidal concentrations of 44 antimicrobial agents against three standard control strains in broth with and without human serum. *Antimicrob Agents Chemother* 1981;19:1050–1055.
185. Reller LB, Schoenknecht FD, Kenny MA, et al. Antibiotic susceptibility testing of *Pseudomonas aeruginosa*: selection of a control strain and criteria for magnesium and calcium content in media. *J Infect Dis* 1974;130:454–463.
186. Rex JH, Pfaller MA. Has antifungal susceptibility come of age? *Clin Infect Dis* 2002;35:982–989.
187. Richmond MH, Sykes RB. The β-lactamases of Gram-negative bacteria and their possible physiological role. In: Rose AH, Tempesti DW, eds. *Advances in microbiology and physiology*. Vol. 9. Academic Press, 1973:31–88.
188. Sabath LD, Lorian V, Gerstein D, et al. Enhancing effect on alkalinization of the medium on the activity of erythromycin against Gram-negative bacteria. *Appl Microbiol* 1968;16:1288–1292.
189. Sabath LD, Wheeler N, Laverdiere M, et al. A new type of penicillin resistance of *S. aureus*. *Lancet* 1977;1:443–447.
190. Sakoulas G, Eliopoulos GM, Moellering RC Jr, et al. *Staphylococcus aureus* accessory gene regulator (agr) group II: is there a relationship to the development of intermediate-level glycopeptide resistance? *J Clin Infect Dis* 2003;187:929–938.

191. Sande MA. Antibiotic therapy of bacterial meningitis: lessons we've learned. *Am J Med* 1981;7:507–510.
192. Sanders CC, Sanders WE. Emergence of resistance to cefamandole: possible role of cefoxitin-inducible β-lactamases. *Antimicrob Agents Chemother* 1979;7: 1521.
193. Sanders CC, Sanders WE. Emergence of resistance during therapy with newer β-lactam antibiotics: role of inducible β-lactamases and implications for the future. *Rev Infect Dis* 1983;5:639–648.
194. Scavizzi MR, Bronner FD. A statistical model for the interpretation of antibiotic susceptibility tests. *Int J Exp Clin Chemother* 1988;1:23–42.
195. Schifman RB, Pindur A, Bryan JA. Laboratory practices for reporting bacterial susceptibility tests that affect antibiotic therapy. *Arch Pathol Lab Med* 1997;121:1168–1170.
196. Schlichter JG, MacLean H. A method of determining the effective therapeutic level in the treatment of subacute bacterial endocariditis with penicillin. *Am Heart J* 1947;34:209–211.
197. Schoenknecht FD, Sabath LD, Thornsberry C. Susceptibility tests: special tests. In: Lennette EH, Balows A, Hausler WH Jr, et al. eds. *Manual of clinical microbiology,* 3rd ed. Washington, DC: American Society for Microbiology, 1985:1000–1008.
198. Sculier JP, Klastersky J. Significance of serum bactericidal activity in gram-negative bacillary bacteremia in patients with and without granulocytopenia. *Am J Med* 1984;76:429–435.
199. Seligman SJ, Hewitt WL. Resistance to penicillins and cephalosporins. *Antimicrob Agents Chemother* 1965; 5:387–391.
200. Sellers W. Antibiotic sensitivity testing. In: Graber CD, ed. *Rapid diagnostic methods in medical microbiology.* Baltimore: Williams & Wilkins, 1970:163–178.
201. Selwyn S, Lam C. Combined effect on protein-binding and β-lactamases on the activity of penicillins and cephalosporins. In: Williams JD, Gedes AM, eds. *Chemotherapy.* Vol. 2. New York: Plenum Press, 1976:325–330.
202. Shapiro HM. *Practical flow cytometry,* 2nd ed. New York: Alan R. Liss, 1988.
203. Sherris JC. Problems in in vitro determination of antibiotic tolerance in clinical isolates. *Antimicrob Agents Chemother* 1986;30:633–637.
204. Sherris JC, Rashad AL, Lighthart GA. Laboratory determination of antibiotic susceptibility to ampicillin and cephalothin. *Ann NY Acad Sci* 1967;145:248–267.
205. Shungu DL. Chemical and physical properties of antibiotics: preparation and control of antibiotic susceptibility disk and other devices containing antibiotics. In: Lorian V. ed. *Antibiotics in laboratory medicine,* 4th ed., Baltimore: William & Wilkins, 1995:766–792.
206. Small PM, Chambers HF. Vancomycin for *Staphylococcus aureus* endocarditis in intravenous drug users. *Antimicrob Agents Chemother* 1990;34:1227–1231.
207. Smith TF. *In vitro* susceptibility of *Ureaplasma urealyticum* to rosaramicin. *Antimicrob Agents Chemother* 1979;16:106–108.
208. Sorensen RH. Rapid antibiotic sensitivity test using a redox indicator. *Med Technol Bull* 1959;10:144–148.
209. Spaepern MS, Kundsin RB. Simple direct broth-disk method for antibiotic susceptibility testing of *Ureaplasma urealyticum*. *Antimicrob Agents Chemother* 1977;11:267–270.
210. Spratt BG. Distinct penicillin binding proteins involved in the division, elongation, and shape of *Escherichia coli*, K 12. *Proc Natl Acad Sci USA* 1975;72:2999–3003.
211. Spratt BG. Properties of the penicillin-binding proteins of *Escherichia coli* K 12. *Eur J Biochem* 1977;72:341–352.
212. Spratt BG. Biochemical and genetical approaches to the mechanism of action of penicillin. *Philos Trans R Soc Lond [Biol]* 1980;289:273–283.
213. Staneck JL, Allen SD, Harris EE, et al. Automated reading of MIC microdilution trays containing fluorogenic enzyme substrates with the Sensititre autoreader. *J Clin Microbiol* 1985;22:187–191.
214. Stevens DL, Higbee JW, Oberhofer TR, et al. Antibiotic susceptibilities of human isolates of *Pasteurella multocida. Antimicrob Agents Chemother* 1979;16:322–324.
215. Stratton CW. The usefulness of the serum bactericidal test in orthopedic infections. *Orthopedics* 1984;7:1579–1580.
216. Stratton CW. Serum bactericidal test. *Clin Microbiol Rev* 1988;1:1926.
217. Stratton CW, Weinstein MP, Reller LB. Correlation of serum bactericidal activity with antimicrobial agent level and minimal bactericidal concentration. *J Infect Dis* 1982;145:160–168.
218. Stull VR. Clinical laboratory use of differential light scattering, I: Antibiotic susceptibility testing. *Clin Chem* 1973;19:883–890.
219. Swenson JM, Hindler JF, Jorgensen JH. Special phenotypic methods for detecting antibacterial resistance. In: Murray PR, Baron EJ, Pfaller MA, et al., eds. *Manual of clinical microbiology,* 8th ed. Washington, DC: ASM Press, 2003:1178–1195.
220. Syriopoulou V, Scheifele DW, Sack CM, et al. Effect of inoculum size on the susceptibility of *Haemophilus influenzae* b to β-lactam antibiotics. *Antimicrob Agents Chemother* 1979;16:510–513.
221. Taylor PC, Schoenknecht FD, Sherris JC, et al. Determination of minimum bactericidal concentration of oxacillin for *Staphylococcus aureus*: influence and significance of technical factors. *Antimicrob Agents Chemother* 1983;23:142–150.
222. Tenover FC. Studies of antimicrobial resistance genes using DNA probes. *Antimicrob Agents Chemother* 1986;29:721–725.
223. Tenover FC, Baker CN, Swenson JM. Evaluation of commerical methods for determining antimicrobial susceptibility of *Streptococcus pneumoniae*. *J Clin Microbiol* 1996;34:10–14.
224. Tenover FC, Popovic T, Olsvik O. Genetic methods for detecting antibacterial resistance genes. In: *Manual of clinical microbiology,* 6th ed. Washington, DC: ASM Press, 1995;1368–1378.
225. Then R. Thymidiine and the assessment of co-trimoxazole. In: Williams JD, Geddes AM, eds. *Chemotherapy.* New York: Plenum Press, 1976:2.
226. Thornsberry C. Methicillin-resistant (heteroresistant) staphylococci. *Antimicrob Newslett* 1984;1:43–47.
227. Thornsberry C, Baker CN, Kirven LA, et al. Susceptibility of ampicillin-resistant *Haemophilus influenzae* to seven ampicillins. *Antimicrob Agents Chemother* 1976;9:70–73.
228. Thornsberry C, Gavan TL, Gerlach EH. *New developments in antimicrobial agent susceptibility testing.* Cumitech 6. Washington, DC: American Society for Microbiology, 1977.
229. Thornsberry C, McDougal LK. Successful use of broth microdilution in susceptibility tests for methicillin-resistant (heteroresistant) staphylococci. *J Clin Microbiol* 1983;18:1084–1091.
230. Thornsberry C, Swensen JM, Baker CN, et al. Susceptibility testing of fastidious and unusual pathogens. *Antimicrob Newslett* 1987;4:47–55.

231. Tilton RC, Lieberman L, Gerlach EH. Microdilution antibiotic susceptibility test: examination of certain variables. *Appl Microbiol* 1973;26:658–665.
232. Tilton RC, Newberg L. Standardization of the microdilution susceptibility test. In: Balows A, ed. *Current techniques for antibiotic susceptibility testing*. Springfield, IL: Charles C Thomas Publisher, 1973:77–87.
233. Tipper DJ. Mode of action of beta-lactam antibiotics. In: Queener SF, Webber JA, Queener SW, eds. *Beta-lactam antibiotics for clinical use.* New York: Marcel Dekker Inc, 1986:17–47.
234. Tipper DJ, Wright A. The structure and biosynthesis of bacterial cell walls. In: Sokatch JR, Ornston LN, eds. *Mechanisms of adaptations*. New York: Academic Press, 1979:291–426.
235. Tomasz A. The mechanism of the irreversible antimicrobial effects of penicillins: how the β-lactam antibiotics kill and lyse bacteria. *Annu Rev Microbiol* 1979;33:113–137.
236. Tomasz A. Penicillin-binding proteins and the antibacterial effectiveness of β-lactam antibiotics. *Rev Infect Dis* 1986;8(Suppl 3):S260–S278.
237. Tomasz A, Albino A, Zanati E. Multiple antibiotic resistance in a bacterium with suppressed autolytic system. *Nature* 1970;227:138–140.
238. Trenholme GM, Kaplan RL, Karakusis PH, et al. Clinical impact of rapid identification and susceptibility testing of bacterial blood culture isolates. *J Clin Microbiol* 1989;27:1342–1345.
239. Trissel LA. *Handbook on injectable drugs*. Bethesda, MD: American Society of Hospital Pharmacists, 1983.
240. Tuomanen E. Phenotypic tolerance: the search for β-lactam antibiotics that kill nongrowing bacteria. *Rev Infect Dis* 1986;8(Suppl):S279–S291.
241. Tuomanen E, Durack DT, Tomasz A. Antibiotic tolerance among clinical isolates of bacteria. *Antimicrob Agents Chemother* 1986;30:521–527.
242. Ur A, Brown D. Monitoring of bacterial activity by impedance measurements. In: Heden C, Illeni T, eds. *New approaches to the identification of microorganisms*. New York: John Wiley and Sons, 1975:61–71.
243. Vanhoof R, Gordts B, Diedickx R, et al. Bacteriostatic and bactericidal activities of 24 antimicrobial agents against *Campylobacter fetus* subsp. *jejuni*. *Antimicrob Agents Chemother* 1980;18:118–121.
244. Van Klingeren B, Rutgers A. Usefulness of commercially available media to MIC determinations of trimethoprim. In: Williams JD, Geddes AM, eds. *Chemotherapy*. Vol. 2. New York: Plenum Press, 1976:2.
245. Vincent JG, Vincent HW. Filter paper modification of the Oxford cup penicillin determination. *Proc Soc Exp Biol Med* 1944;55:162–164.
246. Waisbren BA, Carr C, Dunnette J. The tube dilution method of determining bacterial sensitivity to antibiotics. *Am J Clin Pathol* 1951;21:884–891.
247. Washington JA II, Sutter VL. Dilution susceptibility test: agar and macro-broth dilution procedures. In: Lennette EH, Spaulding EH, Truant JI, eds. *Manual of clinical microbiology.* Washington, DC: American Society for Microbiology, 1980:453–458.
248. Washington JA II. *Laboratory procedures in clinical microbiology.* Boston: Little, Brown and Company, 1974.
249. Waterworth PM. In: Reeves DS, Phillips I, Williams JD, et al., eds. *Laboratory methods in chemotherapy.* Edinburgh: Churchill Livingstone, 1978:4
250. Waterworth PM. Sensitivity tests with trimethoprim-sulphonamide. *S Afr Med J* 1970;44(Suppl):10–12.
251. Waxman DJ, Strominger JL. Penicillin-binding proteins and the mechanisms of action of β-lactam antibiotics. *Annu Rev Biochem* 1983;52:825–869.
252. Weinberg ED. The mutual effects of antimicrobial compounds and metallic cations. *Bacteriol Rev* 1957;21:46–68.
253. Wick WE. Influence of antibiotic stability on the results of in vitro testing procedures. *J Bacteriol* 1964;87:1162–1170.
254. Wick WE. Delineation of the differences of various bacterial susceptibility tests with cephalexin. *Antimicrob Agents Chemother* 1969;1968:435–441.
255. Wicks JH, Nelson RL, Krejcarek GE. Rapid inoculum standardization system: a novel device for standardization of inocula in antimicrobial susceptibility testing. *J Clin Microbiol* 1983;17:1114–1119.
256. Wilson WR, Geraci JE. Antibiotic treatment of infective endocarditis. *Annu Rev Med* 1983;34:413–427.
257. Winslow DL, Damme J, Dieckman E. Delayed bactericidal activity of β-lactam antibiotics against *Listeria monocytogenes*: antagonism of chloramphenicol and rifampin. *Antimicrob Agents Chemother* 1983;23:555–558.
258. Woods DD. The relation of *p*-aminobenzoic acid to the mechanism of action of sulphanilamide. *Br J Exp Pathol* 1940;21:74–90.
259. Woolfrey BF, Fox JMK, Lally RT, et al. Broth microdilution testing of *Pseudomonas aeruginosa* and aminoglycosides: need for employing dilutions differing by small arithmetic increments. *J Clin Microbiol* 1982;16:663–667.
260. Woolfrey BF, Ramadel WA, Quall CO. Evaluation of a semiautomated micro-broth dilution system for determining minimum inhibitory concentrations of antimicrobics. *Am J Clin Pathol* 1980;73:374–379.
261. World Health Organization. *Standardization of methods for conducting microbic sensitivity tests: second report of the Expert Committee on Antibiotics.* World Health Organization technical reports series, no. 210. New York: World Health Organization, 1961.
262. Wyatt PJ. Identification of bacteria by differential light scattering. *Nature* 1969;221:1257–1258.
263. Wyatt PJ. Automation of differential light scattering for antibiotic susceptibility testing. In: Heden CG, Illeni T, eds. *Automation in microbiology and immunology.* New York: John Wiley and Sons, 1975:267–291.
264. Yocum RR, Rasmussin JR, Strominger SL. The mechanism of action of penicillin: penicillin activates the active site of *Bacillus stearothermophilus* D-alanine carboxypeptidase. *J Biol Chem* 1980;255:3977–3986.
265. York MK, Gibbs L, Chehab F, et al. Comparison of PCR detection of *mec*A with standard susceptibility testing methods to determine methicillin resistance in coagulase-negative staphylococci. *J Clin Microbiol* 1996;34:249–253.
266. Yu VL, Chiou CC, Feldman C, et al. An international prospective study of pneumococcal bacteremia: correlation with in vitro resistance, antibiotics administered and clinical outcome. *Clin Infect Dis* 2003;37:230–237.
267. Zanon U. Sub-inhibitory levels of antibiotics. *J Antimicrob Chemother* 1977;3:106–107.
268. Zigheiboin S, Tomasz A. Penicillin binding proteins of multiply antibiotic-resistant South African strains of *Streptococcus pneumoniae*. *Antimicrob Agents Chemother* 1980;17:434–441.

CHAPTER 4

Antimicrobial Susceptibility Testing of Anaerobic Bacteria

David W. Hecht

Anaerobic bacteria, as a source of causing or contributing to infection, has been well established in the literature (24). Some anaerobes can be the singular cause of a specific infection or sequelae, such as tetanus (*Clostridium tetani*), botulism (*Clostridium botulinum*), or food poisoning (*Clostridium perfringens*). However, the majority of infections due to anaerobes occur most often as mixed infections involving intraabdominal, skin and soft tissue, pulmonary, or central nervous system sites (24). Anaerobes are not only recognized as a cause of or contribution to infection, but also treatment is necessary for a good clinical outcome (43,61).

Recently, much attention has been given to antibiotic resistance among numerous aerobic and facultative anaerobic bacteria, with clear evidence of clinical failure when an ineffective antibiotic is used (37,46,47,77). Much less attention has been given to the role of antibiotic resistance among anaerobes and adverse clinical outcome. In fact, clinical trials that assess the efficacy of new antibiotics with good *in vitro* activity against anaerobic bacterial pathogens generally show favorable outcomes when compared with less active agents (56). However, until recently, there have been few studies demonstrating a correlation of antibiotic-resistant anaerobes with poor clinical outcome. Factors that have limited the ability to draw such conclusions from any study include the nature of the infection (mixed aerobes and anaerobes), lack of identification of anaerobic bacteria from specimens, absence of clinical data, effects of surgical drainage or debridement (a major factor that obscures importance of a resistant organism), and previous inaccurate or modified susceptibility testing methods (39,40).

Several retrospective clinical studies were published in the 1980s and early 1990s that supported the association of antibiotic resistance among *Bacteroides* sp. and clinical failure (5,18,58). However, a sentinel prospective, observational, *Bacteroides fragilis* group bacteremia study published in 2000 confirmed these previous suppositions and conclusions (42). In that study, mortality rate for patients receiving ineffective therapy (for resistant *B. fragilis*) was significantly higher than those receiving therapy that was active *in vitro* against the organism. Similarly, clinical failure and microbiological persistence were greater for patients receiving ineffective therapy. These findings, along with numerous reports of increased antibiotic resistance, have prompted a change in the recommendations for susceptibility testing of anaerobic bacteria by the National Committee for Clinical Laboratory Standards (NCCLS) in their most recent standards publication (41). These recommendations are also echoed in other recent publications (14,61).

To arrive at the most recent consensus document, the anaerobe working group of the NCCLS conducted several multicenter collaborative studies to establish a highly reproducible agar dilution reference standard and comparable broth microdilution method (53,54). Coupled with the commercially available Etest (AB BIODISK, Solna, Sweden), there are now three reproducible and reliable methods for susceptibility testing of anaerobic bacteria (15). These different but comparable methods each have their pros and cons, depending on the testing needs.

INDICATIONS FOR SUSCEPTIBILITY TESTING

Susceptibility testing has been rarely employed at most hospitals and medical centers. Despite the increasing prevalence of resistance among anaerobes, the frequency of testing was reported to be declining in the last survey conducted in the early 1990s partly because of budgetary reductions, a concomitant loss of expertise at these institutions, a lack of automated testing for anaerobes, and a failure to consider resistance as important to clinicians (27,29).

The recent and varied trends in antibiotic resistance, spread of resistance genes, and poor clinical outcomes resulting from ineffective antibiotic therapy argue strongly for more susceptibility testing of anaerobes. The most recent NCCLS recommendations include that, at minimum, clinical laboratories should strongly consider susceptibility testing for surveillance purposes (40). In addition, certain clinical situations may warrant individual isolate testing, either in-house or at a reference laboratory. The current major indications for testing individual isolates include persistent infection despite an adequate treatment regimen, difficulty in making empiric decisions based on precedent or confirmation of appropriate therapy for severe infections, the need for long-term therapy, and known resistance of an organism or species. Organisms recognized as highly pathogenic and for which antimicrobial resistance cannot be predicted include members of the *B. fragilis* group, *Prevotella* sp, *Fusobacterium* sp, *Clostridium* sp, *Bilophila wadsworthia*, and *Sutterella wadsworthensis* (40).

Surveillance Testing

Annual surveillance testing is now recommended for clinical laboratories that routinely identify anaerobic bacteria to establish local patterns of resistance for commonly encountered anaerobes (14,40,61). Proper identification of anaerobes is, of course, an important first step in this process. Laboratories should be aware of recent taxonomic changes that have occurred within Gram-negative anaerobic bacteria [based on 16S recombinant DNA (rDNA) techniques] that have resulted in regrouping of some organisms and the identification of new species. The reader is referred to excellent recent descriptions of these changes, as well as a strategy for identification of anaerobic species (13,36,62,63).

Strains to be tested for surveillance purposes should be collected over several months and stored until at least 50 to 100 are available for batch testing, allowing for the most efficient use of time, training, and materials. In general, anaerobic isolates to be tested should reflect the distribution of bacteria isolated in the laboratory. Because of the high frequency of resistance among the *B. fragilis* group, it is recommended that at least 20 isolates be selected from the ten species, with ten isolates tested from among other frequently isolated anaerobic genera. When choosing antibiotics to test, laboratories should consider at least one agent from each antibiotic class, and that should also reflect their respective hospital's formulary (14,40).

Routine Testing

Individual isolate testing may also be appropriate in certain clinical situations. Specific infections for which testing should be strongly considered include cases of brain abscess, endocarditis, osteomyelitis, joint infection, infection of prosthetic devices or grafts, bacteremias, and isolates from normally sterile body sites. Consultation with the physician will be important in deciding on the need for susceptibility testing of these isolates (40).

Strategy for Testing

The anaerobe working group most recently developed a strategy for testing four groups of anaerobes. Priorities for testing various antibiotics against these four groupings are published in the latest NCCLS standard Table 4.1 (40). This includes a listing of primary and supplemental choices for testing *B. fragilis* group and other β-lactamase (BLA)–producing anaerobes, BLA-negative Gram-negative anaerobes, *Clostridium* sp other than *C. perfringens*, and *C. perfringens* and all other Gram-positive anaerobes (40). Examples of primary choices include one each of the β-lactam/BLA-inhibitor combinations, cephamycins, carbapenems, and metronidazole for *B. fragilis* group, and penicillin (or ampicillin), clindamycin, and metronidazole for BLA-negative Gram-negative rods. For Gram-positive anaerobes, penicillin (or ampicillin), β-lactam/BLA inhibitors, cephamycins, clindamycin, carbapenems, and metronidazole are recommended for testing *Clostridium* sp (not *C. perfringens).* Penicillin (or ampicillin), clindamycin, and metronidazole are recommended for all other Gram-positive anaerobes, including *C. perfringens.*

MECHANISMS OF ACTION OF ANTIANAEROBIC ANTIMICROBIAL AGENTS

The mechanism of action for most antianaerobic antimicrobial agents is either proven or presumed the same as that demonstrated for other nonanaerobic organisms. Although many of the pathogenic anaerobic bacteria are Gram-negative, the either high or low degree of activity of some agents does not always closely match that of aerobic or facultative anaerobic bacteria. Cases where differences in activity are known are included in the discussion. The mechanism of action of clindamycin (and lincomycin), metronidazole, quinolones, aminoglycosides, and tetracyclines are discussed here. The mechanism of action of β-lactam antibiotics is not presented in this section, as this has been thoroughly discussed by Dr. Stratton in Chapter 12 of this book.

Clindamycin and lincomycin both work by binding to the 50S ribosomal subunit of bacteria, resulting in a disruption of protein synthesis by interfering with the transpeptidation reaction, preventing peptide chain elongation (11). Of note, chloramphenicol and macrolides compete for binding at the same site and are thought to be potentially antagonistic when used together. In aerobic bacteria, clindamycin may potentiate opsonization

TABLE 4.1

Anaerobic Bacterial Gene Transfer Factors Contributing to Antibiotic Resistance

Bacterial Group	Antibiotic	Gene Designation	Transferable	Transfer Factor
B. fragilis group	Clindamycin	*ermF, ermS*	+	Plasmid
	Tetracycline	*tetQ, tetX**	+	Plasmid
	Cephalosporin	*cepA, cblA*	ND[a]	
	Cefoxitin	*cfxA*	+	Transposon
	Carbapenems	*ccrA, cfiA*	+	Plasmid[b]
	Metronidazole	*nimA, nimB, nimC, nimD, nimE, nimF*	+ *(nimA,C,D)*	Plasmid
	Quinolones	*gyrA, gyrB, parC, parE*	??	
	Streptomycin	*aadS**	+	Transposon
C. perfringens	Chloramphenicol	*catQ,*[c] *catP*	+	Plasmid
	Clindamycin	*ermQ, ermP*	ND	
	Tetracycline	*tetA(P), tetB(P)*	+	Plasmid
C. difficile	Tetracycline	*tcr*	+	Transposon?[d]
	Chloramphenicol	*catD*	+	Transposon
	Clindamycin	*ermZ, ermBZ*	+	Transposon
Clostridium butyricum	Chloramphenicol	*catA, catB*	ND	
Prevotella spp	Tetracycline	*tetQ, tetO, tetM*	+	Transposon *(tetQ)*
Fusobacterium spp	Tetracycline	*tetM*	+	Transposon

*cryptic
[a] Not determined.
[b] A plasmid-borne imipenem resistance determinant has been isolated, but the gene has not been characterized.
[c] *catQ* was characterized from a nonconjugative strain.
[d] The exact nature of the transfer factor is unknown.

and phagocytosis of bacteria, presumably by the resulting changes in the cell wall surface decreasing adherence of bacteria to host cells and increasing intracellular killing (70,71). This phenomenon has not been demonstrated for anaerobes, but could also occur. Clindamycin is considered bactericidal against *B. fragilis,* although its activity can be inconsistent. Resistance to this agent is discussed in the next section.

Metronidazole activity against anaerobes is mediated through a four-step process. In the first step, metronidazole must enter the cell, which it does efficiently as a low molecular weight compound that diffuses easily across cell membranes (22). The second step includes reductive activiation by intracellular transport proteins. Metronidazole is reduced by the pyruvate:ferredoxin oxidoreductase system in the mitochondria of obligate anaerobes altering its chemical structure. Metronidazole is reduced when its nitro group acts as an electron sink, capturing electrons and reducing the compound, which also results in a concentration gradient driving its own uptake as well as forming intermediate compounds and free radicals toxic to the cell (20,38). In the third step, reduced intermediate particles interact with host cell DNA resulting in fatal DNA strand breakage (65,66). Lastly, breakdown of cytotoxic intermediates occurs, resulting in inactive end products (26). Metronidazole is rapidly bactericidal in a concentration-dependent manner, killing *B. fragilis* and *C. perfringens* more rapidly than does clindamycin (50,64).

Fluoroquinolones directly inhibit bacterial DNA synthesis by binding to the complex of both DNA gyrase and topoisomerase IV, which are required for bacterial replication (19). The key event in quinolone action is reversible trapping of gyrase-DNA and topoisomerase

IV–DNA complexes. Complex formation with gyrase is followed by a rapid, reversible inhibition of DNA synthesis and growth, resulting in damage to bacterial DNA and cell death. Thus, quinolones are also bactericidal agents.

Aminoglycosides bind 30s ribosomal subunits of aerobic bacteria, but have no activity against anaerobes. Uptake of aminoglycosides by bacteria requires an energy-dependent phase normally provided by an oxygen- or nitrogen-dependent electron transport system that is absent in strictly anaerobic bacteria (9). Thus, anaerobes do no import aminoglycosides. However, aminoglycosides do bind to the ribosomes of *B. fragilis* and *C. perfringens* from cell-free extracts, indicating likely activity if they could gain entry into cells (8). Tetracyclines, on the other hand, are able to enter bacteria passively, including anaerobes, and also bind the 30S ribosomal subunit, preventing protein synthesis (17). However, resistance to this agent is widespread among anaerobes, and therefore not frequently used. Specific resistance mechanisms are discussed in the next section.

ANTIMICROBIAL RESISTANCE AMONG ANAEROBES

As noted previously, antibiotic resistance among some anaerobes has increased significantly over the last few decades and parallels that of nonanaerobic bacteria (78). Organisms for which the most significant change has occurred are members of the *B. fragilis* group. Three major ongoing surveillance studies have reported significant changes in resistance among these bacteria since the 1980s. The national anaerobe survey, conducted at New England Medical Center, has tracked resistance among the *Bacteroides* sp using the reference standard agar dilution method (59,60), whereas a second national survey, based at Louisiana State University Health Science Center, utilizes the broth dilution method testing the *B. fragilis* group and other anaerobes (2). A third survey, based at Loyola University Medical Center, utilizes agar dilution to test all types of anaerobes from several hospitals in the Chicago area (33,34). All three surveys confirm that resistance is increasing with hospital-to-hospital variation, even within the same geographic area.

Clindamycin Resistance

Clindamycin resistance among *Bacteroides* sp has increased the most significantly in the last two decades. Starting at only 3% in 1987, resistance to clindamycin averaged 26% in 2000 with a range of 16% to 44% resistance among the members of the *B. fragilis* group (34,35,59). For many non-Bacteroides anaerobes, resistance has also increased, albeit not as significantly as in the *B. fragilis* group (35). The most recent report found up to 10% resistance for *Prevotella* sp, *Fusobacterium* sp, *Porphyromonas* sp, and *Peptostreptococcus* sp, with higher rates for some *Clostridium* sp (especially *Clostridium difficile*) (1,2).

β-Lactam Antibiotics

Resistance to β-lactam agents among anaerobes is fairly widespread for the penicillins, cefamycins, and third-generation cephalosporins. Nearly all (more than 97%) of the *B. fragilis* group are resistant to penicillin G by virtue of BLA production. In contrast, cefoxitin retains activity against most *B. fragilis* group members, although resistance has ranged between 8% and 22% over the period of 1987 to 2000. Cefotetan activity is very similar to that of cefoxitin against *B. fragilis*, but is much less potent against other members of the *B. fragilis* group (30% to 87% resistant) (60). Resistance to piperacillin, the most active ureidopenicillin against anaerobes, is also now widespread among members of the *B. fragilis* group (average 25% resistant). Resistance is also found among non-Bacteroides anaerobes (34,35,59).

Fortunately, activity of other more potent β-lactams, the β-lactam/BLA-inhibitor combinations and carbapenems, remains excellent. The three combination agents of ampicillin/sulbactam, ticarcillin/clavulanate, and piperacillin/tazobactam are highly active against members of the *B. fragilis* group, with less than 2% resistance reported in the most recent survey (14,59). However, species-to-species variation in susceptibility has been identified, with the many non-BLA producing *Bacteroides distasonis* demonstrating elevated minimum inhibitory concentrations (MICs) at or approaching the susceptible breakpoint (60). The carbapenems, imipenem, meropenem, and ertapenem remain very potent against all members of the *B. fragilis* group, with only rare (less than 0.1%) resistance identified (2,32,59).

Resistance to β-lactam agents among non-Bacteroides anaerobes is generally much lower than that of *Bacteroides*. However, similar to that of *Bacteroides* organisus, *Prevotella* sp are also potent BLA producers, with more than 50% resistant to penicillin. Aldridge et al. (2) have reported penicillin resistance for *Fusobacterium* sp, *Porphyromonas* sp, and *Peptostreptococcus* sp at 9%, 21%, and 6%, respectively. Resistance to cefoxitin, cefotetan, β-lactam/BLA-inhibitor combinations, and carbapenems was 0% in the same survey, with the exception of *Peptostreptococcus* sp and *Porphyromonas* sp (4% and 5% resistance to ampicillin/sulbactam, respectively).

Metronidazole resistance among Gram-negative anaerobes has been reported in a single case in the United States, from a patient returning from Europe, and occasionally but rarely in European countries (6,68,79). Metronidazole resistance among Gram-positive anaerobes is far more common, especially for most isolates of *Propionibacterium acnes* and *Actinomyces* sp (29).

Fluoroquinolone resistance among anaerobes has increased the most significantly and rapidly. Only one agent in this class, trovafloxacin, has Food and Drug Administration (FDA) approval for treatment of anaerobic infections. Currently, use of this agent is very limited to due to toxicity concerns. Interestingly, trovafloxacin resistance among *Bacteroides* increased from 3% to 8% during the period 1994 to 1996, prior to the antibiotics release in 1997 (59,60). Despite its limited use, resistance increased further to a peak of 25% in 2001 (25). Concomitantly, MICs to newer and experimental quinolones have also been increasing, predicting cross-resistance within this class.

Among other antibiotic classes, tetracycline resistance is now nearly universal among *Bacteroides* sp and many other anaerobes, limiting its use in therapy. Resistance to aminoglycosides is universal among anaerobes, with this antibiotic restricted to combination therapy for mixed infections. Chloramphenicol resistance is very rare, but this agent is also rarely used in the clinical setting (51).

MECHANISMS OF ANTIMICROBIAL RESISTANCE AMONG ANAEROBES

Table 4.1 summarizes the current known mechanisms of resistance and resistance genes for anaerobic bacteria. Not surprisingly, antibiotic resistance mechanisms are quite different for each class of antibiotics. Clindamycin resistance is mediated by a macrolide-lincosamide-streptogramin (MLS) type 23S methylase similar to that of staphylococci (35), and is typically encoded by one of several erythromycin ribosome methylation (*erm*) genes that are typically regulated and expressed at high levels. However, some isolates that contain *erm* genes demonstrate only moderately elevated MICs that would not otherwise be designated as resistant. Some of these latter strains can be detected by testing for erythromycin resistance. It is possible that these isolates could be induced to higher levels of resistance under selective pressure. At the current time, however, there is no specific recommendation to screen for resistance using erythromycin. Transfer of *erm* genes by conjugation in *B. fragilis* group organisms is easily demonstrated in the laboratory, and likely explains the rapid emergence of this resistance phenotype (4,49,73). Of note, clindamycin is no longer recommended as empiric therapy for intraabdominal infections in the latest published guidelines, presumably because of the high rate of resistance (61).

Resistance to β-lactam antibiotics can occur by one of three major mechanisms: inactivating enzymes (BLAs), low-affinity penicillin-binding proteins (PBPs), or decreased permeability. BLA is by far the most common mechanism associated with resistance to β-lactam antibiotics. The most common BLAs found among *Bacteroides* sp and *Prevotella* sp are cephalosporinases of the type 2e class. These BLAs are inhibited by sulbactam, clavulanic acid, or tazobactam, thus the increased potency of the β-lactam/BLA-inhibitor combinations. Cefoxitin- and cefotaxime-inactivating enzymes and other BLAs have also been reported in many *B. fragilis* group species (55). The most potent BLAs are the zinc metalloenzymes encoded by either *ccrA* or *cfiA* genes of the *B. fragilis* group (76). These enzymes are responsible for the rare resistance to carbapenems, are active against all β-lactam antibiotics with known activity against anaerobes, and are not inactivated by current BLA inhibitors. Although resistance to carbapenems is currently quite rare in the United States, up to 3% of *Bacteroides* strains have been found to carry one of the genes expressed at a very low level. These strains can be induced to a higher level of resistance in the laboratory under selective pressure caused by a promoter (contained in an insertion sequence) that has inserted upstream of the *ccrA* or *cfiA* genes (22,48).

Production of BLAs by other anaerobic bacteria has been generally less well studied, but strains of Clostridium, Porphyromonas, and Fusobacterium organisms express resistance by one or more of these enzymes. Penicillin-resistant Fusobacterium and Clostridium organisms express penicillinases that are typically inhibited by clavulanic acid, although exceptions among some *Clostridium* sp have been reported (3,51).

Other mechanisms of resistance to β-lactam antibiotics are far less frequent in occurrence, and less well studied. Decreased binding to PBP2 or PBP1 complex has been reported in rare clinical isolates in cefoxitin resistance among *B. fragilis* strains (23). Alterations in pore-forming proteins of Gram-negative anaerobes are a third type of resistance, with the absence of one or more outer membrane proteins associated with high MICs to ampicillin/sulbactam in some strains of *B. fragilis* (74,75).

Metronidazole resistance occurs by the lack of reduction to its active form in anaerobic bacteria. Metronidazole-resistant *B. fragilis* group organisms, although rare, carry one of six known *nim* genes that appear to encode a nitroimidazole reductase that converts 4- or 5-nitroimidazole to 4- or 5-aminoimidazole, preventing the formation of toxin nitroso residues necessary for the agents' activity (10,30). These genes have been identified on both the chromosome and on transferable plasmids. High-level expression of the *nim* genes requires an insertion sequence with a promoter, similar to that of carbapenem resistance (67). Differential gene expression affecting cell metabolism in *bacteroides* has also been reported as an alternative mechanism for resistance (80). In contrast to *Bacteroides*, the mechanism of resistance to metronidazole for non-*Bacteroides* anaerobes is currently not known. Interestingly, metronidazole resistance in the microaerophilic organism *Helicobacter pylori* has been partially solved for some strains that contain mutations in the *rdxA* gene, an oxygen-insensitive nitroreductase that converts metronidazole to its active form in this organism (69). Other candidate genes for resistance include the flavin oxidoreductase (*frxA*), ferridoxin-like proteins (*fdxA*, *fdxB*), and pyruvate oxidoreductase (*porA*, *porB*) (12). Metronidazole also has activity against *Mycobacterium tuberculosis*, although apparently only in dormant cells, when reduction of the drug can occur. Resistance among actively growing Mycobacterium organisms is presumed secondary to a lack of sufficient reducing potential (72).

Fluoroquinolone resistance among *Bacteroides* sp has been attributed to either a mutation in the quinolone resistance-determining region of the gyrase A gene (*gyrA*) from single or multiple mutations, or an alteration in efflux of the antibiotic (44,45,52,81). High-level resistance may be secondary to both mechanisms in the same cell, although only a few strains have been tested to date. Both of these mechanisms appear to be responsible for the cross-class resistance to newer quinolones.

The lack of activity of aminoglycosides against anaerobes is related to the lack of uptake by the bacteria under anaerobic conditions and a failure to reach their ribosome targets (8). Tetracycline resistance is widespread, especially among *B. fragilis* group and *Prevotella* sp (42). Several genes encoding resistance have been identified among various anaerobes, which encode protective proteins, resulting in protection of the ribosomes. More importantly, however, is the association of tetracycline resistance and the inducible transfer of this resistance determinant upon exposure to low levels of the antibiotic. Chloramphenicol resistance is extremely rare, but when found, is associated with inactivation of the drug by nitroreduction or acetyltransferase (7).

METHODS FOR ANTIMICROBIAL SUSCEPTIBILITY TESTING OF ANAEROBIC BACTERIA

Several different methods, spanning five decades, have been utilized in antimicrobial susceptibility testing (AST) of anaerobic bacteria. During that time, more than 16 methods, 16 different media, and a host of other variables have been described to test susceptibility of anaerobes. NCCLS took the lead in developing a consensus for AST of anaerobes starting with the first approved standard in 1985, along with alternative methods published in a second document the same year. Subsequently, several revisions have been published that modified, added, or eliminated some methods (32). Following extensive multilaboratory collaborative studies sanctioned by the NCCLS in the late 1990s, a consensus was reached culminating in a single agar dilution standard and one broth microdilution method, both using the same medium (40,53,54). In addition to NCCLS methods, a very useful and highly correlated user-friendly method, Etest (AB BIODISK), has been FDA-approved and available for several years (15,57). As a proprietary product, the Etest is not included in the NCCLS documents. Of note, all methods can be performed in ambient air, but require incubation in an anaerobic jar or glove box.

Choosing a method from among these three recognized and approved methods may depend on a number of factors (Table 4.2). The agar dilution standard has a very high degree of reproducibility, but is fairly labor-intensive. A laboratory can test up to 30 isolates plus two controls, making it useful for batch testing. However, individual sets of dilution plates must be pored for each antibiotic, increasing material and labor costs. As the reference standard, agar dilution is most often used for evaluation of new antimicrobial agents. The broth microdilution method is more user-friendly than agar dilution and has the flexibility to test multiple antibiotics using the same microtiter plate, albeit only one isolate at a time. Based on available comparative studies of broth microdilution to the standard, results are considered equivalent when testing members of the *B. fragilis* group. However, results are not as comparable for non-Bacteroides anaerobes because of poor growth, and broth microdilution is not used for this group at this time. It should be noted that previously published studies testing non-Bacteroides

TABLE 4.2

Methods for AST of Anaerobic Bacteria

Method	Medium	Inoculum	Advantages	Disadvantages
Agar dilution	Brucella blood agar	10^5 CFU/spot	Reference method, suitable for surveillance	Labor-intensive
Broth microdilution	Brucella broth supplemented with blood	10^6 CFU/mL	Multiple antibiotics/isolate, commercially available	Limited to *B. fragilis* group, panel shelf life
Etest	Brucella blood agar	1 McFarland swab plate	Precise MIC values, convenient	Expensive for surveillance

anaerobes using a different broth (anaerobe MIC broth) were able to grow non-Bacteroides anaerobes with MIC results within twofold of those for agar dilution. Thus, broth microdilution testing for non-Bacteroides anaerobes can be considered, but only if correlated with the current agar dilution standard. The third method, Etest, is relatively easy to perform and is well suited for testing individual isolates of any anaerobe. For surveillance testing, costs could be prohibitive.

NCCLS REFERENCE AGAR DILUTION METHOD

For the agar dilution reference standard, each test concentration of an antibiotic is mixed into molten agar and poured into separate Petri dishes to which an inoculum of an organism is applied, incubated anaerobically, and examined to determine the MIC for the antimicrobial agent tested. Methods described here are adapted from those of NCCLS standards (40). For laboratories inexperienced with this method and anaerobe AST, a useful time table for setup and testing is provided as an appendix in the NCCLS standards.

Testing Medium

Brucella blood agar supplemented with 5 μg hemin, 1% vitamin K_1, and 5% laked sheep blood is the recommended testing medium. Brucella agar blanks (17 mL) can be prepared in advance containing hemin and vitamin K_1, and flash-autoclaved or microwaved and placed in a ~50°C water bath on the day of use. One milliliter of laked sheep blood is then added to each melted blank while still in the water bath. Two milliliters of each twofold diluted test antibiotic is then added to the agar, mixed by inverting the tubes, and poured into sterile Petri dishes. Following hardening of the plates, and drying briefly in an inverted position in a 37°C incubator, the plates are ready for use. Preferably, plates should be made on the day of testing, but can be at 4°C for periods of up to 72 hours if necessary. Exceptions to storage include plates containing clavulanic acid or imipenem, which must be made on the day of use.

Inoculum Preparation

The inoculum can be prepared by either a direct colony suspension or growth method. Direct colony suspension requires 24- to 48-hour growth on a Brucella blood agar plate. Several colonies are touched lightly with an inoculating needle or cotton swab and suspended in reduced Brucella broth to achieve a turbidity equivalent to a McFarland standard of 0.5. The alternative growth method involves the inoculation of enriched thioglycollate medium (without indicator) with portions of five or more colonies from a Brucella blood agar plate, incubating for 6 to 24 hours at 37°C, and adjusting the turbidity to a McFarland standard of 0.5 by addition of reduced Brucella broth.

Inoculation and Incubation of Plates

Once the inoculum is prepared, it is most often applied using an inoculum-replicating apparatus, such as a Steers-Foltz replicator, to deliver 1 to 2 μL on the agar surface, corresponding to 1×10^5 colony-forming units (CFUs) per spot. Depending on the device, either 32 or 36 wells can be filled with different test organisms and controls using a Pasteur or other pipette. Application of inoculum to plates includes repeated stamping of plates, starting with lowest to highest dilution of each antibiotic set. One plate of supplemented Brucella blood agar without antibiotic should be stamped prior to and after each set of antibiotics for growth control. Contamination by aerobic bacteria during the inoculation procedure can be detected by inoculating a drug-free plate, and incubated aerobically. Once plates are inoculated, they should sit until liquid is absorbed into the medium, and then incubated in an anaerobic environment at 35°C for 42 to 48 hours.

Interpretation of Results

Endpoints are determined by reading each plate against a dark, nonreflecting background and comparing it with the control growth plate. Any growth on the aerobic control should eliminate further interpretation of that test organism. The endpoint for a given test organism is where a marked reduction occurs in the appearance of growth compared with control. A marked change includes a haze, multiple tiny colonies, or one to several normal-sized colonies. These descriptions have been problematic for those inexperienced with using this method. To that end, NCCLS recommends the use of two figures containing eight full-dilution color photographic examples of endpoint readings to illustrate the written descriptions (40).

Interpretative categories approved by NCCLS for MICs derived for anaerobic bacteria are shown in Table 4.3. This table includes agents that are the most frequently used in the clinical setting and were updated through 2003. Interpretative categories for any organism have been determined based on the population distribution of the bacteria, the pharmacokinetics, and pharmacodynamic properties of the antibiotic with verification of efficacy by clinical studies (see an in-depth description in Chapter 1). This works particularly well for single-organism infections. However, this is rarely the case for anaerobic bacteria, which are typically isolated from mixed infections. Many of the published anaerobic breakpoints were determined on the basis of animal models or the result of clinical trials involving patients with polymicrobial infections as well as pharmacokinetic data. Despite these potential limitations, the use of maximum dosages of antibiotics along with appropriate ancillary therapy (debridement

TABLE 4.3

Interpretive Categories for MICs for Anaerobic Bacteria[a]

Antimicrobial Agent	MIC (μg/mL) Susceptible	Intermediate	Resistant
Amoxicillin/clavulanic acid	<4/2	8/4	>16/8
Ampicillin	<0.5	1	>2
Ampicillin/sulbactam	<8/4	16/8	>32/16
Cefotetan	<16	32	>64
Cefoxitin	<16	32	>64
Ceftriaxone	<16	32	>64
Chloramphenicol	<8	16	>32
Clindamycin	<2	4	>8
Ertapenem	<4	8	>16
Imipenem	<4	8	>16
Metronidazole	<8	16	>32
Meropenem	<4	8	>16
Penicillin	<0.5	1	>2
Piperacillin	<32	64	>128
Piperacillin/tazobactam	<32/4	64/4	>128/4
Tetracycline	<4	8	>16
Ticarcillin	<32/2	64/2	>128/2
Trovafloxacin	<2	4	>8

[a] Adapted with permission from NCCLS (40).

or drainage) should be effective for organisms with susceptible breakpoints, although those with intermediate susceptibilities should be monitored closely (40).

NCCLS-RECOMMENDED BROTH MICRODILUTION METHOD

The broth microdilution method has been validated by NCCLS for testing *B. fragilis* group members with results considered equivalent.

Media

Brucella broth supplemented with hemin (5 μg/mL), vitamin K_1, and lysed and cleared horse blood is the recommended medium, which is essentially equivalent to that of agar dilution. Trays can be prepared fresh and then frozen or purchased commercially. Trays should be kept at −70°C. Antibiotics are diluted according to an algorithm recommended by NCCLS in volumes of 15 to 100 mL (40), and delivered using a device that can simultaneously dispense aliquots of 0.1 mL per well (or 0.05 mL per well if a pipette will be used to deliver an equal volume of inoculum). When a pipette is used for inoculation, antibiotic concentrations should be prepared at 2× the final desired concentration. Volumes of less than 0.1 mL are not recommended.

Inoculum Preparation, Inoculation Procedure, and Incubation

Inoculum preparation is the same as for agar dilution to achieve a turbidity of a McFarland standard of 0.5. Commercially available inoculating devices can be used that deliver 10 μL of a 1:10 dilution of the 0.5 McFarland inoculum. For commercially prepared trays, follow the manufacturer's recommendations. The final concentration of inoculum should be 1×10^6 CFU/mL.

Before inoculation, frozen trays should be brought to room temperature and inoculated within 15 minutes of inoculum preparation. It is advisable to perform a colony count and purity check of the inoculum by removing 10 μL from the growth control well and diluting it into 10 mL of saline, streaking 0.1 mL onto the surface of an anaerobic blood agar plate, and incubating anaerobically. One hundred colonies on the plate correspond to 1×10^6 CFUs/mL. Trays are then incubated for 46 to 48 hours at 35°C in an anaerobic atmosphere (see previous discussion), ensuring sufficient humidity to prevent drying.

Interpretation of Results

The MIC values are read by viewing the plates from the bottom using a stand and a mirror. A sufficient growth control is required to interpret results. The MIC endpoint is read as the concentration where no growth, or the most significant reduction of growth, is observed. A trailing effect may be observed for some drug-organism combinations. Again, two figures containing eight examples of broth microdilution endpoints, are provided by NCCLS (40). Breakpoints for broth microdilution interpretation are the same as those for agar dilution (Table 4.3).

QUALITY CONTROL

A quality control program to monitor accuracy of testing, reagents, equipment, and persons conducting tests is essential. The quality control strains chosen for anaerobic bacteria are limited to two *Bacteroides* sp and a *Eubacterium* strain. *B. fragilis* ATCC 25285 and *Bacteroides thetaiotaomicron* ATCC 29741 are appropriate for testing using any of the methods listed, while *Eubacterium lentum* ATCC 43055 would be limited to either agar dilution or Etest. Two of the three quality control strains should be used for each assessment when agar dilution is used. When an individual strain is being tested by broth microdilution or Etest, one strain should be included. Expected values for endpoints for both agar and broth microdilution methods are published by NCCLS. Of note, many laboratories have experienced repeated difficulty reading endpoints for *E. lentum* ATCC 43055. Studies are currently underway to identify a non-Bacteroides, Gram-positive control strain for future testing.

ETEST

The Etest is an excellent and convenient choice for testing individual anaerobic organisms. Several studies have validated this method, demonstrating good correlation with the agar dilution method (15,57). However, Rosenblatt and Gustafson (58) have noted that some *Prevotella* and *Bacteroides* strains show false susceptibility when testing penicillin and ceftriaxone that is minimized if β-lactamase producing strains are eliminated. A more significant warning is potential false resistance to metronidazole as a result of test conditions and medium quality (16). This aberrant result can be avoided by prereducing test plates in an anaerobic chamber the night before testing.

Procedure

The Etest is a familiar technique to most clinical laboratories, and does not differ significantly in its application to anaerobic bacteria. The Etest strips are coated with a gradient of antimicrobial on one side with an MIC interpretative scale on the other. The organism to be tested is prepared to a McFarland standard of 1 and applied to a 150-mm diameter Petri dish of supplemented Brucella blood agar, with the strips applied in a radial fashion. Smaller plates can be used with fewer strips. Incubation is recommended for 48 hours at 35°C, and read where an elliptical zone of inhibition intersects the strip on the scale of MIC values.

β-LACTAMASE TESTING

The BLA testing deserves mention, although it is not a true AST test. Testing for BLA activity can be performed on anaerobic organisms, although it is not recommended for the *B. fragilis* group because of the high prevalence of positivity. This test can be used as a first step to drive additional testing choices (such as those in Table 4.1 in reference 3). Any BLA-producing anaerobe should be considered resistant to penicillin and ampicillin. However, as noted in the section on antimicrobial resistance, alternative mechanisms of resistance to β-lactams are known, and a negative test does not assure susceptibility to penicillin.

The recommended method for testing is chromogenic and cephalosporin-based, either by a nitrocefin disk assay (Cefinase; BBL, Cockeysville, MD) or the S1 chromogenic disk (International BioClinical, Inc., Portland, OR). Tests are performed according to manufacturers' directions. A positive reaction is denoted by a change in color from yellow to red that typically occurs within 5 to 10 minutes. However, some *Bacteroides* strains may react more slowly (up to 30 minutes) (40).

REFERENCES

1. Ackermann G, Degner A, Cohen SH, et al. Prevalence and association of macrolide-lincosamide-streptogramin B (MLS(B)) resistance with resistance to moxifloxacin in Clostridium difficile. *J Antimicrob Chemother* 2003;51:599–603.
2. Aldridge KE, Ashcraft D, Cambre K, et al. Multicenter survey of the changing in vitro antimicrobial susceptibilities of clinical isolates of *Bacteroides fragilis* group, Prevotella, Fusobacterium, Porphyromonas, and Peptostreptococcus species. *Antimicrob Agents Chemother* 2001;45:1238–1243.
3. Appelbaum PC, Spangler SK, Pankuch GA, et al. Characterization of a beta-lactamase from *Clostridium clostridioforme*. *J Antimicrob Chemother* 1994;33:33–40.
4. Bachoual R, Dubreuil L, Soussy CJ, and Tankovic J. Roles of gyrA mutations in resistance of clinical isolates and in vitro mutants of *Bacteroides fragilis* to the new fluoroquinolone trovafloxacin. *Antimicrob Agents Chemother* 2000;44:1842–1845.

5. Bieluch VM, Cuchural GJ, Snydman DR, et al. Clinical importance of cefoxitin-resistant Bacteroides fragilis isolates. *Diagn Microbiol Infect Dis* 1987;7:119–126.
6. Breuil J, Dublanchet A, Truffaut N, et al. Transferable 5-nitroimidazole resistance in the *Bacteroides fragilis* group. *Plasmid* 1989;21:151–154.
7. Britz ML, Wilkinson RG. Chloramphenicol acetyltransferase of *Bacteroides fragilis*. *Antimicrob Agents Chemother* 1978;14:105–111.
8. Bryan LE, Kowand SK, Van Den Elzen HM. Mechanism of aminoglycoside antibiotic resistance in anaerobic bacteria: *Clostridium perfringens* and *Bacteroides fragilis*. *Antimicrob Agents Chemother* 1979;15:7–13.
9. Bryan LE, Van Den Elzen HM. Streptomycin accumulation in susceptible and resistant strains of *Escherichia coli* and *Pseudomonas aeruginosa*. *Antimicrob Agents Chemother* 1976;9:928–938.
10. Carlier JP, Sellier N, Rager MN, et al. Metabolism of a 5-nitroimidazole in susceptible and resistant isogenic strains of *Bacteroides fragilis*. *Antimicrob Agents Chemother* 1997;41:1495–1499.
11. Chang FN, Weisblum B. The specificity of lincomycin binding to ribosomes. *Biochemistry* 1967;6:836–843.
12. Chisholm SA, Owen RJ. Mutations in *Helicobacter pylori* rdxA gene sequences may not contribute to metronidazole resistance. *J Antimicrob Chemother* 2003;51:995–999.
13. Citron DM, Hecht DW. Susceptibility Test Methods: Anaerobic Bacteria. *Manual of clinical microbiology*. 2003:343.
14. Citron DM, Hecht DW. Susceptibility test methods: anaerobic bacteria. In: Murray PR, Baron EJ, Jorgensen JH, Pfaller MA, Yolken RH eds. *Manual of clinical microbiology*. 8th ed. Washington, D.C.: ASM Press, 2003:1141–1148.
15. Citron DM, Ostovari MI, Karlsson A, Goldstein EJ. Evaluation of the E test for susceptibility testing of anaerobic bacteria. *J Clin Microbiol* 1991;29:2197–2203.
16. Cormican MG, Erwin ME, Jones RN. False resistance to metronidazole by E-test among anaerobic bacteria investigations of contributing test conditions and medium quality. *Diagn Microbiol Infect Dis* 1996;24:117–119.
17. Craven GR, Gavin R, Fanning T. The transfer RNA binding site of the 30 S ribosome and the site of tetracycline inhibition. *Cold Spring Harb Symp Quant Biol* 1969;34:129–137.
18. Dalmau D, Cayouette M, Lamothe F, et al. Clindamycin resistance in the *Bacteroides fragilis* group: association with hospital-acquired infections. *Clin Infect Dis* 1997;24:874–877.
19. Drlica K, Zhao X. DNA gyrase, topoisomerase IV, and the 4-quinolones. *Microbiol Mol Biol Rev* 1997;61:377–392.
20. Edwards DI. Reduction of nitroimidazoles in vitro and DNA damage. *Biochem Pharmacol* 1986;35:53–58.
21. Edwards DI. Nitroimidazole drugs—action and resistance mechanisms. I. Mechanisms of action. *J Antimicrob Chemother* 1993;31:9–20.
22. Edwards R, Read PN. Expression of the carbapenemase gene (cfiA) in *Bacteroides fragilis*. *J Antimicrob Chemother* 2000;46:1009–1012.
23. Fang H, Edlund C, Nord CE, et al. Selection of cefoxitin-resistant bacteroides thetaiotaomicron mutants and mechanisms involved in beta-lactam resistance. *Clin Infect Dis* 2002;35:S47–S53.
24. Finegold SM, George WL. *Anaerobic infections in humans*. San Diego, CA: Academic Press, 1989.
25. Golan Y, McDermott LA, Jacobus NV, et al. Emergence of fluoroquinolone resistance among Bacteroides species. *J Antimicrob Chemother* 2003;52:208–213.
26. Goldman P, Koch RL, Yeung TC, et al. Comparing the reduction of nitroimidazoles in bacteria and mammalian tissues and relating it to biological activity. *Biochem Pharmacol* 1986;35:43–51.
27. Goldstein EJ, Citron DM, Goldman RJ. National hospital survey of anaerobic culture and susceptibility testing methods: results and recommendations for improvement. *J Clin Microbiol* 1992;30:1529–1534.
28. Goldstein EJ, Citron DM, Vreni MC, et al. Comparative in vitro activities of ertapenem (MK-0826) against 1,001 anaerobes isolated from human intra-abdominal infections. *Antimicrob Agents Chemother* 2000;44:2389–2394.
29. Goldstein EJC. United States national hospital survey of anaerobic culture and suceptibility methods. *Anaerobe* 1995;1:309–314.
30. Haggoud A, Reysset G, Azeddoug H, et al. Nucleotide sequence analysis of two 5-nitroimidazole resistance determinants from Bacteroides strains and of a new insertion sequence upstream of the two genes. *Antimicrob Agents Chemother* 1994;38:1047–1051.
31. Hecht DW. Evolution of anaerobe susceptibility testing in the United States. *Clin Infect Dis* 2002;35:S28–S35.
32. Hecht DW, Osmolski JR. Activities of garenoxacin (BMS-284756) and other agents against anaerobic clinical isolates. *Antimicrob Agents Chemother* 2003;47:910–916.
33. Hecht DW, Osmolski JR, O'Keefe JP. Variation in the susceptibility of *Bacteroides fragilis* group isolates from six Chicago hospitals. *Clin Infect Dis* 1993;16 (Suppl 4):S357–S360.
34. Hecht DW, Vedantam G. Anaerobe resistance among anaerobes: What now? *Anaerobe* 1999;5:421–429.
35. Jimenez-Diaz A, Reig M, Baquero F, et al. Antibiotic sensitivity of ribosomes from wild-type and clindamycin resistant *Bacteroides vulgatus* strains. *J Antimicrob Chemother* 1992;30:295–301.
36. Jousimies-Somer H, Summanen P. Recent taxonomic changes and terminology update of clinically significant anaerobic gram-negative bacteria (excluding spirochetes). *Clin Infect Dis* 2002;35:S17–S21.
37. Martinez E, Miro JM, Almirante B, et al. Effect of penicillin resistance of *Streptococcus pneumoniae* on the presentation, prognosis, and treatment of pneumococcal endocarditis in adults. *Clin Infect Dis* 2002;35:130–139.
38. Muller M. Reductive activation of nitroimidazoles in anaerobic microorganisms. *Biochem Pharmacol* 1986;35:37–41.
39. National Committee for Clinical Laboratory Standards. *Methods for antimicrobial susceptibility testing of anaerobic bacteria*. 4th ed. M11-A4. Villanova, PA: NCCLS, 1997.
40. National Committee for Clinical Laboratory Standards. *Methods for antimicrobial susceptibility testing of anaerobic bacteria*. 6th ed. M11-A6. Villanova, PA: NCCLS, 2004.
41. Nguyen MH, Yu VL, Morris AJ, et al. Antimicrobial resistance and clinical outcome of Bacteroides bacteremia: findings of a multicenter prospective observational trial. *Clin Infect Dis* 2000;30:870–876.
42. Nikolich MP, Shoemaker NB, Salyers AA. A Bacteroides tetracycline resistance gene represents a new class of ribosome protection tetracycline resistance. *Antimicrob Agents Chemother* 1992;36:1005–1012.
43. North American Congress on Anaerobic Bacteria and Anaerobic Infections. *Clin Infect Dis* 1993;16:S159– S411.
44. Oh H, Hedberg M, Edlund C. Efflux-mediated fluoroquinolone resistance in the *Bacteroides fragilis* group. *Anaerobe* 2002;8:277–282.
45. Onodera Y, Sato K. Molecular cloning of the gyrA and gyrB genes of *Bacteroides fragilis* encoding DNA gyrase. *Antimicrob Agents Chemother* 1999;43:2423–2429.
46. Paterson DL, Ko WC, Von Gottberg A, et al. International

prospective study of *Klebsiella pneumoniae* bacteremia: implications of extended-spectrum beta-lactamase production in nosocomial infections. *Ann Intern Med* 2004;140:26–32.
47. Peres-Bota D, Rodriguez H, Dimopoulos G, et al. Are infections due to resistant pathogens associated with a worse outcome in critically ill patients? *J Infect* 2003;47:307–316.
48. Podglajen I, Breuil J, Collatz E. Insertion of a novel DNA sequence, 1S1186, upstream of the silent carbapenemase gene cfiA, promotes expression of carbapenem resistance in clinical isolates of *Bacteroides fragilis*. *Mol Microbiol* 1994;12:105–114.
49. Privitera G, Dublanchet A, Sebald M. Transfer of multiple antibiotic resistance between subspecies of *Bacteroides fragilis*. *J Infect Dis* 1979;139:97–101.
50. Ralph ED, Kirby WM. Unique bactericidal action of metronidazole against *Bacteroides fragilis* and *Clostridium perfringens*. *Antimicrob Agents Chemother* 1975;8:409–414.
51. Rasmussen BA, Bush K, Tally FP. Antimicrobial resistance in anaerobes. *Clin Infect Dis* 1997;24 (Suppl 1):S110–S120.
52. Ricci V, Piddock L. Accumulation of garenoxacin by *Bacteroides fragilis* compared with that of five fluoroquinolones. *J Antimicrob Chemother* 2003;52:605–609.
53. Roe DE, Finegold SM, Citron DM, et al. Multilaboratory comparison of anaerobe susceptibility results using 3 different agar media. *Clin Infect Dis* 2002;35:S40–S46.
54. Roe DE, Finegold SM, Citron DM, et al. Multilaboratory comparison of growth characteristics for anaerobes, using 5 different agar media. *Clin Infect Dis* 2002;35:S36–S39.
55. Rogers MB, Parker AC, Smith CJ. Cloning and characterization of the endogenous cephalosporinase gene, cepA, from *Bacteroides fragilis* reveals a new subgroup of Ambler class A beta-lactamases. *Antimicrob Agents Chemother* 1993;37:2391–2400.
56. Rosenblatt JE, Brook I. Clinical relevance of susceptibility testing of anaerobic bacteria. *Clin Infect Dis* 1993;16 (Suppl 4):S446–S448.
57. Rosenblatt JE, Gustafson DR. Evaluation of the Etest for susceptibility testing of anaerobic bacteria. *Diagn Microbiol Infect Dis* 1995;22:279–284.
58. Snydman DR, Cuchural GJ Jr, McDermott L, et al. Correlation of various in vitro testing methods with clinical outcomes in patients with *Bacteroides fragilis* group infections treated with cefoxitin: a retrospective analysis. *Antimicrob Agents Chemother* 1992;36:540–544.
59. Snydman DR, Jacobus NV, McDermott LA, et al. National survey on the susceptibility of *Bacteroides fragilis* group: report and analysis of trends for 1997–2000. *Clin Infect Dis* 2002;35:S126–S134.
60. Snydman DR, Jacobus NV, McDermott LA, et al. Multicenter study of in vitro susceptibility of the *Bacteroides fragilis* group, 1995 to 1996, with comparison of resistance trends from 1990 to 1996. *Antimicrob Agents Chemother* 1999;43:2417–2422.
61. Solomkin JS, Mazuski JE, Baron EJ, et al. Guidelines for the selection of anti-infective agents for complicated intra-abdominal infections. *Clin Infect Dis* 2003;37:997–1005.
62. Song Y, Liu C, McTeague M, Finegold SM. 16S ribosomal DNA sequence-based analysis of clinically significant gram-positive anaerobic cocci. *J Clin Microbiol* 2003;41:1363–1369.
63. Song Y, Liu C, McTeague M, et al. Rapid identification of Gram-positive anaerobic coccal species originally classified in the genus Peptostreptococcus by multiplex PCR assays using genus- and species-specific primers. *Microbiology* 2003;149:1719–1727.
64. Stratton CW, Weeks LS, Aldridge KE. Comparison of the bactericidal activity of clindamycin and metronidazole against cefoxitin-susceptible and cefoxitin-resistant isolates of the Bacteroides fragilis group. *Diagn Microbiol Infect Dis* 1991;14:377–382.
65. Tocher JH, Edwards DI. The interaction of reduced metronidazole with DNA bases and nucleosides. *Int J Radiat Oncol Biol Phys* 1992;22:661–663.
66. Tocher JH, Edwards DI. Evidence for the direct interaction of reduced metronidazole derivatives with DNA bases. *Biochem Pharmacol* 1994;48:1089–1094.
67. Trinh S, Haggoud A, Reysset G, et al. Plasmids pIP419 and pIP421 from Bacteroides: 5-nitroimidazole resistance genes and their upstream insertion sequence elements. *Microbiology* 1995;141(Pt 4):927–935.
68. Urban E, Soki J, Brazier JS, et al. Prevalence and characterization of nim genes of *Bacteroides* sp. isolated in Hungary. Anaerobe 2002;8:175–179.
69. van der Wouden EJ, Thijs JC, Kusters JG, et al. Mechanism and clinical significance of metronidazole resistance in *Helicobacter pylori*. *Scand J Gastroenterol Suppl* 2001;10–4.
70. Veringa EM, Ferguson DA Jr, Lambe DW Jr, et al. The role of glycocalyx in surface phagocytosis of Bacteroides spp. in the presence and absence of clindamycin. *J Antimicrob Chemother* 1989;23:711–720.
71. Veringa EM, Verhoef J. Influence of subinhibitory concentrations of clindamycin on opsonophagocytosis of *Staphylococcus aureus*, a protein-A-dependent process. *Antimicrob Agents Chemother* 1986;30:796–797.
72. Wayne LG, Sramek HA. Metronidazole is bactericidal to dormant cells of *Mycobacterium tuberculosis*. *Antimicrob Agents Chemother* 1994;38:2054–2058.
73. Welch RA, Jones KR, Macrina FL. Transferable lincosamide-macrolide resistance in Bacteroides. *Plasmid* 1979; 2:261–268.
74. Wexler HM. Outer-membrane pore-forming proteins in gram-negative anaerobic bacteria. *Clin Infect Dis* 2002; 35:S65–S71.
75. Wexler HM, Halebian S. Alterations to the penicillin-binding proteins in the *Bacteroides fragilis* group: a mechanism for non-beta-lactamase mediated cefoxitin resistance. *J Antimicrob Chemother* 1990;26:7–20.
76. Yang Y, Rasmussen BA, Bush K. Biochemical characterization of the metallo-beta-lactamase CcrA from *Bacteroides fragilis* TAL3636. *Antimicrob Agents Chemother* 1992;36:1155–1157.
77. Yu Y, Zhou W, Chen Y, et al. Epidemiological and antibiotic resistant study on extended-spectrum beta-lactamase-producing *Escherichia coli* and *Klebsiella pneumoniae* in Zhejiang Province. *Chin Med J (Engl)* 2002;115:1479–1482.
78. Hecnt DW. Prevalence of antibiotic resistance in anaerobic bacteria: worrisome developments. *Clin Infect Dis* 2004;39(1):92–97.
79. Ricci V, Peterson ML, Rotschafer JC, Wexler H, Piddock LJ. Role of topoisomerase mutations and efflux in fluoroquinolone resistance of *Bacteroides fragilis* clinical isolates and loboratory mutants. *Antimicrob Agents Chemother* 2004;48(4):1344–1346.
80. Diniz CG, Farias LM, Carvalho MA, Rocha ER, Smith CJ. Differential gene expression in a *Bacteroides fragilis* metronidazole-resistant mutant. *J Antimicrob Chemother* 2004;54(1):100–108.
81. Schapiro JM, Gupta R, Stefansson E, Fang FC, Limaye AP. Isolation of Metronidazole-Resistant *Bacteroides fragilis* Carrying the nimA Nitroreductase Gene from a Patient in Washington State. *J Clin Microbiol* 2004;42(9):4127–4129.

CHAPTER 5

Antimycobacterial Agents: In Vitro Susceptibility Testing and Mechanisms of Action and Resistance

Clark B. Inderlied and Kevin A. Nash

Worldwide, tuberculosis remains a leading cause of morbidity and mortality, with an estimated 9 million new cases of symptomatic disease leading to 2 to 3 million deaths each year. Dwarfing these numbers is the estimated 2 billion people infected by *Mycobacterium tuberculosis,* the primary causative agent of tuberculosis. However, tuberculosis is infrequent in the general population in many Western countries (=20 per 100,000), including North America. This relatively low incidence is offset by the staggering epidemics occurring in many poorer countries. For instance, in the African countries, Botswana, Namibia, and Swaziland, the incidence of tuberculosis is about 600 per 100,000 people (1).

Over the last few years there have been several major advances in our ability to fight tuberculosis globally. In 2000, over half the world's population was in countries with DOTS (directly observed therapy, short course) programs; implementation of DOTS has led to an 80% successful treatment rate of known patients with smear-positive disease (1). And in many countries the numbers of new cases appears to be declining. Despite the successes of the global DOTS program, the World Health Organization (WHO) estimates that it will be 2013 before its goal of 70% case detection is achieved.

As with tuberculosis control, there have been numerous advances in our understanding *M. tuberculosis.* Perhaps the most notable example was in 1998, with the release of the complete genome sequence of *M. tuberculosis* strain H37Rv (2). Since then, the sequencing of nine more mycobacteria, representing five different species, is either finished or nearly complete (Fig. 5.1). These achievements should facilitate the study of the pathogenic mycobacteria, and hasten the development of novel antimycobacterial agents.

The *Mycobacterium avium* complex (MAC) was once a major cause of morbidity and mortality in patients with acquired immunodeficiency disease syndrome (AIDS). However, with the implementation of HAART (highly active antiretroviral therapy) and effective anti-MAC prophylaxis, the incidence of new cases of disseminated MAC disease has been dramatically reduced. Rapidly growing mycobacteria continue to be important causes of respiratory disease and disseminated cutaneous infections, although the antimicrobial armamentarium has improved here, too. Phylogenetically, the rapidly growing mycobacteria are distinct and separate (Fig. 5.1). However, even within the slowly growing mycobacteria there are considerable phylogenetic distinctions. These distinctions are reflected in the diverse relationships between mycobacterial species and susceptibility or resistance to antimicrobial agents. As in the previous edition, the authors of this chapter have strived to integrate conventional wisdom with new knowledge in an effort to provide reliable practical information about antimicrobial agents and mycobacteria for the use of both mycobacteriologists and clinicians.

IN VITRO SUSCEPTIBILITY TESTING METHODS

Mycobacterium tuberculosis Complex

M. tuberculosis is the most clinically important member of the *M. tuberculosis* complex, which includes *M. tuberculosis, Mycobacterium bovis, M. bovis* bacillus Calmette-Guérin (BCG), *Mycobacterium africanum,* and *Mycobacterium microti.* The members of the complex are closely related on the basis of DNA homology (4,5). Indeed, the degree of DNA homology between the species of the complex indicates that the complex is more properly considered a collection of serovars or pathovars of the same species (Fig. 5.1). Disease caused by *M. bovis* and *M. africanum* is clinically indistinguishable from disease

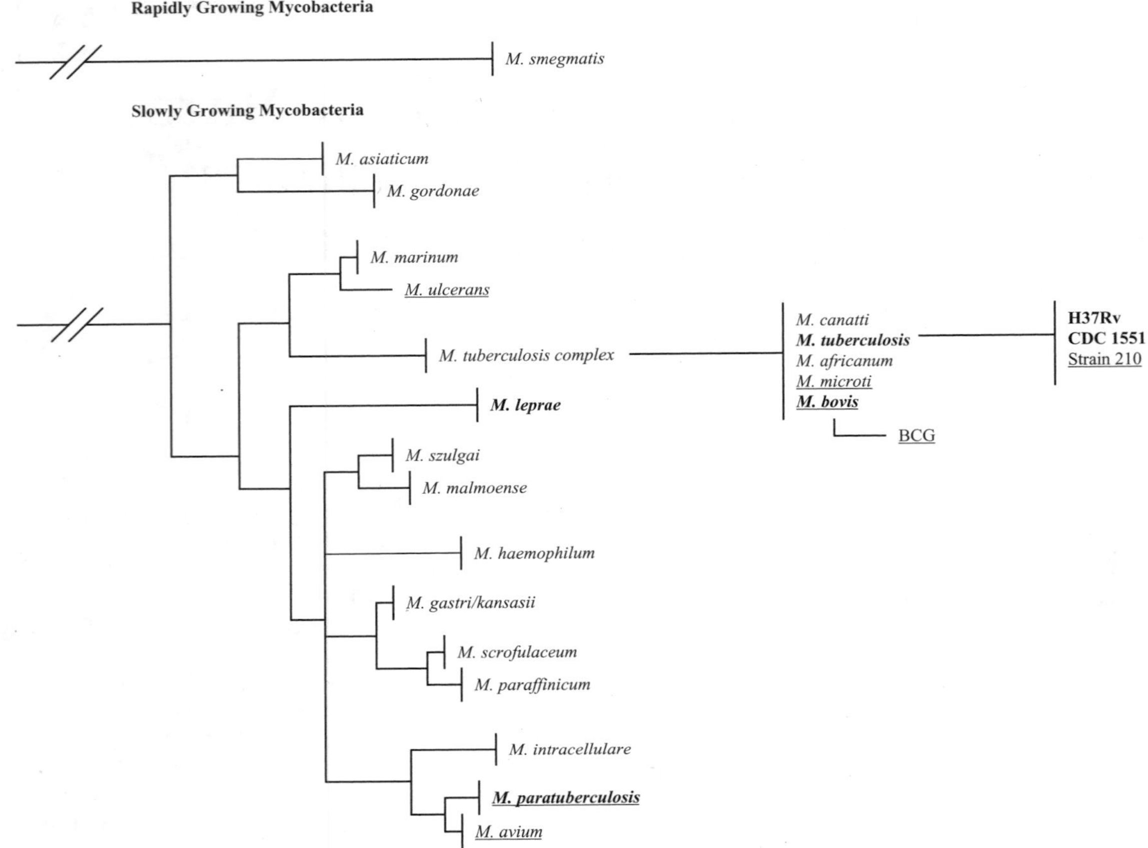

FIGURE 5.1 ● Phylogenetic tree of selected mycobacteria, based on 16S rDNA sequence. Species in **bold** have been sequenced; species underlined, sequencing is in progress or nearly completed. BCG, Bacillus of Calmette-Guérin strain. [Adapted from Brosch et al. (3)]. H37RV, CDC 1551 and Strain 210 are three variant strains of M. tuberculosis.

caused by *M. tuberculosis*, and treatment is the same for all three species. However, since the pasteurization of milk began, the isolation of *M. bovis* is uncommon and *M. africanum* is only rarely isolated from clinical specimens in the United States. *M. microti* causes a tuberculosis-like disease in voles but is not considered pathogenic for humans. Clearly, *M. tuberculosis* is the most common cause of both pulmonary and extrapulmonary tuberculosis in humans.

Treatment

The Centers for Disease Control and Prevention, the American Thoracic Society, and the Infectious Diseases Society of America in the United States now recommend for the initial phase of treatment of *M. tuberculosis* pulmonary disease, a regimen of isoniazid, rifampin, ethambutol, and pyrazinamide for 8 weeks for 5 days per week for 40 doses. The initial phase of treatment may be followed by a continuation phase of isoniazid and rifampin or isoniazid and rifapentine for an additional 18 weeks or 5 days per week for 90 doses (6). While this is considered the standard treatment regimen, it is one of four recommended treatment regimens. Guidelines are provided for appropriate modifications of the initial phase as well as the continuation phase of treatment, including when continuation treatment is appropriate (6). Clearly, the treatment of pulmonary tuberculosis is now greatly influenced by the emergence of multiple-drug resistant (MDR) *M. tuberculosis* and the incidence of tuberculosis in patients with co-infection with human immunodeficiency virus (HIV). The use of four drugs is the preferred regimen for compliant patients with a fully susceptible *M. tuberculosis* isolate. Ethambutol for adults or perhaps streptomycin for children who cannot be monitored for visual acuity should be included in the regimen until susceptibility results are known. At least two additional active agents should be added to failing treatment regimens in any patients with tuberculosis (7–10).

The early detection of drug resistance is essential for the successful management of MDR tuberculosis. In this regard, rifampin resistance may be a useful indicator of an MDR phenotype (minimally, MDR is defined as resistance to isoniazid and rifampin). While the rapid detection of specific mutations in the DNA-dependent RNA polymerase gene (*rpoB* gene) of *M. tuberculosis* is feasible (11–14), rifampin resistance can also be rapidly detected by conventional methods (15,16). In the absence of susceptibility results, patients with suspected MDR tuberculosis should be treated with an injectable drug (e.g., amikacin or kanamycin), a fluoroquinolone, ethambutol, pyrazinamide, and perhaps a fifth drug, (e.g., ethionamide, *p*-aminosalicylic acid, linezolid, clarithromycin, amoxicillin-clavulanate, rifabutin, or cycloserine) (6).

Drug Resistance and Critical Concentrations

An *in vitro* susceptibility test of *M. tuberculosis* is fundamentally a test to detect drug resistance, and the most reliable *in vitro* susceptibility test result that mycobacterial laboratories can report is that an isolate of *M. tuberculosis* is resistant to a drug, because treatment with a drug to which *M. tuberculosis* is resistant invariably leads to therapeutic failure. Drug resistance is defined for *M. tuberculosis* in terms of the critical concentrations of drugs, and this concept is the basis for the methods of susceptibility testing used throughout the world. David (17) showed in the early 1970s that the mutation frequencies for single-drug resistance to isoniazid, rifampin, ethambutol, or streptomycin ranged from 1×10^{-7} to 2×10^{-10}. The clinical significance of these numbers is clear when one considers that a single caseous lesion commonly found in pulmonary tuberculosis can contain 10^8 to 10^{10} tubercle bacilli. Thus, it is apparent why treatment of tuberculosis with a single agent invariably results in relapse due to a resistant isolate. Conversely, two or more agents prevent resistance because the frequency of multiple-drug resistance is the product of the single-drug frequencies of mutation, i.e., 10^{-14} to 10^{-17}. If the frequency of resistant bacilli within a population is greater than 1% (usually much greater than 1%) in a previously untreated patient, this constitutes primary resistance. In most areas of the United States, for example, primary resistance to isoniazid or streptomycin occurs in less than 7% of patients; however, in other areas of the world primary resistance may occur in more than 50% of patients. If resistant bacilli are isolated from a patient in whom the initial isolates were susceptible, this constitutes secondary resistance; the transmission of these resistant organisms represents the most likely source of primary resistance in previously untreated patients.

The MDR phenotype develops as a result of the sequential accumulation of chromosomal mutations (18,19) and neither transposable elements nor plasmids have been associated with a MDR phenotype. In addition, the genetic basis for resistance is the same in MDR *M. tuberculosis* isolates from both HIV-positive and HIV-negative patients (18). No MDR genotypes have been described as being associated with a single genetic event or a novel resistance determinant such as drug efflux.

Thus, the definition of critical concentrations is derived from two important observations. First, 95% or more of wild-type strains of *M. tuberculosis* are fully susceptible to first-line antimycobacterial agents, including isoniazid, rifampin, ethambutol, pyrazinamide, and streptomycin, where a wild-type refers to a strain of *M. tuberculosis* that has never been exposed to antimycobacterial agents. Second, the percentage of a population of tubercle bacilli that would make an isolate different from wild-type strains was defined by the WHO as ranging from 1% (isoniazid and rifampin) to 10% (ethambutol and streptomycin), based, in part, on a correlation with therapeutic efficacy. For reasons of uniformity, 1% was adopted by the Centers for Disease Control and Prevention as the threshold for all drugs tested in the United States. The critical concentration of a drug is then defined as the concentration of drug required to prevent growth above the 1% threshold of the test population of tubercle bacilli. The critical concentration for an antituberculous agent closely approximates the minimal inhibitory concentration (MIC) for wild-type *M. tuberculosis,* because the convention has been to define MICs in terms of an endpoint of 99% inhibition of growth (Table 5.1). Finally, it is important to understand that drugs are used in combination primarily to prevent the emergence of resistance. However, there is some evidence to indicate that first-line agents may act in a synergistic manner. This synergism may reflect combined effects on tubercle bacilli but most likely also reflects the fact that different drugs may act on tubercle bacilli in different physiologic states.

Special (Local) Populations Hypothesis

In considering the susceptibility of *M. tuberculosis* to antimicrobial agents, it is important to appreciate that the organism is likely to exist in the tissue under different physiologic conditions: (a) rapidly growing cells in the aerobic and neutral-pH environment of the pulmonary cavity; (b) slowly growing cells in the oxygen-depleted and low-pH environment of the caseous lesions, where the burden of tubercle bacilli is highest; (c) cells within macrophages; and (d) dormant tubercle bacilli, which are the most intractable to treatment and the likely source of reactivation. Mitchison (21) conceptualized this phenomenon as a special populations hypothesis, which posits that isoniazid, rifampin, and streptomycin are most active against the relatively rapidly dividing bacilli; rifampin is likely to also be active against bacilli that grow in spurts, and pyrazinamide is active against bacilli in the acidic milieu of caseous lesions and in acidified vacuoles of macrophages.

(*text continues on page 160*)

TABLE 5.1

Antimycobacterial Agents Commonly Tested Against *Mycobacterium tuberculosis*[a]

Generic Name	Trade or Other Names	Average MIC (μg/ml) Wild-Type (Susceptible) MTB	Serum and CSF Concentration for Selected Doses			Dosage Recommendations					Half-Life (hr) Normal Adult
				Peak Serum	Peak CSF	Adults		Maximum Daily Dose	Children		
						Dose/Interval			Dose/Interval		
			Dose	Level (μg/ml) @ Time		Oral	Parenteral		Oral	Parenteral	
Primary Agents											
Isoniazid (INH)[a,b]	Niadox, INH, Hyzyd Niconyl	0.05–0.2	0.3 g PO	7 @1–2 hr	3–6	5 mg/kg/day (0.3 g)[c]	5 mg/kg/day IM	0.6 g	10–20 mg/kg/day q 12–24 hr[d]	10–20 mg/kg/day q 12–24 hr IM	0.5–4[b]
Ethambutol (EMB)	Myambutol	1–5	25 mg/kg PO	2–5 @2–4 hr	2–4	15 mg/kg/day[e]		15 mg/kg/day[e]	15 mg/kg/day (not approved)		4–6
Rifampin (RMP)	Rifampicin (United Kingdom), Rifadin, Rimactane	0.5	0.6 g PO (fasting)	10 @2–4 hr	1–2	0.6 g/24 hr		1.2 g	10–20 mg/kg/day q 12–24 hr		2.5–5
Pyrazinamide (PZA)		20	1 g PO	45 @1–4 hr	50	15–30 mg/kg/day		3 g	15–30 mg/kg/day q 12–24 hr		9–10
Secondary Agents											
Amikacin (AN)	Amikin		5 mg/kg IM 7.5 mg/kg IM 7.5 mg/kg IV	16 21 38 @1 hr			5 mg/kg q 8 hr or 7.5 mg/kg q 12 hr	1.5 g		5 mg/kg q 8 hr or 7.5 kg q 12 hr	2–2.5
Streptomycin (SM)		2	1 g IM	25–50 @1–2 hr	9		15 mg/kg/day	2 g		10–15 mg/kg q 12 hr IM	2–3
Ciprofloxacin	Cipro	0.25–3	0.5 g PO 0.75 g PO 0.2 g IV	2.9 4 3.8		0.25–0.75 g q 12 hr	0.2–0.3 g q 12 hr				3.5

Ofloxacin	Floxin	0.5–2.5	0.2 g PO 0.4 g PO 0.6 g PO	2.6 8.6 11		0.2–0.4 g q 12 hr					5.8
Rifabutin	Mycobutin, Ansamycin	0.06[g]–8[h]	0.075–3 g PO	0.2–0.5		0.15–0.3 g/day		0.3 g			
Rifapentine	Priftin	0.125–0.25	600 mg PO	15.05		600 mg q 72 hr					
para-Aminosalicylic acid (PAS)	PAS, Parasal, Para, Pamisyl, Pascorbic, Respias	1	4 g PO (free acid)	75 @1–2 hr		3 g q 6–8 hr		12 g	66.6–75 mg/kg q 6–8 hr		1
Cycloserine (CS)	Oxamycin, Seromycin	5–20	0.25 g PO 0.5 g PO	10 @3–4 hr	8–12	0.25–0.5 g q 12 hr		1 g	3.5–5 mg/kg q 12 hr not approved		10
Ethionamide (ETA)	Trecator-SC	0.6–2.5	0.25–0.5 g PO	2–20 @2–3 hr	1–4	0.25–0.5 g q 12 hr		1 g	5–10 mg/kg q 12 hr not approved		2–4
Kanamycin (KM)	Kantrex		0.5 g IM	14–29 @1 hr	2–10		5 mg/kg q 8 hr or 7.5 mg/kg q 12 hr	1.5 g	150–250 mg/kg/day q 1–6 hr	5–10 mg/kg q 8 hr	2–4
Viomycin	Viocin, Vinactane Tuberactinomycin B	1–10	1 g IM	25–50 @2 hr			1 g q 12 hr twice weekly	2 g			
Capreomycin (CM)[f]	Capastat	1–50	1 g IM	30 @1–2 hr			0.75–1 g q 24 hr 15–20 mg/kg/day IM[i]	20 mg/kg/day		15–30 mg/kg/day IM (not approved)	2
Amithiozone (Not available in USA)	Thiacetazone, Panthrone	1	150 mg PO	1.6–3.2 @4–5 hr							

[a] To minimize the risk of polyneuritis from isoniazid-induced pyridoxine deficiency, pyridoxine (15–50 mg) is often given concurrently. Table adapted (in part) from Norris et al. (20). Please refer to the original reference for additional information. Dosage schedules may change; review the manufacturer's packages information for definitive directions. MIC, minimal inhibitory concentration; CSF, cerebrospinal fluid.

[b] Specific elimination kinetics of isoniazid depend on the acetylator phenotype of the individual; the half-life for rapid acetylators is 0.5–1.5 hr and for slow acetylators, 2–4 hr. For slow acetylators (at least one-half of white Americans), the daily dose should be reduced to 200 mg.

[c] For noncompliant patients, 15 mg/kg can be given twice weekly under supervision. For prophylaxis, isoniazid is usually given for a year in a daily dose of 300 mg for adults and 10/mg/kg (up to 300 mg maximum) for children.

[d] In children with tuberculosis meningitis, some clinicians use 30 mg/kg/day for the first few weeks.

[e] Doses as high as 25 mg/kg/day are occasionally administered during the first 2–3 months of therapy. Intermittent therpay consists of 50 mg/kg/day administered twice weekly.

[f] Pharmacokinetics similar to streptomycin.

[g] Rifampin-susceptible *M. tuberculosis*.

[h] Rifampin-resistant *M. tuberculosis*.

[i] The dosage is 1 g IM daily for 2–4 months and is reduced to 1 g two to three times weekly thereafter.

At present, there are no agents that are known to be active against dormant bacilli. Wayne and Sramek 21a) provided laboratory evidence that metronidazole (a nitroimidazole) is active against dormant bacilli, but nitroimidazoles or similar compounds (22) do not appear to have effective therapeutic activity (23,24).

Detection and Identification

The rapid and accurate detection and identification of *M. tuberculosis* not only is important for the diagnosis of disease, but also for monitoring the response to therapy and for effective control of disease by public health authorities. In addition, the identification of *M. tuberculosis* is essential for accurate and reliable susceptibility testing; for example, the misidentification of *M. avium* as *M. tuberculosis* could result in a false report of MDR *M. tuberculosis,* because *M. avium* is inherently resistant to isoniazid and only variably susceptible to rifampin and ethambutol. Specimens submitted for culture include respiratory, urine, stool, sterile tissue (e.g., bone marrow), and blood samples. There are several semiautomated culture-based methods available for the detection of *M. tuberculosis* and other mycobacteria in clinical specimens including: Bactec 9000MB, Bactec MGIT 960, ESP Culture System II, MB/BacT, and Bactec 460 (25).

The identification of several clinically significant mycobacteria can be achieved within a few hours using commercially available DNA probes (such as AccuProbe, Gen-Probe, Inc., San Diego, CA) that hybridize to species-specific ribosomal RNA (rRNA) sequences (26,27). AccuProbes have proven to be a reliable, fast, and cost-effective method for identifying certain specific mycobacteria isolated from clinical specimens. However, other rapid and reliable methods are available that potentially can identify any mycobacterium. These methods include 16S rDNA sequencing, gas-liquid chromatography of mycolic acid derivatives, multiplex polymerase chain reactions (PCRs), PCR restriction analysis, and others (28–36).

By combining a semiautomated method of detection and one of the newer methods of identification, a definitive laboratory diagnosis of mycobacterial infection should not take longer than 4 weeks. It is not unreasonable for a clinician to expect reliable detection and (at least) presumptive identification of mycobacterial infection within 7 to 14 days. If it is not feasible to use a molecular or other rapid method for identification of mycobacteria, standard methods of identification can be improved by using a strategy that limits the number of biochemical tests (37).

SUSCEPTIBILITY TESTING

Methods and Standardization

There are four well-recognized methods for measuring the susceptibility of *M. tuberculosis* to the antimicrobial agents used for the treatment of tuberculosis (see also Chapter 12, "Molecular Methods"): (a) agar proportion, (b) broth proportion, (c) absolute concentration, and (d) resistance ratio. The proportion methods are widely performed in the United States and western Europe and these methods are the focus of the following discussion. The agar proportion method can be applied as either a direct or indirect test. In the direct test, a specimen that is smear-positive for acid-fast bacilli (AFB) is used as the source of inoculum for the susceptibility test and the specimen is inoculated directly onto the test media with and without drugs. In the indirect test, a pure culture, usually a subculture, of *M. tuberculosis* is used as the source of inoculum for the susceptibility test. On average, the results of the direct test are available 3 to 4 weeks before the results of an indirect test, using agar media. Although the manufacturer indicates that a direct test can be performed using the Bactec broth proportion method, its use is the subject of controversy because of the lack of comparative performance data and the lack of a compelling advantage over the agar-based direct method.

Criteria for Performing Susceptibility Tests

The current recommendation is that all initial isolates of *M. tuberculosis* from a patient, regardless of the source of the specimen, should be tested and the results promptly reported to the health-care provider and the health department (38). Beyond this, susceptibility tests should be performed on subsequent isolates if the patient's cultures fail to convert to negative within 3 months or if there is clinical evidence of a failure to respond to therapy. Other indications for susceptibility testing include: (a) a patient produces specimens that contain an increased number of AFB after an initial decrease; (b) a patient is suspected to have primary resistance, i.e., lives in an area with a high incidence of resistant tuberculosis or was exposed to resistant tuberculosis; or (c) the isolate is from a patient with meningitis or disseminated tuberculosis (38). The susceptibility testing of initial isolates is now recommended for all patients, regardless of the (local) incidence of resistance. The testing of all initial isolates provides for the continuous surveillance of drug susceptibility patterns, which is important because these patterns provide the basis for initial empiric therapy. The issue of laboratory experience in susceptibility testing is controversial. While the original recommendation that susceptibility tests be performed only in laboratories that are capable of species identification and that perform at least 10 susceptibility tests per week (39) was reasonable several years ago, all public health and many private laboratories test primary agents because of the reliability of semiautomated procedures and the compelling need for a rapid turnaround time. Nevertheless, a laboratory that performs susceptibility tests should be able to identify the isolate as to species as a measure of competence. However, testing should be limited to first-line drugs, while the testing of second-line drugs should be referred to a qualified reference laboratory. Indeed, it is prudent to confirm resistance to first-line drugs, especially for initial isolates, by referring the isolate to another laboratory with more experience in susceptibility testing of mycobacteria.

Choice of Antimycobacterial Agents

Primary and secondary antimycobacterial agents are listed in Table 5.1, along with important pharmacokinetic information and the average MIC for susceptible strains of *M. tuberculosis*. Although the recommendation is to test pyrazinamide as a first-line agent, pyrazinamide testing remains somewhat problematic. If pyrazinamide is not routinely tested along with first-line agents, testing must be done as soon as there is evidence for resistance to the other first-line agents. While pyrazinamide monoresistant strains of *M. tuberculosis* are uncommon, the prevalence may be increasing (40). Second-line agents are usually tested only if an isolate is resistant to the primary agents or if the patient has failed therapy with first-line agents. At least one fluoroquinolone should be included as a second-line agent (41,42). Many laboratories do not test second-line agents and refer these requests to an experienced reference laboratory.

Sources of Antimycobacterial Agents

Antimicrobial reference powders can be obtained from commercial sources or from the manufacturer (43). In addition, most antimicrobial reference powders are available from the U.S. Pharmacopeia [Reference Standards Order Department, 12601 Twinbrook Parkway, Rockville, MD 20852; 800–822–8772 or +1−301−881–0666 (international); custsvc@usp.org, marketing@usp.org; or in Europe from the Zentrallaboratorium Deutscher Apotheker, Carl-Mannich-Straβe 20, D-65760 Eschborn, tel., 06196/937–50; fax, 06196/481199; Zentrale@zentrallabor.com].

Antimicrobial agents formulated for therapeutic use in humans or animals should not be used for susceptibility testing. The potency (usually micrograms per milligram of powder) and expiration date must be known for each lot of drug, and the drugs should be stored as recommended by the manufacturer or, in the absence of recommendations, at −20°C in a desiccator under vacuum. The desiccator should be brought to room temperature before opening, in order to avoid condensation and inadvertent hydration of the powders, which may affect the weight and activity of the drugs. The potency of a compound should take into account purity, water content, and active fraction (e.g., free base or acid versus salt) (41).

Stock Solutions of Antimycobacterial Agents

Stock concentrations of drugs should be prepared on the basis of the potency and purity of the drug, which may vary from lot to lot. The required weight (using a fixed volume) or volume (using a fixed weight) for preparing a stock solution can be calculated using one of the following equations:

$$\text{weight (mg)} = [\text{volume (mL)} \times \text{concentration } (\mu\text{g/mL})]/\text{potency } (\mu\text{g/mg})$$

$$\text{volume (mL)} = [\text{weight (mg)} \times \text{potency } (\mu\text{g/mg})]/\text{concentration } (\mu\text{g/mL})$$

Stock solutions should be prepared at a concentration of at least 1000 μg/mL, preferably 10,000 μg/mL or 10-fold higher than the highest concentration to be tested, whichever is greater. The drug should be dissolved in water or the smallest amount of solvent necessary to produce a clear solution. The solvent and diluent should be water, dimethyl sulfoxide, or buffer. In general, it is more accurate to carefully weigh a quantity of drug that is slightly in excess of the desired amount (50 to 100 mg) and adjust the volume of the solvent to achieve the desired final concentration.

If necessary, the stock solution should be sterilized by aseptic filtration through a 0.22-μm pore membrane. Some drug solutions, such as rifampin, autosterilize. The stock solutions should be dispensed into screw-capped polypropylene tubes and stored at 70°C. Thawed tubes of stock drug solution should not be refrozen. Stock solutions prepared and stored in this manner have an expiration date of 1 year (or less) from the time of preparation or a length of time that is in accordance with the manufacturer's recommendations. An important exception is cycloserine, which should be prepared fresh each time (43). Indeed, National Committee for Clinical Laboratory Standards (NCCLS) recommends that cycloserine not be tested because of technical difficulties (41). To add drug to media, a tube of the frozen stock solution is thawed and diluted with water or buffer to yield a solution of 100 to 10,000 μg/mL. The appropriate volume of diluted stock solution is added to 200 mL of sterile 7H10 medium to achieve the desired final concentration (Table 5.2).

Preparation of Media

Three media have been commonly used for *M. tuberculosis* susceptibility testing: Middlebrook and Cohn 7H10 (39) and 7H11 (44) agar supplemented with oleic acid/albumin/dextrose/catalase (OADC), and Löwenstein-Jensen (45) egg-based medium. The Middlebrook 7H10 agar is preferable because of the simple composition and ease of preparation of this medium. Some resistant isolates of *M. tuberculosis* may grow more luxuriantly on Middlebrook 7H11 agar (44,46), but the concentrations of certain drugs must be adjusted if this

TABLE 5.2

Preparation of Stock Concentrations of Antimycobacterial Agents for Use in the Agar Proportion Method

Antimicrobial Agent	Potency[a] (μg/mg)	Solvent[b]	Stock Concentration[c] (μg/mL)	Working Concentration (μg/mL)	Volume to Add[d] (mL)	Final Concentration (μg/mL)
Capreomycin	Varies	SDW	10,000	1,000	2.0	10
Ethambutol HCl	1,000	SDW	10,000	1,000	1.0, 2.0	5, 10
Ethionamide	1,000	DMSO	10,000	1,000	1.0	5
Isoniazid	1,000	SDW	10,000	200	0.2, 1.0	0.2, 1
Kanamycin sulfate	Varies	SDW	10,000	1,000	1.0	5
Ofloxacin	1,000	SDW	10,000	200	2.0	2
Rifabutin	Varies	MEOH	10,000	100	1.0	1
Rifapentine[e]	Varies	DMSO	10,000	100	1.0	1
Rifampin	1,000	DMSO	10,000	1,000	0.2	1
Streptomycin sulfate	Varies	SDW	10,000	1,000	0.4, 2.0	2, 10
p-Aminosalicylic acid	1,000	SDW	10,000	1,000	0.4	2

[a] Calculate weight based on potency (μg/mg) if less than 100%.
[b] SDW, sterile distilled water; DMSO, dimethyl sulfoxide; MEOH, methanol.
[c] Sterilize stock solutions by filtration through 0.22-μm pore membranes, dispense into vials and store at −70°C for up to 12 months, do not re-freeze.
[d] 'Volume to Add' is the mL of 'Working Concentration' added to 200 mL of 7H10 agar to achieve the 'Final Concentration' store at 4°C for up to 1 week.
[e] Proposed breakpoint.

medium is used (42) (Table 5.1). However, routine use of Middlebrook 7H11 medium is not encouraged. Egg-based media, including Löwenstein-Jensen, Wallenstein, and Ogawa media, are not recommended for susceptibility testing.

However, it is important to note that this recommendation (to not use Löwenstein-Jensen) is not universally accepted or perhaps practical. Löwenstein-Jensen medium with or without isoniazid (0.2 mg/L), rifampicin (40 mg/L), dihydrostreptomycin (4 mg/L), and ethambutol (2 mg/L) incorporated into 28 mL universal containers or screw-capped tubes is recommended by the International Union Against Tuberculosis and Lung Disease (IUATLD) for proportion testing of *M. tuberculosis* (47). Indeed, this media may be more readily available where the incidence of tuberculosis is highest and the IUATLD procedures have proven to be valuable in treating and controlling tuberculosis in those parts of the world.

The 7H10 agar medium is prepared according to the manufacturer's directions. The antimicrobial agents are incorporated into 200-mL aliquots of 7H10 agar held at 50°C to 56°C, following the schedule in Table 5.3. The medium is supplemented with OADC and dispensed (in 5-mL aliquots) into sterile plastic quadrant plates. One quadrant is filled with 7H10 medium without drug, which is for the growth control. The medium should be dispensed quickly, the agar allowed to solidify, and either used immediately or stored at 4°C in sealed plastic bags for not more than 28 days (43). The plates should be protected from light during storage and thoroughly equilibrated to room temperature. Check that the agar surface is dry before inoculation.

Disk Elution Alternative

The disk elution alternative method for preparing media for the proportion method of susceptibility testing is both convenient and practical. The disk elution method was originally developed by Wayne and Krasnow (48) and was critically evaluated in comparison with an agar dilution method (43,49). Commercially available disks impregnated with standardized amounts of first-line antimycobacterial drugs are placed in separate quadrants of sterile plastic plates. The amounts of drug contained in the disks, the distribution of disks into the quadrants of the plate, and the final concentrations of drug are shown in Table 5.4. The disks are aseptically placed in the center of the quadrant and 5 mL of 7H10 agar (without drug) at about 52°C is dispensed into each quadrant. The disks

TABLE 5.3

Concentrations of First- and Second-line Drugs Utilizing Agar and Broth Proportion Methods

Drug	Agar Proportion Method		Broth Proportion Methods[a]			
	7H10	7H11	Bactec 460TB	ESP Myco	MGIT 960	BacT/Alert 3D
First-line drugs						
Isoniazid	0.2	0.2	0.1	0.1	0.1	0.09
Isoniazid (high)	1.0	1.0	0.4	0.4	0.4	0.4
Rifampin	1.0	1.0	2.0	1.0	1.0	0.9
Ethambutol	5.0	7.5	2.5	5.0	5.0	2.3
Pyrazinamide	NR	NR	100.0	300	100.0	200.0
Second-line drugs						
Streptomycin	2.0	2.0	2.0	—	1.0	0.9
Streptomycin (high)	10.0	10.0	6.0	—	4.0	—
Ethambutol (high)	10.0	10.0	7.5	—	7.5	—
Capreomycin	10.0	10.0				
Ethionamide	5.0	10.0				
Kanamycin	5.0	6.0				
Ofloxacin	2.0	2.0				
p-Aminosalicylic acid	2.0	8.0				
Rifabutin	0.5	0.5				

[a] Bactec 460TB, the radiometric microbial growth detection system (Becton Dickinson Diagnostic Instruments); ESP Myco, the mycobacteria-adapted ESP Culture System II (Trek Diagnostics); MGIT 960, the Bactec Mycobacteria Growth Indicator Tube (Becton Dickinson Diagnostic Instruments); BacT/ALERT 3D, a semiautomated growth detection system (bioMérieux).

TABLE 5.4

Distribution of Drug-Containing Disks for Disk Elution Susceptibility Test

Plate	Quadrant	Drug	Amount (μg)/ Disk	Final Concentration (μg/ml)
1	I	Control		—
	II	Isoniazid	1	0.2
	III	Isoniazid	5	1.0
	IV	Ethambutol	25	5.0
2	I	Control		—
	II	Rifampin	5	1.0
	III	Streptomycin	10	0.2
	IV	Streptomycin	50	10.0

should remain submerged and centered in the quadrant until the medium solidifies. The plates should be incubated overnight at room temperature to allow for complete diffusion of the drug through the medium. Plates containing antimicrobial agents should be used immediately or stored in plastic bags, in the dark, at 4°C for not more than 4 weeks. At 37°C, more than 50% of the initial concentration of isoniazid, ethambutol, rifampin, ethionamide, and cycloserine in agar plates is lost to deterioration in 2 days (ethambutol) to 1 to 2 weeks (43); these values emphasize the need for proper storage of plates.

Quality Control Strains

No strains of *M. tuberculosis* have been as rigorously standardized for controlling the quality of susceptibility tests as are available for testing rapidly growing gram-negative bacilli and gram-positive cocci. However, there are several strains of *M. tuberculosis* with different resistance phenotypes that can be used for quality control testing. At least one fully susceptible strain should be considered for quality control testing [e.g., *M. tuberculosis* H37Rv, ATCC strain 27294), which is susceptible to the primary agents (isoniazid, rifampin, ethambutol, and pyrazinamide)]. The choice of a resistant strain is more problematic. Many of the resistant strains of *M. tuberculosis* that are available from ATCC have very high levels of resistance, which is not particularly useful when confirming the ability of a method to distinguish resistant from susceptible. Clinical isolates with a stable low-level resistance phenotype may be a preferred quality control strain. Multiply resistant isolates (i.e., MDR *M. tuberculosis*) should *not* be used because of the risk to laboratory staff and others. The quality control strains are grown in liquid medium, diluted to a standard turbidity, dispensed into 1-mL aliquots, and frozen at −70°C. Once each week, or whenever a new lot of medium is prepared, one or more aliquots of the control strains should be thawed and two dilutions prepared according to the standard dilution protocol. One dilution should yield 200 to 300 colonies and the other dilution should yield 20 to 30 colonies on the control plates. In this manner, both the quality of the medium and the dilution technique are tested.

Media Components

Guthertz et al. (50) examined the effects of different lots of Middlebrook 7H10 agar, OADC, and 0.5% glycerol on standard susceptibility test results using a modified proportion method. Three assays were used to measure the comparative quality of the components: (a) a comparative resistance assay to monitor drug stability in solution and in agar, (b) a disk potency assay to monitor the potency of disks impregnated with antimycobacterial agents, and (c) a standard concentration assay to monitor changes in antibiograms caused by changes in the test medium. Rejection criteria included both changes in the size of colonies and changes in the number of colonies; a 20% change in either colony size or number was considered significant. The test strains included *M. tuberculosis* H37Rv (ATCC strain 27294) and several strains of *M. tuberculosis, M. avium,* and other slowly growing mycobacteria. By this method, the authors concluded that 30% of lots of OADC and 15% of lots of Middlebrook 7H10 agar were unacceptable, leading to interpretations of both false susceptibility and false resistance (Fig. 5.2). The primary reasons for rejection were reduced colony size and drug binding. This study emphasizes the importance of recording the lot numbers of all components and testing new lots of medium components, especially OADC and 7H10 powder, with standard strains of *M. tuberculosis* and other slowly growing mycobacteria, to ensure the reliability of results from batch to batch. A convenient protocol for monitoring OADC was described by Butler et al. (51). They established a correlation between the ability of OADC to support the growth of *Bacillus subtilis* (measured as a change in optical density over 24 hours) in a heart infusion broth supplemented with a test lot of OADC and the ability of OADC to support mycobacterial growth. Acceptable lots of OADC support the growth of *B. subtilis* (biomass turbidity increase of 0.2 OD_{650} in 24 hours) and good growth of mycobacteria, whereas failure to support growth of *B. subtilis* correlates with poor growth of mycobacteria.

Sterility Tests

A representative sample (10%) of each lot of plates (agar dilution or disk elution) should be incubated for 48 hours at 35°C and checked for sterility.

Agar Proportion Method: Direct Test

The direct test version of the proportion method should be performed only with specimens that are smear-positive for AFB. The inoculum should be carefully controlled because overinoculation may lead to false resistance and underinoculation may lead to false susceptibility. The direct method may be warranted when there is a high incidence of drug resistance with a patient population, but logically this would require that second-line drugs be tested (52). Therefore, the direct test might best be performed only in a qualified reference laboratory.

1. Digest, decontaminate, and concentrate the specimen, as appropriate, according to an accepted procedure (39, 53).
2. Prepare, stain, and examine a smear using either a fluorochrome or carbol-fuchsin method. Record the number of bacilli in each of 20 fields and calculate the average number per field. Because the test is based on measuring a reduction in colony-forming units (CFU),

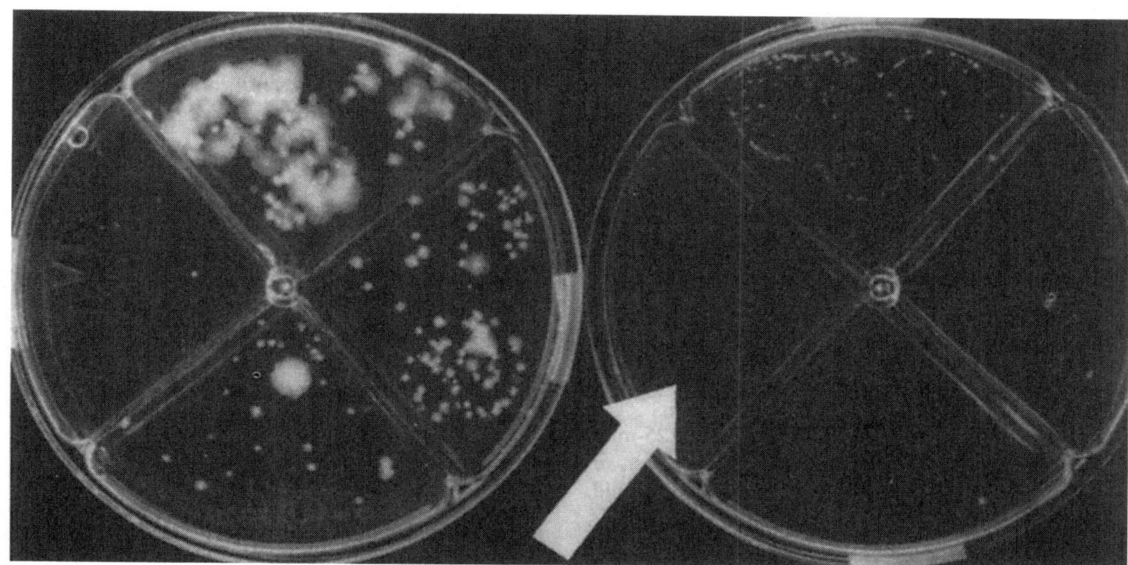

FIGURE 5.2 • Comparative resistance assay. Reduction of colony size by a new medium component and the resulting false drug susceptibility. The standard medium **(left)** contains increasing concentrations of ethionamide in three quadrants and no drug in the fourth quadrant. The test medium **(right)** was prepared using the same method and at the same time, except for a new lot of oleic acid/albumin/destrose/catalase. All quadrants were inoculated with 0.1 mL of a suspension of *M. tuberculosis. Arrow* indicates the quadrant where colony size was not visible (50). (Photo courtesy of Sharon Kurashige, Microbial Diseases Laboratory, California Department of Health Sciences.)

count any clumps as a single organism; however, it is important to emphasize that the suspension should be completely homogenized. Dilute the specimen in water (e.g., 0.5 mL of specimen in 4.5 mL of water) based on the stain, using the dilution scheme shown in Table 5.5 as a guide. Choose two concentrations so there is a 100-fold difference between the concentrations of the two inocula.

TABLE 5.5

Dilution of Sputum Concentrate for Inoculation of Susceptibility Test Medium-Direct Proportion Method[a]

Dilution	Fluorochrome Stain[b]
Undiluted	<25[c]
Undiluted, 1:10	25–50
Undiluted, 1:100	50–250
1:100, 1:1,000	>250

[a] Table adapted from National Committee for Clinical Laboratory Standards (54).
[b] Number of fluorochrome-positive bacilli observed at 200–400X.
[c] Increase inoculum to 0.2 mL if <5 bacilli per 200–400X field.

3. Use a sterile safety pipette to inoculate 0.1 mL of each dilution onto each quadrant of duplicate plates and use separate sets of plates for each dilution of the inoculum. Let the plates stand for 1 hour to absorb the inoculum. If the patient has received antituberculosis medications, include an undiluted inoculum regardless of the smear results, because AFB observed in the smears of specimens from treated patients may be nonviable.
4. Place the plates into CO_2-permeable polyethylene bags (6 × 8 inches) with the medium on the bottom, i.e., do not invert the plates. Heat-seal the bags and incubate the plates at 35°C to 37°C in 5% to 10% CO_2.
5. Read the plates weekly for 3 weeks; however, do not report a result as susceptible before 3 weeks. Colonies of resistant isolates often develop more slowly than the colonies of susceptible isolates. If growth is not apparent, examine each quadrant with a dissecting microscope (30× to 60× magnification) for the presence of slowly growing microcolonies; however, take care not to overinterpret the results because the deterioration of drugs may lead to the appearance of microcolonies (43). Grade the results, at both dilutions, according to the following criteria: confluent (too numerous to count), record 3+ to 4+; in the range of 100 to 200 colonies, record 2+; in the range of 50 to 100 colonies, record 1+; less than 50 colonies, record the actual number (note the presence of microcolonies). The control plate, at one dilution or the other, should contain 50 to

100 colonies, and the percentage of resistant colonies is based on this number. If the control plate contains insufficient growth or confluent growth, the test must be repeated unless the isolate is fully susceptible to all drugs tested. The susceptibility test should be terminated at 3 weeks because even susceptible isolates may eventually grow in the presence of bacteriostatic drugs.

6. Retain the control plate (quadrant) as an additional source of the isolate because this plate was directly inoculated with the specimen.

Agar Proportion Method: Indirect Test

The indirect test is used for testing pure cultures of *M. tuberculosis* after isolation from clinical specimens. As with the direct test, the preparation of the inoculum should be carefully controlled to avoid over- or underinoculation.

1. Prepare the inoculum by scraping colonies from the surface of a solid drug-free medium. Attention should be given to sampling all colony types. Use primary cultures whenever possible and avoid liquid cultures where faster growing and more susceptible bacilli may predominate.
2. Transfer the bacterial mass to a sterile 16 ×125-mm, screw-capped tube containing six to eight glass or plastic beads and 3 to 5 mL of a Tween-albumin liquid medium such as Middlebrook 7H9.
3. Homogenize the mixture using a vortex mixer for 1 to 2 minutes. Swirl, do not churn. This step must be performed in a biologic safety cabinet, ideally with a proper face mask in place.
4. Allow the mixture to stand undisturbed for 30 minutes to allow the large particles to settle and to diminish the release of aerosols when the tube is opened.
5. Withdraw the supernatant suspension and adjust the turbidity to be equivalent to a McFarland no. 1 standard, using 7H9 broth. The suspension should contain approximately 10^7 CFU/mL.
6. Prepare 10^{-2} and 10^{-4} dilutions of the standardized suspension using 7H9 broth. Starting with the 10^{-4} dilution, inoculate 0.1 mL (three drops) to each corner of each quadrant of one set of plates. Then inoculate the 10^{-2} dilution in the same manner using the second set of plates. The plates should contain drugs in quadrants 2, 3, and 4, but no drug in quadrant 1.
7. Proceed with the test as described for the direct test, i.e., steps 3 to 5.
8. If the culture is old, it may be necessary to subculture the isolate by transferring a portion of each colony type into a tube of drug-free 7H9 broth and incubating the tube at 35°C for 7 days or until the turbidity matches that of the McFarland no. 1 standard. Alternatively, use lower dilutions (e.g., 10^{-1} and 10^{-3}) for the inoculum.

Broth Proportion Method: Bactec Indirect Test

The Bactec radiometric method (BD Bactec 460TB system; BD Diagnostic Systems, Sparks, MD), based on the work of Cummings and Rostraph (55) and Middlebrook et al. (56), is a reliable and comparatively rapid method of susceptibility testing (57,58). The radiometric method is based on the fact that mycobacteria actively metabolize fatty acids to CO_2. If these fatty acids are radioactively labeled with ^{14}C, the CO_2 end product can be easily detected in a quantitative manner by the Bactec instrument. The result is a rapid and sensitive method for detecting the growth of mycobacteria. The adaptation of this method for *in vitro* susceptibility testing was a straightforward extension of the growth–detection method.

Principles of the Method

The Bactec 12B (Middlebrook 7H12) broth consists of 0.47% (w/v) 7H9 broth supplemented with 0.5% (weight per volume) bovine serum albumin (fraction V), 192 units of catalase, 0.1% (weight per volume) casein hydrolysate, and 4 μCi of (^{14}C)palmitic acid at a pH of 6.8 $\pm$ 0.2, in a final volume of 4.0 mL. The medium is contained in a 20-mL glass vial sealed with a rubber septum and a crimp cap. The Bactec 460TB instrument automatically evacuates the headspace above the culture medium, replaces the gas with 5% to 10% CO_2 in air, and simultaneously measures the amount of radioactivity in the evacuated gas in terms of a growth index (GI). The GI units are arbitrary units of radioactivity that relate to the actual disintegrations per minute detected by the instrument. The amount of $^{14}CO_2$ released is a direct measure of the amount of growth; for example, if the cumulative GI values are plotted as a function of time, the resulting curve approximates a standard growth curve (108). The susceptibility of mycobacteria to drugs, therefore, can be defined in terms of decreased GI values, compared with an appropriate control. The interpretive criteria used with the Bactec method are based on the same principles as those for the proportion method. Thus, the growth of a clinical isolate of *M. tuberculosis* in the presence of an antimycobacterial drug is measured and compared with the growth of the same organism in the absence of drug, but with a starting inoculum that is diluted 10^{-2}.

Antimycobacterial Agents

Lyophilized preparations of the primary agents (streptomycin, isoniazid, rifampin, and ethambutol) are available from Becton Dickinson (BD Diagnostic Systems) or can be prepared using standard reference powders. The lyophilized preparations are rehydrated by adding 10 mL of POES solvent to the isoniazid stock vial (40 μg) and 5 mL of sterile, distilled, deionized water to all other drug stock vials to yield 40X stock solutions, i.e., the amount of drug in each vial is adjusted such that, when 0.1 mL of the reconstituted stock solution is injected into a Bactec vial (4 mL of medium), the final concentrations will be as shown in Table 5.3. Note that the concentration of rifampin is higher (2.0 μg/mL), that of isoniazid is lower (0.1 μg/mL), and that of ethambutol is lower (2.5 μg/mL) in the Bactec method compared with the proportion method. The lower drug concentrations must be tested because these concentrations yield results that are equivalent to the critical concentrations used in the proportion method. Additional concentrations can be tested; however, the test report should include the interpretation along with the concentration of the drug tested (e.g., susceptible at 7.5 μg/mL ethambutol) (58,59). The stock solutions can be dispensed into smaller aliquots in polypropylene tubes and stored at −70°C for 6 months, at −20°C for 3 months, or at 4°C for 7 days. The lyophilized drugs should be stored unopened at 4°C until the expiration date on the vial. Secondary agents, if tested by this method, should be tested at the concentrations shown in Table 5.3, using standard reference powders.

Drugs are added to the Bactec vials by transferring 0.1 mL of the drug stock solution, either freshly prepared or thawed from frozen stock, using a single-use 1-mL syringe. Once diluted, the vial can be stored at 4°C for 7 days. The vials should be pretested on the Bactec 460TB system in order to replace the gas in the headspace, and any vials with a GI reading of 20 or greater should be discarded.

Inoculum

The source of the inoculum can be either a pure culture of fresh growth on solid medium or a positive Bactec vial containing actively growing bacilli. Preparation of the inoculum using growth from solid medium is the same as previously described except for the use of a special diluting fluid. The use of this special fluid is important in order to avoid diluting the radiospecific activity of the ^{14}C-labeled palmitic acid. The fluid is available from the supplier in aliquots of 9.9 mL and consists of 0.2% fatty acid-free bovine serum albumin and 0.02% polysorbate 80 in distilled deionized water, filter sterilized through a 0.22-μm pore membrane.

Suspensions of the test and control organisms adjusted to be equivalent to a McFarland no. 1 turbidity standard are used with the daily test schedule. Suspensions adjusted to a McFarland no. 0.5 turbidity standard are used for the nonweekend schedule (see later). The purity of the suspension should be checked by inoculating a small amount of the suspension onto a nonselective medium and performing an AFB stain on a smear of the suspension. Dilution of the suspension should be adjusted for the presence of clumps of medium that are likely to contribute to the turbidity of the suspension. If the culture is old or the growth is insufficient, 0.1 mL of the suspension should be inoculated into a Bactec 12B vial and the vial incubated until the GI equals or exceeds 500 (see later).

If the source of the inoculum is a positive Bactec vial, the GI should be 300 to 800 (some workers prefer to use vials with a GI of 999). If the GI is 300, the vial should be incubated for an additional 1 day; however, if the GI is between 500 and 800, one should proceed directly to the susceptibility test. Bactec vials with GI values of 500 to 800 may be held at 4°C for a few days (less than 7 days) to facilitate batch susceptibility testing. If the GI is more than 800, the suspension should be diluted 1:1 with the special diluting fluid as described.

Inoculation

The headspace of each Bactec vial should be replaced by testing the vials in the Bactec 460TB instrument and any vials with GI values of 20 or higher should be discarded. Then 0.1 mL of each appropriately prepared drug stock is added to separate Bactec vials, with one vial for each drug concentration tested and one vial for each control. One-tenth milliliter of the suspension of mycobacteria is inoculated into each vial, using a 1-mL syringe with a fixed needle.

To inoculate the control vial, each suspension should be diluted 1:100 by transferring 0.1 mL into 9.9 mL of special diluting fluid. The dilution should be thoroughly mixed by repetitive (six times) aspiration with a needle and syringe and then 0.1 mL should be transferred into the control vial without drug. An additional control of undiluted inoculum in a vial without any drug may be helpful for interpreting the results for poorly or erratically growing isolates. The top of each vial should be swabbed with disinfectant followed by 70% alcohol. The vials should be incubated at 37°C ± 1°C and protected from sunlight (light may cause the production of formaldehydes in the growth medium, which inhibit the growth of mycobacteria).

Daily Testing

The vials should be tested in the Bactec 460TB instrument daily (including weekends and holidays) within 2 hours of the same time of day. They should be tested for at least 4 days but not more than 12 days.

Nonweekend Testing

A convenient schedule for susceptibility testing using the Bactec radiometric method was described by Hawkins (60,61). Accordingly, susceptibility tests are performed in batches such that all tests are initiated on Friday. The inoculum can be a Bactec vial (1 day after reaching a GI of 300) or a suspension of growth from solid media adjusted to be equivalent to a McFarland no. 0.5 standard. The vials should be tested for the first time on the following Monday and tested each day for a minimum total incubation period of 5 days (Wednesday). As with daily testing, the vials should be tested within 2 hours of the same time each day.

Interpretation

The interpretation of radiometric (Bactec) results is based on measuring the daily change in GI values of the organism incubated in the presence of drug, compared with the daily change in GI values of the organism incubated in the absence of drug but starting with an inoculum that was diluted 1:100. Incubation is continued until the daily change in GI values for the control vial is 30. The interpretive criteria are as follows: daily change in GI values of control more than daily change in GI values with drug, susceptible; daily change in GI values of control less than? daily change in GI values with drug, resistant; daily change in GI values of control equal to daily change in GI values with drug, borderline.

If the daily change in GI values of the control vial is 30 or greater before day 4 with daily testing, the incubation is continued for an additional 1 day before interpretation of the results. If the daily change in GI values is 30 or greater on Tuesday using the nonweekend schedule (GI values on Monday are disregarded), testing is continued until Wednesday regardless of the Tuesday reading. The daily change in GI values value must equal or exceed 30 on Wednesday before the results can be interpreted.

In summary, for interpretation of Bactec susceptibility test results the daily change in GI values must equal or exceed 30 after a period of not less than 4 days of testing (5 days of incubation) using the daily schedule and not less than 3 days of testing (5 days of incubation) using the nonweekend schedule. The borderline interpretation is potentially misleading and the test should be repeated in an effort to clarify whether the isolate is resistant or susceptible.

Broth Proportion Method: Semiautomated Systems

Three semiautomated microbial growth systems have been developed and evaluated for susceptibility testing of *M. tuberculosis:* BacT/ALERT 3D (bioMérieus, Inc., Durham, NC) (62), ESP Myco Culture System II (Trek Diagnostic Systems, Cleveland, OH) (63–65), and MGIT 960 (BD Diagnostic Systems) (66–72). Each system is in essence a broth proportion method that varies in the technology used to continuously monitor metabolic activity as an indicator of growth or the absence of growth (Table 5.6). The BacT/ALERT 3D system can be used to test isoniazid, rifampin, ethambutol, and streptomycin while the ESP Myco and MGIT systems can be used to test these same drugs plus pyrazinamide. None of the systems have been adequately evaluated for testing second-line drugs. The ESP Myco and MGIT systems have been evaluated in multicenter studies and were found to provide results that compared well with either the Bactec 460TB or the agar proportion methods (67,70). The BacT/Alert 3D system is less well studied, but performed well in comparison with the Bactec 460TB (73) and the agar proportion method (74), but was found to be deficient using the manufacturer's new protocol (62).

Broth Proportion Method: Bactec Direct Test

The Bactec method of susceptibility testing also can be employed as a direct test; however, there is only a limited amount of information on the performance characteristics of the Bactec method when used in this manner, and many experienced mycobacteriologists do not advocate using the Bactec direct test and the use of the Bactec 460TB as a direct test will not be described further.

METHODS FOR TESTING PYRAZINAMIDE

Pyrazinamide should be tested only against *M. tuberculosis* because the agent is inactive against all other mycobacteria, including rapidly growing strains. *In vitro* testing of pyrazinamide is more difficult because the drug is active only in the acidic pH range (i.e., pH 5.5) and most strains of *M. tuberculosis* grow poorly at this pH; some strains fail to grow at all. Agar and broth methods have been described for testing pyrazinamide, but broth methods are more convenient, and preferred by many laboratories.

Low pH Agar Method

Butler and Kilburn (75) showed that 90% of *M. tuberculosis* isolates, including pyrazinamide-resistant isolates, can be successfully tested against pyrazinamide using the proportion method with a low-pH Middlebrook 7H10 agar supplemented with albumin/dextrose/catalase (ADC) but not OADC. One should be alert to the fact that oleic acid at pH 5.5 inhibits the growth of 17% to 25% of *M. tuberculosis* isolates that otherwise grow at pH 5.5. The ADC lots should be quality-control tested using the previously described *B. subtilis* assay (30). Pyrazinamide is available from the sources listed earlier and the drug should be tested at 25 to 200 μg/mL; usually 25 and 50 μg/mL are sufficient for routine testing. Colonies are counted after 3 to 6 weeks of incubation at 35°C. The inhibitory effect of pyrazinamide (in low-pH 7H10 agar) is diminished by the partial pressures of CO_2 that are required for the growth of *M. tuberculosis,* and the degree of this effect is strongly influenced by the inoculum size (75). It is important to emphasize that, despite the modifications and controls employed with the low-pH agar method, approximately 10% of *M. tuberculosis* isolates fail to grow on this medium. Heifets and Sanchez described an alternate low pH (pH 6.0) agar medium containing animal serum rather than OADC (76). Pyrazinamide is tested at 900 to 1,200 μg/mL using this medium.

TABLE 5.6

Comparison of Semiautomated Systems for *In Vitro* Susceptibility Testing of *M. tuberculosis* and Other Mycobacteria

	ESP Culture System II	Bactec MGIT 960	BacT/Alert 3D
Growth detection	Gas partial pressure changes due to production and/or consumption of gas	Fluorescence increase as dissolved oxygen is consumed using a fluorescence quenching-based oxygen sensor (ruthenium pentahydrate)	CO_2 production by is detected with a gas-permeable sensor/indicator embedded in the culture tube
Medium	Middlebrook 7H9 broth plus glycerol, casitone, cellulose sponge disks, and OADC[a]	"Modified" Middlebrook 7H9 broth	Middlebrook 7H9 broth plus bovine serum albumin, catalase, casein disks, and OADC
Inoculum	0.5 mL of a 1:10 dilution from a McFarland no. 1 standard	0.5 mL of a 1:5 dilution from a McFarland no. 0.5 standard or a "positive" MGIT growth tube	0.5 mL of a "positive" BacT/Alert bottle prepared by inoculating 0.5 mL of a McFarland no. 1 standard
"Susceptible" criterion	No growth or no growth within 3 days after no drug control turns positive	No growth as interpreted by an automated algorithm and analysis of fluorescence differences between tests and control	No growth before 1:100 no drug control turns positive
Days to result	4–5 days	6–7 days	4–8 days

[a] OADC, oleic acid/albumin/destrose/catalase.

Low-pH Bactec Method

Several modifications of the Bactec 12A radiometric method have been developed to test pyrazinamide. Heifets and Iseman (77) showed good correlation of results from a modified low-pH Bactec method with those from a low-pH 7H11 agar method, as well as with an assay for pyrazinamidase activity. In this method, pyrazinamide was added simultaneously with a solution of phosphoric acid, bovine serum albumin, and Tween 80 to exponentially growing cultures of *M. tuberculosis*. Tarrand et al. (78) used a buffered phosphoric acid solution to lower the pH of the 7H12 Bactec medium and used a 1:10 dilution of the standard inoculum used in the Bactec procedure. Using this method, 1% to 2% pyrazinamide resistance was detected in artificial mixtures of resistant and susceptible isolates of *M. tuberculosis*. Woodley and Smithwick (79) obtained 100% agreement between the low-pH 7H10 agar method and a pH 5.5 Bactec radiometric method where the Bactec 12A medium was supplemented with 0.1 mL of fresh egg yolk, using the 2-mL Bactec 12A vials. Finally Salfinger and Heifets (80), using the pH 5.95 Bactec 12A medium, showed that the susceptibility results with pyrazinamide tested at pH 5.95 could be reliably extrapolated to the results at pH 5.5. This method avoids the problem of adjusting the pH of the growth medium with acid.

Pyrazinamidase Activity

Detection of pyrazinamidase activity has been used to screen for pyrazinamide-resistant strains of *M. tuberculosis* (81); however, a later study showed that there was no direct correlation between loss of pyrazinamidase activity and resistance (82). Indeed, using low-pH Middlebrook 7H10 medium, 11 of 11 strains with pyrazinamide resistance levels of 100 to 150 g/mL and 3 of 10 strains with resistance levels of 200 to 300 μg/mL retained pyrazinamidase activity (29). Virtually all *M. tuberculosis* isolates that are susceptible to pyrazinamide produce detectable pyrazinamidase (83).

Absolute Concentration Method

The absolute concentration method consists of inoculating media, with or without antimycobacterial agents, with a carefully controlled inoculum containing 2×10^3 to 1×10^4 CFU of mycobacteria (84). Resistance is defined as growth that is greater than a certain number of CFUs (usually 20) at a particular drug concentration. The drug concentrations must be precisely confirmed for each batch of medium.

1. To prepare the inoculum, a loop containing 2 μL of growth is evenly suspended in 2 mL of Dubos broth without albumin. The turbidity is adjusted to a McFarland no. 1 standard and the suspension is diluted 1:50 in the same Dubos broth to yield 2×10^5 to 10^6 CFU/mL.
2. Tubes of Löwenstein-Jensen medium containing antimycobacterial agents at the concentrations shown in Table 5.7 are inoculated with a 3-mm loop (2,000 to 10,000 CFU) and then incubated at 37°C for 4 weeks.
3. For interpretation, a control wild-type strain should be tested in parallel with the test strain. The critical concentrations are 0.2 μg/mL for isoniazid, 5 μg/mL for streptomycin, 0.5 μg/mL for *p*-aminosalicylic acid (PAS), and 20 μg/mL for ethionamide. The test isolate of *M. tuberculosis* is considered resistant to a drug if there are 20 CFU on the surface of the Löwenstein-Jensen medium containing a drug at the critical concentration.

Resistance Ratio Method

The resistance ratio method is similar to the absolute concentration method except that a second identical series of tubes are inoculated with the standard *M. tuberculosis* H37Rv strain. The susceptibility test results are expressed in terms of the ratio of the MIC of drug necessary to inhibit the growth of the test isolate of *M. tuberculosis* to that for the standard H37Rv strain. The advantage of this method is that small batch-to-batch variations in the test media can be disregarded because the results are normalized using the H37Rv strain.

1. To prepare the inoculum, 2 μL of growth of the test isolate is evenly suspended in 0.4 mL of sterile distilled water in a 7-mL, screw-capped bottle containing six (3-mm) glass beads. The suspension is vigorously shaken to disperse the cells. A suspension of strain H37Rv is prepared in the same manner.
2. Tubes of Löwenstein-Jensen medium containing antimycobacterial agents at the concentrations shown in Table 5.7 are inoculated with a 3-mm loop suspension of the test strain and then incubated at 37°C for 4 weeks. A second set of tubes are inoculated with strain H37Rv and incubated as previously described.
3. Sufficient growth is defined as 20 CFU or more. The resistance ratio is the MIC of the test strain divided by the MIC of strain H37Rv; for example, if the MIC of the test strain is 8 μg/mL and the MIC of H37Rv is 4 μg/mL, the resistance ratio is 2.
4. Interpretation is as follows: resistance ratio of 2, susceptible; resistance ratio of 8, resistant; and resistance ratio of 4, doubtful. These interpretations are based on the description of the method by Canetti et al. (34). One study where this method was used interpreted a resistance ratio of 4 as resistant (85).

NONTUBERCULOUS, RAPIDLY GROWING MYCOBACTERIA

The rapidly growing mycobacteria include at least 30 species; however, the majority (90%) of infections

TABLE 5.7

Concentrations of Antimycobacterial Agents Used in the Absolute Concentration and Resistance Ratio Methods

Antimycobacterial Agent	Absolute Concentration Method (μg/mL)	Resistance Ratio Method: Test Strain (μg/mL)	Resistance Ratio Method: H37Rv Control Strain (μg/mL)
Isoniazid	0.01, 0.05, 0.2, 1	0.2, 1	0.05–2
Rifampin	—	5–16	5–16
Ethambutol	—	0.5–16	0.5–16
Streptomycin	1, 2, 5, 10	8–32	2–8
Ethionamide	5, 10, 20, 50	—	—
p-Aminosalicylic acid	0.1, 0.2, 0.5, 2	2–8	0.5–2

in humans are caused by three species: *Mycobacterium fortuitum*, *Mycobacterium chelonae*, and *Mycobacterium abscessus* (86,87). These species are important causes of cutaneous, pulmonary, wound, and nosocomial infections, especially following catheter insertions, augmentation mammaplasty, and cardiac bypass surgery. Disseminated disease is rare and is usually associated with immunodeficiency, including that associated with corticosteroid therapy but not HIV infection (88). Other rapidly growing mycobacteria have been implicated in human disease, however, such infections are rare.

The term "rapid grower" refers to the uniform observation that these mycobacteria form visible colonies on solid media within 7 days when inoculated with a dilute suspension of the organism. However, it may take much longer than 7 days for rapid growers to be detected during primary isolation from clinical specimens.

It is important to quickly distinguish the rapidly growing mycobacteria from other mycobacteria because conventional antituberculous drugs (with the exception of rifampin and amikacin) are ineffective for the treatment of infections caused by the rapid growers (25,86,87). This is because rapidly growing mycobacteria are resistant to common antituberculous agents (86), which may not always be appreciated by the clinician with limited experience in treating these infections. Wallace (89) recommended alerting physicians to the clinical significance and the appropriateness of susceptibility testing of rapidly growing mycobacteria by amending the laboratory report with a statement such as the following:

> "The rapidly growing mycobacteria (*M. fortuitum, M. chelonae,* and *M. abscessus*) are resistant to all of the common antituberculosis agents; therefore, routine susceptibility testing is inappropriate for these isolates. Isolates from wounds are almost certainly of clinical significance and susceptibility testing with agents that are likely to be therapeutically effective is appropriate and should be routinely performed with these isolates. Rapidly growing mycobacteria that are isolated from respiratory specimens are rarely clinically significant and routine susceptibility testing is inappropriate. However, testing may be appropriate if large numbers of these mycobacteria are isolated from respiratory tract specimens, especially in repeat specimens, such as from HIV infected patients."

In order to optimize the susceptibility testing and facilitate interpretation of the susceptibility results, the NCCLS recommends that isolates be identified at least to differentiate the *M. fortuitum* group from the *M. abscessus-chelonae* group. Preferably, identification should be to the species level.

Several studies showed that the rapidly growing mycobacteria are susceptible to a variety of antimicrobial agents and that these agents are clinically effective (Table 5.8) (25,86,87). In addition, the macrolides, clarithromycin and azithromycin, are important agents for the treatment of pulmonary and cutaneous infections caused by *M. chelonae* and *M. abscessus* and perhaps 80% of *M. fortuitum* (87). However, the apparent susceptibility of many *M. fortuitum* isolates may be misleading as this species harbors an inducible erythromycin ribosome methylation (*erm)* gene, *erm*(39), that can confer high-level clarithromycin resistance (90,91). Most isolates of *M. chelonae* have clarithromycin MICs of 0.25 μg/mL, but resistance develops quickly with monotherapy (92); in these cases resistance is conferred by mutation in the 23S rRNA gene (93).

SUSCEPTIBILITY TESTING

Several methods have been described for measuring the *in vitro* susceptibility of rapidly growing mycobacteria, including (a) agar dilution (94–96), (b) agar disk elution (97), (c) Etest (AB BIODIS Solne, Swaden) (98–101), (d) disk diffusion (95,102), and (e) broth microdilution (94,103). However, the standard recommended by the NCCLS is a broth microdilution assay using cation-supplemented Mueller-Hinton broth as the preferred medium (41) and only this method is discussed further.

Antimicrobial Agents

Antimicrobial standard reference powders can be obtained commercially from the manufacturer, from United States Pharmacopeia or the Zentrallaboratorium Deutscher Apotheker (see previous contact information). Drug stock solutions, based on the potency of the drug, should be prepared as specified by the NCCLS procedure (41) or as specified by the manufacturer.

The agents that should be tested are shown in Table 5.8. However, there are several provisos that need to be considered. Clarithromycin is considered a class representative for newer macrolides (e.g., azithromycin and roxithromycin). Although ciprofloxacin is representative of other fluoroquinolones, it cannot be used to indicate susceptibility to the newer 8-methoxyfluoroquinolones (e.g., gatifloxacin and moxifloxacin). If these agents are considered for clinical use, we recommend that susceptibility to them is tested directly (no tentative nontuberculous mycobacterium break points available). Testing of imipenem for *M. abscessus* and *M. chelonae* is probably not warranted because the results for these species are difficult to reproduce and thus cannot be considered reliable. Conversely, MIC of tobramycin only needs to be reported for *M. chelonae*.

The drug-containing, 96-well plates can be prepared fresh for each susceptibility assay or batch-prepared ahead of time and stored until needed. Two approaches are recommended for the batch production and storage of drug-containing plates.

TABLE 5.8

Susceptibility Testing of Rapidly Growing Mycobacteria: Recommended Test Ranges, Interpretive Criteria, and Suggested Quality Control Reference Ranges

Antimicrobial Agent	Recommended Test Ranges (μg/ml)	MIC (μg/ml) breakpoint[a]			Reference Range Endpoints (μg/ml) for Quality Control Strains	
		Susceptible	Intermediate	Resistant	*M. peregrinum* ATCC 700686	*S. aureus* ATCC 29213
Amikacin	1–128	≤16	32	≥64	≤1–4	1–4
Cefoxitin	2–256	≤16	32–4	≥128	16–32	1–4
Ciprofloxacin	0.125–16	≤1	2	≥4	≤0.125–0.5	0.125–0.5
Clarithromycin	0.06–64	≤2	4	≥8	≤0.06–0.5	0.125–0.5
Doxycyliine	0.25–32	≤1	2–8	≥16	0.125–0.5	0.125–0.5
Imipenem	1–64	≤4	8	≥16	2–16	—
Linezolid	2–64	≤8	16	≥32	≤2–4	1–4
Sulfamethoxazole	1–64	≤32	—	≥64	≤1–4	32–128
Tobramycin	1–32	≤4	8	≥16	4–8	0.125–1

[a] MIC, minimal inhibitory concentration.

First, drug dilution series can be prepared in broth and 0.1-mL aliquots added to the wells of a 96-well microplate; the plates should then be sealed in plastic bags and stored at –70°C for up to 6 months. The plates should not be stored in a frost-free freezer because such freezers have defrost cycles, and thawed plates should not be refrozen. Commercial systems are available that automatically fill the plates (e.g., Quick Spense II; Dynatech Laboratories, Inc., Chantilly, VA).

Second, drug dilution series can be prepared in sterile distilled water (or other suitable dilutent but it should not significantly affect the constituents of the broth medium when reconstituted), aliquoted, and the material lyophilized in situ. With this approach, the amount of drug added per well should give the required concentration in a final volume of 0.1 mL.

The NCCLS guidelines are based on the use of flat-bottomed, 96-well microplates, which allow the quantitation of microcolonies or bacterial clumps in wells with-low level growth. This ability may aid in determining the endpoint for some antimicrobial agents. Alternatively, U- or V-bottomed plates can be used. The benefit of these styles of plate is that all the sedimented bacteria collect in a small area, which help distinguish wells with low-level grow from wells with no growth. The disadvantage of U- or V-bottom wells is that quantitation of microcolonies or bacterial clumps is not feasible.

Inoculation

Susceptibility tests should be performed only on pure cultures. The organisms can be stored on Löwenstein-Jensen slants before testing and then subcultured to a nonselective medium such as trypticase soy or blood agar plates and incubated in air for 2 to 4 days at 30°C to 35°C to obtain discrete colonies. A sterile swab should be used to transfer a sweep of organisms to tubes containing 4.5 mL of sterile water to give a turbidity equivalent to a McFarland no. 0.5 standard. To aid the dispersion of bacteria clumps, 3-mm glass beads (seven to ten should be sufficient) should be added to the tube and the suspensions vortexed aggressively for 15 to 20 seconds. Any remaining large bacterial clumps should be allowed to settle. Rapidly growing mycobacteria that are adjusted to a McFarland no. 0.5 standard contain 1×10^7 to 2×10^8 CFU/mL (94).

The final inoculum preparation depends on the nature of the drug-containing plates. If plates containing lyophilized agents are used, then the bacterial suspension described must be diluted 200-fold to give a final density of approximately 5×10^5 CFU/mL; for example, 50 μL of suspension (turbidity equivalent to a McFarland no. 0.5 standard) mixed with 10-mL of broth. Aliquots of 0.1-mL per well (approximately 5×10^4 CFU) are then dispensed in to the assay plate using a disposable inoculator (to avoid aerosols). If the plates contain drugs already reconstituted in medium (0.1-mL per well), the inoculum should be diluted to a density of approximately 5×10^5 CFU/mL. Aliquots of 0.01 mL per well (approximately 5×10^4 CFU) are then dispensed in to the assay plate.

The plates are sealed in plastic bags or placed in another sealed storage container and incubated in room air for 3 to 5 days at 30°C ± 2°C.

Reading of Results

The plates should be examined after 3 days (72 hours) and then daily up to day 5 (120 hours). Usually, the MICs can be read at day 3 with most *M. fortuitum* group isolates. In contrast, some strains of *M. chelonae* may require an incubation time of 4 days (96 hours). Minimally, the no-drug controls should be visibly turbid with clumps of bacteria at the bottom of the wells. The most reliable results are likely to be obtained with the shortest incubation period that gives acceptable growth in control wells. This is especially important for drugs that are unstable in broth media, such as imipenem. It is advisable to repeat the testing of isolates that have MIC interpreted as being indicative of resistance, either in-house or sent out to a reference laboratory (recommended for amikacin, imipenem, and tobramycin).

Readers should be cautious when interpreting trailing endpoints when testing *M. fortuitum* isolates against clarithromycin. In such cases, this probably indicates expression of the *erm*(39) rRNA methylase (90,91), which confers macrolide resistance. Consequently, trailing endpoints with clarithromycin should be considered as indicative of resistance.

The MIC is the lowest concentration of antimicrobial agent that completely inhibits the growth of the organism as detected by the unaided eye. Endpoints are easy to read for most drugs; however, a faint haze of growth is common with sulfonamides. Consequently, the sulfamethoxazole MIC is usually determined from the well showing approximately 80% inhibition of growth compared to the no-drug control well.

Quality Control

The NCCLS recommends the use of *M. peregrinum* ATCC 700686 as the QC strain (41). The endpoints for this organism can be read after 4 days (96 hours) at 30°C ±2°C (suggested reference range MICs for this organism are shown Table 5.8). An alternative quality control strain is *Staphylococcus aureus* ATCC 29213. Quality control strains should be set up at least weekly for laboratories that perform more than one test per week. In laboratories performing fewer tests, the quality control strain should always be included. With stored drug-containing microplates, each batch should be validated with the quality control strain and tested for sterility before use.

As with all clinical tests, reliability and reproducibility are critical. Thus, laboratory personnel who score susceptibility assays should be monitored by comparing endpoints with that determined by an experienced reader. All personnel should agree ± 1 dilution with the experienced reader.

NONTUBERCULOUS, SLOWLY GROWING MYCOBACTERIA

In many metropolitan areas of the United States, the incidence of nontuberculous infections may exceed that of *M. tuberculosis* infections. Even before the impact of AIDS-associated mycobacterial infections, MAC isolates constituted nearly 25% of the mycobacterial isolates reported to the Centers for Disease Control and Prevention. Wayne and Sramek (104), in a study of nearly 20,000 isolates of potentially pathogenic environmental mycobacteria, reported that 35% were MAC and at least 50% of these were associated with disease. The isolation of other species of nontuberculous mycobacteria is typically infrequent, but sometimes with significant differences in geographic distribution; for example, *Mycobacterium kansasii* is more frequently isolated in the southeastern, southwestern, and central states than in the northeastern and northwestern states of the United States (105,106), and *Mycobacterium malmoense* is more frequently isolated from patients in the United Kingdom and northern Europe than in southern Europe and the United States (107). Other nontuberculous isolates, such as *M. haemophilum, Mycobacterium celatum,* and *Mycobacterium genavense,* have emerged as mycobacterial pathogens, but the epidemiology of these species is not well understood.

In general, the *in vitro* susceptibility testing of *M. avium* and most of the other nontuberculous mycobacteria, using the methods and interpretive criteria described for *M. tuberculosis,* has little value in guiding the treatment of patients with nontuberculous disease. One important exception is *M. kansasii,* where there is good evidence that *in vitro* susceptibility results based on the *M. tuberculosis* interpretive criteria correlates with clinical efficacy (108). None of the *M. avium* therapeutic efficacy trials were specifically designed to correlate susceptibility test results with clinical efficacy or outcome (109–111), but there is some general agreement on the interpretive criteria for clarithromycin and azithromycin, a macrolide and an azalide, respectively, with proven efficacy in the treatment of *M. avium* and other nontuberculous mycobacteria (41). For many uncommon species of nontuberculous mycobacteria (e.g., *Mycobacterium simiae* and *Mycobacterium szulgai*), there have been exceedingly few clinical cases, and in many instances the initial clinical presentation was confused with tuberculosis. The common difficulty of distinguishing between contamination, colonization, and disease with many of the nontuberculous mycobacteria confounds the situation further.

Salient features of the susceptibility patterns of several species of nontuberculous mycobacteria follow in the next section; however, readers are encouraged to consult publications by Woods and Washington (106), Davidson (108), Wayne and Sramek (104), and Henriques et al. (107) for additional information about the treatment of nontuberculosis mycobacterial infections. Inderlied et al. (112) reviewed the microbiology of MAC including the diagnosis and treatment of MAC disease, a monograph on MAC was edited by Korvick and Benson (113), and Falkinham (114) has discussed the epidemiology of non-tuberculous mycobacterial infections.

THE *MYCOBACTERIUM AVIUM* COMPLEX

The MAC has been traditionally defined as a serologic complex divided into 30 or more serovars (115), based on the composition of the cell surface oligosaccharide linked to a peptidoglycolipid core that is produced by all members of the complex (116). Studies with DNA probes that hybridize to species-specific rRNA sequences of *M. avium* and *Mycobacterium intracellulare* confirmed the predominant role of *M. avium* in AIDS-associated infections (70 to 90% of isolates), whereas only 50% of isolates from non-AIDS patients react with the *M. avium* probe (117,118). The MAC has been divided into three subspecies: *M. avium* subsp. *avium, M. avium* subsp. *paratuberculosis,* and *M. avium* subsp. *silvaticum* (104).

Mycobacterium avium Resistance

MAC isolates are predictably resistant to isoniazid and only variably susceptible to rifampin and ethambutol, and the susceptibility patterns in general are considerably more variable than those of *M. tuberculosis* (119, 120), emphasizing the potential importance of susceptibility testing. The inherent antimicrobial resistance is most likely due to the impermeability of the MAC cell wall and membrane (121), and *in vitro* cell-free studies confirmed that drug targets (e.g., ribosomes, ribosomal subunits, and RNA polymerase) in MAC cells bind the drugs and the corresponding target functions are inhibited. MAC isolates, like most mycobacteria, produce low levels of β-lactamase (122), but there is no evidence that MAC isolates actively degrade or inactivate β-lactams or possess inactivating enzymes for other antimicrobials. Most MAC isolates have plasmids of varying size (114,123) and, while plasmids have been associated with antimicrobial resistance in some MAC isolates (124), specific resistance transfer factors have not been identified.

Colony Variants

Susceptibility testing of the MAC is complicated by the observation that MAC isolates display two colony variants on agar-based media (125). One colony variant is flat, spreading, and translucent in appearance, while the second colony variant is raised, condensed, and opaque (Fig. 5.3). The translucent variant is more resistant to antimicrobial agents (125) and is more virulent in animal models of infection (126). Stormer and Falkinham (127) showed that nonpigmented variants of *M. avium,* isolated from both the environment and patients with disseminated *M. avium* disease, are significantly more resistant to a variety of antimicrobial agents than are pigmented segregants of the same strains. Because the pigmented and more susceptible variants appear more quickly and are more prominent on culture plates, nonpigmented variants could be overlooked in the selection of *M. avium* colonies for susceptibility testing.

When to Test

In most situations, it is unnecessary to perform *in vitro* susceptibility tests on initial MAC isolates from patients with disseminated or localized infections. However, establishing baseline MIC values may assist in interpreting susceptibility test results weeks or months after the start of therapy. Testing is appropriate for patients formerly taking macrolide therapy or patients who develop bacteremia while taking macrolide prophylaxis for MAC. Also, susceptibility testing may be useful if a patient relapses or if the infection is intractable and the clinical situation is desperate. Testing for macrolide resistance may help in deciding whether to add drugs to a treatment regimen. However, it is not clear whether the macrolide should be withdrawn in the face of resistance. Little is known about the effects of multiple-drug regimens on such resistant strains, and the chance of polyclonal MAC infections leads to the possibility of mixed susceptible and resistant strains (3). Susceptibility testing should be repeated 3 months after the start of treatment for disseminated disease or after 6 months for patients with pulmonary disease (41).

Antimicrobial Agents

While MAC infections are usually treated with a combination of antimicrobial agents, *in vitro* susceptibility testing is often restricted to clarithromycin or azithromycin (Table 5.9). Clarithromycin is more convenient to test and the results can be applied to azithromycin, since macrolide/azalide resistance cross. In addition to either clarithromycin or azithromycin, the following drugs have been used to treat disseminated MAC infections: ethambutol, a quinolone (e.g., moxifloxacin), and amikacin. There are animal (129,130) and limited human (131) data

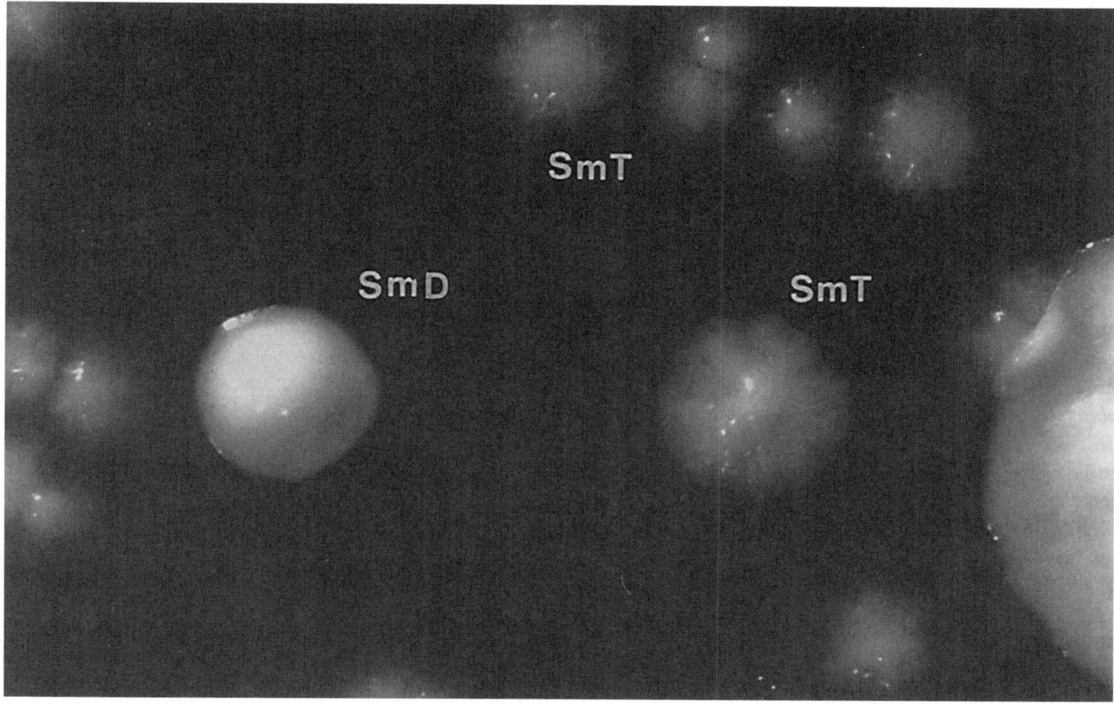

FIGURE 5.3 ● Smooth-domed (*SmD*) and smooth-transparent (*SmT*) colony variants of *M. avium*. [Reprinted with permission from Inderlied and Nash (128).]

on the use of mefloquine. However, no clinical trials have been performed to validate *in vitro* susceptibility testing methods or interpretive criteria for these agents.

Methods

MAC can be tested using either a broth macrodilution method using Bactec 460 12B medium or a broth microdilution method using Middlebrook 7H9 broth with casein and OADC or Mueller-Hinton broth supplemented with cations and OADC; either media can be used at pH 6.8 (standard) or adjusted to pH 7.3 to 7.4 (Table 5.9). These two methods have been evaluated in a multisite study, which found good agreement between laboratories and within a laboratory, but there was more variation with the microdilution method than with the Bactec method (132).

In vitro susceptibility testing of MAC is based on the following generally accepted observations: (a) a broth medium is more reliable than agar; (b) Bactec radiometric broth macrodilution and broth microdilution methods yield consistent and reproducible results; (c) extensive subcultures should be avoided to prevent the selection of more susceptible variants; (d) transparent colonies are more likely to display resistance than opaque colonies; (e) drugs should be tested at three to five concentrations (at least) and the activity measured as a MIC; and (f) Tween 80 or other surfactants should not be used to disperse clumps of bacilli, since these agents may make the bacilli more permeable.

Inoculum

For the Bactec 460TB method, collect colonies (especially transparent colony variants, if present) from the surface of a Middlebrook 7H11 plate and suspend in sterile saline. Mix vigorously and adjust to match a McFarland no. 1 turbidity standard. Prepare a 1:100 dilution of this suspension to make a working inoculum and another 1:100 dilution to inoculate the control vials. Test vials are inoculated with 0.1 mL of the working inoculum to yield $\sim 7.5 \times 10^4$ CFU/mL and control vials are inoculated with 0.1 mL of the 1:100 diluted working inoculum. For the broth microdilution method, suspend sufficient MAC colonies in 5.0 mL of sterile deionized water to match a McFarland no. 0.5 turbidity standard. Transfer 25 μL of the suspension to 5 mL of Middlebrook 7H9 broth with casein or Mueller-Hinton broth with 5% OADC to yield $\sim 5 \times 10^5$ CFU/mL in each well of a microtiter plate.

Bactec 460TB Method

Pre-run the Bactec 12B vials through the Bactec 460TB instrument to replace the headspace with 5% carbon dioxide as well as to detect any contaminated vials. Add

TABLE 5.9

Interpretive Criteria for *M. avium* Complex *In Vitro* Testing of Clarithromycin and Azithromycin Including Quality Control

Antimicrobial Agent	Method[a]	Concentration Range[b]	Limited Concentration Range[c]	pH[d]	Susceptible (μg/mL)	Intermediate (μg/mL)	Resistant (μg/mL)	Quality Control[e]
Clarithromycin	Bactec 460TB	2–64	4, 16, 64	6.8	≤ 16	32	≥ 64	1–4
	Bactec 460TB	2–64	4, 8, 32	7.3–7.4	≤ 4	8–16	≥ 32	0.5–2
	Broth microdilution	0.25–256	1–64	7.3–7.4	≤ 8	16	≥ 32	0.5–2
Azithromycin	Bactec 460TB	16–512	32, 128, 512	6.8	≤ 128	256	≥ 512	8–32

[a] Bactec 460TB using Bactec 12B medium without pH adjustment (pH 6.8) or with pH adjustment (7.3–7.4). Broth microdilution using cation-supplemented Mueller-Hinton broth (pH 7.3–7.4) or Middlebrook 7H9 broth with pH adjusted (pH 7.3–7.4) with 1 M KOH.
[b] Ideal concentration range.
[c] A more limited number of concentrations can be tested to control cost.
[d] Macrolides and azalides are more active at pH 7.3–7.4, but *M. avium* complex grows more poorly at this pH range. However, testing at either pH reliably detects macrolide/azalide resistance, but testing must be performed consistently at one pH. It is more convenient to test at pH 6.8, since the pH of the test medium does not need to be adjusted.
[e] Expected minimal inhibitory concentration ranges for *M. avium* (ATCC 700898).

0.1 mL of drugs at the appropriate and varied concentrations. Add 0.1 mL of the working inoculum to each vial with drug and 0.1 mL of the 1:100 diluted control inoculum to a vial without drug. Additional controls include (a) a vial without drug or inoculum, (b) a vial without drug and 0.1 mL of heat-killed inoculum, and (c) a vial with no drug and 0.1 mL of the working inoculum (to monitor for overinoculation). Vials are incubated at 37°C and read each day for 7 days (8 days of incubation). Results are read when the 1:100 control vial reads 30 or more for 3 days. The MIC is defined as the lowest concentration of drug necessary to yield a final reading of less than 50.

Broth Microdilution Method

Microtiter trays should be inoculated (100 μL per well) within 30 minutes of preparing the inoculum. The trays are sealed with adhesive and incubated at 35°C in ambient air. The plates are first read at 7 days, but read with interpretation only when there is siufficient growth in the growth control well. If necessary, the plates are incubated for an additional 7 days. The MIC is defined as the lowest concentration of drug necessary to inhibit visible growth.

Quality Control

M. avium (ATCC 700898) is recommended for quality control of both Bactec broth macrodilution and the broth microdilution methods (Table 5.9). MAC strains used for quality control should be stored at −70°C or for 3 months at −20°C or at ambient temperature for 30 days and subcultured each week or at the time of testing. Bactec 12B vials adjusted to pH 7.3 to 7.4 should be incubated overnight at 37°C in 5% carbon dioxide and the pH confirmed.

OTHER NONTUBERCULOUS MYCOBACTERIA

Mycobacterium kansasii

M. kansasii is closely related to *Mycobacterium gastri*; however, the isolation of the former is nearly always clinically significant, while isolation of the latter is rarely of clinical importance (104). In general, the incidence of *M. kansasii* disease is low and usually responds well to therapy (133,134). *M. kansasii* isolates from patients who have not been previously treated with rifampin are likely to be susceptible to rifampin at 1 μg/mL (106), and infections have been successfully treated with a combination of rifampin, isoniazid, and a third agent (e.g., ethambutol) (135,136). A 1994 study by the British Thoracic Society of nearly 175 patients with *M. kansasii* pulmonary disease concluded that 9 months of treatment with rifampin and ethambutol alone were effective for the majority of patients (the mortality rate for the patients was high because of other reasons) (133). The group also found that all *M. kansasii* isolates were resistant to isoniazid and pyrazinamide, by the standard proportion method, and concluded that neither drug appears to have a role in the treatment of this disease. *M. kansasii* pulmonary infection in a patient with AIDS also has been successfully treated with isoniazid, rifampin, and ethambutol, but rifabutin should be substituted for rifampin in

TABLE 5.10

Antimicrobial Agents for Potential Testing Against *M. kansasii*[a]

Antimicrobial Agent	Resistant[b] at (μg/mL)		Quality Control[c] (μg/mL)		
	M. kansasii	*M. marinum*	*M. kansasii* ATCC 12478	*M. marinum* ATCC 927	*E. faecalis* ATCC 29212[d]
Primary					
Rifampin	1–2	1	≤ 1	≤ 0.25–1	0.5–4
Secondary					
Amikacin	32	12–32			64–256
Ciprofloxacin	2				0.25–2
Clarithromycin	16	16			—
Doxycycline	—	4–6			—
Ethambutol HCl	5	5			—
Isoniazid	5				—
Rifabutin	2				—
Streptomycin	10				—
Sulfamethoxazole	32	20–32			—
Trimethoprim/ sulfamethoxazole	2/38	2/38			$\leq 0.5/9.5$

[a] Table adapted from the National Committee for Clinical Laboratory Standards (41).
[b] Suggested resistant breakpoints for *M. kansasii* and *M. marinum* (41). Routine susceptibility testing of *M. marinum* is usually unnecessary and not advised.
[c] Methods include agar proportion, Bactec 460TB, and broth microdilution (97,187).
[d] *Enterococcus faecalis* can be used to quality control drug solutions using the NCCLS method for aerobic rapidly growing bacteria.

HIV-infected patients treated with a protease inhibitor (137). Wallace et al. (138) reported that rifampin resistance can be a problem with this mycobacterium; however, most patients responded well to a four-drug regimen. Use of a modified proportion method and the *M. tuberculosis* interpretive criteria may provide useful information for treating *M. kansasii* infections, and a test method that yields an MIC may be more helpful (Table 5.10). However, initial testing should be restricted to rifampin, since treatment failure is mostly associated with rifampin resistance and most *M. kansasii* isolates will test resistant to isoniazid at 0.2 μg/mL and many test resistant to 1.0 μg/mL (41).

Mycobacterium xenopi

Pulmonary infections caused by *M. xenopi* have been described, and the disease occurs more frequently in immunocompromised patients (104, 134). Pseudo-outbreaks of *M. xenopi* infections have been reported and the significance of the isolation of this species, especially from a nonsterile body site, should be carefully examined (139, 140), especially because *M. xenopi* can be mistakenly identified as *M. avium* if biochemical tests only are used for identification. *In vitro* susceptibility test results appear to be important in the management of this disease (141); however, the correlation between *in vitro* susceptibility test results and therapeutic response has been reported to be inconsistent (106). Some indicate that *M. xenopi* is susceptible to isoniazid, rifampin, streptomycin, and cycloserine, while others dispute these results (108). The NCCLS recommends that *in vitro* susceptibility test of *M. xenopi* follow the guidelines for *M. kansasii* (described previously) (41).

Mycobacterium szulgai

M. szulgai is a scotochromogen at 37°C and a photochromogen at 25°C. It was first reported to cause pulmonary disease in the early 1970s. Along with the other uncommon species of slowly growing, nontuberculous mycobacteria, *M. szulgai* appears to cause disease primarily in persons with a history of chronic lung disease (134). These infections are reported to respond to isoniazid, rifampin, and ethambutol (108). Woods and Washington (106) characterized *M. szulgai* as only slightly more resistant than *M. tuberculosis* to antituberculosis agents, and they suggested that streptomycin, capreomycin, and viomycin are potential alternatives to the three previously mentioned first-line agents.

Mycobacterium malmoense

M. malmoense is a nonpigmented environmental mycobacterium that is closely related to *Mycobacterium shimoidei,* but in clinical laboratories it may be more important to distinguish *M. malmoense* from *M. gastri* and *Mycobacterium terrae* because of the difference in clinical significance (104). *M. malmoense* has been reported as a frequent cause of pulmonary infection mostly in elderly patients with underlying lung disease, including tuberculosis and malignancy, but disseminated disease was reported in an HIV-infected patient (134,142). Although *M. malmoense* is reported to be variably susceptible to antimycobacterial agents, it is generally considered to be more susceptible than *M. avium.* Although there are some recommendations for treatment (143) and there are conflicting reports regarding the susceptibility of *M. malmoense* to isoniazid (144) and rifampin (108), Hoffner et al. (145) showed that combinations of ethambutol with aminoglycosides, quinolones, or rifamycins were synergistic against *M. malmoense.* This observation is in agreement with reports on the clinical effectiveness of ethambutol, rifampin, and isoniazid in combination in the treatment of pulmonary disease (146). Banks and Jenkins (143) showed that, although *M. malmoense* was resistant to rifampin and ethambutol, all strains were susceptible to the combination of these drugs at the lowest concentration.

Mycobacterium simiae

M. simiae is regarded as highly resistant to antimycobacterial agents, perhaps with the exception of ethionamide and cycloserine (106); however, there are exceedingly few cases of disease caused by *M. simiae* on which to base any firm conclusions about susceptibility to antimycobacterial agents. In an animal test system, clarithromycin in combination with ethambutol and perhaps a quinolone such as ofloxacin was potentially effective (147). As with *M. szulgai,* disease in humans appears to occur mostly in persons with a history of chronic lung disease, and persons with pulmonary lesions are probably predisposed to colonization with potentially pathogenic environmental mycobacteria (104).

Mycobacterium marinum

This photochromogen is a cause of skin, joint, and deeper infections, primarily of the hand or limbs; infection is usually associated with exposure to water (148,149). The successful management of *M. marinum* infections requires rapid diagnosis and the avoidance of steroid treatments (148,149). *M. marinum* is largely considered predictably susceptible to rifampin and ethambutol, although most infections spontaneously resolve or respond to localized treatment without chemotherapy. Disseminated cutaneous infections respond to rifampin and ethambutol; alternative agents are tetracycline, doxycycline, minocycline, trimethoprim-sulfmethoxazole, ciprofloxacin, and clarithromycin (150,151). Routine susceptibility testing using methods and interpretive criteria described for *M. tuberculosis* is inappropriate, and the methods and interpretive criteria for testing rapidly growing mycobacteria are more likely to provide clinically useful results (Table 5.10).

Mycobacterium ulcerans

Chemotherapy plays a role secondary to surgical treatment in infections caused by *M. ulcerans* (106); however, amikacin combined with rifampin may be a useful adjunct to excision (152) or streptomycin combined with rifampin or dapsone. The potential role of macrolides and azalides is not clear (153). *In vitro* susceptibility testing is inappropriate, but it appears that rifampin resistance is likely to develop with monotherapy (154).

Mycobacterium haemophilum

M. haemophilum is a slowly growing, nonpigmented mycobacterium that requires hemin or ferric ammonium citrate for growth. Early reports on the *in vitro* susceptibility of *M. haemophilum* were inconsistent, and the role of chemotherapy in the treatment of *M. haemophilum* infections was unclear. Woods and Washington (106) concluded that this species is resistant to isoniazid, streptomycin, and ethambutol but susceptible to rifampin and/or PAS. *M. haemophilum* emerged as an important cause of disseminated skin infections in immunocompromised patients, including patients with renal transplant, lymphoma, and AIDS (155). The organism also causes disease in immunocompetent hosts, where it causes mild, self-limited skin infections (156). Correlations have been established between susceptibility test results and clinical efficacy, although virtually all treatment regimens examined included combinations of agents (157). Wild-type isolates of *M. haemophilum* appear to be susceptible to quinolones, rifamycins, clarithromycin, and azithromycin and resistant to pyrazinamide and ethambutol and are likely to be resistant to isoniazid and streptomycin (155, 157).

Mycobacterium gordonae

M. gordonae is commonly found in the environment and is readily isolated from water supplies and ice machines. Wayne and Sramek (104) pointed out that, because *M. gordonae* is so common (30% of nearly 20,000 nontuberculous mycobacteria studied) and disease is so rare (cases of *M. gordonae* infection with clear and compelling clinical correlations are difficult, if not impossible, to find), the pathogenic potential of this species must be extremely low, even in patients with AIDS (158). Nevertheless, it is not uncommon for clinical mycobacteriology laboratories to receive requests for susceptibility testing of *M. gordonae* isolates. In response to such requests, one could pose the questions offered by Wayne and Sramek (104): (a) Is the isolate truly *M. gordonae?* (b) Is there convincing evidence that the isolate is playing a role in the disease? In most cases, susceptibility testing is inappropriate and may only further mislead the clinician as to the true cause of the disease. The rare occurrence of true *M. gordonae* infection in patients with AIDS makes this decision more difficult. *Mycobacterium interjectum* emerged as a potential pathogen and it has been confused with both *M. gordonae* and *Mycobacterium scrofulaceum* (159,160).

Table 5.11, which appears at the end of this chapter, provides a summary of information about the *in vitro* activity of a variety of antimicrobial agents tested against *M. tuberculosis, M. avium,* and several other species of mycobacteria.

ANTIMYCOBACTERIAL AGENTS: MODES OF ACTION AND MECHANISMS OF RESISTANCE

There are several recent reviews of drug resistance mechanisms in mycobacteria (194–196); therefore, the objective of this section is not to simply reiterate these publications. Rather, we aimed to provide an update, and expand on areas not covered or superficially covered in previous reviews.

Isoniazid

The inhibitory activity of isoniazid or isonicotinic acid hydrazide against *M. tuberculosis* is remarkably specific and potent. Indeed, no other single antimycobacterial agent has proved to be as active against the *M. tuberculosis* complex, with such comparatively low toxicity, as isoniazid. However, the activity of isoniazid is less for other mycobacteria, and the drug has little or no role in the treatment of certain types of infections, such as disease caused by rapidly growing mycobacteria and disseminated *M. avium* infection. In addition, isoniazid has no activity against nonacid-fast bacteria and eukaryotic cells. The activity against *M. tuberculosis* is bactericidal; however, the drug is active only against growing organisms (197–199). In addition, the effect of isoniazid is irreversible within only a few hours of exposure of tubercle bacilli to the drug. Isoniazid can bind irreversibly to protein, which is an important interfering factor in the measurement of isoniazid concentrations in biologic fluids.

Isoniazid Activation

Isoniazid is a prodrug that the target organism must activate in order for it to exert an antibacterial effect. Indeed, the relative inability of most bacteria to activate isoniazid is the primary underlying reason for the selective action of this agent against the *M. tuberculosis* complex.

Until recently, little was known about isoniazid activation, with the most significant insight being that it required the *M. tuberculosis* catalase-peroxidase KatG; i.e., the nature of the active form of isoniazid was unknown. However, over the last 5 years, several studies have provided a significant insight of the activation process and of the active form of isoniazid. The first step in isoniazid activation is oxidization by KatG (Fig. 5.4A later in this chapter). This process is enhanced by presence of manganese ions, probably involving a shift in redox state from Mn^{2+} to Mn^{3+} and back (200). In fact, activation of isoniazid can occur in an enzyme-free system in the presence of Mn^{3+} ions and nicotinamide coenzymes (201). The derivative generated by this oxidation is either an isonicotinic acyl radical or anion; evidence supporting the production of the free acyl radical (as well as the hydrazyl, peroxo, and pyridyl radicals) was reported by Wengenack and Rusnak (202). The oxidized isoniazid forms a covalent link to the carbon at position 4 of the nicotinamide moiety of NAD(H) (Fig. 5.4A). The resulting entities are termed isoniazid-NAD(H) adducts. The kinetics of isoniazid activation and InhA inhibition suggests that the isoniazid-NAD(H) adducts form outside InhA and then compete with NAD(H) for the InhA binding site (203).

A possible structure of the active form of isoniazid (Fig. 5.4B) was proposed from the x-ray crystal structure of the primary drug target, InhA, an enoyl-acyl carrier protein reductase (204). However, it is possible that there is more than one active form of isoniazid. Nguyen et al. (201) isolated another isoniazid-NAD(H) adduct with significant inhibitory activity for InhA (Fig 5.4C).

Isoniazid Mechanism of Action

The first insights into the mechanism of action of isoniazid were made by studying the sequence of events that occur after exposure of mycobacteria to this drug. Within 15 minutes of exposure to isoniazid, radioactively labeled drug is taken into the cells and there is a decrease in the ratio of nicotinamide adenine dinucleotide (NAD) to protein and inhibition of mycolic acid synthesis (205). Within 30 minutes there is noticeable production of yellow pigment (peroxidase product), and by 60 to 90 minutes there is a decline in cell viability (205). The bactericidal activity of isoniazid is decreased in growth media depleted of trace

(*text continues on page 190*)

TABLE 5.11

Activity of Antimycobacterial Agents[a]

Agent	MIC 50% (μg/mL)	MIC 90% (μg/mL)	Reference
	M. abscessus		
Amoxicillin-clavulanate	64	64	162
Azithromycin	2	8	161
Cefmetazole	32	64	162
Cefoxitin	32	64	162
Clarithromycin	0.125	0.25	161
Erythromycin	8	>8	161
Imipenem	8	16	162
Linezolid	32	64	163
Roxithromycin	0.5	2	161
	M. asiaticum		
Cycloserine	30	—	164
Ethambutol	5–10	—	164
Isoniazid	5	—	164
Kanamycin	5	—	164
Streptomycin	10	—	164
	M. avium complex		
Amifloxacin	10	=16	165,166
Amikacin	4	16	120,167
Ampicillin	8	16	168
Azithromycin	16	32–16	120,169
Capreomycin	4–8	12	167,170
Ciprofloxacin	4–8	≥16	120
Clarithromycin	2	4	166,169
Clofazimine	—	1	171
Cycloserine	—	50	164
Erythromycin	32	64	172
Ethambutol	4	8	164,120
Ethionamide	4	—	164
Gatifloxacin	8	16	173
Gentamicin	4–8	—	174
Imipenem	8–16	≥32	168
Isoniazid	R	R	164
Kanamycin	4	12	164
Linezolid	32	64	175
Moxifloxacin	2	4	173
Minocycline	>25	>25	172
Norfloxacin	16	>16	176
Ofloxacin	8	>16	171

(continued)

TABLE 5.11 (Continued)

Activity of Antimycobacterial Agents[a]

Agent	MIC 50% (μg/mL)	MIC 90% (μg/mL)	Reference
p-Aminosalicylic acid (PAS)	R	R	170
Pyrazinamide	R	R	164
Rifabutin	0.25	2	171
Rifampin	4	≥8	164
Streptomycin	4–8	8	164
Sulfisoxazole	10	20	174
Vancomycin	25	>25	165
	M. bovis		
Capreomycin	—	10	164
Cycloserine	—	30	164
Ethambutol	—	5–10	164
Ethionamide	—	5–10	164
Isoniazid	0.2	0.2–1	164
Kanamycin	—	5–10	164
PAS	—	2–10	164
Pyrazinamide	R	R	164
Rifampin	—	1	164
Streptomycin	—	2	164
	M. bovis-BCG		
Capreomycin	—	10	164
Cycloserine	—	≥30	164
Ethambutol	—	5	164
Ethionamide	5	—	164
Isoniazid	0.2	0.2–1	164
Kanamycin	—	5	164
PAS	—	2	164
Pyrazinamide	R	R	164
Rifampin	—	1	164
Streptomycin	—	2	164
	M. celatum		
Gatifloxacin	1	1	173
Moxifloxacin	1	1	173
	M. chelonae		
Amikacin	1	1	177
Amoxicillin/clavulanate	64	64	162
Azithromycin	1	2	161
Cefmetazole	≥256	≥256	162
Cefoxitin	≥256	≥256	162,94

(continued)

TABLE 5.11 (Continued)

Activity of Antimycobacterial Agents[a]

Agent	MIC 50% (μg/mL)	MIC 90% (μg/mL)	Reference
Ciprofloxacin	12	12	165
Clarithromycin	0.125	0.125	161
Clofazimine	1	1	178
Cycloserine	R	R	164
Erythromycin	2	8	161
Ethambutol	R	R	164
Ethionamide	R	R	164
Gatifloxacin	4	8	173
Gentamicin	8	32	94
Imipenem	16	32	162
Isoniazid	R	R	164
Linezolid	8	16	163
Minocycline	>25	>25	165
Moxifloxacin	8	16	173
Norfloxacin	8	>16	176
Ofloxacin	12	50	179
PAS	R	R	164
Pyrazinamide	R	R	164
Rifabutin	2	4	177
Rifampin	8	gt;8	164
Roxithromycin	1	2	161
Tobramycin	8	16	94
Trimethoprim	>16	>16	94
Vancomycin	25	>25	165
	M. flavescens		
Capreomycin	—	10	164
Cycloserine	30	—	164
Ethambutol	5	—	164
Ethionamide	R	R	164
Gatifloxacin	0.06	0.06	173
Isoniazid	1	5	164
Kanamycin	—	5	164
Moxifloxacin	0.06	0.06	173
PAS	R	R	164
Pyrazinamide	R	R	164
Rifampin	1	—	164
Streptomycin	2	>10	164
	M. fortuitum		
Amikacin	1	8	94

(continued)

TABLE 5.11 (Continued)

Activity of Antimycobacterial Agents[a]

Agent	MIC 50% (μg/mL)	MIC 90% (μg/mL)	Reference
Azithromycin	8	>8	161
Capreomycin	16	16	94
Cefoxitin	32	64	162
Ciprofloxacin	1	2	165
Clarithromycin	2	4	161
Clofazimine	0.5	0.5	178
Cycloserine	R	R	164
Doxycycline	8	32	94
Erythromycin	6	>25	165
Ethambutol	16	≥64	94
Ethionamide	R	R	164
Gatifloxacin	0.25	0.25	173
Gentamicin	8	16	94
Imipenem	2	4	162
Isoniazid	R	R	164
Kanamycin	5–10	—	164
Linezolid	4	16	163
Minocycline	4	16	94
Moxifloxacin	0.25	0.5	173
Norfloxacin	1	4	176
PAS	R	R	164
Pyrazinamide	R	R	164
Rifabutin	1	2	177
Rifampin	R	R	164
Roxithromycin	4	>8	161
Streptomycin	R	R	164
Sulfamethoxazole	5	152	94
Tetracycline	8	16	94
Tobramycin	16	32	94
Vancomycin	32–64	≥64	165
	M. gastri		
Capreomycin	10	—	164
Cycloserine	30	—	164
Ethambutol	5	—	164
Ethionamide	5	—	164
Isoniazid	—	5	164
Kanamycin	5	—	164
PAS	R	R	164
Pyrazinamide	R	R	164

(continued)

TABLE 5.11 (Continued)

Activity of Antimycobacterial Agents[a]

Agent	MIC 50% (μg/mL)	MIC 90% (μg/mL)	Reference
Rifampin	1	—	164
Streptomycin	2	—	164
	M. gordonae		
Capreomycin	10	—	164
Cycloserine	30	—	164
Ethambutol	5	—	164
Ethionamide	R	—	164
Gatifloxacin	0.5	1	173
Isoniazid	5	—	164
Kanamycin	—	5	164
Linezolid	≤2	4	175
Moxifloxacin	0.25	0.5	173
PAS	R	R	164
Pyrazinamide	R	R	164
Rifabutin	0.5	0.5	164
Rifampin	1	1	164
Streptomycin	10	—	164
	M. immunogenum		
Linezolid	32	50	163
	M. haemophilum		
Rifabutin	≤0.03	≤0.03	157
Rifampin	0.5	1	157
Clarithromycin	≤0.25	≤0.25	157
Erythromycin	2	4	157
Azithromycin	4	8	157
Clofazimine	2	2	157
Amikacin	4	4	157
Ciprofloxacin	2	8	157
Ofloxacin	4	8	157
Sparfloxacin	2	4	157
Isoniazid	8	>32	157
	M. intracellulare		
Ciprofloxacin	1	2	181
Gatifloxacin	4	4	173
Isoniazid	50	>100	182
Moxifloxacin	1	2	173
Ofloxacin	4	12	181,182
Rifabutin	0.25	1	183

(continued)

TABLE 5.11 (Continued)

Activity of Antimycobacterial Agents[a]

Agent	MIC 50% (μg/mL)	MIC 90% (μg/mL)	Reference
Rifampin	≥2	>2	182
Rifapentine	0.5	2	183
Streptomycin	25	>100	182
	M. kansasii		
Amifloxacin	2	4	165
Amikacin	2	4	177
Capreomycin	10		164
Ciprofloxacin	4	8	165,184
Cycloserine	—	20–30	164
Erythromycin	3	6	165
Ethambutol	5	10	164
Ethionamide		5 (68)	164
Gatifloxacin	1	4	173
Isoniazid	1	5	164
Kanamycin	R	R	164
Linezolid	≤2	≤2	164
Minocycline	6	12	164
Moxifloxacin	0.125	2	173
Norfloxacin	8	16	176
Ofloxacin	2	3	182
PAS	—	5–10	164
Pyrazinamide	R	R	164
Rifabutin	0.5	1	177
Rifampin	—	0.5–1	164
Streptomycin	12	50	164
Vancomycin	12	50	165
	M. kansasii (Rifampin-resistant)		
Amikacin	4	8	138
Ciprofloxacin	1	2	138
Clarithromycin	≤0.125	≤0.25	138
Isoniazid	1	16	138
Rifabutin	2	>16	138
Streptomyciin	2	4	138
Sulfamethoxazole	≤1	4	138
	M. malmoense		
Amikacin	—	4	145
Capreomycin	10	—	164
Ciprofloxacin	—	2–4	145
Cycloserine	30	—	164

(continued)

TABLE 5.11 (Continued)

Activity of Antimycobacterial Agents[a]

Agent	MIC 50% (μg/mL)	MIC 90% (μg/mL)	Reference
Ethambutol	5–10	—	164
Ethionamide	5	—	164
Gatifloxacin	0.25	0.25	173
Isoniazid	R	R	164
Kanamycin	5	—	164
Moxifloxacin	0.25	0.25	173
PAS	R	R	164
Pyrazinamide	R	R	164
Rifampin	1	—	164
Streptomycin	2	—	164
	M. marinum		
Amifloxacin	12.5	25	165
Amikacin	1	2	177
Capreomycin	—	10	164
Ciprofloxacin	1	2	165
Cycloserine	—	30	44
Doxycycline	4	4	185
Erythromycin	—	>25	165
Ethambutol	—	5	44
Ethionamide	—	5	44
Gatifloxacin	4	8	186
Gentamicin	20	40	151
Isoniazid	R	R	44
Kanamycin	2	5	164
Linezolid	≤2	2	175,186
Moxifloxacin	4	8	186
Minocycline	2	8	185
Pyrazinamide	R	R	164
Rifabutin	0.25	0.5	177
Rifampin	1	1	164
Streptomycin	—	10	164
Tetracycline	4	16	185
Tobramycin	32	64	185
Vancomycin	>25	>25	165
	M. mucogenicum		
Linezolid	4	100	163
	M. scrofulaceum		
Amikacin	1	8	177
Capreomycin	10	—	164

(continued)

TABLE 5.11 (Continued)

Activity of Antimycobacterial Agents[a]

Agent	MIC 50% (μg/mL)	MIC 90% (μg/mL)	Reference
Ciprofloxacin	4	8	177
Cycloserine	30	—	164
Ethambutol	10	—	164
Ethionamide	10	—	44
Gatifloxacin	1	1	173
Isoniazid	R	R	44
Kanamycin	5	—	44
Moxifloxacin	1	1	173
Pyrazinamide	R	R	164
Rifabutin	<0.12	<0.12	177
Rifampin	1	≥2	177
Streptomycin	10	—	44
	M. simiae		
Cycloserine	30	—	164
Ethambutol	R	R	164
Ethionamide	R	R	164
Isoniazid	R	R	164
Kanamycin	R	R	164
Linezolid	32	>32	175
Pyrazinamide	R	R	164
Rifabutin	R	R	187
Rifampin	R	R	164
Streptomycin	R	R	164
	M. szulgai		
Capreomycin	10	—	164
Cycloserine	30	—	164
Ethambutol	5	—	164
Isoniazid	5	—	164
Linezolid	≤2	4	175
Pyrazinamide	R	R	164
Rifampin	1	—	164
Streptomycin	4	10	164
	M. terrae complex		
Capreomycin	10	—	164
Cycloserine	30	—	164
Ethambutol	5–10	—	164
Gatifloxacin	0.25	32	173
Isoniazid	R	—	164
Moxifloxacin	0.25	16	173

(continued)

TABLE 5.11 (Continued)

Activity of Antimycobacterial Agents[a]

Agent	MIC 50% (μg/mL)	MIC 90% (μg/mL)	Reference
Linezolid	16	32	175
Pyrazinamide	R	R	164
Rifabutin	0.5	R	164
Rifampin	1	1	164
Streptomycin	10	—	164
	M. triplex		
Linezolid	≤4	8	175
	M. triviale		
Capreomycin	10	—	164
Cycloserine	30	—	164
Ethionamide	5	—	164
Isoniazid	R	R	164
Kanamycin	—	5	164
Pyrazinamide	R	R	164
Rifampin	—	1	164
Streptomycin	—	2	164
	M. tuberculosis (Susceptible Wild Type)		
Amifloxacin	4	8	181
Amikacin	0.5	1	177
Azithromycin	>8	>8	188
Capreomycin	—	10	164
Ceftizoxime	64	>64	189
Ciprofloxacin	2	4	181
Clarithromycin	>10	>10	188,190
Clinafloxacin	0.125	0.25	188
Cycloserine	—	30	44
Difloxacin	4	8	189
Erythromycin	>25	>25	165
Ethambutol	2.5	5	44
Ethionamide	—	5	44
Gatifloxacin	0.25	0.25	191,192
Isoniazid	0.2	1	182
Kanamycin	—	5	44
Levofloxacin	0.25	0.25	188
Linezolid	0.5	1	191
Minocycline	>25	>25	165
Moxifloxacin	≤0.25	1	188
Norfloxacin	4	8	176
Ofloxacin	0.5	1	181,188

(continued)

TABLE 5.11 (Continued)

Activity of Antimycobacterial Agents[a]

Agent	MIC 50% (μg/mL)	MIC 90% (μg/mL)	Reference
PAS	—	2	44
Pyrazinamide	—	25	164
Rifabutin	0.5	1	187,188
Rifampin	1	2	182
Sparfloxacin	0.25	0.5	184
Streptomycin	—	2	182
Vancomycin	25	>25	165
	M. tuberculosis (Resistant)		
Azithromycin	>8	>8	188
Ciprofloxacin	0.25	0.5	188
Clarithromycin	>8	>8	188
Clinafloxacin	0.125	0.5	188
Levofloxacin	0.25	0.25	188
Linezolid	0.5	1	193
Ofloxacin	0.5	1	188
Sparfloxacin	0.06	0.125	188
	M. tuberculosis (Multidrug resistant)		
Azithromycin	>8	>8	188
Ciprofloxacin	2	4	188
Clarithromycin	>8	>8	188
Clinafloxacin	1	2	188
Levofloxacin	2	4	188
Ofloxacin	4	8	188
Sparfloxacin	0.5	1	188
	M. ulcerans		
Amikacin	<0.12	0.25	177
Ciprofloxacin	0.25	0.5	177
Rifabutin	<0.12	<0.12	177
Rifampin	<0.12	<0.12	177
	M. xenopi		
Amifloxacin	25	>25	165
Capreomycin	—	10	164
Ciprofloxacin	1	4	165
Cycloserine	30	—	164
Ethambutol	5	—	164
Ethionamide	—	5	164
Gatifloxacin	0.06	0.06	173
Isoniazid	0.2	1	164

(continued)

TABLE 5.11 (Continued)

Activity of Antimycobacterial Agents[a]

Agent	MIC 50% (μg/mL)	MIC 90% (μg/mL)	Reference
Kanamycin	—	5	164
Minocycline	25	>25	165
Moxifloxacin	0.06	0.06	173
Norfloxacin	2	8	176
PAS	2	—	164
Pyrazinamide	R	R	164
Rifabutin	—	1	187
Rifampin	—	1	164
Streptomycin	—	2	164
Vancomycin	25	>25	165

[a] MIC, minimal inhibitory concentration; R, resistant at all concentrations tested.

metals, and the lethal action of isoniazid appears to be suppressed under anaerobic conditions (205).

Over 2 decades ago, the demonstration that isoniazid exposure leads to the inhibition of mycolic acid synthesis led to the hypothesis that this is the major cause of mycobacterial cell death. The evidence supporting this hypothesis was reviewed at that time by Winder (206), who summarized the effects of isoniazid as follows: (a) cells become more fragile and cellular material, including polysaccharides normally acylated to mycolic acids, leaks into the growth medium; (b) intracellular viscosity increases, perhaps due to an increase in cell volume or accumulation of cell wall precursors; (c) cell hydrophobicity decreases; and (d) cells lose the property of acid-fastness. These observations, while largely descriptive and not conclusive, suggest that the exposure of susceptible strains of mycobacteria to isoniazid leads to a loss of cell wall structural integrity and physiologic function that results in cell death.

Takayama et al. (207) demonstrated that isoniazid did indeed inhibit mycolic acid synthesis in *M. tuberculosis,* leading to the accumulation of saturated C_{26} fatty acids. Furthermore, in a later review, Takayama and Qureshi (208) identified a possible site of inhibition by isoniazid in the initial desaturation step to produce the monosaturated C_{24} fatty acid. Isoniazid may also inhibit the elongation of the very long-chain fatty acids and hydroxy lipids.

Since that time, our understanding of mycolic acid synthesis has dramatically increased, and a detailed, overall system of the formation of these long chain fatty acids has been proposed (209). Central to this process are the fatty acid synthesis (FAS) I and II enzyme systems.

The FAS I enzyme system synthesizes saturated fatty acid chains of 16 and 24 carbon atoms. Interestingly, the FAS I system involves a single, multisubunit protein. The FAS II system modifies the $C_{16:0}$ and $C_{24:0}$ FAS I products, leading to the formation of mycolic acid chains of up to C_{56}. Unlike FAS I, the FAS II system involves a series of independent enzymes. The range of structures of the α-mycolic acids produced vary between species; consequently, mycolic acid profiling (by HPLC) has become a standard method of speciating mycobacteria.

One of the FAS II enzymes, the enoyl-acyl carrier protein (ACP) reductase or InhA, was found to be a target for activated isoniazid (210). The enoyl-ACP reductase catalyzes the saturation of terminal $C = C$ double bond of the growing lipid chain prior to chain elongation by the β-ketoacyl-ACP synthases, KasA and KasB. However, the characteristic accumulation of saturated C_{26} fatty acids (bound to ACP) in isoniazid-treated organisms did not appear to be consistent with InhA being the primary target for this drug. Theoretically, inhibition of InhA should lead to the accumulation of monounsaturated fatty acids. This led Mdluli et al. (211) to propose that KasA may also be a target for isoniazid as this enzyme is responsible to elongating fatty acid chains upto C_{40} (212). Furthermore, *kas*A gene mutations were found in isoniazid-resistant clinical isolates of *M. tuberculosis* that lacked mutations in other resistance-associated genes (211), although some *kas*A mutations have been found in isoniazid-susceptible isolates (213,214). Selected KasA mutants have been shown experimentally to confer reduced susceptibility to isoniazid (212).

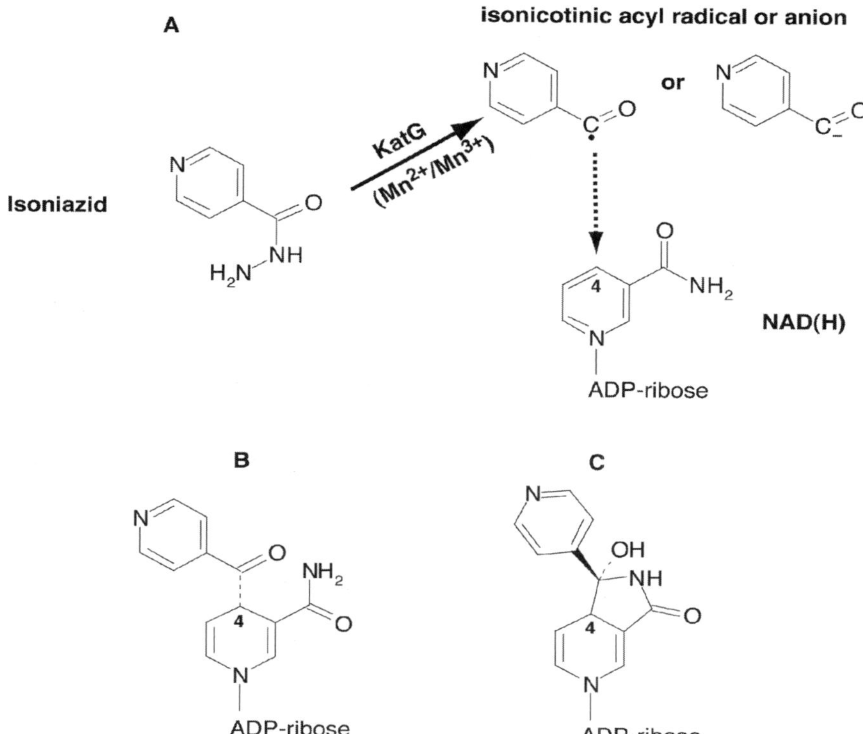

FIGURE 5.4 ● Activation of isoniazid. **A:** The catalase/peroxidase enzyme, KatG, oxidizes isoniazid, probably forming either a free radical or anion. This catalysis is enhanced by the presence of manganese (Mn) ions. The oxidized isoniazid reacts with the nicotinamide moiety of nicotinamide adenine dinucleotide [NAD(H)]. The consequence of this is the formation of a covalent bond between the reactive carbon of the oxidized isoniazid and carbon at position 4 of the nicotinamide ring; the resulting molecule is referred to as an isoniazid-NAD(H) adduct. **B:** The isoniazid-NAD(H) adduct predicted from the crystal structure of the isoniazid target enzyme, InhA. **C:** An alternative isoniazid-NAD(H) adduct produced by the reaction of oxidized isoniazid and NAD(H); this adduct is inhibitory to InhA. [Structures adapted from Nguyen et al. (201) and Rozwarski et al. (204)].

The controversy over the primary target for activated isoniazid is far from being resolved, as several recent studies appear to contradict one another. In one study, the experimental inactivation of InhA alone (i.e., with a functional KasA) in *Mycobacterium smegmatis* led to the accumulation of saturated fatty acids equivalent to that seen in isoniazid-treated cells (215). In contrast, another study reported that isoniazid and thiolactomycin (a KasA-inhibitor), but not triclosan (an InhA-inhibitor), caused the accumulation of $C_{26:0}$ saturated fatty acids in *M. tuberculosis* (216). Perhaps supporting these latter findings, the changes in global gene expression in *M. tuberculosis* caused by isoniazid more closely resemble those caused by thiolactomycin than triclosan (217).

Using purified InhA and KasA proteins from *M. smegmatis,* Kremer et al. (218) demonstrated that KatG-activated isoniazid inhibited the *in vitro* activity of InhA, but not KasA, and Larsen et al. (219) found that overexpression of *inh*A in *trans,* but not *kas*A, increased resistance to isoniazid. Whereas, Slayden et al. (216) found that overexpression of either gene increased resistance (interestingly, overexpression of both genes together resulted in a higher level of isoniazid resistance than either gene alone).

The interaction of isoniazid-NAD(H) adducts with the FAS II pathway is further complicated by the formation of complexes containing both InhA and KasA in isoniazid-treated organisms (218). In addition, most of the functional studies pointing to InhA as the primary target for isoniazid have been with the rapidly growing mycobacterium, *M. smegmatis,* and it is possible that this organism represents an imperfect model of *M. tuberculosis*. For instance, activation of isoniazid by the *M. smegmatis* KatG requires Mn^{2+} ions (220), whereas, the *M. tuberculosis* KatG does not (221). In the latter case, absence of Mn^{2+} ions decreased the yield of the isoniazid-NAD(H) adduct,

InhA inhibitor by only approximately 30% (221). With this in mind, it is possible that the oxidized derivatives of isoniazid that bind to and inhibit InhA and KasA are different.

Whether the primary target of isoniazid is InhA or KasA, or both, the mycolic acid anabolic pathways are a focus of antituberculosis drug development.

Other Effects of Isoniazid

Isoniazid may have other direct effects on mycobacteria as well as inhibiting mycolic acid synthesis. However, the reader should keep in mind that disrupting the cell wall will eventually lead to secondary changes in the cell.

Some of the earliest studies of the effects of isoniazid on mycobacteria demonstrated that levels of nicotinamide nucleotides decreased (222,223). Furthermore, enzymes from mycobacteria and mammalian sources that cleave NAD also catalyze an exchange reaction in which the nicotinamide moiety is replaced by isoniazid to form an NAD analog (224). It was proposed that isoniazid interferes with NAD metabolism as a result of the formation of a similar NAD analog of isonicotinic acid, the major metabolite of isoniazid (225). Thus, isoniazid or an isoniazid metabolite may directly affect reactions catalyzed by NADH and NAD phosphate-dependent dehydrogenases (226). In addition to the formation of analogs of NAD, relatively high concentrations of isoniazid inhibit NAD synthesis in cell-free extracts of isoniazid-sensitive and isoniazid-resistant strains of *M. tuberculosis* H37Rv (227), and it was proposed that isoniazid could affect NAD levels as a result of an indirect influence on the activity of NAD-glycohydrolase (228). Isoniazid was found to bind to and inactivate a heat-labile protein inhibitor of this enzyme.

Davis and Weber (229) found that isoniazid inhibited the regulation of the electron transport system by NAD in *Mycobacterium phlei* but had no effect on the electron transport system in an isoniazid-resistant strain. The NADH dehydrogenases of both isoniazid-sensitive and isoniazid-resistant strains of *M. phlei,* however, are sensitive to inhibition by isoniazid (230). The levels of NAD in *M. tuberculosis* H37Rv treated with isoniazid were measured using a very sensitive method, and the results did not support the hypothesis that NAD depletion is the primary effect of isoniazid (231). First, the growth of cells treated with 62.5 ng of isoniazid was inhibited, but there was no depletion of NAD. Second, the bactericidal activity of isoniazid, but not the level of NAD, was proportional to the product of the period of exposure and the concentration of isoniazid (232). Third, brief exposures to isoniazid are bactericidal, and a postantibiotic effect after the removal of isoniazid did not correlate with changes in NAD levels. It was suggested that NAD was lost as a result of leaks in the cell wall and membrane due to inhibition of mycolate synthesis (233); however, NAD levels recovered in cells exposed to isoniazid for 24 hours, despite the continued inhibition of growth (231). Finally, Krishna Murti (226) proposed that the reduction of NAD levels in tubercle bacilli treated with isoniazid may cause the inhibition of DNA synthesis.

More recently, a link between isoniazid effects and non-InhA NAD(H) metabolism was proposed by Miesel et al. (234), who found that mutations of the *M. smegmatis ndh* gene that reduce NADH dehydrogenase activity conferred increased resistance to isoniazid. In addition, mutations in the *ndh* gene may be present in isoniazid-resistant *M. tuberculosis* that lack mutations in other resistance-associated genes (235). Similarly, mutations in another NAD(H) metabolizing enzyme, Glf (a UDP-galactopyranose mutase), were also found to marginally increase resistance to isoniazid in *M. bovis* (236). However, the causal link between isoniazid resistance and NAD(H) metabolism was probably because of an increase in the NADH/NAD+ ratio leading to a reduction in the activation of isoniazid.

As mentioned previously, an intermediate in the activation of isoniazid is a isonicotinic acyl radical (Fig. 5.4), which could react with other molecules than NAD(H) or potentiate the generation of other reactive species. Evidence for this was presented by Shoeb et al. (237), who showed that crude extracts of *M. tuberculosis* H37Ra catalyzed the production of catechol from phenol in the presence of isoniazid and hydrogen peroxide. This reaction was potentiated by the addition of superoxide dismutase and the reaction was inhibited by hydroxyl radical (^{-}OH) scavengers such as dimethyl sulfoxide and mannitol. Furthermore, superoxide anion (O_2^{-}) was produced by the peroxidase-catalyzed oxidation of isoniazid, as well as by the nonenzymatic reaction of isoniazid with NAD at an alkaline pH, which was produced by the autooxidation of isoniazid (in addition to the superoxide anion) (238). Generation of reactive oxygen species by isoniazid-enhanced reactions may lead to the damage of cellular components, including DNA (239).

Isoniazid Resistance

The activity of isoniazid depends on its activation, binding to its target, and exerting an inhibitory effect on that target. Thus, changes at any of these steps may lead to a change in susceptibility to this drug. However, a critical issue is whether the changes are clinically relevant.

An early observation of isoniazid-resistant clinical isolates of *M. tuberculosis* was the changes in the catalase/peroxidase system of a significant proportion of these organisms (240), and these changes were mapped subsequently to the *kat*G gene (hydroperoxidase I) (241). Such changes in the *kat*G gene prevent or reduce activation of isoniazid. The changes in the *kat*G gene range from point mutations to small deletions, through to loss of most or all of the gene (242), although the latter case is rare. However, the reader should note that an arginine-to-leucine change at codon 463 of the "standard" KatG sequence (i.e., *M. tuberculosis* H37Rv) is a natural polymorphism, and unrelated to isoniazid resistance (243–245). To date, there are numerous studies showing that 36% to 100% (median ~70%) of isoniazid-resistant *M. tuberculosis* worldwide have a resistance enabling mutation in the *kat*G gene (245–266). Interestingly, the majority of isolates have a change at codon 315.

The presence of a nonfunctional *kat*G gene increases susceptibility of *M. tuberculosis* to oxidative damage. Consequently, in such organisms, compensatory mutations in the regulatory region of the *ahp*C gene may be present (267,268). However, increased expression of *ahp*C plays little or no direct role in isoniazid resistance (267).

Although mutations in *kat*G account for the majority of isoniazid resistance in *M. tuberculosis,* in approximately 30% of isolates mutations in other genes must be involved. Several studies have shown that resistance to isoniazid can be associated with mutations within the *inhA* gene (18,210,269–271). Such mutations appear to alter the hydrogen bonding within the NADH binding site, explaining the reduced affinity of NADH for the inhA protein. However, mutations within the *inhA* gene of the *M. tuberculosis* complex appear to cause only low-level isoniazid resistance (272,273). Furthermore, the most common *inh*A-associated mutations in clinical isolates of *M. tuberculosis* were found to be in the promoter region of the *inh*A operon (242). There is some evidence that overexpression of the *inh*A gene can confer increased resistance to isoniazid (216,219). In *M. tuberculosis,* the *inh*A gene is expressed as an operon with its upstream partner, *mab;* the Mab protein is a 3-ketoacyl reductase involved in mycolic acid synthesis, but not in isoniazid resistance (274).

As stated previously, mutations in *kas*A, *ndh,* and *glf* have been linked with increased resistance to isoniazid (211,234–236). Furthermore, recent studies showed that experimental overexpression of the arylamine *N*-acetyltransferase (NAT) encoded by the *nho*A gene may activate isoniazid and cause low-level isoniazid resistance (275,276). Intriguingly, an extensive genetic study of isoniazid-resistant *M. tuberculosis* (251) demonstrated that some organisms can have multiple mutations or polymorphisms in a range of genes (including *kat*G, *inh*A, *kas*A, and *ndh*). Finally, there is evidence that mycobacteria may have an efflux pump that can transport isoniazid out of the cell (277, 278), although the genetic basis of this process is unknown.

With the exception of mutations in *kat*G, the clinical significance of changes in these genes is not clear. However, despite the low-level resistance conferred by mutations in genes such as *inh*A and *kas*A, such changes may increase the likelihood of the acquisition of mutations that confer high-level resistance. For instance, any reduction in the inhibitory effects of an antimicrobial agent may allow an increase in metabolism of the target organisms and hence an increase in DNA synthesis. DNA synthesis is required for mutagenesis.

Rifamycins

The rifamycins (e.g., rifampicin, rifabutin, and rifapentine) are potent inhibitors of prokaryotic DNA-dependent RNA polymerases (279), with little activity against the equivalent mammalian enzymes. This group of antimicrobial agents are compounds composed of aromatic rings linked by an aliphatic bridge. Most likely, the lipophilic properties of the molecule are important for binding of the drug to the polymerase and aid in the penetration of the drug across the mycobacterial cell wall.

The susceptibility of mycobacteria to rifampin is well documented, and the drug is a standard component of antituberculosis therapy, including DOTS and DOTS-plus (280–282). However, there is significant variation in susceptibility to rifampin between MAC isolates, with the majority being intrinsically resistant. Despite this, the DNA-dependent RNA polymerases isolated from *M. intracellulare* and *M. avium* are to be sensitive to rifampin (283,284). Furthermore, substances believed to increase the permeability of the mycobacterial cell wall, such as Tween 80, also cause a significant increase in susceptibility to rifampin. Thus, it appears that the impermeability of the cell wall plays a role in rifampin resistance in the MAC.

Recently, rifapentine was approved by the Food and Drug Administration for use in treating tuberculosis (285). Against *M. tuberculosis in vitro*, rifapentine is more active than rifampin (286,287), and its metabolite, 25-*O*-desacetylrifapentine, has equivalent activity to rifampin (287). Moreover, both rifapentine and 25-*O*-desacetylrifapentine have longer half-lives than rifampin (288–291), and consequently, rifapentine-containing antituberculosis regimens have focused on a reduced dosing regimen compared with rifampin; for instance, twice-weekly dosing during the induction phase of therapy (i.e., the first 2 months) and once-weekly dosing during the continuation phase (292). Furthermore, rifapentine is a weaker inducer of the cytochrome P450 CYP3A system than rifampin (289) and thus rifapentine should interfere less with drugs metabolized by this system (e.g., protease inhibitors). Despite the theoretical benefits of rifapentine, current studies have not shown superior efficacy in treating tuberculosis with this agent compared with rifampin, and may lead to higher relapse rates (289,292–294). These disappointing results are probably related, at least partly, to rifapentine having a greater propensity to bind to proteins than rifampin does. Further studies are required to optimize rifapentine-containing regimens.

Rifabutin has potent activity *in vitro* against MAC (295) and has equivalent activity as rifapentine against *M. tuberculosis* (287). In a series of uncontrolled clinical trials, however, rifabutin failed to demonstrate efficacy in the treatment of MAC disease, although the dosages of rifabutin used may have been too low (112). Rifabutin has been shown to reduce the incidence of MAC disease in HIV-infected patients when used as a prophylactic agent, and the drug has been approved for this use (296,297). Although the basis of the prophylactic activity of rifabutin is not known, this drug has been shown to inhibit the binding of MAC to HT-29 human intestinal carcinoma cells in vitro (298). Thus, rifabutin may prevent colonization of the gastrointestinal tract, which is believed to be a major portal of entry for MAC. Compared with rifampin, rifabutin also has a longer half-life *in vivo* and is concentrated in tissues, especially the lungs, where levels can be 10 times higher than in serum.

Another rifamycin with potential for treating tuberculosis and other mycobacterioses is rifalazil or KRM-1648. Rifalazil is more active *in vitro* than rifampin against *M. tuberculosis* (299–302), and is highly active against MAC (301,303,304). Furthermore, animal studies indicate that rifalazil has better efficacy than rifampin in treating mycobacterioses (299,302,305–308). Like rifapentine and rifabutin, rifalazil accumulates in tissues, and has a long half-life (up to 20 hours) (309). This holds the promise of reduced dosing regimens. Perhaps the most significant potential benefit of rifalazil is that it does not induce the cytochrome P450 CYP3A system [although it is metabolized by this system (310,311)], thus reducing the potential for interfering with drugs metabolized by this pathway (e.g., protease inhibitors).

Based largely on studies with *Escherichia coli*, the target site of rifamycins was found to be the β-subunit of the RNA polymerase. The β-subunit is one of the five subunits that comprise the polymerase and is believed to be the catalytic center of the enzyme. Rifampin (and presumably, the other rifamycins) does not appear to bind in the catalytic center of the β-subunit, but rather the DNA/RNA channel (312,313). This is consistent with the observation that rifampin inhibits the initiation of RNA synthesis, but not RNA elongation once initiation has occurred. Thus, rifampin probably acts as a physical "plug" rather than a direct catalytic inhibitor. In this respect, rifamycins have similarity to macrolides (discussion follows).

Resistance to rifamycins in mycobacteria (and other microorganisms) is the result of mutations within the *rpoB* gene (11). These mutations cluster in a hot spot (Fig. 5.5) and usually result in a single amino acid change in the protein sequence, and reduce the binding affinity of rifamycins to the RNA polymerase. Since the original study by Telenti et al. (11), there have been numerous reports describing the *rpoβ* gene mutations in rifampin-resistant *M. tuberculosis* isolated in different regions of the world. Mutations in or near the hot spot of the *rpoβ* gene mutations account for all but a small percentage of rifampin-resistant *M. tuberculosis*. However, an interesting recent finding was a *rpoβ* mutation at the beginning of the gene (codon 176) that may account for a significant proportion of rifampin-resistant *M. tuberculosis* without hot spot-associated mutations (314). Although previously undescribed mutations are often reported, a common finding in most studies is that the approximately 80% of rifampin-resistant clinical isolates have a mutation in codons 526 or 531 of the β-subunit (194,195), especially mutations causing a serine-to-leucine change at codon 531 (S531L). Intriguingly, the predominant rifampin-resistant *M. tuberculosis* mutants selected *in vitro* also tend have S531L substitutions (315). This suggests that pressures other than rifampin-inhibition of RNA synthesis are involved in the appearance of stable resistant mutants. In support of this is the finding that a S531L substitution has a smaller impact on the activity of the RNA polymerase than other less common mutations (316).

Interestingly, the mutations associated with resistance to different rifamycins do not always match, an observation that appears to explain why rifamycins such as rifapentine, rifabutin, and rifalazil are active *in vitro* against some *M. tuberculosis* strains that are resistant to rifampin (317–320). However, the most common *rpoβ* mutations in rifampin-resistant *M. tuberculosis* (i.e., codons 526 and 531) also confer high-level resistance to the other rifamycins.

Unlike most other antimycobacterial agents, evidence suggests that active rifamycin efflux from mycobacteria is minimal at best (321). Thus, increased efflux is unlikely to be a significant mechanism of clinically significant rifamycin resistance.

Macrolides and Ketolides

The development of new-generation macrolides has had a significant impact on the treatment of mycobacterial diseases, especially those caused by MAC, *Mycobacterium leprae*, and the rapidly growing species; however, macrolides appear to be of little benefit in the treatment of tuberculosis (9,322,323). Azithromycin (an azalide macrolide), clarithromycin, and roxithromycin are structurally related to erythromycin, with modifications that improve acid stability, tissue accumulation, bioavailability, and lengthen elimination half-life without increasing toxicity. Although adverse drug effects are less frequent, compared to erythromycin, gastrointestinal intolerance (abdominal pain, nausea, and diarrhea) does occur with the new macrolides.

Of the macrolides, clarithromycin is the most active against MAC isolates *in vitro* (on a weight basis), with 90% of MAC isolates having MICs of 0.5 to 4 μg/mL under mildly acidic conditions (pH 6.8). Under similar conditions, the MIC values for azithromycin and roxithromycin are both 8 to 32 μg/mL. The activity of macrolides *in vitro*, however, is strongly affected by pH, with MICs being one to two dilutions lower at pH 7.4 compared with at pH 6.8 (41,324).

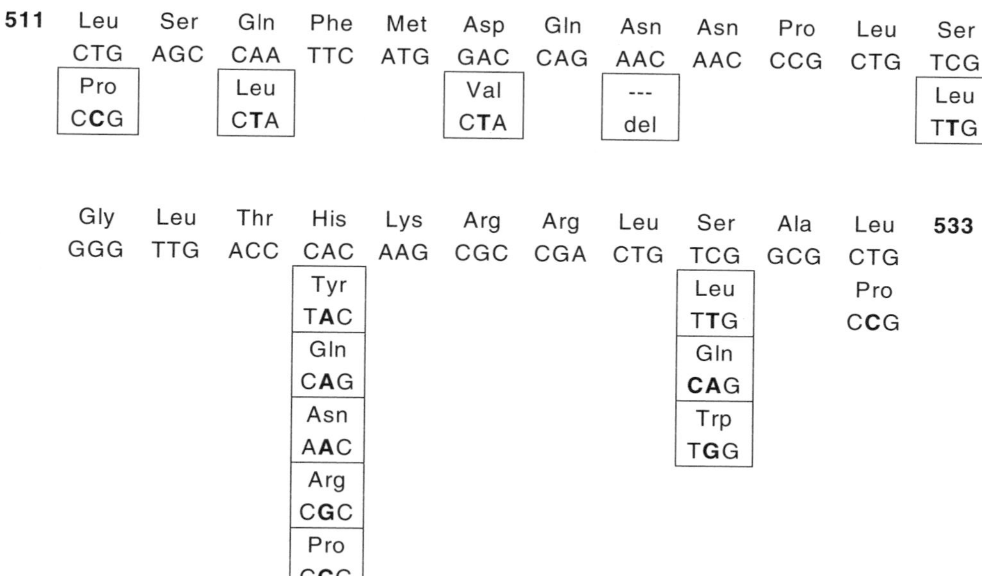

FIGURE 5.5 ● Clustering of mutations in the β-subunit (*rpoβ* gene) of the RNA polymerase found in more than 90% of rifampin-resistant *M. tuberculosis*. Shown is the *rpoβ* gene of *M. tuberculosis* from codon 511 to codon 535. The *boxes* below the sequence show the positions of 15 common gene mutations (specific base changes are shown in *bold*) and the resulting amino acid changes that result in the production of a rifampin-resistant RNA polymerase. [Adapted from Telenti et al. (11)].

This phenomenon has caused some controversy in establishing interpretive standards for assessing susceptibility to macrolides *in vitro*. Testing of macrolides under sightly alkaline conditions, however, may be misleading because MAC strains grow more slowly under such conditions and, thus, MIC values may reflect synergy between pH and drug (295). The conditions within the phagolysosomes of MAC-infected macrophages (i.e., pH 6.0 to 6.5) suggest that susceptibility testing of macrolides under mildly acidic conditions would be more clinically relevant. That said, the NCCLS provides reference range MICs for macrolides at acidic and neutral pH (41).

Although clarithromycin appears to be considerably more active than the other macrolides *in vitro*, the comparative pharmacokinetics suggest a sightly different picture *in vivo*. Following a 500-mg dose of clarithromycin, the maximum serum level achieved is 2 to 3 μg/mL, with an elimination half-life of 7 hours. Tissue concentrations are usually four to five times those in serum, with the levels in macrophages being 20 to 30 times higher. After a similar dose of azithromycin, the maximum serum level is 0.4 to 0.6 μg/mL; however, accumulation within leukocytes approaches 200 to 800 times serum concentrations (325). This high tissue accumulation reflects the extraordinarily long elimination half-life (68 hours) of azithromycin. Roxithromycin achieves the highest serum levels of the three macrolides (11 μg/mL), with a half-life of 19 hours. Little is known about tissue accumulation of roxithromycin, although evidence suggests that roxithromycin achieves poor tissue-to-serum concentration ratios (326–328).

The ketolides represent a class of semisynthetic erythromycin derivatives, with the replacement of the neutral L-cladinose with a keto group at position 3 of the macrolatone ring (329,330). In addition, many ketolides have other changes to the basic erythromycin framework. These changes were introduced to improve the activity and pharmacokinetics of macrolides. Furthermore, ketolides may be active against some macrolide-resistant bacteria (331). For instance, most ketolides do not upregulate expression of inducible *erm* genes (332), and may have some activity against methylated ribosomes that are refractory to macrolides (331,333). This activity may result from the higher binding affinity of ketolides than macrolides for ribosomes (329,330,333). Currently, the ketolide, telithromycin, is approved for clinical use in the United States and Europe.

Telithromycin and other ketolides have been tested against mycobacteria with some success. Telithromycin MICs against mycobacteria tend to be higher than clarithromycin (334–336), and mycobacteria with acquired macrolide resistance are also resistant to ketolides (337). However, studies with ketolides using mouse models of mycobacterioses suggest that these agents are efficacious (337–339). This discrepancy between *in vitro* susceptibility and activity *in vivo* is reminiscent of azithromycin, and is based at least in part on the accumulation of these agents in tissues and their long half-lives *in vivo*.

Macrolides (and ketolides) are bacteriostatic agents that bind to the 50S subunit of the prokaryotic ribosome and block protein synthesis. Within the 50S subunit, the critical macrolide binding site is at the peptidyltransferase region (340), and the agents appear to interact with the adenine residues at positions 2058 and 2059 (A2058 and A2059, *E. coli* numbering) of the 23S rRNA. Macrolides appear to bind to the ribosome in the cleft where the growing peptide chain exits the peptidyltransferase region. Thus, inhibition may be the result of a physical obstruction rather than a direct inhibition of peptidyltransferase activity; such an indirect mode of action is similar to that of rifamycins (see previous discussion). That said, there is some evidence that 16-membered macrolides (e.g., spiramycin) may inhibit peptidyltransferase reactions and that 14-membered macrolides (e.g., clarithromycin) may prevent the translocation of transfer RNA (tRNA) and increase tRNA dissociation from the ribosome (341). However, it is not clear if these are direct or indirect effects of macrolide binding. Macrolides reversibly bind to the ribosome, which is probably a major reason why these agents are primarily bacteriostatic.

Resistance to macrolides has been studied with a range of microorganisms, and three basic mechanisms have been identified (342,343), ribosome modification, drug efflux, and drug inactivation. The predominant mechanism of clinically significant resistance is ribosome modification by methylation of the A2058 residue within the 23S rRNA. This methylation occurs prior to assembly of the 50S ribosomal subunit, which means that organisms must replace their susceptible ribosomes with nascently methylated ribosomes in order to express resistance. The methylase activity is rRNA sequence-specific and encoded by *erm* genes. Methylation of A2058 reduces the binding affinity of macrolides to the ribosome, thus explaining the resistance. Other agents, such as lincosamides and streptogramin B, associate with the A2058 residue; thus, methylation of this site usually confers cross-resistance to these agents (i.e., MLS resistance). Another important mechanism of macrolide resistance in clinically important bacteria is drug efflux, for example, conferred by expression of the *mef*A gene of streptococci or the *msr*A gene of staphylococci (343).

There are several other potential mechanisms of macrolide resistance, including inactivating enzymes and mutations of the ribosomal proteins (342,343); however, their association with clinically significant resistance is unclear.

Unlike most other bacterial pathogens, clinically acquired macrolide resistance in mycobacteria is conferred by point mutations at residue A2058 or A2059 within the 23S rRNA gene (93,344,345), and like rRNA methylation, such mutations reduce the binding of macrolides to the ribosome (346). In mycobacteria, macrolide resistance-associated mutations also confer resistance to ketolides (337). The importance of 23S rRNA gene mutations in macrolide-resistant mycobacteria is because these organisms have only a limited number of copies of the rRNA gene operon per genome, with slowly growing mycobacteria having only a single copy, and most rapidly growing mycobacteria have two copies. Most other bacterial pathogens have multiple copies of the *rrn* operon; a notable exception is *Helicobacter pylori* which only has two copies, and clinically acquired macrolide resistance is also conferred by 23S rRNA gene mutation (347–349).

Although macrolides are the foundation of treatment regimens for many mycobacterioses, innate resistance to macrolides is expressed by some pathogenic mycobacteria, including *M. tuberculosis* (322,323). This resistance does not appear to be due to sequence divergence in the peptidyltransferase region of the 23S rRNA. Recent studies showed that the intrinsic macrolide resistance of *M. fortuitum* (91), *M. smegmatis* (90), and *M. tuberculosis* (350,351) was conferred by novel *erm* genes, *erm*(39), *erm*(38), and *erm*(37). These rRNA methylase genes are chromosomal and inducible with macrolide and lincosamide agents, but not streptogramin B. In addition to ribosome methylases, there is evidence for active macrolide efflux in mycobacteria (352), although the clinical significance of this is unknown.

Aminoglycosides and Peptide Antibiotics

The mechanism of action of aminoglycosides and peptide antibiotics is well accommodated by the allosteric three-site model for the ribosomal elongation cycle (353). According to the model, the ribosome contains three binding sites: the A-site or aminoacyl-transfer RNA (tRNA) site; the P-site or peptidyl-tRNA site; and the E-site or exit site for deacylated tRNA (Fig. 5.6). The A- and E-sites are allosterically linked, such that occupation of one site decreases the affinity for the other site. The result is that the A- and P-sites have high affinity for tRNA before translocation, while the P- and E-sites have high affinity after translation. Deacylated tRNA is released on occupation of the A-site, not during translocation. Thus, during initiation reactions, the E-site is not occupied and the A-site is said to undergo an initiation-type occupation equivalent to formation of the 70S initiation complex; however, once translocation occurs and the E-site is occupied, the A-site undergoes an elongation-type occupation. During the initiation reaction only the P-site carries a tRNA, while during the elongation cycle the ribosome complex carries two tRNAs, i.e., a peptidyl-tRNA and deacylated tRNA. The mechanism of action of aminoglycosides and peptide antibiotics can be understood in terms of the allosteric interactions involving these binding sites (see the following discussion). There is also compelling evidence to support the conclusion that protein synthesis and the effects of protein synthesis inhibitors occur in an identical manner in mycobacteria and rapidly growing bacteria such as *E. coli* (354–356).

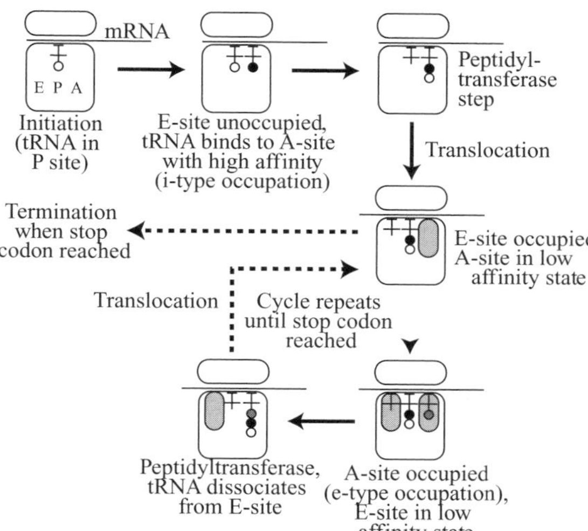

FIGURE 5.6 ● Two types of A-site occupation, according to the allosteric three-site model. The i-type occupation follows the initiation reactions, with the e-site remaining unoccupied. The e-type occupation occurs after an elongation cycle and is characterized by an occupied E-site (357). *EPA*, elongation, peptidyl-transfer, and aminoacyl-binding sites. For simplicity, ribosome accessory factors (e.g., EF-Tu and EF-G) are not shown.

Viomycin and capreomycin are basic peptides with similar structures and are generally considered to share a common mechanism of action; however, few studies have been performed with capreomycin. Viomycin resistance is reported to cross to capreomycin resistance in mycobacteria (357), and viomycin blocks the binding of capreomycin to ribosomes. Viomycin and capreomycin are bacteriostatic agents with potent activity against mycobacteria, with little activity against Gram-negative bacteria. Nevertheless, viomycin is an active inhibitor of cell-free protein synthesis using extracts of Gram-negative bacteria. Viomycin blocks translocation and, surprisingly, impedes elongation type A-site binding; therefore, in the presence of viomycin, the ribosome cannot be transferred back to the pretranslocational state via A-site binding of the elongation type (353). Viomycin and capreomycin are thus inhibitors of translocation that block both allosteric transitions of the ribosome elongation cycle. Little is known about the mechanisms of resistance to basic peptides; however, there is evidence that ribosome mutation is involved (358).

The primary antimycobacterial aminoglycosides are streptomycin for treating tuberculosis and amikacin for treating disseminated *M. avium* infections. In 1943, streptomycin became one of the first effective antimicrobial agent to be used to treat tuberculosis, however, trials with p-aminosalicylic acid were also completed that year, and there is some controversy as to which was actually first used clinically (359). Other aminoglycosides, such as kanamycin and gentamycin, have been used to treat mycobacterioses, although their therapeutic indices are less favorable than streptomycin and amikacin. The aminoglycosides are generally less bactericidal for mycobacteria than for other types of bacteria (167).

Streptomycin and dihydrostreptomycin are derivatives of streptamine, and kanamycin is a glycoside of 2-deoxystreptamine. Amikacin is a semisynthetic kanamycin derivative with a butyric acid moiety at the R3-position of kanamycin. All of the aminoglycosides reduce A-site binding of aminoacyl-tRNA of the elongation type, while A-site binding of the initiation type is minimally affected, as is the puromycin reaction (chain termination). Thus, the primary mechanism of action of the aminoglycosides is to inhibit the posttranslocational-to-pretranslocational transition, with only variable effects on the pretranslocational-to-posttranslocational transition. Aminoglycosides, particularly streptomycin, affect the proofreading function of the A site, leading to the misstranslation of proteins. The pleiotropic effects of the aminoglycosides that are more difficult to explain include irreversible uptake, membrane damage, and ribosomal blockage. However, Hausner et al. (360) hypothesized that the primary molecular mechanism of aminoglycoside bactericidal activity is ribosomal blockage, with the pleiotropic effects occurring as a consequence of the disruption of protein synthesis.

Since aminoglycosides, capreomycin, and viomycin target the ribosome, it is not surprising that modification of this organelle confers high-level acquired resistance (361–370). For instance, the mechanism of resistance to streptomycin in *M. tuberculosis* is associated with mutations within the 16S rRNA gene and the *rpsL* gene, which encodes the S12 ribosomal protein (358,366–369, 371–375). The most common mutations are in codon 43 of the *rpsL* gene, being found in approximately 45% of streptomycin-resistant *M. tuberculosis* isolates (372, 373). These mutations tend to confer high-level resistance (streptomycin MIC more than 500 μg/ml). The other common site for *rpsL* mutations is in codon 88. The 16S rRNA gene mutations tend to cluster in or near the loop 18 region (positions 500 to 545) and the loop 27 region (positions 888 to 912) for the 16S rRNA structure, as shown by Brimacombe et al. (376). Other mutations have been described as mostly in-between these two loop regions. Although base substitution at position 491 of the 16S rRNA gene has been found in streptomycin-resistant *M. tuberculosis* (369), this position appears to be a polymorphism that does not confer resistance (377). The 16S rRNA mutations tend to confer a lower level of streptomycin resistance than *rpsL* mutations. The localizing of resistance-associated mutations in the loop 18 and 27 regions and the *rpsL* gene (i.e., the S12 ribosomal protein) suggests that streptomycin binds in or near the A-site.

The known *rpsL* and 16S rRNA gene mutations account for 60% to 90% of streptomycin resistance. *M. tuberculosis* isolates with low-level streptomycin resistance (MIC ~10 μg/mL) tend to have wild-type *rpsL* and 16S rRNA genes (at least in the loop 18 and 27 regions) (372,378). This suggests that there is a third mechanism of streptomycin resistance, which may be based on changes in cell wall permeability (378).

Despite the similarity between aminoglycosides, the mechanisms of resistance may not completely overlap. For instance, clinically acquired resistance to 2-deoxystreptamine aminoglycosides (e.g., amikacin and kanamycin) in *M. abscessus* is associated with 16S rRNA gene mutation at position 1408 (370). This position is equivalent to the 16S rRNA methylation site that confers resistance to the aminoglycoside-producing bacteria (379). However, this mutation does not confer resistance to streptomycin.

Resistance to aminoglycosides in bacteria can be due to the presence of aminoglycoside-modifying enzymes (380). From studies 2 decades ago, rapidly growing mycobacteria are known to produce aminoglycoside-acetylating enzymes (381), and a substrate profile analysis revealed two patterns of 3-*N*-acetyltransferase, with broad and narrow specificities (382). The broad-specificity enzyme was found only in *M. fortuitum,* while the narrow-specificity enzyme was found in *M. smegmatis, Mycobacterium vaccae,* and *M. phlei*. However, the ubiquitous presence and activity of these enzymes in rapidly growing mycobacteria does not correlate with acquired aminoglycoside resistance (383).

More recently, DNA homology studies identified putative aminoglycoside acetyltransferases in the chromosomes of both rapidly growing and slowly growing mycobacteria, including *M. tuberculosis* (384). Cloning and overexpression of the aminoglycosides acetyltransferase gene, aac(2′)-Id, of *M. smegmatis* conferred a fourfold to 16-fold increase in MIC for a range of aminoglycosides, and disrupting the gene resulted in a drop in MIC of an equivalent magnitude (384). However, expression of the *M. tuberculosis* putative aminoglycosides acetyltransferase in *M. smegmatis* did not increase resistance to this class of agent. Thus, the role of these enzymes in either intrinsic or acquired resistance to aminoglycosides is not clear.

Ethambutol

Ethambutol is active against *M. tuberculosis,* with MICs in the range of 1 to 5 μg/mL, although its antimicrobial activity requires active growth of susceptible cells. The drug has much more variable activity against the other species of slowly growing mycobacteria and is significantly less active against rapidly growing mycobacteria. On the whole, ethambutol is inactive against other microorganisms. Studies of the mechanism of action of ethambutol have focused on two targets: polyamine metabolism and cell wall synthesis. The influence of ethambutol on polyamine metabolism was inferred, in part, from the similarity of the chemical structures of ethambutol (*d*-2,2-[ethylenediimino]di[1-butanol]) and spermine (*N,N′*-bis(3-aminopropyl)1,4-butanediamine) (Fig. 5.7). In addition, early studies showed that the growth inhibition caused by ethambutol could be reversed by the addition of spermidine or Mg^{2+} and that cells could be protected from the effect of ethambutol by the addition of high concentrations of Mg^{2+} or by increases in the ionic strength of the growth medium. Additional studies suggested that the effect of ethambutol was on the synthesis and stability of RNA. However, a later study showed that ethambutol caused a disaggregation of cells, which most likely reflected a reduction in the lipid content of the cell wall (385). Indeed, Takayama et al. (386) showed that ethambutol inhibited the transfer of mycolic acid into the cell wall and stimulated trehalose dimycolate synthesis.

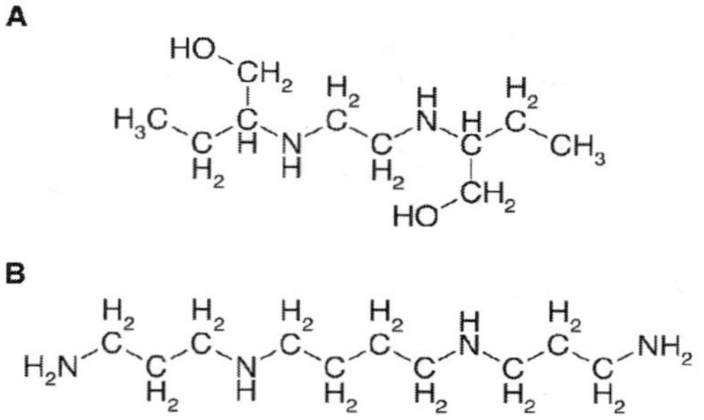

FIGURE 5.7 ● Structures of ethambutol **(A)** and spermine **(B)**.

The problem with many of these studies was that the time between the addition of the drug and the observed effect was often long (hours), thus preventing distinction between primary and secondary effects. Subsequently, several studies demonstrated that the spermidine synthase enzyme from mycobacteria was inhibited by ethambutol (387,388), specifically the *dextro*-isomer and not the *levo*-isomer (only the *dextro*-isomer inhibits the growth of mycobacteria). The synthases from a *Pseudomonas* sp and an *E. coli* isolate (both are ethambutol-resistant) were not inhibited by either form of ethambutol. In addition, the spermidine synthase from a strain of *M. fortuitum,* with an ethambutol MIC of 8 μg/mL, required 80 μmol/L of *d*-ethambutol to inhibit 50% of enzyme activity, compared with 30 μmol/L for the enzymes from strains of *M. bovis* and *Mycobacterium flavescens* with ethambutol MICs of 1 μg/mL. However, using an *M. bovis* strain, the effect of ethambutol on polyamine metabolism *in vivo* required an ethambutol concentration eightfold above the MIC in order to achieve a 46% reduction in spermidine synthesis after 48-hour exposure to the drug. This casts doubt on the relevance of inhibition of polyamine metabolism as the primary antimycobacterial activity of ethambutol, although it may lead to secondary effects.

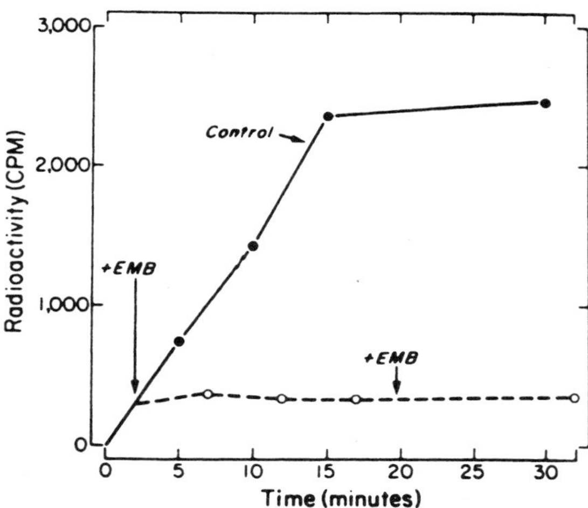

FIGURE 5.8 • Effect of ethambutol *(EMB)* on the time course of incorporation of label from [^{14}C]glucose into the arabinose residues of arabinomannan and arabinogalactan in ethambutol-susceptible *M. smegmatis*. EMB was added (3 μg/mL) to the culture at 2.5 minutes *(arrow)* (390).

In contrast, the effect of ethambutol on cell wall synthesis and, more specifically, trehalose dimycolate synthesis was later shown to occur within 15 minutes of exposure to the drug (389). In that study, precursors such as monomycolate, dimycolate, and mycolic acid began to accumulate within 1 to 12 minutes. These observations led Takayama and Kilburn (390) to identify a more specific metabolic target for ethambutol. They showed a decrease in the incorporation of [^{14}C]glucose into a 55% to 85% ethanol-insoluble fraction of whole cells of an ethambutol-sensitive strain of *M. smegmatis,* within 15 minutes of the addition of 3 μg/mL ethambutol. The ethanol-insoluble fraction was shown to contain cell wall arabinomannan and arabinogalactan. The effect of ethambutol on the incorporation of [^{14}C]glucose into the arabinose residue of these complex sugars was virtually instantaneous (Fig. 5.8). High-performance liquid chromatography analysis of [^{14}C]alditol acetates derived from the polysaccharide fraction of treated and control cells showed 90% and 53% inhibition of the transfer of [^{14}C]glucose label into arabinose and mannose, respectively. Maximal inhibition of glucose incorporation was observed with 5 μg/mL ethambutol, which was in contrast to the 60 μg/mL required to achieve an equivalent level of inhibition in an isogenic ethambutol-resistant strain of *M. smegmatis*. The *in vivo* studies were complemented by preliminary cell-free assays for the effect of ethambutol on arabinose metabolism. Thus, the primary mechanism of action of ethambutol appears to be the inhibition of arabinogalactan synthesis and, to a lesser degree, the inhibition of arabinomannan synthesis (391). The intermediates that accumulate in the presence of inhibitory concentrations of ethambutol include decaprenyl-*P*-arabinose (392), which suggests that this drug inhibits transfer of arabinose from its donor molecule to the relevant polysaccharide the cell wall (393). The proposed disruptive effects of ethambutol on cell wall synthesis are consistent with evidence for a synergistic effect of ethambutol on the activity of other antimycobacterial agents (394,395).

The target(s) of ethambutol in mycobacteria is believed to be one or more of the putative arabinosyl transferases encoded by the *emb* operon. Inhibition of these enzymes would be consistent with the accumulation of arabinosyl-donor molecules in ethambutol-treated cells. The *emb* operon comprises either two genes in *M. avium* (*emb*A and *emb*B) or three genes in *M. tuberculosis, M. leprae,* and *M. smegmatis* [*emb*C, *emb*A, and *emb*B (in this order)] (396,397), and the product of the *emb*R gene probably regulates expression of this operon (396). Mutations in the *emb*B gene confer high-level resistance to ethambutol (398), suggesting that this encodes the primary target for this drug. Although mutations in other regions associated with the *emb* operon have been described (399), perhaps as many as 65% of *M. tuberculosis* isolates with acquired ethambutol resistance have mutations in the *emb*B gene (398), particularly at codon 306. Furthermore, polymorphisms in the *emb*B gene appear to be linked with intrinsic resistance to ethambutol in mycobacteria (400). However, mutations in the codon 306 region have been reported in MDR *M. tuberculosis* that are still susceptible to ethambutol (401). The significance of this is unclear, but may suggest that ethambutol has a target other than *embB*.

Early studies of the frequency of resistance to ethambutol in *M. tuberculosis* cultures showed that low-level resistance occurs relatively frequently (approximately one in 10^5 organisms), but that high-level resistance was extremely rare (402). This suggested that high-level resistance is most likely is the result of a multistep process. Further evidence of a stepwise acquisition of high-level ethambutol resistance was reported recently by Telenti et al (397). The first step appears to be an increase in expression of the *emb* operon, followed by a mutation in *emb*B. Alternatively, the second step may involve a further increase in *emb* expression (397).

Pyrazinamide

Pyrazinamide in combination with isoniazid is considered to be rapidly bactericidal for *M. tuberculosis,* and consequently this agent is a critical component to short-course treatments such as DOTS. However, pyrazinamide has no activity against other mycobacteria, including other members of the *M. tuberculosis* complex and the MAC (403).

The study of the antituberculosis activity of pyrazinamide *in vitro* is problematic in that it is active only at

A

Pyrazinamide (PZA) Pyrazinoic acid (POA)

PZase

B

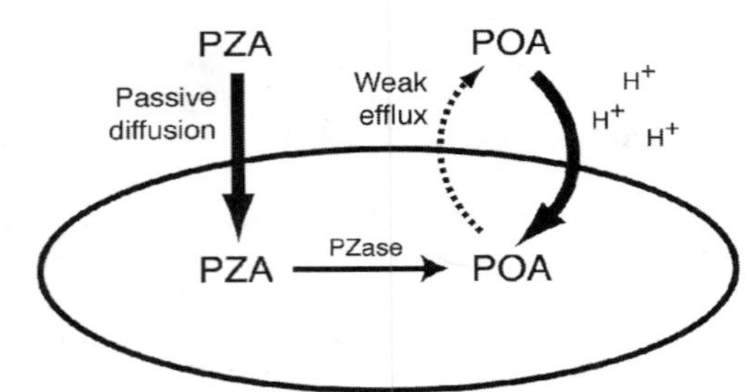

FIGURE 5.9 ● Activation and mobilization of pyrazinamide.
A: Pyrazinamde (*PZA*) is converted to pyrazinoic acid (*POA*) by the cytosolic enzyme, pyrazinamidase/nicotinamidase or *PZase* (encoded by the *pnc*A gene).
B: PZA enters the bacterium by passive diffusion and is converted to POA, which leaves the bacterium by diffusion aided by a weal efflux pump. Under acidic extracellular conditions, approximately 50% of the exported POA may exist in its protonated (i.e., undissociated) form; i.e., at a concentration several orders of magnitude higher than intracellular concentration of this form. Thus, protonated POA will readily reenter the cell down this concentration gradient. [Based on a model proposed by Zhang and Telenti (194)].

an acidic pH (pH 5.6), which itself suppresses growth of mycobacteria. Furthermore, pyrazinamide is a prodrug, the active derivative being pyrazinoic acid (pyrazinecarboxylic acid; Fig. 5.9A). The conversion of pyrazinamide to pyrazinoic acid was shown to be catalyzed by human enzymes, and thus it was suggested that pyrazinamide activation occurs within the acidic environment of the caseous lesion and phagolysosome (404). However, it was subsequently shown that pyrazinamidase activity in mycobacteria was associated with susceptibility to pyrazinamide (81,82); most strains of *M. tuberculosis* that are resistant to pyrazinamide lack pyrazinamidase activity. Thus, pyrazinamide activation most likely occurs inside the bacillus. The gene encoding the pyrazinamidase, *pnc*A, was later identified in the *M. tuberculosis* genome (405). The product of the *pnc*A gene has both pyrazinamidase and nicotimamidase activity, which explains previously reported association between these two enzyme activities (406). Furthermore, Speirs et al. (407) showed that *M. tuberculosis* isolates resistant to pyrazinamide were generally still susceptible to the pyrazinamide derivatives pyrazinoic acid and *n*-propyl pyrazinoate, thus supporting the hypothesis that the primary mechanism of inherent resistance in the other mycobacteria involves the lack of an appropriate pyrazinamide-modifying enzyme.

The activity of pyrazinamide not only depends on the presence of a pyrazinamidase, but also the organism needs to be in an acidic environment (external pH = 5). This is likely because intracellular accumulation of pyrazinoic acid, but not pyrazinamide, is inversely related to the pH outside the bacterium (408). In addition, the relative resistance of *M. smegmatis* to pyrazinoic acid is at least partly the result of active efflux of this compound. Intriguingly, *M. tuberculosis* also has an efflux system for pyrazinoic acid, but this appears with be weak compared with *M. smegmatis* (408).

These findings led Zhang and Telenti (194) to propose a model of pyrazinamide/pyrazinoic acid dynamics in *M. tuberculosis* (Fig. 5.9B). Briefly, pyrazinamide enters the bacterium by passive diffusion and is converted to pyrazinoic acid by the *pnc*A pyrazinamidase (PZase). Independent of external pH, the internal pH of *M. tuberculosis* is maintained at approximately pH 7 (408), and thus pyrazinoic acid will be predominantly (more than 99.9%) in its dissociated form, $C_4H_3N_2$-COO^-(i.e., minus its H^+ ion or proton). Once formed, the pyrazinoic acid diffuses out of the cell (aided by a weak efflux system). If the extracellular and intracellular conditions are comparable (i.e., pH neutral), then the total pyrazinoic acid concentration (ionic and protonated) inside and outside the bacterium will be equivalent. However, if the extracellular environment is acidic, the protonated form of pyrazinoic acid ($C_4H_3N_2$-COOH) may represent 50% of the total extracellular pyrazinoic acid. Thus, there will be a large concentration gradient of protonated pyrazinoic acid between the outside and the inside of the bacterium (perhaps more than 1,000-fold), leading to a net intracellular diffusion of this form of pyrazinoic acid. The weak pyrazinoic acid efflux pump of *M. tuberculosis* would have little impact on this influx, and thus the internal concentration of total pyrazinoic acid will be considerably higher than outside. This model provides a rational explanation for why the activity of pyrazinamide and pyrazinoic acid depends on an acidic environment.

The inhibitory mechanism of pyrazinoic acid is not known, and attempts to isolate pyrazinoic acid-resistant mutants of *M. tuberculosis* have largely failed. It is likely that this compound affects multiple systems. Recently, Zhang et al. (409) demonstrated that pyrazinoic acid disrupts the membrane potential or proton motif force of *M. tuberculosis*. This will have a profound effect on processes that depend on the proton motif force, such as some types of active transmembrane transport (409).

As stated previously, acquired resistance to pyrazinamide in *M. tuberculosis* is primarily the result of loss of PZase-activity, conferred by mutation in the *pnc*A gene or its promoter. The known resistance-conferring *pnc*A mutations are strewn throughout the gene, and unlike isoniazid-resistance associated *kat*G mutations, there does not seem to be a restricted number of principal genotypes. Interestingly, *M. bovis,* which is intrinsically resistant to pyrazinamide and is PZase-negative, has a characteristic polymorphism in the *pnc*A gene leading to a histidine-to-aspartic acid change at codon 57 (410).

Although there have been reports of pyrazinamide-resistant *M. tuberculosis* without *pnc*A mutations, pyrazinamide susceptibility testing is problematic and can lead to an inaccurate indication of resistance. Thus, it is unclear whether mutations in other genes are associated with the acquisition of pyrazinamide resistance. However, the relatively strong efflux of pyrazinoic acid in intrinsically resistant *M. smegmatis* (408) suggests that mutations that enhance efflux in *M. tuberculosis* may lead to increased resistance to pyrazinamide.

Quinolones

Although not routinely considered as first-line agents in the treatment of tuberculosis, the quinolones have emerged as important drugs in the treatment of drug-resistant disease and for patients intolerant of first-line agents. The quinolones that have been studied the most in terms of treating mycobacterioses are ciprofloxacin, ofloxacin, levofloxacin (the L-isomer of ofloxacin), and sparfloxacin (411). These quinolones are bactericidal for most bacteria and are moderately active against rapidly growing and slowly growing mycobacteria (176,412–414). The MICs of these quinolones against *M. tuberculosis* isolates range from 0.01 to 4 μg/mL, with sparfloxacin being the most active on a per weight basis (411). The respective MICs of these quinolones are at or below their maximum serum concentrations. Moreover, the quinolones show good tissue penetration (415), and can reach concentrations several times those in serum in lung tissue, especially alveolar macrophages. The elimination half-life is approximately 5 hours for ciprofloxacin, ofloxacin, and levofloxacin, and 16 to 30 hours for sparfloxacin. Thus, the activity *in vitro* and the pharmacokinetics suggest that these four quinolones should be useful in the treatment of *M. tuberculosis,* and there is clinical evidence in humans to support this conclusion (9,411,416,417). Currently, the recommendation is to use a quinolone as a second-line agent with at least two other agents to which the infecting isolate is susceptible (411).

The role of quinolones in the treatment of disease caused by nontuberculous mycobacteria is unclear, due to the broad range of susceptibilities expressed by clinical isolates. For example, most isolates of *M. fortuitum* are susceptible to ciprofloxacin, whereas there is a high degree of inherent resistance among isolates of *M. chelonae*. Only 30% of MAC isolates are susceptible to ciprofloxacin at 2 μg/mL, and the MIC 90% for MAC is 16 μg/mL (295).

New quinolones, such as moxifloxacin, gatifloxacin, and gemifloxacin, are under evaluation as antimycobacterial agents, with an encouraging level of activity *in vitro* and *in vivo* (191,418–423).

The main target of quinolones is bacterial DNA gyrase or topoisomerase II, which is the enzyme that relaxes and recoils DNA during transcription, replication, and recombination. The binding of a quinolone to the gyrase results in the inhibition of these functions but principally impairs DNA synthesis. The DNA gyrase is encoded by two genes, *gyrA* and *gyrB,* and acquired resistance to quinolones in mycobacteria primarily maps to the *gyrA* gene. Within this gene, mutations tend to cluster in the region of codon 80 (the so-called quinolone-resistance determining region or QRDR), leading to amino acid substitutions within the translated polypeptide chain (249,424–427). The QRDR region of the mycobacterial *gyrA* gene corresponds to the region associated with acquired quinolone resistance in other bacteria. However, there is some evidence that natural polymorphisms exist in this region (195), and these may be associated with low-level natural resistance in some mycobacteria (428). The resistance-conferring substitutions within the *gyrA* polypeptide chain are believed to cause a significant change in the binding of quinolones to the assembled DNA gyrase.

Although mutations in the QRDR of *gyr*A are the predominant basis of high-level acquired resistance in mycobacteria, mutations in the *gyr*B gene have been described in laboratory-selected, quinolone-resistant *M. tuberculosis* (429). Mutations in *gyr*B of *M. tuberculosis* with clinically acquired resistance are infrequent (430) and of unknown clinical significance. Indeed, rather than a role in acquired resistance, the QRDR of *gyr*B may be associated with intrinsic, low-level quinolone-resistance in mycobacteria (428).

Although the DNA gyrase appears to be the main target of quinolones, there is other evidence for an alternative site of action (431). In other bacteria, mutations that confer resistance to quinolones have been mapped to the topoisomerase IV gene (*par*C or *grl*A). However, mycobacteria do not appear to possess a homolog of this gene. Recently, there has been much interest in resistance to quinolones conferred by active efflux pumps, especially in *Pseudomonas* species (432). A quinolone efflux pump (LfrA) has been described for *M. smegmatis,* however, the action of this pathway confers only accounts for low-level resistance (433–435). Currently, there is no functional evidence supporting the role of a quinolone efflux system in resistance to this class of agents in *M. tuberculosis.*

Oxazolidinones

The oxazolidinones are a new class of antimicrobial agent that target the ribosome, causing an inhibition of protein synthesis. Several oxazolidinones show promising activity against slowly growing and rapidly growing mycobacteria, based on *in vitro* susceptibilities (163,175,186,191,193,436), and linezolid may act synergistically with rifampin against *M. tuberculosis* (437). Several oxazolidinones, including linezolid, were shown to significantly reduce bacterial loading in a murine model of tuberculosis (438). In addition, linezolid has been used successfully in treatment regimens for human mycobacterioses (131, 439).

Oxazolidinones bind to the 50S ribosomal subunit in the vicinity of the P-site and block the formation of the 70S ribosome initiation complex (440–445). This complex comprises the 50S and 30S subunits, fMet-tRNA, initiating factors (IF1, IF2, and IF2), and the mRNA. Since the initiation complex is a transitory structure, the oxazolidinones are primarily bacteriostatic.

This mode of action is distinct from that of other protein synthesis inhibitors, such as macrolides and aminoglycosides, and thus resistance to these agents should be independent. In enterococci and straphylococci, acquired resistance to oxazolidinones is conferred by mutations in the 23S rRNA gene at several possible guanidine residues between positions 2447 and 2610 (*E. coli* numbering) for mutants selected *in vitro*, and at position 2576 for mutants selected *in vivo* (443). Selection of mutants *in vitro* is difficult probably because the genomes of these organisms have multiple rRNA gene operons, and more than one operon must be mutated for significant resistance to be expressed. A recent study by Sander et al. (446) showed that oxazolidinone-resistant mycobacteria could be selected *in vitro* using an *M. smegmatis* variant with only a single functional rRNA gene operon. Two classes of mutant were found, with class I mutants having a G- to T-base-substitution at the 2447 residue, and class II having a wild-type rRNA gene operon and susceptible ribosomes. The basis of the class II mutants is currently unknown. The class I mutants are consistent with the findings for enterococci and staphylococci.

Clearly, the oxazolidinones represent a promising class of agents with clinically useful activity against mycobacteria.

p-Aminosalicylic Acid

PAS is active against *M. tuberculosis;* however, nontuberculous mycobacteria and most other microorganisms are considered resistant to this agent. The mechanism of action of PAS in mycobacteria is not entirely clear; however, two targets have been considered: inhibition of folic acid synthesis and inhibition of salicylic acid metabolism (206). PAS inhibits the synthesis of folic acid, and *p*-aminobenzoic acid reverses the effect of PAS in *M. tuberculosis.* Thus, the mechanism of action of this agent appears to be analogous to that of the sulfonamides and other antifolates (447). Winder (206) argued, however, that these and other observations indicating that PAS was an antifolate agent could be attributed to effects other than those on folic acid metabolism.

Ratledge and Brown (448) suggested that the mechanism of action of PAS may be to inhibit mycobactin synthesis. Mycobactins are lipid-soluble iron chelators (449) that contain a salicylate or a 6-methylsalicylate moiety; therefore, PAS may act as a salicylate analog and block mycobactin biosynthesis. However, salicylic acid itself may be involved in iron transport, and with mycobactin-dependent strains of *M. smegmatis* mycobactin does not overcome the effect of PAS (450,451). Brown and Ratledge (451) proposed that PAS interfered with salicylic acid metabolism, perhaps by inhibiting the transfer of iron from mycobactin to the sites of heme synthesis. Winder (206) concluded that the evidence that PAS acts as an antifolate in mycobacteria is inconclusive and, at the same time, there is good evidence that PAS interferes with salicylic acid metabolism, but probably not by inhibiting mycobactin synthesis.

The mechanism of PAS resistance is unclear; however, there is evidence that PAS is acetylated by mycobacteria to yield acetyl-PAS, a compound that is not biologically active (452).

Cycloserine

D-Cycloserine (4-amino-3-isooxazolidinone) is a rigid cyclic analog of D-alanine and is active against all mycobacteria as well as a number of other microorganisms. D-Cycloserine irreversibly inhibits pyridoxal phosphate-dependent enzymes competitively inhibits the enzymes D-alanylalanine synthetase, D-alanine racemase, and D-alanine permease (453). These latter enzymes catalyze the conversion of L-alanine to D-alanine and of D-alanine to D-alanyl-D-alanine. The dipeptide is essential for the biosynthesis of mycobacterial cell walls, and inhibition of its synthesis leads to lysis and cell death. The effect of D-cycloserine is antagonized by exogenous D-alanine (454,455).

Resistance to D-cycloserine is conferred by overexpression of the D-alanine racemase (encoded by the *alr*A gene) (456), whereas, organisms with a defective gene are hypersusceptible to this agent (457). Low-level resistance to D-cycloserine may be conferred by mutations in the D-alanine permease, which is involved in the transport of both D-alanine and D-cycloserine. However, the D-alanine racemase is most likely the primary target for D-cycloserine.

Cross-resistance between D-cycloserine and vancomycin appears to be conferred by alterations in the mycobacterial homolog of the penicillin-binding protein 4 (PBP4) (458), although it is not known if these agents directly inhibit this protein. Other effects of D-cycloserine on mycobacterial cell wall synthesis include the inhibition of D-peptidoglycolipid synthesis in *M. tuberculosis* (459).

Mammalian enzymes such as serine hydroxymethyltransferase are inhibited by D-cycloserine, and these are most likely the targets for the antineoplastic activity of this compound. D-Cycloserine has a high toxic-to-therapeutic ratio for the treatment of mycobacterial disease; therefore, the drug is considered a choice of last resort (460,461).

Ethionamide

Isonicotinyl thioamide and a variety of derivatives, including ethionamide (2-ethylpyridine-4-carbonic acid thioamide), are potent inhibitors of *M. tuberculosis* and other mycobacteria. Ethionamide inhibits the synthesis of mycolic acids and stimulates oxidation-reduction reactions. Treated cells lose acid fastness, and overall the mechanism of action of ethionamide appears to be similar to that of isoniazid (233). Mutations within the *inhA* gene that confer low-level resistance to isoniazid also confer resistance to ethionamide (210). Furthermore, overexpression of the wild-type *inh*A protein in *M. tuberculosis* increased the MIC of ethionamide. This suggests that, like isoniazid, a target for ethionamide is the *inh*A protein. However, unlike isoniazid, mutations within the *katG* gene do not confer resistance to ethionamide, which explains why most *M. tuberculosis* isolates with clinically acquired isoniazid resistance are still susceptible to ethionamide. Thus, by inference, ethionamide is not activated by KatG.

Recently, two groups independently identified the gene (*Rv3854c*) that activates ethionamide in *M. tuberculoisis* strain H37Rv (462,463). The activation pathway of ethionamide is inducible, with *Rv3854c* gene expression being regulated by an adjacent gene, *Rv3855*. The proposed activation pathway (Fig. 5.10) may generate a radical similar to the isonicotinic acyl radical derivative of isoniazid. However, it is unclear whether ethionamide-NAD(H) aducts are formed.

ASSAYS FOR ACTIVITY IN BIOLOGIC FLUIDS

There are a variety of reasons to measure the concentrations of antimycobacterial drugs in biologic fluids, especially serum, including (a) to prevent toxicity reactions that occur with drugs with such as aminoglycosides and cycloserine; (b) to determine whether the concentration in fluids or tissue is adequate for effective therapy; (c) to monitor patient compliance; (d) to monitor the metabolism of certain drugs, such as in the assessment of isoniazid acetylator phenotype; and (e) for research purposes. Patients with malabsorption syndromes, renal impairment (the excretion of isoniazid, rifampin, and PAS is relatively unaffected by renal impairment), or liver function abnormalities, patients who are not responsive to therapy for disease caused by susceptible isolates, or patients with particularly serious disease may require monitoring to assess the toxicity or efficacy of a treatment regimen. The emergence of MDR tuberculosis and the realization that patients with AIDS can develop impaired intestinal absorption as their disease progresses clearly fit these criteria (465,466). Therapeutic drug monitoring is routinely performed in all cases of MDR tuberculosis at the National Jewish Center for Immunology and Respiratory Medicine because of the need to ensure that maximal concentration levels exceed the MICs of the infecting MDR *M. tuberculosis* (467). Other than the aforementioned situations, however, there is only an infrequent need to measure the levels of antimycobacterial agents in the serum of patients with tuberculosis or other mycobacterial infections, and assays such as those described in this section are best performed in reference laboratories that specialize in these procedures. Also, it is important to point out that the procedures described here are based on published information and that other proprietary procedures used in reference laboratories are likely to differ from these procedures or to accommodate the need to assay antimycobacterial drugs in serum and fluids containing multiple other drugs.

In the past, the accurate measurement of antimycobacterial drugs in biologic fluids and tissues was confounded by (a) the use of time-consuming methods with inadequate sensitivity; (b) reliance on bioassays that failed to distinguish metabolites or required the withholding of components of a multiple-drug treatment regimen; (c) metabolism of the drug; and (d) interaction of the drug, especially protein binding. Many of these problems have been overcome with the development of new

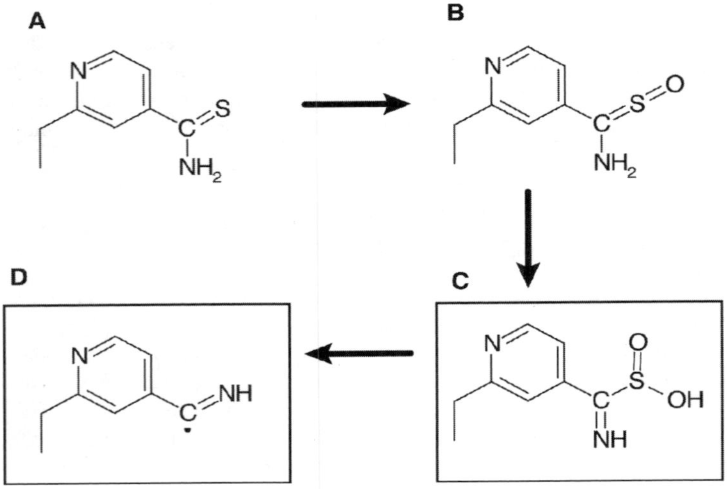

FIGURE 5.10 ● Proposed activation pathway of ethionamide. Ethionamide **(A)** is converted to ethionamide-S-oxide **(B)** by the (FAD)–dependent EtaA enzyme (encoded by gene Rv3854bc). This enzyme then converts the oxide further, possibly to sulfinic acid **(C)** and radical **(D)** species. These later forms are unstable, and probably represent the active derivative of ethionamide. [Pathway adapted from DeBarber et al. (463) and Vannelli et al. (464)].

chromatographic and nonchromatographic methods for the identification and quantitation of virtually all of the primary and secondary antimycobacterial agents. Holdiness (468) has reviewed the analytic methods, and Holdiness (469) and Peloquin (467) have reviewed the pharmacology of antimycobacterial agents.

There are three analytical methods for measuring the concentrations of antituberculous agents in biologic material: (a) bioassays, (b) spectrophotometric and fluorometric methods, and (c) chromatographic methods. Serum should be collected at the time of peak serum concentration; however, one should be aware that a variety of factors may influence the absorption and bioavailability of these drugs, including surgical procedures, food, and pharmacologic formulations of the drug. In addition to the problems created by the simultaneous administration of several drugs, the metabolism of antimycobacterial agents can vary considerably from patient to patient. Most of the metabolites of antimycobacterial drugs lack antimicrobial activity; however, there are important exceptions, i.e., desacetylrifampin, the acetylated and glycylated forms of PAS, and the sulfoxide metabolites of ethionamide are all active against *M. tuberculosis*.

Sample Preparation

Improper specimen preparation can result in the loss of drug activity as a consequence of protein binding or conversion of drugs to inactive or labile derivatives. Deproteination of serum samples is necessary to ensure the stability of isoniazid even at −20°C because in the presence of protein, isoniazid activity is rapidly lost as a consequence of irreversible protein binding. Furthermore, protein frequently interferes with fluorometric methods for the detection and quantitation of isoniazid. Depending on the analytic method, protein can be removed by treatment with 5% to 10% trichloroacetic acid or ammonium sulfate. The protein should be extracted on the day the sample is obtained, and the sample can then be stored at 4°C for up to 2 weeks or frozen at −20°C (or lower) for indefinite periods. Samples collected for rifampin analysis should be treated with ascorbic acid and then stored at −20°C for up to 3 months. Ethambutol, pyrazinamide, pyrazinoic acid, ethionamide, and prothionamide are unlikely to be affected by either protein binding or oxidation, and samples can be stored frozen for indefinite periods. Samples collected for PAS determination should first be chromatographed on a weak cation-exchange column to remove the breakdown product *m*-aminophenol, which can interfere with certain assays. Thiacetazone is acid-labile but is stable at −20°C if extracted with ethyl acetate. Alternatively, thiacetazone can be completely hydrolyzed with 2 mol/L HCl to the stable hydrolysis product *p*-aminobenzaldehyde. There is little information about the stability of the other primary and secondary antituberculous drugs.

Assays

Bioassays and certain nonchromatographic assays for measuring the concentrations of isoniazid, ethionamide, ethambutol, and rifampin in biologic fluids and tissues have been described (44). Bioassays are both sensitive and inexpensive, but require experience, frequently take several days to complete, and are relatively imprecise. Furthermore, bioassays cannot distinguish between the various species of active and inactive metabolites. The remainder of this section contains descriptions of relatively new methods for detecting and quantifying antimycobacterial drugs and the clinically important metabolites of these drugs. The emphasis is on HPLC methods, which is the most common method for measuring therapeutic serum or plasma concentrations of probably most anti-infective agents. It is beyond the scope of this chapter to provide detailed information about these methods. Indeed, the accurate and precise measurement of antimycobacterial agents is a subspecialty within the field of clinical mycobacteriology and an area of expertise for a relatively small number of investigators. Simple and convenient qualitative methods for detecting isoniazid, PAS, pyrazinamide, cycloserine, ethionamide, and ethambutol in urine are described at the end of this section. These latter methods are primarily designed for monitoring patient adherence to treatment.

Isoniazid

Isoniazid or isonicotinic acid hydrazide is metabolized to a variety of products, as shown in Fig. 5.11. Acetylation of isoniazid is the primary and clinically most significant pathway of metabolism. The major products of isoniazid metabolism are *N*-acetylisoniazid, pyruvic hydrazone, a-ketoglutaric hydrazone, isonicotinic acid, isonicotinoyl glycine, monoacetylhydrazine, and 1,2-diacetylhydrazine. The enzyme *N*-acetyltransferase (EC 2.3.1.5) catalyzes the acetylation reaction and is located primarily in the liver and intestine. The activity of *N*-acetyltransferase can vary significantly from person to person, with a bimodal distribution within populations, and genetic analysis showed that the distribution of enzyme activity type is autosomal and dominant (470).

None of these metabolites of isoniazid possesses antimicrobial activity; however, monoacetylhydrazine is considered hepatotoxic when hydroxylated by the cytochrome P-450 mixed-function oxidase. Nevertheless, individuals with a rapid isoniazid acetylator phenotype do not appear to be at greater risk for hepatotoxicity (471,472). The level of *N*-acetyltransferase in a patient

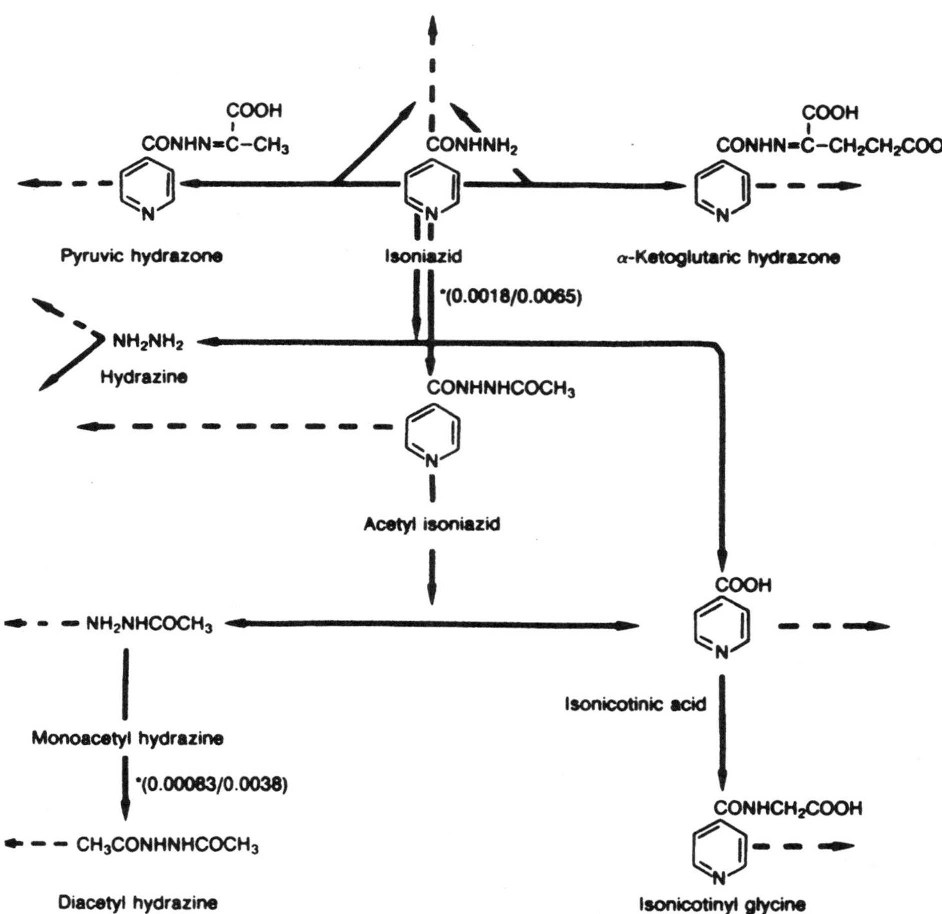

FIGURE 5.11 ● Pathways for the metabolism of isoniazid in humans. First-order rate constants (minutes^{-1}) form the polymorphic acetylation steps (*) are shown for one slow and one rapid acetylator. *Dashed lines* indicate renal elimination (469).

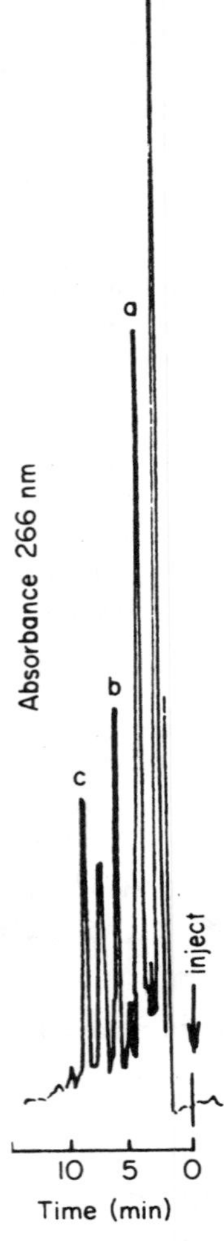

FIGURE 5.12 ● Liquid chromatogram of a patient's urine sample (slow acetylator) in which the isoniazid concentration is 36.5 μg/mL and the *N*-acetylisoniazid concentration is 63.5 μg/mL (inactivation index of 1.7). *Peak a, N*-acetylisoniazid; *peak b*, internal standard; *peak c*, isoniazid (473).

(acetylator status) does influence the concentration of monoacetylhydrazine and diacetylhydrazine in the urine, and this is the basis for assays to determine the acetylator status (phenotype) of patients (473–475).

Several HPLC assays for measuring the concentrations of isoniazid and acetylisoniazid in fluids and tissues have been described (473,476–480). The specific assay that is used to measure isoniazid and/or acetylisoniazid may depend on the purpose of the assay. The method of El-Sayed and Islam (473) was used to specifically measure the concentrations of isoniazid and acetylisoniazid in urine for acetylator phenotyping (Fig. 5.12), and the assays described by Moulin et al. (481) used small volumes of serum and may be particularly useful for testing pediatric patients. In a typical assay, Saxena et al. (482) measured isoniazid and acetylisoniazid in serum and urine using a Bondapak C_{18} column and a mobile phase of methanol/water (3:2), with dioctyl sodium sulfosuccinate as the ion-pairing reagent. The lower limit of detection for this assay was 200 ng for isoniazid and 50 ng for acetylisoniazid, using 1-benzoyl-2-isonicotinoylhydrazine as the internal standard. Moulin et al. (481) used a μBondapak C_{18} column and nicotinic amide as the internal standard (Fig. 5.13). The mobile phase was 5% methanol/95% 0.1 mol/L KH_2PO_4, pH 6.9, degassed and run in an isocratic mode at 2 mL per minute. The serum sample was prepared by adding 2.5 μg of internal standard to 500 μL of serum in a 10-mL, screw-capped, glass tube. The mixture was treated in gradual increments with 150 μL of 0.1 mol/L NaOH and 0.5 g of $(NH_2)\ _2SO_4$, with gentle shaking. The mixture was shaken with 3 mL of chloroform and centrifuged (520 × *g* for 5 minutes) to separate the aqueous and organic phases. An aliquot of the organic phase (2.5 to 3 mL) was transferred to a tapered glass tube and mixed with 200 μL of 0.05 mol/L H_2SO_4. The mixture was shaken and centrifuged, and 30 μL was loaded onto the HPLC column. The extraction and chromatography steps were completed within 30 minutes, and

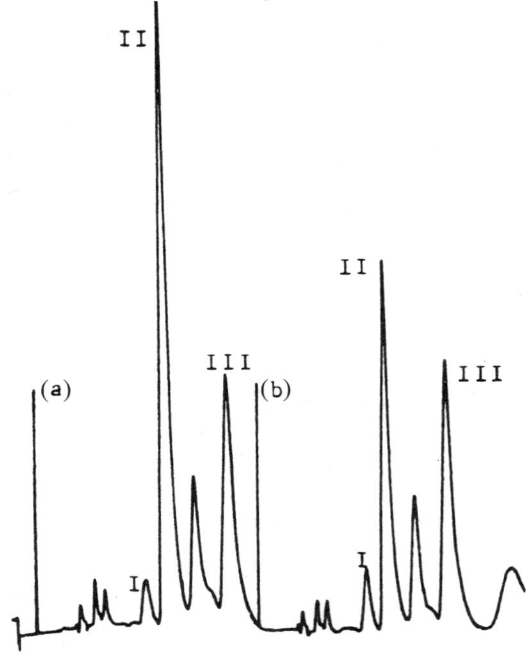

FIGURE 5.13 ● Elution profiles of acetylisoniazid (*peak I*) and isoniazid (*peak II*) from a patient's serum at 2 hours (*peak a*) and 4.5 hours (*peak b*) after an oral dose of isoniazid using nicotinamide (*peak III*) as the internal standard (481).

the lower limits of detection for isoniazid and acetylisoniazid were 300 and 100 ng/μL, respectively. Holdiness (477), using essentially the same procedure as Moulin et al. (481), found it necessary to use dioctyl sodium sulfosuccinate (an ion-pairing reagent) to achieve good separation of profile components. Rifampin, pyrazinamide, streptomycin, and ethambutol have not been reported to interfere with these HPLC assays.

Rifampin

Rifampin or 3-(4-methyl-1-piperazinyliminomethyl) rifamycin is a relatively unstable compound in water, and at pH 2 to 3 rifampin is readily hydrolyzed to 3-formylrifamycin SV and 1-amino-4-methylpiperazine. At alkaline pH, in the presence of atmospheric oxygen, rifampin is slowly oxidized to rifampin-quinone. However, aqueous solutions of rifampin can be stabilized by the addition of sodium ascorbate (200 μg/mL), and solutions of rifampin in dimethylsulfoxide (10 mg/mL) are stable for several weeks. Rifampin is metabolized in the liver to yield 25-*O*-desacetylrifampin, which is readily excreted by the biliary system. In urine, rifampin is hydrolyzed to yield 3-formylrifampin (483). The pathways of rifampin metabolism are shown in Fig. 5.14. Desacetylrifampin is the major metabolite of rifampin; the other metabolites are infrequently detected in fluids or tissues. Cocchiara et al. (484) showed that the major urinary metabolite of rifabutin, a spiropiperidylrifamycin with broad-spectrum antimycobacterial activity (including activity against rifampin-resistant *M. tuberculosis*), was 25-*O*-desacetylrifabutin; the minor metabolites of rifabutin were oxidized and oxidized/deacetylated forms of 25-*O*-desacetylrifabutin.

Ratti et al. (485) described a reverse-phase HPLC method for the quantitation of rifampin and 25-*O*-desacetylrifampin in serum. In this method, 0.5 mL of heparinized serum was added to a tube with butyl-*p*-hydroxybenzoate in acetonitrile/2-propanol (1:1) as an internal standard. The mixture was diluted 1:10 with 1 mol/L KH_2PO_4 containing 1 mg/mL sodium ascorbate and adjusted to pH 4 with 1 N HCl. The sample was extracted into 15 mL of ethyl acetate and the phases were separated by centrifugation. The organic phase was concentrated by evaporation under a stream of nitrogen, resuspended in 3.5 mL of 90% aqueous acetonitrile, and then extracted with 3 mL of *n*-heptane. The *n*-heptane phase was discarded, the acetonitrile phase was concentrated by evaporation under a stream of nitrogen, and the residue was resuspended in 25 to 100 μL

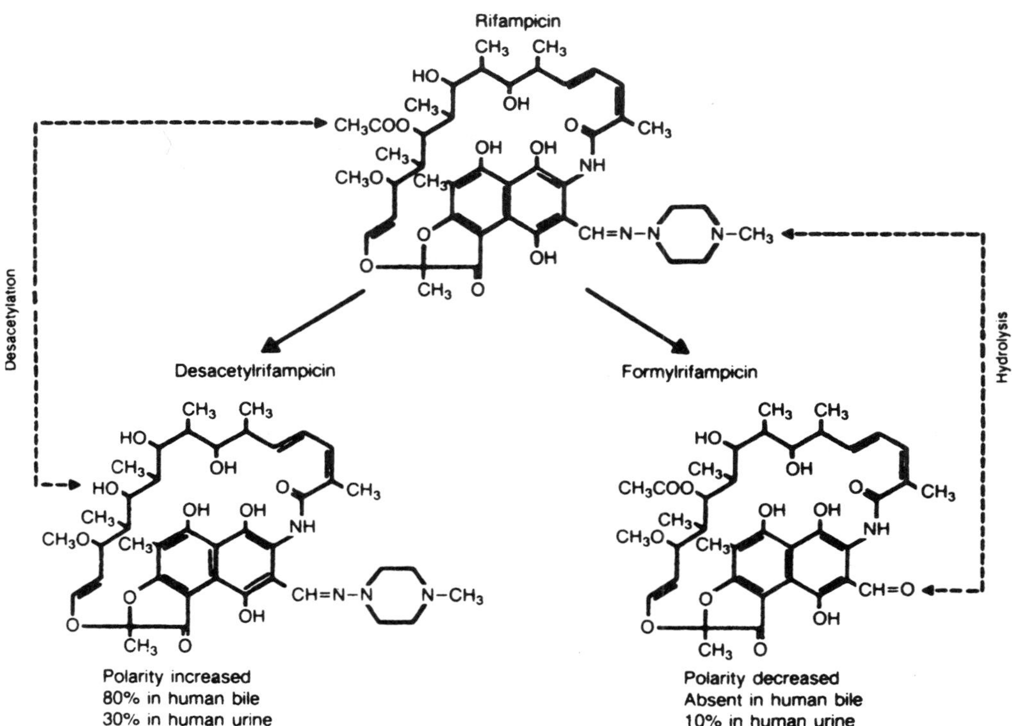

FIGURE 5.14 • Principal metabolic derivatives of rifampin in humans, polarity, and percentage recovery in bile and urine (469).

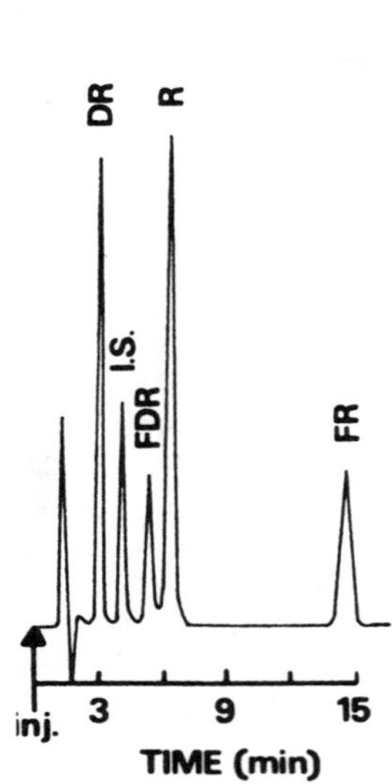

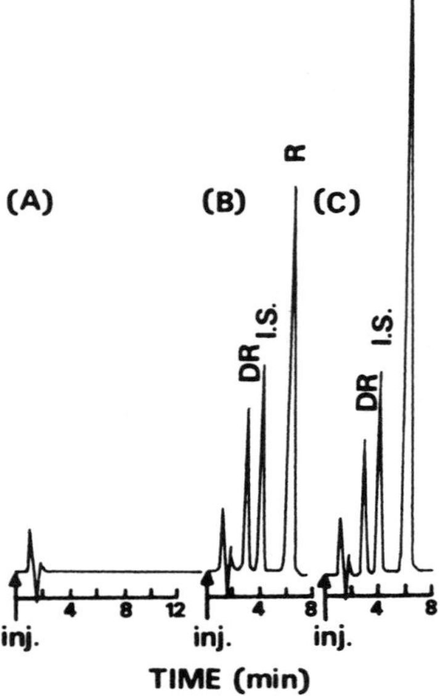

FIGURE 5.15 ● **Left chromatogram,** rifampicin (*R*), 25-desacetyl rifampicin (*DR*), 3-formyl-25-desacetylrifamycin SV (*FDR*), 3-formylrifamycin SV (*FR*), and papaverine as the internal standard (*I.S.*). **Right chromatogram: (A)** blank plasma extract; **(B)** rifampicin (*R*), 25-desacetylrifampicin (*DR*), and papaverine as the internal standard (*I.S.*), spiked to a blank plasma sample. The spiked concentrations of rifampicin and 25-desacetylrifampicin were 3 and 1 μg/mL in plasma, respectively. **(C)** Chromatogram of plasma extracted from a tuberculosis patient treated with 450 mg of rifampicin, 300 mg of isoniazid, and 1.0 g of ethambutol. The concentrations of rifampicin and 25-desacetylrifampicin were estimated at 5.46 and 0.85 μg/mL, respectively (486).

of acetonitrile/2-propanol (1:1) and loaded onto the HPLC column. The column was a 10-m RP-8 column (Brownlee Laboratories, Santa Clara, CA), using an isocratic mobile phase of 0.1 mol/L KH_2PO_4, pH 3.5, with 0.2 mol/L H_3PO_4 and acetonitrile. The conditions varied slightly depending on the type of instrument, and compounds were detected by ultraviolet absorbance at 254 nm. The method allowed for the separation of rifampin, 25-*O*-desacetylrifampin, 3-formylrifamycin SV, 3-formyl-25-*O*-desacetylrifamycin, and *N*-desmethylrifampicin with a sensitivity of 0.2 μg/mL.

Ishii and Ogata (486) described an improved HPLC method that used a single extraction step and detection at 340 nm (Fig. 5.15). In this method, 3 mL of heparinized blood was drawn directly into a tube containing 10 mg of ascorbic acid. The plasma was separated and stored at −20°C in the dark. To an aliquot of 0.5 mL of plasma was added 2 mL of 0.5 mol/L phosphate buffer, pH 7.2, containing 100 L of papaverine HCl (20 μg/mL) as an internal standard. This mixture was extracted with chloroform, the phases were separated by centrifugation, and the lower organic phase was drawn off and concentrated under a stream of nitrogen at 50°C. The residue was dissolved in 300 μL of acetonitrile/2-propanol (1:1) and loaded onto the column. The HPLC column was a 7-μm Nucleosil C_{18} column and the mobile phase was acetonitrile/0.1 mol/L potassium phosphate buffer, pH 4.0 (38:62). This method readily separated rifampin, 25-*O*-desacetylrifampin, 3-formyl-25-descetylrifamycin SV, 3-formylrifamycin, and the internal standard over a period of less than 10 minutes. There was excellent baseline separation of all peaks, and detection at 340 nm obviated the influence of many plasma-derived interfering substances. The sensitivity of the assay was 0.1 μg/mL for rifampin and 0.06 μg/mL for 25-*O*-desacetylrifampin, with good accuracy and precision. Isoniazid and ethambutol did not interfere with the detection of rifampin or the rifampin metabolites using this method (486).

Ethambutol

Ethambutol or dextro-2,2′-(ethylenediimino)-di(1-butanol) is presumably metabolized in the liver to a dicarboxylic acid and a dialdehyde (487); however, the drug is generally considered not to be extensively metabolized in humans. Neither of the known metabolites is active against *M. tuberculosis*, nor are the metabolites noted to be toxic to humans. Spectrophotometric assays have been described for the quantitation of ethambutol in cerebrospinal fluid (488) and urine (489). Samples were extracted with chloroform and reacted with bromthymol blue, with a lower limit of detection of 500 ng/mL. A variety of gas chromatographic and gas chromatographic-mass spectrometric methods have been described for measuring the concentration of ethambutol in biologic fluids (490–493).

Pyrazinamide

Pyrazinamide, which is the amide of pyrazinoic acid, is rapidly absorbed from the gastrointestinal tract and

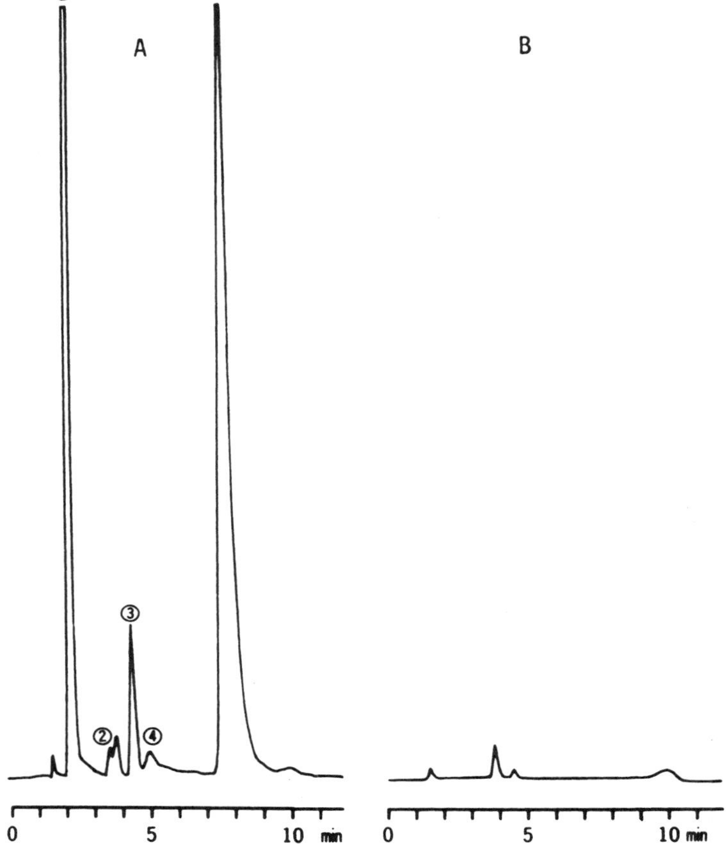

FIGURE 5.16 • **A:** Chromatogram of plasma extract containing pyrazinamide and its metabolites 4 hours after administration. **B:** Chromatogram of blank plasma. *Peak* 1, 2,3-pyrazinedicarboxamide; *peak 2,* 5-hydroxypyrazinoic acid (0.36 μg/mL); *peak* 3, 5-hydroxypyrazinamide (5.74 μg/mL); *peak 4,* pyrazinoic (6.14 μg/mL); *peak 5,* pyrazinamide (73.91 μg/mL) (495).

metabolized to 5-hydroxypyrazinamide, which probably undergoes microsomal deamination to 5-hydroxypyrazinoic acid and pyrazinoic acid, which can be hydroxylated to 5-hydroxypyrazinoic acid. pyrazinamide alone has no activity against *M. tuberculosis;* however, pyrazinamide-susceptible strains of *M. tuberculosis* readily deaminate pyrazinamide to the active metabolite pyrazinoic acid. It can be of value to monitor the concentrations of both pyrazinamide and pyrazinoic acid to prevent side effects, especially hyperuricemia. Yamamoto et al. (494, 495) described an HPLC method for the rapid determination of pyrazinamide and the various metabolic products, to levels as low as 3 ng (5-hydroxypyrazinoic acid and 5-hydroxypyrazinamide) or 30 ng (pyrazinoic acid and pyrazinamide), in plasma and urine (Fig. 5.16). The method employed a 10-μm μBondapak C_{18} column (Waters Associates, Milford, MA), using a mobile phase of 0.02 mol/L KH_2PO_4, pH 2.56, and a fluorescence detector at 410/265 nm. Serum samples (0.5 mL) were treated with 2 mol/L perchloric acid and centrifuged, and an aliquot of the supernatant was neutralized with NaOH and loaded onto the column. Urine was stored at −20°C, thawed, and centrifuged, and a 1:10 dilution of the supernatant was loaded onto the column without further treatment. The internal standard was 2,3-pyrazinedicarboxamide and the chromatogram was developed over 10 minutes.

Woo et al. (496) described another HPLC method for the simultaneous detection of pyrazinamide and rifampin in the serum of patients with tuberculous meningitis. Samples were treated with ascorbic acid and extracted into dichloromethane/diethyl ether (2:3). The treated samples were concentrated and loaded onto a reverse-phase, 5-μm, C_8 analytical column, using a mobile phase of 6% to 48% acetonitrile in 10 mmol/liter KH_2PO_4, pH 3.5, and compounds were detected at 215 nm. Donald and Seifart (497) described an HPLC method for the determination of pyrazinamide in cerebrospinal fluid from patients receiving three additional antimycobacterial drugs (isoniazid, rifampin, and ethionamide) and phenobarbitone. This method used a Whatman Partisil 5-C_8 column, with a gradient of phosphate buffer, acetonitrile, and isopropanol and ultraviolet detection at 280/254 nm. Cerebrospinal fluid was loaded directly onto the column, and the chromatogram was developed over a period of 20 minutes, using prazepam as the internal standard.

Ethionamide

Ethionamide (2-ethylthiosonicotinamide) and the propyl analog of ethionamide, prothionamide, are readily converted to their sulfoxide metabolites. Both the analogs and the sulfoxide metabolites are active against *M. tuberculosis;* however, the 2-ethyl- and 2-propyl-nicotinamide derivatives of the sulfoxides, as well as the corresponding nicotinic acids (the end products of ethionamide and prothionamide metabolism), are inactive against *M. tuberculosis.* Jenner et al. (498) described HPLC methods that distinguish between ethionamide, prothionamide, and the sulfoxide metabolites and showed that these methods are capable of measuring concentrations as low as 10 to 50 ng/mL. Aliquots of plasma or urine (3 mL) were added to tubes containing 0.1 mL of either 150 g or 600 ng of the appropriate internal standard. Prothionamide was used as the internal standard for the ethionamide assay and vice versa. The samples were extracted with 6 mL of diethyl ether and centrifuged to separate the organic and aqueous phases. The organic phase was extracted with 1 mL of 0.1 mol/L HCl, transferred to another tube, treated with 0.1 mL of ammonium phosphate, and then adjusted to pH 7 to 8 with 10% aqueous ammonia. The thionamides were extracted with 2 mL of ethyl acetate and concentrated by evaporation under a stream of nitrogen at 50°C. The residue was dissolved in 1 mL of dichloromethane and dried under nitrogen. Prior to chromatography, the residue was dissolved in 100 μL of the mobile phase. The chromatographic methods employed a Hypersil column of 5-m spherical silica (Shandon Southern Products Ltd., Runcorn, UK), with a mobile phase of chloroform/2-propanol/water (916:8:4) to separate the thionamides and sulfoxide metabolites (method 1) or a mobile phase of diethyl ether/methanol (96:4) to separate the thionamides alone (method 2). The internal standard was 2-methylthioisonicotinamide, and detection was by ultraviolet absorption at 340 or 280 nm, respectively. Separation of the four compounds in plasma can be achieved in approximately 8 minutes using method 1. Method 2 is suitable for distinguishing ethionamide and prothionamide in urine; interfering substances prevent determination of the two sulfoxides in urine.

p-Aminosalicylic Acid

PAS, an analog of *p*-aminobenzoic acid, is metabolized in urine to an acetylated derivative and in plasma to a glycylated derivative, and both of these metabolites are active against *M. tuberculosis.* With high doses of PAS, the glycylated metabolite predominates, probably because the glycylating enzyme competes with the acetylating enzyme for limiting amounts of coenzyme A. This may also explain why isoniazid levels are increased in the presence of PAS. Several HPLC assays for 5-aminosalicylic acid may be used to detect and quantitate PAS (499–501), because PAS is commonly used as an internal standard in these assays (126). A nonextractive fluorometric HPLC assay for PAS in plasma was described by Honigberg et al. (502). In the latter method, protein was removed prior to chromatography by mixing the sample with an equal volume of absolute methanol and centrifuging the flocculent precipitate. An aliquot (50 μL) of the supernatant was mixed with 100 μL of the mobile phase containing internal standard, and this mixture was directly loaded onto the column. The column was a LiChrosorb C_{18} column, with a mobile phase of absolute methanol/distilled water (20:80) containing 0.005 mol/L tetrabutylammonium hydroxide and 0.01 mol/L disodium acid phosphate, pH 5.5. Tetrabutylammonium was added as an ion-pairing reagent to increase the capacity factor for PAS and to improve resolution. The internal standard was anthranilic acid, and detection was by fluorometry using an excitation wavelength of 270 nm and an emission wavelength of 385 nm, based on the native fluorescence of PAS. Plasma volumes as small as 100 μL could be tested, and the lower limit of detection was 500 pg of PAS.

Conclusions

Holdiness (468) concluded that stability studies should always be performed when evaluating an assay for antimycobacterial agents in order to ensure the stability of the agent during storage and under the conditions of the assay. Furthermore, the extraction of samples appears to generally improve the sensitivity and precision of most assays, by either eliminating interfering substances contained in the biologic matrix, increasing the concentration of the agent, or separating the agent from other drugs or metabolites. Finally, the reliability of the assays, in particular the HPLC assays, depends on the expertise of the laboratory staff and on the type and quality of instruments. Thus, the same admonition applies to the analysis of antimycobacterial agents in biologic tissues and fluids as to the susceptibility testing of mycobacteria: experience is the most compelling factor in ensuring that assays are performed in an accurate and precise manner.

QUALITATIVE TESTS FOR ANTIMYCOBACTERIAL AGENTS IN URINE

Simple and reliable qualitative tests can be used to detect antimycobacterial agents in urine. These tests are primarily useful for monitoring patient compliance with treatment.

Isoniazid

Acetylisoniazid can be detected in urine by mixing four drops of urine with four drops of potassium cyanide (10% in water) and 10 drops of chloramine-T (10% in water), in a well of a white porcelain plate. Development of a red color within 1 minute indicates a positive test for acetylisoniazid; a pink color indicates traces of acetylisoniazid.

Ethambutol

One milliliter of urine and 1.0 mL of bromthymol blue are pipetted into a glass-stoppered test tube. If the initial green color of the mixture turns blue, 0.1 N HCl should be added until the green color is restored. If the urine/bromthymol green color turns yellow, 0.1 N NaOH should be added until the initial green color is restored. Then, 4.0 mL of benzene is added to the test tube, which is shaken vigorously. If ethambutol is present in the urine, a yellow color appears in the benzene (organic) phase. A negative control (ethambutol-free urine) and a positive control (urine containing 50 μg/mL ethambutol) should be tested simultaneously with the unknown sample.

Cycloserine and Pyrazinamide

Cycloserine and pyrazinamide react with alkaline sodium nitroprusside to produce either a blue (cycloserine) or orange (pyrazinamide) color. In a well of a white porcelain plate, three drops of urine are mixed with one drop of freshly prepared (used within 1 hour) alkaline sodium nitroprusside solution (equal volumes of 2% aqueous sodium nitroprusside and 2 N sodium hydroxide). If pyrazinamide is present, the yellow color of the reagent changes to orange in 2 to 3 minutes. After 3 to 5 minutes, two drops of 1 N HCl are added to the same well. The presence of cycloserine is indicated by the development of an intense blue color.

p-Aminosalicylic Acid

Phenistix test strips (Phenistix strip test; Miles Inc., Diagnostics Division, Elkhart, IN) is a convenient method for detecting PAS in urine. The presence of PAS is indicated by the development of a beige to reddish-brown color; however, salicylates and phenothiazine derivatives give similar reactions.

Ethionamide

Three grams of sodium citrate (crystals) are dissolved in 8 mL of the urine to be tested. The urine/citrate is extracted with 10 mL of chloroform, and the organic and aqueous phases are separated by low-speed centrifugation for 10 minutes. The chloroform layer is removed and filtered through Whatman no. 52 filter paper. Then, 0.8 mL of 0.1 N HCl is added to the filtrate and vigorously shaken in a 15- × 125-mm, screw-capped test tube. The aqueous phase separates without centrifugation. Ten drops of the clear aqueous supernatant are placed into a well of a white porcelain plate. The presence of ethionamide is indicated by the development of a distinctive yellow color.

ADDENDUM

Recently, a new compound (R207910) was described with potent anti-tuberculosis activity both *in vitro* and *in vivo* (Andries et al 2004, A Diarylquinoline Drug Active on the ATP Synthase of *Mycobacterium tuberculosis*, www.sciencemag.org/cgi/content/abstract/1106753v1). R207910 is a diarylquinoline, with some structural similarity with other quinolines with antimycobacterial activity (e.g., mefloquin). However, quinolines, such as mefloquin, have a 4′ linkage to the side groups, whereas, R207910 has a 3′ linkage, which may be important to its greater activity against *M. tuberculosis*.

REFERENCES

1. World Health Organization. *WHO report 2002, global tuberculosis control*. Geneva: World Health Organization, 2002.
2. Cole ST, Brosch R, Parkhill J, et al. Deciphering the biology of *Mycobacterium tuberculosis* from the complete genome sequence. *Nature* 1998;393:537–544.
3. Brosch R, Pym AS, Gordon SV, Cole ST. The evolution of mycobacterial pathogenicity: clues from comparative genomics. *Trends Microbiol* 2001;9:452–458.
4. Imaeda T. Deoxyribonucleic acid relatedness among selected strains of *Mycobacterium tuberculosis, Mycobacterium bovis BCG, Mycobacterium microti*, and *Mycobacterium africanum*. *Int J Syst Bacteriol* 1985;35:147–150.
5. van Soolingen D, Hoogenboezem T, de Haas PE, et al. A novel pathogenic taxon of the *Mycobacterium tuberculosis* complex, Canetti: characterization of an exceptional isolate from Africa. *Int J Syst Bacteriol* 1997;47:1236–1245.
6. Centers for Disease Control and Prevention ATS, Infectious Diseases Society of America. Treatment of tuberculosis. *MMWR Morb Mortal Wkly Rep* 2003;52:1–77.
7. Ellner JJ. Multidrug-resistant tuberculosis. *Adv Intern Med* 1995;40:155–196.
8. Bradford WZ, Daley CL. Multiple drug-resistant tuberculosis. *Infect Dis Clin North Am* 1998;12:157–172.
9. Iseman MD. Treatment of multidrug-resistant tuberculosis. *N Engl J Med* 1993;329:784–791.
10. Johnson MP, Chaisson RE. Tuberculosis and HIV disease. *AIDS Clin Rev* 1993–94:73–93.
11. Telenti A, Imboden P, Marchesi F, et al. Detection of rifampicin-resistance mutations in *Mycobacterium tuberculosis*. *Lancet* 1993;341:647–650.
12. Mikhailovich V, Lapa S, Gryadunov D, et al. Identification of rifampin-resistant *Mycobacterium tuberculosis* strains by hybridization, PCR, and ligase detection reaction on oligonucleotide microchips. *J Clin Microbiol* 2001;39:2531–2540.
13. Abate G, Aseffa A, Selassie A, et al. Direct colorimetric assay for rapid detection of rifampin-resistant *Mycobacterium tuberculosis*. *J Clin Microbiol* 2004;42:871–873.
14. Williams DL, Waguespack C, Eisenach K, et al. Characterization of rifampin-resistance in pathogenic mycobacteria. *Antimicrob Agents Chemother* 1994;38:2380–2386.
15. Salfinger M, Morris AJ. The role of the microbiology laboratory in diagnosing mycobacterial diseases. *Am J Clin Pathol* 1994;101:S6–S13.

16. Salfinger M, Pfyffer GE. The new diagnostic mycobacteriology laboratory. *Eur J Clin Microbiol Infect Dis* 1994;13:961–979.
17. David HL. Probability distribution of drug-resistant mutants in unselected populations of *Mycobacterium tuberculosis*. *Appl Microbiol* 1970;20:810–814.
18. Cole ST. *Mycobacterium tuberculosis*: drug-resistance mechanisms. *Trends Microbiol* 1994;2:411–415.
19. Heym B, Honore N, Truffot-Pernot C, et al. The implications of multidrug resistance for the future of short course chemotherapy of tuberculosis: a molecular study. *Lancet* 1994;344:293–298.
20. Norris S, Nightingale CH, Mandell GLL. Tables of antimicrobial agent pharmacology. In: Mandell GL, Douglas RG Jr, Bennett JE, eds. *Principles and practices of infectious diseases,* 2nd ed. New York: Churchill Livingstone, 1990.
21. Mitchison DA. The Garrod lecture. Understanding the chemotherapy of tuberculosis—current problems. *J Antimicrob Chemother* 1992;29:477–493.
21a. Wayne LG, Sramek HA. Metronidazole is bactericidal to dorman cells of *Mycobacterium tuberculosis*. *Antimicrob Agents Chemother* 1994;38:2054–2058.
22. Stover CK, Warrener P, VanDevanter DR, et al. A small-molecule nitroimidazopyran drug candidate for the treatment of tuberculosis. *Nature* 2000;405:962–966.
23. Brooks JV, Furney SK, Orme IM. Metronidazole therapy in mice infected with tuberculosis. *Antimicrob Agents Chemother* 1999;43:1285–1288.
24. Dhillon J, Allen BW, Hu YM, et al. Metronidazole has no antibacterial effect in Cornell model murine tuberculosis. *Int J Tuberc Lung Dis* 1998;2:736–742
25. Inderlied CB. Mycobacteria. In: Cohen J, Powderty W, eds. *Infectious diseases*. Vol II. London: Mosby, 2004:2285–2308.
26. Picken RN, Plotch SJ, Wang Z, et al. DNA probes for Mycobacteria. I. Isolation of DNA probes for the identification of *Mycobacterium tuberculosis* complex and for mycobacteria other than tuberculosis (MOTT). *Mol Cell Probes* 1988;2:111–124.
27. Sherman I, Harrington N, Rothrock A, George H. Use of a cutoff range in identifying mycobacteria by the Gen-Probe Rapid Diagnostic System. *J Clin Microbiol* 1989;27:241–244.
28. Wong DA, Yip PC, Tse DL, et al. Routine use of a simple low-cost genotypic assay for the identification of mycobacteria in a high throughput laboratory. *Diag Microbiol Infect Dis* 2003;47:421–426.
29. Tortoli E, Nanetti A, Piersimoni C, et al. Performance assessment of new multiplex probe assay for identification of mycobacteria. *J Clin Microbiol* 2001;39:1079–1084.
30. Wong DA, Yip PC, Cheung DT, Kam KM. Simple and rational approach to the identification of *Mycobacterium tuberculosis, Mycobacterium avium* complex species, and other commonly isolated mycobacteria. *J Clin Microbiol* 2001;39:3768–3771.
31. Suffys PN, da Silva Rocha A, de Oliveira M, et al. Rapid identification of mycobacteria to the species level using INNO-LiPA Mycobacteria, a reverse hybridization assay. *J Clin Microbiol* 2001;39:4477–4482.
32. Kellogg JA, Bankert DA, Withers GS, et al. Application of the Sherlock Mycobacteria Identification System using high-performance liquid chromatography in a clinical laboratory. *J Clin Microbiol* 2001;39:964–970.
33. Petrini B. 16S rDNA sequencing in the species identification of non-tuberculous mycobacteria. *Scand J Infect Dis* 2003;35:519–520.
34. Tanaka II, Anno IS, Leite SR, et al. Comparison of a multiplex-PCR assay with mycolic acids analysis and conventional methods for the identification of mycobacteria. *Microbiol Immunol* 2003;47:307–312.
35. Cook VJ, Turenne CY, Wolfe J, et al. Conventional methods versus 16S ribosomal DNA sequencing for identification of nontuberculous mycobacteria: cost analysis. *J Clin Microbiol* 2003;41:1010–1015.
36. Hall L, Doerr KA, Wohlfiel SL, et al. Evaluation of the MicroSeq system for identification of mycobacteria by 16S ribosomal DNA sequencing and its integration into a routine clinical mycobacteriology laboratory. *J Clin Microbiol* 2003;41:1447–1453.
37. Wayne LG. The "atypical" mycobacteria: recognition and disease association. *CRC Crit Rev Microbiol* 1985;12:185–222.
38. Centers for Disease Control and Prevention. Initial therapy for tuberculosis in the era of multidrug resistance. Recommendations of the Advisory Council for the Elimination of Tuberculosis [published erratum appears in *MMWR Morb Mortal Wkly Rep*1993;42(27):536]. *MMWR Morb Mortal Wkly Rep* 1993;42:1–8.
39. Kent PA, Kubica GP. *Public health mycobacteriology—a guide for the level III laboratory.* Atlanta: US Department of Health and Human Services, Public Health Service, Centers for Disease Control, 1985.
40. Hannan MM, Desmond EP, Morlock GP, et al. Pyrazinamidemonoresistant *Mycobacterium tuberculosis* in the United States. *J Clin Microbiol* 2001;39:647–650.
41. National Committee for Clinical Laboratory Standards. *Susceptibility testing of mycobacteria, Nocardiae, and other aerobic actinomycetes; approved standard.* NCCLS document M24-A. Wayne, PA: National Committee for Clinical Laboratory Standards, 2003.
42. Heifets LB. *Drug susceptibility in the chemotherapy of mycobacterial infections.* Boca Raton, FL: CRC Press, 1991.
43. Griffith ME, Bodily HL. Stability of antimycobacterial drugs in susceptibility testing. *Antimicrob Agents Chemother* 1992;36:2398–2402.
44. McClatchy JK. Antimycobacterial drugs: mechanisms of action, drug resistance, susceptibility testing, and assays of activity in biological fluids. In: Lorian V, ed. *Antibiotics in laboratory medicine,* 2nd ed. Baltimore: Williams & Wilkins, 1986:181–222.
45. David HL. *Bacteriology of the Mycobacterioses.* Vol. DHEW Publication No. (CDC) 76–8316. Washington, DC: US Government Printing Office, 1976.
46. Hawkins JE. Drug susceptibility testing. In: Kubica GP, Wayne LG, eds. *The mycobacteria: a sourcebook (part A).* New York: Marcel Dekker, Inc, 1984:177–193.
47. Rieder HL, Chonde TM, Myking H, et al. The Public Health Service National Tuberculosis Reference Laboratory and the National Laboratory Network: minimum requirements, role and operation in low-income country. Paris: International Union Against Tuberculosis and Lung Disease, 1998.
48. Wayne LG, Krasnow I. Preparation of tuberculosis susceptibility testing mediums by means of impregnated disks. *Am J Clin Pathol* 1966;45:769–771.
49. Griffith M, Barrett HL, Bodily HL, et al. Drug susceptibility tests for tuberculosis using drug impregnated discs. *Am J Clin Pathol* 1967;47:812–817.
50. Guthertz LS, Griffith ME, Ford EG, et al. Quality control or individual components used in Middlebrook 7H10 medium for mycobacterial susceptibility testing. *J Clin Microbiol* 1988;26:2338–2342.
51. Butler WR, Warren NG, Kubica GP, et al. Modified method for testing the quality of albumin-containing enrichments used in growth media for mycobacteria. *J Clin Microbiol* 1990;28:1068–1070.

52. American Thoracic Society. Diagnostic standards and classification of tuberculosis in adults and children. *Am J Respir Crit Care Med* 2000;161:1376–1395.
53. Pfyffer GE, Brown- Elliott BA, Wallace RJ Jr. Mycobacterium: general characteristics, isolation, and staining procedures. In: Murray PR, ed. *Manual of clinical microbiology,* 8th ed. Vol 1. Washington, DC: ASM Press, 2003.
54. National Committee for Clinical Laboratory Standards. Susceptibility testing of Mycobacteria, Nocardiae, and other aerobic actinomycetes; approved standard. NCCLS document M24-A. Wayne, PA: 2003.
55. Cummings DM, Rostraph D. Radiometric detection of metabolic activity of *Mycobacterium tuberculosis. J Nucl Med* 1975;16:1189–1191.
56. Middlebrook G, Reggiardo Z, Tigertt WD. Automatable radiometric detection of growth of *Mycobacterium tuberculosis* in selective media. *Am Rev Respir Dis* 1977;115:1066–1069.
57. Roberts GD, Goodman NL, Heifets L, et al. Evaluation of the BACTEC radiometric method for recovery of mycobacteria and drug susceptibility testing of *Mycobacterium tuberculosis* from acid-fast smear-positive specimens. *J Clin Microbiol* 1983;18:689–696.
58. Siddiqi SH, Hawkins JE, Laszlo A. Interlaboratory drug susceptibility testing of *Mycobacterium tuberculosis* by a radiometric procedure and two conventional methods. *J Clin Microbiol* 1985;22:919–923.
59. Woodley CL. Evaluation of streptomycin and ethambutol concentrations for susceptibility testing of *Mycobacterium tuberculosis* by radiometric and conventional procedures. *J Clin Microbiol* 1986;23:385–386.
60. Hawkins JE. Nonweekend schedule for BACTEC drug susceptibility testing of *Mycobacterium tuberculosis. J Clin Microbiol* 1986;23:934–937.
61. Hawkins JE. Rapid mycobacterial susceptibility tests. *Clin Microbiol Newsltr* 1986;8:101–104.
62. Ängeby KA, Werngren J, Toro JC, et al. Evaluation of the BacT/ALERT 3D system for recovery and drug susceptibility testing of *Mycobacterium tuberculosis. Clin Microbiol Infect* 2003;9:1148–1152.
63. Ruiz P, Zerolo FJ, Casal MJ. Comparison of susceptibility testing of *Mycobacterium tuberculosis* using the ESP culture system II with that using the BACTEC method. *J Clin Microbiol* 2000;38:4663–4664.
64. LaBombardi VJ. Comparison of the ESP and BACTEC systems for testing susceptibilities of *Mycobacterium tuberculosis* complex isolates to pyrazinamide. *J Clin Microbiol* 2002;40:2238–2239.
65. Bergmann JS, Woods GL. Evaluation of the ESP culture system II for testing susceptibilities of *Mycobacterium tuberculosis* isolates to four primary antituberculous drugs. *J Clin Microbiol* 1998;36:2940–2943.
66. Ardito F, Posteraro B, Sanguinetti M, et al. Evaluation of BACTEC Mycobacteria Growth Indicator Tube (MGIT 960) automated system for drug susceptibility testing of *Mycobacterium tuberculosis. J Clin Microbiol* 2001;39:4440–4444.
67. Bemer P, Palicova F, Rusch-Gerdes S, et al. Multicenter evaluation of fully automated BACTEC Mycobacteria Growth Indicator Tube 960 system for susceptibility testing of *Mycobacterium tuberculosis. J Clin Microbiol* 2002;40:150–154.
68. Kontos F, Nicolaou S, Kostopoulos C, et al. Multicenter evaluation of the fully automated Bactec MGIT 960 system for susceptibility testing of *Mycobacterium tuberculosis* to pyrazinamide: comparison with the radiometric Bactec 460TB system. *J Microbiol Methods* 2003;55:331–333.
69. Reisner BS, Gatson AM, Woods GL. Evaluation of mycobacteria growth indicator tubes for susceptibility testing of *Mycobacterium tuberculosis* to isoniazid and rifampin. *Diag Microbiol Infect Dis* 1995;22:325–329.
70. Rusch-Gerdes S, Domehl C, Nardi G, et al. Multicenter evaluation of the mycobacteria growth indicator tube for testing susceptibility of *Mycobacterium tuberculosis* to first-line drugs. *J Clin Microbiol* 1999;37:45–48.
71. Pfyffer GE, Palicova F, Rusch-Gerdes S. Testing of susceptibility of *Mycobacterium tuberculosis* to pyrazinamide with the nonradiometric BACTEC MGIT 960 system. *J Clin Microbiol* 2002;40:1670–1674.
72. Aono A, Hirano K, Hamasaki S, et al. Evaluation of BACTEC MGIT 960 PZA medium for susceptibility testing of *Mycobacterium tuberculosis* to pyrazinamide (PZA): compared with the results of pyrazinamidase assay and Kyokuto PZA test. *Diag Microbiol Infect Dis* 2002;44:347–352.
73. Brunello F, Fontana R. Reliability of the MB/BacT system for testing susceptibility of *Mycobacterium tuberculosis* complex isolates to antituberculous drugs. *J Clin Microbiol* 2000;38:872–873.
74. Diaz-Infantes MS, Ruiz-Serrano MJ, Martinez-Sanchez L, et al. Evaluation of the MB/BacT mycobacterium detection system for susceptibility testing of *Mycobacterium tuberculosis. J Clin Microbiol* 2000;38:1988–1989.
75. Butler WR, Kilburn JO. Improved method for testing susceptibility of *Mycobacterium tuberculosis* to pyrazinamide. *J Clin Microbiol* 1982;16:1106–1109.
76. Heifets L, Sanchez T. New agar medium for testing susceptibility of *Mycobacterium tuberculosis* to pyrazinamide. *J Clin Microbiol* 2000;38:1498–1501.
77. Heifets LB, Iseman MD. Radiometric method for testing susceptibility of mycobacteria to pyrazinamide in 7H12 broth. *J Clin Microbiol* 1985;21:200–204.
78. Tarrand JJ, Spicer AD, Groschel DHM. Evaluation of a radiometric method for pyrazinamide susceptibility testing of *Mycobacterium tuberculosis. Antimicrob Agents Chemother* 1986;30:852–855.
79. Woodley CL, Smithwick RW. Radiometric method for pyrazinamide susceptibility testing of *Mycobacterium tuberculosis* in egg-yolk-enriched BACTEC 12A medium. *Antimicrob Agents Chemother* 1988;32:125–127.
80. Salfinger M, Heifets LB. Determination of pyrazinamide MICs for *Mycobacterium tuberculosis* at different pHs by the radiometric method. *Antimicrob Agents Chemother* 1988;32:1002–1004.
81. McClatchy JK, Tsang AY, Cernich MS. Use of pyrazinamidase activity in *Mycobacterium tuberculosis* as a rapid method for determination of pyrazinamide susceptibility. *Antimicrob Agents Chemother* 1981;20:556–557.
82. Butler WR, Kilburn JO. Susceptibility of *Mycobacterium tuberculosis* to pyrazinamide and its relationship to pyrazinamidase activity. *Antimicrob Agents Chemother* 1983;24:600–601.
83. Salfinger M, Kafader FM. Susceptibility testing of *Mycobacterium tuberculosis* to pyrazinamide. *Zentralbl Bakteriol Mikrobiol Hyg* 1987;265:404–407.
84. Canetti G, Froman S, Grosset J, et al. Mycobacteria: laboratory methods for testing drug sensitivity and resistance. *Bull WHO* 1963;29:565–578.
85. Nilsson LE, Hoffner SE, Ansehn S. Rapid susceptibility testing of *Mycobacterium tuberculosis* by bioluminescence assay of mycobacterial ATP. *Antimicrob Agents Chemother* 1988;32:1208–1212.
86. Brown-Elliott BA, Griffith DE, Wallace RJ Jr. Newly described or emerging human species of nontuberculous mycobacteria. *Infect Dis Clin North Am* 2002;16:187–220.

87. Brown-Elliott BA, Wallace RJ Jr. Clinical and taxonomic status of pathogenic nonpigmented or late-pigmenting rapidly growing mycobacteria. *Clin Microbiol Rev* 2002;15:716–746.
88. McFarland EJ, Kuritzkes DR. Clinical features and treatment of infection due to mycobacterium fortuitum/chelonae complex. *Curr Clin Top Infect Dis* 1993;13:188–202.
89. Wallace RJ. The rapidly growing mycobacteria: characterization and susceptibility testing. *Antimicrob Newsltr* 1985;2:85–92.
90. Nash KA. Intrinsic macrolide resistance in *Mycobacterium smegmatis* is conferred by a novel *erm* gene, *erm*(38). *Antimicrob Agents Chemother* 2003;47:3053–3060.
91. Nash KA, Zhang Y, Brown-Elliott BA, Wallace Jr RJ. Identification of an rRNA methylase gene, erm(39), which confers inducible macrolide resistance to *M. fortuitum,* abstr# 4-017, 104th ASM General Meeting, New Orleans, LA, May 23–27, 2004.
92. Tebas P, Sultan F, Wallace RJ, Jr et al. Rapid development of resistance to clarithromycin following monotherapy for disseminated *M. chelonae* infection in a heart transplant patient. *Clin Infect Dis* 1995;20:443–444.
93. Wallace RJ Jr, Meier A, Brown BA, et al. Genetic basis for clarithromycin resistance among isolates of *Mycobacterium chelonae* and *Mycobacterium abscessus*. *Antimicrob Agents Chemother* 1996;40:1676–1681.
94. Swenson JM, Thornsberry C, Silcox VA. Rapidly growing mycobacteria: testing of susceptibility to 34 antimicrobial agents by broth microdilution. *Antimicrob Agents Chemother* 1982;22:186–192.
95. Wallace RJ Jr, Daloviso JR, Pankey GA. Disk diffusion testing of susceptibility of *Mycobacterium fortuitum* and *Mycobacterium chelonei* to antibacterial agents. *Antimicrob Agents Chemother* 1979;16:611–614.
96. Welch DF, Kelly MT. Antimicrobial susceptibility testing of *Mycobacterium fortuitum* complex. *Antimicob Agents Chemother* 1979;15:754–757.
97. Stone MS, Wallace RJ Jr, Swenson JM, et al. Agar disk elution method for susceptibility testing of *Mycobacterium marinum* and *Mycobacterium fortuitum* complex to sulfonamides and antibiotics. *Antimicrob Agents Chemother* 1983;24:486–493.
98. Woods GL, Bergmann JS, Witebsky FG, et al. Multisite reproducibility of Etest for susceptibility testing of *Mycobacterium abscessus, Mycobacterium chelonae,* and *Mycobacterium fortuitum*. *J Clin Microbiol* 2000;38:656–661.
99. Biehle JR, Cavalieri SJ, Saubolle MA, et al. Evaluation of Etest for susceptibility testing of rapidly growing mycobacteria. *J Clin Microbiol* 1995;33:1760–1764.
100. Hoffner SE, Klintz L, Olsson-Liljequist B, et al. Evaluation of Etest for rapid susceptibility testing of *Mycobacterium chelonae* and *M. fortuitum*. *J Clin Microbiol* 1994;32:1846–1849.
101. Koontz FP, Erwin ME, Barrett MS, et al. Etest for routine clinical antimicrobial susceptibility testing of rapid-growing mycobacteria isolates. *Diag Microbiol Infect Dis* 1994;19:183–186.
102. Casal MJ, Rodriguez FC. In vitro susceptibility of *Mycobacterium fortuitum* and *M. chelonei* to sisomicin, gentamicin and tobramycin. *Ann Microbiol (Paris)* 1983;134B:451–454.
103. Swenson JM, Wallace RJ Jr, Silcox VA, et al. Antimicrobial susceptibility of five subgroups of *Mycobacterium fortuitum* and *Mycobacterium chelonae*. *Antimicrob Agents Chemother* 1985;28:807–811.
104. Wayne LG, Sramek HA. Agents of newly recognized or infrequently encountered mycobacterial diseases. *Clin Microbiol Rev* 1992;5:1–25.
105. Saubolle MA. Nontuberculous mycobacteria as agents of human disease in the United States. *Clin Microbiol Newsltr* 1989;11:113–117.
106. Woods GL, Washington JAI. Mycobacteria other than *Mycobacterium tuberculosis:* review of microbiologic and clinical aspects. *Rev Infect Dis* 1987;9:275–294.
107. Henriques B, Hoffner SE, Petrini B, et al. Infection with *Mycobacterium malmoense* in Sweden: report of 221 cases. *Clin Infect Dis* 1994;18:596–600.
108. Davidson PT. The diagnosis and management of disease caused by *M. avium* complex, *M. kansasii,* and other mycobacteria. In: Snider DE Jr, ed. *Clinics in chest medicine.* Vol 10. Philadelphia: WB Saunders, 1989:431–443.
109. Husson RN, Ross LA, Sandelli S, et al. Orally administered clarithromycin for the treatment of systemic *Mycobacterium avium* complex infection in children with acquired immunodeficiency syndrome. *J Pediatr* 1994;124:807–814.
110. Benson CA, Williams PL, Currier JS, et al. A prospective, randomized trial examining the efficacy and safety of clarithromycin in combination with ethambutol, rifabutin, or both for the treatment of disseminated *Mycobacterium avium* complex disease in persons with acquired immunodeficiency syndrome. *Clin Infect Dis* 2003;37:1234–1243.
111. Koletar SL, Berry AJ, Cynamon MH, et al. Azithromycin as treatment for disseminated *Mycobacterium avium* complex in AIDS patients. *Antimicrob Agents Chemother* 1999;43:2869–2872.
112. Inderlied CB, Kemper CA, Bermudez LEM. The *Mycobacterium avium* complex. *Clin Microbiol Rev* 1993;6:266–310.
113. Korvick J, Benson C. *Mycobacterium avium complex infection: progress in research and treatment.* New York: Marcel Dekker, 1995.
114. Falkinham JO, 3rd. Epidemiology of infection by nontuberculous mycobacteria. *Clin Microbiol Rev* 1996;9:177–215.
115. Tsang AY, Drupa I, Goldberg M, et al. Use of serology and thin layer chromatography for the assembly of an authenticated collection of serovars within the *Mycobacterium avium-Mycobacterium intracellulare-Mycobacterium scrofulaceum* complex. *Int J Sys Bact* 1983;33:285–292.
116. Brennan PJ. Structure of mycobacteria: recent developments in defining cell wall carbohydrates and proteins. *Rev Infect Dis* 1989;11:S420–S430.
117. Drake TA, Herron RM, Hindler JA, et al. DNA probe reactivity of *Mycobacterium avium* complex isolates from patients without AIDS. *Diagn Microbiol Infect Dis* 1988;11:125–128.
118. Kiehn TE, Edwards FF. Rapid identification using a specific DNA probe of *Mycobacterium avium complex* from patients with acquired immunodeficiency syndrome. *J Clin Microbiol* 1987;25:1551–1552.
119. Heifets L. MIC as a quantitative measurement of the susceptibility of *Mycobacteriam avium* strains to seven antituberculosis drugs. *Antimicrob Agents Chemother* 1988;32:1131–1136.
120. Inderlied CB, Young LS, Yamada JK. Determination of in vitro susceptibility of *Mycobacterium avium* complex isolates to antimicrobial agents by various methods. *Antimicrob Agents Chemother* 1987;31:1697–1702.
121. Rastogi N, Frehel C, Ryter A, et al. Multiple drug resistance in *Mycobacterium avium*: is the wall architecture responsible for the exclusion of antimicrobial agents? *Antimicrob Agents Chemother* 1981;20:666–677.
122. Mizuguchi Y, Ogawa M, Udou T. Morphological changes induced by beta-lactam antibiotics in *Mycobacterium*

avium-intracellulare complex. *Antimicrob Agents Chemother* 1985;27:541–547.

123. Crawford JT, Falkinham JO III. Plasmids of the *Mycobacterium avium* complex. In: McFadden J, ed. *Molecular biology of the mycobacteria*. London: Surrey University Press, 1990:97–119.
124. Franzblau SG, Takeda T, Nakamura M. Mycobacterial plasmids: screening and possible relationship to antibiotic resistance in *Mycobacterium avium/Mycobacterium intracellulare*. *Microbiol Immunol* 1986;30:903–907
125. Saito H, Tomioka H. Susceptibilities of transparent, opaque, and rough colonial variants of *Mycobacterium avium* complex to various fatty acids. *Antimicrob Agents Chemother* 1988;32:400–402.
126. Schaefer WB, Davis CL, Cohn ML. Pathogenicity of transparent, opaque and rough variants of *Mycobacterium avium* in chickens and mice. *Am Rev Respir Dis* 1970;102:499–506.
127. Stormer RS, Falkinham JOI. Differences in antimicrobial susceptibility of pigmented and unpigmented colonial variants of *Mycobacterium avium*. *J Clin Microbiol* 1989;27:2459–2465.
128. Inderlied C, Nash KA. Microbiology and in vitro susceptibility testing. In: Korvick J, ed. *Mycobacterium avium complex infection: progress in research and treatment*. New York: Marcel Dekker, 1995:109–140.
129. Bermudez LE, Kolonoski P, Petrofsky M, et al. Mefloquine, moxifloxacin, and ethambutol are a triple-drug alternative to macrolide-containing regimens for treatment of *Mycobacterium avium* disease. *J Infect Dis* 2003;187:1977–1980.
130. Bermudez LE, Kolonoski P, Wu M, et al. Mefloquine is active in vitro and in vivo against *Mycobacterium avium* complex. *Antimicrob Agents Chemother* 1999;43:1870–1874.
131. Nannini EC, Keating M, Binstock P, et al. Successful treatment of refractory disseminated *Mycobacterium avium* complex infection with the addition of linezolid and mefloquine. *J Infect* 2002;44:201–203.
132. Woods GL, Williams-Bouyer N, Wallace RJ Jr, et al. Multisite reproducibility of results obtained by two broth dilution methods for susceptibility testing of *Mycobacterium avium* complex. *J Clin Microbiol* 2003;41:627–631.
133. British Thoracic Society. *Mycobacterium kansasii* pulmonary infection: a prospective study of the results of nine months of treatment with rifampicin and ethambutol. Research Committee, British Thoracic Society. *Thorax* 1994;49:442–445.
134. Hoffner SE. Pulmonary infections caused by less frequently encountered slow-growing environmental mycobacteria. *Eur J Clin Microbiol Infect Dis* 1994;13:937–941.
135. Johanson WGJ, Nicholson DP. Pulmonary disease due to *Mycobacterium kansasii*. An analysis of some factors effecting prognosis. *Am Rev Respir Dis* 1969;99:73–85.
136. Pezzia W, Raleigh JW, Bailey MC, et al. Treatment of pulmonary disease due to *Mycobacterium kansasii*: recent experience with rifampin. *Rev Infect Dis* 1981;3:1035–1039.
137. American Thoracic Society. Diagnosis and treatment of disease caused by nontuberculous mycobacteria. *Am J Respir Crit Care Med* 1997;156:S1–S25.
138. Wallace RJ Jr, Dunbar D, Brown BA, et al. Rifampin-resistant *Mycobacterium kansasii*. *Clin Infect Dis* 1994;18:736–743.
139. Bennett SN, Peterson DE, Johnson DR, et al. Bronchoscopy-associated *Mycobacterium xenopi* pseudoinfections. *Am J Respir Crit Care Med* 1994;150:245–250.
140. Sniadack DH, Ostroff SM, Karlix MA, et al. A nosocomial pseudo-outbreak of *Mycobacterium xenopi* due to a contaminated potable water supply: lessons in prevention. *Infect Control Hosp Epidemiol* 1993;14:636–641.
141. Terashima T, Sakamaki F, Hasegawa N, et al. Pulmonary infection due to *Mycobacterium xenopi*. *Intern Med* 1994;33:536–539.
142. Zaugg M, Salfinger M, Opravil M, et al. Extrapulmonary and disseminated infections due to *Mycobacterium malmoense*: case report and review. *Clin Infect Dis* 1993;16:540–549.
143. Banks J, Jenkins PA. Combined versus single antituberculosis drugs on the in vitro sensitivity patterns of nontuberculous mycobacteria. *Thorax* 1987;42:838–842.
144. Hoffner SE, Hjelm U. Increased growth of *Mycobacterium malmoense* in vitro in the presence of isoniazid. *Eur J Clin Microbiol Infect Dis* 1991;10:787–788.
145. Hoffner SE, Hjelm U, Kallenius G. Susceptibility of *Mycobacterium malmoense* to antibacterial drugs and drug combinations. *Antimicrob Agents Chemother* 1993;37:1285–1288.
146. Banks J, Jenkins PA, Smith AP. Pulmonary infection with *Mycobacterium malmoense*—a review of treatment and response. *Tubercle* 1985;66:197–203.
147. Valero G, Moreno F, Graybill JR. Activities of clarithromycin, ofloxacin, and clarithromycin plus ethambutol against *Mycobacterium simiae* in murine model of disseminated infection. *Antimicrob Agents Chemother* 1994;38:2676–2677.
148. Edelstein H. *Mycobacterium marinum* skin infections. Report of 31 cases and review of the literature. *Arch Intern Med* 1994;154:1359–1364.
149. Kozin SH, Bishop AT. Atypical Mycobacterium infections of the upper extremity. *J Hand Surg* 1994;19:480–487.
150. Forsgren A. Antibiotic susceptibility of *Mycobacterium marinum*. *Scand J Infect Dis* 1993;25:779–782.
151. Sanders WJ, Wolinsky E. In vitro susceptibility of *Mycobacterium marinum* to eight antimicrobial agents. *Antimicrob Agents Chemother* 1980;18:529–531.
152. Marsollier L, Prevot G, Honore N, et al. Susceptibility of *Mycobacterium ulcerans* to a combination of amikacin/rifampicin. *Int J Antimicrob Agents* 2003;22:562–566.
153. Bentoucha A, Robert J, Dega H, et al. Activities of new macrolides and fluoroquinolones against *Mycobacterium ulcerans* infection in mice. *Antimicrob Agents Chemother* 2001;45:3109–3112.
154. Marsollier L, Honore N, Legras P, et al. Isolation of three *Mycobacterium ulcerans* strains resistant to rifampin after experimental chemotherapy of mice. *Antimicrob Agents Chemother* 2003;47:1228–1232.
155. Straus WL, Ostroff SM, Jernigan DB, et al. Clinical and epidemiologic characteristics of *Mycobacterium haemophilum*, an emerging pathogen in immunocompromised patients. *Ann Intern Med* 1994;120:118–125.
156. Kiehn TE, White M. *Mycobacterium haemophilum*: an emerging pathogen. *Eur J Clin Microbiol Infect Dis* 1994;13:925–931.
157. Bernard EM, Edwards FF, Kiehn TE, et al. Activities of antimicrobial agents against clinical isolates of *Mycobacterium haemophilum*. *Antimicrob Agents Chemother* 1993;37:2323–2326.
158. Lessnau KD, Milanese S, Talavera W. *Mycobacterium gordonae*: a treatable disease in HIV-positive patients. *Chest* 1993;104:1779–1785.
159. Emler S, Rochat T, Rohner P, et al. Chronic destructive lung disease associated with a novel mycobacterium. *Am J Respir Crit Care Med* 1994;150:261–265.

160. Springer B, Kirschner P, Rost-Meyer G, et al. *Mycobacterium interjectum,* a new species isolated from a patient with chronic lymphadenitis. *J Clin Microbiol* 1993;31:3083–3089.
161. Brown BA, Wallace RJ Jr, Onyi GO. Activities of clarithromycin against eight slowly growing species of nontuberculous mycobacteria, determined by using a broth microdilution MIC system. *Antimicrob Agents Chemother* 1992;36:1987–1990.
162. Wallace RJ Jr, Brown BA, Onyi GO. Susceptibilities of *Mycobacterium fortuitum* biovar. fortuitum and the two subgroups of *Mycobacterium chelonae* to imipenem, cefmetazole, cefoxitin, and amoxicillin-clavulanic acid. *Antimicrob Agents Chemother* 1991;35:773–775.
163. Wallace RJ Jr, Brown-Elliott BA, Ward SC, et al. Activities of linezolid against rapidly growing mycobacteria. *Antimicrob Agents Chemother* 2001;45:764–767.
164. Good RC, Silcox VA, Kilburn JO, et al. Identification and drug susceptibility test results for Mycobacterium spp. *Clin Microbiol Newsltr* 1985;7:133–136.
165. Collins CH, Uttley AH. In-vitro activity of seventeen antimicrobial compounds against seven species of mycobacteria. *J Antimicrob Chemother* 1988;22:857–861.
166. Khardori N, Rolston K, Rosenbaum B, et al. Comparative in-vitro activity of twenty antimicrobial agents against clinical isolates of *Mycobacterium avium* complex. *J Antimicrob Chemother* 1989;24:667–673.
167. Heifets L, Lindholm-Levy P. Comparison of bactericidal activities of streptomycin, amikacin, kanamycin, and capreomycin against *Mycobacterium avium* and *M. tuberculosis. Antimicrob Agents Chemother* 1989;33:1298–1301.
168. Cynamon MH, Palmer GS, Sorg TB. Comparative in vitro activities of ampicillin, BMY 28142, and imipenem against *Mycobacterium avium* complex. *Diagn Microbiol Infect Dis* 1987;6:151–155.
169. Naik S, Ruck R. In vitro activities of several new macrolide antibiotics against *Mycobacterium avium* complex. *Antimicrob Agents Chemother* 1989;33:1614–1616.
170. Woodley CL, Kilburn JO. In vitro susceptibility of *Mycobacterium avium* complex and *Mycobacterium tuberculosis* strains to a spiro-piperidyl rifamycin. *Am Rev Respir Dis* 1982;126:586–587.
171. Salfinger M, Stool EW, Pito D, et al. Comparison of three methods for recovery of *Mycobacterium avium* complex from blood specimens. *J Clin Microbiol* 1988;26:1225–1226.
172. Collins CH, Uttley AH. In-vitro susceptibility of mycobacteria to ciprofloxacin. *J Antimicrob Chemother* 1985;16:575–580.
173. Rodriguez Diaz JC, Lopez M, Ruiz M, et al. In vitro activity of new fluoroquinolones and linezolid against non-tuberculous mycobacteria. *Int J Antimicrob Agents* 2003;21:585–588.
174. Davis CEJ, Carpenter JL, Trevino S, et al. In vitro susceptibility of *Mycobacterium avium* complex to antibacterial agents. *Diagn Microbiol Infect Dis* 1987;8:149–155.
175. Brown-Elliott BA, Crist CJ, Mann LB, et al. In vitro activity of linezolid against slowly growing nontuberculous mycobacteria. *Antimicrob Agents Chemother* 2003;47:1736–1738.
176. Leysen DC, Haemers A, Pattyn Sr. Mycobacteria and the new quinolones. *Antimicrob Agents Chemother* 1989;33:1–5.
177. Ernst F, van der Auwera P. In-vitro activity of fleroxacin (Ro 23–6240), a new fluoroquinolone, and other agents, against mycobacterium spp. *J Antimicrob Chemother* 1988;21:501–504.
178. Ausina V, Condom MJ, Mirelis B, et al. In vitro activity of clofazimine against rapidly growing nonchromogenic mycobacteria. *Antimicrob Agents Chemother* 1986;29:951–952.
179. Tomioka H, Saito H, Sato K. Comparative antimycobacterial activities of the newly synthesized quinolone AM-1155, sparfloxacin, and ofloxacin. *Antimicrob Agents Chemother* 1993;37:1259–1263.
180. Bernard EM, Edwards FF, Kiehn TE, et al. Activities of antimicrobial agents against clinical isolates of *Mycobacterium haemophilum. Antimicrob Agents Chemother* 1993;37:2323–2326.
181. Fenlon CH, Cynamon MH. Comparative in vitro activities of ciprofloxacin and other 4-quinolones against *Mycobacterium tuberculosis* and *Mycobacterium intracellulare. Antimicrob Agents Chemother* 1986;29:386–388.
182. Haneishi T, Nakajima M, Shiraishi A, et al. Antimycobacterial activities in vitro and in vivo and pharmacokinetics of dihydromycoplanecin A. *Antimicrob Agents Chemother* 1988;32:125–127.
183. Cynamon MH. Comparative in vitro activities of MDL 473, rifampin, and ansamycin against *Mycobacterium intracellulare. Antimicrob Agents Chemother* 1985;28:440–441.
184. Garcia-Rodriguez JA, Gomez G-AC. In-vitro activities of quinolones against mycobacteria. *J Antimicrob Chemother* 1993;32:797–808.
185. Wallace RJJ, Wiss K. Susceptibility of *Mycobacterium marinum* to tetracyclines and aminoglycosides. *Antimicrob Agents Chemother* 1981;20:610–612.
186. Braback M, Riesbeck K, Forsgren A. Susceptibilities of *Mycobacterium marinum* to gatifloxacin, gemifloxacin, levofloxacin, linezolid, moxifloxacin, telithromycin, and quinupristin-dalfopristin (Synercid) compared to its susceptibilities to reference macrolides and quinolones. *Antimicrobl Agents Chemother* 2002;46:1114–1116.
187. Heifets LB, Iseman MD. Determination of in vitro susceptibility of mycobacteria to ansamycin. *Am Rev Respir Dis* 1985;132:710–711.
188. Yew WW, Piddock LJ, Li MS, et al. In-vitro activity of quinolones and macrolides against mycobacteria. *J Antimicrob Chemother* 1994;34:343–351.
189. Byrne SK, Crawford CE, Geddes GL, et al. In vitro susceptibilities of *Mycobacterium tuberculosis* to 10 antimicrobial agents. *Antimicrob Agents Chemother* 1988;32:1441–1442.
190. Gorzynski EA, Gutman SE, Allen W. Comparative antimycobacterial activities of difloxacin, temafloxacin, enoxacin, pefloxacin, reference fluoroquinolones, and a new macrolide, clarithromycin. *Antimicrob Agents Chemother* 1989;33:591–592.
191. Rodriguez JC, Ruiz M, Lopez M, et al. In vitro activity of moxifloxacin, levofloxacin, gatifloxacin and linezolid against *Mycobacterium tuberculosis. Int J Antimicrob Agents* 2002;20:464–467.
192. Alvirez-Freites EJ, Carter JL, Cynamon MH. In vitro and in vivo activities of gatifloxacin against *Mycobacterium tuberculosis. Antimicrob Agents Chemother* 2002;46:1022–1025.
193. Alcala L, Ruiz-Serrano MJ, Perez-Fernandez Turegano C, et al. In vitro activities of linezolid against clinical isolates of *Mycobacterium tuberculosis* that are susceptible or resistant to first-line antituberculous drugs. *Antimicrob Agents Chemother* 2003;447:416–447.
194. Zhang Y, Telenti A. Genetics of drug resistance in *Mycobacterium tuberculosis.* In: Hatfull GF, Jacobs WR Jr, eds. *Molecular genetics of mycobacteria.* Washington, DC: American Society of Microbiology, 2000:235–254.
195. Ramaswamy S, Musser JM. Molecular genetic basis of

antimicrobial agent resistance in *Mycobacterium tuberculosis:* 1998 update. *Tuberc Lung Dis* 1998;79:3–29.

196. Riska PF, Jacobs WR Jr, Alland D. Molecular determinants of drug resistance in tuberculosis. *Int J Tuberc Lung Dis* 2000;4:S4–S10.
197. Betts JC, Lukey PT, Robb LC, et al. Evaluation of a nutrient starvation model of *Mycobacterium tuberculosis* persistence by gene and protein expression profiling. *Mol Microbiol* 2002;43:717–731.
198. Herbert D, Paramasivan CN, Venkatesan P, et al. Bactericidal action of ofloxacin, sulbactam-ampicillin, rifampin, and isoniazid on logarithmic- and stationary-phase cultures of *Mycobacterium tuberculosis*. *Antimicrob Agents Chemother* 1996;40:2296–2299.
199. Yamori S, Ichiyama S, Shimokata K, et al. Bacteriostatic and bactericidal activity of antituberculosis drugs against *Mycobacterium tuberculosis*, *Mycobacterium avium-Mycobacterium intracellulare* complex and *Mycobacterium kansasii* in different growth phases. *Microbiol Immunol* 1992;36:361–368.
200. Magliozzo RS, Marcinkeviciene JA. The role of Mn(II)-peroxidase activity of mycobacterial catalase-peroxidase in activation of the antibiotic isoniazid. *J Biol Chem* 1997;272:8867–8870.
201. Nguyen M, Quemard A, Broussy S, et al. Mn(III) pyrophosphate as an efficient tool for studying the mode of action of isoniazid on the InhA protein of *Mycobacterium tuberculosis*. *Antimicrob Agents Chemother* 2002;46:2137–2144.
202. Wengenack NL, Rusnak F. Evidence for isoniazid-dependent free radical generation catalyzed by *Mycobacterium tuberculosis* KatG and the isoniazid-resistant mutant KatG(S315T). *Biochemistry* 2001;40:8990–8996.
203. Rawat R, Whitty A, Tonge PJ. The isoniazid-NAD adduct is a slow, tight-binding inhibitor of InhA, the *Mycobacterium tuberculosis* enoyl reductase: adduct affinity and drug resistance. *Proc Natl Acad Sci USA* 2003;100:13881–13886.
204. Rozwarski DA, Grant GA, Barton DH, et al. Modification of the NADH of the isoniazid target (InhA) from *Mycobacterium tuberculosis*. *Science* 1998;279:98–102.
205. Takayama K, Davidson LA. Isonicotinic acid hydrazide. In: Hahn FE, ed. *Mechanism of action of antibacterial agents.* Vol V. Berlin: Springer-Verlag, 1979:98–119.
206. Winder FG. Mode of action of the antimycobacterial agents and associated aspects of the molecular biology of the mycobacteria. In: Ratledge C, Stanford J, eds. *The biology of the mycobacteria.* Vol 1 (Physiology, Identification and Classification). New York: Academic Press, 1982:353–438.
207. Takayama K, Schnoes HK, Armstrong EL, et al. Site of inhibitory action of isoniazid in the synthesis of mycolic acids in *Mycobacterium tuberculosis*. *J Lipid Res* 1975;16:308–317.
208. Takayama K, Qureshi N. Structure and synthesis of lipids. In: Kubica GP, Wayne LG, eds. *The Mycobacteria: a sourcebook (part A).* New York: Marcel Dekker, Inc, 1984.
209. Asselineau C, Asselineau J, Laneelle G, et al. The biosynthesis of mycolic acids by Mycobacteria: current and alternative hypotheses. *Prog Lipid Res* 2002;41:501–523.
210. Banerjee A, Dubnau E, Quemard A, et al. inhA, a gene encoding a target for isoniazid and ethionamide in *Mycobacterium tuberculosis*. *Science* 1994;263:227–230.
211. Mdluli K, Slayden RA, Zhu Y, et al. Inhibition of a *Mycobacterium tuberculosis* beta-ketoacyl ACP synthase by isoniazid. *Science* 1998;280:1607–1610.
212. Slayden RA, Barry CE 3rd. The role of KasA and KasB in the biosynthesis of meromycolic acids and isoniazid resistance in *Mycobacterium tuberculosis*. *Tuberculosis* 2002;82:149–160.
213. Piatek AS, Telenti A, Murray MR, et al. Genotypic analysis of *Mycobacterium tuberculosis* in two distinct populations using molecular beacons: implications for rapid susceptibility testing. *Antimicrob Agents Chemother* 2000;44:103–110.
214. Lee ASG, Lim IHK, Tang LLH, et al. Contribution of kasA analysis to detection of isoniazid-resistant *Mycobacterium tuberculosis*in Singapore. *Antimicrob Agents Chemother* 1999;43:2087–2089.
215. Vilcheze C, Morbidoni HR, Weisbrod TR, et al. Inactivation of the inhA-encoded fatty acid synthase II (FASII) enoyl-acyl carrier protein reductase induces accumulation of the FASI end products and cell lysis of *Mycobacterium smegmatis*. *J Bacteriol* 2000;182:4059–4067.
216. Slayden RA, Lee RE, Barry CE 3rd. Isoniazid affects multiple components of the type II fatty acid synthase system of *Mycobacterium tuberculosis*. *Mol Microbiol* 2000;38:514–525.
217. Betts JC, McLaren A, Lennon MG, et al. Signature gene expression profiles discriminate between isoniazid-, thiolactomycin-, and triclosan-treated *Mycobacterium tuberculosis*. *Antimicrob Agents Chemother* 2003;47:2903–2913.
218. Kremer L, Dover LG, Morbidoni HR, et al. Inhibition of inha activity, but not kasa activity, induces formation of a kasa-containing complex in Mycobacteria. *J Biol Chem* 2003;278:20547–20554.
219. Larsen MH, Vilcheze C, Kremer L, et al. Overexpression of inhA, but not kasA, confers resistance to isoniazid and ethionamide in *Mycobacterium smegmatis, M. bovis* BCG and *M. tuberculosis*. *Mol Microbiol* 2002;46:453–466.
220. Zabinski RF, Blanchard JS. The requirement for manganese and oxygen in the isoniazid-dependent inactivation of *mycobacterium tuberculosis* enoyl reductase. *J Am Chem Soc* 1997;119:2331–2332.
221. Lei B, Wei CJ, Tu SC. Action mechanism of antitubercular isoniazid. Activation by *Mycobacterium tuberculosis* KatG, isolation, and characterization of inha inhibitor. *J Biol Chem* 2000;275:2520–2526.
222. Winder FG, Collins PB. The effect of isoniazid on nicotinamide nucleotide levels in *Mycobacterium bovis*strain BCG. *Am Rev Respir Dis* 1968;97:719–720.
223. Winder FG, Collins PB. The effect of isoniazid on nicotinamide nucleotide concentrations in tubercle bacilli. *Am Rev Respir Dis* 1969;100:101–103.
224. Seydel JK, Tono-oka S, Schaper KJ, et al. Mode of action of isoniazid (INH). *Arzneimittelforsch* 1976;26:477–478.
225. Kruger-Thiemer E. Isonicotinic acid hypothesis of the antituberculous action of isoniazid. *Am Rev Tuberc Pulm Dis* 1958;77:364–367.
226. Krishna Murti CR. Isonicotinic hydrazide. In: Corcoran JW, Hahn FE, eds. *Antibiotics: mechanism of action of antimicrobial and antitumor agents.* Vol 3. New York: Springer-Verlag, 1975:623–652.
227. Sriprakash KS, Ramakrishnan T. Isoniazid and nicotinamide adenine dinucleotide synthesis in *M. tuberculosis*. *Indian J Biochem* 1969;6:49–50.
228. Bekierkunst A, Bricker A. Studies on the mode of action of isoniazid on mycobacteria. *Arch Biochem Biophys* 1967;122:385–392.
229. Davis WB, Weber MM. Specificity of isoniazid on growth inhibition and competition for an oxidized nicotiniamide adenine dinucleotide regulatory site on the electron

transport pathway in *Mycobacterium phlei. Antimicrob Agents Chemother* 1977;12:213–218.
230. Davis WB. Identification of an nicotinamide adenine dinucleotide glycohydrolase and an associated inhibitor in isoniazid-susceptible and -resistant *Mycobacterium phlei. Antimicrob Agents Chemother* 1980;17:663–668.
231. Jackett PS, Aber VR, Mitchison DA. The relationship between nicotinamide adenine dinucleotide concentration and antibacterial activity of isoniazid in *Mycobacterium tuberculosis. Am Rev Respir Dis* 1977;115:601–607.
232. Beggs WH, Jenne JW. Isoniazid uptake and growth inhibition of *Mycobacterium tuberculosis* in relation to time and concentration of pulsed drug exposures. *Tubercle* 1969;50:377–385.
233. Winder FG, Collins PB, Whelan D. Effects of ethionamide and isoxyl on mycolic acid synthesis in *Mycobacterium tuberculosis* BCG. *J Gen Microbiol* 1971;66:379–380.
234. Miesel L, Weisbrod TR, Marcinkeviciene JA, et al. NADH dehydrogenase defects confer isoniazid resistance and conditional lethality in *Mycobacterium smegmatis. J Bacteriol* 1998;180:2459–2467.
235. Lee AS, Teo AS, Wong SY. Novel mutations in ndh in isoniazid-resistant *Mycobacterium tuberculosis* isolates. *Antimicrob Agents Chemother* 2001;45:2157–2159.
236. Chen P, Bishai WR. Novel selection for isoniazid (INH) resistance genes supports a role for NAD+-binding proteins in mycobacterial INH resistance. *Infect Immun* 1998;66:5099–5106.
237. Shoeb HA, Bowman BU Jr, Ottolenghi AC, et al. Evidence for the generation of active oxygen by isoniazid treatment of extracts of *Mycobacterium tuberculosis* H37Ra. *Antimicrob Agents Chemother* 1985;27:404–407.
238. Shoeb HA, Bowman BU Jr, Ottolenghi AC, et al. Enzymatic and nonenzymatic superoxide-generating reactions of isoniazid. *Antimicrob Agents Chemother* 1985;27:408–412.
239. Ito K, Yamamoto K, Kawanishi S. Manganese-mediated oxidative damage of cellular and isolated DNA by isoniazid and related hydrazines: non-Fenton-type hydroxyl radical formation. *Biochemistry* 1992;31:11606–11613.
240. Middlebrook G. Isoniazid-resistance and catalase activity of tubercle bacilli. A preliminary report. *Am Rev Tuberc* 1954;69:471–472.
241. Zhang Y, Heym B, Allen B, et al. The catalase-peroxidase gene and isoniazid resistance of *Mycobacterium tuberculosis* (see comments). *Nature* 1992;358:591–593.
242. Musser JM, Kapur V, Williams DL, et al. Characterization of the catalase-peroxidase gene (katG) and inhA locus in isoniazid-resistant and -susceptible strains of *Mycobacterium tuberculosis* by automated DNA sequencing: restricted array of mutations associated with drug resistance. *J Infect Dis* 1996;173:196–202.
243. Lee AS, Tang LL, Lim IH, et al. Lack of clinical significance for the common arginine-to-leucine substitution at codon 463 of the katG gene in isoniazid-resistant *Mycobacterium tuberculosis* in Singapore. *J Infect Dis* 1997;176:1125–1127.
244. van Doorn HR, Kuijper EJ, van der Ende A, et al. The susceptibility of *Mycobacterium tuberculosis* to isoniazid and the Arg→Leu mutation at codon 463 of katG are not associated. *J Clin Microbiol* 2001;39:1591–1594.
245. Haas WH, Schilke K, Brand J, et al. Molecular analysis of katG gene mutations in strains of *Mycobacterium tuberculosis* complex from Africa. *Antimicrob Agents Chemother* 1997;41:1601–1603.
246. Marttila HJ, Soini H, Huovinen P, katG mutations in isoniazid-resistant *Mycobacterium tuberculosis* isolates recovered from Finnish patients. *Antimicrob Agents Chemother* 1996;40:2187–2189.
247. Marttila HJ, Soini H, Eerola E, et al. A Ser315Thr substitution in KatG is predominant in genetically heterogeneous multidrug-resistant *Mycobacterium tuberculosis* isolates originating from the St. Petersburg area in Russia. *Antimicrob Agents Chemother* 1998;42:2443–2445.
248. Mokrousov I, Narvskaya O, Otten T, et al. High prevalence of KatG Ser315Thr substitution among isoniazid-resistant *Mycobacterium tuberculosis* clinical isolates from northwestern Russia, 1996 to 2001. *Antimicrob Agents Chemother* 2002;46:1417–1424.
249. Siddiqi N, Shamim M, Hussain S, et al. Molecular characterization of multidrug-resistant isolates of *Mycobacterium tuberculosis* from patients in North India. *Antimicrob Agents Chemother* 2002;46:443–450.
250. Bakonyte D, Baranauskaite A, Cicenaite J, et al. Molecular characterization of isoniazid-resistant *Mycobacterium tuberculosis* clinical isolates in Lithuania. *Antimicrob Agents Chemother* 2003;47:2009–2011.
251. Ramaswamy SV, Reich R, Dou SJ, et al. Single nucleotide polymorphisms in genes associated with isoniazid resistance in *Mycobacterium tuberculosis. Antimicrob Agents Chemother* 2003;47:1241–1250.
252. Wu X, Zhang J, Zhuang Y, et al. Molecular mechanisms of drug resistance in *Mycobacterium tuberculosis* clinical isolates. *Chin Med J (Engl)* 1999;112:524–528.
253. Abate G, Hoffner SE, Thomsen VO, et al. Characterization of isoniazid-resistant strains of *Mycobacterium tuberculosis* on the basis of phenotypic properties and mutations in katG. *Eur J Clin Microbiol Infect Dis* 2001;20:329–333.
254. Ahmad S, Fares E, Araj GF, et al. Prevalence of S315T mutation within the katG gene in isoniazid-resistant clinical *Mycobacterium tuberculosis* isolates from Dubai and Beirut. *Int J Tuberc Lung Dis* 2002;6:920–926.
255. Torres MJ, Criado A, Gonzalez N, et al. Rifampin and isoniazid resistance associated mutations in *Mycobacterium tuberculosis* clinical isolates in Seville, Spain [comment]. *Int J Tuberc Lung Dis* 2002;6:160–163.
256. Telenti A, Honore N, Bernasconi C, et al. Genotypic assessment of isoniazid and rifampin resistance in *Mycobacterium tuberculosis*: a blind study at reference laboratory level. *J Clin Microbiol* 1997;35:719–723.
257. Van Rie A, Warren R, Mshanga I, et al. Analysis for a limited number of gene codons can predict drug resistance of *Mycobacterium tuberculosis* in a high-incidence community. *J Clin Microbiol* 2001;39:636–641.
258. Tracevska T, Jansone I, Broka L, et al. Mutations in the rpoB and katG genes leading to drug resistance in *Mycobacterium tuberculosis* in Latvia. *J Clin Microbiol* 2002;40:3789–3792.
259. Cingolani A, Antinori A, Sanguinetti M, et al. Application of molecular methods for detection and transmission analysis of *Mycobacterium tuberculosis* drug resistance in patients attending a reference hospital in Italy [comment]. *J Infect Dis* 1999;179:1025–1029.
260. van Soolingen D, de Haas PE, van Doorn HR, et al. Mutations at amino acid position 315 of the katG gene are associated with high-level resistance to isoniazid, other drug resistance, and successful transmission of *Mycobacterium tuberculosis* in the Netherlands. *J Infect Dis* 2000; 182:1788–1790.
261. Imwidthaya P, Mieskes K, Rienthong S. Evaluation of katG codon 315 mutations among isoniazid sensitive and resistant *Mycobacterium tuberculosis* isolates from Thailand. *J Med Assoc Thai* 2001;84:864–869.
262. Abal AT, Ahmad S, Mokaddas E. Variations in the occurrence of the S315T mutation within the katG gene

in isoniazid-resistant clinical *Mycobacterium tuberculosis* isolates from Kuwait. *Microb Drug Resist* 2002;8:99–105.

263. Viader-Salvado JM, Luna-Aguirre CM, Reyes-Ruiz JM, et al. Frequency of mutations in rpoB and codons 315 and 463 of katG in rifampin- and/or isoniazid-resistant *Mycobacterium tuberculosis* isolates from northeast Mexico. *Microb Drug Resist* 2003;9:33–38.
264. Escalante P, Ramaswamy S, Sanabria H, et al. Genotypic characterization of drug-resistant *Mycobacterium tuberculosis* isolates from Peru. *Tuberc Lung Dis* 1998;79:111–118.
265. Gonzalez N, Torres MJ, Aznar J, et al. Molecular analysis of rifampin and isoniazid resistance of *Mycobacterium tuberculosis* clinical isolates in Seville, Spain. *Tuberc Lung Dis* 1999;79:187–190.
266. Kiepiela P, Bishop KS, Smith AN, et al. Genomic mutations in the katG, inhA and aphC genes are useful for the prediction of isoniazid resistance in *Mycobacterium tuberculosis* isolates from Kwazulu Natal, South Africa. *Tuberc Lung Dis* 2000;80:47–56.
267. Sreevatsan S, Pan X, Zhang Y, et al. Analysis of the oxyR-ahpC region in isoniazid-resistant and -susceptible *Mycobacterium tuberculosis* complex organisms recovered from diseased humans and animals in diverse localities. *Antimicrob Agents Chemother* 1997;41:600–606.
268. Wilson TM, Collins DM. ahpC, a gene involved in isoniazid resistance of the *Mycobacterium tuberculosis* complex. *Mol Microbiol* 1996;19:1025–1034.
269. Morris S, Bai GH, Suffys P, et al. Molecular mechanisms of multiple drug resistance in clinical isolates of *Mycobacterium tuberculosis*. *J Infect Dis* 1995;171:954–960.
270. Zhang Y, Young D. Molecular genetics of drug resistance in *Mycobacterium tuberculosis*. *J Antimicrob Chemother* 1994;34:313–319.
271. Basso LA, Zheng R, Musser JM, et al. Mechanisms of isoniazid resistance in *Mycobacterium tuberculosis*: enzymatic characterization of enoyl reductase mutants identified in isoniazid-resistant clinical isolates. *J Infect Dis* 1998;178:769–775.
272. Heym B, Alzari PM, Honore N, et al. Missense mutations in the catalase-peroxidase gene, katG are associated with isonaizid resistance in *Mycobacterium tuberculosis*. *Mol Microbiol* 1995;15:235–245.
273. Wilson TM, Lisle D, Collins DM. Effect of inhA and katG on isoniazid resistance and virulence of *Mycobacterium bovis*. *Mol Microbiol* 1995;15:1009–1015.
274. Banerjee A, Sugantino M, Sacchettini JC, et al. The mabA gene from the inhA operon of *Mycobacterium tuberculosis* encodes a 3-ketoacyl reductase that fails to confer isoniazid resistance. *Microbiology* 1998;144:2697–2704.
275. Payton M, Auty R, Delgoda R, et al. Cloning and characterization of arylamine N-acetyltransferase genes from *Mycobacterium smegmatis* and *Mycobacterium tuberculosis:* increased expression results in isoniazid resistance. *J Bacteriol* 1999;181:1343–1347.
276. Upton AM, Mushtaq A, Victor TC, et al. Arylamine N-acetyltransferase of *Mycobacterium tuberculosis* is a polymorphic enzyme and a site of isoniazid metabolism. *Mol Microbiol* 2001;42:309–317.
277. Viveiros M, Portugal I, Bettencourt R, et al. Isoniazid-induced transient high-level resistance in *Mycobacterium tuberculosis*. *Antimicrob Agents Chemother* 2002;46:2804–2810.
278. Choudhuri BS, Sen S, Chakrabarti P. Isoniazid accumulation in *Mycobacterium smegmatis* is modulated by proton motive force-driven and ATP-dependent extrusion systems. *Biochem Biophys Res Commun* 1999;256:682–684.
279. Levin ME, Hatfull GF. *Mycobacterium smegmatis* RNA polymerase: DNA supercoiling, action of rifampicin and mechanism of rifampicin resistance. *Mol Microbiol* 1993;8:277–285.
280. Bastian I, Stapledon R, Colebunders R. Current thinking on the management of tuberculosis. *Curr Opin Pulm Med* 2003;9:186–192.
281. Farmer P. DOTS and DOTS-plus: not the only answer. *Ann NY Acad Sci* 2001;953:165–184.
282. Frieden TR, Sterling TR, Munsiff SS, et al. Tuberculosis. *Lancet* 2003;362:887–899.
283. Hui J, Gordon N, Kajioka R. Permeability barrier to rifampin in mycobacteria. *Antimicrob Agents Chemother* 1977;11:773–779.
284. Fuji K, Saito H, Tomioka H, et al. Mechanism of action of antimycobacterial activity of the new benzoxazinorifamycin KRM-1648. *Antimicrob Agents Chemother* 1995;39:1489–1492.
285. Roehr B. FDA approves rifapentine for the treatment of pulmonary tuberculosis.... Food and Drug Administration. *J Int Assoc Physicians AIDS Care* 1998;4:19–25.
286. Bemer-Melchior P, Bryskier A, Drugeon HB. Comparison of the in vitro activities of rifapentine and rifampicin against *Mycobacterium tuberculosis* complex. *J Antimicrob Chemother* 2000;46:571–576.
287. Rastogi N, Goh KS, Berchel M, et al. Activity of rifapentine and its metabolite 25-O-desacetylrifapentine compared with rifampicin and rifabutin against *Mycobacterium tuberculosis, Mycobacterium africanum, Mycobacterium bovis* and *M. bovis* BCG. *J Antimicrob Chemother* 2000;46:565–570.
288. Conte JE Jr, Golden JA, McQuitty M, et al. Single-dose intrapulmonary pharmacokinetics of rifapentine in normal subjects. *Antimicrob Agents Chemother* 2000;44:985–990.
289. Burman WJ, Gallicano K, Peloquin C. Comparative pharmacokinetics and pharmacodynamics of the rifamycin antibacterials. *Clin Pharmacokinet* 2001;40:327–341.
290. Keung A, Eller MG, McKenzie KA, et al. Single and multiple dose pharmacokinetics of rifapentine in man: part II. *Int J Tuberc Lung Dis* 1999;3:437–444.
291. Keung AC, Owens RC Jr, Eller MG, et al. Pharmacokinetics of rifapentine in subjects seropositive for the human immunodeficiency virus: a phase I study. *Antimicrob Agents Chemother* 1999;43:1230–1233.
292. Temple ME, Nahata MC. Rifapentine: its role in the treatment of tuberculosis. *Ann Pharmacother* 1999;33:1203–1210.
293. Tam CM, Chan SL, Kam KM, et al. Rifapentine and isoniazid in the continuation phase of a 6-month regimen. Final report at 5 years: prognostic value of various measures [comment]. *Int J Tuberc Lung Dis* 2002;6:3–10.
294. Benator D, Bhattacharya M, Bozeman L, et al. Rifapentine and isoniazid once a week versus rifampicin and isoniazid twice a week for treatment of drug-susceptible pulmonary tuberculosis in HIV-negative patients: a randomised clinical trial. *Lancet* 2002;360:528–534.
295. Inderlied CB. Antimycobacterial susceptibility testing: present practices and future trends. *Eur J Clin Micrbiol Infect Dis* 1994;13:980–993.
296. Masur H. Recommendations on prophylaxis and therapy for disseminated *Mycobacterium avium* complex disease in patients infected with the human-immunodeficiency-virus. *N Engl J Med* 1993;329:898–904.
297. Nightingale SD, Cameron WD, Gordin FM, et al. Two controlled trials of rifabutin prophylaxis against *Mycobacterium avium* complex infection in AIDS. *N Engl J Med* 1993;329:828–833.

298. Bermudez LE, Young LS, Inderlied CB. Rifabutin and sparfloxacin but not azithromycin inhibit binding of *Mycobacterium avium* complex to HT-29 intestinal mucosal cells. *Antimicrob Agents Chemother* 1994;38:1200–1202.
299. Hirata T, Saito H, Tomioka H, et al. In vitro and in vivo activities of the benzoxazinorifamycin KRM-1648 against *Mycobacterium tuberculosis. Antimicrob Agents Chemother* 1995;39:2295–2303.
300. Luna-Herrera J, Reddy MV, Gangadharam PR. In vitro activity of the benzoxazinorifamycin KRM-1648 against drug-susceptible and multidrug-resistant tubercle bacilli. *Antimicrob Agents Chemother* 1995;39:440–444.
301. Mor N, Simon B, Heifets L. Bacteriostatic and bactericidal activities of benzoxazinorifamycin KRM-1648 against *Mycobacterium tuberculosis* and *Mycobacterium avium* in human macrophages. *Antimicrob Agents Chemother* 1996;40:1482–1485.
302. Yamamoto T, Amitani R, Suzuki K, et al. In vitro bactericidal and in vivo therapeutic activities of a new rifamycin derivative, KRM-1648, against *Mycobacterium tuberculosis. Antimicrob Agents Chemother* 1996;40:426–428.
303. Inderlied CB, Barbara B-L, Wu M, et al. Activities of the benzoxazinorifamycin KRM 1648 and ethambutol against *Mycobacterium avium* complex in vitro and in macrophages. *Antimicrob Agents Chemother* 1994;38:1838–1843.
304. Tomioka H, Saito H, Fujii K, et al. In vitro antimicrobial activity of benzoxazinorifamycin, KRM-1648, against *Mycobacterium avium* complex, determined by the radiometric method. *Antimicrob Agents Chemother* 1993;37:67–70.
305. Klemens SP, Cynamon MH. Activity of KRM-1648 in combination with isoniazid against *Mycobacterium tuberculosis* in a murine model. *Antimicrob Agents Chemother* 1996;40:298–301.
306. Reddy MV, Luna-Herrera J, Daneluzzi D, et al. Chemotherapeutic activity of benzoxazinorifamycin, KRM-1648, against *Mycobacterium tuberculosis* in C57BL/6 mice. *Tuber Lung Dis* 1996;77:154–159.
307. Shoen CM, Chase SE, DeStefano MS, et al. Evaluation of rifalazil in long-term treatment regimens for tuberculosis in mice. *Antimicrob Agents Chemother* 2000;44:1458–1462.
308. Emori M, Saito H, Sato K, et al. Therapeutic efficacy of the benzoxazinorifamycin KRM-1648 against experimental *Mycobacterium avium* infection induced in rabbits. *Antimicrob Agents Chemother* 1993;37:722–728.
309. Hosoe K, Mae T, Konishi E, et al. Pharmacokinetics of KRM-1648, a new benzoxazinorifamycin, in rats and dogs. *Antimicrob Agents Chemother* 1996;40:2749–2755.
310. Mae T, Inaba T, Konishi E, et al. Identification of enzymes responsible for rifalazil metabolism in human liver microsomes. *Xenobiotica* 2000;30:565–574.
311. Mae T, Hosoe K, Fujii K, et al. In vitro metabolism of a rifamycin derivative by animal and human liver microsomes, whole blood and expressed human CYP3A isoform. *Xenobiotica* 1996;26:793–802.
312. Korzheva N, Mustaev A, Kozlov M, et al. A structural model of transcription elongation. *Science* 2000;289:619–625.
313. Campbell EA, Korzheva N, Mustaev A, et al. Structural mechanism for rifampicin inhibition of bacterial rna polymerase. *Cell* 2001;104:901–912.
314. Heep M, Brandstatter B, Rieger U, et al. Frequency of rpoB mutations inside and outside the cluster I region in rifampin-resistant clinical *Mycobacterium tuberculosis* isolates. *J Clin Microbiol* 2001;39:107–110.
315. Morlock GP, Plikaytis BB, Crawford JT. Characterization of spontaneous, In vitro-selected, rifampin-resistant mutants of *Mycobacterium tuberculosis* strain H37Rv. *Antimicrob Agents Chemother* 2000;44:3298–3301.
316. Billington OJ, McHugh TD, Gillespie SH. Physiological cost of rifampin resistance induced in vitro in *Mycobacterium tuberculosis. Antimicrob Agents Chemother* 1999;43:1866–1869.
317. Moghazeh SL, Pan X, Arain T, et al. Comparative antimycobacterial activities of rifampin, rifapentine, and KRM-1648 against a collection of rifampin-resistant *Mycobacterium tuberculosis* isolates with known rpoB mutations. *Antimicrob Agents Chemother* 1996;40:2655–2657.
318. Williams DL, Spring L, Collins L, et al. Contribution of rpoB mutations to development of rifamycin cross-resistance in *Mycobacterium tuberculosis. Antimicrob Agents Chemother* 1998;42:1853–1857.
319. Yang B, Koga H, Ohno H, et al. Relationship between antimycobacterial activities of rifampicin, rifabutin and KRM-1648 and rpoB mutations of *Mycobacterium tuberculosis. J Antimicrob Chemother* 1998;42:621–628.
320. Park YK, Kim BJ, Ryu S, et al. Cross-resistance between rifampicin and KRM-1648 is associated with specific rpoB alleles in *Mycobacterium tuberculosis. Int J Tuberc Lung Dis* 2002;6:166–170.
321. Piddock LJ, Williams KJ, Ricci V. Accumulation of rifampicin by *Mycobacterium aurum, Mycobacterium smegmatis* and *Mycobacterium tuberculosis. J Antimicrob Chemother* 2000;45:159–165.
322. Luna-Herrera J, Reddy V, Daneluzzi D, et al. Antituberculosis activity of clarithromycin. *Antimicrob Agents Chemother* 1995;39:2692–2695.
323. Truffot-Pernot C, Lounis N, Grosset JH, et al. Clarithromycin is inactive against *Mycobacterium tuberculosis. Antimicrob Agents Chemother* 1995;39:2827–2828.
324. Rastogi N, Goh KS, Bryskier A. Activities of roxithromycin used alone and in combination with ethambutol, rifampin, amikacin, ofloxacin, and clofazimine against *Mycobacterium avium* complex. *Antimicrob Agents Chemother* 1994;38:1433–1438.
325. Bonnet M, Van de Auwera P. In vitro and in vivo intraleukocytic accumulation of azithromycin (CP-62, 993) and its influence on ex vivo leukocyte chemiluminescence. *Antimicrob Agents Chemother* 1992;36:1302–1309.
326. Costa P, Desclaux d-F, Gouby A, et al. Disposition of roxithromycin in the epididymis after repeated oral administration. *J Antimicrob Chemother* 1992;30:197–201.
327. Fraschini F, Scaglione F, Pintucci G, et al. The diffusion of clarithromycin and roxithromycin into nasal mucosa, tonsil and lung in humans. *J Antimicrob Chemother* 1991;27(Suppl A):61–65.
328. Nilsen OG. Pharmacokinetics of macrolides. Comparison of plasma, tissue and free concentrations with special reference to roxithromycin. *Infection* 1995;23 (Suppl)1:S5–S9.
329. Zhanel GG, Walters M, Noreddin A, et al. The ketolides: a critical review. *Drugs* 2002;62:1771–1804.
330. Douthwaite S, Champney WS. Structures of ketolides and macrolides determine their mode of interaction with the ribosomal target site. *J Antimicrob Chemother* 2001;48:1–8.
331. Leclercq R. Overcoming antimicrobial resistance: profile of a new ketolide antibacterial, telithromycin. *J Antimicrob Chemother* 2001;48:9–23.
332. Rosato A, Vicarini H, Bonnefoy A, et al. A New Ketolide, HMR 3004, Active against streptococci inducibly resistant to erythromycin. *Antimicrob Agents Chemother* 1998;42:1392–1396.
333. Capobianco JO, Cao Z, Shortridge VD, et al. Studies of the

novel ketolide ABT-773: transport, binding to ribosomes, and inhibition of protein synthesis in *Streptococcus pneumoniae*. *Antimicrob Agents Chemother* 2000;44:1562–1567.

334. Yang SC, Hsueh PR, Lai HC, et al. High prevalence of antimicrobial resistance in rapidly growing mycobacteria in Taiwan. *Antimicrob Agents Chemother* 2003;47:1958–1962.
335. Rastogi N, Goh KS, Berchel M, et al. In vitro activities of the ketolides telithromycin (HMR 3647) and HMR 3004 compared to those of clarithromycin against slowly growing mycobacteria at pHs 6.8 AND 7.4. *Antimicrob Agents Chemother* 2000;44:2848–2852.
336. Fernandez-Roblas R, Esteban J, Cabria F, et al. In vitro susceptibilities of rapidly growing mycobacteria to telithromycin (HMR 3647) and seven other antimicrobials. *Antimicrob Agents Chemother* 2000;44:181–182.
337. Cynamon MH, Carter JL, Shoen CM. Activity of ABT-773 against *Mycobacterium* avium complex in the beige mouse model. *Antimicrob Agents Chemother* 2000;44:2895–2896.
338. Consigny S, Bentoucha A, Bonnafous P, et al. Bactericidal activities of HMR 3647, moxifloxacin, and rifapentine against *Mycobacterium leprae* in mice. *Antimicrob Agents Chemother* 2000;44:2919–2921.
339. Bermudez LE, Inderlied CB, Kolonoski P, et al. Telithromycin is active against *Mycobacterium avium* in mice despite lacking significant activity in standard in vitro and macrophage assays and is associated with low frequency of resistance during treatment. *Antimicrob Agents Chemother* 2001;45:2210–2214.
340. Douthwaite S, Aagaard C. Erythromycin binding is reduced in ribosomes with conformational alterations in the 23 S rRNA peptidyl transferase loop. *J Mol Biol* 1993;232:725–731.
341. Zhanel GG, Dueck M, Hoban DJ, et al. Review of macrolides and ketolides: focus on respiratory tract infections. *Drugs* 2001;61:443–498.
342. Weisblum B. Erythromycin resistance by ribosome modification. *Antimicrob Agents Chemother* 1995;39:577–585.
343. Roberts MC, Sutcliffe J, Courvalin P, et al. Nomenclature for macrolide and macrolide-lincosamide-streptogramin B resistance determinants. *Antimicrob Agents Chemother* 1999;43:2823–2830.
344. Meier A, Kirschner P, Springer B, et al. Identification of mutations in 23S rRNA gene of clarithromycin-resistant *Mycobacterium intracellulare*. *Antimicrob Agents Chemother* 1994;38:381–384.
345. Nash KA, Inderlied CB. Genetic basis of macrolide resistance in *Mycobacterium avium*. *Antimicrob Agents Chemother* 1995;39:2625–2630.
346. Doucet-Populaire F, Capobianco JO, Zakula D, et al. Molecular basis of clarithromycin activity against *Mycobacterium avium* and *Mycobacterium smegmatis*. *J Antimicrob Chemother* 1998;41:179–187.
347. Debets-Ossenkopp YJ, Sparrius M, Kusters JG. Mechanism of clarithromycin resistance in clinical isolates of *Helicobacter pylori*. *FEMS Microbiol Lett* 1996;142:37–42.
348. Stone GG, Shortridge D, Flamm RK, et al. Identification of a 23S rRNA gene mutation in clarithromycin-resistant *Helicobacter pylori*. *Helicobacter* 1996;1:227–228.
349. Versalovic J, Shortridge D, Kibler K, et al. Mutations in 23S rRNA are associated with clarithromycin resistance in *Helicobacter pylori*. *Antimicrob Agents Chemother* 1996;40:477–480.
350. Buriankova K, Doucet-Populaire F, Dorson O, et al. Molecular basis of intrinsic macrolide resistance in the *Mycobacterium tuberculosis* complex. *Antimicrob Agents Chemother* 2004;48:143–150.
351. Andini N, Nash KA. Species distribution, functional characterization, and expression analysis of erm(37), a macrolide-resistance determinant of the *M. tuberculosis* complex. In: *Proceedings of the 104th General Meeting of the American Society for Microbiology*. Washington, DC: American Society for Microbiology, 2004.
352. Nash KA. Mycobacterial factors that effect susceptibility to macrolides. In: *Proceedings of the 103rd General Meeting of the American Society for Microbiology*. Washington, DC: American Society for Microbiology, 2003.
353. Rhienberger H-J, Giegenmuller U, Gnirke A, et al. Allosteric three-site model for the ribosomal elongation cycle. In: Hill WE, Dahlberg A, Garrett RA, et al. eds. *The ribosome: structure, function and evolution*. Washington, DC: American Society for Microbiology, 1990:318–330.
354. Shaila MS, Gopinathan KP, Ramakrishnan T. Protein synthesis in *Mycobacterium tuberculosis* H37Rv and the effect of streptomycin in streptomycin-susceptible and -resistant strains. *Antimicrob Agents Chemother* 1971;4:205–213.
355. Yamada T, Nagata A, Ono Y, et al. Alteration of ribosomes and RNA polymerase in drug-resistant clinical isolates of *Mycobacterium tuberculosis*. *Antimicrob Agents Chemother* 1985;27:921–924.
356. Yamada T. The role of ribosomes in the sensitivity of mycobacteria to tuberactinomycin. *Microbiol Immunol* 1987;31:179–181.
357. Verbist L, Gyselen A. Capreomycin susceptibility of strains resistant to streptomycin and/or viomycin. *Am Rev Respir Dis* 1964;90:640–641.
358. Böttger EC. Resistance to drugs targeting protein synthesis in mycobacteria. *Trends Microbiol* 1994;2:416–421.
359. Dubovsky H. Correspondence with a pioneer, Jurgen Lehmann (1898–1989), producer of the first effective antituberculosis specific. *S Afr Med J* 1991;79:48–50.
360. Hausner T-P, Geigenmuller U, Nierhaus KH. The allosteric three-site model for the ribosomal elongation cycle. *J Biol Chem* 1988;263:13103–13111.
361. Yamada T, Masuda K, Shoji K, et al. Analysis of ribosomes from viomycin-sensitive and -resistant strains of *Mycobacterium smegmatis*. *J Bacteriol* 1972;112:1–6.
362. Yamada T, Mizugichi Y, Nierhaus KH, et al. Resistance to viomycin conferred by RNA of either ribosomal subunit. *Nature* 1978;275:460–461.
363. Choi EC, Misumi M, Nishimura T, et al. Viomycin resistance: alterations of either ribosomal subunit affect the binding of the antibiotic to the pair subunit and the entire ribosome becomes resistant to the drug. *Biochem Biophys Res Commun* 1979;87:904–910.
364. Mizuguchi Y, Suga K, Yamada T. Interaction between 30S ribosomal components in a viomycin resistant mutant of *Mycobacterium smegmatis*. *Microbiol Immunol* 1979;23:595–604.
365. Mizuguchi Y, Suga K, Yamada T. Interactions between viomycin resistance and streptomycin resistance on ribosomes of *Mycobacterium smegmatis*. *Microbiol Immunol* 1979;23:581–594.
366. Finken M, Kirschner P, Meier A, et al. Molecular basis of streptomycin resistance in *Mycobacterium tuberculosis:* alterations of the ribosomal protein S12 gene and point mutations within a functional 16S ribosomal RNA pseudoknot. *Mol Microbiol* 1993;9:1239–1246.
367. Nair J, Rouse DA, Bai GH, et al. The rpsL gene and streptomycin resistance in single and multiple drug-resistant strains of *Mycobacterium tuberculosis*. *Mol Microbiol* 1993;10:521–527.

368. Honore N, Cole ST. Streptomycin resistance in mycobacteria. *Antimicrob Agents Chemother* 1994;38:238–242.
369. Meier A, Kirschner P, Bange FC, et al. Genetic alterations in streptomycin-resistant *Mycobacterium tuberculosis*: mapping of mutations conferring resistance. *Antimicrob Agents Chemother* 1994;38:228–233.
370. Prammananan T, Sander P, Brown BA, et al. A single 16S ribosomal RNA substitution is responsible for resistance to amikacin and other 2-deoxystreptamine aminoglycosides in *Mycobacterium abscessus* and *Mycobacterium chelonae*. *J Infect Dis* 1998;177:1573–1581.
371. Kenney TJ, Churchward G. Cloning and sequence analysis of the rpsL and rpsG genes of *Mycobacterium smegmatis* and characterization of mutations causing resistance to streptomycin. *J Bacteriol* 1994;176:6153–6156.
372. Cooksey RC, Morlock GP, McQueen A, et al. Characterization of streptomycin resistance mechanisms among *Mycobacterium tuberculosis* isolates from patients in New York City. *Antimicrob Agents Chemother* 1996;40:1186–1188.
373. Sreevatsan S, Pan X, Stockbauer KE, et al. Characterization of rpsL and rrs mutations in streptomycin-resistant *Mycobacterium tuberculosis* isolates from diverse geographic localities. *Antimicrob Agents Chemother* 1996;40:1024–1026.
374. Springer B, Kidan YG, Prammananan T, et al. Mechanisms of streptomycin resistance: selection of mutations in the 16S rRNA gene conferring resistance. *Antimicrob Agents Chemother* 2001;45:2877–2884.
375. Nachamkin I, Kang C, Weinstein MP. Detection of resistance to isoniazid, rifampin, and streptomycin in clinical isolates of *Mycobacterium tuberculosis* by molecular methods. *Clin Infect Dis* 1997;24:894–900.
376. Brimacombe R, Greuer B, Mitchell P, et al. Three-dimensional structure and function of *Escherichia coli* 16S and 23S rRNA as studied by cross-linking techniques. In: Hill WE, Dahlberg A, Garrett RA, et al. eds. *The ribosome: structure, function and evolution*. Washington, DC: American Society for Microbiology, 1990:73–92.
377. Victor TC, van Rie A, Jordaan AM, et al. Sequence polymorphism in the rrs gene of *Mycobacterium tuberculosis* is deeply rooted within an evolutionary clade and is not associated with streptomycin resistance. *J Clin Microbiol* 2001;39:4184–4186.
378. Meier A, Sander P, Schaper KJ, et al. Correlation of molecular resistance mechanisms and phenotypic resistance levels in streptomycin-resistant *Mycobacterium tuberculosis*. *Antimicrob Agents Chemother* 1996;40:2452–2454.
379. Cundliffe E. Recognition sites for antibiotics within rRNA. In: Hill WE, Dahlberg A, Garrett RA, et al. eds. *The ribosome: structure, function and evolution*. Washington, DC: American Society for Microbiology, 1990:479–490.
380. Shaw KJ, Rather PN, Hare RS, et al. Molecular genetics of aminoglycoside resistance genes and familial relationships of the aminoglycoside-modifying enzymes. *Microbiol Rev* 1993;57:138–163.
381. Hull SI, Wallace RJ Jr, Bobey DG, et al. Presence of aminoglycoside acetyltransferase and plasmids in *Mycobacterium fortuitum*. Lack of correlation with intrinsic aminoglycoside resistance. *Am Rev Respir Dis* 1984;129:614–618.
382. Udou T, Mizuguchi Y, Wallace RJ Jr. Patterns and distribution of aminoglycoside-acetylating enzymes in rapidly growing mycobacteria. *Am Rev Respir Dis* 1987;136:338–343.
383. Wallace RJ Jr, Hull SI, Bobey DG, et al. Mutational resistance as the mechanism of acquired drug resistance to aminoglycosides and antibacterial agents in *Mycobacterium fortuitum* and *Mycobacterium chelonei*. Evidence is based on plasmid analysis, mutational frequencies, and aminoglycoside-modifying enzyme assays. *Am Rev Respir Dis* 1985;132:409–416.
384. Ainsa JA, Perez E, Pelicic V, et al. Aminoglycoside 2′-N-acetyltransferase genes are universally present in mycobacteria: characterization of the aac(2′)-Ic gene from *Mycobacterium tuberculosis* and the aac(2′)-Id gene from *Mycobacterium smegmatis*. *Mol Microbiol* 1997;24:431–441.
385. Kilburn JO, Greenberg J. Effect of ethambutol on the viable cell count in *Mycobacterium smegmatis*. *Antimicrob Agents Chemother* 1977;11:534–540.
386. Takayama K, Armstrong EL, Kunugi KA, et al. Inhibition by ethambutol of mycolic acid transfer into the cell wall of *Mycobacterium smegmatis*. *Antimicrob Agents Chemother* 1979;16:240–242.
387. Poso H, Paulin L, Brander E. Specific inhibition of spermidine synthase from Mycobacteria by ethambutol. *Lancet* 1983;ii:1418.
388. Paulin LG, Brander EE, Poso HJ. Specific inhibition of spermidine synthesis in *Mycobacteria* spp. by the dextro isomer of ethambutol. *Antimicrob Agents Chemother* 1985;28:157–159.
389. Kilburn JO, Takayama K. Effects of ethambutol on accumulation and secretion of trehalose mycolates and free mycolic acid in *Mycobacterium smegmatis*. *Antimicrob Agents Chemother* 1981;20:401–404.
390. Takayama K, Kilburn JO. Inhibition of synthesis of arabinogalactan by ethambutol in *Mycobacterium smegmatis*. *Antimicrob Agents Chemother* 1989;33:1493–1499.
391. Deng L, Mikusova K, Robuck KG, et al. Recognition of multiple effects of ethambutol on metabolism of mycobacterial cell envelope. *Antimicrob Agents Chemother* 1995;39:694–701.
392. Wolucka BA, McNeil MR, de Hoffmann E, et al. Recognition of the lipid intermediate for arabinogalactan/arabinomannan biosynthesis and its relation to the mode of action of ethambutol on mycobacteria. *J Biol Chem* 1994;269:23328–23335.
393. Lee RE, Mikusova K, Brennan PJ, et al. Synthesis of the mycobacterial arabinose donor β-D-arabinofuranosyl-1-monophosphoryldecaprenol, development of a basic arabinosyl-transferase assay, and identification of ethambutol as an arabinosyl transferase inhibitor. *J Am Chem Soc* 1995;117:11829–11832.
394. Hoffner SE, Kallenius G, Beezer AE, et al. Studies on the mechanisms of the synergistic effects of ethambutol and other antibacterial drugs on *Mycobacterium avium* complex. *Acta Leprol* 1989;7 (Suppl. 1):195–199.
395. Rastogi N, Barrow WW. Cell envelope constituents and the multifaceted nature of *Mycobacterium avium* pathogenicity and drug resistance. *Res Microbiol* 1993;145:243–252.
396. Belanger AE, Besra GS, Ford ME, et al. The embAB genes of *Mycobacterium avium* encode an arabinosyl transferase involved in cell wall arabinan biosynthesis that is the target for the antimycobacterial drug ethambutol. *Proc Natl Acad Sci USA* 1996;93:11919–11924.
397. Telenti A, Philipp WJ, Sreevatsan S, et al. The emb operon, a gene cluster of *Mycobacterium tuberculosis* involved in resistance to ethambutol. *Nature Med* 1997;3:567–570.
398. Sreevatsan S, Stockbauer KE, Pan X, et al. Ethambutol resistance in *Mycobacterium tuberculosis*: critical role of embB mutations. *Antimicrob Agents Chemother* 1997;41:1677–1681.
399. Ramaswamy SV, Amin AG, Goksel S, et al. Molecular genetic analysis of nucleotide polymorphisms associated with

ethambutol resistance in human isolates of *Mycobacterium tuberculosis*. *Antimicrob Agents Chemother* 2000;44:326–336.

400. Alcaide F, Pfyffer GE, Telenti A. Role of embB in natural and acquired resistance to ethambutol in mycobacteria. *Antimicrob Agents Chemother* 1997;41:2270–2273.
401. Mokrousov I, Otten T, Vyshnevskiy B, et al. Detection of embB306 mutations in ethambutol-susceptible clinical isolates of *Mycobacterium tuberculosis* from Northwestern Russia: implications for genotypic resistance testing. *J Clin Microbiol* 2002;40:3810–3813.
402. Tsukamura M. Resistance pattern of *Mycobacterium tuberculosis* and *Mycobacterium bovis* to ethambutol. *Acta Tuberc Scand* 1965;46:89–92.
403. Heifets LB, Iseman MD, Crowle AJ, et al. Pyrazinamide is not active in vitro against *Mycobacterium avium* complex. *Am Rev Respir Dis* 1986;134:1287–1288.
404. Lowrie DD. The macrophage and mycobacterial infections. *Trans R Soc Trop Med Hyg* 1983;77:646–655.
405. Scorpio A, Zhang Y. Mutations in pncA, a gene encoding pyrazinamidase/nicotinamidase, cause resistance to the antituberculous drug pyrazinamide in tubercle bacillus. *Nature Med* 1996;2:662–667.
406. Tarnok I, Pechmann H, Krallmann-Wenzel U, et al. Nikotinamidase und die sogenannte Pyrazinamidase in Mycobakterien; gekoppeltes Auftreten der beiden Enzymaktivitaten. *Zentralbl Bakteriol [Orig A]* 1979;244:302–308.
407. Speirs RJ, Welch JT, Cynamon MH. Activity of *n*-propyl pyrazinoate against pyrazinamide-resistant *Mycobacterium tuberculosis:* investigations into mechanism of action of and mechanism of resistance to pyrazinamide. *Antimicrob Agents Chemother* 1995;39:1269–1271.
408. Zhang Y, Scorpio A, Nikaido H, et al. Role of acid pH and deficient efflux of pyrazinoic acid in unique susceptibility of *Mycobacterium tuberculosis* to pyrazinamide. *J Bacteriol* 1999;181:2044–2049.
409. Zhang Y, Wade MM, Scorpio A, et al. Mode of action of pyrazinamide: disruption of *Mycobacterium tuberculosis* membrane transport and energetics by pyrazinoic acid. *J Antimicrob Chemother* 2003;52:790–795.
410. Scorpio A, Collins D, Whipple D, et al. Rapid differentiation of bovine and human tubercle bacilli based on a characteristic mutation in the bovine pyrazinamidase gene. *J Clin Microbiol* 1997;35:106–110.
411. Berning SE. The role of fluoroquinolones in tuberculosis today. *Drugs* 2001;61:9–18.
412. Rastogi N, Goh KS, Bryskier A, et al. In vitro activities of levofloxacin used alone and in combination with first- and second-line antituberculous drugs against *Mycobacterium tuberculosis*. *Antimicrob Agents Chemother* 1996;40:1610–1616.
413. Rastogi N, Goh KS, Bryskier A, et al. Spectrum of activity of levofloxacin against nontuberculous mycobacteria and its activity against the *Mycobacterium avium* complex in combination with ethambutol, rifampin, roxithromycin, amikacin, and clofazimine. *Antimicrob Agents Chemother* 1996;40:2483–2487.
414. Rastogi N, Labrousse V, Goh KS, et al. Antimycobacterial spectrum of sparfloxacin and its activities alone and in association with other drugs against *Mycobacterium avium* complex growing extracellularly and intracellularly in murine and human macrophages. *Antimicrob Agents Chemother* 1991;35:2473–2480.
415. Zhanel GG, Noreddin AM. Pharmacokinetics and pharmacodynamics of the new fluoroquinolones: focus on respiratory infections. *Curr Opin Pharmacol* 2001;1:459–463.
416. Kennedy N, Fox R, Kisyombe GM, et al. Early bactericidal and sterilizing activities of ciprofloxacin in pulmonary tuberculosis. *Am Rev Respir Dis* 1993;148:1547–1551.
417. Peloquin CA, Berning SE, Huitt GA, et al. Levofloxacin for drug-resistant *Mycobacterium tuberculosis*. *Ann Pharmacother* 1998;32:268–269.
418. Gozalbes R, Brun-Pascaud M, Garcia-Domenech R, et al. Prediction of quinolone activity against *Mycobacterium avium* by molecular topology and virtual computational screening. *Antimicrob Agents Chemother* 2000;44:2764–2770.
419. Hu Y, Coates AR, Mitchison DA. Sterilizing activities of fluoroquinolones against rifampin-tolerant populations of *Mycobacterium tuberculosis*. *Antimicrob Agents Chemother* 2003;47:653–657.
420. Gillespie SH, Billington O. Activity of moxifloxacin against mycobacteria. *J Antimicrob Chemother* 1999;44:393–395.
421. Gillespie SH, Morrissey I, Everett D. A comparison of the bactericidal activity of quinolone antibiotics in a *Mycobacterium fortuitum* model. *J Med Microbiol* 2001;50:565–570.
422. Rodriguez JC, Ruiz M, Climent A, et al. In vitro activity of four fluoroquinolones against *Mycobacterium tuberculosis*. *Int J Antimicrob Agents* 2001;17:229–231.
423. Ruiz-Serrano MJ, Alcala L, Martinez L, et al. In vitro activities of six fluoroquinolones against 250 clinical isolates of *Mycobacterium tuberculosis* susceptible or resistant to first-line antituberculosis drugs. *Antimicrob Agents Chemother* 2000;44:2567–2568.
424. Cambau E, Sougakoff W, Besson M, et al. Selection of a gyrA mutant of *Mycobacterium tuberculosis* resistant to fluoroquinolones during treatment with ofloxacin. *J Infect Dis* 1994;170:479–483.
425. Cambau E, Sougakoff W, Jarlier V. Amplification and nucleotide sequence of the quinolone resistance-determining region in the gyrA gene of mycobacteria. *FEMS Microbiol Lett* 1994;116:49–54.
426. Revel V, Cambau E, Jarlier V, et al. Characterization of mutations in *Mycobacterium smegmatis* involved in resistance to fluoroquinolones. *Antimicrob Agents Chemother* 1994;38:1991–1996.
427. Takiff HE, Salazar L, Guerrero C, et al. Cloning and nucleotide sequence of *Mycobacterium tuberculosis* gyrA and gyrB genes and detection of quinolone resistance mutations. *Antimicrob Agents Chemother* 1994;38:773–780.
428. Guillemin I, Jarlier V, Cambau E. Correlation between quinolone susceptibility patterns and sequences in the A and B subunits of DNA gyrase in mycobacteria. *Antimicrob Agents Chemother* 1998;42:2084–2088.
429. Kocagoz T, Hackbarth CJ, Unsal I, et al. Gyrase mutations in laboratory-selected, fluoroquinolone-resistant mutants of *Mycobacterium tuberculosis* H37Ra. *Antimicrob Agents Chemother* 1996;40:1768–1774.
430. Lee AS, Tang LL, Lim IH, et al. Characterization of pyrazinamide and ofloxacin resistance among drug resistant *Mycobacterium tuberculosis* isolates from Singapore. *Int J Infect Dis* 2002;6:48–51.
431. Howard BM, Pinney RJ, Smith JT. Function of the SOS process in repair of DNA damage induced by modern 4-quinolones. *J Pharm Pharmacol* 1993;45:658–662.
432. Aeschlimann JR. The role of multidrug efflux pumps in the antibiotic resistance of *Pseudomonas aeruginosa* and other gram-negative bacteria. Insights from the Society of Infectious Diseases Pharmacists. *Pharmacotherapy* 2003;23:916–924.
433. Sander P, De Rossi E, Boddinghaus B, et al. Contribution of the multidrug efflux pump LfrA to innate mycobacterial drug resistance. *FEMS Microbiol Lett* 2000;193:19–23.

434. Liu J, Takiff HE, Nikaido H. Active efflux of fluoroquinolones in *Mycobacterium smegmatis* mediated by LfrA, a multidrug efflux pump. *J Bacteriol* 1996;178:3791–3795.
435. Takiff HE, Cimino M, Musso MC, et al. Efflux pump of the proton antiporter family confers low-level fluoroquinolone resistance in *Mycobacterium smegmatis*. *Proc Natl Acad Sci USA* 1996;93:362–326.
436. Brickner SJ, Hutchinson DK, Barbachyn MR, et al. Synthesis and antibacterial activity of U-100592 and U-100766, two oxazolidinone antibacterial agents for the potential treatment of multidrug-resistant gram-positive bacterial infections. *J Med Chem* 1996;39:673–679.
437. Rodriguez Diaz JC, Ruiz M, Lopez M, et al. Synergic activity of fluoroquinolones and linezolid against *Mycobacterium tuberculosis*. *Int J Antimicrob Agents* 2003;21:354–356.
438. Cynamon MH, Klemens SP, Sharpe CA, et al. Activities of several novel oxazolidinones against *Mycobacterium tuberculosis* in a murine model. *Antimicrob Agents Chemother* 1999;43:1189–1191.
439. Brown-Elliott BA, Wallace RJ Jr, Blinkhorn R, et al. Successful treatment of disseminated *Mycobacterium chelonae* infection with linezolid. *Clin Infect Dis* 2001;33:1433–1434.
440. Aoki H, Ke L, Poppe SM, et al. Oxazolidinone antibiotics target the p site on *Escherichia coli* ribosomes. *Antimicrob Agents Chemother* 2002;46:1080–1085.
441. Colca JR, McDonald WG, Waldon DJ, et al. Cross-linking in the living cell locates the site of action of oxazolidinone antibiotics. *J Biol Chem* 2003;278:21972–21979.
442. Patel U, Yan YP, Hobbs FW Jr, et al. Oxazolidinones mechanism of action: inhibition of the first peptide bond formation. *J Biol Chem* 2001;276:37199–37205.
443. Livermore DM. Linezolid in vitro: mechanism and antibacterial spectrum. *J Antimicrob Chemother* 2003;51:ii9–ii16.
444. Kloss P, Xiong L, Shinabarger DL, et al. Resistance mutations in 23 S rRNA identify the site of action of the protein synthesis inhibitor linezolid in the ribosomal peptidyl transferase center. *J Mol Biol* 1999;294:93–101.
445. Shinabarger DL, Marotti KR, Murray RW, et al. Mechanism of action of oxazolidinones: effects of linezolid and eperezolid on translation reactions. *Antimicrob Agents Chemother* 1997;41:2132–2136.
446. Sander P, Belova L, Kidan YG, et al. Ribosomal and non-ribosomal resistance to oxazolidinones: species-specific idiosyncrasy of ribosomal alterations. *Mol Microbiol* 2002;46:1295–1304.
447. Hedgecock LW. Antagonism of the inhibitory action of aminosalicylic acid on *Mycobacterium tuberculosis* by methionine, biotin and certain fatty acids, amino acids and purines. *J Bacteriol* 1956;72:839–846.
448. Ratledge C, Brown KA. Inhibition of mycobactin formation in *Mycobacterium smegmatis* by p-aminosalicylate. A new proposal for the mode of action of p-aminosalicylate. *Am Rev Respir Dis* 1972;106:774–776.
449. Snow GA. Mycobactins: iron-chelating growth factors from mycobacteria. *Bacteriol Rev* 1970;34:99–125.
450. Brown KA, Ratledge C. The effect of p-aminosalicylic acid on iron transport and assimilation in mycobacteria. *Biochim Biophys Acta* 1975;385:207–220.
451. Brown KA, Ratledge C. Iron transport in *Mycobacterium smegmatis*: ferrimycobactin reductase (NAD(P)H: ferrimycobactin oxidoreductase), the enzyme releasing iron from its carrier. *FEBS Lett* 1975;53:262–266.
452. Kuntz E. Die heutige Bedeutung der PAS fur die Basis-Behandling der Lungentuberkulos. Klinische Ergebnisse bei 20000 iv. PAS-streptomycin-INH infusionen. *Prax Pneumol* 1965;19:610–615.
453. David HL, Takayama K, Goldman DS. Susceptibility of mycobacterial D-alanyl-D-alanine synthetase to D-cycloserine. *Am Rev Respir Dis* 1969;100:579–582.
454. Hawkins JE, McClean VR. Comparative studies of cycloserine inhibition of mycobacteria. *Am Rev Respir Dis* 1966;93:594–602.
455. Zygmunt WA. Antagonism of D-cycloserine inhibition of mycobacterial growth by D-alaine. *J Bacteriol* 1963;85:1217–1220.
456. Caceres NE, Harris NB, Wellehan JF, et al. Overexpression of the D-alanine racemase gene confers resistance to D-cycloserine in *Mycobacterium smegmatis*. *J Bacteriol* 1997;179:5046–5055.
457. Chacon O, Feng Z, Harris NB, et al. *Mycobacterium smegmatis* D-alanine racemase mutants are not dependent on D-alanine for growth. *Antimicrob Agents Chemother* 2002;46:47–54.
458. Peteroy M, Severin A, Zhao F, et al. Characterization of a *Mycobacterium smegmatis* mutant that is simultaneously resistant to D-cycloserine and vancomycin. *Antimicrol Agents Chemother* 2000;44:1701–1704.
459. David HL, Goldman DS, Takayama K. Inhibition of the synthesis of wax D-peptidoglycolipid of *Mycobacterium tuberculosis* by D-cycloserine. *Infect Immun* 1970;1:74–77.
460. Neuhaus FC, Lynch JL. The enzymatic synthesis of D-alanyl-D-alanine. 3. On the inhibition of D-alanyl-D-alanine synthetase by the antibiotic D-cycloserine. *Biochemistry* 1965;3:471–480.
461. Strominger JL, Threnn RH, Scott SS. Oxamycin, a competitive antagonist of the incorporation of D-alanine into a uridine nucleotide in *Staphylococcus aureus*. *J Am Chem Soc* 1959;81:3803–3804.
462. Baulard AR, Betts JC, Engohang-Ndong J, et al. Activation of the pro-drug ethionamide is regulated in mycobacteria. *J Biol Chem* 2000;275:28326–28331.
463. DeBarber AE, Mdluli K, Bosman M, et al. Ethionamide activation and sensitivity in multidrug-resistant *Mycobacterium tuberculosis*. *Proc Natl Acad Sci USA* 2000;97:9677–9682.
464. Vannelli TA, Dykman A, Ortiz de Montellano PR. The antituberculosis drug ethionamide is activated by a flavoprotein monooxygenase. *J Biol Chem* 2002;277:12824–12829.
465. Gordon SM, Horsburgh CR Jr, Peloquin CA, et al. Low serum levels of oral antimycobacterial agents in patients with disseminated *Mycobacterium avium* complex disease. *J Infect Dis* 1993;168:1559–1562.
466. Peloquin CA, MacPhee AA, Berning SE. Malabsorption of antimycobacterial medications. *N Engl J Med* 1993;329:1122–1123.
467. Peloquin CA. Pharmacology of the antimycobacterial drugs. *Med Clin North Am* 1993;77:1253–1262.
468. Holdiness MR. Chromatographic analysis of antituberculosis drugs in biological samples. *J Chromatog* 1985;340:321–359.
469. Holdiness MR. Clinical pharmacokinetics of the antituberculosis drugs. *Clin Pharmacol* 1984;9:511–544.
470. Lunde PKM, Frislid K, Hansteen V. Disease and acetylation polymorphism. *Clin Pharmacokinet* 1977;2:182–197.
471. Gangadharam PRJ. Isoniazid, rifampin, and hepatotoxicity. *Am Rev Respir Dis* 1986;133:963–965.
472. Singapore Tuberculosis Service, Council BMR. Controlled trial of intermittent regimen of rifampicin plus isoniazid for pulmonary tuberculosis in Singapore: the results up to 30 months. *Am Rev Respir Dis* 1977;116:807–820.

473. El-Sayed YM, Islam SI. Acetylation phenotyping of isoniazid using a simple and accurate high-performance liquid chromatography. *J Clin Phar Ther* 1989;14:197–205.
474. Hanson A, Melander A, Wahlin-Boll E. Acetylator phenotyping: a comparison of the isoniazid and dapsone tests. *Eur J Clin Pharmacol* 1981;20:233–234.
475. Hutchings A, Routledge PA. A simple method for determining acetylator phenotype using isoniazid. *Br J Clin Pharmacol* 1986;22:343–345.
476. Guillaumont M, Leclercq M, Forbert Y, et al. Determination of rifampicin, desacetylrifampicin, isoniazid and acetylisoniazid by high-performance liquid chromatography; application to human serum extracts, polymorphonucleocytes and alveolar macrophages. *J Chromatogr* 1982;232:369–376.
477. Holdiness MR. High pressure liquid chromatographic determination of isoniazid and acetyisoniazid in human plasma. *J Liq Chromatogr* 1982;5:707–714.
478. Hutchings A, Monie RD, Spragg B, et al. High performance liquid chromatographic analysis of isoniazid and acetyisoniazid in biological fluids. *J Chromatogr* 1983;227:385–390.
479. Kimerling ME, Phillips P, Patterson P, et al. Low serum antimycobacterial drug levels in non-HIV-infected tuberculosis patients. *Chest* 1998;113:1178–1183.
480. Peloquin CA, Jaresko GS, Yong CL, et al. Population pharmacokinetic modeling of isoniazid, rifampin, and pyrazinamide. *Antimicrob Agents Chemother* 1997;41:2670–2679.
481. Moulin MA, Albessard F, Lacotte J, et al. Hydrophilic ion-pair reversed-phase high- performance liquid chromatography for the simultaneous assay of isoniazid and acetylisoniazid in serum: a microscale procedure. *J Chromatogr* 1981;226:250–254.
482. Saxena SJ, Stewart JT, Honigsberg IL, et al. Liquid chromatography in pharmaceutical analysis. VIII. Determination of isoniazid and acetyl derivative in plasma and urine samples. *J Pharmaceut Sci* 1977;6:813–816.
483. Kenny MT, Strates B. Metabolism and pharmacokinetics of the antibiotic rifampin. *Drug Metab Rev* 1981;12:159–218.
484. Cocchiara G, Benedetti MS, Vicario GP, et al. Urinary metabolites of rifabutin, a new antimycobacterial agent, in human volunteers. *Xenobiotica* 1989;19:769–780.
485. Ratti B, Parenti RR, Toselli A, et al. Quantitative assay of rifampicin and its main metabolite 25-desacetylrifampicin in human plasma by reversed-phase high-performance liquid chromatography. *J Chromatogr* 1981;225:526–531.
486. Ishii M, Ogata H. Determination of rifampicin and its main metabolites in human plasma by high-performance liquid chromatography. *J Chromatogr* 1988;426:412–416.
487. Peets EA, Sweeney WM, Place VA, et al. The absorption, excretion and metabolic fate of ethambutol in man. *Am Rev Respir Dis* 1964;88:51–58.
488. Gundert-Remy U, Klett M, Weber E. Concentration of ethambutol in cerebrospinal fluid in man as a function of the non-protein-bound drug fraction in serum. *Eur J Clin Pharmacol* 1973;6:133–136.
489. Strauss I, Erhardt F. Ethambutol absorbtion, excretion and dosage in patients with renal tuberculosis. *Chemotherapy* 1970;15:148–157.
490. Holdiness MR, Israili ZH, Justice JB. Gas chromatographic-mass spectrophotometric determination of ethambutol in human plasma. *J Chromatogr* 1981;224:415–422.
491. Lee CC, Varughese A. Disposition kinetics of ethambutol in nephrectomized dogs. *J Pharma Sci* 1984;73:787–789.
492. Lee CS, Benet LZ. Gas-liquid chromatographic determination of ethambutol in plasma and urine of man and monkey. *J Chromatogr* 1976;128:188–192.
493. Ohya K, Shintani S, Sano M. Determination of ethambutol in plasma using selected ion monitoring. *J Chromatogr* 1980;221:293–299.
494. Yamamoto T, Moriwaki Y, Takahashi S, et al. Study of the metabolism of pyrazinamide using a high-performance liquid chromatographic analysis of urine samples. *Anal Biochem* 1987;160:346–349.
495. Yamamoto T, Moriwaki Y, Takahashi S, et al. Rapid and simultaneous determination of pyrazinamide and its major metabolites in human plasma by high-performance liquid chromatography. *J Chromatogr* 1987;413:342–346.
496. Woo J, Wong CL, Teoh R, Liquid chromatographic assay for the simultaneous determination of pyrazinamide and rifampicin in serum samples from patients with tuberculous meningitis. *J Chromatogr* 1987;420:73–80.
497. Donald PR, Seifart H. Cerebrospinal fluid pyrazinamide de concentrations in children with tuberculous meningitis. *Pediatr Infect Dis J* 1988;7:469–471.
498. Jenner PJ, Ellard GA, Gruer PJK, et al. A comparison of the blood levels and urinary excretion of ethionamide and prothionamide in man. *J Antimicrob Chemother* 1984;13:267–277.
499. Brendel E, Meineke I, Stuwe E, et al. Stability of 5-aminosalicylic acid and 5-acetylaminosalicylic acid in plasma. *J Chromatogr* 1988;432:358–362.
500. Brendel E, Meineke I, Witsch D, et al. Simultaneous determination of 5-aminosalicylic acid and 5-acetylaminosalicylic acid by high-performance liquid chromatography. *J Chromatogr* 1987;385:299–304.
501. Lee EJD, Ang SB. Simple and sensitive high-performance liquid chromatographic assay for 5-aminosalicylic acid and acetyl-5-aminosalicylic acid in serum. *J Chromatogr* 1987;413:300–304.
502. Honigberg IL, Stewart JT, et al. Non-extractive fluorometric measurement of p-aminosalicylic acid in plasma by ion-pairing techniques and high-performance chromatography. *J Chromatogr* 1980;181:266–271.

CHAPTER 6

Antifungal Drugs: Mechanisms of Action, Drug Resistance, Susceptibility Testing, and Assays of Activity in Biological Fluids

Michael A. Pfaller, Daniel J. Diekema, Michael G. Rinaldi

Antifungal therapy has undergone a remarkable transformation in recent years. Once the domain of agents such as amphotericin B and 5-fluorocytosine, which were toxic and difficult to use, the treatment of serious fungal infections has now been advanced by the availability of several new, systemically active agents and new formulations of other agents that provide comparable, if not superior, efficacy with significantly less toxicity (Table 6.1) (3,8,50,55,60,80,90,92,98,103,105,106,110, 114,130,170,175,224,250).

The timing of the introduction of these new agents is fortunate because modern medical therapies often produce profound immunocompromise, leaving patients at high risk for invasive fungal infections. The acquired immunodeficiency disease syndrome (AIDS) epidemic has also added large numbers of individuals to this high-risk population. These factors have combined to produce an unprecedented number of serious fungal infections with accompanying morbidity and mortality (7,11,21,30,46a, 97,133,147,164,172,173,180,230,247,252,260,278). The need for better antifungal agents with expanded spectrum and potency and decreased toxicity has never been greater (46a,90,133,147,170,172,180,230,247,252).

In this chapter we will review the antifungal agents, both systemic and topical (Table 6.1). We will discuss their spectrum, potency, mode of action, and clinical indications for their use as well as what is known of their pharmacokinetic and pharmacodynamic parameters. Furthermore, we will discuss the mechanisms of resistance to the various classes of antifungal agents and the *in vitro* methods for determining the susceptibility and resistance of fungi to the available agents. Finally, we will provide an overview of the methods for measuring the concentration of antifungal agents in clinical samples and, where appropriate, discuss the indication for performing such analysis.

SYSTEMICALLY ACTIVE ANTIFUNGAL AGENTS

Polyenes

Conventional amphotericin B and its lipid formulations (Table 6.1) are polyene macrolide antifungal agents used in the treatment of systemic and life-threatening fungal infections. Another polyene, nystatin, is a topical agent and is discussed elsewhere. A lipid formulation of nystatin has been developed for systemic use but has not been approved for use in humans (92).

The polyenes possess a large lactone ring, with a rigid lipophilic chain containing three to seven double bonds, and a flexible hydrophilic portion bearing several hydroxyl groups. Amphotericin B contains seven conjugated double bonds and may be inactivated by heat, light, and extremes of pH. It is poorly soluble in water and is not orally or intramuscularly absorbed. The commercially available preparation of amphotericin B for parental use is amphotericin B deoxycholate (AmB). Largely because of the nephrotoxic nature of conventional amphotericin B, lipid formulations of amphotericin B have been developed (Table 6.1) and in many instances have replaced AmB (170). The lipid-based formulations of AmB include amphotericin B lipid complex (ABLC), liposomal amphotericin B (L-AmB), and amphotericin B cholesteryl sulfate complex (ABCD).

TABLE 6.1

Systemic and Topical Antifungal Agents in Use and in Development[a]

Antifungal Agents	Route	Mechanism of Action	Comments
Allylamines			
Naftifine Terbinafine	Topical Oral, topical	Inhibition of squalene epoxidase	Terbinafine has very broad spectrum activity and acts synergistically with other antifungals
Antimetabolite			
Flucytosine	Oral	Inhibition of DNA and RNA synthesis	Used in combination with amphotericin B and fluconazole; toxicity and secondary resistance are problems
Imidazoles			
Ketoconazole, Bifonazole, Clotrimazole, Econazole, Miconazole, Oxiconazole, Sulconazole, Terconazole, Tioconazole	Oral, topical	Inhibits lanosterol 14-α-demethylase cytochrome P-450-dependent enzymes	Ketoconazole has modest broad spectrum activity and toxicity problems
Triazoles			
Fluconazole	Oral, IV[b]	Same as imidazoles but more specific binding to target	Limited spectrum (yeasts); good central nervous system penetration; good *in vivo* activity; primary and secondary resistance seen with *C. krusei* and *C. glabrata*, respectively
Itraconazole	Oral, IV	Same as imidazoles but more specific binding to target enzyme	Broad-spectrum activity; erratic absorption; toxicity and drug interactions are problems
Voriconazole	Oral, IV	Same as imidazoles but more specific binding to target enzyme	Broad spectrum including yeasts and molds; active vs. *C. krusei*; many drug interactions
Posaconazole	Oral	Same as imidazoles but more specific binding to enzyme	Investigational; broad spectrum including activity vs. Zygomycetes
Ravuconazole	Oral, IV	Same as imidazoles but more specific binding to target enzyme	Investigational; broad spectrum including yeasts and molds
Echinocandins			
Caspofungin Anidulafungin Micafungin	IV IV IV	Inhibition of fungal cell wall glucan synthesis	Caspofungin is approved for treatment of invasive candidiasis and aspergillosis; others are investigational; fungicidal activity against *Candida*
Polyenes			
Amphotericin B	IV, topical	Binds to ergosterol causing direct oxidative membrane damage	Established agent; broad spectrum; toxic

(continued)

TABLE 6.1 (Continued)

Systemic and Topical Antifungal Agents in Use and in Development[a]

Antifungal Agents	Route	Mechanism of Action	Comments
Lipid formulations (amphotericin B lipid complex or colloidal dispersion, liposomal amphotericin B)	IV	Same as amphotericin B	Broad spectrum; less toxic, expensive
Nystatin	Oral suspension, topical	Same as amphotericin B	Liposomal formulation (IV) under investigation
Chitin synthesis inhibitor			
Nikkomycin Z	IV	Inhibition of fungal cell wall chitin synthesis	Investigational agent; possibly useful in combination with other antifungals
Other			
Amorolfine	Topical	Miscellaneous, varied	
Butenafine HCl	Topical		
Ciclopirox olamine	Topical		
Griseofulvin	Oral		
Haloprogin	Topical		
Tolnaftate	Topical		
Undecylenate	Topical		

[a] Adapted from Espinel-Ingroff and Pfaller (73) and Revankar and Graybill (224).
[b] IV, intravenous.

AmB, and its lipid formulations, acts by at least two different mechanisms (8,92,224). The first, and primary, mechanism involves binding to ergosterol, the principal membrane sterol of most fungi. This binding produces ion channels that destroy the osmotic integrity of the membrane and leads to the leakage of intracellular constituents and cell death (148). AmB binds less avidly to cholesterol, the main membrane sterol of mammalian cells, and this binding accounts for most of the toxicity observed when this agent is administered to humans. A second mechanism of action of AmB may involve direct membrane toxicity due to the generation of a cascade of oxidative reactions triggered by the oxidation of AmB itself. This process results in the generation of toxic-free radicals and may be a major contributor to the rapid fungicidal activity of AmB (24,25).

The spectrum of activity of AmB is broad and includes most strains of *Candida, Cryptococcus neoformans, Aspergillus* spp, the Zygomycetes (such as *Mucor* and *Rhizopus*) *Blastomyces dermatitidis, Coccidioides immitis, Histoplasma capsulatum,* and *Paracoccidiodes brasiliensis* (Tables 6.2 to 6.5) (8,92,224). Reduced susceptibility to AmB has been noted among *Candida guilliermondii, C. glabrata, C. krusei,* and *C. lusitaniae* (8,92,186,196) . Likewise, *Aspergillus terreus, Fusarium* spp, *Pseudallescheria boydii, Scedosporium prolificans, Trichosporon beigleii,* and certain dematiaceous fungi may be resistant to AmB (97,252). Primary resistance to AmB has been associated with alterations in membrane sterols but also may be related to decreased susceptibility to oxidative damage secondary to increased catalase activity (92).

AmB must be administered parenterally because of its poor solubility and poor absorption when administered orally. It is widely distributed in various tissues and organs, including liver, spleen, bone marrow, kidney, and lung. Despite negligible concentration in cerebrospinal fluid, AmB is effective in treating fungal infections of the central nervous system, although some instances may require intrathecal administration (93). The tissue distribution of L-AmB is similar to that of AmB; however, ABLC is highly concentrated in the liver, spleen, and lungs but not in the kidney (92). AmB displays concentration-dependent fungicidal activity against many fungi with an optimal maximal concentration-to-minimal inhibitory concentration (C_{max}-to-MIC) ratio of 4–8:1 (5,93–96) and a postantifungal effect of up to 12 hours (3,63,93–96). These findings suggest that the antifungal

(text continues on page 231)

TABLE 6.2

In Vitro Susceptibility of *Candida* spp to Systemically Active Antifungal Agents Determined by NCCLS M27-A2 Broth Dilution MIC Methods[a]

Species	Antifungal Agent	No. Tested	MIC (μg/mL)[b] 50%	90%	% Susceptible
Candida albicans	Amphotericin B[c]	4,195	0.5	1	
	Flucytosine	4,195	0.25	1	97
	Fluconazole	4,195	0.25	0.5	97
	Itraconazole	4,195	0.03	0.12	93
	Posaconazole	2,359	0.03	0.03	
	Ravuconazole	4,195	0.007	0.03	
	Voriconazole	4,195	0.007	0.03	
	Anidulafungin	733[d]	0.03	0.03	
	Caspofungin	733[d]	0.5	0.5	
	Micafungin	733[d]	0.03	0.03	
C. glabrata	Amphotericin B[c]	949	2	4	
	Flucytosine	949	0.12	0.12	99
	Fluconazole	949	8	32	60
	Itraconazole	949	1	2	4
	Posaconazole	607	1	2	
	Ravuconazole	949	0.25	2	
	Voriconazole	949	0.25	1	
	Anidulafungin	458[d]	0.03	0.13	
	Caspofungin	458[d]	0.5	1	
	Micafungin	458[d]	0.03	0.06	
C. parapsilosis	Amphotericin B[c]	814	2	4	
	Flucytosine	814	0.12	0.25	99
	Fluconazole	814	0.5	2	99
	Itraconazole	814	0.12	0.25	54
	Posaconazole	439	0.12	0.25	
	Ravuconazole	814	0.03	0.12	
	Voriconazole	814	0.03	0.06	
	Anidulafungin	391[d]	2	2	
	Caspofungin	391[d]	2	2	
	Micafungin	391[d]	1	2	
C. tropicalis	Amphotericin B[c]	597	1	2	
	Flucytosine	597	0.25	1	93
	Fluconazole	597	0.5	2	98
	Itraconazole	597	0.12	0.5	58
	Posaconazole	319	0.06	0.25	
	Ravuconazole	597	0.03	0.12	
	Voriconazole	597	0.06	0.12	
	Anidulafungin	307[d]	0.03	0.13	

(continued)

TABLE 6.2 (Continued)

In Vitro Susceptibility of *Candida* spp to Systemically Active Antifungal Agents Determined by NCCLS M27-A2 Broth Dilution MIC Methods[a]

Species	Antifungal Agent	No. Tested	MIC (μg/mL)[b]		
			50%	90%	% Susceptible
	Caspofungin	307[d]	0.5	1	
	Micafungin	307[d]	0.03	0.06	
C. krusei	Amphotericin B[c]	234	4	8	
	Flucytosine	234	16	32	4
	Fluconazole	234	32	64	0[e]
	Itraconazole	153	0.5	1	1
	Posaconazole	153	0.5	0.5	
	Ravuconazole	234	0.5	0.5	
	Voriconazole	133	0.25	0.5	
	Anidulafungin	50[d]	0.06	0.13	
	Caspofungin	50[d]	1	2	
	Micafungin	50[d]	0.13	0.25	
C. dubliniensis	Amphotericin B[c]	88	0.25	0.5	
	Flucytosine	88	0.06	0.06	100
	Fluconazole	88	0.12	0.5	94
	Itraconazole	88	0.06	0.25	89
	Posaconazole	70	0.03	0.06	
	Ravuconazole	88	0.007	0.03	
	Voriconazole	88	0.007	0.03	
	Anidulafungin	18[d]	0.03	0.06	
	Caspofungin	18[d]	0.5	0.5	
	Micafungin	18[d]	0.03	0.03	
C. guilliermondii	Amphotericin B[c]	102	0.25	1	
	Flucytosine	102	0.12	0.25	100
	Fluconazole	102	4	16	85
	Itraconazole	85	1	1	7
	Posaconazole	48	0.25	0.5	
	Ravuconazole	102	0.25	1	
	Voriconazole	85	0.12	0.25	
	Anidulafungin	9[d]	1		
	Caspofungin	9[d]	1		
	Micafungin	9[d]	0.5		
C. lusitaniae	Amphotericin B[c]	103	0.25	1	
	Flucytosine	103	0.06	8	89
	Fluconazole	103	0.5	2	96
	Itraconazole	67	0.25	0.25	46
	Posaconazole	67	0.06	0.12	
	Ravuconazole	103	0.06	0.06	

(continued)

TABLE 6.2 (Continued)

In Vitro Susceptibility of *Candida* spp to Systemically Active Antifungal Agents Determined by NCCLS M27-A2 Broth Dilution MIC Methods[a]

Species	Antifungal Agent	No. Tested	MIC (μg/mL)[b] 50%	90%	% Susceptible
	Voriconazole	67	0.06	0.06	
	Anidulafungin	20[d]	0.06	0.25	
	Caspofungin	20[d]	1	2	
	Micafungin	20[d]	0.06	2	
C. kefyr	Amphotericin B[c]	29	2	4	
	Flucytosine	29	0.12	1	100
	Fluconazole	29	0.25	0.5	100
	Itraconazole	10	0.12	0.25	50
	Posaconazole	10	0.12	0.12	
	Ravuconazole	29	0.06	0.06	
	Voriconazole	10	0.06	0.06	
	Anidulafungin[d]	4	0.06		
	Caspofungin[d]	4	0.5		
	Micafungin[d]	4	0.06		
C. rugosa	Amphotericin B[c]	13	1	32	
	Flucytosine	13	0.5	16	85
	Fluconazole	13	4	16	77
	Itraconazole	5	0.12		60
	Posaconazole	7	0.03		
	Ravuconazole	13	0.06	0.25	
	Voriconazole	7	0.03		
	Anidulafungin[d]	7	0.03		
	Caspofungin[c]	7	2		
	Micafungin[d]	7	0.06		

[a] Adapted from Ostrosky-Zeichner et al. (171) and Pfaller et al. (185,186,191,195,199). NCCLS, National Committee for Clinical Laboratory Standards.

[b] MIC, minimum inhibitory concentration. 50%, MIC encompassing 50% of all isolates tested; 90%, MIC encompassing 90% of all isolates tested; % Susceptible: fluconazole MIC, ≤8 μg/mL; itraconazole MIC, ≤0.12 μg/mL; flucytosine MIC, ≤4 μg/mL. There are no established breakpoints for the other agents at the present time.

[c] Amphotericin B MICs determined by Etest.

[d] MICs for echinocandins determined using partial inhibition endpoint criteria (MIC-2) at 48-h incubation.

[e] All isolates of *C. krusei* are considered resistant to fluconazole irrespective of MIC.

efficacy of AmB may be maximized by the administration of large doses at less frequent intervals in order to achieve optimal peak concentrations with decreased toxicity because of a prolonged drug-free interval (92).

The primary clinical indications for AmB administration include invasive candidiasis, cryptococcosis, aspergillosis, zygomycosis, histoplasmosis, coccidioidomycosis, blastomycosis, sporotrichosis, and paracoccidioidomycosis (8,92,224). In addition, AmB is indicated for empirical therapy of febrile, neutropenic patients refractory to broad-spectrum antibacterial agents (7). The lipid formulations of AmB offer an improved efficacy-toxicity profile and are mainly recommended for the treatment of documented fungal infections in individuals failing conventional AmB or having impaired renal function (103). L-AmB is also approved for empirical therapy of suspected fungal infection in febrile, neutropenic patients (103,170). The standard dose of AmB is 0.5 to 0.6 mg/kg

TABLE 6.3

In Vitro Susceptibility of Cryptococcus neoformans to Systemically Active Antifungal Agents Determined by NCCLS M27-A2 Broth Dilution Minimum Inhibitory Concentration (MIC) Methods[a]

Antifungal Agent	No. Tested	MIC (μg/mL)[b]		
		Range	50%	90%
Amphotericin B[c]	732[c]	0.25–2	1	1
Flucytosine	732	0.06–>128	8	16
Fluconazole	732	0.12–>64	8	16
Itraconazole	732	0.03–2	0.5	1
Posaconazole	373	0.015–1	0.12	0.25
Ravuconazole	541	0.007–4	0.12	0.25
Voriconazole	237	0.007–1	0.03	0.12

[a] Adapted from Brandt et al. (27), Pfaller et al. (195, 201), and Yamazumi et al. (280). NCCLS, National Committee for Clinical Laboratory Standards.
[b] 50%, MIC encompassing 50% of all isolates tested; 90%, MIC encompassing 90% of all isolates tested.
[c] Amphotericin B MICs determined by Etest.

per day in cases of febrile neutropenia (92); 0.8 mg/kg per day for cases of cryptococcal meningitis; 0.6 mg/kg per day for candidiasis due to *C. albicans;* 1 mg/kg per day for candidiasis due to *C. glabrata, C. krusei,* and *C. tropicalis* (227); and 1 to 1.5 mg/kg per day for cases of aspergillosis or zygomycosis (253). Lipid formulations are given at higher doses, ranging from 3 to 5 mg/kg per day (92,103).

The main adverse effects of AmB are well known and include nephrotoxicity as well as infusion-related side effects such as fever, chills, myalgia, hypotension, and bronchospasm. The major advantage of the lipid formulations of AmB are the significantly reduced side effects, especially nephrotoxicity (103,170).

Azoles

The antifungal azoles include the imidazoles and the triazoles, which differ in terms of their chemical structure. Among the imidazoles (two nitrogens in the azole ring), only ketoconazole has systemic activity. The triazoles (three nitrogens in the azole ring) all have systemic activity and include fluconazole, itraconazole, and voriconazole. Two additional triazoles, posaconazole and ravuconazole, are still under development and will be discussed in a later section.

All of the azoles act by inhibiting the fungal cytochrome P-450–dependent enzyme lanosterol 14-α-demethylase. This enzyme functions to convert lanosterol to ergosterol, and its inhibition disrupts membrane synthesis in the fungal cell. Depending on the organism and compound, inhibition of ergosterol synthesis results in decreased fungal cell growth and development or cell death. Generally, these agents exhibit fungistatic activity against yeasts such as *Candida* spp and *Cryptococcus neoformans;* however, voriconazole appears to be fungicidal against *Aspergillus* spp (80,90,110,175).

Ketoconazole

Ketoconazole is a lipophilic, orally absorbed imidazole antifungal agent. Its spectrum of activity includes *B. dermatitidis, C. immitis, H. capsulatum, P. brasiliensis,* and *Penicillium marneffei*. It also has *in vitro* activity against most *Candida* species, *C. neoformans,* and *Malassezia* spp (8,224); however, its activity is less than that of the triazoles. It has variable activity against *Scedosporium apiospermum* (*P. boydii*) and little or no activity against *S. prolificans, Aspergillus* spp, *Fusarium* spp, or the Zygomycetes (224).

Ketoconazole requires a normal (acidic) gastric pH for optimal oral absorption and is highly (more than 99%) protein-bound. Its lipophilicity ensures penetration and concentration into fatty tissues and purulent exudates; however, it poorly penetrates the central nervous system (250).

Because of the availability of less toxic and more potent agents, ketoconazole now has very limited clinical indications. It is at best a second-line agent for the treatment of immunocompetent individuals with

(text continues on page 236)

TABLE 6.4

In Vitro Susceptibility of Filamentous Fungi to Systemically Active Antifungal Agents Determined by NCCLS M38-A Broth Dilution Minimum Inhibitory Concentration (MIC) Methods[a]

Species	Antifungal Agent	No. Tested	MIC (μg/mL)[b]	
			50%	90%
Aspergillus fumigatus	Amphotericin B	256	1	1
	Itraconazole	256	1	1
	Posaconazole	256	0.25	0.5
	Ravuconazole	256	0.25	0.5
	Voriconazole	256	0.25	0.5
	Caspofungin	256	0.03	0.06
	Anidulafungin	12	0.03	0.06
	Micafungin	NA[c]	0.007	0.015
A. flavus	Amphotericin B	30	1	2
	Itraconazole	30	0.5	1
	Posaconazole	30	0.25	0.5
	Ravuconazole	30	0.5	1
	Voriconazole	30	0.5	1
	Caspofungin	30	0.03	0.06
	Anidulafungin	10	0.015	0.03
	Micafungin	NA[c]	0.007	0.015
A. niger	Amphotericin B	29	1	1
	Itraconazole	29	2	2
	Posaconazole	29	0.5	1
	Ravuconazole	29	0.5	2
	Voriconazole	29	1	2
	Caspofungin	29	0.03	0.06
	Anidulafungin	NA[c]	0.06	0.12
	Micafungin	NA[c]	0.004	0.008
A. versicolor	Amphotericin B	20	1	2
	Itraconazole	20	1	2
	Posaconazole	20	0.5	1
	Ravuconazole	20	0.25	1
	Voriconazole	20	0.5	1
	Caspofungin	20	0.03	0.12
A. terreus	Amphotericin B	16	2	2
	Itraconazole	16	0.5	0.5
	Posaconazole	16	0.12	0.25
	Ravuconazole	16	0.25	0.5
	Voriconazole	16	0.25	1
	Caspofungin	16	0.03	0.06
	Anidulafungin	NA[c]	0.03	0.03
	Micafungin	NA[c]	0.004	0.008

(continued)

TABLE 6.4 (Continued)

In Vitro Susceptibility of Filamentous Fungi to Systemically Active Antifungal Agents Determined by NCCLS M38-A Broth Dilution Minimum Inhibitory Concentration (MIC) Methods[a]

Species	Antifungal Agent	No. Tested	MIC (μg/mL)[b]	
			50%	90%
Fusarium spp	Amphotericin B	28	NA[c]	4
	Itraconazole	28	NA[c]	>8
	Posaconazole	11	>8	>8
	Ravuconazole	11	8	>8
	Voriconazole	28	NA[c]	4
	Caspofungin	13	>8	>8
	Anidulafungin	NA[c]	>8	>8
	Micafungin	NA[c]	>8	>8
Scedosporium apiospermum	Amphotericin B	13	2	4
	Itraconazole	13	0.5	2
	Posaconazole	13	0.5	1
	Voriconazole	13	0.12	0.25
	Caspofungin	5	0.5	ND[d]
	Anidulafungin	5	1	ND[d]
S. prolificans	Amphotericin B	55	16	>16
	Itraconazole	55	>32	>32
	Posaconazole	55	>8	>8
	Voriconazole	55	4	4
Paecilomyces spp	Amphotericin B	6	0.5	ND[d]
	Itraconazole	6	0.25	ND[d]
	Posaconazole	6	0.12	ND[d]
	Ravuconazole	6	0.25	ND[d]
	Voriconazole	6	0.25	ND[d]
	Caspofungin	6	0.06	ND[d]
Scopulariopsis brevicaulis	Amphotericin B	32	16	ND[d]
	Itraconazole	32	>8	ND[d]
	Voriconazole	32	32	ND[d]
Absidia corymbifera	Amphotericin B	10	0.12	0.12
	Itraconazole	10	0.06	0.25
	Posaconazole	10	0.06	0.12
	Voriconazole	10	16	16
	Caspofungin	NA[c]	>8	>8
	Anidulafungin	NA[c]	>8	>8
	Micafungin	NA[c]	>8	>8
Mucor spp	Amphotericin B	6	0.12	ND[d]
	Itraconazole	6	8	ND[d]
	Posaconazole	6	1	ND[d]
	Ravuconazole	3	>8	ND[d]

(continued)

TABLE 6.4 (Continued)

In Vitro Susceptibility of Filamentous Fungi to Systemically Active Antifungal Agents Determined by NCCLS M38-A Broth Dilution Minimum Inhibitory Concentration (MIC) Methods[a]

Species	Antifungal Agent	No. Tested	MIC (μg/mL)[b]	
			50%	90%
	Voriconazole	6	32	ND[d]
	Caspofungin	3	>8	ND[d]
	Anidulafungin	NA[c]	>8	ND[d]
	Micafungin	NA[c]	>8	ND[d]
Rhizopus spp	Amphotericin B	15	0.5	1
	Itraconazole	15	0.5	4
	Posaconazole	15	0.25	0.5
	Ravuconazole	4	>8	ND[d]
	Voriconazole	15	8	16
	Caspofungin	5	>8	ND[d]
	Anidulafungin	NA[c]	>8	ND[d]
	Micafungin	NA[c]	>8	ND[d]

[a] Adapted from Cuenca-Estrella et al. (39a), Dannaoui et al. (42), Diekema et al. (58), Espinel-Ingroff (66), Johnson and Kauffman (110), Meletiadis et al. (150a), Pearson et al. (175), and Pfaller et al. (207a). NCCLS, National Committee for Clinical Laboratory Standards.
[b] The MIC is given for all agents except caspofungin, anidulafungin, and micafungin, for which the MEC is given (58). MIC/MEC at which 50% or 90% of the isolates were inhibited.
[c] NA, not available.
[d] ND, not done.

TABLE 6.5

Antifungal Spectrum of Activity and Drug of Choice Against the Endemic Dimorphic Fungal Pathogens

Pathogen	Drug of Choice[a]				
	Amphotericin B	Fluconazole	Itraconazole	Voriconazole	Caspofungin[b]
Coccidioides immitis	S[c]	S[c]	S	S	S/R
Blastomyces dermatitidis	S[c]	S/R[c]	S[c]	S	S/R
Histoplasma capsulatum	S[c]	S/R[c]	S[c]	S	S/R
Paracoccidioides braziliensis	S[c]	S/R	S[c]		S/R
Sporothrix schenckii	S[c]	S/R[d]	S[c]		
Penicillium marneffei	S[c]	S/R	S[c]	S	

[a] S, isolates are generally susceptible to the drug; S/R, isolates may be either susceptible (S) or resistant (R).
[b] Echinocandins appear more active against the mycelial phase than the yeast phase of these organisms.
[c] Treatment of choice or first alternative.
[d] Alternative treatment, clinical failure, or resistance has been documented.

nonlife-threatening, nonmeningeal forms of histoplasmosis, blastomycosis, coccidioidomycosis, and paracoccidioidomycosis, as well as mucocutaneous candidiasis and lymphocutaneous sporotrichosis (250).

In addition to erratic absorption, ketoconazole may cause serious adverse effects, including hepatotoxicity, gastric toxicity, nausea, vomiting, and rash (256). At high doses, suppression of testosterone and cortisol levels, with resultant endocrinological side effects, have been observed (256).

Fluconazole

Fluconazole is a very widely used triazole antifungal agent with excellent oral bioavailability and low toxicity (8,92,224,232). Fluconazole is active against most species of *Candida*, *C. neoformans*, dermatophytes, *Trichosporon* spp, *H. capsulatum*, *C. immitis*, and *P. brasiliensis* (Tables 6.2–6.5) (96,191,224,232). Among *Candida* spp, there is decreased susceptibility to fluconazole with *C. glabrata* and *C. krusei* (191). Whereas *C. krusei* is intrinsically resistant to fluconazole, most strains of *C. glabrata* are either susceptible (MIC, less than 8 μg/mL) or susceptible-dose dependent (MIC, 16 to 32 μg/mL) and approximately 10% exhibit high-level resistance (MIC, more than 64 μg/mL). Only limited activity is seen against *B. dermatitidis* and resistance may develop when fluconazole is used to treat histoplasmosis (271). Fluconazole has no useful activity against molds including *Aspergillus* spp, *Fusarium* spp, or the Zygomycetes (250).

Fluconazole is a water-soluble compound and is available in both oral and intravenous formulations. It has an excellent bioavailability (approximately 90%) when given orally and exhibits linear pharmacokinetics that are independent of doses and formulation (26). Protein binding is low and it is distributed to virtually all organs and tissues including the central nervous system (250). Fluconazole is renally excreted with approximately 80% recovered in the urine as an active, unchanged drug. Doses as high as 2 g per day have been used; however, the standard dose in adults is 400 to 800 mg per day and in children it is 6 to 12 mg/kg per day (1,92).

Fluconazole exhibits concentration-independent fungistatic activity against *Candida* and *C. neoformans* (119, 120). The area under the concentration-time curve (AUC) and MIC ratio (AUC/MIC) appears to be the most predictive pharmacodynamic parameter for fluconazole (134).

Fluconazole has an important role in the treatment of candidiasis, cryptococcosis, and coccidioidomycosis. Fluconazole is used as primary therapy for candidemia and mucosal candidiasis, as well as prophylaxis in selected high-risk populations (227,232). It is used in maintenance therapy of cryptococcal meningitis in patients with AIDS (238) and is the agent of choice in treatment of coccidioidal meningitis (86,87). Fluconazole is a second-line agent in the treatment of histoplasmosis, blastomycosis, and sporotrichosis (250). Severe side effects such as exfoliative dermatitis and liver failure are extremely uncommon (96).

Itraconazole

Itraconazole is a lipophilic triazole that may be administered orally as capsules or in a solution, and also intravenously (92). The antifungal activity of itraconazole is broad and includes *Candida* spp, *C. neoformans*, *Aspergillus* spp, dermatophytes, dematiaceous molds, *P. boydii*, *Penicillium marneffei*, *B. dermatitidis*, *C. immitis*, *H. capsulatum*, *P. brasiliensis*, and *S. schenckii* (Tables 6.2–6.5) (224,248–250). Itraconazole has activity against some, but not all, fluconazole-resistant strains of *C. krusei* and *C. glabrata*. Although rare, strains of *Aspergillus fumigatus* that are resistant to itraconazole have been reported (42–44). The Zygomycetes, most strains of *Fusarium*, and *Scedosporium prolificans* are resistant to itraconazole (96).

Itraconazole is available as capsules, as an oral solution in hydroxypropyl-β-cyclodextrin (HP-β-CD), and as an intravenous solution that also uses HP-β-CD. Absorption of the capsular form is erratic and requires an acidic gastric pH and administration with food. The oral solution is much better absorbed and bioavailability is enhanced when given in the fasting state (92). The intravenous formulation provides optimal bioavailability with peak plasma levels obtained within 1 hour of administration. The HP-β-CD carrier is cleared renally and caution is recommended when administering the intravenous formulation to patients with impaired renal function (92,224). The high protein binding and lipophilic nature of itraconazole results in poor penetration into the central nervous system and high concentrations in fatty tissues and purulent exudates (250).

Itraconazole exhibits concentration-independent fungistatic activity against *Candida* spp and *C. neoformans* (96). In contrast, itraconazole has been shown to exert a time- and concentration-dependent fungicidal effect against *Aspergillus* spp (140).

Itraconazole is useful in the treatment of dermatophytic infections and cutaneous and mucosal forms of candidiasis; however, its efficacy in the treatment of hematogenous candidiasis has not been adequately assessed (96). It is the treatment of choice for lymphocutaneous sporotrichosis and nonlife-threatening, nonmeningial forms of histoplasmosis, paracoccidioidomycosis, and blastomycosis (32,155,223,249,272). It is a second-line agent for the treatment of invasive aspergillosis (28,52,53), and may be useful for cases of nonmeningeal coccidioidomycosis (86), for maintenance treatment of cryptococcal meningitis (238), and for some forms of phaeohyphomycosis (248). It has no activity against *Fusarium* spp, the Zygomycetes, or *S. prolificans* (224).

Side effects due to itraconazole may occur and include gastrointestinal intolerance, hypokalemia, edema, rash, and elevated transaminases (92). Severe hepatotoxicity is rare (249,250). In contrast to fluconazole, drug interactions are relatively common with itraconazole because of the inhibition of the oxidative metabolism of agents that are metabolized by hepatic cytochrome-P-450 enzymes (224).

Voriconazole

Voriconazole is a new extended-spectrum triazole that is available in both oral and intravenous formulations (80,90,110,175). Voriconazole has a very broad spectrum that includes *Candida* spp, *C. neoformans, Trichosporon* spp, *Aspergillus* spp, *Fusarium* spp, and other hyaline molds, dematiaceous fungi, and the endemic dimorphic fungi (Tables 6.2–6.5) (58,70,185,196,199,203,206). The anticandidal activity of voriconazole encompasses *C. krusei* and most, but not all, strains of *C. albicans* and *C. glabrata* with decreased susceptibility to fluconazole (185,198,199). Voriconazole is also active against fungi that are resistant to amphotericin B, including *A. terreus* and *P. boydii* (58,70). The Zygomycetes do not appear to be susceptible to voriconazole (45,58).

The oral formulation of voriconazole is well absorbed with a bioavailability of more than 90% (110,175). The intravenous form is solubilized in sulfobutyl ether β-cyclodextrin sodium (SBECD) and is administered twice daily at a dose of 3 to 6 mg/kg (106). Steady-state plasma levels range from 2 to 3 μg/mL following oral administration and 3 to 6 μg/mL after intravenous infusion (106). Voriconazole is 58% protein-bound and has excellent penetration into the central nervous system as well as other tissues (92). It is metabolized in the liver via the cytochrome P-450 enzyme family and less than 5% of a dose of voriconazole is excreted unchanged in urine (92,110).

Voriconazole exhibits concentration-independent fungistatic activity against *Candida* spp. and *C. neoformans* with no apparent postantifungal effect (3,4,118). Recent *in vivo* studies of disseminated *C. albicans* infection indicates that an AUC:MIC ratio of 20–25:1 predicts treatment success (4). In contrast, voriconazole appears to exert a dose-dependent fungicidal effect on *Aspergillus* based on both time-kill studies (140) and clearance of fungal burden in target organs of animal models of invasive aspergillosis (31,190).

Voriconazole is approved for the primary treatment of invasive aspergillosis (51,102) and for treatment of infections due to *P. boydii* (*S. apiospermum*) and *Fusarium* spp in patients intolerant of, or with infections refractory to, other antifungal agents (110). Importantly, voriconazole was shown to be more effective than amphotericin B (53% versus 32% complete or partial response at week 12 of treatment and 71% versus 58% survival, respectively) for primary treatment of invasive aspergillosis (102). Likewise, successful treatment of a variety of fungal infections due to emerging or refractory pathogens, including brain abscesses due to *P. boydii* (164), have been documented. Voriconazole has also been shown to have good efficacy in the treatment of various forms of candidiasis (175,180). Voriconazole has not been approved for empirical treatment of febrile, neutropenic patients despite documented efficacy in the treatment of invasive aspergillosis and in the prevention of breakthrough fungal infections in this same patient population (102,110,265).

As with other triazoles, voriconazole is generally well tolerated (92,110,175). The most common side effect is a reversible disturbance of vision, which occurs in approximately 30% of patients but is transient and rarely leads to discontinuation of the drug (110,175,265). Other adverse effects include transient liver enzyme abnormalities (10% to 20%), skin reactions (less than 10%), and hallucinations or confusion (less than 10%) (92,102). Because voriconaozle is metabolized by the hepatic cytochrome P-450 enzyme system, drug interactions requiring dosage adjustment and/or monitoring are common (92).

Echinocandins

The echinocandins are a novel class of semisynthetic lipopeptides that exert selective antifungal activity through inhibition of the synthesis of 1,3-β-glucans, important constituents at the level of the fungal cell wall (50,55,92,105,114,130). The glucans are important in maintaining the osmotic integrity of the fungal cell and play a key role in cell division and cell growth (88,125). Selective inhibition of the glucan synthesis enzyme complex results in fungicidal activity against *Candida* spp and fungistatic activity against *Aspergillus* spp (3,50). Currently, three echinocandins are in various stages of development (92): caspofungin (Merck) is licensed for use in patients with candidiasis and aspergillosis (55,92,105,114,130), and approval of anidulafungin (Versicor) and micafungin (Fujisawa) by regulatory authorities is expected in the near future.

In addition to activity against *Candida* and *Aspergillus* spp, the echinocandins have variable activity against dematiaceous fungi and the endemic dimorphic pathogens (Tables 6.2 to 6.5) (55,92,105,130). They are inactive against *Fusarium* and other hyalohyphomycetes, *C. neoformans, Trichosporum* spp, and the Zygomycetes (55,58,114). Primary resistance to echinocandins appears to be extremely uncommon among *Candida* spp (130,189,192,197) and *Aspergillus* spp (58,130). Notably, echinocandins are active against fluconazole-resistant strains of *Candida* spp (152,192).

The oral bioavailability of the echinocandins is limited and only intravenous formulations are currently available or under development. The echinocandins exhibit dose-dependent linear pharmacokinetics and are highly (more than 95%) protein bound (50,92). The echinocandins are broadly distributed to all major organs, including the brain, although concentrations in cerebrospinal fluid are low (114). Metabolism occurs in the liver by a cytochrome P-450 independent mechanism and the inactive metabolites are excreted in the feces and urine; less than 2% of a dose is excreted in the urine in active form (114).

Both *in vitro* and *in vivo* studies in *Candida* spp have shown a concentration-dependent fungicidal effect that is optimized at a peak-to-MIC ratio of approximately 8:1 (3,62,64,64a) and a postantifungal effect of up to 12 hours (3,63). In contrast, activity against *Aspergillus* spp is fungistatic, with activity localized to the growing hyphal tips and branch points with resultant inhibition of growth and angioinvasion but only a modest effect on the fungal burden in tissues (23,95,181,183).

At the present time, only caspofungin is licensed for use in patients. The approved clinical indications for caspofungin include primary therapy of invasive candidiasis including candidemia (114,130,152) and treatment of patients with invasive aspergillosis refractory to, or intolerant of, other approved therapies (114). Caspofungin has been shown to have similar activity to amphotericin B in treatment of patients with candidemia and other forms of invasive candidiasis (152). A favorable overall response occurred in 73.4% of caspofungin recipients and in 61.7% of amphotericin B recipients. Caspofungin was significantly better tolerated than amphotericin B (152). In a study of salvage therapy for invasive aspergillosis, favorable response (complete plus partial responses) occurred in 37 of 83 patients (45%) (114).

The standard dosing of caspofungin in adults consists of a loading dose of 70 mg followed by 50 mg daily thereafter, administered intravenously over 1 hour (114). This dosing regimen results in peak plasma concentrations of 8 μg/mL or greater and trough concentrations of 1 μg/mL or greater (114).

All of the echinocandins are extremely well tolerated at the currently investigated dosing regimens (92,114). The most frequently reported adverse effects include increased liver transaminases, gastrointestinal upset, and headache (114,152). Drug interactions are rare; however, concomitant administration of caspofungin and cyclosporin is not recommended because of reports of transient elevations of hepatic transaminases (92). Cyclosporin has been noted to increase the AUC of caspofungin by approximately 35%, but these alterations are not sufficient to suggest dosage modifications (114,152).

Antimetabolites

The only available antifungal agent that functions as a true antimetabolite is 5-fluorocytosine (flucytosine; 5-FC).

Flucytosine

Flucytosine is a water-soluble, synthetic, fluorinated pyrimidine analogue that exerts antifungal activity by interfering with the synthesis of DNA, RNA, and proteins in the fungal cell. Flucytosine is taken up into the cell by a fungus-specific cytosine permease and converted in the cytoplasm to 5-fluorouracil (5-FU) by cytosine deaminase. The 5-FU is converted by uracil monophosphate (UMP) pyrophosphorylase into 5-fluorouridylic acid, which then competes with uracil in the synthesis of RNA and ultimately causes RNA miscoding and inhibition of DNA and protein synthesis (262).

Flucytosine has a relatively narrow spectrum of activity, including *Candida* spp, *C. neoformans, Saccharomyces cerevisiae,* and selected dematiaceous molds (Tables 6.2 and 6.3). Primary resistance to flucytosine is uncommon among most species of *Candida* (200); however, resistance may develop among *Candida* spp and *C. neoformans* during flucytosine monotherapy (27,200). Flucytosine has no meaningful activity against *Aspergillus* spp or other hyaline molds (200).

Flucytosine is available in an oral formulation with excellent bioavailability. Unfortunately, the intravenous formulation is no longer widely available. High concentrations of flucytosine may be achieved in serum, cerebrospinal fluid, and other body fluids (262,263). Recent *in vitro* pharmacodynamic studies have determined that flucytosine exhibits concentration-independent fungistatic activity against *Candida* spp that is optimized at concentrations four times the MIC (131). Furthermore, flucytosine exerts a significant postantifungal effect of 2.5 to 4 hours against *Candida* spp (131). These findings have been confirmed *in vivo* by Andes and van Ogtrop (6), who showed that time above the MIC was the pharmacodynamic parameter that correlated best with outcome in flucytosine treatment of murine candidiasis. Furthermore, maximum efficacy was seen when flucytosine blood levels exceeded the MIC for only 20% to 25% of the dosing interval (6). The later observation may be accounted for by the postantifungal effect of flucytosine.

Because of its propensity for secondary resistance (81), flucytosine is not usually used as monotherapy but in combination with either amphotericin B (20,82,260) or fluconazole (144). These combinations have been shown to be efficacious in treating both cryptococcosis and candidiasis (92,279).

The major adverse effects of flucytosine therapy are bone marrow suppression, gastrointestinal intolerance, and hepatotoxicity (262,263). Flucytosine is renally excreted and nephrotoxicity due to concomitant administration of amphotericin B may result in the accumulation of toxic blood levels of flucytosine. Monitoring plasma concentrations of flucytosine is essential to avoid toxicity. Peak plasma levels of 40 μg/mL easily exceed the MICs of most *Candida* spp and *C. neoformans* (27,200) and provide optimal antifungal activity while minimizing hematologic adverse effects (263).

Allylamines

The allylamine class of antifungal agents is composed of terbinafine and naftifine. Only terbinafine has systemic activity. Naftifine is a topical agent and will be discussed in a subsequent section. Both terbinafine and naftifine inhibit the enzyme squalene epoxidase, which results in the accumulation of squalene and blocks the synthesis of ergosterol (91). The accumulation of high concentrations of squalene results in increased membrane permeability and, ultimately, cell death.

Terbinafine

Terbinafine is a lipophilic antifungal agent that is available in oral and topical formulations. Terbinafine has a rather broad spectrum of activity that includes dermatophytes, *Candida* spp, *Malassezia furfur, Aspergillus* spp, *C. neoformans, Trichosporon* spp, *Sporothrix schenckii,* and *P. marneffei* (98,109,146,236,237).

Terbinafine is well absorbed orally and achieves high concentrations in fatty tissues, skin, hair, and nails (98,258).

Terbinafine exhibits low toxicity and good efficacy in the treatment of virtually all dermatomycoses, including onychomycosis (22). The combination of terbinafine and fluconazole has shown promise for the treatment of infections due to fluconazole-resistant *Candida* spp (89). Terbinafine also has shown clinical efficacy in cases of sporotrichosis, aspergillosis, and chromoblastomycosis (78,179).

There are very few adverse effects associated with terbinafine therapy. The most commonly reported side effects include gastrointestinal upset and cutaneous reactions (99). Reversible agranulocytosis has been reported but is rare (99,168).

Griseofulvin

Griseofulvin is a long-standing oral agent used for the treatment of dermatomycoses. Its mechanism of action is thought to involve interaction with microtubules within the fungal cell and inhibition of mitosis.

Griseofulvin is active against most dermatophytes (268); however, newer agents, such as itraconazole and terbinafine, appear to be more potent and exhibit greater efficacy (122,123).

Griseofulvin is best absorbed orally when administered in an ultramicrocrystalline form with a heavy meal. It is deposited primarily in keratin precursor cells.

Griseofulvin is currently a second-line agent in the treatment of dermatomycosis. Although more expensive, both itraconazole and terbinafine are more rapid acting and provide greater efficacy (101). Administration of griseofulvin is associated with a number of mild side effects including nausea, diarrhea, headache, cutaneous disruptions, hepatotoxicity, and neurological side effects (123).

ANTIFUNGAL AGENTS FOR TOPICAL USE

There are numerous topical antifungal preparations available for the treatment of superficial cutaneous and mucosal fungal infections (Table 6.1). The available preparations encompass a wide variety of antifungal classes including polyenes (amphotericin B, nystatin, pimaricin), allylamines (naftifine and terbinafine), and numerous imidazoles and other miscellaneous agents. Preparations for use in cutaneous disease and onychomycosis include creams, lotions, ointments, powders, and sprays, whereas suspensions, tablets, troches, and suppositories are used for treatment of various forms of mucosal candidiasis (222,250,258).

The selection of topical versus systemic therapy for cutaneous or mucosal fungal infections depends on the status of the host and the type and extent of the infection. The refractory nature of infections such as onychomycosis or tinea capitis usually mandates long-term systemic therapy, whereas most cutaneous dermatophytic infections and oral or vaginal thrush will respond well to topical therapy. Systemic agents are generally recommended for chronic, recurrent oral or vaginal candidiasis and for candidal esophagitis.

ANTIFUNGAL AGENTS UNDER DEVELOPMENT

Currently, several different antifungal agents are under active development, including those with established modes of action as well as some novel new classes of antifungal agents (Table 6.1). These include a liposomal formulation of nystatin, novel triazole agents (posaconazole and ravuconazole), echinocandins (anidulafungin and micafungin), a chitin synthase inhibitor (nikkomycin Z), and sordarin and azasordarin derivatives. The mechanisms of action and spectra of activity of liposomal nystatin, the novel triazoles, and the echinocandins are essentially the same as the polyenes, triazole, and echinocandin agents currently available (Tables 6.2 to 6.5). In each case, the newer agents in the respective classes offer the potential of fewer toxicities and drug interactions, more favorable pharmacokinetic and pharmacodynamic properties, and possible improved activity against selected refractory pathogens (92). The sordarins and azasordarins offer the potential of a completely unique class of antifungal agent, whereas the existing antifungal agents act on either the fungal cell membrane (polyenes and azoles) or the cell wall (echinocandins), the sordarins and azasordarins block elongation factor 3, which is essential for fungal protein synthesis (60,104). Nikkomycin Z, which inhibits chitin synthesis in the fungal cell wall, provides another novel mode of action that may act in concert with other inhibitors of cell wall or cell membrane synthesis (35). The introduction of several of these new agents into clinical practice appears imminent (posaconazole, anidulafungin, micafungin) and should augment our available antifungal resources. The development of agents with novel modes of action is both necessary and promising for future antifungal therapy.

MECHANISMS OF RESISTANCE TO ANTIFUNGAL AGENTS

Resistance to antimicrobial agents is an issue of concern worldwide with important implications for morbidity, mortality, and the costs of health care. Although much attention has been focused on antibacterial resistance (111,112), innate or acquired resistance to antifungal agents is now recognized among pathogenic fungi (198,247). This recognition has spurred the development of new antifungal agents as well as intensive efforts to define the molecular mechanisms of resistance to various agents (91,247,275,277). The extensive utilization of fluconazole has been coupled with increasing reports of azole resistance (198,230) and some of the most elegant investigations of antifungal resistance mechanisms have involved the azole class of antifungals and *Candida* spp (247,275–277). In this section we will review what is known of the molecular and cellular mechanisms of resistance to antifungal agents as well as the clinical factors that may result in resistance to antifungal therapy.

Molecular and Cellular Mechanisms of Resistance to Antifungal Agents

Most fungal infections are caused by *Candida* spp and most of our understanding of the mechanisms of resistance comes from studies of *C. albicans* and other species of *Candida* (247,275–277). Although *Aspergillus* spp and *C. neoformans* constitute a significant proportion of opportunistic mycoses, fewer studies have been performed on these organisms, and almost no information on antifungal resistance mechanisms is available for other opportunistic fungal pathogens (91,177).

Although there are many parallels that exist between antibacterial resistance mechanisms and antifungal resistance mechanisms (91), there are no data to suggest that destruction or modification of antifungal agents is an important component of antifungal resistance. Likewise, it does not appear that fungi can employ the genetic exchange mechanisms that allow rapid transmission of antimicrobial resistance in bacteria (91). On the other hand, it is apparent that multidrug efflux pumps, target alterations, and reduced access to targets are important mechanisms of resistance to antifungal agents, just as they are important in antibacterial resistance (Table 6.6) (91,247,275–277). In contrast to the rapid emergence of high-level antimicrobial resistance that occurs among bacteria, antifungal resistance usually develops slowly and involves the emergence of intrinsically resistant species or a gradual, stepwise alteration of cellular structures or functions that results in resistance to an agent to which there has been prior exposure (91).

Polyenes

Resistance to amphotericin B remains uncommon despite extensive utilization over more than 30 years. Among the *Candida* spp, decreased susceptibility to amphotericin B has been reported in *C. lusitaniae, C. glabrata, C. krusei*, and *C. guilliermondii* (Table 6.2) (79,91,186,196,202, 231,247). Although primary resistance to amphotericin B may be seen among *C. lusitaniae, C. krusei*, and *C. guilliermondii* (177,186,196), most reports of amphotericin B resistance in *Candida* spp appear to be secondary to amphotericin B exposure during treatment (79,247,276). Most isolates of *Aspergillus* spp appear susceptible to amphotericin B (Table 6.4); however, *A. terreus* seems to be resistant to amphotericin B both *in vitro* and *in vivo* (44,58,127,266). Likewise, primary resistance to amphotericin B among *C. neoformans* has not been reported and secondary resistance appears rare (Table 6.3) (27,115,279).

Our understanding of the mechanism of resistance to amphotericin B stems largely from studies of mutants of *Candida* spp and *C. neoformans* derived from sequential passage in varying concentrations of amphotericin B (12,99a) and from characterization of serial isolates from patients failing amphotericin B therapy (56,57,79,115,217,239,277,281). The mechanism of amphotericin B resistance appears to be from a qualitative or quantitative alteration in the sterol content of cells (91). Because ergosterol is the primary sterol target for amphotericin B in the fungal cell membrane, resistant cells with altered sterol content should bind smaller amounts of amphotericin B than do susceptible cells (91). Accordingly, mutants of *Candida* spp and *C. neoformans* resistant to amphotericin B have been shown to have a reduced total ergosterol content (56,115), replacement of polyene-binding sterols (ergosterol) by ones that bind polyenes less well (fecosterol) (84,115), or masking of ergosterol in the cell membrane so that binding with polyenes is hindered by steric or thermodynamic factors (85,91,116). One or more of these factors may account for decreased susceptibility to amphotericin B (Table 6.6). This resistance is often specific for amphotericin B, but cross-resistance to azoles has also been reported (79). The molecular mechanisms of amphotericin B resistance in *Candida* and *C. neoformans* have not been determined; however, sterol analyses of resistant isolates suggest that they are defective in *erg*2 or *erg*3, genes encoding for the C-8 sterol isomerase and C-5 sterol desaturase enzymes, respectively (277).

Azoles

The excellent safety profile of fluconazole has led to extensive utilization of this agent worldwide (91,177). Concomitant with this utilization has come reports of emerging resistance to fluconazole and other azoles (230). Despite these reports, primary resistance to fluconazole is unusual among most species of *Candida* causing bloodstream infections (191). Among the five most common species of *Candida* isolated from blood (*C. albicans, C. glabrata, C. parapsilosis, C. tropicalis*, and *C. krusei*), the overall frequency of resistance (MIC more than

TABLE 6.6

Mechanisms Involved in the Development of Resistance to Antifungal Agents in Pathogenic Fungi[a]

Fungus	Amphotericin B	Flucytosine	Itraconazole	Fluconazole	Caspofungin
A. fumigatus			Altered target enzyme, 14-α-demethylase Decreased azole accumulation		
C. albicans	Decrease in ergosterol Replacement of polyene-binding sterols Masking of ergosterol	Loss of permease activity Loss of cytosine deaminase activity Loss of uracil phosphoribosyl-transferase activity		Overexpression or mutation of 14-α-demethylase Overexpression of efflux pumps, *CDR* and *MDR* genes	Mutation in *FKS*1 gene
C. glabrata	Alteration or decrease in ergosterol content	Loss of permease activity		Overexpression of efflux pumps (*CgCDR* genes)	
C. krusei	Alteration or decrease in ergosterol content			Active efflux Reduced affinity for target enzyme, 14-α-demethylase	Mutation in *FKS*1 gene
C. lusitaniae	Alteration or decrease in ergosterol content Production of modified sterols				
C. neoformans	Defects in sterol synthesis Decreased ergosterol Production of modified sterols			Alterations in target enzyme Overexpression of MDR efflux pump	

[a] Adapted from Ghannoum and Rice (91), Perea and Patterson (177), White (275), and White et al. (277).

64 μg/mL) to fluconazole is less than 3% (Table 6.2) (191). Resistance is rare among bloodstream infections of *C. albicans* (0% to 2%), *C. parapsilosis* (0% to 1%), and *C. tropicalis* (0% to 1%), whereas approximately 9% of *C. glabrata* isolates exhibit primary resistance to this agent (Table 6.2) (191,193,194). *Candida krusei* is considered intrinsically resistant to fluconazole and MICs are usually more than 32 μg/mL for this species (Table 6.2). Notably, the frequency of resistance to fluconazole among bloodstream infection isolates of *Candida* spp has not increased substantially after more than a decade of utilization worldwide (191).

The new triazoles (posaconazole, ravuconazole, and voriconazole) exhibit more potent activity against *Candida* spp than that of fluconazole, including activity against *C. krusei* and some fluconazole-resistant strains of *Candida* (185,186,194–196,199,201,202). Isolates of *C. glabrata* for which fluconazole MICs are 16 to 32 μg/mL (susceptible-dose dependent) appear susceptible (MICs, less than 1 μg/mL) to voriconazole, posaconazole, and ravuconazole (185,194,199,201,202); however, those isolates for which fluconazole MICs exceed 64 μg/mL (resistant) also tend to be less susceptible to the new triazoles with MICs more than 2 μg/mL (185,194,199,201,202). In general among *Candida* isolates, there is a strong positive correlation between fluconazole MICs and those of voriconazole, posaconazole, and ravuconazole, suggesting some degree of cross-resistance (185,199, 201).

Similar to *Candida* spp, primary resistance to fluconazole is uncommon among isolates of *C. neoformans* (27), although secondary resistance has been described among individuals with AIDS and relapsing cryptococcal meningitis (27,29,174). Despite these reports, the susceptibility profile of this organism to fluconazole has remained unchanged over the past 10 years (Table 6.3) (27,185,201,206,280).

Although *Aspergillus* spp are intrinsically resistant to fluconazole, most isolates appear susceptible to itraconazole and the new triazoles (Table 6.4) (58). MICs greater than 1 μg/mL for these azoles are very unusual among clinical isolates of *Aspergillus* (58,70). Only a small number of *A. fumigatus* isolates have been shown to demonstrate resistance to itraconazole *in vitro* and *in vivo* (42,43,46, 54,69,70). In contrast to *Candida,* cross-resistance between itraconazole and the new triazoles is not complete: cross-resistance between itraconazole and posaconazole, but not voriconazole, was observed in two strains (69).

The mechanism of azole resistance in *Candida* has been well worked out for fluconazole and *C. albicans* (Table 6.6) (177,247,277). Resistance can be from a modification in the quality or quantity of the target enzyme, reduced access of the drug to the target, or some combination of these mechanisms (91,275,277). In the first instance, point mutations in the gene (*ERG11*) encoding for the target enzyme, 14-α-demethylase, leads to an altered target with decreased affinity for azoles. Overexpression of *ERG11* results in the production of high concentrations of the target enzyme, creating the need for higher intracellular azole concentrations to inhibit all of the enzyme molecules in the cell. Loss of allelic variation in the *ERG11* promoter may also result in a resistant strain that is homozygous for the mutated gene (276).

The second major mechanism involves active efflux of azole antifungal agents out of the cell through the action of two types of multidrug efflux transporters: the major facilitators (encoded by *MDR* genes) and those of the ATP-binding cassette superfamily (encoded by *CDR* genes) (91,177,247,277). Upregulation of the *MDR1* gene leads to fluconazole resistance, whereas upregulation of *CDR* genes leads to resistance to multiple azoles (243–246, 276, 277). Evidence that these mechanisms may act individually, sequentially, and in concert has been derived by studying serial isolates of *C. albicans* from AIDS patients with oropharyngeal candidiasis (135,136,221,276). An example of the evolution of fluconazole resistance from these mechanisms in a single patient is shown graphically in Figure 6.1 (221,276,277).

It appears that the mechanisms of resistance to azoles in *C. glabrata* involve upregulation of *CDR1* genes, resulting in resistance to multiple azoles (242). Azole resistance in *C. krusei* appears to be mediated by reduced susceptibility of the target enzyme to inhibition by fluconazole and itraconazole (169). This does not seem to be the case with the new triazoles, given their potent activity against *C. krusei*. (Table 6.2) (186,196,199,201,202).

The mechanisms of azole resistance in *Aspergillus* spp has not been as extensively characterized given the paucity of documented resistant strains (177). Both increased drug efflux and alterations in the 14-α-demethylase target were identified in two isolates of itraconazole-resistant *A. fumigatus* (42,43,46).

The *C. neoformans* isolates that have developed secondary resistance to fluconazole have been shown to have an altered target enzyme as well as overexpression of MDR efflux pumps (113,126). The ABC transporter cdr1 has also been described in *C. neoformans* (177).

Echinocandins

Among the echinocandin antifungal agents, caspofungin has been approved for primary therapy for invasive candidiasis, including candidemia, and for salvage therapy for invasive aspergillosis (92,152). Caspofungin, anidulafungin, and micafungin all exhibit potent fungicidal activity against all species of *Candida,* including azole-resistant strains (3,62–64a,95,182,183,189,190,192,197). Isolates for which caspofungin MICs exceed 1 μg/mL rarely occur in clinical infections (Table 6.2) (152,189,197). Efforts to produce laboratory mutants of *Candida* spp with reduced susceptibility to caspofungin have demonstrated that the

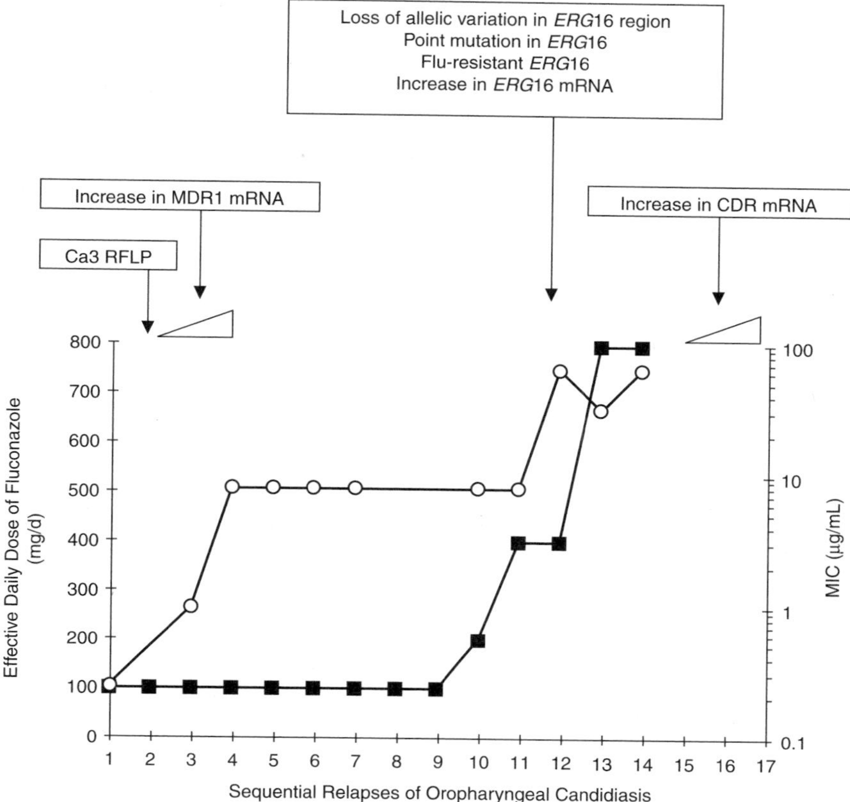

FIGURE 6.1 ● Relationship between minimum inhibitory concentration (MIC), dose of fluconazole, and emergence/expression of specific resistance mechanisms in oropharyngeal candidiasis.○, MIC of fluconazole for the clinical isolate; ■, effective daily dose of fluconazole. MICs are represented on the secondary y-axis, in logarithmic scale. Boxes above the graph represent genetic changes identified at each stage. Based on data from Redding et al. (221), White (275,276), and White et al. (277). (From Ghannoum and Rice [91], with permission.)

frequency of these mutants is extremely low (1 in 10^8 cells), suggesting a very low potential for the emergence of resistance in the clinical setting (61,124). Likewise, isolates of *Aspergillus* spp from clinical sources with reduced susceptibility to echinocandins are virtually unheard of to date (58) and efforts to obtain laboratory-derived mutants with decreased susceptibility to these agents have been unsuccessful (92).

Studies of laboratory-derived mutants of *C. albicans* with reduced *in vitro* and *in vivo* susceptibility to caspofungin have documented point mutations in the *FKS1* gene encoding for the FKS1 integral membrane protein, which is the catalytic subunit of the glucan-synthesis enzyme complex (61,124,130). These mutant strains demonstrate an increased IC_{50} (50% Inhibitory Concentration) for inhibition of the glucan synthesis enzyme complex and reduced susceptibility to all echinocandins *in vitro* and *in vivo* in animal models (18, 61,124). These strains remain susceptible to polyenes and azole antifungal agents. Although the *FKS1* gene is essential in *Aspergillus* spp as well (19), similar mutations have not been demonstrated to date (92,130).

Flucytosine

Despite reports in the older literature of a higher frequency of primary resistance to flucytosine among *Candida* spp and *C. neoformans* (49,254), more recent studies using validated, standardized test methods indicate that primary resistance is actually uncommon among bloodstream infection isolates of *Candida* spp (200) and isolates of *C. neoformans* (27) (Tables 6.2 and 6.3). Furthermore, studies of an international collection of bloodstream infection isolates of *C. albicans* reveal that resistance to flucytosine is restricted to a single genetic clade (DNA group I) (219). Secondary resistance to flucytosine, on the other hand, is well documented to occur among both *Candida* spp and *C. neoformans* during monotherapy with this agent (273).

Resistance to flucytosine may develop from decreased uptake (loss of permease activity) or by loss of enzymatic activity required for the conversion of flucytosine to 5-FU (cytosine deaminase) and 5-fluorouridylic acid (FUMP pyrophosphorylase) (Table 6.6) (91,273,274). Of these possible mechanisms, the most important appear to be the loss of cytosine deaminase activity or the loss of UMP pyrophosphorylase activity. Uracil phosphoribosyltransferase, another enzyme in the primidine salvage pathway, is also important in the formation of FUMP and loss of its activity is sufficient to confer resistance to flucytosine (274).

Allylamines

Allylamine resistance has not been detected among pathogenic fungi despite clinical failures observed with utilization of these agents (91). Sanglard et al. (245) have reported that the CDR1 multidrug efflux pump can use terbinafine as a substrate, thus the possibility of efflux-mediated resistance to allylamines exists.

Clinical Factors Contributing to Antifungal Resistance

Fungal infections may fail to respond to appropriate antifungal therapy, thereby demonstrating "clinical resistance," despite the fact that the drug employed is active against the infecting organism (225). The interaction of the host, the drug, and the fungus is very complex and the clinical outcome may be greatly influenced by a variety of interactions (225,275).

The immune status of the host is without question the most important factor in determining the outcome of antifungal therapy of an invasive mycosis. The presence of neutrophils, utilization of immunomodulating drugs, concomitant infections (e.g., HIV), surgical procedures, age, and nutritional status of the host all may be more important than the ability, or lack thereof, of the antifungal agent to inhibit or kill the infecting organism. Likewise, the site and severity of the infection play a very important role in determining whether or not an infection can be controlled by antifungal therapy alone. The presence of a foreign body, such as catheter, prosthetic valve, or vascular graft material, may allow an otherwise susceptible organism to cause an infection that is recalcitrant to therapy with an otherwise active agent. Finally, an antifungal agent cannot act if the patient does not take it in the prescribed manner. Noncompliance is a major cause of apparent "resistance" to antifungal therapy and may also contribute to the development of resistant strains (275).

The absorption, distribution, and metabolism of an antifungal agent all contribute to the effectiveness of the drug at the site of infection. Insufficient (too low) dosing practices may influence both therapeutic efficacy and the potential for resistance development. The ability of an antifungal agent to exhibit fungicidal activity versus fungistatic activity may be especially important in severe infections, in infections where the organism burden is high, and in the neutropenic host (190). Drug-drug interactions may also affect the activity of an antifungal agent: drugs that are metabolized by the cytochrome-P-450 enzyme system, such as rifamycin, may dramatically decrease the achievable concentrations of azole antifungal agents such as itraconazole and voriconazole.

Fungal properties, aside from the expression of known resistance factors, may also impact the clinical success or failure of antifungal therapy. The different morphologic forms of fungi (e.g., blastospore, hypha, pseudohypha, conidia, chlamydospore) may all have different susceptibilities to various antifungal agents (275). Phenotypic switching in *Candida* has been shown to have a dramatic impact on the susceptibility of various species to polyenes and azoles (79,261). Finally, the rate of growth of a fungus and whether or not it is growing in a planktonic or sessile form can determine whether it will require low or high concentrations of an antifungal to inhibit growth (13). *Candida* spp become much more resistant to antifungals when grown in a biofilm than when they are suspended in solution (29a).

ANTIFUNGAL SUSCEPTIBILITY TESTING

The increasing number and diversity of invasive infections, expanding utilization of new and established antifungal agents, and recognition of antifungal resistance as an important clinical problem have contributed to the need for reproducible, clinically relevant antifungal susceptibility testing, especially for yeasts, but also for the filamentous fungi (68,71,73,77,203a,209,226,230,233). Through the collaborative efforts of numerous investigators and the National Committee for Clinical Laboratory Standards (NCCLS) Subcommittee on Antifungal Susceptibility Testing, antifungal susceptibility testing has been standardized and now plays an increasingly important role in guiding therapeutic decision making, as an aid in drug-development studies, and as a means of tracking the development of antifungal resistance in epidemiologic studies (27,58,70,158,159,185,189,191–193,195–202,225,227,228,230).

Rationale for Antifungal Susceptibility Testing

The central objective of all *in vitro* susceptibility testing is to help predict the likely impact of administration of the tested agent on the outcome of disease caused by the tested organism or similar organisms (203a,225). As such, *in vitro* susceptibility tests of antifungal agents are performed for the same reasons as tests of antibacterial agents are performed (61,111,112,203a,225,226,228): (a) to provide a reliable estimate of the relative activities of two or more agents, (b) to correlate with *in vivo* activity and predict the outcome of the therapy, (c) to provide a means by which to survey the development of resistance among a normally susceptible population of organisms, and (d) to predict the therapeutic potential of newly developed investigational agents. In the clinical microbiology/mycology laboratory, the focus of testing is on a specific isolate from an individual patient. In drug discovery, the focus of testing may be on the selection of the most potent of a series of compounds for further development. In antimicrobial resistance surveillance, the issue may be the tendency of resistance to emerge in initially susceptible isolates or species and to establish local, regional, or national patterns of resistance (191,198,203a). In each of these settings, it is necessary to keep in mind the fact that the prediction of outcome in a complex and dynamic biological system (clinical infection) from results obtained in an artificial and well-defined matrix (antimicrobial susceptibility test) is an inherently error-prone process and that only modest degrees of correlation can be expected (203a,209,225,226). Decades of experience with antibacterial susceptibility testing confirms the limited degree of *in vitro–in vivo* correlation that can be achieved (145,154,225,241,255). Although *in vitro* resistance may often (but not always) predict clinical failure, *in vitro* susceptibility does not always predict successful therapy (225).

Development of Standardized Methods

At the present time, the state-of-the-art method for susceptibility testing of yeasts is comparable with that of bacteria (225). The NCCLS Subcommittee on Antifungal Susceptibility Testing has developed and published approved methods for broth dilution testing of yeasts (159) and for disk diffusion testing of yeasts against fluconazole (157). These methods are reproducible, accurate, and available for use in clinical laboratories (17,157,159,195). Standardized methods have also been developed for broth dilution testing of filamentous fungi but require further refinement and studies to establish the *in vivo* correlation with the *in vitro* data (68,69,71,158,166,167). A great deal of progress has been made since 1982 in the development of standardized methods for antifungal susceptibility testing (Table 6.7).

Standardized Broth Dilution Methods for Yeasts: *NCCLS Document M27-A2*

The NCCLS Subcommittee on Antifungal Susceptibility Testing was established in 1982 and focused on the key *in vitro* testing variables of inoculum preparation and size, medium composition, temperature and duration of incubation, and MIC endpoint determination in an effort to develop a standardized approach to antifungal susceptibility testing of yeasts (*Candida* spp and *C. neoformans*) using a broth dilution format (83,209,215,216). As a result of several collaborative studies, consensus within the subcommittee was achieved on all of the variables, leading to the publication of a proposed broth macrodilution method, *M27-P*, in 1992 (163). This document was revised and published in 1995 as NCCLS document *M27-T* (tentative standard), which described the broth microdilution method and provided reference MIC ranges for two quality control (QC) strains for the available antifungal agents (72,73,162,210,229). In 1997, the subcommittee established interpretive MIC breakpoints for three antifungal agents (fluconazole, itraconazole, and flucytosine) (228) and the NCCLS-approved standard M27-A was published (161). Since then, the subcommittee has developed 24- and 48-hour reference QC MIC ranges for microdilution testing of both established (amphotericin B, flucytosine, fluconazole, itraconazole, and ketoconazole) and newly introduced (voriconazole, posaconazole, and ravuconazole) agents (16). The results of these studies are included in the second edition of NCCLS document M27, *M27-A2*, published in 2002 (Table 6.7) (159).

The NCCLS M27-A2 method has been reviewed in detail in previous publications (73,203a,225,226) and the key features are summarized in Table 6.8. Adherence to the NCCLS M27-A2 method provides excellent intralaboratory and interlaboratory reproducibility (17,18,27,83), and utilization of the recommended QC isolates will further ensure reliable test performance (16,159,210, 229).

Standardized Disk Diffusion Methods for Yeasts: *NCCLS Document M44-A*

Disk diffusion testing has served as a simple, rapid, and cost-effective alternative to broth dilution testing of antibacterial agents for many years (110a,156). Disk diffusion testing of antifungal agents has been slow to develop; however, early studies with fluconazole disks showed promise for testing *Candida* spp (149,214). Further development of this method by Barry and colleagues (14,15,17,187,188,194,195) has documented the precision and accuracy of the fluconazole disk diffusion test and has established QC zone diameter limits for both fluconazole and voriconazole when tested against *Candida* spp (Table 6.9). The method as refined by Barry et al. (17) has been incorporated into the NCCLS approved guideline for antifungal disk diffusion susceptibility testing of yeasts, M44-A (157).

The NCCLS M44-A method uses Mueller-Hinton agar supplemented with 2% glucose and 0.5 μg/mL of methylene blue (14,17,157). The increased glucose and the methylene blue supplementation provides improved growth and sharper zones surrounding the fluconazole and voriconazole disks (17). This method employs an inoculum suspension adjusted to the turbidity of 0.5 McFarland Standard and 24-hour incubation at 35°C. The zone diameters surrounding the 25-μg fluconazole disks and the

TABLE 6.7

Progress Since 1982 in the Development of Antifungal Susceptibility Testing Methods

1. Development of macrodilution and microdilution broth reference methods for *Candida* and *Cryptococcus neoformans* (NCCLS[a] M27-A).
2. Establishment of quality control strains and minimum inhibitory concentration (MIC) reference ranges for amphotericin B, flucytosine, fluconazole, itraconazole, ketoconazole, posaconazole, ravuconazole, voriconazole, anidulafungin, and caspofungin (NCCLS M27-A2).
3. Development of MIC interpretive breakpoints for fluconazole, itraconazole, and flucytosine.
4. Standardized broth microdilution method for testing filamentous fungi (NCCLS M38-A).
5. Standardized disk diffusion susceptibility testing of yeasts (NCCLS M44-A).
6. Method for the determination of MIC by broth dilution of fermentative yeasts (EUCAST[b] E. Dis 7.1).
7. Development of alternative methods
   a. Spectrophotometric endpoint determination
   b. Colorimetric endpoint determination (Sensititre Yeast One, FDA-approved)
   c. Stable gradient agar MIC test (Etest)
   d. Glucose consumption
   e. Ergosterol quantitation
   f. Flow cytometry
   g. Commercial breakpoint methods
   h. Semisolid agar screen
   i. Minimum fungicidal and time-kill determinations
   j. Method for testing dermatophytes
8. Global standardization
   a. NCCLS and EUCAST (yeasts)
   b. Global surveillance
9. Proficiency testing (College of American Pathologists)

[a] NCCLS, National Committee for Clinical Laboratory Standards.
[b] EUCAST, European Committee on Antibiotic Susceptibility Testing.

1-μg voriconazole disks are read using reflected light and measured to the nearest whole millimeter at the point at which there is prominent reduction in growth. Pinpoint microcolonies at the zone edge or large colonies within a zone are ignored.

This method provides qualitative susceptibility results 24 hours sooner than the standard NCCLS M27-A2 MIC method for yeasts (195). The disk test results correlate well with reference MICs for both fluconazole and voriconazole and have allowed the establishment of zone interpretive criteria (breakpoints) for fluconazole (Table 6.9) and QC parameters for both fluconazole and voriconazole (Table 6.10) (15,17,157,187,194,195). The use of supplemented Mueller-Hinton agar in lieu of RPMI 1640 medium should make antifungal susceptibility testing available to a larger number of clinical laboratories at reduced cost. It is expected that disk diffusion testing will be expanded to include other azoles and additional classes of antifungal agents (187) as well as additional fungal genera. Recently, the M44-A disk test method has been shown to be a useful approach for determining the fluconazole susceptibility of *C. neoformans* (188).

Standardized Broth Dilution Methods for Filamentous Fungi: *NCCLS Document M38-A*

Serious infections due to filamentous fungi (molds), especially those due to *Aspergillus* spp, are increasing rapidly, and effective therapy for these infections constitutes an unmet medical need (46a,133,147,172,173). Given the increasing array of antifungal agents with systemic activity against the filamentous fungi (58,103,130,180), it is recognized that antifungal susceptibility testing of those opportunistic pathogens may be important in guiding the

TABLE 6.8

Key Features of NCCLS[a] and EUCAST[b] Methods for Antifungal Susceptibility Testing of Yeasts and Filamentous Fungi

	Standards		
	Yeast		Mold
Variable	*NCCLS M27-A2*[c]	*EUCAST*[d]	*M38-A*[e]
Method	Macrodilution (final vol. 1 mL) Microdilution (final vol. 200 μl)	Microdilution (final vol. 200 μl)	Microdilution (final vol. 200 μl)
Inoculum preparation	Spectrophotometric adjustment with use of 0.5 McFarland turbidity standard	Spectrophotometric adjustment using 0.5 McFarland standard	Spectrophotometric adjustment of spore suspension; 0.09–0.11 Optical density for *Aspergillus* and *Rhizopus* 0.15–0.17 OD for *Fusarium* and *P. boydii*
Inoculum concentration (final)	0.5–2.5 × 10^3 cells/mL	0.5–2.5 × 10^5 cells/mL	0.4–5.0 × 10^4 CFU/mL
Test medium	RPMI 1640	RPMI 1640 with 2% glucose	RPMI 1640
Buffer	MOPS[f]	MOPS[f]	MOPS[f]
PH	7.0	7.0	7.0
Incubation temperature	35°C	35°C	35°C
Incubation Time	48h (72 h for *C. neoformans*) 24 h for echinocandins	24 h	24 h for *Rhizopus* 48 h for *Aspergillus* and *Fusarium* 72 h for *P. boydii*
MIC endpoint determination	Visual Amphotericin B: no visible turbidity Azoles and flucystosine: ≥80% inhibition for macrodilution; ≥50% inhibition for microdilution Echinocandins: ≥50% for microdilution	Spectrophotometric (530 nm) azoles and flucytosine: ≥50% inhibition Amphotericin B: ≥ 90% inhibition	Visual Amphotericin B: no visible turbidity Azoles: no visible turbidity Echinocandins: prominent decrease or lowest concentration with morphologic change (MEC)[g]

[a] NCCLS, National Committee for Clinical Laboratory Standards.
[b] EUCAST, European Committee for Antimicrobial Susceptibility Testing.
[c] Method is published in NCCLS document M27-A2 (159).
[d] Method is published in Rodriguez-Tudela et al. (235).
[e] Method is published in NCCLS document M38-A (158).
[f] MOPS, morpholenepropanesulfonic acid.
[g] MEC, minimum effective concentration.

TABLE 6.9

Interpretive Criteria for Minimum Inhibitory Concentration (MIC) and Disk Testing of Antifungal Agents Against Yeasts Utilizing NCCLS-Recommended Methods

Antifungal Agent	Susceptibility Category[a]	Interpretive Criteria	
		MIC (μg/mL)[b]	Zone (mm)[c]
Fluconazole	S	<8	>19
	S-DD	16–32	15–18
	R	>64	<14
Itraconazole	S	<0.12	NA[d]
	S-DD	0.25–0.5	NA[d]
	R	>1	NA[d]
Flucytosine	S	<4	NA[d]
	I	8–16	NA[d]
	R	>32	NA[d]

NCCLS, National Committee for Clinical Laboratory Standards.
[a] S, susceptible; S-DD, susceptible-dose dependent; I, intermediate; R, resistant.
[b] Method performed as described in NCCLS document M27-A2 (159).
[c] Method performed as described in NCCLS document M44-A (157).
[d] NA, not available.

selection of antifungal agents for treatment of invasive disease (73). This is especially true for the newer triazole (posaconazole, ravuconazole, and voriconazole) and echinocandin (caspofungin, micafungin, and anidulafungin) agents, all of which have varying degrees of activity against the opportunistic molds (Table 6.4) (58,66,70,105,110,130). Based on the achievements in standardizing *in vitro* susceptibility testing of yeasts, the NCCLS antifungal subcommittee has proceeded to develop a standardized method for the broth dilution testing of molds, NCCLS M38-A (158). The NCCLS subcommittee used the M27-A2 microdilution method as a template for the development of the method for filamentous fungi. The approved method, M38-A, is applicable for testing *Aspergillus* spp, *Fusarium* spp, *P. boydii*, and the Zygomycetes (73,158). The key features of the NCCLS M38-A method for testing filamentous fungi are listed in Table 6.8. Several multicenter studies have documented the excellent reproducibility of this method (65,68,69,71), and have shown promise in predicting antifungal efficacy (127,167).

Quality Control

The importance of QC strains in the development and day-to-day performance of antimicrobial susceptibility testing cannot be overemphasized. QC strains for broth dilution antifungal testing of yeasts have been defined for 10 antifungal agents (16,159,210,229). Likewise, QC strains for broth dilution testing of molds (158) and disk diffusion testing of yeasts (14,157,187) have also been defined. The MICs and zone diameters of the various antifungals for these QC strains consistently fall within a relatively narrow range of values when the test is properly performed and, as with bacterial susceptibility testing, QC testing has proven to be of great importance in ensuring the accuracy and reproducibility of antifungal testing. The properties of these strains for broth dilution and disk diffusion testing are summarized in Table 6.10. The QC parameters for the various strains and antifungal agents have been developed by multicenter studies in accordance with the guidelines published in NCCLS document M23-A2 (160). These strains are essential for routine QC of antifungal susceptibility testing in the clinical laboratory. Each new batch of broth medium, lot of microdilution tubes, microdilution trays, agar plates, and antifungal disks should be tested using the available QC strains to ensure that the MICs and zones are within the reference ranges. Furthermore, the overall performance of the test system should be monitored by testing the QC strains each day in which a test is performed for each drug (73,160). These strains are also useful in studying other testing methods and factors that may influence MIC or disk diffusion test results. It is important to realize, however, that the QC strains were selected in part for their stability and consistent performance in the NCCLS MIC and disk diffusion systems and thus may be less affected by minor modifications in the test parameters than fresh clinical isolates (203a).

Progress and New Developments in Antifungal Susceptibility Testing

The availability of the M27 reference method for broth dilution testing of yeasts has paved the way for the development of the reference method for filamentous fungi and was a necessary precursor to the M44 disk diffusion method. In addition, the M27 method has served as a touchstone for further development and evaluation of new and improved methods for performing antifungal testing in the clinical laboratory (Table 6.7) and has facilitated the performance of large-scale national and international surveillance studies of the *in vitro* susceptibility of *Candida* spp and other fungi to both established and investigational antifungal agents (2,11,27,34,41a,47,58,117,129,149,171,191,198,259). Such studies have been useful in generating broad MIC distribution profiles for clinical isolates (Tables 6.2 to 6.4) (198) and for identifying isolates to be used in the characterization of resistance mechanisms (275–277). Finally, the standardization of antifungal susceptibility testing has made it possible to conduct nationwide studies of laboratory proficiency and to begin to establish the

TABLE 6.10

Minimum Inhibitory Concentration (MIC) and Zone Diameter Ranges of Various Antifungal Agents for Four Quality Control Strains of *Candida* Species When Tested by NCCLS Broth Dilution and Disk Diffusion Procedures

		Broth Dilution MIC (μg/mL)[a] and Disk Diffusion Zone Diameter (mm)[b] Ranges for Tests with					
		C. parapsilosis		*C. krusei*		*C. tropicalis*	*C. albicans*
Test Format	**Antifungal Agent**	ATCC 22019 at 24 h	48 h	ATCC 6258 at 24 h	48 h	ATCC 750 at 24 h	ATCC 90028 at 24 h
Macrodilution	Amphotericin B	—	0.25–1	—	0.25–2	—	—
	Flucytosine	—	0.12–0.5	—	4–16	—	—
	Fluconazole	—	2–8	—	16–64	—	—
	Itraconazole	—	0.06–0.25	—	0.12–0.5	—	—
	Ketoconazole	—	0.06–0.25	—	0.12–0.5	—	—
Microdilution	Amphotericin B	0.25–2	0.5–4	0.5–2	1–4	—	—
	Flucytosine	0.06–0.25	0.12–0.5	0.5–2	1–4	—	—
	Fluconazole	0.5–4	1–4	8–64	16–128	—	—
	Itraconazole	0.12–0.5	0.12–0.5	0.12–1	0.25–1	—	—
	Ketoconazole	0.03–0.25	0.06–0.5	0.12–1	0.25–1	—	—
	Voriconazole	0.016–0.12	0.03–0.25	0.06–0.5	0.12–1	—	—
	Posaconazole	0.06–0.25	0.06–0.25	0.06–0.5	0.12–1	—	—
	Ravuconazole	0.016–0.12	0.03–0.25	0.06–0.5	0.25–2	—	—
	Caspofungin	0.25–1	0.5–4	0.12–1	0.25–1	—	—
	Anidulafungin	1–8	1–8	0.03–0.25	0.06–0.5	—	—
Disk diffusion	Fluconazole	22–33	—	—	—	26–37	28–39
	Voriconazole	28–37	—	16–25	—	—	31–42

NCCLS, National Committee for Clinical Laboratory Standards.
[a] As determined in NCCLS document M27-A2 (159) and Barry et al. (16).
[b] As determined in NCCLS document M44-P (157) and Barry et al. (14) and Pfaller et al. (187).

clinical relevance of antifungal susceptibility testing (203a,225,228).

New Test Development

The purpose of reference methods for antimicrobial susceptibility testing is to encourage standardization of the process and improve reproducibility among laboratories; however, the reference method per se may not be optimal for testing all organisms or the most convenient method for use in all clinical laboratories (73,203a,231). Thus, the NCCLS M27 method has been used as a reference, or "touchstone," not only for the development of the M38 and M44 methods, but also for alternative methods that may be easier to perform and to read and that may utilize technology already being utilized for other testing in the clinical laboratory (Table 6.7). The alternative methods most often employ a microdilution format and are read spectrophotometrically (2,9,10,36,40,41,77,211,231,235) or colorimetrically (75,100,108,132,142,150,151,153,212,213,234,257). In addition, novel breakpoint methods (73,153), agar-based methods (37,38,65,67,74,76,128,139,142,143,184,195, 203–205,207,208,218,251,267), and flow cytometry (33, 220,269,270) have been applied with varying degrees of success.

The utilization of colorimetric growth indicators has been applied to the microdilution method in an effort to provide improved ease and precision of MIC endpoint determination and possibly provide a more rapid means of testing clinically important fungi (73,203a). Colorimetric determination of residual glucose (132,234), pH indicator dyes (81), and various tetrazolium salt methods

(100,108) have all shown promise; however, the use of the oxidation reduction indicator alamarBlue (AccuMed International Inc., Chicago, IL) is the best studied and most widely used approach (75,141,153,212,213,257). In a broth, fungal growth causes the alamarBlue indicator to change from blue to pink. In an alamarBlue-containing system, the MIC for an antifungal agent is recorded as the first well to show a change from pink (growth) to purple or blue (growth inhibition). The alamarBlue indicator has been incorporated into a commercially available broth microdilution system, the Sensititre YeastOne colormetric antifungal plate (TREK Diagnostics Systems, Westlake, OH). The YeastOne system has been shown to perform comparably to the NCCLS reference method (75,141,150,153) and is approved by the U.S. Food and Drug Administration for *in vitro* susceptibility testing of yeasts.

The use of spectrophotometry has long been employed to measure the growth of microbes in a broth system. Spectrophotometric determination of fungal growth in the presence and absence of antifungal agents has been utilized to provide a more precise and objective means of MIC endpoint reading, especially for the azole class of antifungal agents (2,137,211,235).

A novel spectrophotometric method for determining the *in vitro* susceptibility of *Candida* spp to azoles was proposed by Arthington-Skaggs and colleagues at the Centers for Disease Control (9,10). They employed quantitation of the ergosterol content of cells following the growth of *Candida* spp in various concentrations of fluconazole and found it to be an excellent method for distinguishing fluconazole-susceptible, fluconazole-resistant, and highly resistant strains. The method was objective, quantitative, and not affected by the trailing that may confound the reading of fluconazole endpoints (9,10). Good agreement was observed between the sterol quantitative method and the M27 broth microdilution method. Unfortunately, this method is only applicable to the testing of azoles and possibly other inhibitors of ergosterol synthesis.

In many clinical settings, determination of precise MICs using a full-range dilution series is not necessary. Testing of the clinical isolate against one or two antimicrobial drug concentrations that distinguish susceptible from resistant strains, so-called "breakpoint testing" is often all that is necessary to allow the selection of optimal antifungal therapy. Various commercial breakpoint broth methods are available outside the United States, including Candifast (International Microbio/Stago Group, Milan, Italy), Mycototal (Behring Diagnostics, Rueil-Malmaison, France), Integral Systems Yeasts (Liofilchem Diagnostics, L'Aquila, Italy), and Fungitest (Bio-Rad SDP, Paris, France) (73,153). In general, the performance of these breakpoint methods has been disappointing, with only the Fungitest system showing acceptable agreement with the M27 reference method (48,153). In most instances, poor agreement with the reference method has been associated with a lack of medium standardization and lack of objective criteria for interpretation of results (153).

The agar-based methods for antifungal susceptibility testing include the previously mentioned disk diffusion method (NCCLS M44), the Etest stable agar gradient method (38,58,67,74,128,138,184,194,195,203–205,207,208,251,267), and the semisolid agar dilution method (218). The Etest method (AB BIODISK, Solna, Sweden) has been widely employed as a means of producing an accurate, reproducible, and quantitative MIC result using an agar diffusion format (240). This method is based on the diffusion of a continuous concentration gradient of an antimicrobial agent from a plastic strip into an agar medium. When an Etest strip is placed on an agar plate inoculated with a test organism, and incubated for 24 to 48 hours, an ellipse of growth inhibition occurs, and the intersection of the ellipse with the numeric scale on the strip allows the reading of the MIC. This test method has been extensively studied for utilization in antibacterial testing and is comparable with the reference broth and agar dilution MIC methods (240). The Etest is also applicable to antifungal susceptibility testing. Numerous studies demonstrate the usefulness of Etest for determining the *in vitro* susceptibility of both yeasts and molds to a variety of antifungal agents including amphotericin B, flucytosine, ketoconazole, itraconazole, voriconazole, posaconazole, and caspofungin (36–38,65,67,74,76,138,142,143,150,184,195,203–205,207,208,267). MICs determined by Etest generally agree quite well with those determined by the NCCLS reference method (17); however, this agreement may vary, depending on the antifungal agent tested, the choice of agar medium, and the organism species (74). The use of RPMI agar supplemented with 2% glucose seems to work well for most organisms and antifungal agents; however, decreased agreement has been reported for fluconazole and itraconazole tested against *C. glabrata* and *C. tropicalis* (194,195). The use of Mueller-Hinton agar supplemented with glucose and methylene blue has been shown to improve the overall agreement of Etest MICs with the reference method when testing *C. glabrata* against fluconazole and voriconazole (194). Of major importance is the fact that Etest is the most sensitive and reliable method for detecting decreased susceptibility to amphotericin B among isolates of *Candida* spp and *C. neoformans* (37,128,138,208,231, 267).

A semisolid agar dilution method was proposed by Provine and Hadley (218) to serve as a rapid, breakpoint screening test to detect isolates of *Candida* spp with decreased susceptibility to fluconazole. The method employs heart infusion broth with 0.5% agar and without glucose. The organism is inoculated into the system by stabbing the agar and the resulting conditions

TABLE 6.11

Fluconazole Resistance Among *Candida* Bloodstream Infection (BSI) Isolates as Determined by Different Surveillance Programs

Surveillance Program[a]	Years	Ref.	No. BSI Tested	% Resistant to Fluconazole[b]			
				C. albicans	*C. glabrata*	*C. parapsilosis*	*C. tropicalis*
Iceland	1980–99	11	170	0	0	0	0
CDC	1992–93	198	394	1	14	0	2
CDC	1998–00	198	944	1	10	0	6
Sweden	1994–98	198	233	0	40	15	0
Quebec	1996–98	198	442	1	9	0	0
Taiwan	1994–95	34	133	1.3	0	0	0
Taiwan	1996–97	34	227	0	0	0	0
Taiwan	1999–00	34	192	0	0	0	0
Argentina	1996–99	41a	230	8.5[c]	50[c]	1.4[c]	6.3[c]
Spain	1996–99	41a	514	1.9[c]	43[c]	0[c]	0[c]
Italy	1997–99	259	261	NA[d]	4	0	5
SENTRY	1997–00	198	2,047	1	7	0	1
EIEIO	1998–01	198	254	0	10	0	0
ARTEMIS	2001–02	185	3,932	1	9	1	1

[a] CDC, Centers for Disease Control; EIEIO, Emerging Infections and the Epidemiology of Iowa Organisms.
[b] Determined by using National Committee for Clinical Laboratory Standards or European Committee for Antimicrobial Susceptibility Testing broth microdilution and interpretive criteria (MIC >64 μg/mL).
[c] Includes both Susceptible-Dose Dependent (MIC, 16–32 μg/mL) and Resistant (MIC >64 μg/mL) categories.
[d] Not available.

are considered to mimic more closely the growth conditions of infected tissue (218). This simple method provides good categorical agreement with the M27 reference method, although the number of isolates tested to date is limited.

Flow cytometric methods have been employed with good success in testing *Candida* spp against fluconazole and amphotericin B (33,220). This approach uses a standard flow cytometer and fluorescent DNA binding dyes to detect fungal cell damage following exposure to an antifungal agent. The method produces results within 6 hours that agree very well with MICs determined by the M27 reference method (33,220).

Surveillance and New Drug Evaluation

One of the important offshoots of the standardization process has been the ability to conduct active surveillance of resistance to antifungal agents (198). Meaningful large-scale studies of antifungal susceptibility and resistance conducted over time would not be possible without a standardized microdilution method for performing the *in vitro* studies (34,191,198,203a). Many such studies have now been published and include studies of isolates from patients in the intensive care unit (21,129, 202) and nosocomial bloodstream infections in the United States and other countries worldwide (11, 27,34,41a,47,58,117,129,149,171,185,189,191,193,195, 197–202,259). Furthermore, studies analyzing resistance trends to commonly utilized antifungal agents such as fluconazole (11,27,34,41a,47,117,171,191,198) and comparative analyses of licensed and established antifungal agents (58,171,191,193,195,197–202, 259) have provided large amounts of useful data and have been greatly facilitated by a standardized microdilution method (Tables 6.2 to 6.4 and 6.11). As new antifungal agents are evaluated in clinical trials, *in vitro* susceptibility testing of the clinical isolates utilizing a reference method will be essential and will allow the establishment of *in vitro*/*in vivo* correlations (225).

Proficiency Testing

The participation of clinical laboratories in proficiency testing programs is considered an important step in ensuring quality and standardization in the performance of antimicrobial susceptibility testing (110a). Prior to the publication of NCCLS document M27-A, little was known of the proficiency of clinical laboratories in performing antifungal susceptibility testing aside from those laboratories actively engaged in NCCLS-conducted studies (68,71,74,75,166,215). Following the publication in 1997 of the NCCLS M27-A reference method for testing yeasts, the College of American Pathologists initiated a proficiency-testing program for antifungal susceptibility testing (203a). Since that time, the number of participants has increased from approximately 50 to 100 laboratories and the performance of laboratories has steadily improved (203a; R.N. Jones, personal communication). The participants are compliant with the NCCLS guidelines and a clear majority report utilizing the commercially available YeastOne colorimetric microdilution panel (203a; R.N. Jones, personal communication).. This program provides important information regarding the performance of antifungal susceptibility testing in the United States and indicates a level of performance that is on par with that of antibacterial testing.

Global Standardization

Subsequent to the development of the NCCLS M27-A method for broth microdilution testing of yeasts, a similar method has been developed under the auspices of the Subcommittee on Antifungal Susceptibility Testing (AFST) of the European Committee on Antibiotic Susceptibility Testing (EUCAST) (235). This method is very similar to the NCCLS M27-A2 method (Table 6.8) and employs a higher inoculum (10^5 CFU/mL), RPMI 1640 medium supplemented with additional glucose (2%), and spectophotometric readings of MIC endpoints following incubation at 35°C to 37°C for 24 hours (235). The efforts of the EUCAST-AFST subcommittee have stimulated a collaboration with the NCCLS subcommittee and recent multicenter studies have documented good intralaboratory reproducibility of the EUCAST method (41) and good agreement between the EUCAST and NCCLS microdilution methods (36,40,77). Such global collaboration in standardization of an antimicrobial susceptibility testing method is rare and marks a very positive step in the improvement of antifungal susceptibility testing worldwide (203a). In addition, global surveillance programs such as the ARTEMIS global antifungal program for disk testing (149,195) and MIC testing (185,195), the European Confederation of Medical Mycology survey of candidemia (117,259), and the SENTRY antifungal surveillance program (59,198,202), promote the use of standardized disk and broth dilution MIC methods and provide useful and consistent antifungal susceptibility data from a broad network of hospitals and laboratories on an international scale (198).

Clinical Relevance of Antifungal Susceptibility Test Results

In order to be useful clinically, *in vitro* susceptibility testing of antimicrobial agents should reliably predict the *in vivo* response to therapy in human infections. However, the *in vitro* susceptibility of an infecting organism to the antimicrobial agent is only one of several factors that may influence the likelihood that therapy for an infection will be successful (225). Factors related to the host immune response and/or the status of the current underlying disease, drug pharmacokinetics and pharmacodynamics, drug interactions, proper patient management, and factors related to the virulence of the infecting organism and its interaction with both the host and the antimicrobial agent administered all influence the outcome of treatment of an infectious episode (225,228). In order to appreciate the clinical value of antifungal susceptibility testing, one must understand that after more than 30 years of study, *in vitro* susceptibility testing can be said to predict the outcome of *bacterial* infections with an accuracy that has been summarized as the "90–60 rule" (225): infections due to susceptible isolates respond to therapy approximately 90% of the time, whereas infections due to resistant isolates respond approximately 60% of the time. There is now a considerable body of data indicating that standardized antifungal susceptibility testing (NCCLS M27-A2) for selected organism-drug combinations (most notably *Candida* spp and azole antifungal agents) provides results that have a predictive utility consistent with the 90–60 rule (Table 6.12).

Antifungal susceptibility testing is now increasingly and appropriately utilized as a routine adjunct to the treatment of fungal infections (225,227). Guidelines for the utilization of antifungal testing, and other laboratory studies, have been developed (Table 6.13) (225). Selective application of antifungal susceptibility testing, coupled with broader identification of fungi to the species level, should prove useful especially in difficult-to-manage fungal infections (225,227). Future efforts will be dedicated to the further validation of interpretive breakpoints for established antifungal agents and developing them for newly introduced, systemically active agents. In addition, procedures must be optimized for testing non-*Candida* yeasts (e.g., *C. neoformans*, *Trichosporon* spp) and molds (166,203a).

QUANTITATION OF ANTIFUNGAL AGENTS IN BIOLOGICAL FLUIDS

The determination of antifungal drug concentrations in serum, cerebrospinal fluid, and other body fluids may provide clinicians with information that can be utilized to adjust chemotherapy. Numerous methods are available to determine drug levels in body fluids including microbiologic bioassay, gas-liquid chromatography, high-performance liquid chromatography (HPLC), fluorometry, spectrophotometry, thin-layer chromatography, and others. Physicochemical assay methods (Table 6.14) tend to be more sensitive, specific, rapid, and less labor-intensive than bioassay methods. They are also capable of separating the parent compound from a biologically

TABLE 6.12

Correlations of Susceptibility Testing with Outcome for Fungal and Bacterial Infections: The 90–60 Rule[a]

Organism Group	No. Studies	No. Patients	Cases with Successful Outcome % (No. Cases/Total) by Susceptibility Class[b]		
			S	R	P Value
Bacteria[c]	12	5,447	89 (4521/5081)	59 (215/366)	<0.001
Fungi[d]	13	1,197	91 (828/923)	48 (131/274)	<0.001

[a] Adapted from Rex and Pfaller (225). Antifungal testing performed according to M27-A2 (159). Susceptibility to antibacterial agents determined by minimum inhibitory concentration (MIC), zone diameter, AUC/MIC ratio, or peak/MIC ratio.
[b] Outcome measurement varied from clinical and/or microbiological response to therapy. S, susceptible; R, resistant.
[c] Includes bacteremia, otitis, and other severe infections treated with various agents, including cephalosporins, β-lactamase inhibitor combinations, aminoglycosides, and fluoroquinolones.
[d] Includes mucosal, fungemia, meningitis, and disseminated infections due to *Candida* treated with fluconazole, itraconazole, or ketoconazole.

active metabolite, whereas bioassays are usually unable to do so (107,164,176,178).

Bioassay methods are available for several of the systemically active antifungal agents (Table 6.15). Bioassays have some advantages over physicochemical assays in that they do not require initial extraction steps or specialized instrumentation. In addition, bioassays evaluate the biological activity of the antifungal agent, as well as any active metabolites, in the body fluid whereas physiochemical determinations do not necessarily indicate biologically active drugs (107,165). The easiest and most practical bioassays to perform in the clinical laboratory are agar diffusion assays (Table 6.15). Amphotericin B levels in body fluids are often determined by using an agar diffusion bioassay method. Briefly, molten agar is seeded with a standardized suspension of *Paecilomyces variotti* (ATCC 36257), poured into 150-mL Petri dishes, and allowed to solidify on a level surface. Known concentrations of the antifungal agent to be tested, as well as the patient's serum, are placed into wells cut from the agar and allowed to diffuse into the medium. The plates are incubated at 30°C for 24 to 48 hours, and the zones of inhibition around the reservoirs are measured to the nearest millimeter. A standard curve is plotted on semilogarithmic paper using the known concentrations of the drug and the corresponding zones of inhibition. The curve should be linear from 0.03 to 1.0 μg/mL (121). Once the standard curve has been constructed, the drug levels in the patient's body fluid may be determined by plotting the zone of inhibition on the standard curve. To ensure intralaboratory reproducibility, internal standards of known concentrations should be included with each assay.

Amphotericin B concentrations may be determined in the presence of flucytosine by substituting a flucytosine-resistant strain of *Chrysosporium pruinosium* (ATCC 36374) for *P. variotii*. The medium may also be supplemented with the flucytosine antagonist cytosine (10 μg/mL). These measures prevent the flucytosine from interfering with the determination of the amphotericin B concentration.

Flucytosine concentrations in body fluids are determined in the same manner as those of amphotericin B except that *S. cerevisiae* (ATCC 36375) is substituted for *P. variotii* and yeast morphology agar is used instead of antibiotic medium 12. To assay for flucytosine in the presence of amphotericin B, the latter is inactivated by heating the sample for 30 minutes at 90°C. Once the serum has been heated and the amphotericin B inactivated, the sample may be assayed to determine the concentration of flucytosine present.

Microbiological bioassays are also available to determine the concentrations of itraconzole and voriconazole in serum or plasma (107,165,178). Importantly, the bioassay for itraconazole reflects the activity of both itraconazole and the hydroxylated metabolite, hydroxyitraconazole (107). The antifungal activity of hydroxyitraconazole is equal to or greater than the parent compound and may contribute approximately four to six times the activity of itraconazole in bioassays. Thus, bioassay results for itraconazole will be highly discrepant when compared with itraconazole concentrations determined by physiochemical methods unless the physiochemical determination of hydroxyitraconazole is also taken into account (107). Hydroxyitraconazole probably contributes importantly to the therapeutic activity of itraconazole and should be taken into account when assays for itraconazole are performed (107,165). In contrast, metabolism of voriconazole results in inactive metabolites and an excellent correlation between bioassay and HPLC determinations of voriconazole in serum has been reported (178).

(text continues on page 256)

TABLE 6.13

Recommendations for Studies of Fungal Isolates in the Clinical Laboratory[a]

Clinical Setting	Recommendation
Routine	• Species level identification of all *Candida* isolates from deep sites (e.g., blood, normally sterile fluids, tissues, abscesses) • Species level identification of *Aspergillus,* genus level for all other molds • Routine antifungal testing of fluconazole against *C. glabrata* isolated from deep sites • Routine testing of fluconazole and flucytosine against other species of *Candida* may be helpful but susceptibility usually predictable (see Table 6.2)
Oropharyngeal candidiasis	• Determination of susceptibility to fluconazole and itraconazole not routinely necessary • Susceptibility testing may be useful for patients unresponsive to azole therapy
Invasive disease with clinical failure of initial therapy	• Consider susceptibility testing as an adjunct *Candida* spp and amphotericin B, flucytosine, fluconazole, voriconazole, caspofungin *C. neoformans* and fluconazole, flucytosine, or amphotericin B *H. capsulatum* and fluconazole • Consultation with an experienced microbiologist recommended
Infection with species with high rates of intrinsic or acquired resistance	• Susceptibility testing not necessary when intrinsic resistance is known *C. krusei* and fluconazole, flucystosine *A. terreus* and amphotericin B Select therapy based on literature • When high rates of acquired resistance, monitor closely for signs of failure and perform susceptibility testing *C. glabrata* and fluconazole *C. glabrata* and amphotericin B *C. krusei* and amphotericin B *C. lusitaniae* and amphotericin B *Candida* spp. and flucytosine
New treatment options (e.g., caspofungin, voriconazole) or unusual organisms	• Select therapy based on published consensus guidelines and review of survey data on the organism-drug combination in question (see Tables 6.2–6.5) • Susceptibility testing may be helpful when patient is not responding to what should effective therapy
Patients who respond to therapy despite being infected with an organism later found to be resistant	• Best approach not clear • Take into account severity of infection, patient immune status, consequences of recurrent infection, etc. • Consider alternative therapy for infections with isolates that appear to be highly resistant to therapy selected
Mold infections	• Susceptibility testing not recommended as a routine • Interpretive criteria have not been established for any agents • Identification to genus and species desirable

(continued)

TABLE 6.13 (Continued)

Recommendations for Studies of Fungal Isolates in the Clinical Laboratory[a]

Clinical setting	Recommendation
Selection of susceptibility testing methods	• Standardized methods • NCCLS broth-based methods Yeasts; M27-A2 Molds; M38-A • NCCLS agar-based methods Disk diffusion; yeasts M44-A • EUCAST broth-based method Yeasts • Other Etest, numerous agents, yeasts, and molds

NCCLS, National Committee for Clinical Laboratory Standards. EUCAST, European Committee for Antimicrobial Susceptibility Testing.
[a] Adapted from Pfaller and Yu (203a) and Rex and Pfaller (225).

TABLE 6.14

Physicochemical Methods for Quantitation of Antifungal Agents in Biological Material

Method	Drug	Specimen	Sensitivity (μg/mL)
Gas-liquid chromatography	Clotrimazole	Skin	0.005–0.01
	Fluconazole	Plasma	0.92
	Griseofulvin	Serum, skin, sweat	0.001–0.05
	Flucytosine	Serum	0.01
	Miconazole	Serum, skin	0.005
High-performance liquid chromatography	Amphotericin B	Serum	0.005–0.02
	Econazole	Serum	0.04
	Flucytosine	Serum	0.8–1
	Fluconazole	CSF,[a] serum urine	0.2–0.5
	Griseofulvin	Serum, urine	0.5–6
	Itraconazole	Serum	0.001
	Ketoconazole	Serum	0.01
	Miconazole	Saliva, serum	0.25–0.5
	Voriconazole	Plasma	0.2
Spectrophotofluorometry	Amphotericin B	Serum	NS[b]
	Flucytosine	Serum	0.5
	Griseofulvin	Serum, sweat, urine	0.1
Thin-layer or paper chromatography	Flucytosine	Serum	0.02
	Griseofulvin	Serum, urine	0.02

[a] CSF, cerebrospinal fluid.
[b] NS, not stated.

TABLE 6.15

Bioassay Determination of Antifungal Agents in Biological Material

Method	Drug	Assay Fungi	Specimen	Sensitivity (μg/mL)
Agar diffusion	Amphotericin B	*C. albicans*	CSF,[a] serum	0.01–0.5
		C. kefyr	urine	
		C. tropicalis		
		S. cerevisiae		
		P. variotii		
	Clotrimazole	*C. kefyr*	Serum, urine	0.2
	Econazole	*C. albicans*	Serum	0.1
	Flucytosine	*C. albicans*	Serum	1
		C. tropicalis		
		S. cerevisiae		
	Griseofulvin	*M. gypseum*	Skin	NS[b]
	Itraconazole	*C. kefyr*	Serum	0.15–0.6
		C. albicans		
	Ketoconazole	*C. albicans*	Serum	0.12–0.5
		C. kefyr		
	Voriconazole	*C. kefyr*	Plasma	0.25
Radiometric potassium or rubidium ion	Amphotericin B	*C. albicans*	Serum	0.2
	Amphotericin B	*C. parapsilosis*	CSF,[a] serum	0.015–0.06
Efflux				

[a] CSF, cerebrospinal fluid.
[b] NS, not stated.

CONCLUSION

The number of systemically active antifungal agents has increased dramatically in recent years in response to the challenge of invasive mycoses. Additional work is needed to better understand the mechanisms of action of these agents as well as the mechanisms of resistance expressed by the fungal pathogens. Antifungal susceptibility testing has been standardized and refined and now may be considered to play an important role in the management of invasive mycoses. More work is needed to optimize the methods for testing new antifungal agents and for testing pathogens other than *Candida*. The ongoing efforts and international collaborations designed to address these issues will provide important information that will improve the management of serious fungal infections.

REFERENCES

1. Anaissie EJ, Kontoyiannis DP, Huls C, et al. Safety, plasma concentrations, and efficacy of high-dose fluconazole in invasive mold infections. *J Infect Dis* 1995;172:599–602.
2. Anaissie E, Paetznick V, Bodey GP. Fluconazole susceptibility testing of *Candida albicans*: microtiter method that is independent of inoculum size, temperature, and the time of reading. *Antimicrob Agents Chemother* 1991;35:1641–1646.
3. Andes D. In vivo pharmacodynamics of antifungal drugs in treatment of candidiasis. *Antimicrob Agents Chemother* 2003;47:1179–1186.
4. Andes D, Marchillo K, Stamstad T, et al. In vivo pharmacokinetics and pharmacodynamics of a new triazole, voriconazole, in a murine candidiasis model. *Antimicrob Agents Chemother* 2003;47:3165–3169.
5. Andes D, Stamsted T, Conklin R. Pharmacodynamics of amphotericin B in a neutropenic-mouse disseminated-candidiasis model. *Antimicrob Agents Chemother* 2001; 45:922–926.
6. Andes D, van Ogtrop M. In vivo characterization of the pharmacodynamics of flucytosine in a neutropenic murine disseminated candidiasis model. *Antimicrob Agents Chemother* 2000;44:938–942.
7. Aoun M. Standard antifungal therapy in neutropenic patients. *Int J Antimicrob Agents* 2000;16:143–145.

8. Arikan S, Rex JH. Antifungal agents. In: Murray PR, Baron EJ, Jorgensen JH, et al. eds. *Manual of clinical microbiology,* 8th ed. Washington, DC: ASM Press, 2003;1859–1868.
9. Arthington-Skaggs BA, Jradi H, Desai T, et al. Quantitation of ergosterol content: novel method for determination of fluconazole susceptibility of *Candida albicans*. *J Clin Microbiol* 1999;37:3332–3337.
10. Arthington-Skaggs BA, Lee-Yang W, Ciblak MA, et al. Comparison of visual and spectrophotometric methods of broth microdilution MIC endpoint determination and evaluation of sterol quantitation method for in vitro susceptibility testing of fluconazole and itraconazole against trailing and nontrailing *Candida* isolates. *Antimicrob Agents Chemother* 2002;46:2477–2481.
11. Asmundsdottir LR, Erlendsdottir H, Gottfredsson M. Increasing incidence of candidemia: results from a 20-year nationwide study in Iceland. *J Clin Microbiol* 2002;40:3489–3492.
12. Athaer MA, Winner HI. Development of resistance by *Candida* species to polyene antibiotics in vitro. *J Med Microbiol* 1971;4:505–517.
13. Baillie GS, Douglas LJ. Matrix polymers of *Candida* biofilms and their possible role in biofilm resistance to antifungal agents. *J Antimicrob Chemother* 2000;46:397–403.
14. Barry A, Bille J, Brown S, et al. Quality control limits for fluconazole disk susceptibility tests on Mueller-Hinton agar with glucose and methylene blue. *J Clin Microbiol* 2003;41:3410–3412.
15. Barry AL, Brown SD. Fluconazole disk diffusion procedure for determining susceptibility of *Candida* species. *J Clin Microbiol* 1996;34:2154–2157.
16. Barry AL, Pfaller MA, Brown SD, et al. Quality control limits for broth microdilution susceptibility tests of ten antifungal agents. *J Clin Microbiol* 2000;38:3457–3459.
17. Barry AL, Pfaller MA, Rennie RP, et al. Precision and accuracy of fluconazole susceptibility testing by broth microdilution, Etest, and disk diffusion methods. *Antimicrob Agents Chemother* 2002;46:1781–1784.
18. Bartizal K, Odds FC. Influences of methodological variables on susceptibility testing of caspofungin against *Candida* species and *Aspergillus fumigatus*. *Antimicrob Agents Chemother* 2003;47:2100–2107.
19. Beauvais A, Bruneau JM, Mol PC, et al. Glucan synthase complex of *Aspergillus fumigatus*. *J Bacteriol* 2001; 183:2273–2273.
20. Bennett JE, Dismukes WE, Duma RJ, et al. A comparison of amphotericin B alone and combined with flucytosine in the treatment of cryptococcal meningitis. *N Engl J Med* 1979;301:126–131.
21. Blumberg HM, Jarvis WR, Soucie JM, et al. Risk factors for candidal bloodstream infections in Surgical Intensive Care Unit patients: the NEMIS prospective multicenter study. *Clin Infect Dis* 2001;33:177–186.
22. Blumer JL. Pharmacologic basis for the treatment of tinea capitis. *Pediatr Infect Dis J* 1999;18:191–197.
23. Bowman JC, Hicks PS, Kurtz MB. The antifungal echinocandin caspofungin acetate kills growing cells of *Aspergillus fumigatus* in vitro. *Antimicrob Agents Chemother* 2002;46:3001–3012.
24. Brajtburg J, Elberg S, Schwartz DR, et al. Involvement of oxidative damage in erythrocyte lysis induced by amphotericin B. *Antimicrob Agents Chemother* 1985;27:172–176.
25. Brajtburg J, Powderly WG, Kobayashi GS, et al. Amphotericin B: current understanding of mechanisms of action. *Antimicrob Agents Chemother* 1990;34:183–188.
26. Brammer KW, Farrow PR, Faulkner JK. Pharmacokinetics and tissue penetration of fluconazole in humans. *Rev Infect Dis* 1990;12(Suppl 3):S318–S326.
27. Brandt ME, Pfaller MA, Hajjeh RA, et al. Trends in antifungal drug susceptibility of *Cryptococcus neoformans* isolates in the United States: 1992 to 1994 and 1996 to 1998. *Antimicrob Agents Chemother* 2001;45:3065–3069.
28. Caillot D, Bassaris H, McGeer A, et al. Intravenous itraconazole followed by oral itraconazole in the treatment in invasive pulmonary aspergillosis in patients with hematologic malignancies, chronic granulomatous disease or AIDS. *Clin Infect Dis* 2001;33:e83–e90.
29. Casadevall A, Spitzer ED, Webb D, et al. Susceptibilities of serial *Cryptococcus neoformans* isolates from patients with recurrent cryptococcal meningitis to amphotericin B and fluconazole. *Antimicrob Agents Chemother* 1993;37:1383–1386.
29a. Chandra J, Kuhn, Mukherjee PK, et al. Biofilm formation by the fungal pathogen *Candida albicans*: development, architecture and drug resistance. *J Bacteriol* 2001;183:5385–5394.
30. Chandrasekar PH, Cutright JL, Manavathu EK. Aspergillus: rising frequency of clinical isolation and continued susceptibility to antifungal agents, 1994–1999. *Diagn Microbiol Infect Dis* 2001;41:211–214.
31. Chandrasekar PH, Cutright JL, Manavathu EK. Efficacy of voriconazole against invasive pulmonary aspergillosis in a guinea pig model. *J Antimicrob Chemother* 2000;45:673–676.
32. Chapman SW, Bradshaw RW Jr, Campbell GD Jr, et al. Practice guidelines for the management of patients with blastomycosis. *Clin Infect Dis* 2000;30:679–683.
33. Chaturvedi V, Ramani R, Pfaller MA. Collaborative study of the NCCLS and flow cytometry methods for antifungal susceptibility testing of *Candida albicans*. *J Clin Microbiol* 2004;45:2252–2254.
34. Chen Y-C, Chang S-C, Luh K-T, et al. Stable susceptibility of *Candida* blood isolates to fluconazole despite increasing use during the past 10 years. *J Antimicrob Chemother* 2003;52:71–77.
35. Chiou CC, Mavrogiorgos N, Tillem E, et al. Synergy, pharmacodynamics, and time-sequenced ultrastructural changes of the interaction between nikkomycin Z and the echinocandin FK463 against *Aspergillus fumigatus*. *Antimicrob Agents Chemother* 2001;45:3310–3321.
36. Chryssanthou E, Cuenca-Estrella M. Comparison of the Antifungal Susceptibility Testing Subcommittee of the European Committee on Antibiotic Susceptibility Testing Proposed Standard and the E-test with the NCCLS broth microdilution method for voriconazole and caspofungin susceptibility testing of yeast species. *J Clin Microbiol* 2002;40:3841–3844.
37. Clancy CJ, Nguyen MH. Correlation between in vitro susceptibility determined by Etest and response to therapy with amphotericin B: results from a multicenter prospective study of candidemia. *Antimicrob Agents Chemother* 1999;43:1289–1290.
38. Colombo AL, Barchiesi F, McGough DA, et al. Comparison of Etest and National Committee for Clinical Laboratory Standards broth macrodilution method for azole antifungal susceptibility testing. *J Clin Microbiol* 1995;33:535–540.
39. Cuenca-Estrella M, Gomez-Lopez A, Mellado E, et al. *Scopulariopsis brevicaulis,* a fungal pathogen resistant to broad-spectrum antifungal agents. *Antimicrob Agents Chemother* 2003;47:2339–2341.

40. Cuenca-Estrella M, Lee-Yang W, Ciblak MA, et al. Comparative evaluation of NCCLS M27-A and EUCAST broth microdilution procedure for antifungal susceptibility testing of *Candida* species. *Antimicrob Agents Chemother* 2002;46:3644–3647.
41. Cuenca-Estrella M, Moore CB, Barchiesi F, et al. Multicenter evaluation of the reproducibility of the proposed antifungal susceptibility testing method for fermentative yeasts of the Antifungal Susceptibility Testing Subcommittee of the European Committee on Antimicrobial Susceptibility Testing (AFST-EUCAST). *Clin Microbiol Infect* 2003;9:467–474.
41a. Cuenca-Estrella M, Rodero L, Garcia-Effron G, et al. Antifungal susceptibilities of *Candida* spp. isolated from blood in Spain and Argentina, 1996–1999. *J Antimicrob Chemother* 2002;49:981–987.
42. Dannaoui E, Borel E, Monier MF, et al. Acquired itraconazole resistance in *Aspergillus fumigatus*. *J Antimicrob Chemother* 2001;47:333–40.
43. Dannaoui E, Borel E, Persat F, et al. In-vivo itraconazole resistance of *Aspergillus fumigatus* in systemic murine aspergillosis. EBGA Network. European research group on Biotypes and Genotypes of *Aspergillus fumigatus*. *J Med Microbiol* 1999;48:1087–1093.
44. Dannaoui E, Borel E, Persat F, et al. Amphotericin B resistance of *Aspergillus terreus* in murine model of disseminated aspergillosis. *J Med Microbiol* 2000;49:601–606.
45. Dannaoui E, Meletiadis J, Mouton JW, et al. In vitro susceptibilities of zygomycetes to conventional and new antifungals. *J Antimicrob Chemother* 2003;51:45–52.
46. Dannaoui E, Persat F, Borel E, et al. Sterol composition of itraconazole-resistant and itraconazole-susceptible isolates of *Aspergillus fumigatus*. *Can J Microbiol* 2001;47:706–710.
46a. Dasbach EJ, Davies GM, Teutsch SM. Burden of aspergillosis-related hospitalizations in the United States. *Clin Infect Dis* 2000;31:1524–1528.
47. Datta K, Jain N, Sethi S, et al. Fluconazole and itraconazole susceptibility of clinical isolates of *Cryptococcus neoformans* at a tertiary care center in India: a need for care. *J Antimicrob Chemother* 2003;52:683–686.
48. Davey KG, Holmes AD, Johnson EM, et al. Comparative evaluation of FUNGITEST and broth microdilution methods for antifungal drug susceptibility testing of *Candida* species and *Cryptococcus neoformans*. *J Clin Microbiol* 1998;36:926–930.
49. Defever KS, Whelan WL, Rogers AL, et al. *Candida albicans* resistance to 5-fluorocytosine: frequency of partially resistant strains among clinical isolates. *Antimicrob Agents Chemother* 1982;22:810–815.
50. Denning DW. Echinocandins: a new class of antifungal. *J Antimicrob Chemother* 2002;49:889–891.
51. Denning DW, Ribaud P, Milpied N, et al. Efficacy and safety of voriconazole in the treatment of acute invasive aspergillosis. *Clin Infect Dis* 2002;34:563–571.
52. Denning DW, Stepan DE, Blume KG, et al. Control of invasive pulmonary aspergillosis with oral itraconazole in a bone marrow transplant patient. *J Infect* 1992;24:73–79.
53. Denning DW, Tucker RM, Hanson LH, et al. Treatment of invasive aspergillosis with itraconazole. *Am J Med* 1989;86:791–800.
54. Denning DW, Venkateswarlu K, Oakely KL, et al. Itraconazole resistance in *Aspergillus fumigatus*. *Antimicrob Agents Chemother* 1997;41:1364–1368.
55. Deresinski SC, Stevens DA. Caspofungin. *Clin Infect Dis* 2003;36:1445–1457.
56. Dick JD, Merz WG, Saral R. Incidence of polyene-resistant yeasts recovered from clinical specimens. *Antimicrob Agents Chemother* 1980;18:158–163.
57. Dick JD, Rosengard BR, Merz WG, et al. Fatal disseminated candidasis due to amphotericin B-resistant *Candida guilliermondii*. *Ann Intern Med* 1985;102:67–68.
58. Diekema DJ, Messer SA, Hollis RJ, et al. Activities of caspofungin, itraconazole, posaconazole, ravuconazole, voriconazole, and amphotericin B against 448 recent clinical isolates of filamentous fungi. *J Clin Microbiol* 2003;41:3623–3626.
59. Diekema DJ, Pfaller MA, Messer SA, et al. In vitro activities of BMS-207147 against over 600 contemporary clinical blood stream isolates of *Candida* species from the SENTRY Antimicrobial Surveillance Program in North American and Latin America. *Antimicrob Agents Chemother* 1999;43:2236–2239.
60. Dominguez JM, Kelly VA, Kinsman OS, et al. Sordarins: a new class of antifungals with selective inhibition of the protein synthesis elongation cycle in yeasts. *Antimicrob Agents Chemother* 1998;42:2274–2278.
61. Douglas CM, Dippolito JA, Shei GJ, et al. Identification of the FKS1 gene of *Candida albicans* as the essential target of 1, 3-β-D-glucan synthase inhibitors. *Antimicrob Agents Chemother* 1997;41:2471–2479.
62. Ernst EJ, Klepser ME, Ernst ME, et al. In vitro pharmacodynamic properties of MK-0991 determined by time-kill methods. *Diagn Microbiol Infect Dis* 1999;33:75–80.
63. Ernst EJ, Klepser ME, Pfaller MA. Postantifungal effects of echinocandin, azole, and polyene antifungal agents against *Candida albicans* and *Cryptococcus neoformans*. *Antimicrob Agents Chemother* 2000;44:1108–1111.
64. Ernst ME, Klepser ME, Wolfe EJ, et al. Antifungal dynamics of LY303366, an investigational echinocandin B analog against *Candida* spp. *Diagn Microbiol Infect Dis* 1996;26:125–131.
64a. Ernst EJ, Roling EE, Petzold CR, et al. In vitro activity of micafungin (FK-463) against *Candida* spp: Microdilution, time-kill and post antifungal effect studies. *Antimicrob Agents Chemother* 2002;46:2846–2853.
65. Espinel-Ingroff A. Evaluation of broth microdilution testing parameters and agar diffusion Etest procedure for testing susceptibilities of *Aspergillus* spp. to caspofungin acetate (MK-0991). *J Clin Microbiol* 2003;41:403–409.
66. Espinel-Ingroff A. In vitro fungicidal activities of voriconazole, itraconazole, and amphotericin B against opportunistic moniliaceous and dematiaceous fungi. *J Clin Microbiol* 2001;39:954–958.
67. Espinel-Ingroff A. Comparison of the E-test with the NCCLS M38-P method for antifungal susceptibility testing of common and emerging pathogenic filamentous fungi. *J Clin Microbiol* 2001;39:1360–1367.
68. Espinel-Ingroff A, Bartlett M, Bowden R, et al. Multicenter evaluation of proposed standardized procedure for antifungal susceptibility testing of filamentous fungi. *J Clin Microbiol* 1997;35:139–143.
69. Espinel-Ingroff A, Bartlett M, Chaturvedi V, et al. Optimal susceptibility testing conditions for detection of azole resistance in *Aspergillus* spp: NCCLS collaborative evaluation. National Committee for Clinical Laboratory Standards. *Antimicrob Agents Chemother* 2001;45:1828–1835.
70. Espinel-Ingroff A, Boyle K, Sheehan DJ. In vitro antifungal activities of voriconazole and reference agents as determined by NCCLS methods: review of the literature. *Mycopatholgia* 2001;150:101–115.
71. Espinel-Ingroff A, Dawson K, Pfaller M, et al. Comparative and collaborative evaluation of standardization

of antifungal susceptibility testing for filamentous fungi. *Antimicrob Agents Chemother* 1995;39:314–319.

72. Espinel-Ingroff A, Kish CW Jr, Kerkering TM, et al. Collaborative comparison of broth macrodilution and microdilution antifungal susceptibility tests. *J Clin Microbiol* 1992;30:3138–3145.
73. Espinel-Ingroff A, Pfaller MA. Susceptibility test methods: yeasts and filamentous fungi. In: Murray PR, Baron EJ, Jorgensen JH, et al., eds. *Manual of clinical microbiology,* 8th ed. Washington, DC: ASM Press, 2003:1880–1893.
74. Espinel-Ingroff A, Pfaller M, Erwin ME, et al. Interlaboratory evaluation of Etest method for testing antifungal susceptibilities of pathogenic yeasts to five antifungal agents by using Casitone agar and solidified RPMI 1640 medium with 2% glucose. *J Clin Microbiol* 1996;34:848–852.
75. Espinel-Ingroff A, Pfaller M, Messer SA, et al. Multicenter comparison of the Sensititre YeastOne Colorimetric Antifungal Panel with the National Committee for Clinical Laboratory Standards M27—A reference method for testing clinical isolates of common and emerging *Candida* spp., *Cryptococcus* spp., and other yeasts and yeast-like organisms. *J Clin Microbiol* 1999;37:591–595.
76. Espinel-Ingroff A, Rezusta A. E-test method for testing susceptibilities of *Aspergillus* spp. to the new triazoles voriconazole and posaconazole and to established antifungal agents: comparison with NCCLS broth microdilution method. *J Clin Microbiol* 2002;40:2101–2107.
77. Espinel-Ingroff A, Rodriguez-Tudela JL, Martinez-Suarez JV. Comparison of two alternative microdilution procedures with the National Committee for Clinical Laboratory Standards reference macrodilution method M27-P for in vitro testing of fluconazole-resistant and -susceptible isolates of *Candida albicans*. *J Clin Microbiol* 1995;33:3154–3158.
78. Esterre P, Inzan CK, Ramarcel ER, et al. Treatment of chromomycosis with terbinafine: preliminary results of an open pilot study. *Br J Dermatol* 1996;134(Suppl 46):33–36.
79. Favel A, Michel-Nguyen A, Peyron F, et al. Colony morphology switching of *Candida lusitaniae* and acquisition of multidrug resistance during treatment of a renal infection in a newborn: case report and review of the literature. *Diagn Microbiol Infect Dis* 2003;47:331–339.
80. Florea NA, Kuti JL, Quintiliani R. Voriconazole: a novel azole antifungal. *Formulary* 2002;37:1–10.
81. Fournier C, Gaspar A, Bordlot F, et al. Evaluation of a broth microdilution antifungal susceptibility test with a pH indicator: comparison with the broth macrodilution procedures. *J Antimicrob Chemother* 1995;35:373–380.
82. Francis P, Walsh TJ. Evolving role of flucytosine in immunocompromised patients: new insights into safety, pharmacokinetics, and antifungal therapy. *Clin Infect Dis* 1992;15:1003–1018.
83. Fromtling RA, Galgiani JN, Pfaller MA, et al. Multicenter evaluation of a macrobroth antifungal susceptibility test for yeasts. *Antimicrob Agents Chemother* 1993;37:39–45.
84. Fryberg M. Sterol biosynthesis in antibiotic-resistant yeasts: nystatin. *Arch Biochem Biophys* 1947;160:83–89.
85. Gale EF, Johnson AM, Kerridge D, et al. Factors affecting the changes in amphotericin B sensitivity of *Candida albicans* during growth. *J Gen Microbiol* 1975;87:20–36.
86. Galgiani JN, Catanzaro A, Cloud A, et al. Comparison of oral fluconazole and itraconazole for progressive, nonmeningeal coccidioidomycosis: a randomized, double-blind trial. Mycoses Study Group. *Ann Intern Med* 2000;133:676–686.
87. Galgiani JN, Catanzaro A, Cloud GA, et al. Fluconazole therapy for coccidioidal meningitis. The NIAID Mycoses Study Group. *Ann Intern Med* 1993;119:28–35.
88. Georgopapadakou NH. Update on antifungals targeted to the cell wall: focus on beta-1,3-glucan synthase inhibitors. *Expert Opin Investig Drugs* 2001;10:269–280.
89. Ghannoum MA, Elewski B. Successful treatment of fluconazole-resistant oropharyngeal candidiasis by a combination of fluconazole and terbinafine. *Clin Diagn Lab Immunol* 1999;6:921–923.
90. Ghannoum MA, Kuhn DM. Voriconazole—better chances for patients with invasive mycoses. *Eur J Med Res* 2002;7:242–256.
91. Ghannoum MA, Rice LB. Antifungal agents: mode of action, mechanisms of resistance, and correlation of these mechanisms with bacterial resistance. *Clin Microbiol Rev* 1999;12:501–517.
92. Groll AH, Gea-Banacloche JC, Glasmacher A, et al. Clinical pharmacology of antifungal compounds. *Infect Dis Clin North Am* 2003;17:159–191.
93. Groll AH, Giri N, Petraitis V, et al. Comparative efficacy and distribution of lipid formulations of amphotericin B in experimental *Candida albicans* infection of the central nervous system. *J Infect Dis* 2000;182:274–282.
94. Groll AH, Gullick BM, Petraitiene R, et al. Compartmental pharmacokinetics of the antifungal echinocandin caspofungin (MK-0991) in rabbits. *Antimicrob Agents Chemother* 2001;45:596–600.
95. Groll AH, Mickiene D, Petraitiene R, et al. Pharmacokinetic and pharmacodynamic modeling of anidulafungin (LY303366): reappraisal of its efficacy in neutropenic animal models of opportunistic mycoses using optimal plasma sampling. *Antimicrob Agents Chemother* 2001;45:2845–2855.
96. Groll AH, Piscitelli SC, Walsh TJ. Clinical pharmacology of systemic antifungal agents: a comprehensive review of agents in clinical use, current investigational compounds, and putative targets for antifungal drug development. *Adv Pharmacol* 1998;44:343–500.
97. Groll AH, Walsh TJ. Uncommon opportunistic fungi: new nosocomial threats. *Clin Microbiol Infect* 2001;7(Suppl 2):8–24.
98. Gupta AK, Shear NH. Terbinafine: an update. *J Am Acad Dermatol* 1997;37:979–988.
99. Hall M, Monka C, Krupp P, et al. Safety of oral terbinafine: results of a post-marketing surveillance study in 25,884 patients. *Arch Dermatol* 1997;133:1213–1219.

99a. Hamilton-Miller JMT. Chemistry and biology of the polyene macrolide antibiotics. *Bacterol Rev* 1973;37:166–196.

100. Hawser SP, Norris H, Jessup CJ, et al. Comparison of a 2,3-bis (2-methoxy-4-nitro-5-sulfophenyl)-5-[(phenylamino) carbonyl]-2H-tetrazolium hydroxide (XTT) colorimetric method with the standardized National Committee for Clinical Laboratory Standards method of testing clinical yeast isolates for susceptibility to antifungal agents. *J Clin Microbiol* 1998;36:1450–1452.
101. Hecker D. Current trends in onychomycosis therapy: a literature review. *Mt Sinai J Med* 1997;64:399–405.
102. Herbrecht R, Denning DW, Patterson TF, et al. Voriconazole versus amphotericin B for primary therapy of invasive aspergillosis. *N Engl Med* 2002;347:408–415.
103. Herbrecht R, Natarajan-Ame S, Nivoix Y, et al. The lipid formulations of amphotericin B. *Expert Opin Pharmacother* 2003;4:1277–1287.

104. Herreros E, Martinez CM, Almela MJ, et al. Sordarins: in vitro activities of new antifungal derivatives against pathogenic yeasts, *Pneumocystis carinii,* and filamentous fungi. *Antimicrob Agents Chemother* 1998;42:2863–2869.
105. Hoang A. Caspofungin acetate: an antifungal agent. *Am J Health-Syst Pharm* 2001;58:1206–1214.
106. Hoffman HL, Rathburn RC. Review of the safety and efficacy of voriconazole. *Expert Opin Investig Drugs* 2002;11:409–429.
107. Hostetler JS, Heykants J, Clemons KV, et al. Discrepancies in bioassay and chromatography determinations explained by metabolism of itraconazole to hydroxyitraconazole: studies in interpatient variations in concentrations. *Antimicrob Agents Chemother* 1993;37:2224–2227.
108. Jahn B, Martin E, Stueben A, et al. Susceptibility testing of *Candida albicans* and *Aspergillus* species by a single microtiter menadione-augmented 3-(4, 5-dimethyl-2-thiazolyl)-2, 5-diphenyl-2H-tetrazolium bromide assay. *J Clin Mcrobiol* 1995;33:661–667.
109. Jessup C, Ryder NS, Ghannoum MA. An evaluation of the in vitro activity of terbinafine. *Med Mycol* 2000;38:155–159.
110. Johnson LB, Kauffman CA. Voriconazole: a new triazole antifungal agent. *Clin Infect Dis* 2003;36:630–637.
110a. Jones RN. Method preferences and test accuracy of antimicrobal susceptibility testing: updates from the College of American Pathologists Microbiology Surveys Program (2000). *Arch Pathol Lab Med* 2001;125:1285–1289.
111. Jones RN. Detection of emerging resistance patterns within longitudinal surveillance systems: data sensitivity and microbial susceptibility. *J Antimicrob Chemother* 2000;46(Topic T2):1–8.
112. Jones RN. The emergent needs for basic research, education, and surveillance of antimicrobial resistance. Problems facing the report from the American Society for Microbiology Task Force on Antibiotic Resistance. *Diagn Microbiol Infect Dis* 1996;25:53–61.
113. Joseph-Horne T, Hollomon D, Loeffler RST, et al. Cross-resistance to polyene and azole drugs in *Cryptococcus neoformans*. *Antimicrob Agents Chemother* 1995;39:1526–1529.
114. Keating GM, Jarvis B. Caspofungin. *Drugs* 2001;61:1121–1129.
115. Kelly SL, Lamb DC, Taylor M, et al. Resistance to amphotericin B associated with defective sterol $\Delta^{8,7}$ isomerase in a *Cryptococcus neoformans* strain from an AIDS patient. *FEMS Microbiol Lett* 1994;122:39–42.
116. Kerridge D, Koh TY, Marriott MS, et al. Microbiology and plant protoplasts. In: Peberdy JF, Rose AH, Rodger HJ, et al., eds. *Microbiology and plant protoplasts.* London: Churchill Livingstone, 1976;23–28.
117. Kibbler CC, Seaton S, Barnes RA, et al. Management and outcome of bloodstream infections due to *Candida* species in England and Wales. *J Hosp Infect* 2003;54:18–24.
118. Klepser ME, Malone D, Lewis RE, et al. Evaluation of voriconazole pharmacodynamics using time-kill methodology. *Antimicrob Agents Chemother* 2000;44:1917–1920.
119. Klepser ME, Wolfe EJ, Jones RN, et al. Antifungal pharmacodynamic characteristics of fluconazole and amphotericin B tested against *Candida albicans*. *Antimicrob Agents Chemother* 1997;41:1392–1395.
120. Klepser ME, Wolfe EJ, Pfaller MA. Antifungal pharmacodynamics of fluconazole and amphotericin B against *Cryptococcus neoformans*. *J Antimicrob Agents Chemother* 1998;41:397–401.
121. Kobayashi GS, Medoff G. Antifungal agents: recent developments. *Annu Rev Microbiol* 1977;31:291–308.
122. Korting HC, Ollert M, Abeck D. The German Collaborative Dermatophyte Drug Susceptibility Study Group. Results of German multicenter study of antimicrobial susceptibilities of *Trichophyton rubrum* and *Trichophyton mentagrophytes* strains causing tinea unguium. *Antimicrob Agents Chemother* 1995;39:1206–1208.
123. Korting HC, Schafer-Korting M, Zienicke H, et al. Treatment of tinea unguium with medium and high doses of ultramicrosize griseofulvin compared with that with itraconazole. *Antimicrob Agents Chemother* 1993;37:2064–2068.
124. Kurtz MB, Abruzzo G, Flattery A, et al. Characterization of echinocandin-resistant mutants of *Candida albicans*: genetic, biochemical, and virulence studies. *Infect Immun* 1996;64:3244–3251.
125. Kurtz MB, Douglas CM. Lipopeptide inhibitors of fungal glucan synthase. *J Med Vet Mycol* 1997;35:79–86.
126. Lamb DC, Corran A, Baldwin BC, et al. Resistant P450 51A1 activity in azole antifungal tolerant *Cryptococcus neoformans* from AIDS patients. *FEBS Lett* 1995;368:326–330.
127. Lass-Florl C, Kofler G, Kropshofer G, et al. In vitro testing of susceptibility to amphotericin B is a reliable predictor of clinical outcome in invasive aspergillosis. *J Antimicrob Chemother* 1998;42:497–502.
128. Law D, Moore CB, Denning DW. Amphotericin B resistance testing of *Candida* spp.: a comparison of methods. *J Antimicrob Chemother* 1997;40:109–112.
129. Leone M, Albanese J, Michel-Nguyen A, et al. Long-term epidemiological survey of *Candida* species: comparison of isolates found in an intensive care unit and in conventional wards. *J Hosp Infect* 2003;55:169–174.
130. Letscher-Bru V, Herbrecht R. Caspofungin: the first representative of a new antifungal class. *J Antimicrob Chemother* 2003;51:513–521.
131. Lewis RE, Klepser ME, Pfaller MA. In vitro pharmacodynamic characteristics of flucytosine determined by time-kill methods. *Diagn Microbiol Infect Dis* 2000;36:101–105.
132. Li RK, Elie CM, Clayton GE, et al. Comparison of a new colorimetric assay with the NCCLS broth microdilution method (M27-A) for antifungal drug MIC determination. *J Clin Microbiol* 2000;38:2334–2338.
133. Lin SJ, Schranz J, Teutsch SM. Aspergillosis case-fatality rate: systematic review of literature. *Clin Infect Dis* 2001;32:358–366.
134. Louie A, Drusano GL, Banerjee P, et al. Pharmacodynamics of fluconazole in a murine model of systemic candidiasis. *Antimicrob Agents Chemother* 1998;42:1105–1109.
135. Lopez-Ribot Al, McAtee RK, Lee LN, et al. Distinct patterns of gene expression associated with development of fluconazole resistance in serial *Candida albicans* isolates from human immunodeficiency virus-infected patients with oropharyngeal candidiasis. *Antimicrob Agents Chemother* 1998;42:2932–2937.
136. Lopez-Ribot JL, McAtee RK, Perea S, et al. Multiple resistant phenotypes of *Candida albicans* coexist during episodes of oropharyngeal candidiasis in human immunodeficiency virus-infected patients. *Antimicrob Agents Chemother* 1999;43:1621–1630.
137. Lozano-Chiu M, Arikan S, Paetznick VL, et al. Optimizing voriconazole susceptibility testing of *Candida*: effects of incubation time, endpoint rule, species of *Candida* and level of fluconazole susceptibility. *J Clin Microbiol* 1999;37:2755–2759.

138. Lozano-Chiu M, Paetznick VL, Ghannoum MA, et al. Detection of resistance to amphotericin B among *Cryptococcus neoformans* clinical isolates: performance of three different media assessed using Etest and National Committee for Clinical Laboratory Standards M27-A methodologies. *J Clin Microbiol* 1998;36:2817–2822.
139. Lozano-Chiu M, Nelson PW, Paetznick VL, et al. Disk diffusion method for determining susceptibilities of *Candida* spp. to MK-0991. *J Clin Microbiol* 1999;37:1625–1627.
140. Manavathu EK, Cutright JL, Chandrasekar PH. Organism-dependent fungicidal activity of azoles. *Antimicrob Agents Chemother* 1998;42:3018–3021.
141. Martin-Mazuelos E, Penman J, Valverde A, et al. Comparison of the Sensititre YeastOne colorimetric antifungal panel and Etest with the NCCLS M38-A method to determine the activity of amphotericin B and itraconazole against clinical isolates of *Aspergillus* spp. *J Antimicrob Chemother* 2003;52:365–370.
142. Maxwell MJ, Messer SA, Hollis RJ, et al. Evaluation of Etest for determining voriconazole and amphotericin B MICs for 162 clinical isolates of *Cryptococcus neoformans. J Clin Microbiol* 2003;41:97–99.
143. Maxwell MJ, Messer SA, Hollis RJ, et al. Evaluation of Etest method for determining fluconazole and voriconazole MICs for 279 clinical isolates of *Candida* species infrequently isolated from blood. *J Clin Microbiol* 2003;41:1087–1090.
144. Mayanja-Kizza H, Oishi M, Mitarai S, et al. Combination therapy with fluconazole and flucytosine for cryptococcal meningitis in Ugandan patients with AIDS. *Clin Infect Dis* 1998;269:1362–1366.
145. McCabe WR, Tredwell TL. In vitro susceptibility tests: correlations between sensitivity testing and clinical outcome in infected patients. In: Lorian V, ed. *Antibiotics in laboratory medicine,* 2nd ed. Baltimore: Williams & Wilkins, 1985;925–937.
146. McGinnis MR, Nordoff NG, Ryder NS, et al. In vitro comparison of terbinafine and itraconazole against *Penicillium marneffei. Antimicrob Agents Chemother* 2000;44:1407–1408.
147. McNeil MM, Nash SL, Hajjeh RA, et al. Trends in mortality due to invasive mycotic diseases in the United States, 1980–1997. *Clin Infect Dis* 2001;33:641–647.
148. Medoff G. The mechanisms of action of amphotericin B. In: Van den Bossche H, ed. International symposium on *Aspergillus* and aspergillosis. New York: Plenum Press, 1988;161–164.
149. Meis J, Petrou M, Bille J, et al. A global evaluation of the susceptibility of *Candida* species to fluconazole by disk diffusion. *Diagn Microbiol Infect Dis* 2000;36:215–223.
150. Meletiadis J, Mouton JW, Meis JFGM, et al. Comparison of the Etest and Sensititre colorimetric methods with the NCCLS proposed standard for antifungal susceptibility testing of *Aspergillus* species. *J Clin Microbiol* 2002;40:2876–2885.
150a. Meletiadis J, Meis JFGM, Mouton JW, et al. In vitro activities of new and conventional antifungal agents against clinical *Scedosporium* isolates. *Antimicrob Agents Chemother* 2002;46:62–68.
151. Meletiadis J, Meis JF, Mouton JW, et al. Comparison of NCCLS and 3-(4,5-dimethy12-thiazolyl)-2,5-diphenyl-2H-tetrazolium bromide (MTT) methods of in vitro susceptibility testing of filamentous fungi and development of a new simplified method. *J Clin Microbiol* 2000;38:2949–2954.
152. Mora-Duarte J, Betts R, Rotstein C, et al. Comparison of caspofungin and amphotericin B for invasive candidiasis. *N Engl J Med* 2002;347:2020–2029.
153. Morace G, Amato G, Bistoni F, et al. Multicenter comparative evaluation of six commercial systems and the National Committee for Clinical Laboratory Standards M27—a broth microdilution method for fluconazole susceptibility testing of *Candida* species. *J Clin Microbiol* 2002;40:2953–2958.
154. Murray PR. Antimicrobial susceptibility tests: testing methods and interpretive problems. In: Poupard JA, Walsh LR, Klegan B, eds. *Antimicrobial susceptibility testing: critical issues for the 90s.* New York: Plenum Press, 1994;15–25.
155. Naranjo MS, Trujillo M, Munera MI, et al. Treatment of paracoccidioidomycosis with itraconazole. *J Med Vet Mycol* 1990;28:67–76.
156. National Committee for Clinical Laboratory Standards. *Performance standards for antimicrobial disk susceptibility tests: approved standard,* 8th ed. National Committee for Clinical Laboratory Standards document M2-A8. Wayne, PA: National Committee for Clinical Laboratory Standards, 2003.
157. National Committee for Clinical Laboratory Standards. *Method for antifingal disk diffusion susceptibility testing of yeasts: approved guideline.* National Committee for Clinical Laboratory Standards document M44-A. Wayne, PA: National Committee for Clinical Laboratory Standards, 2004.
158. National Committee for Clinical Laboratory Standards. *Reference method for broth dilution antifungal susceptibility testing of filamentous fungi: approved standard.* National Committee for Clinical Laboratory Standards document M38-A. Wayne, PA: National Committee for Clinical Laboratory Standards, 2002.
159. National Committee for Clinical Laboratory Standards. *Reference method for broth dilution susceptibility testing of yeasts: approved standard,* 2nd ed. National Committee for Clinical Laboratory Standards document M27-A2. Wayne, PA: National Committee for Clinical Laboratory Standards, 2002.
160. National Committee for Clinical Laboratory Standards. *Development of in vitro susceptibility testing criteria and quality control parameters: approved guideline,* 2nd ed. National Committee for Clinical Laboratory Standards document M23-A2. Wayne, PA: National Committee for Clinical Laboratory Standards, 2001.
161. National Committee for Clinical Laboratory Standards. *Reference method for broth dilution susceptibility testing of yeasts: approved standard.* National Committee for Clinical Laboratory Standards document M27-A. Wayne, PA: National Committee for Clinical Laboratory Standards, 1997.
162. National Committee for Clinical Laboratory Standards. *Reference method for broth dilution susceptibility testing of yeasts: tentative standard.* National Committee for Clinical Laboratory Standards document M27-T. Villanova, PA: National Committee for Clinical Laboratory Standards, 1995.
163. National Committee for Clinical Laboratory Standards. *Reference method for broth dilution susceptibility testing of yeasts: proposed standard.* National Committee for Clinical Laboratory Standards document M27-P. Villanova, PA: National Committee for Clinical Laboratory Standards, 1992.
164. Nesky MA, McDougal EC, Peacock JE Jr. *Pseudallescheria boydii* brain abscess successfully treated with voriconazole and surgical drainage: case report and literature review of central nervous system pseudallescheriasis. *Clin Infect Dis* 2000;31:673–677.

165. Odds FC, Dupont B, Rinaldi MG, et al. Bioassays for itraconazole blood levels: an interlaboratory collaborative study. *J Antimicrob Chemother* 1999;43:723–727.
166. Odds FC, Motyl M, Andrade R, et al. Interlaboratory comparison of results of susceptibility testing with caspofungin against *Candida* and *Aspergillus* species. *J Clin Microbiol* 2004;42:3475–3482.
167. Odds FC, Van Gerven F, Espinel-Ingroff A, et al. Evaluation of possible correlations between antifungal susceptibilities of filamentous fungi in vitro and antifungal treatment outcomes in animal infection models. *Antimicrob Agents Chemother* 1998;42:282–288.
168. Ornstein DL, Ely P. Reversible agranulocytosis associated with oral terbinafine for onychomycosis. *J Am Acad Dermatol* 1998;39:1023–1024.
169. Orozco A, Higginbotham L, Hitchcock C, et al. Mechanisms of fluconazole resistance in *Candida krusei*. *Antimicrob Agents Chemother* 1998;42:2645–2649.
170. Ostrosky-Zeichner L, Marr KA, Rex JH, et al. Amphotericin B: time for a new "Gold Standard." *Clin Infect Dis* 2003;37:415–425.
171. Ostrosky-Zeichner L, Rex JH, Pappas PG, et al. Antifungal susceptibility survey of 2,000 bloodstream *Candida* isolates in the United States. *Antimicrob Agents Chemother* 2003;47:3149–3154.
172. Patterson TF. Invasive mycoses: management and unmet medical needs. *Curr Opin Infect Dis* 2001;14:669–671.
173. Patterson TF, Kirkpatrick WR, White M, et al. Invasive aspergillosis: disease spectrum, treatment practices, and outcomes. I^3 *Aspergillus* Study Group. *Medicine* 2000;79:250–260.
174. Paugam A, Dupovy-Camet P, Gaugeneux JP, et al. Increased fluconazole resistance of *Cryptococcus neoformans* isolated from a patient with AIDS and recurrent meningitis. *Clin Infect Dis* 1994;19:975–976.
175. Pearson MM, Rogers PD, Cleary JD, et al. Voriconazole: a new triazole antifungal agent. *Ann Pharmacother* 2003;37:420–432.
176. Pennick GJ, Clark M. Sutton DA, et al. Development and validation of a high-performance liquid chromatography assay for voriconazole. *Antimicrob Agents Chemother* 2003;47:2348–2350.
177. Perea S, Patterson TF. Antifungal resistance in pathogenic fungi. *Clin Infect Dis* 2002;35:1073–1080.
178. Perea S, Pennick G, Modak A, et al. Comparison of high-performance liquid chromatographic and microbiologic methods for determining voriconazole levels in plasma. *Antimicrob Agents Chemother* 2000;44:1209–1213.
179. Perez A. Terbinafine: broad new spectrum of indications in several subcutaneous and systemic mycotic and parasitic diseases. *Mycoses* 1999;42:111–114.
180. Perfect JF, Marr KA, Walsh TJ, et al. Voriconazole treatment for less-common, emerging, or refractory fungal infections. *Clin Infect Dis* 2003;36:1122–1131.
181. Petraitiene R, Petraitis V, Groll AH, et al. Antifungal efficacy of caspofungin (MK-0991) in experimental pulmonary aspergillosis in persistently neutropenic rabbits: pharmacokinetics, drug disposition, and relationship to galactomannan antigenemia. *Antimicrob Agents Chemother* 2002;46:12–23.
182. Petraitiene R, Petraitis V, Groll AH, et al. Antifungal activity of LY303366, a novel echinocandin B, in experimental disseminated candidiasis in rabbits. *Antimicrob Agents Chemother* 1999;43:2148–2155.
183. Petraitis V, Petraitiene R, Groll AH, et al. Comparative antifungal activities and plasma pharmacokinetics in micafungin (FK 463) against disseminated candidiasis and invasive pulmonary aspergillosis in persistently neutropenic rabbits. *Antimicrob Agents Chemother* 2002;46:1857–1869.
184. Pfaller JB, Messer SA, Hollis RJ, et al. In vitro susceptibility testing of *Aspergillus* spp.: comparison of Etest and reference microdilution methods for determining voriconazole and itraconazole MICs. *J Clin Microbiol* 2003;41:1126–1129.
185. Pfaller MA, Messer SA, Boyken L, et al. In vitro activities of voriconazole, posaconazole, and fluconazole against 4,169 clinical isolates of *Candida* spp. and *Cryptococcus neoformans* collected during 2001 and 2002 in the ARTEMIS global antifungal surveillance program. *Diagn Microbiol Infect Dis* 2004;48:201–205.
186. Pfaller MA, Diekema DJ, Messer SA, et al. In vitro susceptibilities of rare *Candida* bloodstream isolates to ravuconazole and three comparative antifungal agents. *Diagn Microbiol Infect Dis* 2004;48:101–105.
187. Pfaller MA, Barry A, Bille J, et al. Quality control limits for voriconazole disk susceptibility tests on Mueller-Hinton agar with glucose and methylene blue. *J Clin Microbiol* 2004;42:1716–1718.
188. Pfaller MA, Messer SA, Boyken L, et al. Evaluation of the NCCLS M44-P disk diffusion method for determining fluconazole susceptibility of 276 clinical isolates of *Cryptococcus neoformans*. *J Clin Microbiol* 2004;42:380–383.
189. Pfaller MA, Messer SA, Boyken L, et al. Further standardization of broth microdilution methodology for in vitro susceptibility testing of caspofungin against *Candida* species by use of an international collection of more than 3,000 clinical isolates. *J Clin Microbiol* 2004;42:3117–3119.
190. Pfaller MA, Sheehan DJ, Rex JH. Determination of fungicidal activity against yeasts and molds: lessons learned from bactericidal testing and the need for standardization. *Clin Microbiol Rev* 2004;17:268–280.
191. Pfaller MA, Diekema DJ, the International Fungal Surveillance Participant Group. Twelve years of fluconazole in clinical practice: global trends in species distribution and fluconazole susceptibility of bloodstream isolates of *Candida*. *Clin Microbiol Infect* 2004;10(Suppl 1):11–23.
192. Pfaller MA, Messer SA, Boyken L, et al. Caspofungin activity against clinical isolates of fluconazole-resistant *Candida*. *J Clin Microbiol* 2003;41:5729–5731.
193. Pfaller MA, Messer SA, Boyken L, et al. Variation in susceptibility of bloodstream isolates of *Candida glabrata* to fluconazole according to patient age and geographic location. *J Clin Microbiol* 2003;41:2176–2179.
194. Pfaller MA, Diekema DJ, Boyken L, et al. Evaluation of the Etest and disk diffusion methods for determining susceptibilities of 235 bloodstream isolates of *Candida glabrata* to fluconazole and voriconazole. *J Clin Microbiol* 2003;41:1875–1880.
195. Pfaller MA, Diekema DJ, Messer SA, et al. Activities of fluconazole and voriconazole against 1,586 recent clinical isolates of *Candida* species determined by broth microdilution, disk diffusion, and Etest methods: report from the ARTEMIS Global Antifungal Susceptibility Program, 2001. *J Clin Microbiol* 2003;41:1440–1446.
196. Pfaller MA, Diekema DJ, Messer SA, et al. In vitro activities of voriconazole, posaconazole, and four licensed systemic antifungal agents against *Candida* species infrequently isolated from blood. *J Clin Microbiol* 2003;41:78–83.
197. Pfaller MA, Diekema DJ, Messer SA, et al. In vitro activities of caspofungin compared with those of fluconazole and itraconazole against 3,959 clinical isolates of *Candida* spp., including 157 fluconazole-resistant isolates. *Antimicrob Agents Chemother* 2003;47:1068–1071.

198. Pfaller MA, Diekema DJ. Role of sentinel surveillance of candidemia: trends in species distribution and antifungal susceptibility. *J Clin Microbiol* 2002;40:3551–3557.
199. Pfaller MA, Messer SA, Hollis RJ, et al. In vitro activities of ravuconazole and voriconazole compared with those of four approved systemic antifungal agents against 6,970 clinical isolates of *Candida* spp. *Antimicrob Agents Chemother* 2002;46:1723–1727.
200. Pfaller MA, Messer SA, Boyken L, et al. In vitro activities of 5-fluorocytosine against 8,803 clinical isolates of *Candida* spp.: global assessment of primary resistance using National Committee for Clinical Laboratory Standards susceptibility testing methods. *Antimicrob Agents Chemother* 2002;46:3518–3521.
201. Pfaller MA, Messer SA, Hollis RJ, et al. In vitro activities of posaconazole (Sch 56592) compared with those of itraconazole and fluconazole against 3,685 clinical isolates of *Candida* spp. and *Cryptococcus neoformans*. *Antimicrob Agents Chemother* 2001;45:2862–2864.
202. Pfaller MA, Diekema DJ, Jones RN, et al. International surveillance of bloodstream infections due to *Candida* species: frequency of occurrence and in vitro susceptibilities to fluconazole, ravuconazole, and voriconazole of isolates collected from 1997 through 1999 in the SENTRY Antimicrobial Surveillance Program. *J Clin Microbiol* 2001;39:3254–3259.
203. Pfaller MA, Messer SA, Mills K, et al. Evaluation of Etest method for determining caspofungin (MK-0991) susceptibilities of 726 clinical isolates of *Candida* species. *J Clin Microbiol* 2001;39:4387–4389.

203a. Pfaller MA, Yu WL. Antifungal susceptibility testing: new technology and clinical applications. *Infect Dis Clin North Am* 2001;15:1227–1261.

204. Pfaller MA, Messer SA, Mills K, et al. Evaluation of the Etest method for determining posaconazole MICs for 314 clinical isolates of *Candida* species. *J Clin Microbiol* 2001;39:3962–3954.
205. Pfaller MA, Messer SA, Houston A, et al. Evaluation of the Etest method for determining voriconazole susceptibilities of 312 clinical isolates of *Candida* species by using three different agar media. *J Clin Microbiol* 2000;38:3715–3717.
206. Pfaller MA, Zhang J, Messer SA, et al. In vitro activities of voriconazole, fluconazole, and itraconazole against 566 clinical isolates of *Cryptcoccus neoformans* from the United States and Africa. *Antimicrob Agents Chemother* 1999;43:169–171.
207. Pfaller MA, Messer SA, Karlsson A, et al. Evaluation of the Etest method for determining fluconazole susceptibilities of 402 yeast isolates by using three different agar media. *J Clin Microbiol* 1998;36:2586–2589.

207a. Pfaller MA, Marco F, Messer SA, et al. In vitro activity of two echinocandin derivatives, LY 303366 and MK-0991 (L-743,792), against clinical isolates of *Aspergillus, Fusarium, Rhizopus,* and other filamentous fungi. *Diagn Microbiol Infect Dis* 1998;30:251–255.

208. Pfaller MA, Messer SA, Bolmström A. Evaluation of Etest for determining in vitro susceptibility of yeast isolates to amphotericin B. *Diagn Microbiol Infect Dis* 1998;32:223–227.
209. Pfaller MA, Rex JH, Rinaldi MG. Antifungal susceptibility testing: technical advances and potential clinical applications. *Clin Infect Dis* 1997;24:776–784.
210. Pfaller MA, Bale M, Buschelman B, et al. Quality control guidelines for National Committee for Clinical Laboratory Standards recommended broth microdilution testing of amphotericin B, fluconazole, and flucytosine. *J Clin Microbiol* 1995;33:1104–1107.
211. Pfaller MA, Messer SA, Coffmann S. Comparison of visual and spectrophotometric methods of MIC endpoint determinations by using broth microdilution methods to test five antifungal agents, including the new triazole D 0870. *J Clin Microbiol* 1995;33:1094–1097.
212. Pfaller MA, Barry AL. Evaluation of a novel colorimetric broth microdilution method for antifungal susceptibility testing of yeast isolates. *J Clin Microbiol* 1994;32:1992–1996.
213. Pfaller MA, Grant C, Morthland V, et al. Comparative evaluation of alternative methods for broth dilution susceptibility testing of fluconazole against *Candida albicans*. *J Clin Microbiol* 1994;32:506–509.
214. Pfaller MA, Dupont B, Kobayashi GS, et al. Standardized susceptibility testing of fluconazole: an international collaborative study. *Antimicrob Agents Chemother* 1992;36:1805–1809.
215. Pfaller MA, Rinaldi MG, Galgiani JN, et al. Collaborative investigation of variables in susceptibility testing of yeasts. *Antimicrob Agents Chemother* 1990;34:1648–1654.
216. Pfaller MA, Burmeister L, Bartlett MS, et al. Multicenter evaluation of four methods of yeast inoculum preparation. *J Clin Microbiol* 1988;26:1437–1441.
217. Powderly WG, Kobayashi GS, Herzig GP, et al. Amphotericin B-resistant yeast infection in severely immunocompromised patients. *Am J Med* 1988;84:826–832.
218. Provine H, Hadley S. Preliminary evaluation of a semisolid agar antifungal susceptibility test for yeasts and molds. *J Clin Microbiol* 2000;38:537–541.
219. Pujol C, Pfaller MA, Soll DR. Flucytosine resistance is restricted to a single genetic clade of *Candida albicans*. *Antimicrob Agents Chemother* 2004;48:262–266.
220. Ramani R, Chaturvedi V. Flow cytometry antifungal susceptibility testing of pathogenic yeasts other than *Candida albicans* and comparison with the NCCLS broth microdilution test. *Antimicrob Agents Chemother* 2000;44:2752–2758.
221. Redding SJ, Smith J, Farinacci G, et al. Resistance of *Candida albicans* to fluconazole during treatment of oropharyngeal candidiasis in a patient with AIDS: documentation by in vitro susceptibility testing and DNA subtype analysis. *Clin Infect Dis* 1994;18:240–242.
222. Reef SE, Levine WC, McNeil MM, et al. Treatment options for vulvo-vaginal candidiasis. Background paper for development of 1993 STD treatment recommendations. *Clin Infect Dis* 1995;20(Suppl 1):S80–S90.
223. Restrepo A, Robeldo J, Gomez I, et al. Itraconazole therapy in lymphangitic and cutaneous sporotrichosis. *Arch Dermatol* 1986;122:413–417.
224. Revankar SG, Graybill JR. Antifungal therapy. In: Anaissie EJ, McGinnis MR, Pfaller MA, eds. *Clinical mycology*. New York: Churchill Livingstone, 2003;157–192.
225. Rex JH, Pfaller MA. Has antifungal susceptibility come of age? *Clin Infect Dis* 2002;35:982–989.
226. Rex JH, Pfaller MA, Walsh TJ, et al. Antifungal susceptibility testing: practical aspects and current challenges. *Clin Microbiol Rev* 2001;14:643–658.
227. Rex JH, Walsh TJ, Sobel JD, et al. Practice guidelines for the treatment of candidiasis. *Clin Infect Dis* 2000;30:662–678.
228. Rex JH, Pfaller MA, Galgiani JN, et al. Development of interpretive breakpoints for antifungal susceptibility testing: conceptual framework and analysis of in vitro–in vivo correlation data for fluconazole, itraconazole, and *Candida* infections. *Clin Infect Dis* 1997;24:235–247.
229. Rex JH, Pfaller MA, Lancaster M, et al. Quality control guidelines for National Committee for Clinical Laboratory

Standards-recommended broth microdilution testing of ketoconazole and itraconazole. *J Clin Microbiol* 1996;34:816–817.
230. Rex JH, Rinaldi M, Pfaller MA. Resistance of *Candida* species to fluconazole. *Antimicrob Agents Chemother* 1995;39:1–8.
231. Rex JH, Cooper CR Jr, Merz WG, et al. Detection of amphotericin B-resistant *Candida* isolates in a broth-based system. *Antimicrob Agents Chemother* 1995;39:906–909.
232. Rex JH, Bennett JE, Sugar AM, et al. A randomized trial comparing fluconazole with amphotericin B for the treatment of candidemia in patients without neutropenia. *N Engl J Med* 1994;331:1325–1330.
233. Rex JH, Pfaller MA, Rinaldi MG, et al. Antifungal susceptibility testing. *Clin Microbiol Rev* 1993;6:367–381.
234. Reisselman MH, Hazen KC, Cutler JE. Determination of antifungal MICs by using rapid susceptibility assay. *J Clin Microbiol* 2000;38:333–340.
235. Rodriguez-Tudela JL, Barchiesi F, Bille J, et al. Method for the determination of minimum inhibitory concentration (MIC) by broth dilution of fermentative yeasts. *Clin Microbiol Infect* 2003;9:1–8.
236. Ryder NS. Activity of terbinafine against serious fungal pathogens. *Mycoses* 1999;42:115–119.
237. Ryder NS, Wagner S, Leitner I. In vitro activities of terbinafine against cutaneous isolates of *Candida albicans* and other pathogenic yeasts. *Antimicrob Agents Chemother* 1998;42:1057–1061.
238. Saag MS, Cloud GA, Graybill JR, et al. A comparison of itraconazole versus fluconazole as maintenance therapy for AIDS-associated cryptococcal meningitis. National Institute of Allergy and Infectious Diseases Mycoses Study Group. *Clin Infect Dis* 1999;28:291–296.
239. Safe LM, Safe SH, Subden RE. Sterol content and polyene antibiotic resistance in isolates of *Candida krusei, Candida parakrusei,* and *Candida tropicalis. Can J Microbiol* 1977;23:398–401.
240. Sanchez ML, Jones RN. Etest, an antimicrobial susceptibility testing method with broad clinical and epidemiologic application. *Antimicrobic Newsletter* 1992;8:1–7.
241. Sanders WE Jr, Sanders CC. Do in vitro antimicrobial susceptibility tests accurately predict therapeutic responsiveness in infected patients? In: Lorian V, ed. *Significance of medical microbiology in the care of patients,* 2nd ed. Baltimore: Williams & Wilkins, 1982;325–340.
242. Sanglard D, Ischer F, Calabrese D, et al. The ATP binding cassette transporter gene *CgCDR1* from *Candida glabrata* is involved in the resistance of clinical isolates to azole antifungal agents. *Antimicrob Agents Chemother* 1999;43:2753–2765.
243. Sanglard D, Ischer F, Koymans L, et al. Amino acid substitutions in the cytochrome P-450 lanosterol 14α-demethylase (CYP51A1) from azole-resistant *Candida albicans* clinical isolates contribute to resistance to azole antifungal agents. *Antimicrob Agents Chemother* 1998;42:241–253.
244. Sanglard D, Ischer F, Monod M, et al. Cloning of *Candida albicans* resistance genes conferring resistance to azole antifungal agents: characterization of *CDR2,* a new multidrug ABC transporter gene. *Microbiology* 1997;143:405–416.
245. Sanglard D, Ischer F, Monod M, et al. Susceptibility of *Candida albicans* multidrug transporter to various antifungal agents and other metabolic inhibitors. *Antimicrob Agents Chemother* 1996;40:2300–2305.
246. Sanglard D, Kuchler K, Ischer F, et al. Mechanisms of resistance to azole antifungal agents in *Candida albicans* isolates from AIDS patients involve specific multidrug transporters. *Antimicrob Agents Chemother* 1995;39:2378–2386.
247. Sanglard D, Odds FC. Resistance of *Candida* species to antifungal agents: molecular mechanisms and clinical consequences. *Lancet Infect Dis* 2002;2:73–85.
248. Sharkey PK, Graybill JR, Rinaldi MG, et al. Itraconazole treatment of phaeohyphomycosis. *J Am Acad Dermatol* 1990;23:577–586.
249. Sharkey PK, Rinaldi MG, Dunn JF, et al. High-dose itraconazole in the treatment of severe mycoses. *Antimicrob Agents Chemother* 1991;35:707–713.
250. Sheehan DJ, Hitchcock CA, Sibely CM. Current and emerging azole antifungal agents. *Clin Microbiol Rev* 1999;12:40–79.
251. Simor AE, Groswell G, Louie L, et al. Antifungal susceptibility testing of yeast isolates from blood cultures by microbroth dilution and the Etest. *Eur J Clin Microbiol Infect Dis* 1997;16:693–697.
252. Sterling TR, Merz WG. Resistance to amphotericin B: emerging clinical and microbiological patterns. *Drug Resist Updates* 1998;1:161–165.
253. Stevens DA, Kan VL, Judson MA, et al. Practice guidelines for diseases caused by *Aspergillus.* Infectious Diseases Society of America. *Clin Infect Dis* 2000;30:696–709.
254. Stiller RL, Bennett JE, Scholer HJ, et al. Susceptibility to 5-fluorocystsine and prevalence of serotype in 402 *Candida albicans* isolates from the United States. *Antimicrob Agents Chemother* 1982;22:482–487.
255. Stratton CW. In vitro testing: correlations between bacterial susceptibility, body fluid levels, and effectiveness of antibacterial therapy. In: Lorian V, ed. *Antibiotics in laboratory medicine,* 3rd ed. Baltimore: Williams & Wilkins, 1991:847–879.
256. Sugar AM, Alsip SG, Galgiani JN, et al. Pharmacology and toxicity of high-dose ketoconazole. *Antimicrob Agents Chemother* 1987;31:1847–1878.
257. Tiballi RN, He X, Zarins LT, et al. Use of a colorimetric system for yeast susceptibility testing. *J Clin Microbiol* 1995;33:915–917.
258. Torres-Rodriguez JM. New topical antifungal drugs. *Arch Med Res* 1993;24:371–375.
259. Tortorano AM, Rigoni AL, Biraghi E, et al. The European Confederation of Medical Mycology (ECMM) survey of candidaemia in Italy: antifungal susceptibility patterns of 261 non-*albicans Candida* isolates from blood. *J Antimicrob Chemother* 2003;52:679–682.
260. Van der Horst SM, Saag MS, Cloud GA, et al. Treatment of cryptococcal meningitis associated with acquired immunodeficiency syndrome. *N Engl J Med* 1997;337:15–21.
261. Vargas K, Messer SA, Pfaller M, et al. Elevated phenotypic switching and drug resistance of *Candida albicans* from human immunodeficiency virus-positive individuals prior to first thrush episode. *J Clin Microbiol* 2000;38:3595–3607.
262. Vermes A, Guchelaar HJ, Dankert J. Flucytosine: a review of its pharmacology clinical indications, pharmacokinetics, toxicity and drug interactions. *J Antimicrob Chemother* 2000;46:171–179.
263. Vermes A, Van Der Sijs H, Guchelaar HJ. Flucytosine: correlation between toxicity and pharmacokinetic parameters. *Chemotherapy* 2000;46:86–94.
264. Wallace JE, Harris SC, Gallegos J, et al. Assay of fluconazole by high-performance liquid chromatography with

a mixed-phase column. *Antimicrob Agents Chemother* 1992;36:603–606.

265. Walsh TJ, Pappas P, Winston DJ, et al. Voriconazole compared with liposomal amphotericin B for empirical antifungal therapy in patients with neutropenia and persistent fever. *N Engl Med* 2002;346:225–234.
266. Walsh TJ, Petraites V, Petraitiene R, et al. Experimental pulmonary aspergillosis due to *Aspergillus terreus*: pathogenesis and treatment of an emerging fungal pathogen resistant to amphotericin B. *J Infect Dis* 2003;188:305–319.
267. Wanger A, Mills K, Nelson PW, et al. Comparison of Etest and National Committee for Clinical Laboratory Standards broth macrodilution method for antifungal susceptibility: enhanced ability to detect amphotericin B-resistant *Candida* isolates. *Antimicrob Agents Chemother* 1995;39:2520–2522.
268. Weitzman I, Summerbell RC. The dermatophytes. *Clin Microbiol Rev* 1995;8:240–259.
269. Wenisch C, Linnou KF, Parschalk B, et al. Rapid susceptibility testing of fungi by flow cytometry using vital staining. *J Clin Microbiol* 1997;35:5–10.
270. Wenisch C, Moore CB, Krause R, et al. Antifungal susceptibility testing of fluconazole by flow cytometry correlates with clinical outcome. *J Clin Microbiol* 2001;39:2458–2462.
271. Wheat J, Marichal P, Vanden Bossche H, et al. Hypothesis on the mechanism of resistance to fluconazole in *Histoplasma capsulatum*. *Antimicrob Agents Chemother* 1997;41:410–414.
272. Wheat J, Sarosi G, McKinsey D, et al. Practice guidelines for the management of patients with histoplasmosis. Infectious Diseases Society of America. *Clin Infect Dis* 2000;30:688–695.
273. Whelan WL. The genetic basis of resistance to 5-fluorocytosine in *Candida* species and *Cryptococcus neoformans*. *Crit Rev Microbiol* 1987;15:45–56.
274. Whelan Wl, Kerridge D. Decreased activity of UMP pyrophosphorylase associated with resistance to 5-fluorocytosine in *Candida albicans*. *Antimicrob Agents Chemother* 1984;26:570–574.
275. White TC. Mechanisms of resistance to antifungal agents. In: Murray PR, Baron EJ, Jorgensen JH, et al., eds. *Manual of clinical microbiology*, 8th ed. Washington, DC: ASM Press, 2003:1869–1879.
276. White TC. The presence of an R467K amino acid susbstitution and loss of allelic variation correlate with an azole-resistant lanosterol 14 alpha demethylase in *Candida albicans*. *Antimicrob Agents Chemother* 1997;41:1488–1494.
277. White TC, Marr KA, Bowden RA. Clinical cellular, and molecular factors that contribute to antifungal resistance. *Clin Microbiol Rev* 1998;19:382–402.
278. Wilson LS, Reyes CM, Stolpman M, et al. The direct cost and incidence of systemic fungal infections. *Value Health* 2002;5:26–34.
279. Witt MD, Lewis RJ, Larsen RA, et al. Identification of patients with acute AIDS-associated cryptococcal meningitis who can be effectively treated with fluconazole: the role of antifungal susceptibility testing. *Clin Infect Dis* 1996;27:322–328.
280. Yamazumi T, Pfaller MA, Messer SA, et al. In vitro activities of ravuconazole (BMS-207147) against 541 clinical isolates of *Cryptococcus neformans*. *Antimicrob Agents Chemother* 2000;44:2883–2886.
281. Yoon SA, Vazquez JA, Steffan PE, et al. High-frequency, in vitro reversible switching of *Candida lusitaniae* clinical isolates from amphotericin B susceptibility to resistance. *Antimicrob Agents Chemother* 1999;43:836–845.

CHAPTER 7

Antimicrobial Susceptibility Testing for Some Atypical Microorganisms (*Chlamydia, Mycoplasma, Rickettsia, Ehrlichia, Coxiella,* and Spirochetes)

Jean-Marc Rolain, Didier Raoult

This chapter discusses susceptibility testing for fastidious organisms, including mycoplasmas (164), *Borrelia burgdorferi* (8), *Leptospira,* and those that cannot be cultured without the use of animals or tissue culture (*Chlamydia, Rickettsia, Ehrlichia,* and *Coxiella burnetii*). The special testing requirements make it very difficult for all but research laboratories to perform susceptibility testing of these organisms. Thus, the susceptibility testing that has been done has been somewhat limited in terms of both the number of isolates tested and the number of different antiinfective agents evaluated. Furthermore, frequently only well-characterized laboratory strains have been tested rather than recent clinical isolates.

Nonetheless, continual progress is being made in the use of tissue culture for some of these highly fastidious agents, such as *Treponema pallidum* (36), and it should soon be possible to carry out more extensive studies. Expanding the range of studies will certainly be important, because resistance will continue to remain unconfirmed if testing is not carried out (171). This will be true even if resistance is suspected from observations of patients, as was true in the case of a *T. pallidum* infection (168).

The complexity of the methods needed to propagate these organisms argues for an attempt to standardize the methods used for susceptibility testing. In the case of chlamydiae, standardization should be possible, but despite the many different techniques used for the testing of chlamydiae, the results obtained have been remarkably consistent (35). Nonetheless, greater uniformity of testing techniques would make it easier to compare results obtained in different laboratories. The Japan Society of Chemotherapy has published a method for susceptibility testing of *Chlamydia trachomatis* with the obvious intent of having different investigators use the same method. European guidelines for susceptibility testing of intracellular and cell-associated pathogens have been recently published and should be used by laboratories to allow comparison of the results obtained (140).

Since the previous publication of this chapter, much new information has been published on the susceptibility of chlamydiae, mycoplasmas, and rickettsiae. And with the increasing importance of Lyme disease, caused by the spirochete *B. burgdorferi* (172), a considerable quantity of new data on the antimicrobial susceptibility of this important human pathogen has become available.

Resistance to antimicrobials has been infrequent among the organisms considered in this chapter, although resistance of genital mycoplasmas to tetracycline has been reported (107), as well as resistance of *C. trachomatis* to erythromycin and tetracycline (72,114).

CHLAMYDIAE

Chlamydiae are obligate intracellular bacteria that undergo a complex growth cycle. Three human pathogens, *C. trachomatis* (171), *Chlamydia psittaci* (65), and *Chlamydia pneumoniae* (TWAR) (43), occur in this genus of obligate, intracellular parasites. *C. trachomatis* is a major human pathogen and is probably the most prevalent sexually transmitted pathogen in the United States (183),

C. psittaci is a mainly animal pathogen that occasionally causes pneumonia in humans (27), and *C. pneumoniae* is an important cause of community-acquired respiratory infections and is responsible for an average of 10% of cases of pneumonia and 5% of cases of bronchitis and sinusitis (42,43,90). Although many research groups perform antimicrobial susceptibility testing of *Chlamydia* organisms, there is not a standardized methodology or a uniformly accepted interpretation of results. The techniques used for susceptibility testing of these organisms is similar and involve inoculating cell monolayers with the bacteria and incubating them in the presence of serial dilutions of antibiotic (89). However, detection of bacteria varied from enumeration of bacterial inclusions after staining (Giemsa or immunofluorescence) to quantification using RT-PCR (reverse transcriptase-polymerase chain reaction) (26) or flow cytometry (29). Because of the importance of these pathogens in human disease, susceptibility testing of *Chlamydia* has been extensive (Table 7.1).

Cell Lines and Organism

A number of different cell lines have been used to propagate *C. trachomatis,* including McCoy, HeLa 229, and BHK-21 (clone 13). According to a recent study, it seems that the recommended cell line for susceptibility testing for *C. trachomatis* should be the McCoy line, and Hep-2 should be used for *C. pneumoniae* (176). To render these cells more susceptible to infection, a variety of treatments have been employed, including cycloheximide, DEAE-dextran, 5-iodo-2-deoxyuridine, cytochalasin B, and irradiation. However, there is general agreement that the treatment of choice is cycloheximide. Cycloheximide is used at a concentration of 0.5 to 2.0 g/mL. Each lot should be tested for potency by dose-response curve analysis, because this varies and the optimum concentration for any lot can be determined only by experimentation. An acceptable growth medium is Eagle's minimal essential medium (EMEM) supplemented with 2 mmol/L glutamine, 4.4% (wt/vol) sodium bicarbonate, and 10% (vol/vol) fetal bovine serum (5).

McCoy cells should undergo at least two passages in an antibiotic-free medium to ensure that all traces of antibiotic in the growth medium have been removed. Some investigators carry out 10 to 15 passages in antibiotic-free medium before using the cells for susceptibility testing (171). When microdilution plates are used, the cells are seeded at a concentration of 3×10^5 cells per well, and the plates are incubated for 48 to 72 hours, at the end of which time the cells should have formed a subconfluent monolayer (171).

Despite the widespread use of HeLa and McCoy cells for susceptibility studies with *C. trachomatis,* these cells may not provide a relevant *in vitro* environment for such testing. This was demonstrated in a publication by Wyrick et al. (195), who showed that the minimal inhibitory concentration (MIC) for azithromycin was substantially lower with polarized human endometrial-gland epithelial cells than with similar nonpolarized cells (0.125 g/mL and 0.5 g/mL, respectively). This was later confirmed by Paul et al. (122). However, the use of such cells is still not practical for most laboratories, and further work will have to be done to determine whether the extra effort of employing such cell systems is going to yield results that are more clinically relevant.

Chlamydial organisms should undergo at least one passage in antibiotic-free tissue culture cells, and sufficiently high titered pools should be developed so that 10^2 to 10^3 inclusion-forming units (IFU) per coverslip are achieved. Because relatively little variation in susceptibility has been seen among different clinical isolates, investigators either have used well-characterized laboratory isolates (5) or recent clinical isolates (92,149,151,176). The latter are preferable if an attempt is being made to detect whether resistance is developing in current clinical isolates.

Antimicrobial Susceptibility Testing

Some workers prefer 1-dram shell vials, as opposed to microdilution plates, because the larger surface area of the coverslips (diameters vary from 10 to 12 mm) used with the vials makes it somewhat easier to detect low numbers of inclusions. The larger area provides greater assurance that a valid endpoint (MIC) will be obtained. On the other hand, if one uses high-titered pools of chlamydiae so that 10^2 to 10^3 IFU/coverslip are achieved, there is no reason why microdilution plates with 96 wells cannot be used (45,171). An alternative is to use 24-well plates with wells of a 13-mm diameter, which effectively circumvents the problem of too small a surface area (117). Probably perfectly valid results can be obtained with microdilution plates, and if larger numbers of clinical isolates are to be tested or if larger numbers of compounds are to be evaluated, then the use of microdilution plates (or plates with at least 24wells) is the only practical alternative.

Recommended Technique: Microdilution Plate Method

Prior to inoculation, the monolayers are exposed to DEAE-dextran at a concentration of 30 g/mL for 10–30 minutes (22,171). Each of the 24-well plates is inoculated with an inoculum of chlamydiae that yields 5×10^3 IFU/mL. The infectious inoculum (0.1 mL) is centrifuged onto the monolayer at 1200 g for 60 minutes at room temperature. This centrifugation step is essential to infect cells with all *C. trachomatis* strains other than those that cause lymphogranuloma venereum. After centrifugation, the growth medium is removed and replaced with EMEM medium supplemented with glucose (5 mg/L), cycloheximide (generally 1 mg/L), 3% fetal

TABLE 7.1

Antimicrobial Susceptibility of *Chlamydia trachomatis* and *Chlamydia pneumoniae*

Drug	*C. trachomatis*		*C. pneumoniae*	
	MIC (μg/mL)	References	MIC (μg/mL)	References
Aminoglycosides				
Gentamicin	500	(13)	ND	ND
Kanamycin	>100	(64)	ND	ND
Spectinomycin	250	(198)	ND	ND
Trospectomycin	3.5–12.5	(198)	10–20	(89)
Cephalosporins				
CefamaNDole	256–1024	(11)	ND	ND
Cefoperazone	16–32	(47)	ND	ND
Cefotaxime	≥64	(100)	ND	ND
Cefoxitin	1024–2048	(11)	ND	ND
Cefsulodin	≥128	(47)	ND	ND
Ceftriaxone	8–16	(116)	ND	ND
Cephalothin	16	(116)	ND	ND
Moxalactam	≥128	(47)	ND	ND
Macrolides				
Azithromycin	0.03–1 (azi)	(1,157)	0.06–1	(1,193)
Clarithromycin	0.002–0.008	(7)	0.004–0.25	(141)
Erythromycin	0.1–1	(13)	0.01–0.25	(157)
Josamycin	0.032	(9)	0.25	(141)
Roxithromycin	≤0.125	(159,170)	0.125–0.25	(22)
Telithromycin	ND	ND	0.031–0.25	(111)
Cethromycin	ND	ND	0.016–0.031	(113)
Penicillins				
Amoxicillin	2->4	(13)	ND	ND
Ampicillin	0.5–50	(91)	>100	(89)
Penicillin	1–10	(91)	>500	(39)
Piperacillin	≥4096	(11)	ND	ND
Ticarcillin	>960	(12)	ND	ND
Quinolones				
Ciprofloxacin	0.5–2	(112,162)	0.25–4 (cip)	(112)
Difloxacin	0.125–0.25	(162)	ND	ND
Enoxacin	3.13–6.25	(99)	ND	ND
Fleroxacin	3.13–6.25	(99)	2–8	(48)
Garenoxacin	0.007–0.03	(31)	0.015–0.03	(31,150)
Gatifloxacin	0.06–0.25	(145)	0.06–0.25	(46,145)
Gemifloxacin	ND	ND	0.06–0.25	(46)
Grepafloxacin	0.06–0.125	(112)	0.06–0.5	(46,112)
Levofloxacin	0.25–0.5	(112)	0.25–1	(46,112)

(continued)

TABLE 7.1 (Continued)

Antimicrobial Susceptibility of *Chlamydia trachomatis* and *Chlamydia pneumoniae*

Drug	*C. trachomatis* MIC (μg/mL)	*C. trachomatis* References	*C. pneumoniae* MIC (μg/mL)	*C. pneumoniae* References
Moxifloxacin	0.06–0.125	(112)	0.125–1	(46,112)
Nalidixic acid	>50	(53)	ND	ND
Norfloxacin	8–>16	(162)	ND	ND
Ofloxacin	1	(5,170)	0.5–2	(48,50)
Pefloxacin	4	(9)	ND	ND
Sparfloxacin	0.03–0.06	(93,112)	0.06–0.5	(50,112)
Temafloxacin	0.125–0.25	(162)	0.125–4	(50,148)
Trovafloxacin	0.031–1	(71)	0.5–1	(148)
Tetracyclines				
Chlortetracycline	0.125–2.5	(23)	ND	ND
Doxycycline	0.012–0.025	(53)	0.05–0.5	(40,148)
Minocycline	0.025–0.05	(99)	0.0075–0.015	(84)
Tetracycline	0.3	(5)	0.05–1	(22,194)
Sulfamethoxazole	50	(64)	>500	(22)
Miscellaneous				
Chloramphenicol	2–4	(21)	ND	ND
Clindamycin	2–16	(51)	ND	ND
Imipenem	32	(47)	ND	ND
Metronidazole	>5000	(13)	ND	ND
Rifampin	0.005–0.25	(70)	0.005–0.031	(38,39)
Trimethoprim	>100	(64)	>400	(83)
Cotrimoxazole	0.03/0.6–32/640	(45)	>400	(83)
Vancomycin	1.000	(63)	ND	ND

ND, not determined.

bovine serum, and serial twofold dilutions of each antibiotic to be tested (5). All tests are performed in triplicate. The plates are then incubated at 35°C in a CO_2 incubator for 48 to 72 hours. Then the coverslips are removed from the wells, fixed in absolute methanol-acetone, and stained (22,171).

Detection of Inclusions

Most investigators who have done susceptibility testing of *C. trachomatis* have used iodine staining for the detection of inclusions (35). One of the major disadvantages of this stain is that the inclusions may not be detected if they are particularly small or aberrant in shape. Aberrantly shaped inclusions are particularly common when *C. trachomatis* is cultured in the presence of β-lactam antibiotics (56). Giemsa staining has also been used, but it is evident that either direct or indirect fluorescent staining of the monolayers is the most sensitive method for detecting chlamydial antigen in cell monolayers (5,56,171). Initially fluorescent staining for susceptibility testing used an indirect fluorescent antibody technique employing a polyclonal antibody raised in a rabbit against the same serovar E strain used in the susceptibility studies (12). However, with the availability of fluorescein-conjugated monoclonal antibodies (Syva, Palo Alto, CA; Ortho Diagnostics, Raritan, NJ; or Kallestad, Chaska, MN) to *C. trachomatis*, direct fluorescent staining has become the method of choice for detecting chlamydial antigen in tissue culture (22,45,49,92,146,147,149,151,152,161,162,171). In using fluorescent stains, the manufacturers' directions should be followed. When Giemsa staining and direct immunofluorescent (using the Syva monoclonal antibody) techniques were compared, it was evident that the MICs obtainable with the monoclonal antibody were about two times higher than those obtained with Giemsa staining (56). Enzyme-linked immunosorbent assays have also been used to detect chlamydial antigen, and these yield MIC values comparable to those obtained with the immunofluorescent method (21). A commercially available enzyme immunoassay (Chlamydiazyme; Abbott Laboratories, North Chicago, IL) has also been used to detect antigen, and the results were similar to those obtained using a genus-specific monoclonal antibody (Ortho Diagnostics) in an immunoperoxidase test (9).

The MIC is defined as the lowest concentration of antibiotic that completely inhibits inclusion formation after 48 to 72 hours of incubation, and the minimal bactericidal concentration (MBC) is defined as the lowest concentration of antibiotic that completely inhibits the development of inclusions when the cells are disrupted at 48 to 72 hours and passed into tissue culture medium that is free of antibiotics.

Other Assays

Antibiotic susceptibility testing for *Chlamydia* has also been performed using flow cytometry (29). In this assay, evaluation of antibiotic activity was done at the 25-hour time point, and cells were best permeabilized using the Ortho/Permeafix treatment. The mean fluorescence intensity (MFI) of cells was determined by this method after staining of chlamydial inclusions with an anti-*Chlamydia* fluorescent monoclonal antibody. Calculation of the inhibitory concentration 50 (IC_{50}), defined as the antibiotic concentration required to reduce the drug-free control MFI by 50%, by flow cytometry allowed a more objective and precise evaluation of antibiotic activity than MIC (29).

Finally, a RT-PCR–based method has been developed for antimicrobial susceptibility testing of *C. pneumoniae* (83) and *C. trachomatis* (26). The results obtained in these studies were in the range previously reported using immunofluoresent staining, and the MICs obtained by RT-PCR were consistently higher (26,83). The advantage of the RT-PCR technique over ordinary PCR methods is that only viable organisms will produce RNA.

Results of Susceptibility Testing

Table 7.1 presents the results of MICs of antimicrobial agents against *C. trachomatis* and *C. pneumoniae* indicating the intense interest in antimicrobials with activity against these important human pathogens. In Table 7.1, as in all subsequent tables, a range is given for the MIC values, except in those instances when so few isolates were studied that only a single MIC value is available. Aminoglycosides are without any activity and can therefore be incorporated into tissue culture media used for the isolation of this organism. β-Lactamine compounds, chloramphenicol, clindamycin, imipenem, metronidazole, and vancomycin are not active against *Chlamydia*. The β-lactams result in the formation of aberrant inclusions but lack significant activity. Susceptibility of *C. pneumoniae* is similar to that of *C. trachomatis*, except that *C. pneumoniae* is resistant to sulfonamides. The most active agents against *Chlamydia* are the macrolides, tetracyclines, rifampin, and fluoroquinolones. However, rifampin is not used clinically because resistance develops rapidly *in vitro* (160).

Antimicrobial Resistance

The development of significant resistance to currently used antimicrobials has not been a problem, although relative resistance to sulfonamides, erythromycin, rifampin, and fluoroquinolones has been reported for *C. trachomatis* (72,82,110a,114), arguing for the continued surveillance of current clinical isolates. One potential explanation for the lack of resistance by chlamydiae is their unique life cycle (169). Despite the lack of evidence for frequent resistance in chlamydiae, it is clearly possible to induce resistance in the laboratory by serial passages of organisms in subinhibitory concentrations of antimicrobials (28,169).

MYCOPLASMAS

Disease in humans is associated with at least four *Mycoplasma* species: respiratory infections with *Mycoplasma pneumoniae* and urogenital infections with *Mycoplasma hominis, Mycoplasma genitalium,* and *Ureaplasma urealyticum.* Finally, *Mycoplasma fermentans* has been isolated from patients with acquired immunodeficiency syndrome (AIDS), and there has been conjecture about the possible role of these mycoplasmas as cofactors in the disease caused by the human immunodeficiency virus (52). *M. fermentans* has also been detected in some cases of fatal respiratory distress in immunocompetent adults (98).

The main structural characteristic of mycoplasmas is their lack of a cell wall, which makes them naturally resistant to β-lactams and all antibiotics that target the cell wall and agents that interfere with the synthesis of folic acid (107).

The techniques for isolating and identifying these agents are well known (165), but the techniques for performing antimicrobial susceptibility studies are less well defined (163). Both the agar dilution (80) and broth dilution (188) methods have their proponents. The two methods may yield quite disparate results for certain antibiotics, and so it is always important to consider the method used when evaluating the results of susceptibility studies (192).

A particular problem with each is that there is some drift of endpoints with time (a progressive increase in MIC values with prolonged incubation), as long incubation times are required for most mycoplasmas because of their slow growth. One of the probable reasons for the phenomenon of drift is that antibiotic inactivation occurs during incubation.

One advantage of the agar method is that in a mixture of sensitive and resistant strains the two types of strains can be differentiated. With the broth method, differentiation is impossible without the cloning of isolates (80). On the other hand, from a purely clinical standpoint, it is probably of little importance to detect a mixture of resistant and susceptible strains, although it could be of considerable research interest (143).

Tanner et al. (179) adapted commercially available Sensititre broth microdilution plates for the susceptibility testing of *Mycoplasma hyopneumoniae,* and this technique was also successfully employed by Poulin et al. (125) for testing AIDS-associated mycoplasmas. The technique yields results comparable to those obtained with the macrodilution method.

Limb et al. (97) have utilized the measurement of ATP bioluminescence for the susceptibility testing of mycoplasmas. Using this technique, they were able to demonstrate good correlation with conventional methods and could achieve results within 6 hours.

Media and Organisms

Actively growing broth cultures are frozen at −70°C. A suitable medium for *M. pneumoniae, M. fermentans, M. incognitus,* and *M. genitalium* is SP-4 medium (185), and a suitable medium for both of the genital mycoplasmas is 10-B broth. 10-B broth is usually made with penicillin, which should be omitted in susceptibility testing. Commercially prepared 10-B broth, as well as other specialized media for the isolation and propagation of mycoplasmas, may be obtained from commercial sources (e.g., Regional Media Laboratories, Lenexa, KS) and can be ordered without antibiotics for susceptibility testing.

For the culture of *M. hominis,* arginine, rather than urea, is incorporated into the medium (165). An aliquot of the culture is thawed, and serial dilutions are carried out to determine how many color changing units (CCUs) are present per milliliter. One CCU is the minimum inoculum required to produce enough growth to cause a color change in the phenol red indicator.

Antimicrobial Susceptibility Testing

The authors favor the broth dilution technique because it can be carried out in microdilution plates, allowing relatively large numbers of isolates to be tested against a reasonable number of different antimicrobials (187). Furthermore, the technique is adaptable for a variety of mycoplasmas, and when tests are carried out in triplicate, very good reproducibility is noted (187).

In the case of *U. urealyticum,* there has been good agreement noted between the more laborious tube dilution technique and the microdilution technique (144). Furthermore, both the MIC and the MBC can be determined using the broth dilution technique, whereas only the MIC can be determined using the agar dilution technique. Finally, the antibiotic broth dilution technique is really just an adaptation of the metabolic inhibition test (165), which has been used for identifying and serotyping mycoplasmas as well as for serodiagnosis. For this reason, laboratories may already be familiar with the basic components of the broth dilution technique.

The metabolic inhibition technique depends on the presence of either antibodies or, in the case of susceptibility testing, antimicrobials inhibiting the growth of the mycoplasmas. Inhibition of growth is detected by the lack of color change of a pH indicator, generally phenol red. Suitable substrates are included in the growth medium for the varying mycoplasmas: glucose in the case of *M. pneumoniae,* arginine for *M. hominis,* and urea for *U. urealyticum.*

Recommended Technique: Broth Dilution Technique

The broth dilution method is performed in 96-well plates with a volume of 200 μL in each well. Each stock antibiotic is added in a volume of 0.025 mL to a well of a microdilution plate, generally in triplicate (163,187). An aliquot of a previously frozen (−70°C), actively growing broth culture is thawed on the day of the assay and added to 50 mL of the appropriate broth medium (SP-4 for *M. pneumoniae* and 10-B broth for *M. hominis* and *U. urealyticum*) for each antibiotic to be tested. The stock culture is diluted to yield 10^3 to 10^4 organisms per microdilution well. To further establish how many CCUs have been added to each well, tenfold dilutions of the inoculum are made to verify that at least 10^3 CCUs but no more than 10^5 CCUs have been added to each well. Inoculated broths are incubated for 2 hours at 37°C before these broths are added to the microdilution plates. Mycoplasma suspensions are added in 0.175-ml aliquots to each well containing antibiotics. The plates are sealed in plastic bags containing sterile gauze moistened with distilled water and are incubated at 35°C to 37°C under atmospheric conditions.

Three controls are included: (a) a broth control with no mycoplasmas, (b) a drug control consisting of the maximum drug concentration tested in broth alone, and (c) a mycoplasma control consisting of the mycoplasma suspension alone in a total of 0.2 mL of broth. Plates are examined after 17 to 20 hours of incubation and once daily until growth is noted in the mycoplasma control well. The MIC will be generally available for *U. urealyticum* at

24 hours, for *M. hominis* at 48 hours, and for *M. pneumoniae* after 5 or more days.

Determination of MIC and MBC

With SP-4 medium and 10-B broth, growth of *U. urealyticum* sufficient for determination of the MIC occurs overnight. Comparable times are 24 to 48 hours for *M. hominis* and 3 to 5 days for *M. pneumoniae*. Often investigators determine both initial and final MICs (187); the initial MIC is the minimum amount of antibiotic required to inhibit any color change of the broth when the control well (containing organisms but no antibiotic) first shows a color change, and the final MIC is the minimum concentration of antibiotic that prevents a color change over a period of 2 consecutive days. The final MIC is employed with mycoplasmas because of their slow growth characteristics, which result in the drift of the MIC. In fact, the final MIC may be as much as eight times higher than the initial MIC for some antimicrobials (187).

It is also possible to determine the MBC, by diluting the broth from wells showing no color change in antibiotic-free medium. Generally, this is a 20-fold dilution, which is usually sufficient to dilute the antibiotic to a level below the antibiotic's MIC value (163) but hopefully not to a point where organisms can no longer be detected. An alternate method avoids these possible pitfalls by filtering the broth from wells with no color change through a filter with a pore size of 220 nm, washing the filter free of residual antibiotic, and culturing the filter (181). Using the latter technique, Taylor-Robinson and Furr (181) were able to show that the macrolide rosaramicin acted in a purely mycoplasmastatic fashion on some ureaplasmas.

In the case of ureaplasmas, there is a self-sterilizing effect, so that by 24 hours there is often a precipitous fall in the number of organisms (163). Because Taylor-Robinson and Furr (181) showed that there is no change in the MIC values for these organisms between 5 and 25 hours, subculturing for the determination of MBC values can be done as early as 5 hours, which avoids any problems that may be caused by the self-sterilizing phenomenon (163).

Results of Susceptibility Testing

The results of susceptibility testing on mycoplasmas are summarized in Tables 7.2 and 7.3. Mycoplasma lack peptidoglycan and penicillin-binding proteins and thus are naturally resistant to β-lactam antibiotics. Moreover, they are also resistant to rifampin owing to the particular structure of their RNA polymerase, and also to polymyxins, nalidixic acid, sulfonamides, and trimethoprim. Tetracyclines, erythromycin, clindamycin, chloramphenicol, aminoglycosides, and fluoroquinolones have been shown to have activity against one or more mycoplasmal species (158).

TABLE 7.2

Antimicrobial Susceptibility of *Mycoplasma pneumoniae*

Drug	MIC (μg/mL)	References
Aminoglycosides		
Gentamicin	0.3–0.8	(62)
Kanamycin	3.1–6.3	(62)
Streptomycin	0.15–0.2	(62)
Macrolides		
Azithromycin	0.008–0.12	(79,139,158,196)
Clarithromycin	0.015–0.06	(58,79,196)
Erythromycin	0.03–0.12	(79,110,139)
Josamycin	0.03–0.12	(79,110,196)
Roxithromycin	0.06–0.25	(79,197)
Telithromycin	0.008–0.06	(79,197)
Quinolones		
Ciprofloxacin	0.5–4	(20,81,188)
Gatifloxacin	0.25–1	(81)
Grepafloxacin	0.06–0.25	(81)
Levofloxacin	0.06–2	(81,188)
Moxifloxacin	0.016–0.125	(81,188)
Ofloxacin	1	(120)
Sparfloxacin	0.125–0.25	(81,188)
Trovafloxacin	0.12–0.5	(81)
Tetracyclines		
Chloramphenicol	0.8–2.4	(62,188)
Doxycycline	0.016–0.5	(189)
Minocycline	0.25–1	(81)
Tetracycline	0.5–2	(81)

Mycoplasma pneumoniae

Erythromycin and tetracyclines are usually active against *M. pneumoniae*. Resistance to erythromycin has now been described (123a,175), although resistance to tetracycline has not been documented. Azithromycin and telithromycin are more active against *M. pneumoniae in vitro* than erythromycin, clarithromycin, or roxithromycin (49,58,196). Fluoroquinolone compounds are also active against *M. pneumoniae*, but *in vitro* studies have shown that they are not as effective as macrolides (48,73,76).

Mycoplasma hominis

M. hominis is usually naturally susceptible to tetracyclines but tetracycline-resistant isolates containing DNA sequences homologous to the streptococcal determinant

TABLE 7.3

Antimicrobial Susceptibility of *Mycoplasma hominis* and *Ureaplasma urealyticum*

Drug	*M. hominis*		*U. urealyticum*	
	MIC (μg/mL)	References	MIC (μg/mL)	References
Macrolides				
Azithromycin	16–32	(79)	0.125–4	(79,188)
Clarithromycin	>32	(79)	≤0.06–2	(79,188)
Erythromycin	>32	(79)	0.125–8	(79,188)
Josamycin	0.25–0.5	(79)	0.5–2	(79)
Roxithromycin	>32	(79)	1–4	(79)
Telithromycin	16–32	(79)	0.06–0.25	(79)
Quinolones				
Ciprofloxacin	0.016–1	(79,188)	1–16	(188)
Gatifloxacin	0.06–0.25	(79)	1–2	(79)
Grepafloxacin	0.06–0.125	(79)	0.12–1	(142)
Levofloxacin	0.016–2	(79,188)	0.25–2	(79,188)
Moxifloxacin	≤0.008–0.06	(79,88)	0.03–1	(79,188)
Ofloxacin	0.5–1	(78)	1–4	(78,79)
Sparfloxacin	≤0.008–0.125	(79,188)	0.06–2	(79,188)
Trovafloxacin	0.015–0.125	(78,79)	0.06–5	(78)
Tetracyclines				
Chloramphenicol	4–25	(19)	NA	
Doxycycline	0.03–2	(77)	1–2	(77)
Minocycline	0.06–0.5[a]	(79)	0.06–0.5	(79)
Tetracycline	0.5–4[a]	(79)	0.5–4	(79)

[a] Tetracycline-susceptible strains (resistant strains had MICs >32 μg/mL).
NA, not available.

tetM have been reported (143). It has been convincingly demonstrated that *tetM* is not a plasmid and that it is present in both species of genital mycoplasmas. Resistance to tetracycline *in vitro* is associated with failure of tetracycline treatment to eradicate *M. hominis* (107). The new glycylcyclines have been shown to be active *in vitro* against *M. hominis* strains resistant to other tetracyclines. Because of this emerging resistance, it is proving to be increasingly difficult to devise suitable antimicrobial regimens for the effective therapy of genital mycoplasma infections (107,182,190,191). Clindamycin can be used for the treatment of *M. hominis* infections resistant to tetracyclines, and erythromycin or quinolones can be used for tetracycline-resistant *U. urealyticum* infections (107). Usually fluoroquinolone compounds are active against *M. hominis*, but resistance to fluoroquinolones has been reported and is associated with mutations in DNA gyrase (6). *M. hominis* is resistant to erythromycin, roxithromycin, azithromycin, and clarithromycin but remains susceptible to josamycin (Table 7.3).

Ureaplasma urealyticum

Tetracyclines and fluoroquinolone compounds are active against *U. urealyticum*. Erythromycin is generally active against ureaplasmas, but resistance has been noted (183) and is associated with specific mutations in the 23S rRNA gene (123).

RICKETTSIA

All members of the genus *Rickettsia* are obligate, Gram-negative, intracellular bacteria. The genus comprises typhus group rickettsiae, which includes *Rickettsia prowazekii*, the agent of epidemic typhus, and *Rickettsia typhi*, the agent of murine typhus; *Orientia tsutsgamushi*, the agent of scrub typhus (178); and spotted fever group (SFG) rickettsiae. The number of recognized SFG rickettsioses has recently increased. The six SFG rickettsioses previously described are Rocky Moutain spotted fever, caused by *Rickettsia rickettsii;* Mediterranean spotted fever, caused by *Rickettsia conorii;* Siberian tick typhus, caused by *Rickettsia sibirica* israeli; spotted fever, caused by *Rickettsia conorii* serotype israeli; Queensland tick typhus, caused by *Rickettsia australis;* and rickettsialpox, caused by *Rickettsia akari.* Since 1984, 12 new SFG rickettsiosis have been described: the Japanese spotted fever, caused by *Rickettsia japonica* and described in 1984 (186); Flinders Island spotted fever, caused by *Rickettsia honei* and described in 1991 (174); Astrakhan fever, caused by *Rickettsia conorii* serotype Astrakhan and reported in 1991 (180); African tick-bite fever, caused by *Rickettsia africae* and described in 1992 (75); a new spotted fever due to "*Rickettsia mongolotimonae*," reported in France in 1996 (128,197); *Rickettsia slovaca* infection, reported in 1997 (127); *Rickettsia helvetica* infection, described in 2000 (37); flea-borne rickettsioses, caused by *Rickettsia felis* and reported in 2001 (131); *Rickettsia aeschlimannii* infection, reported in 2001 (130); *Rickettsia heilongjlangensis* infection; and *Rickettsia parkeri* infection, reported in 2003 (unpublished data).

All of the members of the genus *Rickettsia* are obligate intracellular pathogens and therefore require either animal models, embryonated eggs, or tissue culture for susceptibility assays (135). It would appear that, of the *in vitro* techniques now available, the plaque assay and a colorimetric assay (135) are the most practical for evaluating antiinfectives for this group of organisms. However, because of the technical difficulties in working with these agents, susceptibility testing will probably be confined to relatively few laboratories. Furthermore, it is evident that when *in vivo* techniques, such as suppression of lethality in chicken embryos, are compared with *in vitro* techniques, such as the plaque assay, the results may be somewhat discrepant (133). The two assays (plaque assay and colorimetric assay) depend on the induction of cytopathic effects and plaque formation in cell cultures by the rickettsiae, but some rickettsiae do not normally cause cytopathic effects in primary cultures (154,155). Recently, Ives et al. (59,60) described a new assay that uses immunofluorescent staining, which avoids the problem of a lack of cytopathic effects. Very recently we have developed a new quantitative PCR DNA assay using the LightCycler system for the evaluation of antibiotic susceptibilities of three rickettsial species, including *R. felis*, a rickettsial species that does not induce plaque in cell cultures (155).

Cell Lines and Organisms

Organisms used for these studies are laboratory strains. For example, in the case of *R. rickettsii*, the Sheila Smith strain is used (135), and for *R. conorii* the American Type Culture Collection VR 141 Moroccan strain (134). Only a few studies on *in vitro* antibiotic susceptibilities of SFG rickettsiae other than *R. conorii*, *R. rickettsii*, and *R. akari* are available. We recently reported an extensive study that investigated the reaction of 27 rickettsiae to 13 antimicrobials (Table 7.4) (154).

Antimicrobial Susceptibility Testing

Reference Method: Plaque Assay

Vero cell monolayers seeded 24 hours before use in round, plastic, tissue culture Petri dishes (60 mm; Corning Glass Works, Corning, NY) are infected with 1 mL of a solution containing 4 $\times$ 10^3 plaque-forming units (PFU) of the desired rickettsial strain (135). After 1 hour of incubation at room temperature (22°C), the plates are overlaid with 4 mL of a medium containing Minimum Essential Eagle Medium (Gibco), 2% newborn calf serum, 2% (*N*-(2-hydroxyethyl) piperazine-*N*′-(2-ethanesulfonic acid)) (HEPES) (Sigma-Aldrich), and 0.5% agar. The antibiotic solutions are added to the medium to obtain the desired final concentrations (an antibiotic-free control plate is also included), and the plates are incubated for 4 to 7 days at 35°C in a CO_2 incubator. All antibiotics are assayed in triplicate, at a minimum. After incubation, the monolayers are fixed with 4% formaldehyde and stained with 1% crystal violet in 20% ethanol. The MIC is the lowest concentration of the agent tested causing complete inhibition of plaque formation, compared with the drug-free controls. Plates may then be photographed to obtain a permanent record of the results. The major problem with this technique is that some rickettsial strains may not induce the formation of plaques in cell cultures. In this case, several passages in various cell lines may allow selection of variants able to produce plaques.

Rickettsiacidal activity can be determined from this assay by staining surviving cells with either Gimenez or immunofluorescent stain (133). The minimal concentration of antibiotic that completely sterilizes the monolayer is defined as the minimum rickettsiacidal concentration.

Dye-Uptake Assay

Flat-bottomed microdilution plates are seeded with 1.5 $\times$ 10^4 Vero cells (suspended in a solution of EMEM, 5% newborn calf serum, and 2 mmol/L L-glutamine) per well and subsequently infected with varying concentrations of a suspension of *Rickettsia* organisms (135). The Vero cell suspension (100 μL) is added to each well. The infectious inoculum is added to individual wells in a final volume of 50 μL. For each 96-well plate, the first horizontal row of 8 wells contains no rickettsiae, the second horizontal row is inoculated with 2000 PFU, the third horizontal row with 200 PFU, and the fourth with 20 PFU (Fig 7.1). Two

TABLE 7.4

Antimicrobial Susceptibility of *Rickettsia*[a]

Strain	Doxy	Thiam	Rifam	Ery	Clar	Josa	Prist	Cip	Ofl	Pef
R. prowazekii	0.06	2	0.06	0.125	0.5	0.5	4	0.5	1	1
R. typhi	0.125	1	0.25	0.5	1	1	2	1	1	1
R. akari	0.06	1	0.25	8	2	1	4	0.5	0.5	1
R. conorii Seven	0.06–0.125	1–2	0.125	8	1	0.5	1–2	0.5	1	0.5–1
R. conorii strain Moroccan	0.06–0.125	1–2	0.25	4	2	1	2	0.25	1	0.5–1
R. conorii serotype Israeli	0.06	1	0.5	4	1	0.5	1	0.5	1	1
R. conorii serotype Astrakhan	0.06	0.5	0.03	8	0.5	0.5	2	0.5	0.5	0.5
R. sibirica	0.06	0.5	0.06	2	2	1	2	1	1	1
R. australis	0.06	2	0.125	8	4	0.5	2	0.5	1	1
R. japonica	0.125	1	0.25	8	1	1	8	1	1	1
R. honei	0.06	2	0.5	4	1	0.5	2	1	1	1
R. africae	0.125	1	0.125	8	2	0.5	2	0.5	1	1
R. "mongolotimonae"	0.125	1	0.125	8	4	1	2	1	1	1
R. slovaca	0.06	1	0.5	2	0.5	1	1	1	1	1
R. felis	0.06–0.125	1–2	0.06–0.25	16	ND	ND	ND	0.05–1	0.05–1	ND
R. bellii	0.125	0.5	0.06	4	4	1	2	0.5	0.5	1
R. canada	0.06	1	0.125	4	1	1	2	0.5	0.5	1
R. helvetica	0.125	1	0.06	2	1	0.5	2	0.25	0.5	1
R. parkeri	0.25	4	0.25	4	1	0.5	2	0.25	0.25	0.5
Thai tick typhus rickettsia	0.06	2	0.125	8	1	1	4	0.5	2	1
Strain Bar29	0.06	1	2	4	2	0.5	4	0.25	0.5	0.5
R. massiliae	0.06	1	2	2	1	1	1	0.25	0.5	0.5
R. aeschlimannii	0.06	1	2	8	1	0.5	2	0.5	0.5	1
R. montana	0.125	2	2	8	1	2	4	1	1	1
R. rhipicephali	0.25	1	2	4	1	1	2	1	1	1

Clar, clarithromycin; Cip, ciprofloxacin; Doxy, doxycycline; Ery, erythromycin; Josa, josamycin; ND, not determined; Ofl, ofloxacin; Pef, pefloxacin; Prist, pristinamycin; Rifam, rifampin; Thiam, thiamphenicol.
[a] Susceptibility is given in terms of MIC (μg/mL).

antibiotics are tested per plate, four concentrations of each antibiotic are tested, and each concentration of antibiotic is replicated 12 times; that is, each row contains the same antibiotic at the same concentration. Antibiotics are added in 50-μL volumes. Incubation is then carried out at 36°C for 4 days in a CO_2 incubator.

After this the medium is removed, 50 μL of neutral red dye (0.15% in saline, pH 5.5; Sigma Chemical Co., St. Louis, MO) is added to each well, and the plate is incubated for 60 minutes at 36°C. Unincorporated dye is then washed (three washes) from the cells using phosphate-buffered saline (pH 6.5). Incorporated dye is removed from the well using 100 μL of phosphate-ethanol buffer (10% ethanol in phosphate-buffered saline, adjusted to pH 4.2).

Finally, the optical density (OD) of the solution is read at 492 nm with a multichannel spectrophotometer designed for use with microdilution plates (EIA Autoreader, model EL310; Bio-Tek Instruments, Winooski, VT). The mean OD of the control wells (containing only Vero cells) is assigned a value of 1, and the mean OD of the wells containing 2000 PFU is assigned a value of 0 (Fig. 7.1). The MIC is considered to be any OD value that falls between the mean OD of the wells containing 20 PFU and the mean OD of the control wells containing only Vero cells.

This assay is an adaptation of an assay used to determine the efficacy of agents against herpes viruses (108) and is dependent on the fact that intact cells take up neutral red dye. Hence, wells that contain fewer cells take

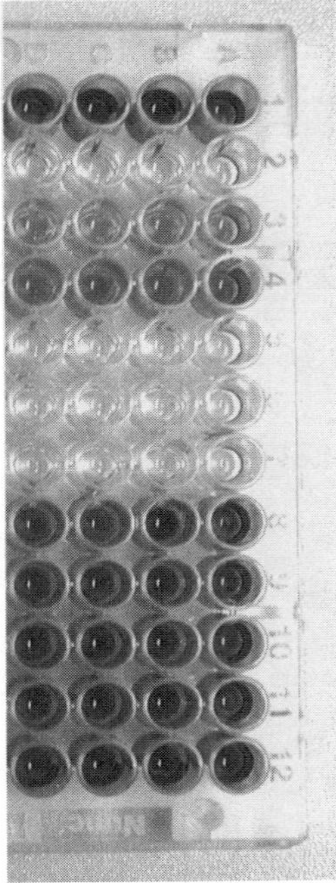

FIGURE 7.1 ● Dye uptake assay for *Rickettsia conorii.* The MIC is considered to be any OD value that falls between the mean OD of the wells containing 20 PFU and the mean OD of the control wells containing only Vero cells. In this example, the doxycycline MIC = 0.125 μg/mL.

up less neutral red and yield lower OD values. This test is therefore a derivative of the plaque assay but has the advantage of using microdilution technology as well as an automated means of reading the plates.

Other Assays

IF Assay. More recently, an immunofluorescence assay was described by Ives (59). In this model, Vero cells cultured in wells of chamber culture microscope slides were infected with rickettsiae. After incubation of cultures for 3 hours at 37°C in a 5% CO_2 atmosphere, cell supernatants were replaced by new medium containing various concentrations of the antibiotics to be tested. Drug-free cultures served as controls. Cell culture monolayers were then fixed with methanol and stained using an immunofluorescence assay to reveal the presence of immunofluorescent foci (clusters of rickettsiae) in 25 random fields for each well. The minimal antibiotic concentration allowing complete inhibition of foci formation as compared with the drug-free controls was recorded as the MIC.

LightCycler PCR Assay. Cells cultured in 24-well plates were infected with rickettsiae and incubated for 7 days at 37°C in a 5% CO_2 atmosphere with medium containing various concentrations of the antibiotics to be tested. Wells were harvested each day for 7 days and stored at −20°C before the PCR assay. Real-time PCR was performed on LightCycler instrumentation (Roche Biochemicals, Mannheim, Germany) (194). The specificity of amplification can be confirmed by melting curve analysis. Single melting peaks can be generated by depicting the negative derivative of fluorescence versus temperature (−dF/dT) over the course of a gradual PCR product melt.

Extraction of DNA. After thawing, harvested tubes were centrifuged at 5000 rpm for 10 minutes, supernatant was discarded, and pellet was washed twice with sterile distilled water and finally resuspended with 200 μL of sterile distilled water. Extraction of the DNA was performed using chelex (biotechnology-grade chelating resin, Chelex 100, Bio-Rad, Richmond, CA) at 20% in sterile water (173). Briefly, 500 μL of chelex was added to each tube, then the tubes were vortex-mixed and placed in a boiling water bath for 30 minutes. The tubes were then centrifuged at 14,000 rpm for 10 minutes, and supernatant was harvested and stored in sterile tubes at 4°C before use.

PCR Master Mix. Master mixes were prepared by following the manufacturer's instructions, using the primers CS877F (5′-GGG GGC CTG CTC ACG GCG G-3′) and CS1258R (5′-ATT GCA AAA AGT ACA GTG AAC A-3′) of the citrate synthase gene previously described (136). The 20-μL sample volume in each glass capillary contained the following: for all single experiments, 2 μL of LightCycler DNA Master SYBR Green (Roche Biochemicals), 2.4 μL of $MgCl_2$ at 4 mM, 1 μL of each primer at 0.5 μM, 11.6 μL of sterile distilled water, and 2 μL of DNA.

PCR Cycling and Melting Curve Conditions. After one-pulse centrifugation to allow mixing and to drive the mix into the distal end of each tube, glass capillaries were placed in the LightCycler instrument. The amplification program included an initial denaturation step consisting of 1 cycle at 95°C for 120 seconds and 40 cycles of denaturation at 95°C for 15 seconds, annealing at 54°C for 8 seconds, and extension at 72°C for 15 seconds, with fluorescence acquisition at 54°C in single mode. Melting curve analysis was done at 45°C to 90°C (temperature transition, 20°C per second), with stepwise fluorescence acquisition by real-time measurement of fluorescence directly in the clear glass capillary tubes. Sequence-specific standard curves were generated using tenfold serial dilutions (10^5 to 10^6 copies) of a standard bacterial concentration of *Rickettsia* organisms. The number of copies of each sample transcript was then calculated from a standard curve using the LightCycler software. The MIC was defined as the first antibiotic concentration allowing the inhibition of growth of bacteria as compared with the number of DNA copies at day 0. Experiments were made twice in duplicate. This technique is specific, reproducible, easy to perform, and rapid. It can also be used to measure the number of DNA copies at any time, and we were able to perform for the first time a kinetic of the growth of *Rickettsia* organisms even if the bacteria did not lead to plaque *in vitro* in cell cultures.

Results of Susceptibility Testing

The results of susceptibility testing of *Rickettsia* species are presented in Table 7.4. Sensitivities to amoxicillin (MICs from 128 to 256 μg/mL), gentamicin (MICs from 4 to 16 μg/mL), and co-trimoxazole were poor (154,155). Doxycycline was the most effective antibiotic against all strains tested, with MICs ranging from 0.06 to 0.25 μg/mL. The MICs of thiamphenicol ranged from 0.5 to 4 μg/mL, and the MICs for fluoroquinolone compounds ranged from 0.25 to 2 μg/mL. Among the macrolide compounds, josamycin was the most effective antibiotic, with MICs ranging from 0.5 to 1 μg/mL. Typhus group rickettsiae were susceptible to erythromycin (MICs from 0.125 to 0.5 μg/mL), whereas SFG rickettsiae were not (MICs from 2 to 8 μg/mL). Recently we demonstrated that the new ketolide compound telithromycin was very effective against typhus group rickettsiae and SFG rickettsiae, with MICs ranging from 0.5 to 1 μg/mL (153). Susceptibilities to rifampin varied: typhus group rickettsiae and most SFG rickettsiae were susceptible (MICs from 0.03 to 1 μg/mL), but a cluster including *Rickettsia massiliae, Rickettsia montana, Rickettsia rhipicephali, Rickettsia aeschlimannii,* and strain Bar 29 were more resistant (MICs from 2 to 4 μg/mL). This relative resistance to rifampin was linked to natural mutations in the *rpoB* gene (32).

EHRLICHIA

Ehrlichioses are emerging infectious diseases caused by obligate, Gram-negative, intracellular bacteria belonging to the *Proteobacteria* α subgroup (34). The genus *Ehrlichia* is divided into three genogroups: the group *Neorickettsia,* with *N. sennetsu*; *N. risticii*; and *N. helminthoeca*; the group *Ehrlichia,* with *E. canis, E. chaffeensis, E. rumitantium, E. muris,* and *E. ewingii*; and the group *Anaplasma* with *A. platys, A. marginale, Ehrlichia equi,* and *A. phagocytophilum* (33,34).

They are responsible of human and animal diseases. *E. chaffeensis* is the agent of human monocytic ehrlichiosis (HME); *A. phagocytophilum,* the agent of human granulocytic ehrlichiosis (HGE); and *E. canis,* the agent of canine ehrlichiosis. *In vitro* and *in vivo* antibiotic susceptibility studies have been carried out on various species of *Ehrlichia.* All have found that doxycycline and rifampin are highly effective against ehrlichiae, and thus they are currently preferred for treating animal and in human ehrlichiosis.

Antimicrobial Susceptibility Testing

Animal Models

E. sennetsu was first isolated in mice (109), and subsequently infections in mice have been used as a model for Sennetsu fever. Although the growth of *E. sennetsu* in mice is much slower than the growth of other rickettsiae, treatment of mice with cyclophosphamide prior to inoculation has been found to enhance the growth of *E. sennetsu* (177), and this technique has been used for the preparation of antigen in mice. The first study of antibiotic susceptibility in mice for *E. sennetsu* has shown that erythromycin, sulfisoxazole, penicillin, streptomycin, polymyxin B, bacitracin, and chloramphenicol were ineffective even at high concentrations (86). Chlortetracycline was more effective than oxytetracycline and tetracycline. Further studies have evaluated the effect of tetracycline therapy on spleen size as a percentage of body weight and on the splenic infectious burden in mice infected with *E. sennetsu* (74,88). In mice in which tetracycline therapy was initiated at the same time as inoculation, there were no detectable ehrlichiae in the spleen (74). Therefore, it would appear that the time of initiation of treatment may be important in controlling the course of infection with

E. sennetsu and that delayed therapy may allow the development of chronic infections.

Cell Culture Model

The susceptibility of *Ehrlichia* species to various antibiotics has been tested using ehrlichiae-infected contact-inhibition-growth cell lines incubated for 48 to 72 hours in the antibiotic concerned. Thereafter, the antibiotic-containing media is removed, and ehrlichiae-infected cells are incubated with antibiotic-free media for at least 3 more days. The number of ehrlichiae-infected cells are counted every day, and an antibiotic is considered ineffective if the number of ehrlichiae-infected cells after exposure to the antibiotic is similar to that of noninfected control cells. If the number of ehrlichiae-infected cells is found to decrease during incubation with an antibiotic, the antibiotic is regarded as being bactericidal. Antibiotics are considered bacteriostatic if there is no increase or decrease in ehrlichiae-infected cells when the antibiotic is present but the number of infected cells increases when antibiotic-free media is provided.

Results of Susceptibility Testing

Results of susceptibility testing for *A. phagocytophilum*, *E. canis*, and *E. chaffeensis* are presented in Table 7.5. The *in vitro* susceptibility of *E. sennetsu* Miyayama strain to eight antibiotics was determined using Diff-Quick staining of infected P388D1 cells over a 5-day period (16). In this study, it was also demonstrated that Diff-Quick staining was as reliable as immunofluorescence assay for detecting infected cells. It was found that *E. sennetsu* was not susceptible to penicillin, gentamicin, co-trimoxazole, erythromycin, and chloramphenicol, whereas rifampin, doxycycline, and ciprofloxacin were effective, with MICs of 0.5, 0.125, and 0.125 μg/mL, respectively.

The *in vitro* antibiotic suceptibility of *E. chaffeensis* was studied recently (17,153) by means of a microplate colorimetric assay using ehrlichiae-infected DH82 cell culture. The percentage of infected cells was determined each day by Diff-Quick staining, which has been found to stain only viable organisms. On the third day of incubation, the antibiotic-containing medium was removed and replaced with antibiotic-free medium. Using these methods, it was found that *E. chaffeensis* was sensitive to 0.5 μg/mL of doxycycline and 0.125 μg/mL of rifampin. Chloramphenicol, co-trimoxazole, erythromycin, telithromycin penicillin, gentamicin, and ciprofloxacin were not effective against *E. chaffeensis*.

The HGE agent is sensitive to doxycycline, ofloxacin, ciprofloxacin, and trovafloxacin but is resistant to clindamycin, co-trimoxazole, erythromycin, azithromycin,

TABLE 7.5

MICs (μg/mL) of Antibiotics against *Anaplasma phagocytophilum, Ehrlichia canis,* and *Ehrlichia chaffeensis* as Determined Using the Diff-Quick (DQ) Assay

	A. phagocytophilum			*E. canis*	*E. chaffeensis*	
Antibiotic	Klein et al. (85) (M, NY, W)	Horowitz et al. (54) (6 strains NY)	Maurin et al. (102) (Webster, W)	Brouqui et al. (18)	Brouqui et al. (17) (Atlanta)	Rolain et al. (153) (Atlanta)
Gentamicin	50	Amiklin >16	Amiklin >64	>100	>32	ND
Ceftriaxone	>64	>64	>128	ND	ND	ND
Amoxicillin	>32	>32	>128	1000	ND	ND
Ofloxacin	2	<2	ND	ND	ND	ND
Ciprofloxacin	2	ND	ND	Pefloxacin > 2	>2[a]	ND
Levofloxacin	ND	<1	0.5	ND	ND	ND
Rifampin	0.5	<0.125	0.03	0.03	0.125	ND
Doxycycline	0.25	<0.125	0.03	0.03	<0.5	ND
Co-trimoxazole	>16	ND	50	>4	>4	ND
Chloramphenicol	>32	>16	2–8[a]	>4	>4	ND
Telithromycin	ND	ND	ND	ND	ND	>1
Erythromycin	>8	>8	>16	>4	>8	ND

M, Minnesota; ND, not done; NY, New York; W, Wisconsin.
[a] MIC = 2–8 μg/mL according to strains tested.

ampicillin, ceftriaxone, and imipenem (54,85,102). Chloramphenicol and aminoglycosides only display a poor bacteriostatic activity and are never bactericidal (85). Fluoroquinolones are more active *in vitro* against *A. phagocytophilum* than against *E. chaffeensis* and *E. canis* (Table 7.5). Fluoroquinolones might represent a potential therapeutic alternative to tetracycline for HGE, but they have not received FDA approval for use in children and pregnant women (121). Moreover, a *Gyr*A-mediated resistance in the related species *E. canis* and *E. chaffeensis* has recently been described and can explain this difference (101).

COXIELLA BURNETII

Coxiella burnetii, the agent of Q fever, is an obligate, intracellular bacterium that multiplies within acidic vacuoles of eukaryotic cells (104). *C. burnetii* is classified in the family of Rickettsiaceae, where it belongs to the *Proteobacteria* γ subgroup based on 16S-rRNA sequence analysis (106). *C. burnetti* is a bioterrorism agent that is resistant to heat and drying and can survive in the environment for months. It is also highly infectious by the aerosol route. Owing to these features, Q fever has been investigated and developed as a bioweapon. If used, it would not generate mass fatalities but rather act as an incapacitating agent (24,44). Acute Q fever is the primary infection, and in specific hosts it may become chronic (132). A few patients (~0.7%) suffer from chronic Q fever, which in most cases corresponds to chronic endocarditis, especially in patients with previous cardiac valve defects and/or with a cardiac valve prosthesis, in immunocompromised patients, and in pregnant women (106).

Antimicrobial Susceptibility Testing and Results

Antibiotic susceptibility testing of *C. burnetii* is difficult because this organism is an obligate, intracellular bacterium. However, three models of infection have been developed: animals, chick embryos, and cell culture. The method currently used to test antibiotic susceptibility of *C. burnetii* is based on cell culture models. Torres and Raoult (185) have developed a shell vial assay with HEL cells for assessment of the bacteriostatic effect of antibiotics.

Recommended Technique: The Shell Vial Assay

In this model, human embryonic lung (HEL) fibroblast cells are grown in shell vials at 37°C in a 5% CO_2 atmosphere. Cell monolayers are infected with a *C. burnetii* inoculum previously determined to induce 30% to 50% infection of HEL cells after 6 days of incubation in the absence of antimicrobial agents, as revealed by an immunofluorescence technique with anti–*C. burnetii* polyclonal antibodies. The percentage of infected cells in antimicrobial-containing cultures is determined after the same incubation time using the same immunofluorescence procedure. MICs correspond to the minimum antimicrobial concentration allowing complete inhibition of growth, that is, 0% infected cells after the 6-day incubation period (Fig. 7.2).

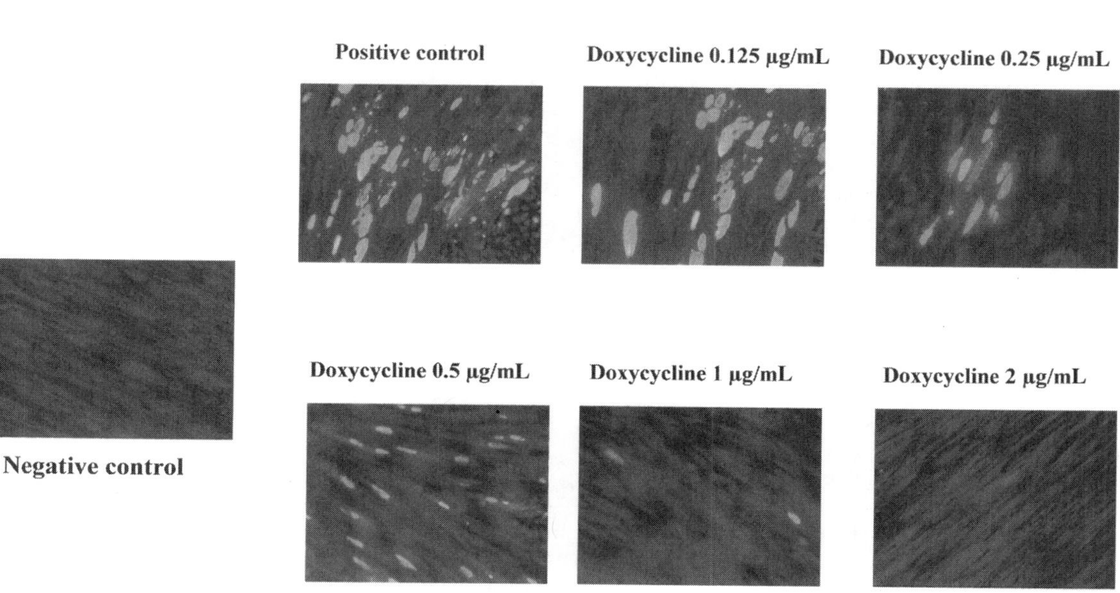

FIGURE 7.2 • Shell vial assay for *Coxiella burnetii.* MICs correspond to the minimum antimicrobial concentration allowing complete inhibition of growth (i.e., 0% infected cells after the 6-day incubation period). In this example, the doxycycline MIC = 2 μg/mL.

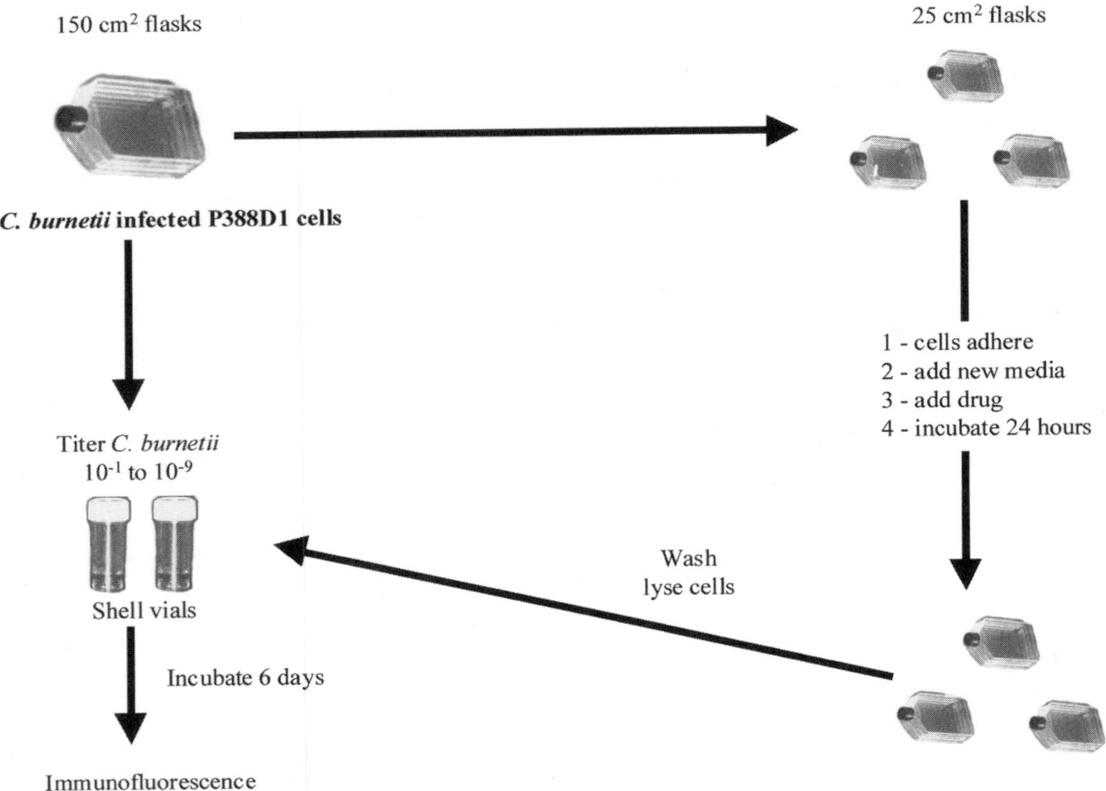

FIGURE 7.3 ● Intracellular *Coxiella burnetii* killing assay.

Amikacin and amoxicillin were not effective, ceftriaxone and fusidic acid were inconsistently active (185), whereas co-trimoxazole, rifampin, doxycycline, clarithromycin, and the quinolones were bacteriostatic (61,105). There was a heterogeneity of susceptibility to erythromycin of the strains tested (137,184). *C. burnetii* can establish a persistent infection in several cell lines, including L929 mouse fibroblasts and J774 or P388D1 murine macrophage-like cells (4). Infected cells can be maintained in continuous cultures for months (156). Raoult et al., using P388D1 and L929 cells, showed that pefloxacin, rifampin, and doxycycline (129) as well as clarithromycin (105) were bacteriostatic against *C. burnetii*. A real-time quantitative PCR assay was recently used for antibiotic susceptibility testing on *C. burnetii* and proved to be more specific and sensitive than the shell vial assay (10,14).

An original model of killing assay has been developed by Maurin to assess the bactericidal activity of antibiotics against *C. burnetii* (103). The bactericidal activity of antibiotics in this technique is directly evaluated by titration of residual viable bacteria in persistently infected P388D1 cell cultures (Fig. 7.3). On the first day of the experiment, P388D1 cells infected with *C. burnetii* were harvested from a 150-cm^2 culture flask and seeded into 25-cm^2 flasks so that each flask received the same primary inoculum. Antibiotics were added to some of the flasks, and all the flasks, with or without antibiotics, were incubated for 24 hours at 37°C. Then cells were lysed, and tenfold serial dilutions of cell lysates were distributed into shell vials containing uninfected HEL cells (138). After 6 days of incubation, *C. burnetii* were stained by indirect immunofluorescence in the shell vials. It was demonstrated that doxycycline, pefloxacin, and rifampin did not show any significant bactericidal activity. The lack of bactericidal activity was related to inactivation by the low pH of the phagolysosomes in which *C. burnetii* survives. Raoult demonstrated that the addition of a lysosomotropic alkalinizing agent, chloroquine, to antibiotics improved the activities of doxycycline and pefloxacin, which then became bactericidal (103).

SPIROCHETES

There are several pathogens of major importance in this group, including the leptospires, *Borrelia* species (including *B. burgdorferi*, the etiologic agent of Lyme disease), and *Treponema* species (including *T. pallidum*, the etiologic agent of syphilis). Whereas *B. burgdorferi* can be grown in a cell-free system (8), *T. pallidum* requires tissue culture for propagation (118). Because of the complexities of working with *T. pallidum,* as well as the fact that it is rarely isolated from clinical material, susceptibility testing for *T. pallidum* will have to be carried out in specialized research laboratories whose personnel have both the interest and the competence to work with this fastidious organism.

Borrelia burgdorferi

Antimicrobial Susceptibility Testing

A modified Kelly bovine serum medium has been developed that will support the growth of laboratory-adapted strains of this organism as well as fresh clinical isolates (8). The *in vitro* susceptibility tests use macro- or microdilution methods and standard Barbour-Stoenner-Kelly (BSK) medium (30). Using this medium, a tube dilution susceptibility test has been developed that yields both MIC and MBC values. The MIC was defined by Berger et al. (8) as the minimum concentration of antibiotic that did not allow the spirochete to multiply, whereas Preac-Mursic et al. (126) defined the MIC as the minimum concentration that prevented growth altogether. The MBC was also determined by Berger et al. (8) by subculturing all tubes that showed inhibition of growth of the spirochete into tubes containing antibiotic-free Kelly bovine serum medium. The minimum antibiotic concentration that yielded no organisms on subculture was defined as the MBC. From these definitions of MIC and MBC, it would appear that what Preac-Mursic et al. defined as the MIC was what Berger et al. defined as the MBC. This indeed seems to be confirmed by the results obtained by the two groups. Thus, the MBCs obtained by Berger et al. (8) for penicillin G ranged from 0.08 to 2.5 units/mL and were comparable to the range of MICs (0.06 to 3.0 g/mL) obtained by Preac-Mursic et al. (126).

Tube Dilution Technique

The procedure developed by Berger et al. (8) is described here. In this technique a serum-free Kelly medium is used. This medium is prepared as follows: 5 g of neopeptone (Difco Laboratories, Detroit, MI) is dissolved in 50 mL of boiling water, and after the solution cools to 37°C, the mixture is filtered through a no. 42 Whatman filter (Whatman Ltd., Maidstone, England). Bovine serum albumin (40 g) (fraction V, no. A2152; Sigma Chemical Co., Saint-Louis, MO) is dissolved in 200 mL of distilled water, filtered through a coarse filter, and then filtered through Whatman no. 42 paper. Next, the albumin and neopeptone solutions are added to sufficient distilled water to make a total of 900 mL.

The remaining ingredients of modified Kelly medium are as follows: 100 mL of CMRL 1066 medium with glutamine and without sodium bicarbonate (10; GIBCO Laboratories, Grand Island, NY), 6.0 g of HEPES (Sigma Chemical Co.), 0.7 g of sodium citrate, 5.0 g of glucose, 0.8 g of sodium pyruvate, 0.4 g of *N*-acetylglucosamine, 2.2 g of sodium bicarbonate, and 1.25 g of yeastolate (Difco). This solution is adjusted to pH 7.2 with 5.0 mol/L NaOH, after which 200 mL of a warm 7% solution of gelatin is added. Finally the medium is sterilized by passing it through a 0.2-m filter (Nalgene sterilization filter unit type LS; Nalge Co., Rochester, NY).

B. burgdorferi, including laboratory-adapted strains, readily grow in modified Kelly medium; by 72 hours, counts as high as 6×10^6 spirochetes can be achieved. Fresh human isolates tend to clump when they grow, which is not as true for the laboratory-adapted strains. Incubation is carried out at 32°C to 33°C, and cell counts are carried out by performing serial tenfold dilutions to 1:1000 and examining 6 μL on a slide by dark-field microscopy. Slides are prepared by covering the sample gently with a coverslip ringed with petrolatum.

Susceptibility testing is carried out in 13 × 100-mm test tubes prepared with 5 mL of modified Kelly medium, 1 mL of antibiotic solution containing seven times the final desired antibiotic concentration, and 1.0 mL of spirochetes at a concentration of 7×10^5/mL. The MIC is determined after 72 hours of incubation and is defined as the antibiotic concentration in which more than 90% of the spirochetes are motile (as determined by examination under dark-field microscopy, as described above) and yet the number of spirochetes is not greater than the original inoculum. The MBC is determined by transferring 50 μL from all tubes showing no growth at 72 hours to 7.0 mL of modified Kelly medium. These tubes are subsequently examined at 11 days by removing 10 μL and viewing this under a dark-field microscope. The MBC is defined as the concentration of antibiotic that prevents growth. It should be noted, however, that the developers of this technique found that the MBC determinations were not reproducible (8).

Dever et al. (31) adapted the macrodilution method to a microdilution method using microtiter trays and demonstrated that the results obtained using this very efficient method were comparable to those obtained with the more laborious macrodilution method.

Recently, Hunfeld et al. developed a new standardized colorimetric assay for the determination of susceptibility to antibiotics of several strains of *Borrelia* (57). This assay is based on color changes that result from actively metabolizing spirochetes after 72 hours of incubation. Briefly, *Borrelia* stock cultures were thawed, cultured in modified BSK medium at 33°C until the log phase of growth, and adjusted to 2.5×10^7 organisms/mL as determined by enumeration with a Kova counting chamber (Hycor, Garden Grove, CA) combined with dark-field microscopy. Final concentrations of the lyophilized antibiotics were reconstituted by adding of 200 μL of the final inoculum suspension (5×10^6 cells) in BSK containing phenol red (25 g/mL) as a growth indicator. Samples and growth controls were sealed with sterile adhesive plastic and cultured at 33°C with 5% CO_2. The presence or absence of growth was examined after 0, 24, 48, and 72 hours by kinetic measurement of indicator color shift at 562/630 nm applying a commercially available ELISA-reader (PowerWave 200, Bio-Tec Instruments, Winooski, VT) in combination with a software-assisted calculation program (Microwin 3.0, Microtek, Overath, Germany). Colorimetric MICs of isolates were measured in triplicate by the quantification of growth achieved through the calculation of growth curves.

Results of Susceptibility Testing

The results of susceptibility testing for *B. burgdorferi* are presented in Table 7.6. *B. burgdorferi* strains of both European and North American origin have been tested against a variety of antimicrobials because of the increasing attention that this pathogen has recently attracted (2,66). It is evident that the macrolides, the tetracyclines, amoxicillin, and the third-generation cephalosporins all have good *in vitro* activity (30,68,95). Penicillin G activity is strain-dependent, with some strains being moderately resistant (69).

TABLE 7.6

Antimicrobial Susceptibility of *Borrelia burgdorferi*

Drug	MIC (μg/mL)	References
Aminoglycosides		
Amikacin	>32	(57,126)
Gentamicin	>32	(126)
Cephalosporins		
Cefixime	0.25–2	(57)
Cefoperazone	0.03–2	(57)
Cefotaxime	0.01–0.25	(57,115)
Ceftriaxone	0.01–0.25	(57,68,115,166)
Macrolides		
Azithromycin	≤0.015–0.06	(57,166)
Erythromycin	0.03–0.125	(25,68,115)
Roxithromycin	≤0.015–0.125	(57)
Penicillins		
Amoxicillin	0.06–2	(57,126,166)
Ampicillin	0.25–1	(126)
Penicillin	0.25–8	(68,115,126)
Piperacillin	≤0.06–0.125	(57)
Quinolones		
Ciprofloxacin	1–4	(115)
Tetracyclines		
Doxycycline	≤0.25–2	(69,166)
Minocycline	0.03–1	(57,69)
Tetracycline	0.06–2	(57,68,69)
Miscellaneous		
Chloramphenicol	1–3	(126)
Imipenem	0.06–1	(115)
Sulfamethoxazole	>1024	(126)

Treponema pallidum

Until recently, it was not possible to cultivate this organism. However, in 1981 Fieldsteel et al. (36) published a technique for the propagation of this treponeme in tissue culture. This cell culture was later confirmed (96) and has been used for drug susceptibility testing (118). Although there is no evidence of the emergence of resistance to benzylpenicillin (the treatment of choice for syphilis), resistance to erythromycin has been documented (168). The failure of penicillin therapy for syphilis has been particularly noted in patients with AIDS. However, this is not because of any demonstrated resistance of the treponeme to penicillin but rather because the therapy probably does not completely eliminate viable treponemes from the host and eradication of the infection depends on host defenses lacking in patients with AIDS (41).

Antimicrobial Susceptibility Testing

It has been shown that 24- to 100-fold multiplication of *T. pallidum* can be obtained in tissue culture using Sf1Ep cottontail rabbit epithelial cells (obtainable from the American Type Culture Collection, Rockville, MD) under 1.5% to 3.0% oxygen at 33°C to 34°C (67,96). However, continuous *in vitro* culture has not yet been achieved (118).

Results of Susceptibility Testing

The results of susceptibility testing of *T. pallidum* are presented in Table 7.7. Using this procedure, antimicrobial susceptibilities have been determined with penicillin, tetracycline, erythromycin, spectinomycin, oral cephalosporins, and quinolones. The MICs achieved with the tissue culture system correlate quite well with the clinical and experimental results obtained with these antimicrobials, with the exception of spectinomycin. The single clinical isolate that has been shown by the method of inhibition of protein synthesis to be resistant to erythromycin (168) had an A to G transition mutation at position 2058 of the 23S rRNA gene (167).

Leptospira

Prior to 1989, the genus *Leptospira* was divided into two species, *L. interrogans* comprising all pathogenic strains, and *L. biflexa,* comprising the strains from the

TABLE 7.7

Antimicrobial Susceptibility of *Treponema pallidum*

Drug	MIC (μg/mL)	References
Amoxicillin	0.42	(41)
Ceftriaxone	0.01	(87)
Erythromycin	0.005	(118)
Penicillin G	0.0005	(118)
Spectinomycin	0.5	(118)
Tetracycline	0.2	(118)

environment (94). Within the species *L. interrogans,* there are approximately 200 serovars. The current classification of *Leptospira* is genotypic and now includes a number of genomospecies containing all serovars (94). A new species, *L. fainei,* has been recently reported to cause infections in humans (3,124). Leptospirosis is a zoonosis acquired from a wide variety of domestic and wild animals. Although penicillin is considered the drug of choice because of its low MIC, there is concern that this antibiotic is not bactericidal for *Leptospira* species. Unfortunately, only limited *in vitro* studies with newer antimicrobials have been carried out.

Organism

Reference organisms obtained from the National Institute of Health (Tokyo, Japan) were used in a recent extensive study of antimicrobial susceptibility (119). These organisms are cultured in Korthof medium at 30°C, as described by Johnson and Harris (67).

Antimicrobial Susceptibility Testing

Tube dilution methodology may be used for determining the MIC and MBC (119). Inocula of 0.5 mL containing 0.5×10^8 to 1.5×10^8 organisms are put in each tube after the *Leptospira* species have been grown in Korthof medium for 5 days at 30°C. Inocula of 0.5 mL are added to tubes containing 4.5 mL of fresh Korthof medium with the desired concentration of antibiotics, and the tubes are incubated for 7 days at 30°C. The MIC is defined as the minimum concentration of antibiotic that inhibits all visible growth. The MBC was determined by taking 10 μL from each clear tube, subculturing this aliquot into 10 mL of fresh Korthof medium, and incubating these tubes for 3 weeks. The MBC is the minimum concentration of antibiotic that allows no growth in these subcultures, as determined by the absence of any visible growth.

Results of Susceptibility Testing

Oie et al. (119) studied the *in vitro* activity of 16 antibiotics against five serovar strains of the genus *Leptospira*. Five antibiotics (ampicillin, cefmetazole, moxalactam, ceftizoxime, and cefotaxime) yielded lower MICs than did penicillin G. Ceftizoxime and cefotaxime demonstrated the lowest MBCs and were more effective than penicillin G, streptomycin, tetracycline, ampicillin, and cefmetazole.

Because of the failure of penicillin to prevent a laboratory-acquired case of leptospirosis due to *L. interrogans* subgroup *icterohaemorrhagiae,* Broughton and Flack (15) determined MIC and MBC values for amoxicillin, erythromycin, lincomycin, tetracycline, oxytetracycline, and minocycline for the infecting strain. Amoxicillin and erythromycin were the most effective, with MBCs of 0.5 μg/mL and 0.1 μg/mL, respectively. Recently, the susceptibilities of 11 serovars (seven species) of *Leptospira* to 14 antibiotics have been reported (55). With the exception of chloramphenicol, all tested agents were at least as potent as penicillin and doxycyline, with the macrolide and ketolide drugs producing the lowest MICs ($\leq$0.01 μg/mL).

CONCLUDING REMARKS

All of the organisms considered in this chapter, with the exception of the mycoplasmas, *B. burgdorferi,* and the *Leptospira* species, require either tissue culture or *in vivo* techniques for their propagation and susceptibility testing. Because of this, they frequently are not isolated from patients in whom they are causing disease.

Thus, two difficulties exist in terms of adequately defining their patterns of susceptibility to both available and experimental antimicrobials: the susceptibility testing procedures are often cumbersome and technically demanding, and recent clinical isolates are not likely to be available for testing. For these reasons, it will be important to further simplify and standardize the susceptibility testing procedures for these organisms to allow additional laboratories to undertake susceptibility testing. If emerging resistance is to be detected, it is essential that recent clinical isolates are also tested, particularly those from patients who appear to be failing, or have failed, appropriate therapy. Our new real-time PCR assay could be useful in the future for the determination of the susceptibility to antibiotics of such fastidious bacteria (155).

Certainly, the appearance of the *tetM* tetracyline resistance determinant in genital mycoplasmas, which probably was acquired from a streptococcal organism, indicates that these organisms are capable of acquiring genetic material from other microbial species and thus possible destroying the utility of an important therapeutic agent such as tetracycline. This fact alone should make us wary of further developments of this sort and encourage laboratories to monitor the emergence of resistance in this group of organisms, despite the often technically demanding methods required for accurate susceptibility testing.

REFERENCES

1. Agacfidan A, Moncada J, Schachter J. In vitro activity of azithromycin (CP-62,993) against *Chlamydia trachomatis* and *Chlamydia pneumoniae*. *Antimicrob Agents Chemother* 1993;37:1746–1748.
2. Agger WA, Callister SM, Jobe DA. In vitro susceptibilities of *Borrelia burgdorferi* to five oral cephalosporins and ceftriaxone. *Antimicrob Agents Chemother* 1992;36:1788–1790.
3. Arzouni JP, Parola P, La Scola B, et al. Human infection caused by *Leptospira fainei*. *Emerg Infect Dis* 2002;8:865–868.
4. Baca OG, Akporiaye ET, Aragon AS, et al. Fate of phase I and phase II *Coxiella burnetii* in several macrophage-like tumor cell lines. *Infect Immun* 1981;33:258–266.
5. Bailey JM, Heppleston C, Richmond SJ. Comparison of the in vitro activities of ofloxacin and tetracycline against *Chlamydia trachomatis* as assessed by indirect immunofluorescence. *Antimicrob Agents Chemother* 1984;26:13–16.
6. Bebear CM, Bove JM, Bebear C, et al. Characterization of *Mycoplasma hominis* mutations involved in resistance to fluoroquinolones. *Antimicrob Agents Chemother* 1997;41:269–273.
7. Benson C, Segreti J, Kessler H, et al. Comparative in vitro activity of A-56268 (TE-031) against Gram-positive and Gram-negative bacteria and *Chlamydia trachomatis*. *Eur J Clin Microbiol* 1987;6:173–178.
8. Berger BW, Kaplan MH, Rothenberg IR, et al. Isolation and characterization of the Lyme disease spirochete from the skin of patients with erythema chronicum migrans. *J Am Acad Dermatol* 1985;13:444–449.
9. Bianchi A, Scieux C, Salmeron CM, et al. Rapid determination of MICs of 15 antichlamydial agents by using an enzyme immunoassay (Chlamydiazyme). *Antimicrob Agents Chemother* 1988;32:1350–1353.
10. Boulos A, Rolain JM, Maurin M, et al. Measurement of the antibiotic susceptibility of Coxiella burnetii using real time PCR. *Int J Antimicrob Agents* 2004;23(2):169–174.
11. Bowie WR. Lack of in vitro activity of cefoxitin, cefamandole, cefuroxime, and piperacillin against *Chlamydia trachomatis*. *Antimicrob Agents Chemother* 1982;21:339–340.
12. Bowie WR. In vitro activity of clavulanic acid, amoxicillin, and ticarcillin against *Chlamydia trachomatis*. *Antimicrob Agents Chemother* 1986;29:713–715.
13. Bowie WR, Lee CK, Alexander ER. Prediction of efficacy of antimicrobial agents in treatment of infections due to *Chlamydia trachomatis*. *J Infect Dis* 1978;138:655–659.
14. Brennan RE, Samuel JE. Evaluation of *Coxiella burnetii* antibiotic susceptibilities by real-time PCR assay. *J Clin Microbiol* 2003;41:1869–1874.
15. Broughton ES, Flack LE. The susceptibility of a strain of *Leptospira interrogans* serogroup Icterohaemorrhagiae to amoxycillin, erythromycin, lincomycin, tetracycline, oxytetracycline and minocycline. *Zentralbl Bakteriol Mikrobiol Hyg [A]* 1986;261:425–431.
16. Brouqui P, Raoult D. In vitro susceptibility of *Ehrlichia sennetsu* to antibiotics. *Antimicrob Agents Chemother* 1990;34:1593–1596.
17. Brouqui P, Raoult D. In vitro antibiotic susceptibility of the newly recognized agent of ehrhlichiosis in humans, *Ehrlichia chaffeensis*. *Antimicrob Agents Chemother* 1992;36:2799–2803.
18. Brouqui P, Raoult D. Susceptibilities of Ehrlichiae to antibiotics. In: Raoult D, ed. *Antimicrobial agents and intracellular pathogens*. Boca Raton, FL: CRC Press, 1993:179–199.
19. Bygdeman SM, Mardh PA. Antimicrobial susceptibility and susceptibility testing of *Mycoplasma hominis*: a review. *Sex Transm Dis* 1983;10:366–370.
20. Cassell GH, Waites KB, Pate MS, et al. Comparative susceptibility of *Mycoplasma pneumoniae* to erythromycin, ciprofloxacin, and lomefloxacin. *Diagn Microbiol Infect Dis* 1989;12:433–435.
21. Cevenini R, Donati M, Sambri V, et al. Enzyme-linked immunosorbent assay for the in-vitro detection of sensitivity of *Chlamydia trachomatis* to antimicrobial drugs. *J Antimicrob Chemother* 1987;20:677–684.
22. Chirgwin K, Roblin PM, Hammerschlag MR. In vitro susceptibilities of *Chlamydia pneumoniae* (*Chlamydia* sp. strain TWAR). *Antimicrob Agents Chemother* 1989;33:1634–1635.
23. Christensen JJ, Holten-Andersen W, Nielsen PB. *Chlamydia trachomatis:* in vitro susceptibility to antibiotics singly and in combination. *Acta Pathol Microbiol Immunol Scand [B]* 1986;94:329–332.
24. Christopher GW, Cieslak TJ, Pavlin JA, et al. Biological warfare: a historical perspective. *JAMA* 1997;278:412–417.
25. Cinco M, Padovan D, Stinco G, et al. In vitro activity of rokitamycin, a new macrolide, against *Borrelia burgdorferi*. *Antimicrob Agents Chemother* 1995;39:1185–1186.
26. Cross NA, Kellock DJ, Kinghorn GR, et al. Antimicrobial susceptibility testing of *Chlamydia trachomatis* using a reverse transcriptase PCR-based method. *Antimicrob Agents Chemother* 1999;43:2311–2313.
27. Crosse BA. Psittacosis: a clinical review. *J Infect* 1990;21:251–259.
28. Dessus-Babus S, Bebear CM, Charron A, et al. Sequencing of gyrase and topoisomerase IV quinolone-resistance–determining regions of *Chlamydia trachomatis* and characterization of quinolone-resistant mutants obtained in vitro. *Antimicrob Agents Chemother* 1998;42:2474–2481.
29. Dessus-Babus S, Belloc F, Bebear CM, et al. Antibiotic susceptibility testing for *Chlamydia trachomatis* using flow cytometry. *Cytometry* 1998;31:37–44.
30. Dever LL, Jorgensen JH, Barbour AG. In vitro antimicrobial susceptibility testing of *Borrelia burgdorferi*: a microdilution MIC method and time-kill studies. *J Clin Microbiol* 1992;30:2692–2697.
31. Donati M, Pollini GM, Sparacino M, et al. Comparative in vitro activity of garenoxacin against *Chlamydia* spp. *J Antimicrob Chemother* 2002;50:407–410.
32. Drancourt M, Raoult D. Characterization of mutations in the rpoB gene in naturally rifampin resistant Rickettsia species. *Antimicrob Agent Chemother* 1999;43:2400–2403.
33. Dumler JS, Bakken JS. Ehrlichial diseases of humans: emerging tick-borne infections. *Clin Infect Dis* 1995;20:1102–1110.
34. Dumler JS, Barbet AF, Bekker CP, et al. Reorganization of genera in the families Rickettsiaceae and Anaplasmataceae in the order Rickettsiales: unification of some species of *Ehrlichia* with *Anaplasma, Cowdria* with *Ehrlichia* and *Ehrlichia* with *Neorickettsia,* descriptions of six new species combinations and designation of *Ehrlichia equi* and "HGE agent" as subjective synonyms

of *Ehrlichia phagocytophila. Int J Syst Evol Microbiol* 2001;51:2145–2165.
35. Ehret JM, Judson FN. Susceptibility testing of *Chlamydia trachomatis*: from eggs to monoclonal antibodies. *Antimicrob Agents Chemother* 1988;32:1295–1299.
36. Fieldsteel AH, Cox DL, Moeckli RA. Cultivation of virulent *Treponema pallidum* in tissue culture. *Infect Immun* 1981;32:908–915.
37. Fournier PE, Gunnenberger F, Jaulhac B, et al. Evidence of *Rickettsia helvetica* infection in humans, Eastern France. *Emerg Infect Dis* 2000;6:389–392.
38. Freidank HM, Losch P, Vogele H, et al. In vitro susceptibilities of *Chlamydia pneumoniae* isolates from German patients and synergistic activity of antibiotic combinations. *Antimicrob Agents Chemother* 1999;43:1808–1810.
39. Gieffers J, Solbach W, Maass M. In vitro susceptibilities of *Chlamydia pneumoniae* strains recovered from atherosclerotic coronary arteries. *Antimicrob Agents Chemother* 1998;42:2762–2764.
40. Gnarpe J, Eriksson K, Gnarpe H. In vitro activities of azithromycin and doxycycline against 15 isolates of *Chlamydia pneumoniae*. *Antimicrob Agents Chemother* 1996;40:1843–1845.
41. Goldmeier D, Hay P. A review and update on adult syphilis, with particular reference to its treatment. *Int J STD AIDS* 1993;4:70–82.
42. Grayston JT, Kuo C-C, Campbell A, et al. *Chlamydia pneumoniae* sp. nov. for *Chlamydia* TWAR. *Int J Syst Bacteriol* 1989;39:88–90.
43. Grayston JT, Kuo C-C, Wang S-P, et al. A new *Chlamydia psittaci* strain called TWAR from acute respiratory tract infections. *N Engl J Med* 1986;315:161–168.
44. Greenfield RA, Drevets DA, Machado LJ, et al. Bacterial pathogens as biological weapons and agents of bioterrorism. *Am J Med Sci* 2002;323:299–315.
45. Hammerschlag MR. Activity of trimethoprim-sulfamethoxazole against *Chlamydia trachomatis* in vitro. *Rev Infect Dis* 1982;4:500–505.
46. Hammerschlag MR. Activity of gemifloxacin and other new quinolones against *Chlamydia pneumoniae*: a review. *J Antimicrob Chemother* 2000;45[Suppl 1]:35–9:35–39.
47. Hammerschlag MR, Gleyzer A. In vitro activity of a group of broad spectrum cephalosporins and other betalactam antibodies against *Chlamydia trachomatis*. *Antimicrob Agents Chemother* 1983;23:493–494.
48. Hammerschlag MR, Hyman CL, Roblin PM. In vitro activities of five quinolones against *Chlamydia pneumoniae*. *Antimicrob Agents Chemother* 1992;36:682–683.
49. Hammerschlag MR, Roblin PM, Bebear CM. Activity of telithromycin, a new ketolide antibacterial, against atypical and intracellular respiratory tract pathogens. *J Antimicrob Chemother* 2001;48[Suppl T1]:25–31.
50. Hardy DJ. Activity of temafloxacin and other fluoroquinolones against typical and atypical community-acquired respiratory tract pathogens. *Am J Med* 1991;91:12S–14S.
51. Harrison HR, Riggin RM, Alexander ER, et al. In vitro activity of clindamycin against strains of *Chlamydia trachomatis, Mycoplasma hominis,* and *Ureaplasma urealyticum* isolated from pregnant women. *Am J Obstet Gynecol* 1984;149:477–480.
52. Hayes MM, Wear DJ, Lo SC. In vitro antimicrobial susceptibility testing for the newly identified AIDS-associated *Mycoplasma, Mycoplasma fermentans* (incognitus strain). *Arch Pathol Lab Med* 1991;115:464–466.
53. Heessen FW, Muytjens HL. In vitro activities of ciprofloxacin, norfloxacin, pipemidic acid, cinoxacin, and nalidixic acid against *Chlamydia trachomatis*. *Antimicrob Agents Chemother* 1984;25:123–124.
54. Horowitz HW, Hsieh T-C, Aguero-Rosenfeld ME, et al. Antimicrobial susceptibility of *Ehrlichia phagocytophila*. *Antimicrob Agents Chemother* 2001;45:786–788.
55. Hospenthal DR, Murray CK. In vitro susceptibilities of seven *Leptospira* species to traditional and newer antibiotics. *Antimicrob Agents Chemother* 2003;47:2646–2648.
56. How SJ, Hobson D, Hart CA, et al. A comparison of the in-vitro activity of antimicrobials against *Chlamydia trachomatis* examined by Giemsa and a fluorescent antibody stain. *J Antimicrob Chemother* 1985;15:399–404.
57. Hunfeld KP, Kraiczy P, Wichelhaus TA, et al. Colorimetric in vitro susceptibility testing of penicillins, cephalosporins, macrolides, streptogramins, tetracyclines, and aminoglycosides against *Borrelia burgdorferi* isolates. *Int J Antimicrob Agents* 2000;15:11–17.
58. Ishida K, Kaku M, Irifune K, et al. In vitro and in vivo activities of macrolides against *Mycoplasma pneumoniae*. *Antimicrob Agents Chemother* 1994;38:790–798.
59. Ives TJ, Manzewitsch P, Regnery RL, et al. In vitro susceptibilities of *Bartonella henselae, B. quintana, B. elizabethae, Rickettsia rickettsii, R. conorii, R. akari,* and *R. prowazekii* to macrolide antibiotics as determined by immuno-fluorescent-antibody analysis of infected Vero cell monolayers. *Antimicrob Agents Chemother* 1997;41:578–582.
60. Ives TJ, Marston EL, Regnery RL, et al. In vitro susceptibilities of Bartonella and *Rickettsia* spp. to fluoroquinolone antibiotics as determined by immunofluorescent antibody analysis of infected Vero cell monolayers. *Int J Antimicrob Agents* 2001;18:217–222.
61. Jabarit-Aldighieri N, Torres H, Raoult D. Susceptibility of *R. conorii, R. rickettsii* and *C. burnetii* to CI-960 (PD 127,391), PD 131,628, pefloxacin, ofloxacin and ciprofloxacin. *Antimicrob Agents Chemother* 1992;36:2529–2532.
62. Jao RL. Susceptibility of *Mycoplasma pneumoniae* to 21 antibiotics in vitro. *Am J Med Sci* 1967;253:639–650.
63. Jenkin HM, Hung SC. Effect of vancomycin on the growth of psittacosis-trachoma agents cultivated in eggs and cell culture. *Appl Microbiol* 1967;15:10–12.
64. Johannisson G, Sernryd A, Lycke E. Susceptibility of *Chlamydia trachomatis* to antibiotics in vitro and in vivo. *Sex Transm Dis* 1979;6:50–57.
65. Johnson FW, Clarkson MJ, Spencer WN. Susceptibility of *Chlamydia psittaci* (ovis) to antimicrobial agents. *J Antimicrob Chemother* 1983;11:413–418.
66. Johnson RC. Isolation techniques for spirochetes and their sensitivity to antibiotics in vitro and in vivo. *Rev Infect Dis* 1989;11[Suppl 6]:S1505–10.
67. Johnson RC, Harris VG. Differentiation of pathogenic and saprophytic letospires: I. Growth at low temperatures. *J Bacteriol* 1967;94:27–31.
68. Johnson RC, Kodner C, Russell M. In vitro and in vivo susceptibility of the Lyme disease spirochete, *Borrelia burgdorferi,* to four antimicrobial agents. *Antimicrob Agents Chemother* 1987;31:164–167.
69. Johnson SE, Klein GC, Schmid GP, et al. Susceptibility of the Lyme disease spirochete to seven antimicrobial agents. *Yale J Biol Med* 1984;57:549–553.
70. Jones RB, Ridgway GL, Boulding S, et al. In vitro activity of rifamycins alone and in combination with other antibiotics against *Chlamydia trachomatis*. *Rev Infect Dis* 1983;5[Suppl 3]:S556–S561.
71. Jones RB, Van der Pol B, Johnson RB. Susceptibility

of *Chlamydia trachomatis* to trovafloxacin. *J Antimicrob Chemother* 1997;39[Suppl B]:63–65.

72. Jones RB, Van der Pol B, Martin DH, et al. Partial characterization of *Chlamydia trachomatis* isolates resistant to multiple antibiotics. *J Infect Dis* 1990;162:1309–1315.
73. Kaku M, Ishida K, Irifune K, et al. In vitro and in vivo activities of sparfloxacin against *Mycoplasma pneumoniae*. *Antimicrob Agents Chemother* 1994;38:738–741.
74. Kelly DJ, LaBarre DD, Lewis GEJ. Effect of tetracycline therapy on host defense in mice infected with *Ehrlichia sennetsu*. In: Winkler HH, Ristic M, eds. *Microbiology*. Washington, DC: American Society for Microbiology, 1986:209–212.
75. Kelly PJ, Beati L, Mason PR, et al. *Rickettsia africae* sp nov, the etiological agent of African tick bite fever. *Int J Syst Bacteriol* 1996;46:611–614.
76. Kenny GE, Cartwright FD. Susceptibility of *Mycoplasma pneumoniae* to several new quinolones, tetracycline, and erythromycin. *Antimicrob Agents Chemother* 1991;35: 587–589.
77. Kenny GE, Cartwright FD. Susceptibilities of *Mycoplasma hominis, Mycoplasma pneumoniae,* and *Ureaplasma urealyticum* to new glycylcyclines in comparison with those to older tetracyclines. *Antimicrob Agents Chemother* 1994;38:2628–2632.
78. Kenny GE, Cartwright FD. Susceptibilities of *Mycoplasma pneumoniae, Mycoplasma hominis,* and *Ureaplasma urealyticum* to a new quinolone, trovafloxacin (CP-99,219). *Antimicrob Agents Chemother* 1996;40:1048–1049.
79. Kenny GE, Cartwright FD. Susceptibilities of *Mycoplasma hominis, M. pneumoniae,* and *Ureaplasma urealyticum* to GAR-936, dalfopristin, dirithromycin, evernimicin, gatifloxacin, linezolid, moxifloxacin, quinupristin-dalfopristin, and telithromycin compared to their susceptibilities to reference macrolides, tetracyclines, and quinolones. *Antimicrob Agents Chemother* 2001;45:2604–2608.
80. Kenny GE, Cartwright FD, Roberts MC. Agar dilution method for determination of antibiotic susceptibility of *Ureaplasma urealyticum*. *Pediatr Infect Dis* 1986;5:S332–S334.
81. Kenny GE, Hooton TM, Roberts MC, et al. Susceptibilities of genital mycoplasmas to the newer quinolones as determined by the agar dilution method. *Antimicrob Agents Chemother* 1989;33:103–107.
82. Keshishyan H, Hanna L, Jawetz E. Emergence of rifampin-resistance in *Chlamydia trachomatis*. *Nature* 1973;244: 173–174.
83. Khan MA, Potter CW, Sharrard RM. A reverse transcriptase-PCR based assay for in-vitro antibiotic susceptibility testing of *Chlamydia pneumoniae*. *J Antimicrob Chemother* 1996;37:677–685.
84. Kimura M, Kishimoto T, Niki Y, et al. In vitro and in vivo antichlamydial activities of newly developed quinolone antimicrobial agents. *Antimicrob Agents Chemother* 1993;37:801–803.
85. Klein MB, Nelson CM, Goodman JL. Antibiotic susceptibility of the newly cultivated agent of human granulocytic ehrlichiosis: promising activity of quinolones and rifamycins. *Antimicrob Agents Chemother* 1997;41:76–79.
86. Kobayashi Y, Ikeda O, Miaso T. Chemotherapy of sennetsu disease. In: *Progress in virology.* Tokyo: Bainukan, 1962:130–142.
87. Korting HC, Walther D, Riethmuller U, et al. Comparative in vitro susceptibility of *Treponema pallidum* to ceftizoxime, ceftriaxone and penicillin G. *Chemotherapy* 1986;32:352–355.
88. Koyama T. Immunological studies of rickettsial infection-analysis of lymphoid cell subpopulations of the spleen of mice infected with *Rickettsia sennetsu* and *Rickettsia tsutsugamushi*. *Kansenshogaku Zasshi* 1979;53:243–257.
89. Kuo CC, Grayston JT. In vitro drug susceptibility of *Chlamydia* sp.strain TWAR. *Antimicrob Agents Chemother* 1988;32:257–258.
90. Kuo CC, Jackson LA, Campbell LA, et al. *Chlamydia pneumoniae* (TWAR). *Clin Microbiol Rev* 1995;8(4):451–461.
91. Kuo CC, Wang SP, Grayston JT. Antimicrobial activity of several antibiotics and a sulfonamide against *Chlamydia trachomatis* organisms in cell culture. *Antimicrob Agents Chemother* 1977;12:80–83.
92. Kutlin A, Roblin PM, Hammerschlag MR. In vitro activities of azithromycin and ofloxacin against *Chlamydia pneumoniae* in a continuous-infection model. *Antimicrob Agents Chemother* 1999;43:2268–2272.
93. Lefevre JC, Bauriaud R, Gaubert E, et al. In vitro activity of sparfloxacin and other antimicrobial agents against genital pathogens. *Chemotherapy* 1992;38:303–307.
94. Levett PN. Leptospirosis. *Clin Microbiol Rev* 2001;14: 296–326.
95. Levin JM, Nelson JA, Segreti J, et al. In vitro susceptibility of *Borrelia burgdorferi* to 11 antimicrobial agents. *Antimicrob Agents Chemother* 1993;37:1444–1446.
96. Levy JA. Confirmation of the successful cultivation of *Treponema pallidum* in tissue culture. *Microbiologica* 1984;7: 367–370.
97. Limb DI, Wheat PF, Hastings JG, et al. Antimicrobial susceptibility testing of mycoplasmas by ATP bioluminescence. *J Med Microbiol* 1991;35:89–92.
98. Lo, SC, Wear DJ, Green SL, et al. Adult respiratory distress syndrome with or without systemic disease associated with infections due to *Mycoplasma fermentans*. *Clin Infect Dis* 1993;17[Suppl 1]:S259–263.
99. Maeda H, Fujii A, Nakata K, et al. In vitro activities of T-3262, NY-198, fleroxacin (AM-833; RO 23-6240), and other new quinolone agents against clinically isolated *Chlamydia trachomatis* strains. *Antimicrob Agents Chemother* 1988;32:1080–1081.
100. Martin DH, Pastorek JG, Faro S. In-vitro and in-vivo activity of parenterally administered beta-lactam antibiotics against *Chlamydia trachomatis*. *Sex Transm Dis* 1986; 13:81–87.
101. Maurin M, Abergel C, Raoult D. DNA Gyrase-mediated natural resistance to fluoroquinolones in *Ehrlichia* spp. *Antimicrob Agents Chemother* 2001;45:2098–2105.
102. Maurin M, Bakken JS, Dumler JS. Antibiotic susceptibilities of *Anaplasma* (Ehrlichia) *phagocytophilum* strains from various geographic areas in the United States. *Antimicrob Agents Chemother* 2003;47:413–415.
103. Maurin M, Benoliel AM, Bongrand P, et al. Phagolysosomal alkalinization and the bactericidal effect of antibiotics: the *Coxiella burnetii* paradigm. *J Infect Dis* 1992;166:1097–1102.
104. Maurin M, Benoliel AM, Bongrand P, et al. Phagolysosomes of *Coxiella burnetii*: infected cell lines maintain an acidic pH during persistent infection. *Infect Immun* 1992; 60:5013–5016.
105. Maurin M, Raoult D. In vitro susceptibilities of spotted fever group rickettsiae and *Coxiella burnetii* to clarithromycin. *Antimicrob Agents Chemother* 1993;37:2633–2637.
106. Maurin M, Raoult D. Q fever. *Clin Microbiol Rev* 1999; 12:518–553.
107. McCormack WM. Susceptibility of mycoplasmas to

antimicrobial agents: clinical implications. *Clin Infect Dis* 1993;17[Suppl 1]:S200–201.

108. McLaren C, Ellis MN, Hunter GA. A colorimetric assay for the measurement of the sensitivity of herpes simplex viruses to antiviral agents. *Antiviral Res* 1983;3:223–234.
109. Misao T, Kobayashi Y. Studies on infectious mononucleosis (glandular fever): isolation of etiologic agent from blood, bone marrow, and lymph node of a patient with infectious mononucleosis by using mice. *Kyushu J Med Sci* 1995;6:145–152.
110. Misu T, Arai S, Furukawa M, et al. Effects of rokitamycin and other macrolide antibiotics on *Mycoplasma pneumoniae* in L cells. *Antimicrob Agents Chemother* 1987;31:1843–1845.

110a. Misyurina OY, Chipitsyna EV, Finashutina YP, et al. Mutations in a 23S rRNA of Chlamydia trachomatis associated with resistance to macrolides. *Antimicrob Agents Chemother* 2004;48:1347–9.

111. Miyashita N, Fukano H, Niki Y, et al. In vitro activity of telithromycin, a new ketolide, against *Chlamydia pneumoniae. J Antimicrob Chemother* 2001;48:403–405.
112. Miyashita N, Fukano H, Yoshida K, et al. In-vitro activity of moxifloxacin and other fluoroquinolones against *Chlamydia* species. *J Infect Chemother* 2002;8:115–117.
113. Miyashita N, Fukano H, Yoshida K. In vitro activity of cethromycin, a novel antibacterial ketolide, against *Chlamydia pneumoniae. J Antimicrob Chemother* 2003;52:497–499.
114. Mourad A, Sweet RL, Sugg N, et al. Relative resistance to erythromycin in *Chlamydia trachomatis. Antimicrob Agents Chemother* 1980;18:696–698.
115. Mursic VP, Wilske B, Schierz G, et al. In vitro and in vivo susceptibility of *Borrelia burgdorferi. Eur J Clin Microbiol* 1987;6:424–426.
116. Muytjens HL, Heessen FW. In vitro activities of thirteen beta-lactam antibiotics against *Chlamydia trachomatis. Antimicrob Agents Chemother* 1982;22:520–521.
117. Nagayama A, Nakao T, Taen H. In vitro activities of ofloxacin and four other new quinoline–carboxylic acids against *Chlamydia trachomatis. Antimicrob Agents Chemother* 1988;32:1735–1737.
118. Norris SJ, Edmondson DG. In vitro culture system to determine MICs and MBCs of antimicrobial agents against *Treponema pallidum* subsp. *pallidum* (Nichols strain). *Antimicrob Agents Chemother* 1988;32:68–74.
119. Oie S, Hironaga K, Koshiro A, et al. In vitro susceptibilities of five *Leptospira* strains to 16 antimicrobial agents. *Antimicrob Agents Chemother* 1983;24:905–908.
120. Osada Y, Ogawa H. Antimycoplasmal activity of ofloxacin (DL-8280). *Antimicrob Agents Chemother* 1983;23:509–511.
121. Owens RC, Ambrose PG. Clinical use of the fluoroquinolones. *Med Clin North Am* 2000;84:1447–1469.
122. Paul TR, Knight ST, Raulston JE, et al. Delivery of azithromycin to *Chlamydia trachomatis*–infected polarized human endometrial epithelial cells by polymorphonuclear leucocytes. *J Antimicrob Chemother* 1997;39:623–630.
123. Pereyre S, Gonzalez P, de Barbeyrac B, et al. Mutations in 23S rRNA account for intrinsic resistance to macrolides in *Mycoplasma hominis* and *Mycoplasma fermentans* and for acquired resistance to macrolides in *M. hominis. Antimicrob Agents Chemother* 2002;46:3142–3150.

123a. Pereyre S, Guyot C, Renaudin H, et al. In vitro selection and characterization of resistance to macrolides and related antibiotics in Mycoplasma pneumoniae. *Antimicrob Agents Chemother* 2004;48:460–5.

124. Petersen AM, Boye K, Blom J, et al. First isolation of *Leptospira fainei* serovar Hurstbridge from two human patients with Weil's syndrome. *J Med Microbiol* 2001;50:96–100.
125. Poulin SA, Perkins RE, Kundsin RB. Antibiotic susceptibilities of AIDS-associated mycoplasmas. *J Clin Microbiol* 1994;32:1101–1103.
126. Preac-Mursic V, Wilske B, Schierz G. European *Borrelia burgdorferi* isolated from humans and ticks: culture conditions and antibiotic susceptibility. *Zentralbl Bakteriol Mikrobiol Hyg [A]* 1986;263:112–118.
127. Raoult D, Berbis P, Roux V, et al. A new tick-transmitted disease due to *Rickettsia slovaca. Lancet* 1997;350:112–113.
128. Raoult D, Brouqui P, Roux V. A new spotted-fever-group rickettsiosis. *Lancet* 1996;348:412.
129. Raoult D, Drancourt M, Vestris G. Bactericidal effect of doxycycline associated with lysosomotropic agents on *Coxiella burnetii* in P388D1 cells. *Antimicrob Agents Chemother* 1990;34:1512–1514.
130. Raoult D, Fournier PE, Abboud P, et al. First documented human *Rickettsia aeschlimannii* infection. *Emerg Infect Dis* 2002;8:748–749.
131. Raoult D, La Scola B, Enea M, et al. A flea-associated Rickettsia pathogenic for humans. *Emerg Infect Dis* 2001;7:73–81.
132. Raoult D, Mege JL, Marrie T. Q fever: queries remaining after decades of research. In: Scheld WM, Craig WA, Hughes JM, eds. *Emerging infections.* Washington, DC: ASM Press, 2001;29–56.
133. Raoult D, Roussellier P, Galicher V, et al. In vitro susceptibility of *Rickettsia conorii* to ciprofloxacin as determined by suppressing lethality in chicken embryos and by plaque assay. *Antimicrob Agents Chemother* 1986;29:424–425.
134. Raoult D, Roussellier P, Tamalet J. In vitro evaluation of josamycin, spiramycin, and erythromycin against *Rickettsia rickettsii* and *R. conorii. Antimicrob Agents Chemother* 1988;32:255–256.
135. Raoult D, Roussellier P, Vestris G, et al. In vitro antibiotic susceptibility of *Rickettsia rickettsii* and *Rickettsia conorii:* plaque assay and microplaque colorimetric assay. *J Infect Dis* 1987;155:1059–1062.
136. Raoult D, Roux R, Ndihokubwaho JB, et al. Jail fever (epidemic typhus) outbreak in Burundi. *Emerg Infect Dis* 1997;3:357–360.
137. Raoult D, Torres H, Drancourt M. Shell-vial assay: evaluation of a new technique for determining antibiotic susceptibility, tested in 13 isolates of *Coxiella burnetii. Antimicrob Agents Chemother* 1991;35:2070–2077.
138. Raoult D, Vestris G, Enea M. Isolation of 16 strains of *Coxiella burnetii* from patients by using a sensitive centrifugation cell culture system and establishment of strains in HEL cells. *J Clin Microbiol* 1990;28:2482–2484.
139. Renaudin H, Bebear C. Comparative in vitro activity of azithromycin, clarithromycin, erythromycin and lomefloxacin against *Mycoplasma pneumoniae, Mycoplasma hominis* and *Ureaplasma urealyticum. Eur J Clin Microbiol Infect Dis* 1990;9:838–841.
140. Ridgway GL, Bebear C, Bebear CM, et al. Antimicrobial susceptibility testing of intracellular and cell-associated pathogens. *Clin Microbiol Infect* 2001;7:1–10.
141. Ridgway GL, Mumtaz G, Fenelon L. The in-vitro activity of clarithromycin and other macrolides against the type strain of *Chlamydia pneumoniae* (TWAR). *J Antimicrob Chemother* 1991;27[suppl A]:43–45.
142. Ridgway GL, Salman H, Robbins MJ, et al. The in-vitro

activity of grepafloxacin against *Chlamydia* spp., *Mycoplasma* spp., *Ureaplasma urealyticum* and *Legionella* spp. *J Antimicrob Chemother* 1997;40[Suppl A]:31–34.

143. Roberts MC, Koutsky LA, Holmes KK, et al. Tetracycline-resistant *Mycoplasma hominis* strains contain streptococcal *tetM* sequences. *Antimicrob Agents Chemother* 1985;28:141–143.
144. Robertson JA, Coppola JE, Heisler OR. Standardized method for determining antimicrobial susceptibility of strains of *Ureaplasma urealyticum* and their response to tetracycline, erythromycin, and rosaramicin. *Antimicrob Agents Chemother* 1981;20:53–58.
145. Roblin PM, Hammerschlag MR. In-vitro activity of gatifloxacin against *Chlamydia trachomatis* and *Chlamydia pneumoniae*. *J Antimicrob Chemother* 1999;44:549–551.
146. Roblin PM, Hammerschlag MR. In vitro activity of GAR-936 against *Chlamydia pneumoniae* and *Chlamydia trachomatis*. *Int J Antimicrob Agents* 2000;16:61–63.
147. Roblin PM, Hammerschlag MR. In vitro activity of a new antibiotic, NVP-PDF386 (VRC4887), against *Chlamydia pneumoniae*. *Antimicrob Agents Chemother* 2003;47:1447–1448.
148. Roblin PM, Kutlin A, Hammerschlag MR. In vitro activity of trovafloxacin against *Chlamydia pneumoniae*. *Antimicrob Agents Chemother* 1997;41:2033–2034.
149. Roblin PM, Kutlin A, Reznik T, et al. Activity of grepafloxacin and other fluoroquinones and newer macrolides against recent clinical isolates of *Chlamydia pneumoniae*. *Int J Antimicrob Agents* 1999;12:181–184.
150. Roblin PM, Reznik T, Hammershlag MR. In vitro activity of garenoxacin against recent clinical isolates of *Chlamydia pneumoniae*. *Int J Antimicrob Agents* 2003;21:578–580.
151. Roblin PM, Reznik T, Kutlin A, et al. In vitro activities of gemifloxacin (SB 265805, LB20304) against recent clinical isolates of *Chlamydia pneumoniae*. *Antimicrob Agents Chemother* 1999;43:2806–2807.
152. Roblin PM, Reznik T, Kutlin A, et al. In vitro activities of rifamycin derivatives ABI-1648 (Rifalazil, KRM-1648), ABI-1657, and ABI-1131 against *Chlamydia trachomatis* and recent clinical isolates of *Chlamydia pneumoniae*. *Antimicrob Agents Chemother* 2003;47:1135–1136.
153. Rolain JM, Maurin M, Bryskier A, et al. In vitro activities of telithromycin (HMR 3647) against *Rickettsia rickettsii, Rickettsia conorii, Rickettsia africae, Rickettsia typhi, Rickettsia prowasekii, Coxiella burnetii, Bartonella henselae, Bartonella quintana, Bartonella bacilliformis,* and *Ehrlichia chaffeensis*. *Antimicrob Agents Chemother* 2000;44:1391–1393.
154. Rolain JM, Maurin M, Vestris G, et al. In vitro susceptibilities of 27 Rickettsiae to 13 antimicrobials. *Antimicrob Agents Chemother* 1998;42:1537–1541.
155. Rolain JM, Stuhl L, Maurin M, et al. Evaluation of antibiotic susceptibilities of three rickettsial species including *Rickettsia felis* by a quantitative PCR DNA assay. *Antimicrob Agents Chemother* 2002;46:2747–2751.
156. Roman MJ, Coriz PD, Baca OG. A proposed model to explain persistent infection of host cells with *Coxiella burnetii*. *J Gen Microbiol* 1986;132:1415–1422.
157. Rumpianesi F, Morandotti G, Sperning R, et al. In vitro activity of azithromycin against *Chlamydia trachomatis, Ureaplasma urealyticum* and *Mycoplasma hominis* in comparison with erythromycin, roxithromycin and minocycline. *J Chemother* 1993;5:155–158.
158. Rylander M, Hallander HO. In vitro comparison of the activity of doxycycline, tetracycline, erythromycin and a new macrolide, CP 62993, against *Mycoplasma pneumoniae, Mycoplasma hominis* and *Ureaplasma urealyticum*. *Scand J Infect Dis Suppl* 1988;53:12–17.
159. Samra Z, Rosenberg S, Soffer Y, et al. In vitro susceptibility of recent clinical isolates of *Chlamydia trachomatis* to macrolides and tetracyclines. *Diagn Microbiol Infect Dis* 2001;39:177–179.
160. Schachter J. Rifampin in chlamydial infections. *Rev Infect Dis* 1983;5[Suppl 3]:S562–564.
161. Segreti J, Kapell KS. In vitro activity of dirithromycin against *Chlamydia trachomatis*. *Antimicrob Agents Chemother* 1994;38:2213–2214.
162. Segreti J, Kessler HA, Kapell KS, et al. In vitro activities of temafloxacin (A-62254) and four other antibiotics against *Chlamydia trachomatis*. *Antimicrob Agents Chemother* 1989;33:118–119.
163. Senterfit LB. Antibiotic sensitivity testing of mycoplasmas. In: Razin S, Tully JG, eds. *Methods in mycoplasmology*. New York: Academic Press, 1983:397–401.
164. Senterfit LB. Tetrazolium reduction. In: Razin S, Tully JG, eds. *Methods in mycoplasmalogy*. New York: Academic Press, 1983:377–378.
165. Senterfit LB. Laboratory diagnosis of mycoplasma infections. *Isr J Med Sci* 1984;20:905–907.
166. Sicklinger M, Wienecke R, Neubert U. In vitro susceptibility testing of four antibiotics against *Borrelia burgdorferi*: a comparison of results for the three genospecies *Borrelia afzelii, Borrelia garinii,* and *Borrelia burgdorferi* sensu stricto. *J Clin Microbiol* 2003;41:1791–1793.
167. Stamm LV, Bergen HL. A point mutation associated with bacterial macrolide resistance is present in both 23S rRNA genes of an erythromycin-resistant *Treponema pallidum* clinical isolate. *Antimicrob Agents Chemother* 2000;44:806–807.
168. Stamm LV, Stapleton JT, Bassford PJ Jr. In vitro assay to demonstrate high-level erythromycin resistance of a clinical isolate of *Treponema pallidum*. *Antimicrob Agents Chemother* 1988;32:164–169.
169. Stamm WE. Potential for antimicrobial resistance in *Chlamydia pneumoniae*. *J Infect Dis* 2000;181[Suppl 3]: S456–459.
170. Stamm WE, Suchland R. Antimicrobial activity of U-70138F (paldimycin), roxithromycin (RU 965), and ofloxacin (ORF 18489) against *Chlamydia trachomatis* in cell culture. *Antimicrob Agents Chemother* 1986;30:806–807.
171. Stapleton JT, Stamm LV, Bassford PJ Jr. Potential for development of antibiotic resistance in pathogenic treponemes. *Rev Infect Dis* 1985;7[Suppl 2]:S314–317.
172. Steere AC. Borrelia burgdorferi (Lyme disease, Lyme borreliosis). In: Mandell GL, Bennett JE, Dolin R, eds. *Principles and practice of infectious diseases*. New York: Churchill Livingstone, 1995:2143–2154.
173. Stein A, Raoult D. A simple method for amplification of DNA from paraffin-embedded tissues. *Nucleic Acids Res* 1992;20:5237–5238.
174. Stewart RS. Flinders Island spotted fever: a newly recognised endemic focus of tick typhus in Bass Strait. I. Clinical and epidemiologiocal features. *Med J Aust* 1991;154:94–99.
175. Stopler T, Branski D. Resistance of *Mycoplasma pneumoniae* to macrolides, lincomycin and streptogramin B. *J Antimicrob Chemother* 1986;18:359–364.
176. Suchland RJ, Geisler WM, Stamm WE. Methodologies and cell lines used for antimicrobial susceptibility testing of *Chlamydia* spp. *Antimicrob Agents Chemother* 2003;47:636–642.
177. Tachibana N, Kobayashi V. Effect of cyclophosphamide

on the growth of *Rickettsia sennetsu* in experimentally infected mice. *Infect Immun* 1975;12:625–629.

178. Tamura A, Ohashi N, Urakami H, et al. Classification of *Rickettsia tsutsugamushi* in a new genus, Orientia gen. nov., as *Orientia tsutsugamushi* comb. nov. *Int J Syst Bacteriol* 1995;45:589–591.
179. Tanner AC, Erickson BZ, Ross RF. Adaptation of the Sensititre broth microdilution technique to antimicrobial susceptibility testing of *Mycoplasma hyopneumoniae*. *Vet Microbiol* 1993;36:301–306.
180. Tarasevich IV, Makarova V, Fetisova NF, et al. Astrakhan fever: new spotted fever group rickettsiosis. *Lancet* 1991;337:172–173.
181. Taylor-Robinson D, Furr PM. The static effect of rosaramicin on *Ureaplasma urealyticum* and the development of antibiotic resistance. *J Antimicrob Chemother* 1982;10:185–191.
182. Taylor-Robinson D, Furr PM. Clinical antibiotic resistance of *Ureaplasma urealyticum*. *Pediatr Inf Dis J* 1986;5[Suppl]:6:335–337.
183. Thompson SE, Washington AE. Epidemiology of sexually transmitted *Chlamydia trachomatis* infections. *Epidemiol Rev* 1983;5:96–123.
184. Torres H, Raoult D. In vitro activities of ceftriaxone and fusidic acid against 13 isolates of *Coxiella burnetii*, determined using the shell vial assay. *Antimicrob Agents Chemother* 1993;37:491–494.
185. Tully JG, Whitcomb RF, Clark HF, et al. Pathogenic mycoplasmas: cultivation and vertebrate pathogenicity of a new spiroplasma. *Science* 1977;195:892–894.
186. Uchida T, Uchiyama T, Kumano K, et al. *Rickettsia japonica* sp. nov., the etiological agent of spotted fever group rickettsiosis in Japan. *Int J Syst Bacteriol* 1992;42:303–305.
187. Waites KB, Cassell GH, Canupp KC, et al. In vitro susceptibilities of mycoplasmas and ureaplasmas to new macrolides and aryl-fluoroquinolones. *Antimicrob Agents Chemother* 1988;32:1500–1502.
188. Waites KB, Crabb DM, Bing X, et al. In vitro susceptibilities to and bactericidal activities of garenoxacin (BMS-284756) and other antimicrobial agents against human mycoplasmas and ureaplasmas. *Antimicrob Agents Chemother* 2003;47:161–165.
189. Waites KB, Crabb DM, Duffy LB. Inhibitory and bactericidal activities of gemifloxacin and other antimicrobials against *Mycoplasma pneumoniae*. *Int J Antimicrob Agents* 2003;21:574–577.
190. Waites KB, Crouse DT, Cassell GH. Antibiotic susceptibilities and therapeutic options for *Ureaplasma urealyticum* infections in neonates. *Pediatr Infect Dis J* 1992;11:23–29.
191. Waites KB, Crouse DT, Cassell GH. Therapeutic considerations for *Ureaplasma urealyticum* infections in neonates. *Clin Infect Dis* 1993;17[Suppl 1]:S208–S214.
192. Waites KB, Figarola TA, Schmid T, et al. Comparison of agar versus broth dilution techniques for determining antibiotic susceptibilities of *Ureaplasma urealyticum*. *Diagn Microbiol Infect Dis* 1991;14:265–271.
193. Welsh LE, Gaydos CA, Quinn TC. In vitro evaluation of activities of azithromycin, erythromycin, and tetracycline against *Chlamidia trachomatis* and *Chlamidia pneumonia*. *Antimicrob Agents Chemother* 1992;36:291–294.
194. Wittwer CT, Ririe KM, Andrew RV, et al. The LightCycler: a microvolume multisample fluorimeter with rapid temperature control. *Biotechniques* 1997;22:176–181.
195. Wyrick PB, Davis CH, Raulston JE, et al. Effect of clinically relevant culture conditions on antimicrobial susceptibility of *Chlamydia trachomatis*. *Clin Infect Dis* 1994;19:931–936.
196. Yamaguchi T, Hirakata Y, Izumikawa K, et al. In vitro activity of telithromycin (HMR3647), a new ketolide, against clinical isolates of *Mycoplasma pneumoniae* in Japan. *Antimicrob Agents Chemother* 2000;44:1381–1382.
197. Yu X, Fan M, Xu G, et al. Genotypic and antigenic identification of two new strains of spotted fever group rickettsiae isolated from China. *J Clin Microbiol* 1993;31:83–88.
198. Zurenko GE, Yagi BH, Vavra JJ, et al. In vitro antibacterial activity of trospectomycin (U-63366F), a novel spectinomycin analog. *Antimicrob Agents Chemother* 1988;32:216–223.

CHAPTER 8

Applications, Significance of, and Methods for the Measurement of Antimicrobial Concentrations in Human Body Fluids

Roger D. Klein, Stephen C. Edberg

The proliferation of antimicrobial agents in recent years presents clinical laboratories with a potentially large number of antibiotics to assay. Many of these new drugs were designed for their particular distribution properties (e.g., penetration through the blood–brain barrier or longer half-lives), confronting laboratorians with the challenges of developing appropriate test methods, interpreting the results produced by those methods, and establishing clinical indications for the therapeutic drug monitoring of antimicrobial drugs.

Automated chemical methods for the determination of antibiotic concentrations in body fluids, most commonly serum or plasma, have become commonplace and can be performed with relative ease at reasonable costs. These automated methods have largely replaced bioassays, which are not routinely performed. Therapeutic drug monitoring of aminoglycosides is generally performed by enzyme (EIA), turbidimetric inhibition (PETINIA), fluorescence polarization (FPIA), or similar labeled immunoassays because of their ease of performance, rapid turnaround times, and reasonable costs.

For example, Abbott Laboratories (Abbott Park, IL) produces fluorescence polarization immunoassays for gentamicin, tobramycin, and amikacin. The latter assay is designed to run on Abbott's TDx and TDxFLx instruments, while gentamicin and tobramycin can be run on the TDx/TDxFLx, or more commonly in clinical laboratories on Abbott's AxSYM, an automated chemistry analyzer that can process up to 120 tests per hour.

The Dade Behring Gentamicin and Tobramycin Flex reagent cartridges (Dade Behring, Inc., Dearfield, IL), which are designed to run on Dade's high throughput Dimension analyzer, are homogeneous particle-enhanced, turbidimetric inhibition immunoassays. These assays use latex particle antibiotic conjugates to compete for monoclonal antibody binding sites with the free, unconjugated antibiotic in the sample. The binding of unbound antibiotic to the antibody decreases the rate of aggregation of the particle-antibody complexes, which is inversely proportional to the concentration of antibiotic in the sample.

Roche Diagnostics' (Indianapolis, IN) CEDIA gentamicin II and tobramycin assays run on several of the company's automated chemistry analyzers. In the CEDIA assays, an inactive fragment of recombinant bacterial β-galactosidase that has been genetically engineered into two inactive fragments is conjugated to the study antibiotic. Under assay conditions, the two enzyme fragments spontaneously reassociate to form a fully active enzyme that cleaves a chromogenic substrate. A color change is generated that is spectrophotometrically measured. Binding of a monoclonal antibody directed at the enzyme-drug conjugate interferes with enzyme reassociation. Free analyte in the sample competes with the conjugated drug for antibody sites. The quantity of enzyme that is formed and the resultant absorbance change are directly proportional to the amount of analyte that is present in the sample.

Vancomycin and chloramphenicol (CAM) levels are routinely obtained through the use of immunoassay or high-performance liquid chromatography (HPLC)-based methods. Determination of sulfonamide, trimethoprim, β-lactam, macrolide, quinolone, tetracycline, and other antimicrobial levels is largely confined to reference laboratories. Methods include HPLC, immunoassay, and bioassay, although this latter method has fallen into disfavor because of assay variability and potential interference when multiple drugs are administered. While radioimmunoassay (RIA) and gas chromatography techniques can also be used for antibiotic concentration analysis, these methods generally confer little advantage over existing immunoassays and are infrequently used.

Interestingly, despite the major advances in technology and the large increase in the number of antimicrobial drugs, the clinical indications for therapeutic monitoring of antibiotic concentrations are limited to a few select drugs and clinical settings. This is largely because of the improved toxicity profiles and large therapeutic windows of the majority of currently used antimicrobials. Most routine antimicrobial therapeutic drug monitoring involves aminoglycoside and glycopeptide (vancomycin) antibiotics, and to a lesser extent CAM. Antituberculosis, antifungal, and antiretroviral therapies present additional applications in which therapeutic drug monitoring may prove to be of value.

The assay of antibiotics or antibiotic material dates back to the demonstration of lysozyme in an agar diffusion assay system by Fleming (119) in 1922. Thus, the first use and many of the other initial uses of assay systems were for the detection of antibiotic activity that resulted from the *in vivo* production of antimicrobial substances. Assays of antibiotics in blood, urine, and other body fluids and tissues were primarily performed in conjunction with the determination of antibiotic pharmacology and pharmacokinetics.

In the late 1960s, accurate, rapid assays to measure blood levels of antimicrobial substances, particularly those with narrow toxic/therapeutic ratios, were sought (28,96,100,109,274,302). The value of such information for the optimal use of certain antibiotics eventually became apparent, but the popularization of rapid serum assays required most of the decade of the 1970s. Data from several laboratories demonstrated that the efficacy of some antibiotics correlated with their peak serum antibiotic levels (183,239; Williams et al., unpublished data, 1984). Primarily as a consequence of this work, the measurement of aminoglycoside levels began to be performed in all seriously ill patients who received these drugs, irrespective of the patients' renal status (93).

Toxicity was also shown to be related to both peak and trough serum levels. Although the study by Line et al. (206) showed a correlation between streptomycin toxicity and trough levels, the concept that trough levels correlated better with toxicity than peak levels for aminoglycoside drugs remained in dispute for some time. Indeed, although it was quite clear from retrospective analyses that toxicity was associated with high serum levels of these antibiotics, it was difficult to prove that toxicity occurred at particular blood levels for a given drug. Table 8.1 demonstrates the toxic/therapeutic ratios of some commonly used aminoglycosides (213).

TABLE 8.1

Toxic/Therapeutic Ratios of Commonly Used Aminoglycoside Antibiotics

Antibiotic	Average Daily Dose (mg/kg)	Therapeutic Concentration (μg/mL)	Toxic Concentrations (μg/mL)	
			Peak	Trough
Amikacin	15	8–16	>35	>10
Gentamicin	3–5	4–8	>12	>2
Kanamycin	15	8–16	>35	>10
Netilmicin	6.5	4–12	>16	>4
Tobramycin	3–5	4–8	>12	>2

The measurement of antibiotic concentrations in various fluids has been a prominent aspect of the evaluation of new antibiotics and the quality control of their manufacture. With the availability of rapid, accurate assays, the measurement of antibiotic material in serum and other body fluids is feasible, desirable, and widely practiced for these purposes. Clinically, such assays have been used primarily for the determination of aminoglycoside levels in serum, for which peak levels primarily establish adequacy of therapy, while trough levels reflect potential drug accumulation and toxicity.

Although the most common reason for performing rapid serum antibiotic assays in hospitals is to regulate therapy with aminoglycoside antibiotics and vancomycin, there are other indications. For patients who have organ dysfunction, such as hepatic or renal failure, it is desirable to know whether or not antibiotics that are metabolized or eliminated (e.g., CAM) by damaged or imperfectly functioning organs accumulate. In some patients who are taking oral antibiotics, it may be important to know the extent to which they are absorbing the drugs from their gastrointestinal tracts (69,114,163,169). Therapeutic monitoring of β-lactam, macrolide, tetracyline, and other antibiotics with wide therapeutic windows occurs infrequently, but may be performed to assess compliance, and/or in patients with renal failure.

Aminoglycoside levels are usually ordered to establish the adequacy of therapy and to prevent toxicity. Retrospectively, there is a correlation between both peak and trough levels and toxicity. In one study, Black et al. (39) found a significant correlation between ototoxicity of amikacin and both peak and trough levels, with the *P* value being slightly lower for the peak than the trough value.

Another indication for the measurement of antibiotics from human body fluids has been the establishment of therapeutic levels of drugs in various body fluids. The field of the pharmacokinetics of antibiotics has developed rapidly, along with the number of drugs that are currently available to treat serious infections. The concept of the "class" or "type" antibiotic that is representative of all related members is no longer valid. For example, we can no longer predict the tissue distribution of all cephalosporins based on the activity of cephalothin. Many of the third-generation cephalosporins appear in extravascular body fluid compartments, while cephalothin does not. Therefore, the ability to assay each cephalosporin level in cerebrospinal fluid is desirable. As pharmaceutical chemists modify currently available antibiotics, additional generations and individual drugs will continue to be developed.

In the 1960s and 1970s, most work concentrated on microbiologic assay systems for the major classes of antibiotics. The 1970s witnessed the evolution of reference methods to rapid procedures that became available in clinical laboratories. By the late 1970s, approximately 75% to 85% of all assays in clinical laboratories were microbiologic in nature, with most of the remainder being RIAs (315). Subsequently, commercially available, nonisotopic immunoassays largely replaced microbiologic assays. Methods for the assay of virtually all classes of antibiotics by HPLC have become available and can be performed in a broad spectrum of laboratories. Immunoassays for aminoglycosides and vancomycin have become routine "black box" procedures because of the widespread availability of commercial kits. Assays for antituberculous, antifungal, and antiviral medications can be found in their respective chapters.

HOW TO CHOOSE AN ASSAY

The selection of an assay method depends on the clinical and research needs, and on the capabilities and resources of the laboratory in which the assay is to be performed. For high-volume assays that require rapid turnaround, commercially sold immunoassays that use specific monoclonal antibodies and are performed on automated chemistry analyzers will be the methods of choice. Low-volume assays for which monoclonal antibodies, commercial kits, or automated chemistry analyzers are unavailable may be performed by HPLC or, in some instances, bioassay. As a rule of thumb, a laboratory that processes ten or more specimens per day should select the most automated, least labor-intensive methods available, even if reagent and equipment costs are increased by doing so. Because the availability of assays to detect minimal deviations from the therapeutic range can be clinically important, sensitivity may take precedence over specificity (181). There remain circumstances in which microbiologic assays may still be useful with particular antibiotics. They have the advantage of being performed without costly or dedicated laboratory equipment. In addition, they determine the concentration of all active metabolites in one step.

There is an extremely broad array of microbiologic agar diffusion assays that are available for use. Each combination of agar, pH, and organism has been chosen to optimize the measurement of a given antibiotic, either alone or in combination with other antibiotics. For clinical purposes, however, the absolute sensitivity of the organism used is of less importance than such factors as the turnaround time of the test, the ability to store plates, and the resistance pattern of the organism. Rarely is it necessary for clinical assays to equal the sensitivity of research assays (198,334). When microbiologic assays in agar are well designed and measurements of zone sizes are made properly, these assays have shown excellent agreement with immunologic techniques (78,79,132,301).

A study was undertaken in Great Britain in the mid-1970s in which salted serum specimens of gentamicin were sent to numerous clinical laboratories that performed microbiologic assays for measurement of the drug in body fluids (265). This study classified the performance of fewer than 20% of laboratories, on average, as "good." Those laboratories with the least experience fared the worst. Radioenzyme assays and RIAs were studied according to similar protocols. Repeated testing of the same laboratories demonstrated marked improvement, because of either increased motivation or reexamination of and improvement in their techniques. Pocket calculators can be programmed to provide linear regression analysis with such factors as slope, intercept, and coefficient of variation, and it is recommended that such records be maintained as an internal quality control check of a bioassay (225). Deviations beyond 2 SD, or 1 SD in the same direction, an inordinate number of times should prompt reexamination of the method.

Proficiency testing samples with serum samples spiked with antibiotics such as amikacin, gentamicin, tobramycin, and vancomycin are available from the College of American Pathologists and other authorized organizations. Participation in Centers for Medicare and Medicaid Services-approved proficiency testing programs for clinically tested antibiotic analytes for which such programs are available is required under the Clinical Laboratory Improvement Amendments of 1988 and for laboratory accreditation by certifying entities, irrespective of the testing method used. For antibiotics for which no Centers for Medicare and Medicaid Services-approved proficiency testing samples are available, laboratories must document biannual verification of the accuracy of their procedures.[a]

Table 8.2 summarizes the general advantages and disadvantages of the agar diffusion assay method. Almost all of the equipment necessary to perform the microbiologic

[a] *12 CFR parts 493.803 and 493.1236 (2003).*

TABLE 8.2
Antibiotic Assay Methods

Factor	Microbiological Assay	Radioenzymatic Assay	RIA	Nonradioactive Immunoassay	HPLC
Mean coefficient of variation (%)[a]	8.9	8.3	8.1	8.5	7.0
Variation range (%)[a]	3.3–17.0	6.0–10.4	4.3–17.3	5–10	5–9
Sensitivity (μg/mL)	0.5	0.5	0.1	0.25	0.1
Time required (h)	3–4	2–3	3–4	1	1
Technical time	10–20 min	1.5–2.5 h	1.5–2.5 h	30 min	30 min
Technical difficulty	Easy	Difficult	Difficult	Easy	Difficult
Availability	General	Specific	Specific	General	Specific
Cost	Inexpensive	Relatively inexpensive[b]	Expensive[b]	Moderate	Expensive

[a] From Stevens et al. (310), in part.
[b] Cost decreases as the number of specimens processed at one time increases.

assay successfully is familiar to microbiology technicians and is readily available in the microbiology laboratory. The only factor that needs to be rigidly controlled is the preparation of the antibiotic standards (278). For those laboratories without sensitive electrical balances or a person experienced in preparing such standards, the hospital pharmacy can be extremely helpful and is often willing to prepare standards. Skilled technical personnel are not required to perform the assay, and it generally takes less than 2 hours to train a technician to successfully complete it. Once the standards are made and familiarity with the calculation of results and preparation of media is attained, an antibiotic blood level can be set up within 10 to 20 minutes of receipt of the specimen. With most *Staphylococcus*, *Enterobacteriaceae*, and *Bacillus* assays, results are available within 2 to 4 hours (255,287,310). Finally, inexpensive equipment is used, limiting the cost of the assay and possible problems with instrument accessibility.

The major disadvantage of the microbiologic assay is the steep slope that is generated, especially for the assay of aminoglycoside antibiotics. As a consequence, a small difference in measurement can significantly alter the apparent concentration (240). Vernier calipers or automated instruments that are designed especially for this purpose, rather than millimeter rulers, should always be used to measure zone sizes. Rather than hand-drawing a "best" straight line, x and y values should be interpolated from a regression curve. The regression curve can be generated with a pocket calculator. A second or third antibiotic that is present in the specimen and unknown to the laboratory can, of course, lead to erroneously high results. Because a large percentage of hospitalized patients receive two or more antibiotics, it is incumbent on the assayist to contact the ward or the pharmacy to inquire as to what antibiotics the patient is receiving, irrespective of the information that is provided on the requisition form (62,270).

It is probably convenient when choosing a microbiologic assay to choose an organism, such as *Klebsiella*, that is inherently resistant to many antibiotics. The technician should be sure that likely combinations of antibiotics will not act synergistically on the organism that is selected. Inordinately high results should be confirmed by repeating the assay with the specimen diluted 1:5 and 1:10 in normal human serum, and by determining whether an unknown second antibiotic is present (53).

Immunoassays are the method of choice for aminocyclitol/aminoglycoside antibiotics. The major advantages of these assays include specificity, automated analysis, microprocessor-controlled calculations, and versatility of analytes that can be measured with the required instrumentation. Immunoassays for aminoglycosides and other antibiotics are invariably competitive assays, in which bound or conjugated drug competes with free drug in the specimen for antibody binding sites. Some assay formats that are commonly used in clinical laboratories to measure aminoglycoside concentrations are listed in Table 8.3. For the measurement of gentamicin and tobramycin concentrations, the Abbott AXSYM fluorescence polarization immunoassay (Abbott Laboratories), the Dade Dimension turbidimetric inhibition immunoassay (Dade Behring, Inc.), and the Beckman Synchron reagent are among the most commonly used assay systems in clinical laboratories. For the analysis of amikacin concentrations, the Abbott TDX/TDX FLEX is a very popular assay format.

Although the material costs per test are higher for immunoassays than for microbiologic assays, the labor costs are significantly less. The necessary instrumentation costs

TABLE 8.3

Assay Formats Commonly Used to Measure Aminoglycoside Concentrations

ACS:180 (Bayer)	Chemiluminescence enzyme immunoassay
ADVIA CENTAUR (Bayer)	Chemiluminescence enzyme immunoassay
AXSYM (Abbott)	Fluorescence polarization immunoassay
CEDIA (Microgenics/Roche)	Homogeneous enzyme immunoassay (cloned donor immunoassay)
COBAS INTEGRA (Roche)	Fluorescence polarization immunoassay
DIMENSION (Dade)	Turbidimetric inhibition immunoassay
DPC IMMULITE 2000	Chemiluminescence enzyme immunoassay
SYNCHRON RGT (Beckman)	Turbidimetric inhibition immunoassay
SYVA EMIT 2000 PLUS (Dade Behring)	Homogeneous enzyme immunoassay (enzyme multiplied immunoassay)
TDX/TDFLX (Abbott)	Fluorescence polarization immunoassay

significantly less than RIA or radioenzymatic assay equipment, and in most cases capital expenditures for instruments can be transferred to the costs of individual tests as disposable items. Because many reagents have refrigerated lifetimes of up to 12 weeks after they are constituted, these methods are applicable to laboratories of any size. Moreover, specialized technologists are not needed to perform immunoassays. In deciding between various assay methods and formats, one often must balance the costs of labor versus the costs of supplies. For clinical purposes, the sensitivity of nonisotopic immunoassays is no different from that of RIAs (9,10,13,45,65,68,102,202).

HPLC is has become the method of choice for analysis of β-lactam concentrations in serum and other body fluids. Again, one must deal with the proviso that the equipment is expensive. However, one can process large numbers of specimens quite accurately in short periods of time (131,311). HPLC technology is the primary method of analysis of antibiotic concentrations in human body fluids in the research setting, especially when new drugs are being investigated. It is the method of choice when one wishes to analyze individual components of an antibiotic or its metabolites (318).

A particular advantage of HPLC is the ability to quantify closely related compounds in a mixture (162,185,191,220,221,224,320). HPLC procedures have been developed for the analysis of almost all antibiotics used for the treatment of human diseases (121,134,188). Unfortunately, the high cost of HPLC instruments makes it impractical for this technique to compete with immunoassays, once a specific antibody has been produced for an antibiotic. In addition to the cost of the HPLC apparatus, the procedure generally requires a trained technologist and dedicated instrument to the analysis of particular antibiotics or classes of antibiotics for a defined period of time. Different antibiotic classes may require different columns and conditions. Unlike gas-liquid chromatography (GLC), however, the basic columns in HPLC technology (C_8 and C_{18}) may be used in the reverse-phase mode for all water-soluble antibiotics. The primary modifications that are required for the measurement of these drug concentrations are to the solvent systems. Because of the ability of HPLC to separate constituents in a mixture (e.g., the three gentamicin components), its analytical capabilities extend beyond those of RIAs (140,282,306,314).

SPECIMEN HANDLING

To achieve optimal results, specimens should be processed as soon as possible after they are obtained. Each antibiotic loses potency at its own rate. For example, aminoglycosides are much more stable than the penicillins.

Serum or EDTA-treated plasma is the recommended specimen for measuring blood concentrations of aminoglycosides. Heparin in the concentrations present in heparin-containing blood collection tubes may inactivate aminoglycoside antibiotics through complex formation. This can cause underestimates of aminoglycoside concentrations. Heparin in therapeutic concentrations does not appear to have *in vivo* effects on aminoglycoside activity, but heparin-containing collection tubes should not be used unless their suitability has been verified by the manufacturer of an assay. Although sera of patients receiving gentamicin can be stored between 20°C and +25°C for up to 2 days without any significant effect, samples that are not tested within 2 hours should be stored at 0°C to 5°C to avoid possible inactivation by co-administered β-lactam antibiotics (173,325).

Acceptable samples for measurement of blood CAM concentrations include serum and EDTA or citrate anticoagulated plasma. These specimens should be kept protected from light and, if not analyzed immediately, stored frozen.

Serum or EDTA anticoagulated plasma are appropriate specimens for analysis of vancomycin concentrations. Heparin-containing samples are generally also considered acceptable. However, reports of vancomycin instability in the presence of heparin recommend exercising caution in testing such samples. Verification of specimen suitability is essential.

In general, if a specimen cannot be processed within 1 to 2 hours of its receipt, steps must be taken to ensure its potency. If it is to be processed the same day, it should be refrigerated at less than 4°C. If it cannot be processed the same day, it should be frozen. If the specimen can be processed within 3 to 4 days, freezing at −20°C should be sufficient. If storage is for a longer period, the specimen should be frozen at −70°C. If a tissue specimen cannot be processed within 2 to 3 hours, it should be frozen at −20°C for processing within 24 hours. If storage will be for more than 24 hours, the specimen should be frozen at −70°C (260).

FLUIDS OTHER THAN BLOOD

The clinical assay of antibiotics from sites other than serum or plasma has generally not been standardized (330). The determination of antibiotic concentrations in fluids other than blood involves all the variability that accompanies the measurement of antibiotic levels in serum, and much more (21,151,261,329). These fluids can contain different types and amounts of proteins, chemical compounds, and cellular compounds, and have different pH values as compared with serum. In order for an assay to be valid, standards must be prepared in the same milieu as the sample, or in a matrix that has has been demonstrated to be equivalent to it. In assaying a fluid, one must be sure that the specimen is not contaminated by blood. Although rather simplistic in practice, the avoidance of such contamination is difficult and sometimes not readily detectable (29).

No universal method is described that can be used for the assay of antibiotic concentrations in all fluids. The key to the assay of antibiotics in body fluids is that the standard antibiotic dilution curves should be prepared in the same media as the patient samples. For example, in assaying the level of an antibiotic in joint fluid, one should prepare standards in normal human joint fluid, or in a solvent with a high protein content. In the determination of gentamicin concentrations in spinal fluid, it was found that if the standards were made in water a 400% error could result. If the standards were made in 0.5% saline, the error was reduced to 50%. Finally, if the suspending medium was 150 mmol/L NaCl per 4.5 mmol/L $CaCl_2$, the results were not significantly different from those for cerebrospinal fluid (86).

One may determine the antibiotic concentration in fluids such as cerebrospinal fluid, joint fluid, or any other nonviscous fluid by diluting the antibiotic standards in normal fluid and performing the microbiologic assay, as described in the section "Elements Influencing Microbiologic Assays," for total biologic activity (150). When assaying an antibiotic that is not readily degraded (e.g., aminoglycosides and CAM), an immunologic or chemical assay is best.

It is important to establish the concentration of antibiotic that was actually present in the fluid under study from that obtained in the presence of contaminating blood. One should analyze the fluid specimen for blood by weighing the fluid and measuring the amount of blood inside it (344). This may be done by spectrophotometric analysis. The fluid should be centrifuged at 3,000 rpm for 15 minutes and the supernatant placed in a 1-cm spectrophotometric cell. After brief aeration, the absorbance at 576 nm is recorded and corrected for turbidity produced by cellular debris by recording the absorbances at 600 and 624 nm. At these latter wavelengths, the hemoglobin absorption is less than 10% of the maximum.

To the absorbance at 600 nm is added the difference between the absorbances at 600 and 624 nm. The resulting absorbance represents the contributions made by the turbidity to the absorbance at 576 nm. This correction is then subtracted from total absorbance at 576 nm, with the remainder providing a measure of the tissue hemoglobin content. The absorbance value so obtained can be standardized in terms of hemoglobin concentration by making similar measurements with a sample of the patient's own blood, diluted 1:150.

Another potential problem in the assay of antibiotic concentrations in tissue is storage. When performing fluid assays one tends to collect the fluid and freeze it until ready for use. In contrast, most clinical assays of antibiotic blood levels are performed soon after the specimen has been received.

The stability of an antibiotic depends on the medium in which it is suspended. An antibiotic that is stable in buffer for long periods of time at 20°C or at 4°C may be quite unstable at the same temperature in serum or tissue (46). One should store all body fluids at −70°C prior to assay. It is incumbent on the assayist, when storing antibiotics in a given tissue medium, to store a standard in parallel to assess any loss of activity (38). At this time it is not possible to definitively predict how an antibiotic's stability will be affected by the particular fluid or tissue in which it is found (38,46). Antibiotics have been assayed successfully from many body sites by employing the principles described. Each fluid and antibiotic must be treated as a unique combination. Procedures that are satisfactory for one fluid and antibiotic pair will not necessarily prove satisfactory for another pair, even if the two are closely related.

Urine should be buffered to the optimum pH of the antibiotic in question, and its protein and sugar content should be recorded. Normal pooled urine from patients who are not receiving antibiotics, buffered in the same way, should be used as controls. The *Bacillus subtilis* technique has been used successfully for the determination of antibiotic concentrations in urine. As described in the section "Elements Influencing Microbiologic Assays," dilutions in a phosphate buffer provide good results. It has been reported that individuals may naturally excrete organic acids that can be antibacterial. Although this scenario is not common, the assayist should be on guard for spuriously high urine antibiotic levels due to the presence of such organic acids. One must filter-sterilize the urine if it contains microorganisms (340,342).

MICROBIOLOGIC ASSAYS

Microbiologic assays are relative rather than absolute (263). In one type of assay, an antibiotic concentration is determined from the microbiologic response of a strain of test organism to a series of standard antibiotic concentrations.

Agar Methods

Assays in agar fall into three broad categories: one-dimensional, two-dimensional, and three-dimensional. The one-dimensional assay employs a test tube or a capillary tube in which seeded agar has been poured and allowed to harden as the agar medium (Fig. 8.1). An antibiotic test suspension is pipetted onto the surface of the hardened agar, and zones of inhibition in one dimension are formed. The one-dimensional assay is especially appropriate for the assay of antibiotics under anaerobic conditions. This method never gained popularity in clinical laboratories in the United States, although it has been used frequently in Japan (128). The method does not lend itself to automation. Its major disadvantages are that is requires complex sample preparation and time-consuming dilution steps. The one-dimensional assay can be useful in determining the antibiotic fluid levels in a pediatric population or in other circumstances in which only a small amount of fluid is available for testing. A procedure for the one-dimensional tube assay is provided later in this chapter.

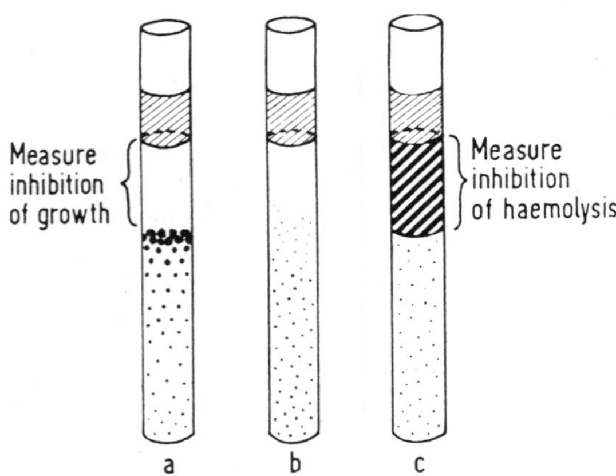

FIGURE 8.1 ● Diagrammatic illustration of the one-dimensional assay. a: Assay of streptomycin with *S. aureus* as test organism. b: Penicillin assay with *S. aureus* as test organism. c: Penicillin assay with *Streptococcus pyogenes* in blood agar. (From Garrod et al. [128], with permission.)

Clinical laboratories have most commonly used two-dimensional or three-dimensional assays. A two-dimensional assay is one in which the antibiotic diffuses directly against a wall of seeded bacteria. This typically involves one of two designs. In the first technique, wells are cut in agar and seeded throughout with the test organism. In the second method, the test organism is swabbed onto the surface of the agar. Antibiotic disks are then placed on the agar surface. The assay is considered two-dimensional because the concentration of antibiotic as it diffuses radially is equal at any given distance from its source. In a three-dimensional assay, the antibiotic diffuses vertically to the bottom of the Petri plate, in addition to migrating along the surface of the agar. At a distance x from the disk, therefore, the concentration of antibiotic may not be identical in all dimensions. As the agar thickness in a three-dimensional system decreases, the likelihood that the antibiotic concentrations are equal at any given distance x from the source increases because the three-dimensional system is physically moving toward a two-dimensional system.

For clinical assays, the differences between the three- and two-dimensional systems are of little significance. In research settings, both systems should be compared to establish that they yield equal results before a three-dimensional system is used. The two-dimensional assay is theoretically somewhat sounder than the three-dimensional assay (182). The three-dimensional assay is one in which cylinders, fishspines, or disks are placed on the surfaces of seeded agar plates. The well-type, two-dimensional assay and paper disk-type, three-dimensional assay have been extensively used clinically. One generally can determine the lower limits of antibiotic concentrations using well-type assays.

Elements Influencing Microbiologic Assays

In performing microbiologic assays, one must carefully account for the many conditions that affect the action of the antibiotic under study and the growth properties of the organism. Deviations from the use of rigid controls result in erroneous assay values (120). The most prominent factors that affect the performance of microbiologic assays follow.

Design

Basic to the assay of antibiotic concentrations is a system design that determines the levels accurately. One must be certain that the zone of inhibition around a source of antibiotic is produced in direct proportion to the amount of antibiotic that is contained within that source. One must also be certain that the response is linear within the range that is normally encountered in clinical specimens. Because dose-response curves are sigmoidal in shape, the assayist must test a sufficient number of specimens to be assured that they fall on the dose-response curve. Environmental factors such as temperature and pH must not affect the assay in either the high or low ranges.

Media

There are a wide variety of media from which to choose for the assay of antibiotic concentrations. Grove and Randall (141) in 1955 described 11 different media that were available for the assay of antibiotic concentrations in human specimens. Almost all subsequently published methods have used some variation of these 11 types of media. The choice of medium is related to the antibiotic under study, the assay design, and the test organism. Although a detailed discussion of the relative merits of each medium–antibiotic-organism combination is not within the scope of this chapter, the medium chosen should be optimized for the assayed antibiotic (182) (Table 8.4). A medium that is satisfactory for use with one antibiotic-organism combination may not be acceptable for the measurement of the same antibiotic concentration in an assay that uses a different organism (333).

The pH of the agar may vary with the mixture of ingredients and the method of preparation. Although the agars are made according to the same formulation, they may not be identical. This variability is the result of the undefined nature of many of the ingredients. For example, yeast extract and animal infusions are in no way standardized. Table 8.4 presents the effects that different agar preparations and pH values have on the results of an assay for the measurement of gentamicin concentrations. Although most researchers have not thought it necessary to use indicators in media, several have found it useful to add fermentable sugars that enable the determination of zones of inhibition by the accompanying pH changes (241). The spraying of plates with tetrazolium blue allows for the ascertainment of zone size more rapidly than by visible inspection alone (203). Agars differ in their susceptibilities to pH changes, crispness of zones, absolute sensitivities, and slopes of the standard curves that they produce (352). Because antibiotic standards and patients' specimens are included on the same plates in most clinical assays, such variations are internally controlled (Fig. 8.2).

Antibiotic Standards

The production of antibiotic standards is the most critical factor in these assays. Because microbiologic assays are relative assays, any inconsistency in the antibiotic standards results in erroneous concentration measurements. Each antibiotic is differentially active at different pH values (128,189). Because it is impractical to make antibiotic standards from powder each time an assay is to be performed, one may produce and store working concentrations of the antibiotic in small aliquots. Practically, the antibiotics are dissolved in appropriate buffers (Table 8.5) at high concentrations. These 1-mL aliquots can be stored at -20°C but should not be kept longer than 3 months. The aminoglycosides are extremely stable and probably can be held longer than the penicillins, which are more labile (182,345,346). Subsequent dilutions from these buffers are made in appropriate body fluids for assay use.

Antibiotics must be weighed using an analytical balance. The potency of the antibiotic should be calculated based on active micrograms per milligram of powder. In addition, the identical antibiotic must be present in the standard and the sample. For example, gentamicin is a compound composed of three molecular elements. They should be present in the same proportion in the assay standards as they are in the pharmacy.

It is also important that there not be a second antibacterial substance present in the antibiotic standard. Because pharmacy materials may contain preservatives, they should not be used as standards except under emergency circumstances. It is necessary to make standards as close in composition to the patient's specimen as possible.

For the determination of antibiotic levels in blood, the specimen should be diluted in plasma or serum (17). As discussed subsequently, this principle also applies to the determination of antibiotic levels from other tissue fluids. Considerable work has been performed to establish the types of sera that may be used for dilution. Horse serum, bovine serum, normal human serum, normal human serum inactivated at 56°C for 30 minutes, bovine serum albumin (BSA), and fetal calf serum have been the most extensively studied (165,173,288,289). It was found that, when antibiotics were suspended in different sera than that used in the test samples, errors of 80% to 367% in measured antibiotic concentrations resulted (274). In assaying antibiotics from cerebrospinal fluid, 150 mmol/L NaCl per 4.5 mmol/L $CaCl_2$ should be added to a phosphate buffer or inaccuracies occur (86). Apparently, it is not necessary to physically buffer the diluent serum (165). It also appears that cations present in sera at physiologic concentrations do not appreciably affect clinical assays (165).

Two factors that are present in sera may, however, exert some effect on microbiologic assays. The gentamicin recovery rate in normal serum has been reported to be between 80% and 90%. However, in uremic serum (blood urea nitrogen levels greater than 50 mg/100 mL),

TABLE 8.4

Discriminatory Power, pH Susceptibility, and Reproducibility of Growth Inhibition Zones for Gentamicin on Five Media

Medium and pH	Discriminatory Power (ZDD, mm)[a]	Lateral Shift of Standard Curve by pH 7.0–8.5 Increase in Standard Solutions (mm)[b]	Reproducibility of Zone Diameters (SD of Mean, mm)[c]
DST (Oxoid)			
6.5	2.9	±0.0	
7.5	3.6	±0.2($P > .05$)	0.21
8.5	(4.8)	0.0	
CAB (Oxoid)			
6.5	2.6	+0.6($P < .05$)	
7.5	2.8	+0.5($P < .01$)	0.24
8.5	(5.1)	+0.3($P > .05$)	
BAB (Oxoid)			
6.5	2.2	+0.6($P < .001$)	
7.5	3.0	+0.5($P < .01$)	0.24
8.5	(5.1)	+0.2($P > .05$)	
AM No. 2 (Oxoid)			
6.5	1.6	+0.9($P < .001$)	
7.5	1.9	+0.9($P < .001$)	0.22
8.5	(2.8)	+0.7($P < .01$)	
AM No. 2 (Difco)			
6.5	1.0	+1.1($P < .001$)	
7.5	1.6	+1.1($P < .001$)	0.20
8.5		+0.3($P > .05$)	

[a] Zone diameter difference (ZDD) between twofold dilutions of antibiotics. At agar pH 8.5, linearity in the semilogarithmic graph at concentrations below 2.0 mg/L was lost.
[b] A gentamicin standard series was divided and pH was adjusted to 7.0 or 8.5. Solutions were randomly distributed in wells 5 mm in diameter. Each value represents the mean of six determinations. Statistical analysis was by Student's test for nonpaired observations.
[c] A solution of 4.0 mg/L gentamicin was applied to 50 wells (3 mm in diameter, filled to the brim) on five plates, and the standard deviation (SD) of mean zone diameters was calculated.

the recovery rate of gentamicin has been shown to be only 50% to 69%. A more drastic decrease in the tobramycin level in the setting of uremia has been demonstrated. There has been some controversy about whether or not high levels of bilirubin in sera can interfere with the results of microbiologic assays of antibiotic concentrations. Blood bilirubin levels of greater than 23 mg/100 mL were shown to cause erroneous determinations of antibiotic concentrations (275). Bilirubin levels of 8 mg/100 mL did not affect the assay under study. Most workers have found that only assays in which bilirubin levels are above 20 mg/100 mL are adversely affected (128,274). These levels are exceedingly rare in clinical samples. Suspending the antibiotic in a matrix equivalent medium that is similar to that from which it came corrects for several factors, the most important of which is protein binding.

Physical Factors

Disks must be known to be effective for assaying antibiotics. Schleicher & Schuell BioScience, Inc. (Keene, NH) 740-E disks have been used extensively. Although individual investigators have used disks of different diameters, the smallest disk that produces good zone sizes in the range of the anticipated antibiotic levels should be used. If one is using the recommended 740-E disk, 20 μL of sample should be used in the assay. The maximum volume that this disk accurately holds is 25 μL. The filter paper must lie flat on the surface of the agar or irregular

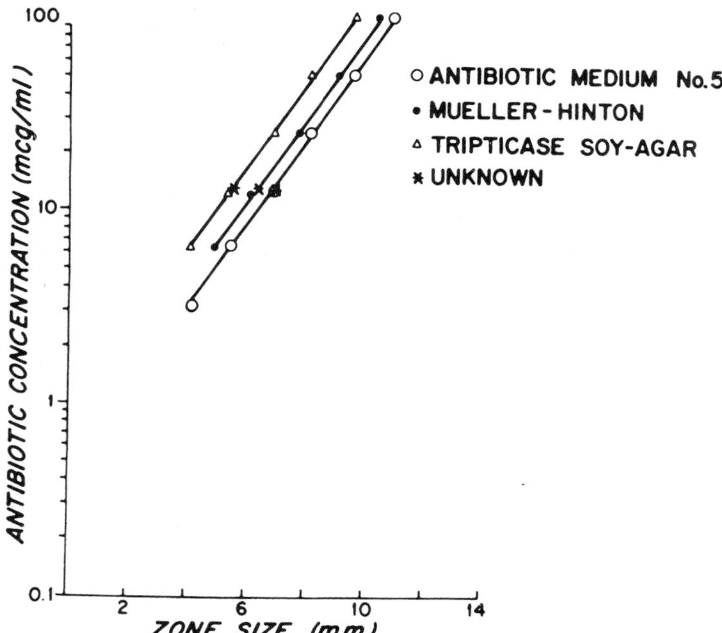

FIGURE 8.2 ● Determination of a CAM blood level using *E. coli* ATCC strain 25922 as the test organism. Although zone of inhibition diameters varied with each agar, all media yielded the same value, 10.4 μg/mL (±5%). (From Edberg and Chu [96], with permission.)

zone sizes will be produced. Supersaturation can lead to surface distortions.

The well technique is approximately five to six times more sensitive than techniques that use paper disks (275). Wells can be conveniently punched in agar with a metal cylinder that is attached to a suction device (35). It is necessary, however, to allow the agar to harden for at least 15 minutes so that cracking does not occur around the wells. The wells can be filled using capillary pipettes because slight overfilling does not produce significant errors in the results obtained (35). Wells should be filled while a low-watt light bulb is maintained at an angle of approximately 30 degrees so that the wells in an assay plate contain uniform amounts of samples or standards. Because the agar depth affects the sensitivity of the test, it is best to add as little agar as possible to the container when a plate is poured.

Choice of Organism

One can use a microbiologic assay to measure the concentration of almost any drug for which a sufficiently susceptible test organism can be isolated (203). It is quite simple to choose an organism for the assay of a sample in which only one antibiotic is present. However, one must exercise considerable caution in organism selection for an assay in which the specimen contains antibiotics in addition to the test drug.

The usual method is to use as the test organism a microorganism that is very sensitive to one of the antibiotics and insensitive to the other (141). This dictum appears simple but is often not reliable in practice (173). One must take into account synergy or antagonism, even though the test organism may appear to be resistant to one of the antibiotics. Thresholds at which one antibiotic interferes with another are published (16). The optimum way to assay antibiotics in a mixture is to chemically separate them by electrophoresis or chromatography prior to their measurement (204). This is probably not practical in clinical laboratories. Many test strains have been isolated that adequately take into account the physiologic levels of antibiotic combinations found in humans.

Organisms used for the clinical measurement of antibiotic blood levels most commonly include *Bacillus* (179,190,203,276,347), *Staphylococcus aureus* (244,275,313,333), *Sarcina lutea* (253,331), *Streptococcus* (177,313), *Clostridium* (200,264,276), *Klebsiella*, *Providencia* (214), and others (Fig. 8.3). Fungi and bacteria have been used for the assay of chemotherapeutic drugs (147,148). Assays that use bioluminescent bacteria (157,212) have also been employed. The actual choice of organism depends on the antibiotic to be measured, its susceptibility pattern, its ability to produce clear and crisp zones on the given agar medium, and its ability to provide results within 4 hours. The organism that is selected impacts upon the minimum level of antibiotic that one can detect. Table 8.6 demonstrates the lower levels of detectability for some common antibiotics with assays that use Kirby-Bauer control strains *S. aureus*, American Type Culture Collection (ATCC) strain 25923, and *Escherichia coli* ATCC strain 25922 as test organisms.

TABLE 8.5

Standard Buffers for Initial Solution and Subsequent Dilution of Most Commonly Used Antibiotics (97)

Antibiotic	Initial Concentration and Solvent[a]
Amikacin	1,000 μg/mL in buffer C
Ampicillin	100 μg/mL in dw
Azlocillin	1,000 μg/mL in dw
Bacitracin	100 μg/mL in buffer B
Cefamandole	1,000 μg/mL in dw
Cefoperazone	1,000 μg/mL in dw
Cefotaxime	1,000 μg/mL in dw
Cefoxitin	1,000 μg/mL in dw
Ceftriaxone	1,000 μg/mL in dw
Cephaloridine	1,000 μg/mL in buffer B
Cephalothin	1,000 μg/mL in buffer B
Chloramphenicol	10,000 μg/mL in ethanol
Clindamycin	1,000 μg/mL in dw
Cycloserine	1,000 μg/mL in dw
Dicloxacillin	1,000 μg/mL in buffer B
Erythromycin	10,000 μg/mL in methanol
Gentamicin	1,000 μg/mL in buffer C
Kanamycin	1,000 μg/mL in buffer C
Methicillin	1,000 μg/mL in buffer B
Mezlocillin	1,000 μg/mL in dw
Moxalactam	1,000 μg/mL in dw
Nafcillin	1,000 μg/mL in buffer B
Neomycin	1,000 μg/mL in buffer C
Netilmicin	1,000 μg/mL in buffer C
Oxacillin	1,000 μg/mL in buffer B
Penicillin G	1,000 units in buffer B
Piperacillin	1,000 μg/mL in dw
Streptomycin	1,000 μg/mL in buffer C
Tetracycline	1,000 μg/mL in 0.1 N HCl
Tobramycin	1,000 μg/mL in buffer C
Vancomycin	1,000 μg/mL in dw

[a] Buffer B, 1% phosphate buffer, pH 6.0 ± 0.05 (2 g of K_2HPO_4 plus 8 g of KH_2PO_4 in 1,000 mL of distilled water); buffer C, 0.1 mol/L phosphate buffer, pH 7.9 ± 0.1 (16.73 g of K_2HPO_4 plus 0.523 g of KH_2PO_4 in 1,000 mL of distilled water); dw, distilled water.

For the rapid determination of antibiotic levels, vegetative organisms must not be more than 24 hours old. The organism can be inoculated the night before the test is run or, more simply, swabbed off a plate, including a Kirby-Bauer sensitivity plate, that is no more than 1 day old (96).

An organism with a particularly unusual sensitivity pattern may be seen infrequently. A 4- to 6-hour growth of bacteria can be diluted 1:1 in either fetal calf serum or 7% BSA, and stored at −20°C to −70°C for up to 3 weeks. These frozen cultures can be thawed and used directly for rapid antibiotic assays (73,97). Although varying the size of the inoculum changes the sensitivity of the test, this also affects the test time, with a large inoculum reducing both test time and sensitivity.

It is not possible in this chapter to detail all conditions for the assay of the large number of antibiotics that are used in humans. Table 8.7 provides references for assays that are based on the previously mentioned microbiologic principles for some commonly used antibiotics. Table 8.7 also presents the conditions that are required for the determination of concentrations by diffusion assay for some of the major classes of antimicrobials. The choices of test organism, test agar, and buffer diluent shown are optimal for the class of antibiotic. One need only substitute the required test organism for *Klebsiella*, use the proper agar and diluent described in Table 8.7, and choose the proper dilution series for the antibiotic standard, as described in Table 8.8.

As with other microbiologic assays, when distinct zone sizes appear around the wells or disks, they may be measured. The concentration of antibiotic is calculated in the same way as described for the *B. subtilis* assay of aminoglycoside concentrations. If one substitutes another test organism, buffer diluent, or test agar for those described here, this would not necessarily invalidate the assay, but would likely decrease its sensitivity. As with all assays, one must obtain a straight line for the standards when plotting zone diameters versus logarithms of the antibiotic concentrations. The *B. subtilis* assay described subsequently can determine the clinically applicable levels of almost all medically used antibiotics (115).

The basic approach used in bioassays is exemplified by the method of Lund et al. (209). This method is typical of those that use organisms that are resistant to all but specific antibiotics for the rapid assay of antibiotic concentrations in clinical material (97,100,130). Although any organism that possesses the appropriate sensitivity and meets the criteria described here can be used, the method of Lund et al. (209) provides a good model. The multiresistant *Klebsiella* strain they described is available from the ATCC. The method has been successfully field-tested. Prior to the substitution of another organism in this method, users should ensure that the new organism meets the criteria previously described. This strain of *Klebsiella* is resistant to most commonly used antibiotics, except gentamicin, tobramycin, and amikacin.

Presence of Aminoglycosides

Because the aminoglycoside antibiotics have broad activity, the assay of other classes of antibiotics that are present in combination with them has proved difficult. There are

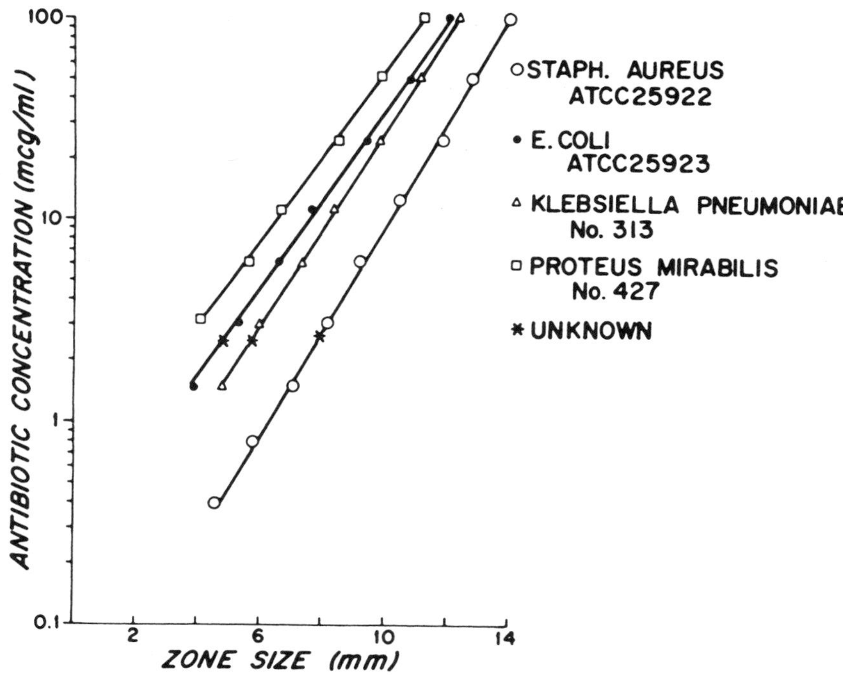

FIGURE 8.3 ● Determination of a gentamicin blood level using members of the family Enterobacteriaceae and *S. aureus* as test organisms. In each case antibiotic medium 5 and an inoculum density of 0.5 McFarland standard was used. The *Proteus mirabilis* was not sensitive enough to yield a direct reading. All other test strains gave a gentamicin level of 2.4 μg/mL (±5%). (From Edberg and Chu [96], with permission.)

few bacteria that are resistant to aminoglycosides but sensitive to other classes of antibiotics. A group B streptococcus has been used that allows the determination of clindamycin (CLD) concentrations in the presence of aminoglycosides (176). Care should be exerted when using any streptococcus if a patient is receiving penicillin-type antibiotics because of possible synergy between penicillin and aminoglycosides with this genus. Because aminoglycoside antibiotics are not active under anaerobic conditions, it is possible to determine the level of CLD in the presence of gentamicin using *Clostridium perfringens* (276). The addition of calcium and other divalent

TABLE 8.6

Approximate Lower Limits of Detectability Utilizing *Staphylococcus aureus* ATCC Strain 25923 and *Escherichia coli* ATCC Strain 25922 as Test Organisms (97)

	Limit of Detectability (μg/mL)[a]															
Organism	Ami	Amp	Carb	Meth	PenG	Ceph	Gm	Km	Col	Nal	Nit	Ery	Te	Tb	Chl	Cli
S. aureus	1	0.25	2	1	0.25	0.5	0.5	1.0	256	128	128	0.3	0.5	0.5	4.0	0.5
E. coli	2	8	8	256	128	8.0	1.5	3.0	1.0	4	4	64	1.0	1.0	8.0	128
B. subtillis	0.1	0.1	0.5	0.8	0.01	0.1	0.1	0.1	—	—	—	0.5	0.1	0.1	0.2	0.2

[a] Ami, amikacin; Amp, ampicillin; Carb, carbenicillin; Meth, methicillin; PenG, penicillin G; Ceph, cephalothin; Gm, gentamicin; Km, kanamycin; Col, colistin; Nal, nalidixic acid; Nit, nitrofurantoin; Ery, erythromycin; Te, tetracycline; Tb, tobramycin; Chl, chloramphenicol; Cli, clindamycin.

TABLE 8.7

Conditions for Assay of Major Classes of Antibiotics by Plate Diffusion Assay[a]

Antibiotic	Test Organism	Agar Type[b]	Dilution Buffer[c]
Penicillin G	*S. aureus* ATCC 6538P	AAM 1	B
Nafcillin	*S. aureus* ATCC 6538P	AAM 1	B
Oxacillin	*S. aureus* ATCC 6538P	AAM 1	B
Other semisynthetics (except ampicillin)	*S. aureus* ATCC 6538P	AAM 1	B
Cephalothins	*S. aureus* ATCC 6538P	AAM 1	B
Ampicillin	*S. lutea* ATCC 9341	AAM 11	C
Chloramphenicol	*S. lutea* ATCC 9341	AAM 1	B
Clindamycin	*S. lutea* ATCC 9341	AAM 11	C
Polymyxins	*Bordetella bronchiseptica* ATCC 4617	AAM 10	Same as B but 10 times as much salt
Erythromycin	*S. lutea* ATCC 9341	AAM 11	C
Rifampin	*B. subtilis* ATCC 6633	AAM 2	B
Tetracycline	*Bacillus cereus* var. *mycoides* ATCC 11778	AAM 8	A
Vancomycin	*B. cereus* var. *mycoides*	AAM 8	A

[a] For aminoglycosides, see the methods described in the text.
[b] Antibiotic media as described by Grove and Randall (141).
[c] Diluent buffers are those described in Table 8.5.

cations to the medium has proved effective (108). However, high levels of calcium may affect bacterial growth and render the medium somewhat turbid. Based on the same principle, cellulose phosphate powder can be incubated with the serum specimen to remove gentamicin (309).

Aminoglycoside antibiotics are inactivated by the polyanionic detergent sodium polyanetholesulfonate in a stoichiometric precipitation reaction (95). The addition of this material to media allows for the rapid determination of the levels of all other classes of antibiotics in the presence of all aminoglycosides (94). Using either nutrient agar or plate count agar, sterile 5% sodium polyanetholesulfonate solution (Grobax; Hoffmann-LaRoche, Nutley, NJ) is added to establish a final concentration of 0.8%. Using the Kirby-Bauer *S. aureus* ATCC strain 25923, or *E. coli* ATCC strain 25922, the standard well-type bioassay is run. For penicillin, cephalosporins, erythromycin, tetracycline, CAM, and vancomycin, *S. aureus* is the better choice. For antibiotics that are more active against Gram-negative bacteria, such as ampicillin or the polymyxins, *E. coli* is preferred. The procedure described for the *Klebsiella* assay can be followed with either of these strains.

One-Dimensional Assays

As previously described, one-dimensional assays can be useful for the determination of antibiotic concentrations under anaerobic conditions, and for assays for which only small amounts of specimen are available.

Medium

Nutrient agar is diluted with an equal amount of 1% peptone in water and brought to pH 7.8 (the pH varies depending on the type of antibiotic to be assayed). It is dispensed for storage in 19-mL amounts.

Procedure

The bacterial test strain (*S. aureus* 658P) is grown overnight in trypticase soy broth. It is diluted 1:100 and mixed well by shaking to break up clumps. Before use, the agar is melted and cooled to 48°C in a temperature-controlled water bath. Then 1 mL of the bacterial suspension is added to 19 mL of the test agar. The bacteria and the test agar are mixed well. The test agar is pipetted into conical test tubes that have an internal diameter of approximately 3 mm (K tubes used for determination

TABLE 8.8

Standard Curve Concentrations for Commonly Used Antibiotics (97)

Antibiotic	Standard Curve Concentration (μg/mL)
Amikacin	5.0, 15.0, 25.0
Ampicillin	1.0, 5.0, 10.0
Aziocillin	2.0, 16.0, 64.0
Bacitracin	1.0, 1.25, 1.56
Cefamandole	2.0, 16.0, 64.0
Cefoperazone	2.0, 16.0, 64.0
Cefotaxime	2.0, 16.0, 64.0
Cefoxitin	2.0, 16.0, 64.0
Ceftriaxone	2.0, 16.0, 64.0
Cephaloridine	4.0, 8.0, 16.0
Cephalothin	2.0, 8.0, 32.0
Chloramphenicol	4.0, 8.0, 16.0
Clindamycin	1.0, 5.0, 10.0
Dicloxacillin	6.0, 12.0, 24.0
Erythromycin	2.0, 8.0, 32.0
Gentamicin	1.0, 5.0, 10.0
Kanamycin	5.0, 15.0, 25.0
Methicillin	1.0, 8.0, 16.0
Mezlocillin	2.0, 16.0, 64.0
Moxalactam	2.0, 16.0, 64.0
Nafcillin	0.5, 2.0, 8.0
Neomycin	2.0, 8.0, 32.0
Netilmicin	1.0, 5.0, 10.0
Oxacillin	1.0, 8.0, 16.0
Penicillin G	1.0, 4.0, 16.0
Piperacillin	2.0, 16.0, 64.0
Streptomycin	5.0, 15.0, 25.0
Tetracycline	1.0, 4.0, 25.0
Tobramycin	1.0, 5.0, 10.0
Vancomycin	5.0, 15.0, 25.0

of complement fixation in the Kolmer test in syphilis serology are satisfactory). The agar is added to a depth of 3 mm from the bottom of the tube. The agar is allowed to harden (at least 5 minutes). Standards for many commonly used antibiotics are described in Table 8.5. Each standard is pipetted into a different tube. Each standard should be repeated three times. The patient's serum is treated identically. The antibiotic standards and patient's serum should be added until they are 1.5 mm above the agar layers. Small deviations from this level do not affect the accuracy of the method. The tubes are incubated at 37°C overnight.

Interpretation

Typical assay results are presented in Figure 8.1. To determine inhibition of growth, each tube is laid on its side. Using an eyepiece with the ability to measure distances, the distance in millimeters from the point where the patient's specimen and the test agar meet (the meniscus of the test agar) to the point where growth of the test strain begins (often it is the place where large colonies are seen) is recorded. This measurement is repeated for each standard and the patient's specimen. The results are calculated as for any dose-response curve. On the ordinate (*y axis*) the logarithm of the antibiotic concentration is plotted. The depth of inhibition is plotted on the abscissa (*x axis*). The concentration of the patient's specimen is found by drawing a vertical line from the depth of inhibition on the *x axis* to the standard line, and drawing a horizontal line from the point of intersection to the *y axis*, where the concentration of the antibiotic is read directly.

Amoxicillin and Clavulanic Acid

β-Lactamase inhibitors protect β-lactam antibiotics from destruction by these enzymes. Clavulanic acid, sulbactam, and tazobactam are those currently used. Because β-lactamase inhibitors are combined with β-lactam antibiotics in the same pharmaceutical preparations, a procedure for the assay of amoxicillin and clavulanic acids is presented (82).

Augmentin consists of amoxicillin trihydrate and the potassium salt of clavulanic acid as the anhydrous free acids in the ratio of two parts amoxicillin to one part clavulanic acid. Amoxicillin may be assayed in the presence of clavulanic acid. A conventional microbiologic assay technique with *S. lutea* as the assay organism can be used to measure amoxicillin concentrations in body fluids after the administration of Augmentin. This is not the case with clavulanic acid because its very low level of antibacterial activity precludes the use of a microbiologic assay technique that depends on measurement of antibacterial activity. Instead, clavulanic acid concentrations in body fluids can be assayed by a microbiologic agar diffusion method involving measurement of the inhibition of β-lactamase activity of a strain of *Enterobacter aerogenes*. In the method subsequently described, clavulanic acid does not interfere with the microbiologic assay of amoxicillin in clinical specimens, and amoxicillin does not influence the measurement of clavulanic acid.

This method uses a large-plate microbiologic assay technique in which samples are added to wells punched in agar. Modifications may be made as required; e.g., Petri dishes may be used instead of large plates, and the specimens may be applied to the plates by assay cylinders, paper disks' fish spines, beads, and others. Moreover, the bacteriologic media used are not critical and individual laboratories may find their own modifications to be more suitable for their purposes than those described.

In principle, specimens should be assayed as soon as possible after collection and should not be stored for more than a few days before assays are performed. As a rule, β-lactam compounds are relatively unstable in aqueous solutions and in body fluids and clavulanic acid is no exception. Consequently, care must be taken in the handling and storage of clinical specimens that contain amoxicillin and clavulanic acid. Serum specimens may be stored for up to 2 days in the refrigerator (4°C) or for up to 3 days in a freezer (−20°C). Clavulanic acid is relatively unstable in undiluted urine, particularly at alkaline pH, and is less stable (in urine) at −20°C than at 4°C. Accordingly, urine specimens for assay should be diluted tenfold in citrate buffer, pH 6.5, as soon as possible after collection, and stored at 4°C. Under these conditions, specimens of urine containing amoxicillin and clavulanic acid may be kept for up to 5 days at 4°C before assay.

The stability of clavulanic acid is influenced by the concentration, pH, and composition of the buffer solution that is used as a diluent. Solutions of clavulanic acid are most stable at pH 6.0 to 7.0, and preparations in citrate buffers or distilled water are more stable than those in phosphate buffers. Also, aqueous solutions that contain amoxicillin and clavulanic acid are more stable at 4°C than at −20°C. Consequently, aqueous solutions of Augmentin, clavulanic acid, or amoxicillin for microbiologic tests should be prepared in 0.1 mol/L of a citrate buffer, pH 6.5. Solutions that are prepared in this medium and contain up to 0.1 mol/L of amoxicillin or clavulanic acid may be stored at 4°C for up to 4 weeks.

Amoxicillin

Apparatus. The following equipment is required:

1. Large glass assay plates
2. Pasteur pipettes (nominally 30 drops/mL) or standard dropping pipettes (0.02 mL per drop)
3. Punches for cutting holes (7- to 8-mm diameter)
4. Lancets or broad needles
5. Test tubes, flasks, and pipettes as required
6. Leveling tripods or a level surface
7. Water bath at 50°C
8. Incubator at 30°C or 37°C
9. Needle-point calipers

Antibiotic medium 2 (141) is obtainable commercially in dehydrated form from Chesapeake Biological Laboratories (Baltimore, MD), Oxoid, Inc. (Ogdensburg, NY), and Difco Laboratories (Sparks, MD). It is prepared by dissolving beef extract (1.5 g), yeast extract (3.0 g), peptone (6.0 g), and agar (15.0 g) in 1,000 mL of distilled water, and adjusting the pH to 6.5 to 6.6. Volumes of 300 mL are distributed in screw-capped bottles and sterilized at 15 psi for 15 minutes.

The required amount of medium is melted and maintained at 50°C in a water bath until the plates are ready to be poured. The assay plates are placed on a level surface or on leveling tripods and adjusted until they are level. The plates are sterilized by swabbing them with alcohol, followed by flaming. The swabbing and flaming procedure is performed twice. The inoculum is added to each bottle of agar and mixed thoroughly. The surface of the plate is flamed and the inoculated medium is poured evenly over the plate. The surface of the agar is again flamed to eliminate air bubbles, and the agar is allowed to solidify with the lid slightly open. The plates may be kept in a refrigerator at 4°C for up to 24 hours.

Buffer. Sorensen's buffer (0.1 mol/L citrate buffer, pH 6.5) is used. Solution A is 0.1 mol/L disodium citrate (21.0 g of citrate acid in water, dissolved in 200 mL of 1 N NaOH [4.0 g/1000 mL] and diluted to 1000 mL). Solution B is 0.1 N NaOH (4.0 g/1,000 mL). Fifty-four milliliters of solution A is added to 46 mL of solution B. The pH of final solution is checked and, if necessary, adjusted by adding the required amounts of solution A or B.

Standard Solutions. Normal pooled human serum is sterilized by filtration and tested for the absence of antibacterial activity. The quantity of laboratory reference standard amoxicillin trihydrate that is equivalent to the required amount of amoxicillin pure, free acid is accurately weighed and dissolved in 0.1 mol/L citrate buffer, pH 6.5. Dilutions are made in pooled human serum for the assay of serum specimens, or in 0.1 mol/L of a citrate buffer, pH 6.5, for the assay of other specimens or urine. Serial dilutions are prepared in the requisite diluent to give the necessary range of standard solutions. Each specimen is diluted to give a concentration that is estimated to fall within the range of the standard line.

Serum specimens are diluted in pooled human serum. Specimens of urine are diluted in 0.1 mol/L citrate buffer, pH 6.5. The required dilution depends on the dose of the drug that was administered and on the time at which the specimen was taken. The mean serum concentrations of amoxicillin and clavulanic acid in fasting volunteer subjects 1 hour after the administration of single oral 375 mg doses of Augmentin are 5.6 μg/mL for amoxicillin and 3.7 μg/mL for clavulanic acid. The mean urine concentration of clavulinic acid is 545 μg/mL.

Bacteria. A suspension of *S. lutea* (National Collection of Type Cultures strain 8340, ATCC strain 9341) is prepared by using a loop to inoculate 100 mL of nutrient broth in a 500 mL Erlenmeyer flask with organisms from a stock culture that has been grown on a nutrient agar slant and stored in the refrigerator at 4°C. The flask is incubated for 48 hours at 37°C and stored at 4°C. Stock cultures on agar slants may be kept for up to 4 months at 4°C. Broth suspensions may be held for 4 to 5 weeks at 4°C. An inoculum of 0.8 mL of the broth suspension into

100 mL of agar usually provides satisfactory growth on the large assay plates.

Procedure. Seeded plates are taken from the refrigerator and the agar surface is blotted dry with filter paper. Holes 8 mm in diameter are cut with a punch. The agar plugs are removed with a lancet or broad needle. The holes are filled with the specimens and standard solutions using a Pasteur or dropping pipette. The pipette is rinsed three times in buffer solution between each sample loading. The plates are incubated overnight at 30°C or 37°C.

Interpretation. The diameters of the inhibition zones are measured and the standard and sample responses are averaged. The mean inhibition zone diameters of the standard solutions are plotted against the logarithm of the antibiotic concentrations using semilogarithmic paper. The best-fitting straight line connecting the points is constructed. The concentration of each dilution of specimen is determined by extrapolation from the straight line.

Clavulanic Acid

Clavulanic acid is a weak antibacterial agent. However, it is a potent inhibitor of certain β-lactamases. This latter property is the basis of a microbiologic assay for clavulanic acid in clinical specimens. In brief, a subinhibitory concentration (60 μg/mL) of benzylpenicillin is added to a nutrient agar that is inoculated with the β-lactamase-producing organism *E. aerogenes* BRL strain 1. Plates are poured and wells are cut in the agar in the usual fashion. At the concentrations tested, clavulanic acid has no inhibitory effect on the growth of the assay organism, but it does inhibit the β-lactamase activity of the enterobacterium, thereby preventing destruction of the benzylpenicillin incorporated in the agar. As a consequence, inhibition zones are produced by the penicillin, the diameters of which are proportional to the concentration of clavulanic acid in the test sample.

The assay for the determination of clavulanic acid is identical to that for amoxicillin, with the following exceptions. The assay medium is adjusted to pH 7.4. The amount of laboratory standard material of potassium clavulanate that is equivalent to the required amount of the pure, free clavulanic acid is accurately weighed and dissolved in 0.1 mol/L of a citrate buffer, pH 6.5. Nutrient broth inoculated with a wire loop from a nutrient agar slant of *E. aerogenes* BRL strain 1 (or *Klebsiella pneumoniae* ATCC strain 29665) and incubated overnight at 37°C is used to inoculate the assay agar. A fresh culture should be used for each assay. An inoculum of 3.0 mL of overnight broth culture in 100 mL of agar produces satisfactory growth on large assay plates.

The inoculum is added to the agar and benzylpenicillin is added to the inoculated agar to give a final concentration of 6 μg of benzylpenicillin per milliliter of agar. The agar is poured into the plates, as described for the assay of amoxicillin. When the agar has set, the plates are stored in the refrigerator at 4°C and are used as soon as possible on the same day. This is essential because the assay organism is able to inactivate the penicillin incorporated in agar plates if they are allowed to stand at room temperature or overnight at 4°C. The results are interpreted as for the amoxicillin assay as previously described.

Three-Dimensional Assays

Antibiotic medium 11 (Difco Laboratories) is adjusted to pH 7.9. This agar may be stored in 25-mL aliquots in the refrigerator for up to 1 month. Prior to performing the assay, an appropriate number of tubes are melted and brought to 50°C; 0.4 mL of an overnight growth of *Klebsiella* in trypticase soy broth is added. The suspension is thoroughly mixed and 9 mL is poured into two 100 × 15 mm plastic Petri plates. Alternatively, 0.4 mL of a heavily inoculated 5-hour broth culture can be added to the agar.

Procedure

For each assay, 0.02 mL of the patient's serum is pipetted with sterile disposable capillary pipettes onto Schleicher & Schuell 740-E disks. Alternatively, wells can be cut in the agar. The method described by Sabath et al. (274,275) is followed, using the same number of standards and samples of the patient's serum.

Calculation of Results

Generally for a given antibiotic, results are obtained from a plot of the logarithm of the antibiotic concentration versus the zone diameter. This is quite adequate for calculations involving limited ranges of antibiotic concentrations. However, if the concentration range is greater than fourfold, it is better to plot the logarithm of the antibiotic concentration versus the square of the zone diameter. Lines that visually appear straight on plots of the logarithm of the antibiotic concentration versus zone diameter have frequently been shown by computer analysis to have low coefficients of variation (179). This caveat is particularly important if the slope of a line is steep. When using logarithmic paper to calculate antibiotic concentrations in this way, very small differences in values can produce large changes in the apparent concentrations, especially in the range of 10 to 100 μg/mL. It is best to use an assay system that provides the flattest possible line. Pocket calculators or handheld computers can provide "best-fit" straight lines, coefficients of variation, standard deviations, and direct interpolations. Keeping permanent records of these calculations provides a strong internal quality control. One may, for example, detect the decay of antibiotic standards by changes in line slopes or differences in coefficients of variation.

When used to perform clinical assays, the microbiologic method produces results in 4 hours or less. Figures 8.4 and 8.5 illustrate that longer incubations affect the zone size only slightly. The size of the zone is, in effect, established approximately 2 to 3 hours after

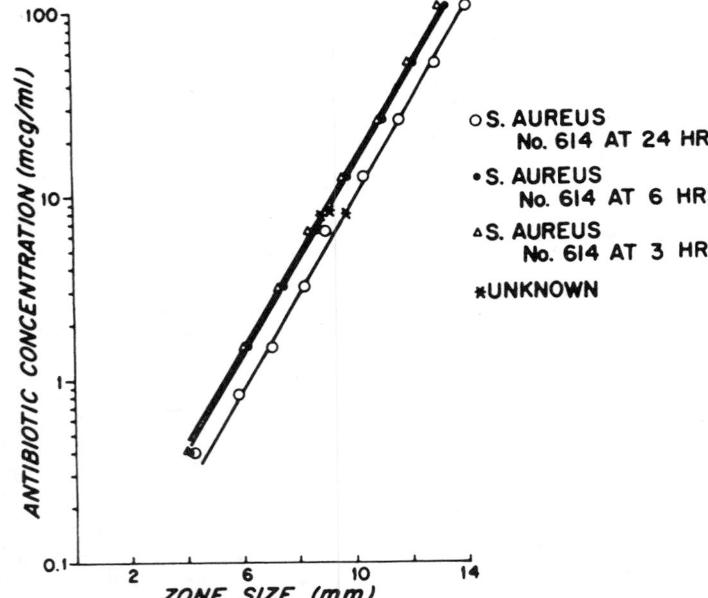

FIGURE 8.4 ● Determination of a gentamicin blood level with only the time of reading varied. All levels were 8.2 μg/mL (±6%). The 2-hour reading was within 15% of the 24-hour reading by zone diameter measurement. (From Edberg and Chu [96], with permission.)

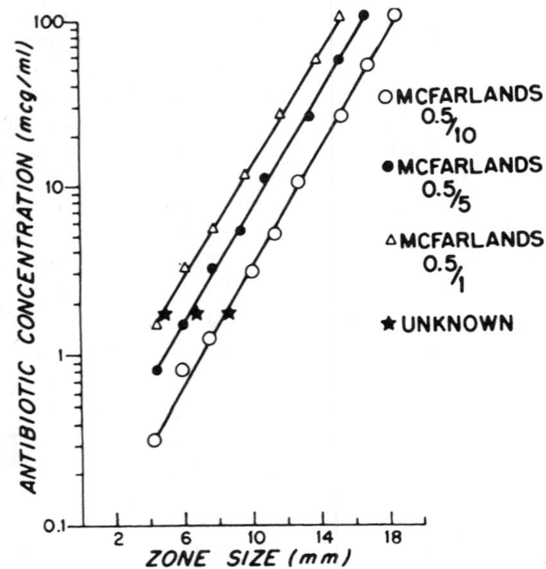

FIGURE 8.5 ● Determination of a gentamicin level with only the inoculum density varied. Antibiotic medium 5 and *S. aureus* were used in all tests. All inoculum densities yielded the same gentamicin level, 1.9 μg/mL (±5%). A large inoculum decreases the time the test requires but also decreases the sensitivity of the assay. (From Edberg and Chu [96], with permission.)

incubation. Small, uniform increases in zone size do not affect the slope of the line or the final calculation of antibiotic concentration.

Electrophoretic Separation of Antibiotics

Methods have been developed to separate antibiotics in a mixture by gel electrophoresis and to assay these separated compounds by covering the gel with an indicator bacterium in agar. After incubation, zones of inhibition are seen in the covering agar slab. These methods were especially useful before HPLC became available and may still have some applicability if one needs to assay for disparate classes of antibiotics in a mixture (6,14).

Broth Methods

Turbidimetric Assays

For completeness, the basic parameters of the assay of antibiotics by turbidimetric means are mentioned. These techniques have largely been relegated to the assay of antibiotic-containing materials in situations in which one wants to screen large numbers of samples in a short period of time. Turbidity is used here to mean any technique in which the growth of bacteria in a liquid medium is used to quantify the amount of antibiotic in a solution. Included under this heading is a consideration of techniques in which the change in the number of bacteria is directly measured photometrically (as numbers or mass of organisms) and, as an extension, those in which a product such as a change in pH or the release of CO_2 is measured.

An examination of the theory of optical methods was explored by Kavanaugh (182). Only the pertinent factors involved in the assay of antibiotics by turbidimetric means are discussed here. The assay of antibiotics by photometry depends on the direct relationship between growth of bacteria in culture and the amount of antibiotic present. Generally, this relationship is displayed in a plot of growth per unit time versus percent transmission or the optical density of the bacterial suspension. It should be noted that absorbance measures mass or volume rather than the concentration of bacteria (182). This relationship can be stated as a form of Beer's law as

$$\log(Io/I) = OD = (N)[Eab/2.3]$$

in which Io is the amount of light leaving a suspension, I is the amount of light entering a suspension, OD is the optical density, N is the mass of bacteria, E is the extinction coefficient of the particles, a is the optically effective area of the particle, and b is the thickness of the suspension. Early work on the assay of antibiotics utilized modifications of this equation from commercial fermentation processes for the assay of antibiotics. Several investigators have attempted to modify it for use in clinical assays (177).

Irrespective of the instrument or technique used, procedures must be employed to straighten the generally curved calibration lines for turbidimetric microbiologic assays. Although it is beyond the scope of this chapter to treat the subject fully, the following relationships should be useful for the applied assay. A theoretical dose-response line for an antibiotic that decreases the growth rate of the test organism is

$$N_t = N_o \exp(k_o + f(v)k_M - k_a C)t,$$

where N_t is the concentration of the test inoculum after an incubation period of t, N_o is the concentration of the test inoculum at the beginning of the assay, k_o is the generation rate constant in the absence of antibiotic, C is the concentration of antibiotic with an inhibitory coefficient of k_a, k_M is the effect of the medium, and the function *f*(v) is a function of the volume of the sample added to the assay. This is a theoretical expression because the major characteristics of the equation, although interrelated, are not absolutely known.

In an individual assay, N_o, k_o, f(v), k_M, k_a, and *t* (time) are constant. Therefore, the variables of the equation may be related as follows:

$$\log N = G + BC,$$

where G and B are constants that are intrinsic to the assay. Because most spectrophotometers use absorbance (A), this equation may be translated into

$$\log A = E + FC.$$

To straighten the line, this equation may be modified as

$$\log(A + M) = O + PC.$$

The algebraic sign M is used to straighten the line over the particular concentration range in question. The constant M compensates for two sources of curvature: the nonlinear relationship between log N and C, and the inherent nonlinear responsiveness of photometers.

Because of this complexity, pure photometry has proven successful only in situations in which all conditions except the quantity of a single antibiotic in solution could be rigidly controlled. The Abbott Laboratories MS-2 instrument, a device that continually monitors bacterial growth in optical density units, has been used to determine antibiotic blood levels under clinical conditions using a growth curve analysis (98). The principle of this technique is that, for any dose-response curve, the response is the turbidity of bacteria in solution. The MS-2 instrument determines turbidity using red light-emitting diodes. The test culture is inoculated into the cuvette. After the culture reaches logarithmic growth phase, the culture is pulled down into compartments, each of which contains a disk. The disks can contain either a patient's serum or a standard. Generally, the patient's serum is tested in two compartments and each standard is repeated twice. After approximately 3 hours of incubation, the optical density (after minor corrections that are required because of the physical nature of the instrument) is plotted on the *y* axis and the logarithm of the antibiotic concentration is plotted on the *x* axis. The instrument has a built-in computer that enables it to continuously monitor the growth of the test cultures. All calculations are automated. In the early 1980s we used this instrument successfully with *S. aureus* as a test organism to determine the concentration of aminoglycosides in blood (98).

Broth Dilution Bioassay for Polymyxins

Broth dilution bioassay is rarely performed. However, this technique may prove useful for the measurement of polymyxin-class antibiotics. It was found that in normal agar, but not agarose, assays of colistin concentration yielded false low blood and urine values (277). This was probably occurring because a highly diffusible precursor was being converted into a poorly diffusible active compound. The turbidimetric technique more accurately reflected what was actually occurring in the body than did agar techniques. Levels of the polymyxin group of antibiotics can be determined by a modification of the standard turbidimetric technique in which the number of viable organisms is counted.

Procedure. A strain of *Pseudomonas aeruginosa* that is sensitive to the polymyxins is employed as the test organism. The inoculum that is used for each antibiotic concentration determination is 0.05 mL of a 1- to 8-hour culture (grown in trypticase soy broth) that has been diluted at a 1:10,000 ratio in normal human serum.

The patient's specimen is diluted in the same fluid that is to be assayed (serum specimens are diluted in serum, cerebrospinal fluid specimens are diluted in cerebrospinal fluid, and so on) to yield final percentage concentrations of 90%, 80%, 70%, 60%, 50%, 40%, 30%, 20%, 10%, and 0%. The final volume of each of these dilutions is 0.5 mL, after the addition of 0.05 mL of the inoculum. Standards should be incubated with normal human serum for 18 hours at 37°C. This preincubation is necessary for activation of the polymyxin type drugs.

Immediately after the addition of the inoculum, all tubes are incubated at 37°C for 30 minutes. After incubation, the tubes are plunged into an ice bath (0°C). The number of bacteria in each tube is determined by performing serial tenfold dilutions with distilled water and plating 0.1 mL of each dilution on the surface of trypticase soy agar plates. The total number of viable bacteria per milliliter of inoculum is calculated from these colony counts after 18 hours of incubation at 37°C.

The endpoint for each titration of the polymyxins in each patient's serum (or other fluid) is the smallest amount of patient's serum that results in a reduction of inoculum to 10% of the original viable count. To increase the precision of the endpoints, the concentration of the subject's serum or the concentration of known antibiotic that causes a reduction of 90% of the viable organisms is read from a curve that is drawn on semilogarithmic paper by plotting the number of organisms on the logarithmic axis versus the concentration on the arithmetic axis. Performing the assay with normal human serum alone accounts for any reduction in bacteria that is caused by nonspecific factors.

Interpretation. The antibacterial activity of the polymyxin standards is compared with the antibacterial activity of the patient's specimen. The calculations are as set forth in the "Turbidimetric Assays" section. The titer of the patient's serum is multiplied by the minimum inhibitory concentration of the organism for the individual polymyxin, to yield the amount of polymyxin type antibiotic in the patient's serum.

pH Change Assays

Antibiotics act on bacteria by halting their growth and/or metabolism. Antibiotic-induced changes bacterial metabolic activity can be used to determine antibiotic concentrations in body fluids and tissues. The methods used are based on the principle that the larger the quantity of antibiotic that is in contact with a bacterial population, the greater will be the modification of the population's metabolic pathways. As with all dose-response assays, one must obtain a standard dose-response curve and calculate from only those points that fit the equation for a straight line.

The most popular method of this type employs a change in the pH of the growth medium as a measure of the amount of antibiotic that is present. If no antibiotic is present, the test strain grows and produces a change in the pH of the growth medium by metabolizing a constituent (e.g., a sugar, which would lower the pH, or urea, which would increase the pH). If an antibiotic is added to the system and the test organism is affected by it, the change in pH is lessened. The urease-based bioassay is representative of this group of assays and can be used by laboratories without special equipment.

Adenosine Triphosphate Measurement Assays

A potentially automatable assay that is a combination of a bioluminescence procedure and a chemical assay uses rates of endogenous adenosine triphosphate (ATP) production by *Klebsiella edwardsii* to determine antibiotic concentrations. The amount of ATP that is present in a broth reflects bacterial growth, which is inversely related to the amount of antibiotic present. Standards are inoculated with the test strain in parallel with the patient's serum. After 2 hours of incubation at 37°C, the tubes are extracted with an ethylenediaminetetraacetate/H_2SO_4 solution. The amount of bacterial ATP that is released is determined by spectrophotometry (91). A plot of the antibiotic concentration versus the relative amount of ATP released is used to calculate the antibiotic blood level. One should heat the serum prior to performing the assay in order to destroy human adenosine triphosphatase. Instruments that enumerate bacteria in urine and other body sites based on this principle are available from a number of vendors, including Celsis International (Newmarket, Suffolk, UK), Coral Biotechnology (San Diego, CA), and New Horizons Diagnostics Corporation (Columbia, MD).

Bioluminescence

Methods that involve the use of luminescent bacteria have been proposed to determine the activity of antibiotics in serum (157,212). One type of assay called the induced test is based on the ability of some antibiotics to inhibit luciferase synthesis by luminescent bacteria (324). Ulitzur's method, described in the following section, is sensitive, rapid, and potentially automatable.

Procedure. The serum is heated at 56°C for 30 minutes to eliminate bacterial activity. To 0.8 mL of serum, 0.2 mL of 10% NaCl containing 0.1 mol/L 3-(*N*-morpholino)propanesulfonic acid buffer and 1.5% glycerol is added. The final pH value of the mixture should be 7.9 for all antibiotics except CAM and tetracycline, which are tested at pH 6. A *Photobacterium leiognathi* 8SD18 cell suspension (200 μL, 3×10^8 cells/mL) is added to 0.8 mL of the serum, as well as to 1 mL of antibiotic-free pooled serum. After 10 minutes of preincubation at 30°C, proflavin is added to give a final concentration of 1.5 μg/mL for pH 7.9, or 25 μg/mL for pH 6.0. The vials are then incubated with gentle shaking at 30°C. Proflavin is a DNA-intercalating agent that induces the luminescence system of dark mutant luminescent bacteria. The results are recorded after 40 to 60 minutes of incubation. Luminescence is measured with a photometer/photomultiplier and is universely proportional to the concentration of the antibiotic in the specimen.

The bioluminescence test specifically determines the activity of the tested antibiotic as a *de novo* protein synthesis inhibitor. Antibiotics that act on DNA or cell wall synthesis are not detected by this test. The bioluminescence test is more sensitive than most available bioassays. This high sensitivity may be attributable to the greater susceptibility of newly synthesized proteins to the inhibitory actions of many antibiotics.

Serum Inhibitory Concentration and Serum Bactericidal Concentration

Broth dilution tests that employ patient serum as the antimicrobial milieu date to the work of Schlichter and McLean (279), who reported on the serum inhibitory concentrations (SIC) in ten patients with streptococcal endocarditis. They obtained serum from these ten patients, geometrically diluted each sample in broth, and inoculated each dilution with the patient's own organism (280). They obtained a titer of each patient's serum that reflected the serum's ability to inhibit macroscopic growth of the microbe. Fisher (118) subsequently extended this procedure by subculturing each tube that failed to exhibit macroscopic evidence of growth after overnight incubation. The highest dilution of a patient's serum, or titer, that was able to kill the microbial inoculum was called the serum bactericidal concentration (SBC). SIC/SBC tests have since been applied to specimens from patients receiving therapy for intravascular and other closed-space infections (312).

Procedure. The patient's infecting microbe is adjusted to yield between 10^5 and 10^6 colony forming units (CFU)/mL in each tube (27). It is important that the actual CFU per milliliter value be determined. To do this, 0.1 mL each of a 1:100 and a 1:1,000 dilution of the inoculum is spread over the surface of the appropriate agar medium. After overnight incubation, the inoculum size is calculated from the number of colonies that are present on the plate that has between 20 and 200 colonies on it. For example, if there are 40 colonies on the plate that was inoculated with a 1:1,000 dilution, the original inoculum contained 4×10^5 CFU/mL.

The serum is diluted geometrically and the test is performed in a manner that is analogous to the minimum inhibitory concentration/minimum bactericidal concentration procedures. For most organisms, the broth can be Mueller-Hinton broth, with brain-heart or Levinthal medium used for fastidious microbes. To each of 12 tubes, 1 mL of broth is added. To the first tube is added 1 mL of serum, followed by thorough mixing. One milliliter from tube 1 is added to tube 2, and is thoroughly mixed. One milliliter from tube 2 is added to tube 3, and so forth. This process is continued through tube 12. However, 2 mL of broth is added to tube 12, rather than 1 mL as in the other tubes. One milliliter is removed from tube 12 and is transferred to a sterile test tube as a sterility control. A geometric dilution of the patient's serum has, therefore, been made from 2^1 to 2^{12}. One should also have a 14th tube that contains only the patient's undiluted serum. To each tube is added 1 mL of the patient's own microbe, diluted to yield a final concentration of 10^5 to 10^6 CFU/mL. All transfers should be made with sterile pipettes. All tubes are incubated in ambient air at 35°C for 18 to 24 hours. The lowest concentration (dilution) of the patient's serum that completely inhibits visible growth is the SIC. Concentration or dilution is converted to titer by the formula: titer = 1 per dilution. As the titer increases, the amount of serum in the tube decreases.

The SBC is determined by spreading 0.1 mL from each tube that does not show turbidity and the first tube that does show turbidity over the entire surface of a 100-mm diameter agar plate that contains the appropriate growth medium. A different pipette should be used for each transfer from a tube. The plates are incubated for 24 hours and preliminary colony counts are performed and recorded. The plates should be incubated for 48 hours when examining staphylococci and for up to 72 hours when examining other microbes. This extended incubation allows the organism to grow on the surface of agar and obviates any effects that transferred antibiotic may exert. The SBC is the lowest concentration (i.e., highest titer) of serum that produces 99.9% killing. For example, if the inoculum in each tube was 2.0×10^5 CFU/mL, killing would be defined as an agar plate that demonstrates no more than 20 colonies from a 0.1 mL subculture.

Interpretation. Much controversy surrounds the use of SIC/SBC tests (262,308). Importantly, few groups have performed the procedure in the same manner. Variations in protocols have involved inoculum size, type of broth, bactericidal endpoint, time of incubation, timing of the blood sample, volume of the broth sample, and the definition of the bactericidal endpoint. For these reasons, this test is no longer performed at Yale.

DIRECT CHEMICAL ASSAYS

Although considerable effort has gone into the determination of antibiotic concentrations in body fluids by direct chemical analysis, there are few instances in the clinical laboratory when one can use these methods. Because these assays are based on reactions that involve specific chemical groups on antibiotic molecules, the concentrations of antibiotics determined by many chemical assays include active drugs as well as metabolic breakdown products that retain the reacting moiety. Consequently, a chemical assay is most satisfactory in a pharmaceutical fermentation process in which one is dealing with a pure substance.

In vivo, from 0% to more than 95% of an adminstered drug may not exist in its native state. Because a clinical assay is intended to determine the amount of active material circulating, chemical assays may yield false high values. In addition, for many antibiotics all their breakdown products may not be known. When chemically assaying the amount of active drug from biologic sources for such antibiotics, it is dangerous to use estimates of average metabolically active fractions. In addition, secondary substances (either other chemotherapeutic agents or normal body constituents) may interfere with these assays. Because it is very difficult to exclude all possible agents in a given assay, falsely elevated values can unpredictably result.

Most chemical assays require extraction of the antibiotic prior to analysis. This extraction leads both to an inordinate number of technical procedures, and to a greater possibility of error. Also, extracted material often requires specialized environmental safety conditions. Although these obstacles are not insurmountable in industry, they may be unwieldy for clinical laboratories.

The advantages of chemical assays for clinical laboratories are, at present, more theoretical than practical. Chemical assays can potentially be automated and should provide rapid turnaround times. Moreover, chemical analysis yields an absolute quantity, as opposed to a relative response, as in the microbiologic assay. This makes the standardization and implementation of controls easier. Only those assays that are useful in the routine and/or clinical research laboratory are discussed in the following paragraphs.

Colorimetric Assays

Aminoglycosides/Aminocyclitols

The thiobarbituric assay of streptomycin has been modified to allow it to determine clinically important levels of many deoxy-sugars (2). Although the chromatogen that is produced when streptomycin and thiobarbituric acid react is quite stable, biologic homogenates that contain glycoproteins, sugars, and plasma proteins have been found to interfere with the assay. Changing the temperature of incubation from 100°C to 37°C eliminates all but plasma protein interference. Automated dialysis and computerized result analysis can potentially be used to design automated assays based on the method.

A crude solution of the enzyme is used in the reaction. The acetylated product, rather than being adsorbed to phosphocellulose paper, is not used at all. Thiol coenzyme A that is produced in the reaction is allowed to react with 5,5′-dithiobis(2-nitrobenzoic acid). The product of this reaction is thionitrobenzoic acid, a compound that has a maximum absorbance at 412 nm. The amount of thionitrobenzoic acid produced is a measure of the aminoglycoside concentration. For successful application of this assay, protein impurities must be removed. One should use a more pure enzyme suspension than that required for radioenzymatic assay procedures. With this assay system, gentamicin blood levels can be obtained within 15 minutes (343). Efforts to increase the sensitivity of the assay and to establish the optimal reaction conditions are underway. It should be noted that vancomycin, which is often used in conjunction with gentamicin and streptomycin, does not interfere in the chemical assays described in this chapter.

β-Lactam Antibiotics

Concentrations of the penicillins and related antibiotics in human specimens have been spectrophotometrically determined by a variety of methods. Most methods rely on a β-lactamase to hydrolyze the β-lactam ring of the drug and involve the measurement of the end products of the reaction (92,125). Historically, these methods have suffered from an inability to distinguish one form of penicillin from another. A relationship can be established between the consumption of iodine by a penicillin and the quantity of the penicillin in solution.

In one useful method, interfering protein is easily removed. Isopropyl alcohol is added to an aliquot of serum to remove the protein. The protein is precipitated by centrifugation (16,000 rpm in a Sorvall RC-2 centrifuge). Two equal volume aliquots of the supernatant are taken. One aliquot is used as the sample, and the other is used as a blank. Iodine solution (0.01 N), buffered at pH 6.5, is added to each aliquot. A measured amount of aqueous penicillinase (Rikker penicillinase, 1,000 units/mL) is added to the sample, while an equal amount of distilled water is added to the blank. After 25 minutes, the excess iodine in each tube is quantitated using a thiosulfate reagent and a starch indicator. The penicillin concentration can be calculated from the difference in iodine uptake between the specimen and the blank. The amounts of base and penicillinase that are required, as well as the incubation times, vary with the penicillins that are being measured. As a general formula, the amount of penicillin-type antibiotic (although susceptibility to penicillinase varies) can be calculated by the general formula:

$$\mu\text{g/mL penicillin} = (V_2 - V_1)(\text{MW/N})/\text{sample weight in mg}$$

where V_2 is the volume of 0.01 N iodine consumed after inactivation with alkali, V_1 is the iodine consumption before inactivation, MW is the molecular weight of the individual penicillin, and N is the number of iodine equivalents (83).

Another technique is to assay for a specific constituent of the penicillin molecule. This approach proved successful in the determination of 6-amino-penicillinoic acid with a glucosamine reagent (285). An additional method of analysis relies on the differential absorption of light a given wavelength by different penicillin molecules to determine antibiotic levels when more than one drug is present. Ampicillin has a higher absorbance at 268 nm in a solution of pH 5 than in one at pH 9. This property has been used to measure concentrations of ampicillin in the presence of cloxacillin (149).

To avoid the difficulties inherent in the alkalized starch-iodine method, a procedure was developed that substituted chloroplatinic acid for base in the assay. Chloroplatinic acid degrades penicillin to penicillinoic acid, which can be measured colorimetrically. The color generated is more stable than that produced with the alkaline method. In the assay, 0.13 mL of 0.2% chloroplatinic acid is added to the penicillin-containing specimen and brought to a final volume of 4 mL with distilled water. The mixture is kept at room temperature for 30 minutes, after which time 1.5 mL of starch-iodine color reagent is added. The starch-iodine color reagent is prepared by adding equal volumes of water-soluble starch solution (0.8%) and 480 mol/L of a 4.8 mmol/L potassium iodine solution. After incubation for 5 minutes at room temperature, the amount of penicillin may be calculated from the absorbance measurement at 260 nm (244).

Active Sulfonamides

The body fluid is extracted into ethyl acetate from a nondeproteinized sample, yielding active unchanged sulfonamide and an acetylated inactive component. The acetylated component does not react in this assay.

Reagents. The following reagents are used:

1. McIlvain buffer, pH 5.5, which is made by mixing 8.6 volumes of a 0.2 mol/L aqueous solution of citric acid with 11.4 volumes of a 0.4 mol/L aqueous solution of disodium phosphate
2. Ethyl acetate
3. 2 N solution of HCl in acetone/water. The required quantity of this reagent must be freshly prepared immediately before each series of analyses by mixing 1 volume of 8 N HCl with 3 volumes of acetone. This product should not be kept for more than a few hours and should be discarded as soon as a brown color develops.
4. 0.1% sodium nitrate in a mixture of 3:1 acetone/distilled water
5. 5% solution of sulfaminic acid in 3:1 acetone/distilled water
6. 0.1% solution of α-naphthylethylenediamine dihydrochloride in a 3:1 mixture of acetone/distilled water
7. Methanol

Procedure. For plasma samples, 1 mL of McIlvain buffer is pipetted into a 10- to 15-mL shaking tube that is sealed by either an ether-tight glass or polyethylene stopper. Plasma (0.1 mL) and ethyl acetate (5 mL) are added. The tube is mixed by shaking for 10 minutes for extraction and simultaneous partial deproteinization and centrifuged 5 minutes at 3,000 rpm. The proteins settle between the two liquid phases as a fine precipitate.

Three milliliters of the supernatant is transferred to a test tube and 0.5 mL of HCl is added and mixed. Then 0.5 mL of 0.1% sodium nitrite solution is added, mixed, and allowed to stand for 6 minutes. One-half milliliter of sulfaminic acid solution is added and mixed well by shaking until there is no further liberation of gas bubbles. After 3 minutes, 0.5 mL of α-naphthylethylenediamine dihydrochloride solution is added and mixed. 0.5 mL of absolute methanol is then added. The tube is mixed until a homogeneous liquid phase is achieved. The tube is closed with a polyethylene stopper. In 20 minutes to 1 hour, one can determine the concentration of the product photometrically, as described below.

Total Sulfonamides

Reagents. The following reagents are used:

1. 20% trichloroacetic acid
2. 3 N aqueous HCl
3. 0.1% aqueous sodium nitrite
4. 0.5% aqueous sulfaminic acid
5. 0.1% aqueous solution of α-naphthylethylenediamine dihydrochloride (Note that all reagents can be stored at −20°C for up to 1 year. Some reagents may freeze and should be well mixed after defrosting.)

Procedure. Four milliliters of distilled water is pipetted into a shaking tube that holds 10 to 15 mL and can be closed with either an ether-tight glass or polyethylene stopper. Then 0.2 mL of plasma is added and the tube is mixed well. The tube is placed in a boiling water bath for 4 minutes. One milliliter of 20% trichloroacetic acid is immediately added, followed by thorough mixing of the tube. The tube is centrifuged for 10 minutes at 3,000 rpm. Three milliliters of the supernatant is transferred to a test tube and 0.5 mL of 3 N HCl is added and mixed. The tubes are sealed and placed in a boiling water bath. After 1 hour, hydrolysis is complete. The tubes are allowed to cool and any condensation drops that may have formed along the walls are washed down. One-half milliliter of 0.1% sodium nitrite is added, mixed, and allowed to stand for 6 minutes. Sulfaminic acid (0.5%) is added to the tube, which is mixed by shaking until no gas bubbles are released. One-half milliliter of 0.1% aqueous α-naphthylethylenediamine dihydrochloride is added and mixed. The solution can be measured spectrophotometrically, as described later, in approximately 20 to 60 minutes.

For urine samples, the procedure is the same as that described for plasma, except that in the assay for active sulfonamides 0.15 mL of urine is mixed with 5 mL of McIlvain buffer, and 1 mL of this mixture is added to ethyl acetate. In the assay for total sulfonamides, 0.5 mL of urine is diluted with 20 to 50 mL of distilled water (depending on the amount of sulfonamide present). Standards in a similar solvent should be prepared to cover the range of sulfonamide concentrations that are expected in the sample and run in parallel with the patient samples. In addition, distilled water and a sample of the same type of specimen (e.g., plasma or urine) from a patient who has not received sulfonamides are also run as negative controls. All tubes are assayed at 554 nm. The value for each tube is determined by subtracting from the reading for each patient sample the reading obtained from the body fluid that does not contain sulfonamides. A standard Beer's law type of curve is constructed. One can interchange standard curves among the sulfonamides.

Occasionally, there may be so much sulfonamide present in a sample that it may not fall on the straight portion of the line. In these instances, samples should be diluted in the same body fluid from which they were collected and the assay should be repeated. If the identical body fluid is not available, distilled water can be used as a diluent with little error for all body fluids except bile. These methods are satisfactory for all sulfonamides.

Trimethoprim

Trimethoprim (TMP) can be extracted from body fluids with chloroform at a basic pH, extracted back into dilute H_2SO_4, and oxidized with $KMnO_4$ in an alkaline milieu to yield the fluorescent trimethoxybenzoic acid (TMBA) (281).

Reagents. The following reagents are used:

1. 0.1 N sodium carbonate solution
2. analytical-grade chloroform
3. 0.01 N H_2SO_4
4. 0.1 mol/L $KMnO_4$ in 0.1 N NaOH
5. 35% formaldehyde
6. 1 N H_2SO_4

Procedure. For the production of standard solutions of TMP, (a) 29.24 mg of TMBA is weighed in a 100-mL volumetric flask, which is then filled with chloroform; and (b) 5 mL of the solution from step (a) is added to a 100-mL volumetric flask, which is then filled with chloroform (this yields 20 μg/mL TMP). From this working standard solution, dilutions can be made in chloroform to cover the range of TMP that is encountered in biologic material.

To extract the antibiotic, 8 mL of Na_2CO_3, 10 mL of chloroform, and 1 or 2 mL of biologic fluid are added to a 25-mL shaking tube. The tube is stoppered and, to avoid emulsion, inverted gently head-over-tail for 4 minutes. The tube is centrifuged for 10 minutes at 3,000 rpm. As much of the aqueous phase as possible is aspirated into a new shaking tube and 4 mL of 0.01 N H_2SO_4 and 4 mL of the chloroform extract from the previous step are added. The tube is mixed by shaking for 10 minutes and centrifuged as described.

For oxidation of TMP to TMBA, 3 mL of the H_2SO_4 extract and 2 mL of the alkaline $KMnO_4$ solution are added to a shaking tube. The tube is mixed and placed in a 60°C water bath for 20 minutes. Then 0.3 mL of formaldehyde is added and the tube is mixed. One milliliter of 1 N H_2SO_4 is added, and the tube is placed in a 60°C water bath for 20 minutes. The tube is mixed and cooled to room temperature.

For extraction of TMBA, 2 mL of chloroform is added and the tube is mixed by vigorous shaking for 10 minutes, followed by centrifugation at 3,000 rpm. The clear chloroform phase is transferred into a quartz cuvette and fluorescence is measured at an activation wavelength of 375 nm and a fluorescence wavelength of 360 nm. The amount of TMP is determined by

$$C = (Ma)(Cs)(F)/Ms,$$

where C is the concentration of TMP in the sample, Cs is the concentration of drug in the standard, Ma is the fluorescence of the TMP-containing sample after blank subtraction, Ms is the fluorescence reading of the standard after subtraction of the chloroform bank, and F is a constant that takes into account the conversion yield of TMP in TMBA (for 1 mL of body fluid it is 5.442 and for 2 mL it is 2.721).

Plotting the amount of TMBA and TMP (obtained through the conversion factor) versus fluorescent intensity should yield straight lines. The method is useful for the determination of TMP in samples from all body fluids. It has a sensitivity of 20 ng of TMP/mL of plasma. Other drugs, including the sulfonamides, do not react in this procedure. The method determines the concentration of unmetabolized, active TMP.

Chloramphenicol

CAM is used for the therapy of acute bacterial meningitis, rickettsial infections, typhoid fever, and brain abscesses. However, CAM may cause hematologic toxicity. Rarely, aplastic anemia with a high fatality rate occurs. In addition, CAM can cause bone marrow suppression, which is reversible and dose-related. Toxicity occurs in relation to dose when plasma levels exceed 80 mol/L (25 μg/mL). Therapeutic monitoring of serum CAM concentrations may be helpful in evaluating and maintaining effective levels of this potentially toxic antibiotic. This may be particularly important for patients with compromised liver status. In premature neonates, metabolism of the drug is unpredictable. High serum levels in these infants can produce the fatal gray baby syndrome.

In one useful chemical method for the determination of CAM concentrations, the drug is extracted from clinical specimens in isoamyl acetate. After extraction, the CAM concentration can be determined by analysis of the yellow color that develops when the extract reacts with isonicotinic acid hydrazine and sodium hydroxide (245). It appears that many of the biologic breakdown products of CAM are not extractable by this procedure.

Duplicate standards are prepared at 10, 20, and 30 μg/mL. Two milliliters of a phosphate buffer (0.1 mol/L;

2.21 μg of $NaH_2PO_4 \cdot H_2O$ and 7.61 g of $Na_2HPO_4 \cdot H_2O$ in 1 liter of distilled water) is added to all tubes. Then 0.5 to 1.0 mL of serum or a standard solution is added. Distilled water is added to an additional tube as a negative control. Three milliliters of isoamyl acetate (Fisher Scientific Co., Hampton, NH) is pipetted into each tube. Each tube is tightly stoppered, mixed well by shaking for approximately 10 minutes, and centrifuged (16,000 rpm in a Sorvall RC-2 centrifuge is optimal). To each tube that contains 2 mL of the supernatant solvent, 1.0 mL each of 1.5 N NaOH and 3% isonicotinic acid hydrazide (Eastman Kodak Co., Rochester, NY) are added. The tubes are then stoppered and incubated in a water bath at approximately 30°C for 45 minutes. The tubes are agitated periodically to ensure good mixing. After the incubation step has been completed, the yellow underlayer is aspirated with a Pasteur pipette and the absorbance is measured with a spectrophotometer at 430 nm. The blank is read as the negative control. The standard dose-response curve is then constructed by plotting the absorbance at 430 nm (the reading obtained from the test less the reading obtained with the blank) on the x axis versus the logarithm of antibiotic concentration on the y axis. Another colorimetric assay for CAM is described next.

Reagents. The enzyme reagent includes 200 mmol/L glycylglycine, pH 8, 1 mmol/L magnesium chloride, 7 mmol/L oxamic acid, 0.09 mmol/L acetyl coenzyme A, 60 U/L CAM acetyltransferase (CAT), 90.5 mmol/L nicotinamide adenine dinucleotide (NAD), 0.2 mmol/L thiamine pyrophosphate (TPP), 0.6 mmol/L 2-oxoglutarate, 20 U/L 2-oxoglutarate dehydrogenase (2-OGDH), and 0.01% GAFAC RE610. This reagent must be used within 2 hours of preparation. However, if the acetyl coenzyme A is omitted, the reagent can be stored at 4°C for 24 hours without a significant loss in activity of either enzyme. The color reagent, a solution of 0.2 mmol/L 2-(2-benzothiazolyl)-5-styryl-3-(4-phthalhydrazidyl)tetrazolium chloride in 12 mmol/L citric acid, that contains 0.02 mmol/L MPMS, 0.04% Nonidet P-40, and 0.1% sodium azide, is stored in a dark bottle at 4°C. Citric acid provides maximum reagent stability.

Procedure. The enzymatic reactions are individually optimized with respect to buffer type, pH, and substrate and cofactor concentrations. To facilitate a rapid reaction, acetyl coenzyme A is required by CAT at a concentration that is in excess of the sample CAM concentration. The 2-OGDH reaction requires the substrate 2-oxoglutarate and the cofactors NAD, TPP, and magnesium ions. Oxamic acid is included as an inhibitor of endogenous serum lactate dehydrogenase activity. When the two enzymatic reactions are combined, glycylglycine buffer (200 mmol/L, pH 8) facilitates rapid reactions and gives maximum enzyme stability.

Dehydrogenase activity is detected by using reduction of the tetrazolium salt 2-(2-benzothiazolyl)-5-styryl-3-(4-phthalhydrazidyl)tetrazolium chloride (180) to a formazan dye, with the highest molar extinction coefficient under the prevailing assay conditions. CAT activity is determined by measuring the increase in absorbance at 412 nm of an assay mixture containing 100 mmol/L Tris-HCl, pH 8.0, 0.1 mmol/L acetyl coenzyme A, 0.1 mmol/L CAM, and 1 mmol/L 5,5-dithiobis(2-nitrobenzoic acid) (Ellman's reagent). The reaction is initiated by adding 25 μL of CAT to 1 mL of assay mixture in a semimicrocuvette (path length of 1 cm).

2-OGDH (EC 1.2.4.2) activity is determined by measuring the increase in absorbance at 340 nm at 30°C of an assay mixture (1 mL) that contains 50 mmol/L of potassium phosphate buffer, pH 8.0, 1 mmol/L $MgCl_2$, 2.5 mmol/L NAD, 0.2 mmol/L TPP, 0.1 mmol/L coenzyme A, 2.5 mmol/L cysteine, and 2 mmol/L 2-oxoglutarate. The reaction is initiated with 25 μL of 2-OGDH.

The serum sample or CAM standard (0.1 mmol/L, 32 mg/L, 0.1 mL) is added to the enzyme reagent (0.5 mL) in a semimicrocuvette (path length of 1 cm), mixed well, and incubated at room temperature for 4 minutes. Color reagent (0.5 mL) is added and, after incubation at room temperature for exactly 2 minutes, the absorbance of the reaction mixture is measured at 575 nm. After 2 minutes, the reaction mixture exhibits a gradual increase in absorbance. A sample blank is prepared and its absorbance is measured by following the same procedure, except that glycylglycine buffer (200 mmol/L, pH 8) is substituted for the enzyme reagent.

The method is based on the reduction of a pale tetrazolium salt to a strongly colored formazan dye by NADH. The thiol groups of 2-OGDH also act as reducing agents, causing formazan production independent of the NADH reaction. Therefore, a reagent blank is required in addition to the sample blank, the absorbance of which is added to the sample blank value. The absorbance of the reagent blank is constant.

Performance. The assay is linear over the CAM range of 5 to 200 mol/L. The intra- and interbatch coefficients of variation (precision) are 1.4% to 4.9% and 4.3% to 6.3%, respectively. Mean recoveries (accuracy) from CAM-spiked (0.1 mmol/L and 0.025 mmol/L) serum samples from normal individuals and patients with renal failure, were 98.4% and 105.6% for serum from normal individuals and 100.9% and 106.8% for serum from patients with renal failure. The method does not detect the inactive prodrug forms of CAM, i.e., CAM succinate (intravenous preparations) and CAM palmitate (oral suspensions). Of the metabolites tested (CAM base, reduced base, and glycolic acid), only glycolic acid is recognized by CAT, with a cross-reactivity of 81%. However, this is a minor metabolite (less than 3%) and its detection is not considered important to the clinical utility of the assay.

Previous work indicates that CAT does not recognize CAM glucuronide (226). The method correlates well with reverse-phase HPLC, which is specific for microbiologically active CAM. The assay also detects thiamphenicol, a

CAM analog, with similar sensitivity and with a linear response up to a serum concentration of 100 mol/L. The endogenous colored compounds bilirubin and hemoglobin interfere with the color reaction when they are present in serum at concentrations above 200 mol/L and 0.2 mg/dL, respectively, because of a shift in the optimum wavelength of the final color. Thus, because of colorimetric interference, this assay is not recommended for use with grossly hemolyzed samples, or when bilirubin concentrations exceed 200 μM.

A main advantage of this procedure is the speed with which an accurate CAM measurement can be obtained. The method requires no pretreatment of the sample such as heating or solvent extractions, as is required for HPLC, the more commonly employed assay for CAM. Moreover, a result is available within 6 minutes. The precision of the assay described here, when performed manually, is similar to that of the automated enzyme-multiplied immunoassay technique (EMIT) (80). However, it has the advantages of producing a linear response (allowing a single-point calibration) and requiring only a simple spectrophotometer to measure absorbance. Because it is a two-reagent system, the assay may also be adapted for a wide range of discrete analyzers. The method is specific and shows no significant interference by high concentrations of urea, creatinine, or phenolic compounds, which may be present in the serum of patients with renal failure (226).

RADIOENZYME ASSAYS

Bacteria are often resistant to antibiotics because they produce inactivating enzymes. Benveniste and colleagues (36,84) provided the basis for radioenzymatic techniques in their description of a method by which they could determine the types of enzymes that inactivated certain antibiotics. Their basic method is used for the theoretical study of bacterial resistance.

Radioenzyme assays have been largely replaced. They were originally a byproduct of the study of how enzymes destroy aminoglycosides and CAM. Table 8.2 presents the general advantages and disadvantages of radioenzymatic assays. Radioactive ATP in the presence of adenylating enzyme transfers radioactive ^{14}C to the aminoglycoside. Aminoglycosides, which are positively charged, stick to negatively charged phosphocellulose papers. By enumerating the radioactive counts on these phosphocellulose papers, the extent to which adenylation occurred can be measured. Acetylating enzymes, which transfer acetyl groups from radioactive acetyl coenzyme A to aminoglycosides, can be similarly employed, with the measured counts on phosphocellulose paper reflecting the amount of acetylation that took place. (36,84).

These adenylation and acetylation reactions provide the basis for radioenzymatic assays. It should be noted that the reactions are stoichiometric in that the amount of transfer in both adenylation and acetylation reactions is directly related to the quantity of antibiotic in the solution. The reaction takes place in several steps.

Many authors have used a method by which periplasmic enzymes are released from bacteria due to changes in osmotic pressure (154,243). By this method, less than 4% of the intracellular bacterial contents are released. However, the method is time-consuming and technically involved. Sonication has been investigated as a faster and easier method of obtaining the enzyme (54). The enzymes obtained by sonication appear to be as effective as those produced by osmotic shock. However, enzymes obtained by sonication may be somewhat more contaminated and unstable because of the release of proteolytic enzymes inside the bacteria (123). This could limit the length of time that the enzyme can be stored, a critical factor in the long-term usage of radioenzymatic techniques (296).

One may prepare the sonicate as follows. A 16-hour culture of *E. coli* RS/W677 is centrifuged at 14,000 × g for 5 minutes. The sediment is washed twice in 30 mmol/L NaCl plus 10 mmol/L Tris-HCl, pH 7.8. After the second wash, the pellet is suspended in 0.5 mmol/L $MgCl_2$ at 4°C (5 mL of 0.5 mmol/L $MgCl_2$ per 100 mL of original culture volume). The suspension is then sonicated for 20 seconds using a Dawe-type 3057A Soniprobe (Dawe Instruments Ltd., London, UK) set to give a 4 amp current. The cellular debris is removed by centrifugation at 25,000 × g for 20 minutes. The supernatant is divided into 0.1-mL aliquots and stored at 20°C (35).

Because it is undesirable to have to prepare the enzyme frequently, its stability has been studied under various conditions (123). Several methods have been developed to decrease enzyme lability. Keeping the enzyme frozen and in an ice bath are effective techniques (9,286). The enzyme has been shown to be stable for 24 hours at 4°C, and 30 days at −20°C with BSA (300). Storing partially purified enzyme in reducing agents appears to increase its life span (299). Freezing the enzyme at low temperatures, such as −70°C, in quantities that will be used in a day's run, appears to be the most efficient and effective technique (59,317). It increases the storage life of the enzyme and significantly decreases the amount of technician time that is required to set up the assays.

DIRECT FLUORESCENT CHEMICAL ANALYSIS

A molecule is fluorescent when it can receive light at one wavelength and emit it at another wavelength. The wavelengths at which a given molecule receives and emits light are often specific to the molecule, a reactive group on a molecule, or a class of molecules. One major disadvantage of these assays is that other material present in the specimen, particularly radiologic fluorescein dyes and certain proteins, can fluoresce and interfere with the test. However, fluorescent assays typically are much more sensitive than chemical assays and can quantify compounds in the nanogram and often picogram per milliliter range.

Fluorescence can be determined in one of two ways. First, one may use the inherent fluorescent properties of the molecule. Second, for antibiotics that are either weakly fluorescent or nonfluorescent, one may covalently link a strongly fluorescent moiety to the drug in question. Because of the need for an extraction step, the possible need for coupling steps, the need for rather specialized equipment, the lack of standardized techniques, and the frequent inability to distinguish between active and inactive antibiotics, fluorescence methods have not been widely used in clinical laboratories, although they have been used in industry and US Public Health Service laboratories. The reader is referred to the book by Undenfriend (326) for a general view of fluorescent analysis.

Although penicillins and cephalosporins are not generally inherently fluorescent, many produce fluorescent compounds under hydrolysis in the presence of acid (178). Attempts to simplify the extraction procedures and the number of technical manipulations that are required to generate such reactions have led to methods for measurement that can be clinically useful (24,83). For example, ampicillin concentrations can be determined in the absence of ampicillinoic acid by extraction. Standards should be prepared to cover the expected range of concentrations and serum blanks should be run to obtain measurements of background fluorescence.

Tetracyclines

Different tetracyclines require different fluorescent reagents to enhance their light-emitting properties (231). Each tetracycline should be tested individually to optimize these assays. Hall (146) has expanded the technique to measure the concentrations of tetracycline mixtures in plasma by using acid hydrolysis or alkaline degradation to convert the tetracycline into a fluorescent form. In these methods, aluminum salts are used to enhance the fluorescence of the end products. This fluorescence is measured with a spectrofluorometer. Each tetracycline exhibits a different structural arrangement of the chemical groups that surround the fluorescent nucleus of the anhydrous salts, creating individual fluorescent characteristics (146). A general method for the fluorometric determination of tetracyclines follows (199).

Apparatus

An Aminco-Bowman spectrophotofluorometer (American Instrument Company, Silver Spring, MD) fitted with a xenon arc lamp and an R 136 photomultiplier, or its equivalent, should be employed. Mirrors and 1-mm slits are placed in the cell housing.

Reagents

For most tetracyclines, one can use 0.5 mol/L magnesium acetate tetrahydrate plus 0.3 mol/L sodium barbitone in ethanedial. Minocycline, and other 7-aminotetracyclines, can be measured with a mixture of 0.2 mol/L magnesium acetate and 0.2 mol/L citric acid in ethanedial.

Procedure

A 0.2-mL aliquot of the sample (serum or other fluid) is mixed with 0.4 mL of a phosphate buffer (3 mol/L NaH_2PO_4 plus 1 mol/L Na_2SO_3) and thoroughly extracted with 2.5 mL of amyl acetate. The phases are separated by allowing them to settle, or centrifuging the tube (approximately 500 $\times$ g). Two milliliters of the organic (top) phase are transferred to a Brown fluorometer cuvette. A suitable fluorescence reagent (0.6 mL) is added. (Fluorescence reagents are described later.) The tubes are mixed by shaking for 5 minutes. The turquoise fluorescence in the lower phase is read 20 minutes or more after shaking. If the lower phase is cloudy, the tubes are centrifuged (500 $\times$ g for 2 to 3 minutes) before reading. Standards (0.2 mL of a 10 mmol/L solution of the appropriate tetracycline) and blanks (0.2 mL of water) are also made.

For the determination of minocycline, a pH 6.5 buffer (0.5 mol/L NaH_2PO_4 plus 0.5 mol/L Na_2HPO_4) should be used instead of the phosphate sulfite buffer (2). Fluorescence is measured with excitation at 405 nm and emission at 490 nm. The fluorescence of 7-aminotetracyclines is read with excitation at 380 nm and emission at 480 nm (199).

IMMUNOLOGIC ASSAYS

Immunologic assays came into use in the mid-1970s. These assays were based largely on existing equipment and merely exploited procedures available for the assay of hormones. However, for the first time, the assay of antibiotics was removed from the realm of the specialist. These assays could be performed in a central location, with the instrument playing the primary role. The development of the means to elicit specific, high-titered antibodies to hapten antibiotics also allowed RIA techniques to deliver specificity that uses impossible with biologic assays. As with any nonbiologic assay, however, one always had to be particularly careful not to measure a nonactive metabolite.

Because RIA equipment was expensive, the measurement of antibiotics was often mixed in with the assay of other drugs, resulting in significant delays in processing. The requirement to maintain a stock of highly active radioisotopes (often with short half-lives) gave impetus to the development of nonisotopic immunoassays. Unlike hormones, which are present in extremely small amounts and require highly sensititive methods of detection, antibiotics are generally present in levels above 0.5 μg/mL.

Because other small molecules, such as antiepileptics and drugs of abuse, are also present in these levels, a technology was developed to measure small molecules by somewhat less sensitive, nonisotopic means. Unlike the stimulatory role played by existing RIA equipment in the development of RIA, the impetus for the development of the new nonisotopic immunoassays was largely the need to assay the aminoglycoside class of antibiotics.

Before the application of this technique to the measurement of antibiotic concentrations in 1975, RIA had been used for a number of years for the quantitation of hormonal substances (174). All RIAs of antibiotics employ three broad reaction steps. The first step involves three components: radiolabeled antigen (antibiotic), high titer, high avidity antibody to that antigen, and unlabeled antigen (antibiotic obtained from the patient's serum). The reaction with either labeled or unlabeled antigen produces antibody combined with labeled antigen, or antibody combined with unlabeled antigen. The more unlabeled antigen that is present in the reaction mixture, the less radiolabeled antigen combines with antibody.

After equilibrium is reached, one must quantify the amount of bound antibody in the mixture. This step involves either the removal of the bound antigen-antibody complex from solution by a precipitating agent, or the removal of the unbound antigen from solution by chemical means. Because antigen/antibody reactions are stoichiometric in nature, the quantification of either the bound radiolabeled or the free radiolabeled antigen is directly proportional to the antibiotic level in a sample (55–57).

Although there are individual modifications, the test procedures follow a basic course (174). First, one incubates a known quantity of tritiated antibiotic with antibody (of known potency) to that antibiotic. A given amount of patient's serum is added and the mixture is allowed to come to equilibrium. These assays are heterogeneous and produce sigmoidal co-precipitation curves. Early investigators were hampered because only the relatively linear part of the sigmoidal curve could be used for the calculation of antibiotic concentrations. Robard et al. (268) devised a method in which the sigmoidal curve was converted to a straight line, thereby permitting the calculation of results over a much wider range of values. They found that the plot of $y = 100$ (B/B°) may be linearized by the equation representing a straight line in which logit $(y) = A + B \log x$, where x is the amount of unlabeled or patient drug, and y represents the percentage of antibiotic that is bound.

This logit conversion not only allowed a much wider range of antibiotic concentrations to be measured, but also permitted the development of standard curves. As a result, one did not have to repeat all the controls each time a specimen was run. An advantage of immunologic assays is their within-class specificity. Although there may be cross-reactivity among members of the same drug class, there is no cross-reactivity among members of different classes (e.g., gentamicin and vancomycin).

Nonisotopic Immunoassays

The development of enzyme immunoassays by Engvall and Perlmann (105,106) laid the foundation for design of nonradioisotopic immunoassays. In these immunoassays, an enzyme or fluorometric substance is coupled to the antigen or antibody in such a way that the activity of the parent compound is not appreciably affected. The significant difference between nonisotopic immunoassays and RIAs is the means of counting the label. In nonisotopic assays, the quantity label present is estimated from enzyme or fluorescence activity, which changes under the assay conditions.

Generally, when an enzyme-substrate reaction is used in an immunoassay, enzyme activity is measured as reaction velocity. In this situation, the reaction velocity must be proportional to the number of enzyme molecules that catalyze the reaction (230). In fluorescence immunoassays, a change in the nature of the interaction of light with the substrate is measured (34).

In many nonisotopic immunoassays, the label, whether fluorescent or nonfluorescent, is an enzyme. In order to distinguish RIAs from nonisotopic immunoassays, we must consider the characteristics of an enzyme label. First, it must be recognized easily as the label. The enzyme must be attached to the substrate in such a way that it maintains activity, yet performs satisfactorily under the assay conditions. Second, the label must be stable. The label must not disintegrate when the assay is in process and it must be stable during storage. Invariably, the enzyme is covalently bound to the labeled molecule. Third, the enzyme must be quantitatively measurable. In nonisotopic immunoassays, one measures a secondary reaction product (i.e., produced by a substrate acting on the enzyme), rather than direct release of a radioisotope (210,219). Therefore, we do not measure the enzyme molecules themselves, but instead measure the catalyzed reaction processes. With any enzymatic label, the product that is produced must be proportional to the amount of enzyme that catalyzes the reaction.

In considering the theory of enzyme activity and its relationship to the clinical assay, we must remember the Michaelis-Menten equation:

$$v = V[S/(S + K_m)],$$

where v is the measured reaction velocity, S is the concentration of substrate, and K_m is the calculated constant. In practice, one attempts to design the assay conditions so that S is much greater than K_m. In this case we may assume that v is approximately equal to V, and that

$$v = (k)E_2,$$

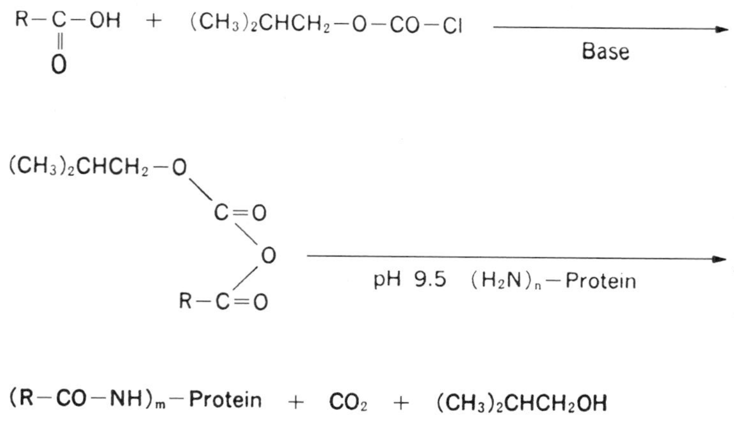

$$R-C(=O)-OH + (CH_3)_2CHCH_2-O-CO-Cl \xrightarrow{\text{Base}}$$

$$(CH_3)_2CHCH_2-O-C(=O)-O-C(=O)-R \xrightarrow{\text{pH 9.5} \quad (H_2N)_n-\text{Protein}}$$

$$(R-CO-NH)_m-\text{Protein} + CO_2 + (CH_3)_2CHCH_2OH$$

FIGURE 8.6 ● Mixed-anhydride reaction to label hapten antibiotics. (From Kitagawa et al. [187], with permission.)

where E_2 is the total amount of enzyme that is present in the reaction mixture. It should be noted that this equation implies that the reaction velocity is independent of time.

The equations just described require that the reactions be followed continuously as they occur. One must measure the accumulation of product or the change in fluorescence as it occurs over time. There have been three primary means of quantitatively following enzyme reactions for the assay of haptens, including antibiotics, under these conditions. First is the spectrophotometric assay. The spectrophotometer is useful when the product of the reaction can be measured between 190 and 800 nm. Most workers have attempted to measure the release of the product directly. However, the product may first have to be transformed into a colored product. The advantage of using a spectrophotometer is that this instrument is readily available in clinical laboratories.

Much work has involved the study of fluorometric methods, which is the second approach. The outstanding feature of fluorometry is its high degree of sensitivity. Fluorometic methods are generally 100 to 1,000 times more sensitive than spectrophotometric methods. This sensitivity is especially manifested either when the initial substrate is nonfluorescent and becomes so during the reaction or when there is a change in fluorescence polarization as the reaction proceeds.

The third method, which employs electrodes, offers several advantages. Hydrogen ion concentrations and automatic titration apparatus may be employed to continuously measure a reaction as it proceeds. Considerable work has been performed on an oxygen electrode, which is a type of polarography (121).

Fundamental to nonisotopic immunoassays is the preparation of hapten-protein conjugates, in which haptens (antibiotic) and proteins (generally an enzyme) both function naturally. Most of the described methods have attached the hapten to the protein by free amino, hydroxyl, or carboxyl groups. Haptens with hydroxyl groups may be conjugated to a carrier protein by activation of the carboxyl group, followed by acylation of amino groups in the protein. The mixed-anhydride procedure has been commonly used for this purpose. Figure 8.6 demonstrates the principles of the reaction. The procedure is performed directly with the hapten and the conjugate.

Alternatively, one may use the carbodiimide procedure, in which uridine-5-carboxylic acid is coupled directly to poly-DL-alanyl-poly-L-lysine with dicyclohexylcarbodiimide in 95% dimethylformamide. The carrier or enzyme, excess hapten, and reagent are simply stirred together in water for 30 minutes each day for several days.

Haptens with amino groups, which include the aminocyclitol/aminoglycoside class of antibiotics, may be coupled to proteins. The reactions that are used to conjugate these haptens depend on whether the groups are aromatic or aliphatic amines. If the amino group is an aromatic amine, the hapten may be conjugated to proteins by the classic diazotization procedure. For example, CAM may be conjugated by this means (187). With this method, one must reduce the nitro group to an amino group before the conjugation reaction can occur. If the hapten contains an aliphatic amine, it can be reacted with carboxyl groups by the carbodiimide reagent. The conditions of this reaction are straightforward and similar to those employed for the conjugation of carboxyl groups. Optimally, amino groups of the hapten molecule can be acetylated by the hetero-bifunctional reagent *N*-(*m*-maleimidebenzoyloxy)succinimide to introduce a maleimide residue. As shown in Figure 8.7, the maleimide residue may be coupled with thiol groups, which are converted from the disulfide bonds of cystine residues by reductive cleavage.

Few enzymes have been used to label antibiotics. Peroxidase was coupled to gentamicin by a modified Nakne's method (183). One of the first enzymes used, which is still commonly employed in the EMIT system, is glucose-6-phosphate dehydrogenase. The means of covalently linking this enzyme to antibiotics is, however, a proprietary secret. β-D-Galactosidase has also been commonly

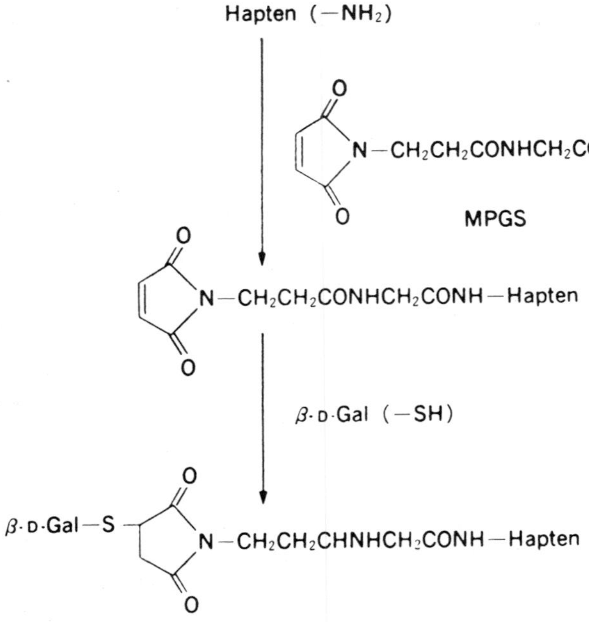

Hapten (—NH2)
N—CH2CH2CONHCH2COO—N
MPGS
N—CH2CH2CONHCH2CONH—Hapten
β-D-Gal (—SH)
β-D-Gal—S
N—CH2CH2CHNHCH2CONH—Hapten

FIGURE 8.7 ● Reaction with antibiotic and protein for the production of high-titered antibody. *β-D-Gal, β-D-galactosidase*. (From Kitagawa et al. [187], with permission.)

employed. This reaction has been made possible through the use of hetero-bifunctional reagents such as *N*-(3-maleimidopropionylglycyloxy)succinimide (MPGS). A number of these reagents are equally useful. The general method is shown in Figure 8.8.

The bonding of ampicillin serves as a useful model of this type of antibiotic labeling. Fifty micromoles of ampicillin are dissolved in 0.05 mol/L of a phosphate buffer, pH 7.0. This is incubated with MPGS for 50 minutes at 30°C. After lyophilization, the powder is washed three times with 10 mL of ether/methylene chloride solution (2:1) to remove excess MPGS. Following desiccation, the powder is dissolved in 0.5 mol/L of a phosphate buffer, pH 6.0. Approximately 30% to 40% of the ampicillin is acetylated by MPGS. The acetylated ampicillin is coupled to the β-D-galactosidase enzyme by dissolving 1 mol in 1 mL of 0.05 mol/L phosphate buffer, pH 6.0, with 93 pmol of β-D-Galactosidase, and incubating the mixture overnight at room temperature. This the conjugate is separated chromatigraphically using a Sepharose 6B column (1.8 × 30 cm) with 0.02 mol/L phosphate-buffered saline (PBS), pH 7.0, that contains 0.1% NaN_3, as the eluent. One unit of enzyme activity may be defined as the amount of enzyme that hydrolyzes 1 μmol of 7-β-D-galactopyanosyloxy-4-methylcoumarin per minute (187).

Nonisotopic immunoassays invariably use competition between labeled and unlabeled drug for antibody binding sites to derive the antimicrobial concentration in a specimen. These assays may be divided into two types: heterogeneous and homogeneous. The heterogeneous type was the first to be developed and is best exemplified by the enzyme-linked immunosorbent assay.

Hapten—NH2
COO—N
MBS
Hapten—NH—OC
Reduced
BSA—(SH)n
BSA
Hapten—NH—OC
S—BSA

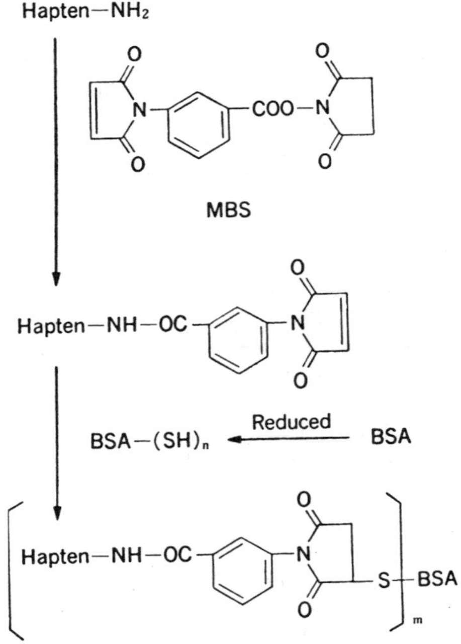

FIGURE 8.8 ● Mixed-anhydride reaction for the production of high-titered antibody to aminoglycoside antibiotics. *MBS, N-(m-maleimidebenzoyloxy)succinimide*. (From Kitagawa et al. [187], with permission.)

Heterogeneous assays require wash steps to separate the bound and free ligands. Most commonly, these assays have been used to measure and detect large molecules. Homogeneous assays do not require the removal of unbound ligand from the reaction mixture, and therefore may be performed as single step assays.

If an antibody is bound to the antigen, the substrate is unable to gain access to the catalytic site of the enzyme. Accordingly, the enzyme's activity is inhibited. When unlabeled antigen is added, it competes with the enzyme-labeled antigen for binding to the antibody and the free form of the enzyme labeled antigen is increased. As a result, enzyme activity is increased. Consequently, enzyme activity is proportional to the concentration of unlabeled antigen and can be used to quantitatively assay small hapten molecules.

Most commonly, the inhibition of enzyme activity on binding to antibody is caused by steric modification of the enzyme. Homogeneous assays are inherently more easily automated than are heterogeneous assays. These assays have been extensively developed for the measurement of a wide variety of molecules. The elimination in homogeneous assay of the need to remove unbound ligand from the reaction has made possible the generation of machinery that requires minimal technical input from the clinical laboratory. Automated instruments can measure enzyme activity through detection of reaction products and, with internally programmed computer analysis, derive the concentrations of the antibiotics in question.

Heterogeneous Nonisotopic Immunoassays

An assay for ampicillin is presented as a representative heterogeneous nonisotopic immunoassay. A mixture of 18 units of enzyme-labeled ampicillin (the production of which is described in the previous section) and 50 μL of 104-fold diluted rabbit ampicillin antiserum is incubated. 0.1 mL of sample or standard is added to 0.1 mL of the diluted ampicillin antiserum. To the sample or standard plus antiserum is added 0.5 mL of ampicillin-β-D-galactosidase conjugate, and 0.05 mL of a 0.05 mol/L phosphate buffer, pH 6.0. This final volume of reactants is incubated for 6 to 8 hours at 4°C. Following incubation, 0.05 mL of normal rabbit serum, which has been diluted 1:500, is added to 0.05 mL of goat antirabbit IgG serum, which has been diluted 1:5 and incubated with the reactant solution for 8 to 16 hours at 4°C. After this incubation period, 1 mL of 0.05 mol/L phosphate buffer, pH 6.0, is added and the entire mixture is centrifuged at 2,500 rpm for 20 minutes. The centrifugation step is repeated twice. To the reactant phase, 0.15 mL of substrate solution is added, with incubation at 30°C for 60 minutes. The amount of ampicillin present is calculated in a fluorometer, with excitation wavelength of 365 nm and emission wavelength of 448 nm (Fig. 8.9) (71,72,187).

To avoid the requirement for a centrifugation step, a method was developed that used antibody that was covalently linked to magnetizable particles (306). The sample is incubated with fluorescein-labeled gentamicin and antigentamicin serum to which has been attached magnetic particles. The magnetic particles are rapidly sedimented from the reaction mixture through contact with a polarized surface.

Receptor Antibody Sandwich Assay for Teicoplanin

Teicoplanin, a glycopeptide antibiotic with activity similar to that of vancomycin, is currently used in Europe, Japan, and other countries to treat severe infections caused by Gram-positive bacteria. Traditional methods for measuring concentrations of teicoplanin include microbiologic assays, HPLC, and solid-phase enzyme receptor assays (249). These methods have several limitations. First, the microbiologic assay is not specific for teicoplanin in the presence of other antibiotics and is of low accuracy when it is performed on biologic fluids. HPLC requires specialized equipment and laborious extraction procedures for sample preparation. Finally, the solid-phase enzyme receptor assay does not always yield accurate results in complex specimens such as bronchial expectorates or skin homogenates. The following method is a receptor antibody sandwich assay that is able to quantify teicoplanin in complex matrices. The method is based on bioselective adsorption of teicoplanin onto microtiter plates coated with BSA-ε-aminocaproyl-D-alanyl-D-alanine, a synthetic analog of the antibiotic's biologic target, followed by reaction with antiteicoplanin antibodies. The sandwich complexes are detected by incubation with peroxidase-labeled goat antibodies to rabbit IgGs and a chromogenic reaction with *o*-phenylenediamine.

Procedure

Polyvinylchloride microtiter plates (96-well, Falcon Micro Test III flexible assay plates; Becton-Dickinson, Oxnard, CA) are coated with BSA-ε-aminocaproyl-D-alanyl-D-alanine. The wells of the last vertical row of each plate are coated with BSA alone at a concentration of 10 mg/L and serve as blank wells. Each well in the microtiter plate contains fixed volumes (0.1 mL) of a standard solution of teicoplanin in PBS (0.15 mol/L NaCl and 0.05 mol/L sodium phosphate buffer, pH 7.3). The plates are incubated for 2 hours at 30°C in a covered, humidified box, washed eight times with PBS that contains 0.5 mL of Tween 201, and dried by shaking.

The wells are then filled with 0.1 mL of rabbit antiteicoplanin antiserum (diluted 250-fold with PBS/Tween 201 containing 3 g/L BSA) and allowed to react for 1 hour at room temperature. Microtiter plates are again washed with PBS/Tween 201. Each well is filled with 0.1 mL of peroxidase-conjugated goat antirabbit

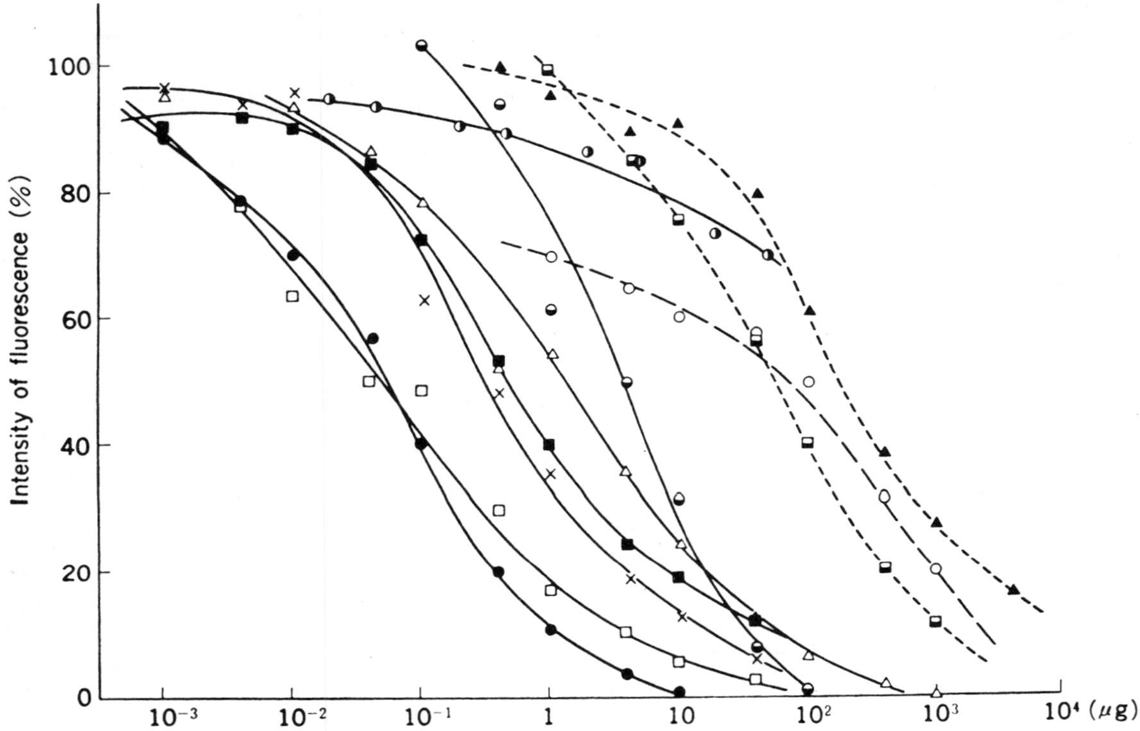

FIGURE 8.9 ● Heterologous nonisotopic immunoassay of ampicillin using an ampicillin-β-galactosidase conjugate. ●, Ampicillin; ■, penicillin G; ×, carbenicillin; □, sulbenicillin; ⊖, flucloxicillin; ⊟, cephalexin; ▲, cephaloglycin; ○, penicilloic acid. (From Kitagawa et al. [187], with permission.)

antibodies (diluted 1,500-fold with PBS/Tween 201/BSA). After reaction for 1 hour at room temperature and a wash step with PBS/Tween 201, 0.15 mL of chromogenic peroxidase substrate solution (1 g/L *o*-phenylenediamine and 3.5 mmol/L hydrogen peroxide, in 0.1 mol/L sodium citrate buffer, pH 5) is added to each microtiter well. After 30 minutes of color development at 30°C, the reaction is stopped by adding 50 μL of 4.5 mol/L sulfuric acid to each well. Ten minutes later, the absorbance at 492 nm is measured in a Titertek Multiskan photometer (Titertek, Huntsville, AL). The binding curves are obtained by plotting, on semilogarithmic paper, the absorbances at 492 nm as a function of the teicoplanin concentration.

Performance

This assay has been used to detect teicoplanin in serum, ascitic fluid, skin homogenates, bronchial expectorates, pleural fluid, and prostate homogenates. Wells coated with only BSA, without BSA-ε-aminocaproyl-D-alanyl-D-alanine, have shown that nonspecific binding is negligible. A dose-response curve that is linear in the teicoplanin range of 0.004 to 0.15 mg/L indicates that the sandwich complex is formed despite the low molecular mass of the antibiotic.

The interaction of teicoplanin with BSA-ε-aminocaproyl-D-alanyl-D-alanine and the antiteicoplanin antibodies is highly specific for teicoplanin because the receptor antibody sandwich assay does not give a response when other glycopeptide antibiotics are present in the concentration range of 0.001 to 100 mg/L. However, when teicoplanin solutions are assayed in the presence of vancomycin, recoveries of teicoplanin are lower than expected. Because similar effects are likely with other antibiotics of the same class, receptor antibody sandwich assays should not be used to determine teicoplanin concentrations in the presence of other glycopeptide antibiotics without performing studies that investigate possible interferences. The mean analytical recovery of teicoplanin with this assay is 99.5%. The interassay coefficient of variation is 5.13% for all samples. The detection limit is 0.03 mg/L. Receptor antibody sandwich assays of this type detect the total amount of immunoreactive material that is present in the sample, irrespective of biologic activity (71).

Homogeneous Nonisotopic Immunoassays

Fluorescence Quenching

Fluorescence quenching was the first widely available, homogeneous, nonisotopic immunoassay procedure for the assay of antibiotic concentrations. The method is based on the decrease in fluorescence that results from the combination of antibody with fluorescein-labeled antibiotic. This technique is rapid, sensitive, does not require an extraction step, and is automatable (291–293). The procedure is based on the same competitive binding principle that governs RIA.

Gentamicin

In a fluorescence-quenching assay for gentamicin, a drug that has been made fluorescent through a reaction with fluorescein thiocarbamyl (FTC), is mixed with a serum specimen that contains both gentamicin and antigentamicin antiserum. Antigentamicin antiserum combines with FTC-gentamicin and stoichiometrically decreases the fluorescence of the conjugated antibiotic. As the amount of unconjugated gentamicin in the serum sample increases, the amount of antigentamicin antiserum available for binding to the FTC-gentamicin conjugate decreases, causing a proportional rise in the emitted fluorescence (8,292).

Apparatus

Fluorometric measurements are made with a xenon arc lamp in standard 1 × 1 cm glass cells.

Reagents

FTC-gentamicin is produced by the reaction of 0.425 g/L gentamicin free base with 0.50 g/L fluorescein isothiocyanate isomer (Sigma Biochemicals, Sigma-Aldrich, St. Louis, MO) in 50 nmol/L sodium carbonate-bicarbonate buffer, pH 9.0. The mixture is incubated for 2 hours at room temperature. Two milliliters of the reaction mixture is chromatographed on a 1 × 97 cm Sephadex G-15 column eluted at 1.8 mL/minute with a carbonate-bicarbonate buffer. The purity of the eluate can be determined by electrophoresing the products on Whatman no. 1 paper in 20 nmol/L of sodium carbonate-bicarbonate buffer, pH 9.0, at 10 V/cm for 2 hours. The band is visualized under shortwave ultraviolet (UV) light. Antigentamicin antiserum is prepared in rabbits, as for the RIA method (211).

Procedure

Excitation is at 495 nm and emission at 540 nm. In constructing a standard curve, the fluorescence value of a serum sample without gentamicin should be subtracted from both the patient serum and standard readings.

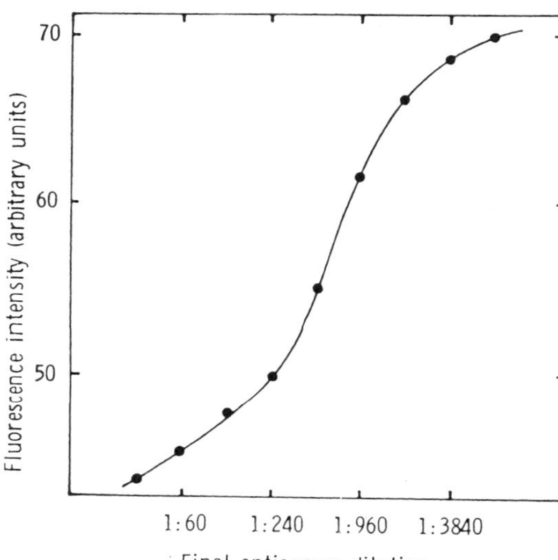

FIGURE 8.10 ● Standard curve for antibody dilution in the fluorescent quenching assay. (From Shaw [291], with permission.)

Antigentamicin antibody dilution curves are determined by making doubling dilutions in buffer of antigentamicin antiserum and pipetting 1-mL aliquots into two series of tubes. A 0.5-mL aliquot of a 1:200 dilution of stock FTC-gentamicin solution in buffer is added to each tube of one series and mixed. To each tube of the other series, 0.5 mL of the buffer is added. The tubes of the latter series serve as blanks that allow estimation of the fluorescence produced by the antiserum itself. Incubation is at room temperature for 5 minutes. The fluorescence of the test mixture and blanks is then measured. The corresponding blank signal is subtracted from the total signal of each test mixture. Figure 8.10 presents a typical antibody dilution curve.

The quenching-fluorescence assay method is performed by diluting 50 μL of serum specimen 1:50 in buffer. To prepare standards, gentamicin concentrations are made in a geometric series from 0.25 to 32 μg/mL and diluted 1:50 in buffer. Aliquots of 0.5 mL of the diluted samples or standards are pipetted in duplicate into two series of small tubes. To each tube of one series, 0.5 mL of the 1:200 dilution in buffer of the stock FTC-gentamicin solution is added and mixed. Then 0.5 mL aliquots of a 1:80 dilution in buffer or antigentamicin serum are added to each tube and the contents are immediately mixed. To each tube of the other series, 1 mL of buffer is added and mixed. This latter series serves for estimation of the fluorescence blank signals contributed by the intrinsic fluorescence of the serum samples or standards themselves.

The assay mixtures and blanks are incubated at room temperature for at least 5 minutes. All tubes are read in the

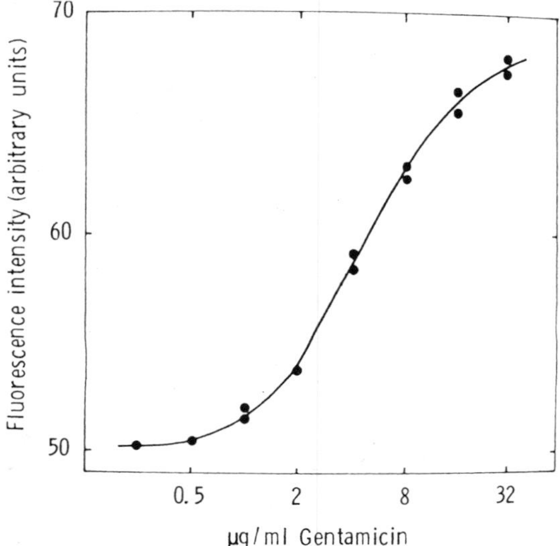

FIGURE 8.11 ● Quenching fluorescence immunoassay curve for the determination of a gentamicin blood level. One must extrapolate on the straight portion of the curve. (From Shaw [291], with permission.)

fluorometer. The corresponding blank signal is subtracted from the total signal of each assay mixture tube. The relationship between the amount of gentamicin present in the sample and the fluorescent intensity is presented in Figure 8.11.

Performance

The fluorescence-quenching method correlates with the RIA procedure at a correlation coefficient of 0.98. FTC-gentamicin is stable for more than 1 year. Once the antibody has been standardized, minimal technical manipulation is required for the method. Results are available within 15 minutes of receipt of a specimen. Also, the procedure is amenable to automation using continuous flow-type chemical analysis (8,292).

PARTICLE AGGLUTINATION ASSAY FOR GENTAMICIN

In an effort to develop a rapid and simple assay, the cost of which approaches that of the microbiologic assay, a hemagglutination inhibition assay for gentamicin was developed (212). The technique applies to gentamicin that is covalently linked to BSA, which is covalently linked to sheep erythrocytes and fixed in formaldehyde. This preparation is stable for up to 8 months in a refrigerator. The test is performed in Linbro microtiter trays (Flow Laboratories) with V wells. In principle, one drop of the patient's diluted serum is mixed with one drop of antiserum and, after 5 minutes at room temperature, one drop of gentamicin-bound sheep erythrocytes is added. The mixture is then incubated for 60 to 90 minutes at room temperature. Each of the reagents is standardized. If the patient's serum contains more gentamicin than is neutralized by the antiserum, agglutination of the gentamicin-coated sheep erythrocytes occurs. The lowest dilution of a patient's serum that causes agglutination is recorded.

A gentamicin standard containing 10 ng/mL is diluted to produce final concentrations of 0.31, 1.86, 2.97, 4.96, 6.51, 9.61, and 18.9 μg/mL in each microwell. Appropriate controls are added to adjacent wells. A given amount of reconstituted antiserum is added to all wells except the control well and the tray is mixed by gentle rotation. After 5 to 10 minutes, 50 μL of reconstituted cells is added to each well and the tray is mixed again by shaking. After 1 hour, the well number showing a pellet of cells equal to that of the control well is recorded. In effect, a titer, similar to cross-over broth dilution assays, is obtained. Although one can obtain only discontinuous values (values for which standard individual control wells are available), the method may prove effective if produced cheaply enough for clinical purposes. Based on the principle stated here, latex particles as carriers have also been marketed for the rapid semiquantitation of the major aminoglycoside/aminocyclitol antibiotics (184).

ENZYME-MULTIPLIED IMMUNOASSAY TECHNIQUE (EMIT)

The EMIT technique was developed from a free radical assay method that employed a spin label and detected drugs by electron spin resonance spectrometry. Electron spin resonance spectrometry requires expensive and very specialized equipment. EMIT was developed to bring the advantages of EIAs to clinical laboratories, without the requirement for large capital expenditures.

The heart of the EMIT is the attachment of an enzyme to the hapten. Commonly, lysozyme from egg whites, glucose-6-phosphate dehydrogenase from the bacterium *Leuconostoc mesenteroides*, malate dehydrogenase from pig heart mitochondria, and β-D-galactosidase from *E. coli* have been used as enzymes in EMIT assays. All these enzymes maintain significant activity after conjugation to the assayed drug.

Binding of antibody to the drug enzyme conjugate inhibits the activity of the enzyme. The large protein antibody sterically hinders the association of the substrate with the active site of the enzyme, resulting in a reduction in the quantity of the product that is produced. The EMIT assay employs the stoichiometric competition between the antibiotic in the serum sample and the enzyme-conjugated drug for antibody binding sites to derive the serum antibiotic concentration. The activity of the conjugated enzyme is decreased on antibody binding and the amount of enzyme activity is directly proportional to the concentrations

TABLE 8.9

Major Characteristics of the EMIT Nonisotopic Immunoassay System

Parameter	Characteristic
Analysis time	>1 min
Technologist time	<1 min
Sample volume	<10 μL
Number of samples/time	30–40 samples/h
Reagent stability, lyophilized	1 yr
Reagent stability, reconstituted	12 wk
Standard curve stability	8–72 h

of free and bound enzymes present in the assay mixture. Therefore, one can derive the concentration of antibiotic in a sample from quantitative measurements of the reaction products by relating them to a standard curve. The major steps in immunoassay by EMIT are as follows:

1. Drug of unknown concentration + antibody → antibody-drug
2. Drug enzyme conjugate + antibody → drug-enzyme-antibody
3. Substrate + antibiotic-enzyme → product

No separation step is required and the product is measured directly. Table 8.9 presents the major characteristics of the EMIT immunoassay. Table 8.10 lists the major advantages and disadvantages of the EMIT system.

TABLE 8.10

Advantages and Disadvantages of the EMIT System

Advantages
1. Small sample volume
2. Same technique for all antibiotics
3. Minimum technical skill and sample manipulation
4. Automatable
5. Results available quickly

Disadvantages
1. High cost of reagents
2. Analyzes drugs one at a time
3. May have interference from metabolites or similar compounds
4. May measure inactive metabolites

EMIT procedures have been modified for a wide variety of automated instruments. For example, Dade Behring's Syva EMIT Gentamicin 2000 homogeneous immunoassays are designed for used with most chemistry analyzers, including the company's Dimension combined chemistry/immunochemistry workstations. Many automated instruments automatically analyze the rate of change in absorbance of the sample or standard, correct for the absorbance from the drug-free control, and fit the data to a log-logit curve. In most cases, the coefficients of variation of the instruments range from 2% to 3%, but generally 5% should be expected. It must be noted that, because the standard curves are not linear, small analytical errors may cause relatively large concentration errors at their limits. Thus, accurate timing and pipetting are crucial. For this reason, automated systems, even though they require larger capital investments and cost more per test, are less labor-intensive and require fewer repeat assays than manual procedures (31,328,398).

As with immunoassays in general, there are few limitations on the use of EMIT or interferences with its performance. The most common interference is the presence of the unconjugated enzyme in the specimen. For example, lysozyme and malate dehydrogenase may be endogenous in urine specimens. Lipemia, hemolysis, and hyperbilirubinemia do not interfere significantly with EMIT assays. When using EMIT to measure antibiotic concentrations in urine, changes in the pH or ionic strength may introduce errors into the system. This can be particularly pronounced when urease-splitting microbes in the urine increase its pH. It had been noted with the EMIT, as well as with other nonisotopic immunoassay systems, that the reproducibility of standard curves diminished when most of the reagent in a bottle had been used. Since this phenomenon appeared to have been caused by reagent evaporation, many manufacturers began packaging their reagents in smaller vessels (229).

The labor cost per test in the EMIT system is relatively small compared with the microbiologic assay. Approximately 20% of EMIT and 60% of biologic assay costs are for labor. In general, for the assay of antibiotics, the rapid availability of the assays overcomes the requirement for single-drug analysis (37,332).

The basic apparatus for EMIT includes as ultraviolet/visible light spectrophotometer with a temperature-controlled cuvette, a timer/printer, and a pipette/diluter. In general, serum or urine samples are diluted with buffer before the antibody-substrate and enzyme-antibiotic reagents are added. The mixture is aspirated into a spectrophotometer and absorbance is measured at two time points.

Amikacin

The assay of amikacin by EMIT is presented as a model for the assay of aminoglycoside/aminocyclitol antibiotics by this method. The principles, apparatus, and procedures are identical for other antibiotics. In the EMIT procedure, serum or plasma is mixed with reagent antibiotic that is coupled to glucose-6-phosphate dehydrogenase (reagent A). After incubation, antibodies to the particular drug are added. Glucose-6-phosphate serves as the substrate for the enzyme, and NAD is used as a cofactor.

The antidrug antibody competitively binds to both the free antibiotic and the enzyme-labeled drug. Antibody binding to the antibiotic-enzyme conjugate inactivates the enzyme. Consquently, as the antibiotic concentration in the specimen increases, the activity of glucose-6-phosphate dehydrogenase proportionally increases. Enzyme activity is reflected in the conversion of NAD to NADH. This reduction reaction produces a color change that is spectrophotometrically measured. Since NAD serves as a cofactor with bacterial, but not human glucose-6-phosphate dehydrogenase, interferences due to the presence of the human form of the enzyme are avoided by using bacterial glucose-6-phosphate dehydrogenase (from *L. mesenteroides*) in the assay.

Apparatus

A spectrophotometer that is capable of measurement at 340 nm at a constant temperature of 30°C must be used. A data-handling device must be attached to the spectrophotometer to analyze and print absorbance readings. In the past, recommended spectrophotometers have included the Syva S-111 (Dade Behring, Inc.) and Gilford Stasar 111 (Gilford Instrument Laboratories, Inc., Oberlin, OH). Each of these spectrophotometers should be set in the absorbance mode, with distilled water set to an optical density of 1.000. The switch mode control is set to concentration, and the set display is placed at 2.667 with the concentration calibrator knob. The display is zeroed with the zero control knob. Data handling has been performed with a Syva CP-5000 clinical processor, Syva CP-1000 timer/printer, or Syva timer/printer model 2400. Automatic sample handling has been accomplished with the Syva pipette/diluter model 1500. Any semiautomatic pipette/diluter that is capable of sampling 50 μL and delivering this sample along with 250 mL of assay buffer with sufficient force to ensure that there adequate mixing of the reactants is satisfactory.

Reagents

Reagent A is amikacin to which has been covalently coupled glucose-6-phosphate dehydrogenase (the means of coupling is proprietary). This reagent, when reconstituted in buffer, is standardized to work with reagent B. Reagent A is reconstituted from the lyophilized form by adding 6.0 mL of distilled water. Following reconstitution, the reagent may be stored in the refrigerator overnight, but it must remain at room temperature for at least 2 hours before use. Reagent A should always be stored at 2°C to 8°C; it has a shelf life of 12 weeks.

Reagent B contains sheep antiamikacin antibody. This antibody-substrate reagent contains a standardized preparation of sheep γ-globulin, enzyme substrate glucose-6-phosphate, the coenzyme NAD, and preservatives in Tris buffer, pH 5.2. The lyophilized reagent is reconstituted with 6 mL of distilled water and must be allowed to remain at room temperature for at least 2 hours before use. Reagent B may be reconstituted and allowed to remain at 28°C overnight, but must come to room temperature before use. It must be stored at 2°C to 8°C and is stable for 12 weeks.

The standard buffer solution used for dilution in the EMIT assay is 0.055 mol/L Tris-HCl buffer, pH 8.0, with a small amount of surfactant. The buffer solution is stable at room temperature for up to 12 weeks. Six amikacin calibrators and a control must be used. The calibrators are reconstituted with 1.0 mL of distilled water and the controls are reconstituted with 3.0 mL of distilled water. After reconstitution, the calibrators and controls must remain at room temperature for at least 2 hours before use. The calibrators and controls may be reconstituted and refrigerated overnight before use, but must be at room temperature when the assays are run. The calibrators and controls must be stored at 2°C to 8°C and are stable for 12 weeks. The calibrators contain amikacin concentrations of 0, 2.5, 10, 20, and 50 μg/mL. The controls contain 15 μg/mL amikacin.

Procedure

Preparations for the test are made as follows: (a) all reagents are prepared as previously described, (b) all reagents must be well mixed and brought to room temperature, (c) all instruments must be properly calibrated, (d) the spectrophotometer must be zeroed with distilled water to 0.000, (e) the pipetter/diluter should be primed and flushed with buffer to ensure that there are no air bubbles in the lines, and (f) there must be a sufficient number of beakers present in the work rack. For calibrating, and for assaying unknowns, measurements should be made in duplicate and the results averaged. Duplicate readings that differ by more than six absorbance units should be repeated. The pipette tips must be carefully wiped with laboratory tissues both before and after the delivery of each solution. Solutions should not be held in the tubing for more than 5 seconds before delivery. The samples are analyzed as follows:

1. The calibrator, control, or specimen is diluted by delivering 50 μL of the appropriate solution and 250 μL of buffer to a 2.0-mL disposable beaker.
2. The sample is diluted again by adding 50 μL of the diluted sample from no. 1 to 250 μL of buffer solution and delivering this mixture to a second 2.0-mL disposable beaker.
3. Fifty microliters of reagent A is mixed with 250 μL of buffer solution, with delivery to the second beaker.

4. The spectrophotometer flow cell is purged.
5. Fifty microliters of reagent B plus 250 μL of buffer solution is added to the second beaker.
6. Immediately after the addition of reagent B, the contents of the second beaker are aspirated into the spectrophotometer flow cell. The printer/recorder should be automatically activated.
7. For the remaining samples, controls, and calibrators, steps 1 through 6 are repeated.
8. The spectrophotometer flow cell must be cleaned with the cleaning solution supplied with the instrument and the pipette/dilution lines must be stored in distilled water. After a 15-second delay, absorbance readings are made for each sample. The change in absorbance over a 30-second measurement period is used to calculate results.

The difference between the average calibrator zero reading (A_0) and the reading of each of the other calibrators (A), known as A - A_0, must be determined to plot a standard curve and to calculate the concentrations of the unknown samples. The Syva CP-5000 clinical processor automatically calculates the concentration of amikacin. The Syva CP-1000 timer/printer and Syva timer/printer model 2400 have built-in memory functions that store the A_0 reading so that the technologist may perform the necessary calculations on log-logit paper. The technologist derives the amikacin concentrations by preparing a standard curve and plotting A - A_0 for each calibrator against the calibrator concentrations on the lot-specific graph paper that is supplied with each reagent kit. A best-fit line is constructed. Each time a new bottle of reagent A, reagent B, or buffer is used, a new standard line must be prepared. Furthermore, new standard lines must be drawn whenever duplicate controls vary by more than 10% or if any calibrator point lies more than six absorbance units off the line.

Performance

The EMIT amikacin assay is designed to measure the concentration of this antibiotic in serum or plasma. The major form of nontechnical error is generated by cross-reactivity with other compounds. Kanamycin significantly cross-reacts with the amikacin assay. Table 8.11 lists the concentration of a number of antibiotics that are required to produce a 30% measurement error in a sample that contains 10 μg/mL kanamycin. The assay range of quantitation is between 2.5 and 50 μg/mL. The coefficient of variation between runs is typically approximately 10%.

The EMIT has proven accuracy in clinical settings with the following limitations: (a) when β-lactam antibiotics are present in addition to amikacin, specimens must be assayed immediately or stored frozen; (b) severely hemolytic, lipemic, or icteric samples may interfere with the assay; and (c) kanamycin shows significant cross-reactivity with the amikacin assay. Table 8.9 describes the major performance characteristics of the EMIT immunoassay system (43,354).

TABLE 8.11

Antibiotic Serum Concentrations Required to Produce 30% Error in a Specimen Containing 10 μg/mL Kanamycin (31)

Antibiotic	Concentration (μg/mL)
Carbenicillin	500
Cephalothin	500
Chloramphenicol	500
Clindamycin	500
Erythromycin	500
Gentamicin	100
Neomycin	500
Netilmicin	100
Penicillin	1000
Tetracycline	1000
Ticarcillin	500
Tobramycin	100
Sisomicin	100
Streptomycin	500
Sulfonamide	500

Chloramphenicol

The recommended peak CAM concentration is from 10 to 20 mg/L (15 to 25 mg/L for meningitis). Because of CAM's potential toxicity, therapeutic monitoring of blood levels may be desirable with its use. Bioassays involve tedious preparation and lengthy incubation times. HPLC uses expensive equipment, and highly trained personnel are needed to perform HPLC assays. The following method describes a Syva EMIT assay (Dade Behring, Inc.) that was developed for measurement of CAM in human serum (282).

The Syva EMIT kit may be purchased from Dade Behring, Inc. Calibrators and buffers are reconstituted according to the manufacturer's instructions. The assay has been performed with a Cobas-Bio centrifugal analyzer (Roche Analytical Instruments, Nutley, NJ) that was equipped with DENS (Data Reduction for Nonlinear Standard Curves) program version 8326. A standard curve for CAM is stored in the Cobas-Bio analyzer and the results from the individual serum samples are compared with the standard curve.

The sensitivity of the assay, defined as the smallest amount of CAM that can be accurately measured, is 2.5 mg/L (7.7 mol/L) for EMIT. Lower concentrations of CAM can be detected, but not accurately quantified. The within-day precision coefficient of variation for EMIT is 4.0% at 5.0 mg/L, and the between-day coefficient of variation is less than 5.5%. When compared with HPLC and bioassay methods, the EMIT is specific for CAM and correlates well by regression analysis. The EMIT measures only the biologically active base form of the drug, uses a small sample size (0.2 mL), and provides rapid results. However, the reagents are expensive, and personnel need special training to perform the assay.

SUBSTRATE-LABELED IMMUNOFLUORESCENT ASSAY

The substrate-labeled immunofluorescent assay (SLIFA), like other immunoassays that are used to measure antibiotic concentrations, is based on competitive inhibition of the label of conjugated drug by drug that is present in the specimen. In the SLIFA procedure, the fluorescent moiety umbelliferone is generated from β-galactosylumbelliferone that is covalently bound to the antibiotic. In its usual state, the labeled antibiotic does not fluoresce. However, if the antibiotic-substrate reagent is cleaved by β-galactosidase, umbelliferone is released. When the β-galactosylumbelliferone-drug conjugate binds to the antidrug antibody, the conjugate is prevented from interacting with the enzyme. As in any competitive binding assay, the free antibiotic in serum sample competes with the conjugate for binding sites on the antibodies. The amount of conjugate available for the reaction is, therefore, directly related to the amount of free drug in the serum sample. In the SLIFA, the rate of increase in the intensity of fluorescence is proportional to the amount of antibiotic in the sample.

The reaction to label the aminoglycoside class of antibiotics with β-galactosylumbelliferone is a carbodiimide procedure. The reaction sequence proceeds in the same manner with all aminoglycoside/aminocyclitol antibiotics. For the aminoglycoside amikacin, the β-galactosylumbelliferone reaction is performed by adding 50 mg of the potassium salt of β-[7-(3-carboxycoumarinoxyl)]-β-galactoside to 171 mg of amikacin sulfate in 2 mL of water. The pH is adjusted to 3.8 and the mixture is cooled to 0°C (in an ice bath). Thirty milligrams of 1-ethyl-[3-(3-dimethylaminopropyl)]carbodiimide hydrochloride are added.

After 2 hours the mixture is chromatographed at 25°C on a 2.5 × 50 cm column of CM-Sephadex C-25. The effluent is monitored at 345 nm. The column is washed with 200 mL of 50 mmol/L ammonium formate to elute the unreacted β-galactosylumbelliferone-amikacin. A linear gradient is formed with 400 mL of 50 mmol/L and 400 mL of 1.8 mol/L ammonium formate solution and applied to the column. A peak of material is eluted at a concentration of approximately 1.4 mol/L ammonium formate. The column is washed with 600 mL of 1.8 mol/L ammonium formate. The carbodiimide reaction appears to lead to the formation of amide bonds between the carboxylic acid of 1β-[7-(3-carboxycoumarinoxyl)]galactoside and the primary amino groups of the aminoglycoside antibiotic.

Amikacin

In the past, SLIFA kits have been commercially available for the assay of aminoglycoside/aminocyclitol antibiotics, including gentamicin, tobramycin, and amikacin (85,192). In addition, noncommercial antibiotic SLIFA kits have been produced for other aminoglycoside/aminocyclitol antibiotics. The procedure for the assay of amikacin in human serum or plasma is identical to other aminoglycoside/aminocyclitol assays. Only the absolute amounts of some of the reactants differ.

Apparatus

The SLIFA may be performed with any fluorescence spectrophotometer. Most commonly, either an Aminco-Bowman spectrophotofluorometer (American Instrument Company) or an Ames fluorocolorimeter (Miles Laboratories, Elkhart, IN) has been employed. The Aminco instrument is set for excitation at 400 nm and emission at 450 nm. The Ames instrument requires a 450 nm, narrow bandpass, interference filter for excitation, and a glass 5–56 (blue) filter on top of a glass 3–73 (yellow) filter for emission light. The described SLIFA is not completely hands off in the sense that there are no microprocessors and flow-through apparatus available to interpret the data. Accessory equipment includes: (a) disposable fluorescence polystyrene cuvettes (Evergreen Scientific, Los Angeles, CA), (b) a pipetter/diluter equipped with a 250 μL reagent syringe and a 2.5 mL buffer syringe, (c) an accurate timer, and (d) 13 × 100 mm test tubes. It should be noted that aminoglycoside/aminocyclitol antibiotics may adsorb from dilute solutions onto glass. Therefore, plastic test tubes should always be used. (This physicochemical guideline applies to all assays, not just the SLIFA.)

Reagents

The antibody-enzyme reagent is composed of 1.5 units of β-galactosidase and antiserum-to-amikacin in 50 mmol/L bicine/0.1% sodium azide buffer (Worthington Biochemical, Inc., Freehold, NJ). Bicine buffer ([*N*,*N*-bis[2-hydroxyethyl]glysine) (grade A; Calbiochem, La Jolla, CA) is used at pH 8.5. The enzyme should be standardized at 25°C in 3 mL bicine buffer, pH 8.5, containing 3 mmol/L *o*-nitrophenyl-β-D-galactoside. The molar extinction coefficient for the product of this reaction, *o*-nitrophenyl, is 4.27 at 415 nm. One unit of enzyme activity hydrolyzes 1.0 mmol of substrate per minute. The antiserum has been commercially available (316). The antiserum must be of potency to inhibit the fluorescence to 10% to 20% of that in the absence of antiserum.

The antibiotic-drug conjugate consists of β-galactosylumbelliferyl-amikacin (0.007 absorbance units at 343 nm) in 5 mmol/L formate with 0.1% sodium azide buffer, pH 3.5. Each reaction mixture must contain 0.00035 absorbance units at 343 nm.

Standard amikacin concentrations should be made in normal human serum in the range of 0, 10, 20, 30, and 40 μg/mL amikacin. The range adjustment solution consists of a mixture of 7-hydroxycoumarin-3-(*N*-hydroxyethyl)carboxamide in 5 mmol/L formate, pH 3.5, with a final concentration of 0.1% sodium azide buffer. When 50 μL of the range adjustment solution is mixed with 1.5 mL of bicine buffer, the fluorescence intensity must be comparable to that absorbed with the high calibration samples at the end of a 20-minute incubation. The fluorescent antibiotic reagent must absorb maximally at 343 nm. However, on hydrolysis by β-galactosidase, the absorbance at 343 nm must decrease and a new maximum must appear at 405 nm. The absorbance of the enzyme-antibiotic conjugate at 405 nm after hydrolysis should be 1.6 times that at 343 nm before hydrolysis.

Procedure

After reconstitution, all components can be stored at 2°C to 3°C for up to 10 weeks. All components must be at room temperature before the assay is performed. The assay proceeds as follows.

1. Using a pipette/diluter, 1:50 dilutions of the calibrators and samples are made by diluting 50 μL of each specimen with 2.5 mL of diluted bicine buffer.
2. Fifty microliters of the antibody-enzyme reagent and 500 μL of buffer are dispensed, using the pipette/diluter, into the reaction cuvettes that are required for duplicate determinations of the calibrators and samples.
3. Fifty microliters of each of the diluted calibrators and samples is mixed with 500 μL of buffer and added to the reaction cuvettes.
4. Starting in the same calibrator sequence, the reactions are initiated at timed intervals by dispensing 50 μL of the amikacin fluorogenic reactant and 500 μL of buffer to each cuvette. The reactants must be thoroughly mixed.
5. After approximately 19 minutes, the reactions are read in sequence by zeroing the instrument with buffer and reading the first specimen in the fluorometer after adjusting the fluorescence reading to 90% of full scale.
6. At 20 minutes, the fluorescence intensity of the highest calibrator is read and recorded. Then the fluorescence intensity of the remaining cuvettes is read and recorded in the same sequence as that in which the reactions were initiated.

TABLE 8.12

Performance Characteristics for the Assay of Amikacin by the SLIFA Technique (259)

Characteristic	Parameter
Intraassay precision (15 μg/mL)	
Mean	15 μg/mL
Coefficient of variation	2.4%
Interassay precision (15 μg/mL control)	
Mean	15.5 μg/mL
Coefficient of variation	1.6%
Sensitivity	1.0 μg/mL
Correlation with RIA	
Correlation coefficient	0.99
Slope	0.95
Intercept	0.2 μg/mL
Standard error of estimate	1.6 μg/mL

7. The concentration of amikacin in the assay is determined by constructing a standard line by plotting the average fluorescence readings for duplicate calibrators versus the amikacin concentrations.

The SLIFA performs comparably with other radiometric and nonisotopic immunoassays. Table 8.12 presents the salient performance characteristics of the assay for amikacin. As demonstrated in Figure 8.12, kanamycin and tobramycin cross-react at 2.4% and 0.2%, respectively, changing the response to the maximum dose by 50%. Other aminoglycoside/aminocyclitol antibiotics, including gentamicin, netilmicin, sisomicin, and streptomycin, do not significantly interfere with the assay. Additional antibiotics that have been tested, including carbenicillin, cephalothin, CAM, erythromycin, methicillin, and tetracycline, do not appear to affect the assay (257).

The assay of amikacin by the SLIFA technique is accurate from 5 to 50 μg/mL. The accuracy of the SLIFA is affected by the same factors as other immunoassays of antibiotics (257).

Cycling Enzyme Assay

Cycling procedures are inherently appealing because they do not consume reagents during the course of reactions and can, therefore, use the same reagents for extended periods of time. Historically, the coenzymes NAD^+ and flavin adenine dinucleotide have been most frequently used as reaction co-factors. The assays have traditionally

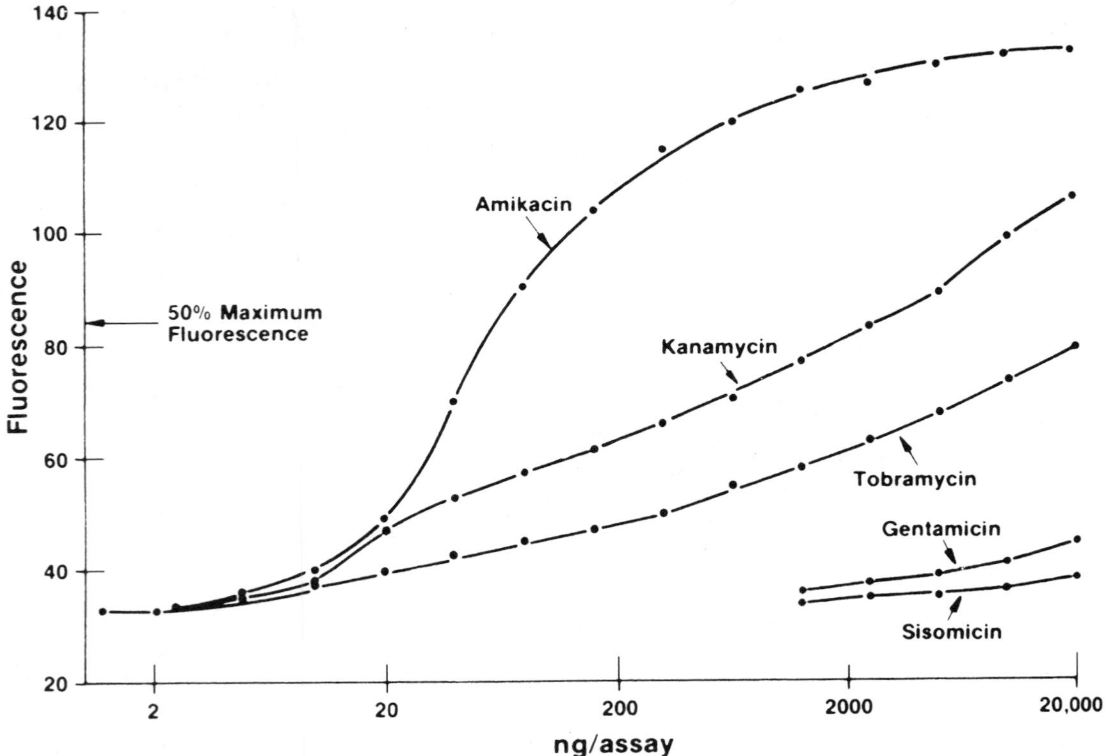

FIGURE 8.12 ● Cross-reactivity of aminoglycoside/aminocyclitol antibiotics in the SLIFA nonisotopic immunoassay. (From Thompson and Burd [316], with permission.)

suffered from a lack of suitable detection systems for biologic samples. Cycling procedures have been described that use alcohol dehydrogenase and malate dehydrogenase as reagents. These assays are of limited use with biologic specimens because significant interference is generally present during the enzymatic cycling steps and in the final fluorometric measurements. An enzymatic cycling procedure with two irreversible reactions that are catalyzed by NAD^+ peroxidase and glucose-6-phosphate dehydrogenase has been devised. This cycling procedure is not adversely affected in an appreciable way by biologic fluids.

The reaction has been designed to proceed as follows:

1. Gentamicin + (NAD^+-gentamicin) + antibody → gentamicin-antibody + (NAD^+-gentamicin)-antibody.
2. (NAD^+-gentamicin) + glucose-6-phosphate + glucose-6-phosphate dehydrogenase → (NADH-gentamicin) + H^+ + 6-phosphogluconate (cycling step).
3. 6-Phosphogluconate + NADP + glucose-6-phosphate dehydrogenase → NADPH + H^+ + ribulose-5-phosphate + CO_2 (indicator reaction).

Apparatus

A Perkin-Elmer model 555 ultraviolet/visible spectrophotometer (Perkin Elmer, Norwalk, CT) has been used for determining absorbance. This gentamicin assay has been performed with an Eppendorf model 1101M spectrophotometer (Eppendorf, Hamburg, Germany) that is equipped with a 334-nm filter.

Reagents

NAD^+ peroxidase (EC 1.11.1.1), glucose-6-phosphate dehydrogenase (EC 11.1.49), NAD phosphate ($NADP^+$) 1-oxoreductase from *L. mesenteroides*, 6-phosphogluconate dehydrogenase (EC 1.1.1.44), $NADP^+$ 2-oxoreductase, and β-D-glucose-6-phosphate crystallized monosodium salt were all obtained from Boehringer-Mannheim (Mannheim, Germany). Antigentamicin antibodies were obtained from Atlantic Antibodies (Scarborough, ME).

Procedure

For synthesis of NAD^+-labeled gentamicin, 5 g of gentamicin sulfate is dissolved in 15 mL of water. The pH of the solution is adjusted to 11.5 with 5 mol/L NaOH. The mixture is lyophilized and extracted in 2 liters of boiling methanol. Free gentamicin base is dried in a vacuum. Gentamicin is conjugated to NAD^+ after the coenzyme has been converted to N^6-(2-carboxyethyl)-NAD^+. One gram of gentamicin base is dissolved in 5 mL of water, with the pH adjusted to 7.0 using 6 mol/L HCl. One hundred milligrams of N^6-(2-carboxyethyl)-NAD^+ and 500 mg of 1-ethyl-3-(3-dimethylaminopropyl)carbodiimide are dissolved in 2 mL of water. The pH is kept constant at 4.7 for a 3-hour incubation period. After incubation, the pH is adjusted to 7.0 and the mixture is applied to a Dowex 1-X2 column (chloride form, 2.6 × 40 cm) and eluted with water (100 mL/hour). The UV-absorbing fraction is concentrated on a rotary evaporator. The mixture is desalted on a Sephadex G-15 column (2.6 × 60 cm), with water as the eluent. The UV-absorbing material is applied to a BioRex 70 column (2.6 × 40 cm) that has been previously washed with 20 mmol/L ammonium acetate. The void volume is washed out at 100 mL/hour with 60 mmol/L ammonium acetate. Elution is accomplished with a linear gradient of ammonium acetate (20 to 50 mmol/L) over a period of 4 hours. The UV-absorbing fraction contains both NAD^+ and gentamicin.

The fraction that contains both NAD^+ and gentamicin is concentrated and fractionated on a Bio-Gel P4 column (2.6 × 60 cm) with water flowing at 40 mL/hour. After volume reduction to 10 mL, the two NADH and gentamicin peaks are stored at −30°C. These two peaks are analyzed for NAD^+content using ethanol and alcohol dehydrogenase. Peak 1 has a molar absorbtivity at 265 nm of 24.1×10^3/mol/L/cm in the oxidized form and 20.7×10^3/mol/L/cm in the reduced form. Peak 2 has absorbtivity of 2.9×10^3/mol/L/cm in the oxidized form and 19.2×10^3/mol/L/cm in the reduced form. Peak 1 has a gentamicin content by RIA of 1.45 μg/mL and peak 2 a gentamicin content of 0.99 μg/mL.

Fifty microliters of sample is added to 50 μL of the ice-cooled cycling reagent that contains 0.2 mol/L Tris, 0.28 mol/L potassium acetate, 12 mmol/L β-D-glucose-6-phosphate, 12 mmol/L hydrogen peroxide, 200 μg/mL NAD^+ peroxidase, and 200 μg/mL glucose-6-phosphate dehydrogenase, pH 8.5. The solution is mixed for 2 hours at 30°C. After cooling, 0.5 mL of 20 mmol/L Tris, 30 mmol/L ammonium acetate, 0.1 mmol/L ethylenediaminetetraacetate, 0.2 g/L BSA, 0.6 mmol/L $NADP^+$, and 10 μg/mL 6-phosphogluconate dehydrogenase, pH 7.7 (the spectrophotometric indicator reagent), is added. The absorbance at 334 nm is recorded after the mixture is incubated for 30 minutes at 25°C.

Interpretation

Figure 8.13 demonstrates the inhibition of NAD^+-gentamicin peak 2 by antigentamicin antiserum at various gentamicin levels. A standard curve for gentamicin was calculated from these values and is displayed in Figure 8.14. The absorbance values for gentamicin standards and patient specimens are measured at 334 nm, and after subtracting blank absorbance values, related to the gentamicin concentrations.

Performance

The spectrophotometric enzyme cycling procedure is able to detect 5 ng of gentamicin (0.1 μg/mL). The method is equal to other nonisotopic immunoassays and RIA in the range of 1 to 10 μg/mL. The intraassay coefficient of variation is 6.1% with a mean at 7.4 μg/mL. The intraassay coefficient of variation is 3.4% at a concentration of 13.1 μg/mL. The specificity and performance of the spectrophotometric cycling enzyme assay are equal to those of other nonisotopic immunoassays and the standard RIA method. In addition, reagents are not rapidly consumed and measurements may be made on a simple spectrophotometer (116).

FLUORESCENCE POLARIZATION IMMUNOASSAY

Like the other nonradioactive immunoassay techniques such as SLIFA and EMIT, the FPIA method was developed as a technology to assay small molecules. The theoretical basis for FPIA was described in the early 1970s by Dandliker et al. (81). Subsequently, Abbott Laboratories accelerated the entry of this technology into clinical laboratories by developing an automated fluorescence polarization analyzer system (41).

A molecule naturally gravitates toward its lowest energy state, but becomes excited after exposure to light. This excitation is the result of electrons moving from a lower energy shell to a higher energy shell. The leap to higher energy levels, governed by the laws of quantum mechanics, is temporary. The electron naturally returns to its original energy shell. The amount of energy gained during the first jump to a higher energy shell is greater than the amount of energy that the molecule loses when the electron returns to its normal orbit. The wavelength of light that is emitted during the return trip (emitted light) is longer than that which is absorbed during the primary jump (excitation light) and is measured as fluorescence. Ordinary (white) light contains a spectrum of wavelengths (white light). The electrical vectors of light waves that are produced by standard sources are randomly oriented. Excitation sources that are used in flurorimeters can emit light at one, several, or a range of wavelengths of interest depending on the applications for which the instrument is used. The intensity of the emitted fluorescent light is related to the excitation intensity of the initially absorbed light at the absorption wavelength.

Plane-polarized light is generated when light is passed through crystalline materials known as "polarizers." A polarizer orients the electrical vectors of incoming light waves in a single plane. Fluorescence polarization occurs when fluorophores that have been excited by polarized

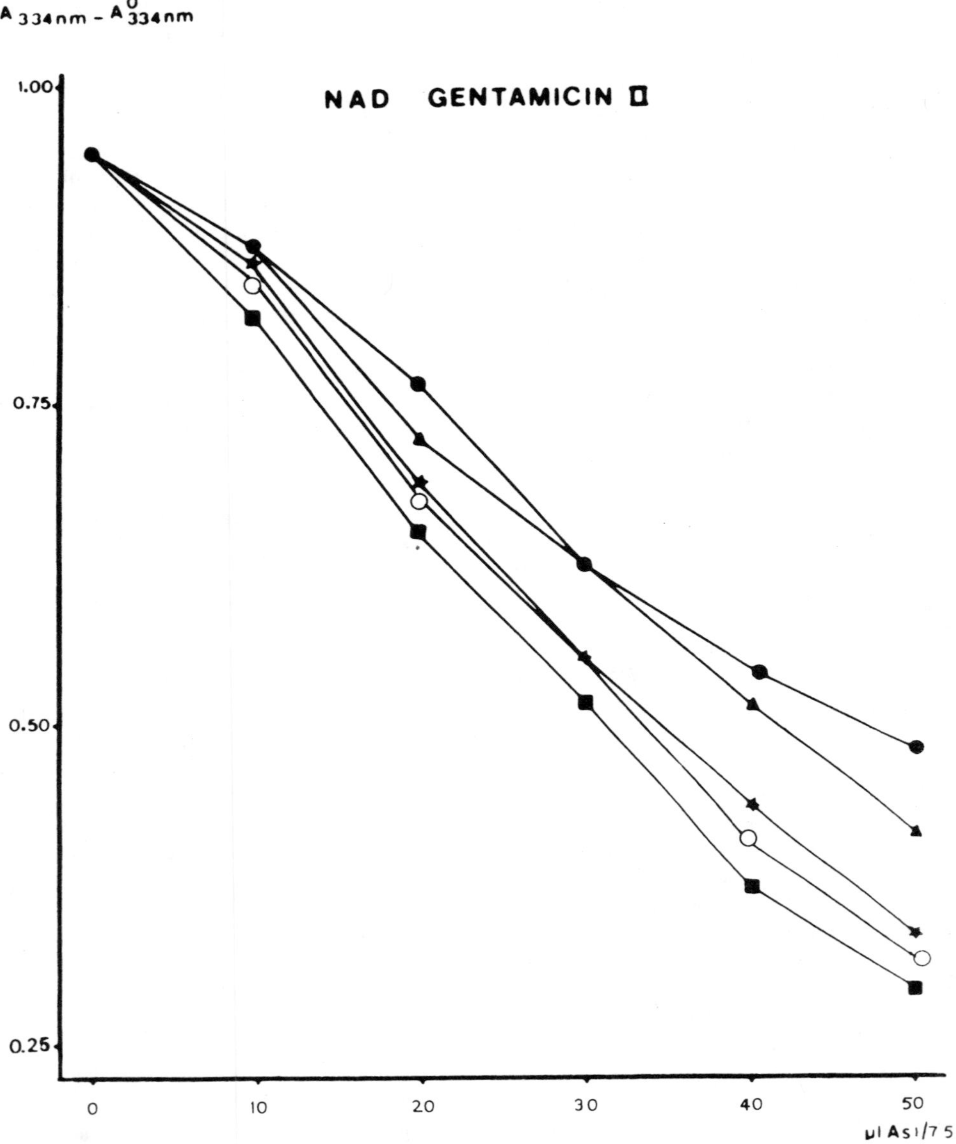

FIGURE 8.13 ● Inhibition of NAD$^+$-gentamicin by antigentamicin antiserum for various levels of gentamicin (■, 0 μg/mL; ○, 0.3 μg/mL; ★, 0.5 μg/mL; ▲, 1 μg/mL; ●, 1.5 μg/mL).

light also emit polarized light. This occurs when the Brownian movement (rotational relaxation) of the fluorophores under analysis is slower than their fluorescence decay times. Small molecules rotate rapidly, such that their rotational relaxation times are much shorter than their fluorescence decay times. Consequently, small fluorophores emit depolarized fluorescent light, while large fluorophores emit polarized fluorescent light (107a).

In developing the FPIA technique, the fluorescence decay times and rotational relaxation times of the molecules under study needed to be considered. The fluorescence decay time of the molecule is the time interval from the moment it is struck by polarized light until it releases its emitted light (336). The rotational relaxation time describes the molecule's Brownian motion and is the time an oriented molecule takes to leave alignment after an incoming burst of polarized light. To effectively determine analyte concentrations with an FPIA assay that uses routine equipment, the rotational relaxation time of the molecule under analysis must be 1 nanosecond or

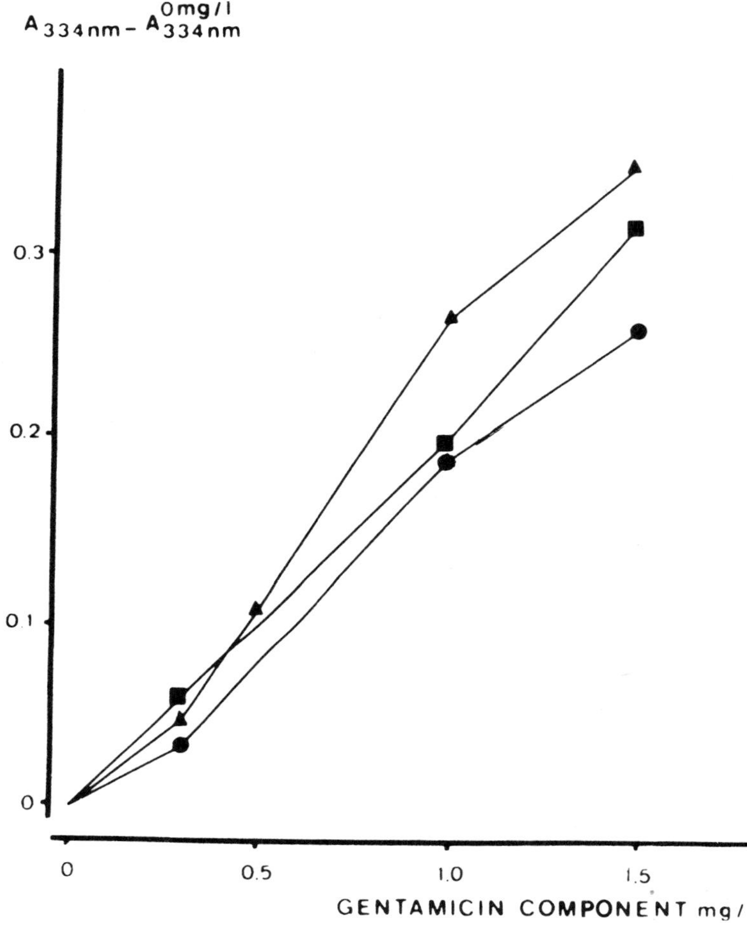

FIGURE 8.14 • Standard curves for gentamicin components by the cycling immunoassay. ▲, C_1; ●, C_{1a}; ■, C_2.

less. This limits the use of the technique to the analysis of small molecules. For example, immunoglobulins have rotational relaxation times of approximately 100 nanoseconds.

The fluorescent light intensity that is produced by the sample is measured both parallel to and perpendicular to the plane of the polarized excitation light. The fluorescence polarization is measured by the following formula:

$$P = (I_{PAR} - I_{PERP})/(I_{PAR} + I_{PERP}),$$

where I_{PAR} (parallel) is the intensity of fluorescence parallel to the plane of the excitation light and I_{PERP} (perpendicular) is the intensity of fluorescence perpendicular to the plane of the excitation light.

In practice, the antibiotic is labeled with fluorescein. When the antibiotic binds to a specific antibody, the rotational relaxation time of the large antigen-antibody complex is increased so that it exceeds the fluorescence decay time of the label. The concentrations of antibody and fluorescent-labeled antigen are kept constant, with the only variable being the concentration of the antibiotic (unlabeled antigen) in the specimen. The higher the concentration of free antibiotic in the sample, the more this antigen limits binding of the labeled antibiotic to antibody, resulting in a proportional decrease in fluorescence polarization (127,170,227,321,322). Conversely, as the concentration of unlabeled antibiotic decreases, the amount of fluorescence polarization proportionately increases.

Fluorescence Immunoassay Method

Apparatus

A specially designed fluorometer with microprocessor controls is available from Abbott Laboratories. Figure 8.15 presents the instrument and specimen flow pathways.

The filament of a General Electric EFM 50W tungsten/halogen lamp is focused through a 3-mm diameter

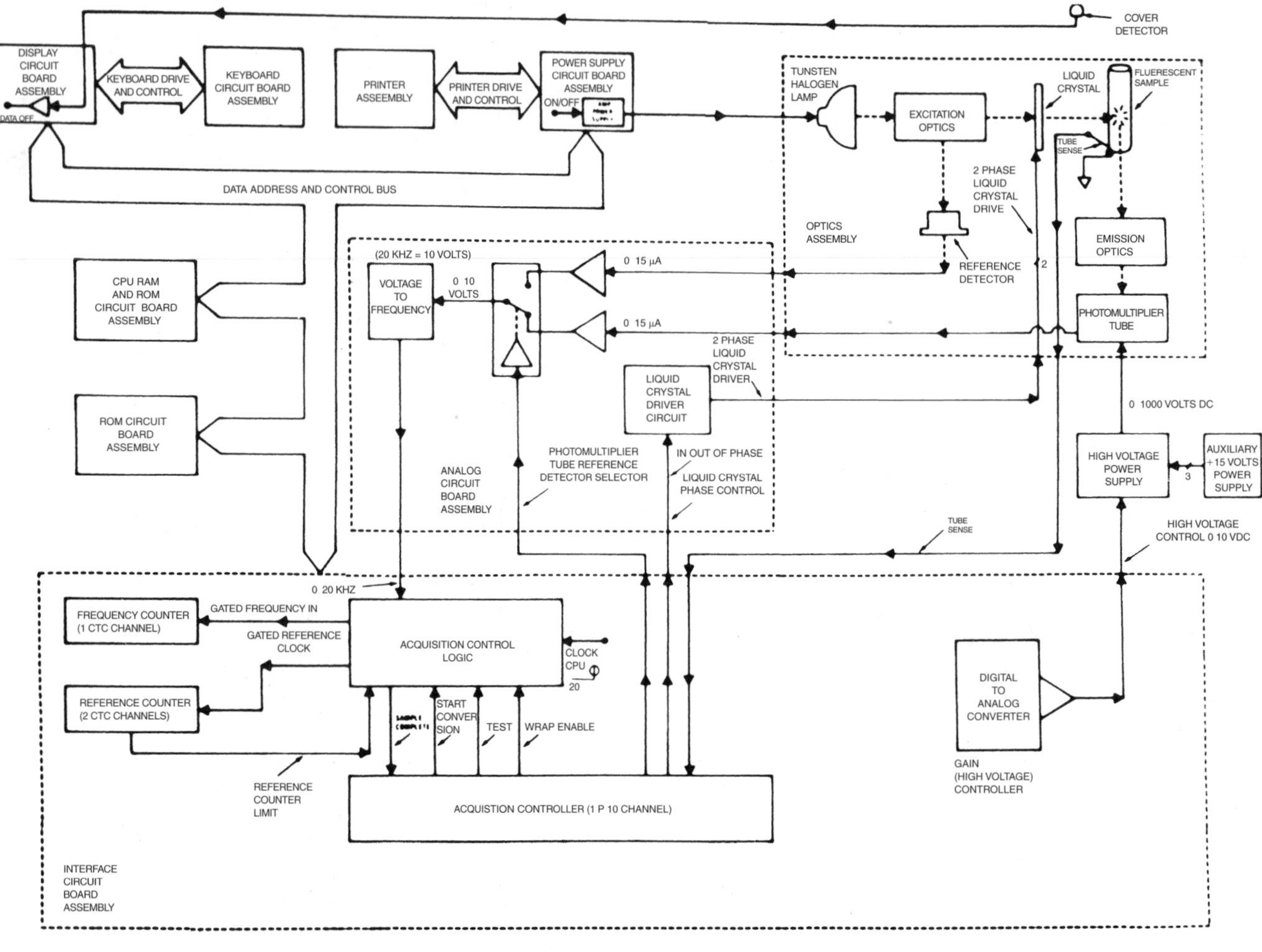

FIGURE 8.15 ● Schematic representation of the analysis of aminoglycoside antibiotics by FPIA, using an automated instrument. (From Popelko et al. [258], with permission.)

entrance aperture. After passing through heat-absorbing glass (BD-38; Corion Corp., Holliston, MA), the light is collimated. All lenses in the system are Mellesgriot plano-convex lenses that have a focal length of 18 mm and a diameter of 15 mm. The collimated light is directed through a 10-nm bandwidth, 485-nm center wavelength, excitation filter (Corion). Light reflected from the transparent glass beam splitter (Corning coverglass no. 1, Corning, NY) is focused onto a UV 215 B reference silicon detector (EG & G, Salem, MA). The reference detector signal is used to monitor the intensity of the lamp. The light transmitted through the beam splitter passes through a HN38S polarizer/crystalloid transmission type liquid crystal combination (Polaroid, Cambridge, MA). This beam splitter also serves to rotate the plane of polarization. The excitation light is directed onto the sample, which is contained in a 12 × 75 mm glass tube. The emitted light is collimated through a lens, passed through a 10-nm band with a 525-nm interference filter, and then directed through a vertical HN38S polarizer. The emitted light is focused onto a 3 × 8 mm aperture and R928 photomultiplier tube (Hamamatsu Corp., Middlesex, NJ). The excitation optics and the emission optics are perpendicular. The polarizer/liquid crystal combination is rotated in an electric field applied to the liquid crystal. When voltage is directed through the liquid crystal, no rotation occurs and horizontal light passes through the sample. When there is no voltage, the liquid crystal rotates by 90% and the sample is excited by vertical light (254,339).

Measurements are made as directed by the microprocessor through emission fluorescence intensity measured by the photomultiplier tube. The gain of the photomultiplier tube is controlled by a model PMT-20 A/N high-voltage power supply (Bertran Associates, Syosset, NY). Both the excitation and fluorescent polarization intensities are captured in the vertical and horizontal modes and converted from voltages to frequencies, which are measured by a counter timer. Intensity values are presented as the ratio of the frequency channel counts to the reference clock channel counts (258).

Reagents

The fluorescein conjugate of amikacin is prepared by reacting the antibiotic with 5-[(4,6-dichlorotriazian-2-yl)amino] fluorescein. The fluorescein compound is dissolved in methanol and added to amikacin in water at pH 9.0. The final concentration of the fluorescein reagent is 16 mol/L and that of amikacin is 160 mol/L. After 1 hour at room temperature, the mixture is applied to a diethylaminoethyl-cellulose chromatography column with 0.1 mol/L phosphate buffer, pH 8, as the eluent.

The amikacin-fluorescein conjugate is diluted in 0.1 mol/L Tris(hydroxymethyl)methylamine buffer, pH 7.5, that contains 1.212 g/L sodium dodecyl sulfate, 0.1 g/L bovine γ-globulin, and 0.1 g/L sodium azide. The concentration of the conjugate is approximately 100 nmol/L. Antiserum is diluted in a phosphate buffer, pH 7.5, that contains 0.1 g/L bovine γ-globulin, 0.1 g/L sodium azide, and 50 mg/L benzalkonium chloride. Standards and controls of amikacin are made as described for the SLIFA procedure.

Procedure

Amikacin is assayed by transferring 20 μL of sample or control into 1 mL of buffer. This step is repeated. After 20 μL of the diluted sample is dispensed into a 12 × 75-mm disposable culture tube, 200 μL of dilution buffer is added. To this solution, 40 μL of conjugate is added, followed by 700 μL of buffer. Finally, 40 μL of antiserum solution is added and dispensed into the reaction vessel, followed by 1.0 mL of buffer.

Performance

Table 8.13 presents the salient characteristics of the FPIA for amikacin. The following antibiotics cross-react at a rate of less than 0.1% in the FPIA of amikacin: ampicillin, amphotericin, carbenicillin, cefamandole, cephalexin, cephaloglycin, cephaloridine, cephalothin, CAM, CLD, erythromycin, ethacrynic acid, 5-fluorocytosine, fortimicin A, fortimicin B, furosemide, fusidic acid, lincomycin, methicillin, methotrexate, oxytetracycline, penicillin, rifampin, sulfadiazine, sulfamethoxazole, tetracycline, ticarcillin, TMP, and vancomycin.

Table 8.14 presents the cross-reactivity of closely related compounds with the FPIAs of the aminoglycosides gentamicin, tobramycin, and amikacin. Figure 8.16 compares the FPIA results for amikacin with those of RIA, bioassay, and SLIFA. Discrepancies between the slopes for the different assays are most likely attributable to the sources of the standards or their preparation and storage.

TABLE 8.13

Expected Performance of Assay of Amikacin by the FPIA Technique (170,171)

Parameter	3 μg/mL	15 μg/mL	30 μg/mL
Mean (μg/mL)	2.8	15.14	30.68
Standard deviation within run (μg/mL)	0.17	0.30	0.65
Coefficient of variation within run (%)	6.11	2.01	2.12
Standard deviation between runs (μg/mL)	0.21	0.52	1.00
Coefficient of variation between runs (%)	7.50	3.51	3.26

TABLE 8.14

Cross-reactivity of Aminoglycosides Gentamicin, Tobramycin, and Amikacin in the FPIA (170,171)

Drug	Cross-reactivity (%)		
	Gentamicin	Tobramycin	Amikacin
Sagamicin sulfate	55.0	<0.1	<0.1
Sisomicin	30.0	<0.1	<0.1
Netilmicin	7.0	<0.1	<0.1
Gentamicin	100.0	<0.1	<0.1
Kanamycin A	<0.1	44.0	30.0
Kanamycin B	<0.1	43.0	3.0
3′,4′-Dideoxykanamycin B	<0.1	60.0	2.5
Tobramycin	<0.1	100.0	3.5
Amikacin	<0.1	1.5	100.0
Neomycin	<0.1	<0.1	<0.1
Spectinomycin	<0.1	<0.1	<0.1
Streptomycin	<0.1	<0.1	<0.1

Coefficients of variation between the immunoassays were 6.96% or greater. Results seen here with amikacin are also applicable to the aminoglycosides gentamicin and tobramycin (170,171).

Micromethod Fluorescence Polarization Immunoassay of Aminoglycosides

Gentamicin and netilmicin are aminoglycoside antibiotics that are used to treat Gram-negative bacterial infections. Monitoring the concentrations of these drugs, usually in venous blood samples, helps optimize care by limiting the incidence of toxicity and therapeutic failure. However, venous samples are often difficult to obtain from infants and children. Capillary blood spotted on filter paper has been used successfully for detection of inborn errors of metabolism and for monitoring drug concentrations. For example, this technique has been used with an HPLC assay that has been previously described in this chapter to detect netilmicin and sisomicin. The following method is an FPIA that determines the gentamicin and netilmicin concentrations from blood samples spotted on filter paper.

Procedure

One hundred microliters of the standard aqueous solutions (0 to 20 μg/mL prepared in distilled water) and the gentamicin and netilmicin blood standards (0 to 20 μg/mL prepared with antibiotic-free pooled blood) are spotted onto filter paper. The spots are dried at 50°C for 10 minutes in an air-circulating oven or at room temperature for 5 hours. Using scissors, the blood-containing area is cut into five or six pieces and all are placed into one tube. Addition of 500 μL of warmed (35°C) 0.5 mol/L Na_2HPO_4 buffer to the tube is followed by incubation of the sample in an oven (35°C) for 60 minutes and centrifugation for 15 minutes (3000 × g). The colorless clear filtrate is transferred to a well of a TDx cartridge (Abbott Laboratories) for measurement by FPIA.

The measurement of hemoglobin in extracts can be performed using a hemoglobin assay kit (Wako Pure Chemical Industries, Osaka, Japan). Twenty microliters of each extracted sample is mixed with 5 mL of cyanmethemoglobin reagent. After 5 minutes, the absorbance is measured at 540 nm and compared with that of the standard solution containing 3.58 of cyanmethemoglobin/5 mL.

Performance

Hemoglobin levels below 8.6 g/L do not affect the FPIA gentamicin assay. Ultrafiltration of a gentamicin-free sample with a hemoglobin level greater than 8.6 g/L gives a clear, colorless filtrate, demonstrating that the hemoglobin in the filtrate is almost completely removed by the ultrafiltration procedure. Maximum elution time from the spotted paper for both gentamicin and netilmicin is 60 to 90 minutes under the given extraction conditions.

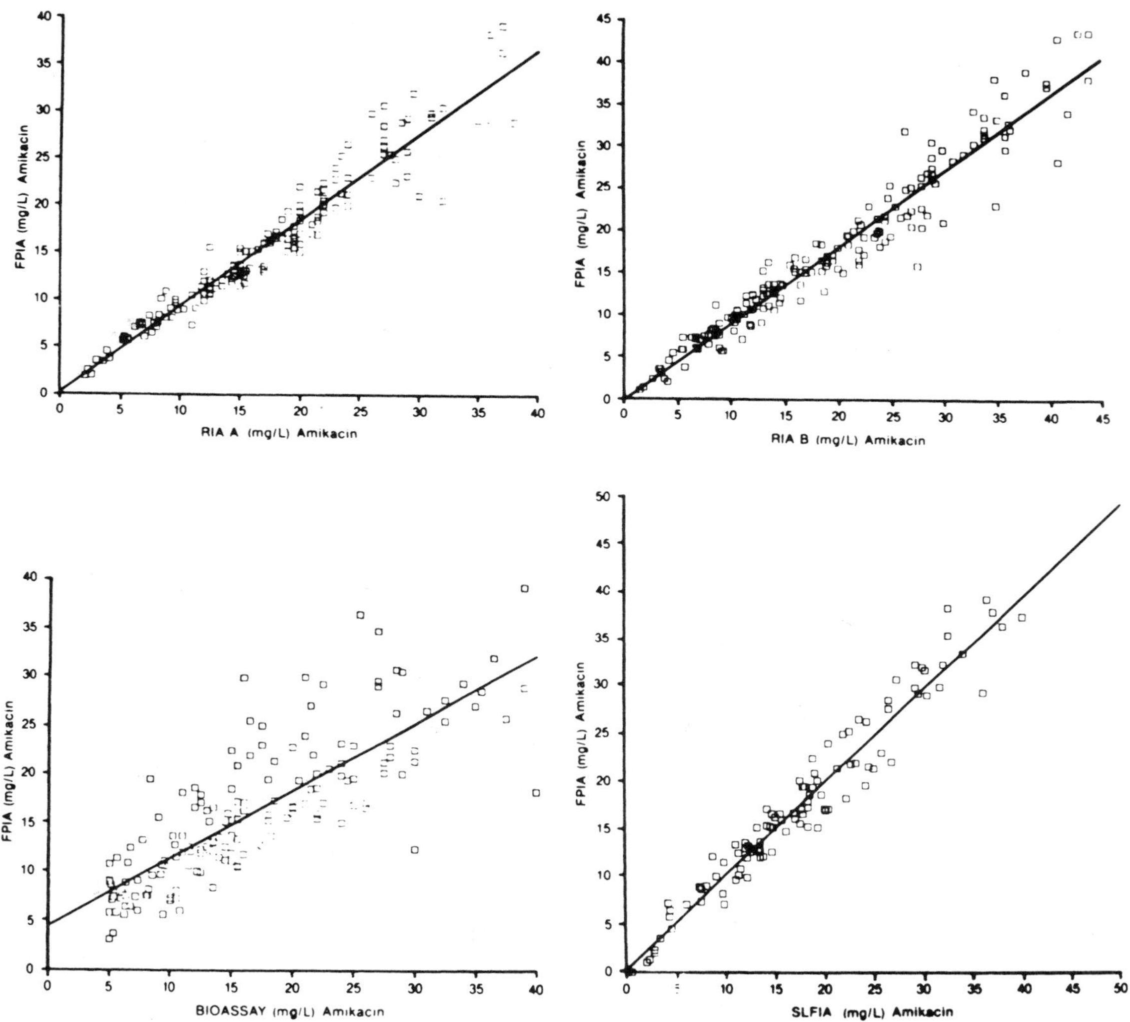

FIGURE 8.16 ● Comparison of the analysis of amikacin by RIA, bioassay, and fluorescent nonisotopic immunoassay. (From Jolley [170], with permission.)

Recovery of gentamicin from dried blood-spotted samples in the concentration range of 1.5 to 20 μg/mL is from 92% to 115%. The lower limit of detection of gentamicin or netilmicin with the FPIA reagent kits is 1 μg/mL each for samples spotted with 100 μL of whole blood.

The calibration curve for gentamicin or netilmicin in dried blood spots is linear over the concentration range of 1.0 to 20 μg/mL. The intraassay coefficients of variation are 5.6% and 6.3% for gentamicin concentrations of 5 and 10 μg/mL, and 4.6% and 1.6% for netilmicin concentrations of 10 and 20 μg/mL, respectively. The interassay coefficient of variation is 4.5% for a gentamicin concentration of 5 μg/mL and 9.7% for a netilmicin concentration of 10 μg/mL. Clinical samples from pediatric patients treated with netilmicin show excellent linear correlation when corrected for hematocrit levels. The applicability of the determination of gentamicin or netilmicin concentrations in dried blood spots by FPIA is limited because the quantification limit exceeds the effective range of the antibiotics (127).

Teicoplanin

Teicoplanin levels in serum can be determined by FPIA using fluorescein-labeled teicoplanin, which competes with unlabeled teicoplanin for antibody (272).

Procedure

For the generation of the calibration curve, standards containing 0, 5.0, 10.0, 25.0, 50.0, and 100.0 μg/mL

TABLE 8.15

Specificity of Teicoplanin FPIA (272)

Drug	Interference (%)
Cefazolin	3.1
Ciprofloxacin	4.4
Daptomycin	3.0
Erythromycin	1.4
Gentamicin	0.2
Nafcillin	3.6
Piperacillin	2.8
Rifampin	6.3
Vancomycin	2.8

teicoplanin are prepared. The International Bioclinical reagent system is used to prepare standards and serum samples for measurement by the American Bioclinical FP analyzer. This instrument calculates the millipolarization values and extrapolates the teicoplanin concentration for each sample by comparing the values to those of the calibration curve.

Performance

The lower limit of detection of teicoplanin is 0.5 μg/mL. Other antibiotics that interfere in this assay are shown in Table 8.15. The results of the FPIA agree well with those of bioassay, with a correlation coefficient of 0.901.

RADIOIMMUNOASSAYS

The general advantages and disadvantages of the RIA technique are shown in Table 8.2 (3,284) (Fig. 8.17). Because it is no longer in routine clinical use, it is not discussed further in this chapter.

CHROMATOGRAPHIC ASSAYS

Chromatography uses the ability of a compound in one type of medium to be selectively removed from that medium onto an adsorbent and to be quantitatively assayed. Most commonly, the compound is in a liquid and is adsorbed onto a solid (liquid chromatography) or is in the gas phase and is adsorbed onto a liquid (GLC). Inherent in any chromatographic method is the requirement for specialized adsorbent columns (which may be different for different antibiotics), the use of expensive equipment (especially in GLC), the use of various extraction procedures, and the requirement for a skilled technician to perform the assay.

The advantages of the procedure are that chromatography can separate even closely related compounds and analyze them separately. Generally, the method is quite sensitive, i.e., able to quantitate between 1.0 and 0.5 μg/mL for most antibiotics, and is quite rapid, requiring 30 to 60 minutes per specimen. The principles of chromatography have evolved from the early decades of the 20th century, with the most exciting applications occurring within the last 40 years.

Modern chromatography dates to 1941 when Martin and Synge (216) published their classic paper on liquid-liquid partition chromatography. They described individual rates of migration of substances that were a consequence of differing partition ratios between mobile and stationary liquid phases. Gas chromatography (GC) and

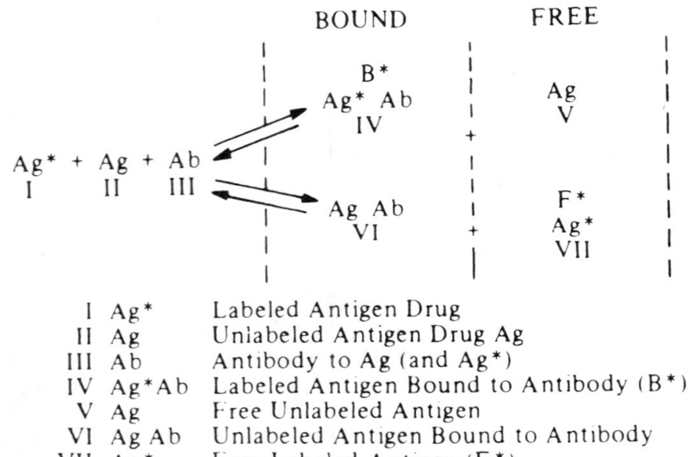

FIGURE 8.17 ● Reaction series of the RIA *, radiolabeled substances. (From Monitor Science Corp. [129], with permission.)

thin-layer chromatography (TLC) appeared in the 1950s and were received enthusiastically. However, the time-consuming, crudely quantitative characteristics of TLC and the requirements of molecule volatility and thermostability for GC are disadvantages of these techniques. Building on chromatographic principles that evolved over five or more decades and experience gained from GC and TLC in particular, researchers developed HPLC in the late 1960s. The debut of HPLC was largely from the pioneering work of Horvath and Lipsky (159).

Although homogeneous and heterogeneous enzyme FPIA techniques may be viewed as competitive with HPLC, a more global view of the subject reminds us that each method has its own strengths and weaknesses, and that the fields of therapeutic monitoring and pharmacokinetic assessment of antibiotics are strengthened by the appropriate application of each of these technologies. The advantages of HPLC are many. These will be amplified as improvements in instrumentation, packing materials, and method are made. As with GC, mass spectroscopy (MS) is now being applied to HPLC (89). GC-MS will undoubtedly remain the method of choice for the most accurate identification and most sensitive quantitation of small, volatile, thermostable molecules. However, for many larger, nonvolatile, thermosensitive molecules, HPLC-MS has major potential as an analytic method. In this technique, HPLC is a preparatory step prior to MS, and allows the identification and quantification of molecules in the picogram range. Several papers have demonstrated the application of HPLC to MS, and have presented instrument modifications to reduce MS contamination (107,153).

HIGH-PERFORMANCE LIQUID CHROMATOGRAPHY

HPLC is a reference method, if not the major reference method, by which all new antimicrobial agents are studied, from discovery to clinical application. It plays a major role in drug preparation, pharmacologic assessment, and clinical monitoring (216,217,220,288,330). Thus, an understanding of the analysis of antimicrobial agents by HPLC is essential in clinical laboratory practice.

HPLC as a technology has assumed a central role in the analysis of all water-soluble molecules in clinical laboratories. This technique is the method of choice for the analysis of penicillin and cephalosporin antibiotics. HPLC is especially useful clinically in the measurement of third-generation cephalosporins in the nonblood body compartments (304). It is also being used more frequently to measure parent antibiotics and their metabolites. This section discusses this powerful tool and provides specific examples of how it is used to determine concentrations of most of the major classes of antibiotics in use today.

Many antibiotics have been analyzed successfully by HPLC, including aminoglycosides (11,223,251,252), cephalosporins and penicillins (58,64,70,194), tetracyclines (60,237), and others (131,294,341). The interested reader is referred to reviews by Nilsson-Ehle (236) and Jehl et al. (166) for discussions of the general method and its application to the analysis of drugs.

A number of factors stimulated the application of HPLC, a technique that was already in common use in science and industry, to the quantitation of antibiotics in biologic fluids (5,12,18). This technology was commonly used in modern laboratories to measure antiarrhythmic and anticonvulsant agents. The equipment and expertise were thus available. Several HPLC methods, using standard chromatographic equipment, have been developed that allow the simultaneous quantitation of multiple, closely related antibiotics (44,47,49,290). Others permit simultaneous quantitation of parent drugs and some metabolites (20,61,113,135,137,150,185,195,196,239). Simultaneous analysis of mixtures of antibiotics can be performed with small changes in operating conditions (158). Once the equipment has been obtained, the cost of quantifying antibiotics by HPLC is competitive with other methods (205,207,242,248,349). Finally, the rapidity with which assays may be performed by HPLC is crucial for seriously ill patients who are receiving drugs with narrow toxic/therapeutic ratios or that have potentially severe side effects (77). HPLC methods can detect quantities of antibiotics as low as 500 ng/L, reflecting levels of sensitivity beyond what is needed in clinical practice (158).

Using the HPLC technique, highly reproducible, difficult separations are achieved rapidly and quantitatively (67,110,134,152). The majority of HPLC separations are accomplished in less than 1 hour, with many requiring only a few minutes. A wide variety of molecular species may be separated and quantitated by HPLC, including both large and small molecules, ions, isomers, polymers, polar molecules, and nonpolar molecules (117,283,323). Because HPLC is often performed at low or ambient temperatures, thermosensitive molecules are easily handled (208,233,259). After the analyte molecules pass the instrument detector, they may be collected quantitatively in unaltered form for further purification or investigation.

Prior to reviewing the practical application of the liquid-liquid partition principle in HPLC, let us first briefly consider its theoretical basis. All HPLC methods use the same basic steps:

1. Extraction of the drug with a specific solvent
2. Separation of the drug on the solid phase by HPLC
3. Detection of the effluent from the solid phase by spectrometry
4. Quantitation of the amount of antibiotic present by peak height analysis or peak area analysis

The aim of chromatography in general is the resolution or separation of different molecular species. To

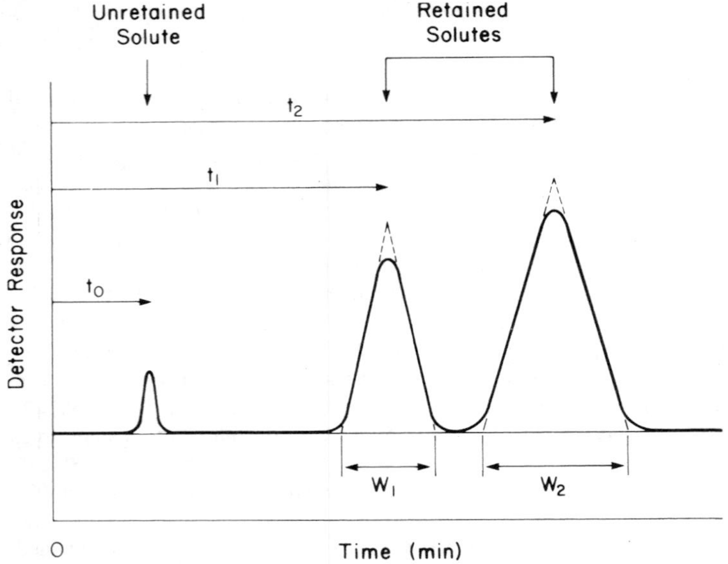

FIGURE 8.18 ● Theoretical chromatogram of unretained and retained solutes.

understand resolution in the context of HPLC, we must consider a few explanatory equations. These equations and a more in-depth discussion may be found in an excellent concise paper by Guiochon (142) or in the work of Giddings (133). First, let us assume that the groups of molecules eluting from the chromatographic column or peaks on the chromatogram are Gaussian in distribution (not entirely true, but adequate for mathematical interpretation). The resolution (R) of two Gaussian peaks is defined by the equation

$$R = 2(t_{R2} - t_{R1})/(W_1 + W_2),$$

where t_{R1} and t_{R2} are the retention times of the first and second peaks, respectively, and W_1 and W_2 are the widths at the base of the chromatographic peaks. If the two peaks are close, the resolution is defined by the equation

$$R = (\text{sq rt. } [N/4)[(\alpha - 1)/\alpha][k'_2/(1 + k'_2)]$$

To understand this equation, let us look at its component factors. First, remember that the width at the base of a Gaussian distribution is equal to 4 SD (σ). N, or the plate number of the column (a standard measure of its efficiency), is defined as

$$N = (16_{tR}/W)^2 = (t_R/\sigma_t),$$

where σ_t is the standard deviation of the peak in units of time and t_R and W are the retention time and base width of the peak, respectively. The relative retention of the two compounds being considered, σ, is described by the equation

$$\alpha = (t_{R2} - t_0)/(t_{R1} - t_0) = t'_{R2}/t'_{R1} = k'_2/k'_1,$$

where t_0 is the retention of an inert molecular species that theoretically is not retained by the column, t'_{R1} and t'_{R2} are the adjusted retention times, and k′ is the capacity factor of the column (how retentive it is in terms of these particular molecular species). The capacity factor, k, for each molecular species, may be redefined as

$$k = (t_R - t_0)/t_0 = r'_R/t_0$$

This factor, k, is important because it is proportional to the equilibrium constant that describes the distribution of molecules between the chromatographic phases.

Applying these formulas to HPLC, the mobile solvent phase passes over the stationary phase at a constant rate. The two phases possess different chemical polarities. As the analyte molecules in the mobile phase pass over the stationary phase, those with polarity closer to that of the stationary phase are retained selectively for a time on the column. Conversely, the analyte molecules with polarity closer to that of the mobile phase tend to remain in the mobile phase, passing through the column faster. Passing through the instrument monitor sequentially, these groups of molecules give rise to peaks on the chromatogram (Fig. 8.18).

The term "high-performance liquid chromatography" encompasses several different types of chromatography. Systems that have a polar stationary phase with a nonpolar mobile phase are termed "normal phase" or "straight phase," while those having a nonpolar stationary phase with a polar mobile phase are termed "reverse phase." A popular variant of reverse-phase HPLC is ion-pair chromatography, where the polarity (and thus the retention) of the analyte is changed by adding a second ion of opposite charge (counter-ion). Ion-exchange chromatography

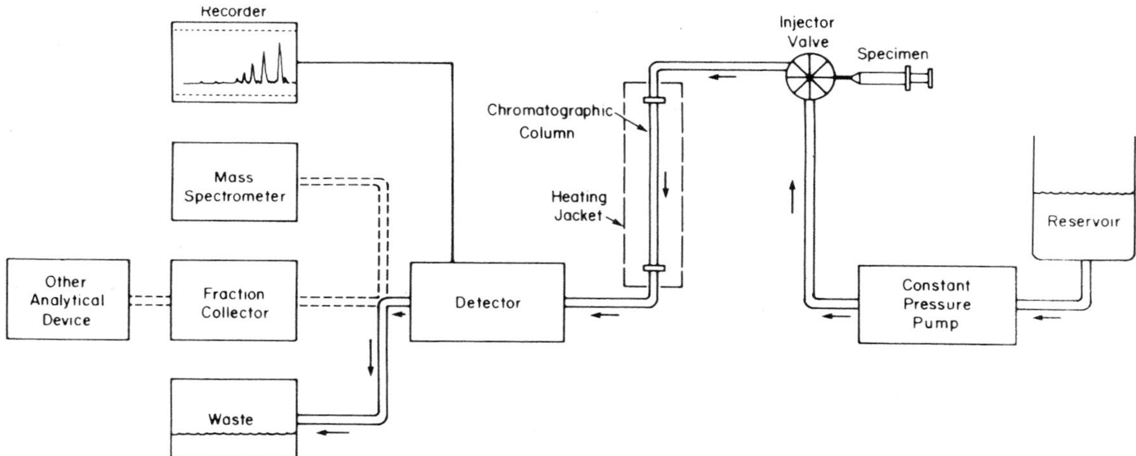

FIGURE 8.19 • Diagrammatic representation of HPLC.

is based on competition between the analyte ion and a second, similarly charged molecule for oppositely charged sites on the exchange resin. An early form of HPLC using a solid stationary phase that separates molecules on the basis of differing size and weight is termed "size-exclusion" or "gel-permeation chromatography." Gel-permeation chromatography has wide industrial and research applications but is rarely used for antimicrobial determinations in clinical laboratories.

Much of the versatility of HPLC is because of the wide variety of instrument components and chromatographic conditions from which to choose. In its simplest form (Fig. 8.19), the HPLC system is a closed system composed of an injector, pump, chromatographic column, and detector, with a reservoir for the mobile phase liquid. The composition of the mobile phase selected depends on the physical characteristics of the analyte, the complexity of the sample mixture, and the column packing employed. Although initially the mobile phase was usually nonpolar (straight phase), most recent applications use a buffered aqueous mobile phase containing acetonitrile, methanol, or some other relatively polar organic (reverse-phase) compound. For an extensive review of solvent phase selection, the reader is referred to the work of Snyder and Kirkland (303).

The injector, either manual or automatic, is a simple but very important component that allows the sample to be placed into the mobile phase stream without disrupting the flow. The HPLC pump is critical in that it must present the mobile-phase liquid to the chromatographic column at a constant pressure (usually less than 2,000 psi) to provide acceptable and reproducible analyte separations in a timely fashion. Pumps are available over a broad price range, with considerable variations in design that serve mainly to minimize pressure fluctuations.

Progress in the field of HPLC has been made through improvements in the chromatographic packing materials themselves and the consistency with which the columns are packed. High-quality, commercially prepared columns are available that offer improved batch-to-batch reliability and a wide selection of column lengths, efficiencies, types of support phases, particle sizes, shapes, pore sizes, pH ranges, and chemical specificities of the liquid stationary phase (186). The column sleeve is usually made of stainless steel, although the radial compression technology uses polyethylene (19).

In practice, most HPLC systems use a polar mobile phase and nonpolar stationary phase (reverse phase). In order to eliminate false peaks (bubbles) and to remove microparticulate matter, the mobile phase is degassed and filtered. The organic stationary phase is commonly composed of C_8 or C_{18} aliphatic chains bonded chemically to microparticulate porous silica of 5 to 10 μm mean particle diameter, densely and uniformly packed into a stainless steel sleeve. A rule of thumb for column efficiency is that for an efficient column a single theoretical plate should be two to five times the mean particle diameter of the support phase, with an overall efficiency of 3,000 to 5,000 theoretical plates. The internal diameter of the sleeve is usually 2 to 5 mm, with the column length varying from 3 cm to several meters, although typically it is less than 30 cm. The rate of flow of the mobile phase is usually 1 to 3 mL/minute, requiring a pressure of up to about 2,000 psi to maintain the flow and to attenuate chromatographic time.

Most current methods are performed at ambient temperature or at up to approximately 50°C. Above this, silica-based packing materials begin to deteriorate. The pH of the mobile phase is kept below 7 to 7.5 for the same reason, although nonsiliceous packing materials are available that work well in the basic region.

The selection of the means by which the HPLC instrument "sees" the analyte molecules as they proceed in groups from the chromatographic column allows one to further tailor the instrument and the analysis for particular needs. Commonly used detectors include UV/visible, fluorescence, refractive index, electrochemical, infrared, and radiometric instruments. UV detectors are most commonly used to monitor the effluent from the column, although fluorescence detectors, because of increased sensitivity and elimination of interfering peaks, are often preferred. State-of-the-art detectors tend to be microprocessor-controlled, with flow-cell volumes down to 1 μL. However, less sophisticated detectors with flow cells of 10 μL are adequate for the majority of applications. Typically, 5 to 100 μL of the prepared sample is injected. The chromatographic time is usually less than 20 minutes. Current HPLC systems routinely work in the nanogram range. Between-day coefficients of variation are usually less than 5% to 7%. An internal standard is commonly used to minimize errors inherent in the system, particularly if some form of sample pretreatment is employed. For a concise review of the use of internal standards, the reader is referred to the work of Snyder and Kirkland (303).

Biologic fluids are typically complex mixtures that are composed of a wide variety of proteins, carbohydrates, lipids, and others. Beyond the deleterious effects these materials have on the injector, column packing material, and pump, their presence frequently interferes with the separation and quantitation of the analyte molecules under study. Consequently, some form of sample preparation is almost always required prior to the chromatography. Four major techniques are commonly employed to prepare samples for injection.

In most assays of biologic fluids, including antibiotic assays, it is essential to remove as much protein from the fluid under study as possible. Most directly, one can precipitate the protein, for example, with trichloroacetic acid. However, acid precipitation leaves many interfering materials in the sample and the resultant pH change may be deleterious to the analyte molecules, metabolites, packing material, or other equipment components.

Alternatively, one may remove the protein with an ultrafilter such as those available from Amicon (7), but not all low molecular weight proteinaceous material can be removed. Other interfering materials may pass through the filter as well. Additionally, analyte is lost if there is significant protein binding. In spite of its limitations, this method has been gaining popularity (76).

Solvent extraction has been the most common preparatory technique. Organic solvents extract specific organic molecules selectively from the specimen by solvent partitioning. In this process, protein in the sample is usually denatured and left at the liquid-liquid interface. By appropriate solvent selection and manipulation of the specimen pH, a satisfactory separation of the analyte from most of the other materials in the specimen can frequently be achieved. For example, piperacillin can be extracted into chloroform/1-pentanol at an acidic pH (50). The organic solvent containing the drug can be removed by evaporation, or the drug can be extracted back into an aqueous solution with a pH of 7, where the drug is ionized and water-soluble. This latter step further cleans the specimen and may be used to concentrate the analyte if a reduced quantity of the aqueous phase is used.

Many compounds may be isolated by first adsorbing them either onto an ion-exchange resin (215), if they are charged, or onto a bonded reverse-phase packing material if they are not charged (155), followed by elution. For example, the aminoglycoside/aminocyclitol antibiotics are very polar and difficult to extract with an organic solvent. However, they may be easily adsorbed onto Amberlite resin (215) or silicic acid (213), eluted, and analyzed.

The advantages of HPLC—rapid availability of results, sensitivity, specificity, and the ability to measure several drugs and their metabolites simultaneously—allow for easy therapeutic monitoring of antibiotics. At the same time, they enhance antibiotic development and pharmacokinetic evaluation. Nearly all of the antibiotics in use today have been assessed by HPLC. Concurrent with improvements in HPLC equipment and packing materials, methods have been developed for the quantitation of certain antibiotics by EMIT, RIA, fluorescence assays, FPIA, and other nonisotopic immunoassays. When a choice of technique is possible, some factors that should be considered before a selection is made include the equipment and expertise that is available within the laboratory, the positive and negative attributes of the specific methods under consideration, the laboratory's test volumes and costs, and the institution's clinical requirements (26,32,67,75,88,90,143,156,160, 167,168,175,188,193,201,217,232,267,298,350).

Chloramphenicol

At present, CAM is probably the antibiotic most commonly quantified by HPLC in clinical laboratories. Several relatively simple methods are available that give sensitive and reproducible results rapidly and require only small quantities of specimen. Additionally, CAM and its succinate or palmitate prodrug esters may be measured simultaneously. HPLC conditions for their measurement are similar to those employed for quantitation of theophylline, acetaminophen, and some anticonvulsants, thus requiring minimal method modification for the many laboratories already measuring these drugs by HPLC (305). Radioenzymatic assays (269,299) are available to measure CAM, and a modification of these has been compared with HPLC (338). Table 8.16 presents a summary of the HPLC methods available for measuring CAM. The authors have preferred the method of Velagapudi et al. (327) because the procedure employs ethyl acetate

(text continues on page 345)

TABLE 8.16

HPLC Methods

Author	Antimicrobial Compound Measured[a]	Sample Preparation[b]	Internal Standard	Mobile Phase	Stationary Phase (Reverse-Phase Unless Otherwise Indicated)	Temperature[c]	Derivatization	Detection
Aravind et al. (14)	CAM, CAM-S	Ethyl acetate	5-Ethyl-5-*p*-toly-barbituric acid	ACN/H_2O (15:85)	C_{18} (PE) ODS-HC-SIL-X-1	50°C	None	UV, 280 nm
Weber et al. (337)	CAM, CAM-S	ACN pptn	*P*-Nitropropionanilide	Methanol/H_2O (35:65)	C_{18} μBondapak	RT	None	UV, 280/254 nm
Velagapudi et al. (327)	CAM, CAM-S	Ethyl acetate	Thlamphenicol	ACN/H_2O (20:80)	C_{18} μBondapak	RT	None	UV, 278 nm
Brisson and Fourtillian (51)	Cefazolin, cephalothin, cefoxitin, cefotaxime, cefamandole, cefuroxime, cefoperazone	Chloroform/pentanol (3:1)	None	Methanol or ACN	C_{18} μBondapak	RT	None	UV, 240/275 nm
Lecaillon et al. (196)	Cefsulodin, cefotiam, cephalexin, cefotaxime, deacetyl-cefotaxime, cefuroxime, cefroxadin	Methanol/TCA pptn	None, cephalexin or cefoxadin	Methanol/H_2O ± TBHS	LiChrosorb RP-8 or RP-18	RT	None	UV, 254 nm
Aravind et al. (15)	Moxalactam	Methanol pptn	8-Chlorotheophylline	Methanol/H_2O (4:96)	C_{18}(PE) HC-SIL-X	RT	None	UV, 230 nm
Brisson and Fourtillan 50	Piperacillin	Chloroform/pentanol	None	Methanol/H_2O (40:60)	C_{18} μBondapak	40°C	None	UV, 254 nm
Hildebrandt and Gundert-Remy (155)	Aziocillin, meziocillin	Sep-Pak C_{18}	None	ACN/H_2O (27:73)	C_{18} μBondapak	RT	None	UV, 220 nm

(continued)

TABLE 8.16 (Continued)

HPLC Methods

Author	Antimicrobial Compound Measured[a]	Sample Preparation[b]	Internal Standard	Mobile Phase	Stationary Phase (Reverse-Phase Unless Otherwise Indicated)	Temperature[c]	Derivatization	Detection
Maltra et al. (213)	Gentamicin	Silicic acid column	None	Methanol/H_2O (79:21)	C_{18} μBondapak	RT	Precolumn o-phthalaldehyde	Fluorescence, 36/430 nm
Bawdon and Madsen (33)	Sulbactum	Derivation: Imidazole reagent + specimen; extraction: ACN/dichloro-methane procedure	None	89% 0.1 mol/L phosphate buffer/11% ACN	Beckman ODS-5, stainless steel	RT	Imidazole	UV, 313 nm
LaFollette et al. (193)	Clindamycin	ACN	Triazolam	ACN/H_2O/phosphoric acid/76 mmol/L TMA (30:70:0.2:0.075), pH 6.7	Nova-Pak C_{18}	RT	None	UV, 198 nm
Jones and Chmel (172)	Meziocillin	TBAP	Piperacillin	Methanol/TBAP (25:75)	Econosphere C_{18}	RT	Precolumn	UV, 220 nm
Godbillon et al. (136)	(5*R*,6*S*)2-Amino-6-[(1*R*)-hydroxyethyl]-2-penem-3-carboxylic acid	Serum: ammonium sulfate/phosphate buffer; urine: 25x dilution with phosphate buffer, pH 6.0	(5*R*,6*S*)2-Amino-6-[(1*R*)-hydroxyethyl]-2-penem-3-carboxylic acid	Phosphate buffer, pH 6.0	LiChrosorb RP-8	RT	None	UV, 320 nm
Pilkiewicz et al. (256)	Aztreonam	Serum: ACN; urine: 10x dilution with $TBAHSO_4$, pH 3.0	None	$TBAHSO_4$/ACN (80:20)	C_{18} μBondapak on Corasll	RT	None	UV, 293 nm

Yamamoto et al. (353)	Pyrazinamide + metabolites (2,3-pyrazinedicarboxamide, 5-hydroxypyrazinoic acid, 5-hydroxypyrazinamide, pyrazinoic acid, pyrazinamide)	Perchloric acid	2,3-pyrazine dicarboxamide	KH_2PO_4	C_{18} μBondapak	RT	None	Fluorescence, 410/365 nm
McAteer et al. (222)	Cefbdme, cefaclor, cefadroxil, cephalexin, cephradine	ACN	Ceflxime for other four cephalosporins; cephalexin for cefixime	Methanol/K_2HPO_4 (20:80)	C_{18} Altex Ultrasphere	RT	None	UV, 240 nm
Leeder et al. (197)	Ceftazidime	Serum: methanol; urine: dilution with distilled H_2O within concentration range of standards	8-Chlorotheophyllin	Serum: KH_2PO_4/methanol (82:18); urine: KH_2PO_4/methanol (88:12)	C_{18} μBondapak	RT	None	UV, 225 nm
Barbhaiya et al. (23)	BMY-28142 (cephalosporin)	Plasma: ACN/TCA; urine: 3 × dilution with sodium buffer	Cefadroxil	ACN/octane sulfonic acid (12:88)	C_{18} Partisil 5 ODS-3RAC	RT	None	UV, 280 nm
			Ceftazidime	Methanol/sodium dodecyl sulfate/TCA/phosphoric acid/tetrahydrofuran (49.7:40.4:3.9:0.7:5.3)				
Granich and Krogstad (139)	Ceftriaxone	Serum: ACN, CSF: ACN; urine; dilution 1:10 with normal saline	Moxalactam	ACN/H_2O (46:54) + ion-pairing agent (hexadecyltrimethylammonium bromide dibasic potassium phosphate)	C_{18} μBondapak	RT	None	UV, 274 nm
Chan et al. (66)	Cephalothin, cefoxitin, cefamandole, cefuroxime, cefotaxime, moxalactam, ceftriaxone, ceftazidime	Plasma, serum, CSF, bile, peritoneal fluid, pleural fluid, ascitic fluid: ACN	Ceftazidime	*N*-Cetyl-*N*,*N*,*N*-trimethyl ammonium bromide, Titrisol/phosphate buffer, glacial acetic acid/ACN (350 mL)	LiChrosorb RP-18	RT	None	UV, 240 nm
		Urine, peritoneal dialysis fluid: diluted + ACN	Ceftazidime	As above with 600 mL ACN				

(continued)

TABLE 8.16 (Continued)

HPLC Methods

Author	Antimicrobial Compound Measured[a]	Sample Preparation[b]	Internal Standard	Mobile Phase	Stationary Phase (Reverse-Phase Unless Otherwise Indicated)	Temperature[c]	Derivatization	Detection
Demotes-Mainaird et al. (88)	Roxithromycin	Plasma, urine: dilution in phosphate buffer/ dichloromethane	Erythromycin	ACN/ammonium acetate/methanol (55:23:22), pH 7.5	C_{18} μBondapak	RT	None	Dual coulometric electrodes operated in oxidative screen mode (screen electrode = E1 + 0.7 V; sample electrode = E2 + 0.9 V)
Croteau et al. (75)	Erythromycin + esters (ethylsuccinate, estolate)	Plasma, saliva: diethylether, with residue reconstituted with ACN; urine: K_2HPO_4/diethylether, with residue reconstituted with ACN	Roxithromycin	Sodium acetate buffer/ACN/methanol (56:50:4), pH 7.0	C_{18} μNovapak	RT	None	Single electrode cell in oxidative mode with amperometric cell potential at +0.9 V
Georgopoulos et al. (131)	Telcoplanin	SAX Bond Elut/Columns	Teicoplanin	Methanol/water (5:95)/*n*-heptane-sulfonate, pH 4.0	LiChrosorb RP-8	30°C	None	UV, 240 nm

[a] CAM-S, CAM succinate.
[b] ACN, acetonitrile; pptn, precipitation; TCA, trichloroacetic acid; TBAP, tetrabutylammonium phosphate; TBHS, tetrabutylammonium hydrogen sulfate; TMA, tetramethylammonium chloride; $TBAHSO_4$, tetrabutylammonium hydrogen sulfate; CSF, cerebrospinal fluid.
[c] RT, room temperature.

extraction, is performed at ambient temperature, is monitored at the absorption maximum of CAM (278 nm), and uses a closely related compound (thiamphenicol) as the internal standard (40). Table 8.16 presents recent useful HPLC methods (103).

Cephalosporins

Factors to consider when deciding whether or not to monitor blood concentrations of cephalosporin drugs include the potential for toxicity and concerns about patient compliance (for the oral preparations), possible failure to reach or sustain therapeutic concentrations for other reasons, or inappropriate use of expensive medications. Blood concentrations of these drugs may also be monitored for the purposes of pharmacokinetic studies (349). Table 8.16 summarizes a number of available HPLC procedures for many of the cephalosporins (4,18,23,42,49, 66,74,104,111,126,139,197,218,222,234,248,319,351). Several clinically important cephalosporin antibiotics are reviewed in this chapter.

Oral cephalosporins (cefaclor, cefadroxil, cephalexin, and cephradine) are widely used antibiotics. Cefixime, a newer member of this class of drugs, offers broader pharmacokinetic properties than older cephalosporin drugs, with enhanced Gram-negative activity. Cefixime can be used for the treatment of otitis media, urinary tract infections, and respiratory tract infections. In the past, HPLC methods were limited to the detection of one or two cephalosporins with the same assay system and in their ability to measure drug concentrations in clinically significant ranges. The method described here uses a single HPLC system to measure the five oral cephalosporins mentioned in a clinically significant range of drug concentrations.

Equipment

One Waters HPLC system (Millipore, Waters Division, Milford, MA) consists of a model 590 pump used to deliver the mobile phase and a model 481 variable wavelength detector set at 240 nm. Analysis may be performed using a 4.6 mm × 15 cm Altex Ultrasphere octyl C_8 column (5 μm particles; Beckman Instruments, Berkeley, CA) with a silica RCSS Guard Pak precolumn (Waters). Linear least-squares regression analysis is performed using a laboratory automation system (model 3357; Hewlett-Packard, Paramus, NJ).

Chromatographic Conditions

The mobile phase consists of methanol/12.5 mmol/L monobasic sodium phosphate buffer (20:80, by volume), adjusted to pH 2.6 with concentrated phosphoric acid. The mobile phase is filtered, degassed before use, and delivered at ambient temperature at a flow rate of 2 mL/minute. The order of elution for the five cephalosporins is cefadroxil, cefaclor, cefixime, cephalexin, and cephradine, between the times of 3 to 20 minutes.

Five milligrams of cefixime or 5 mg of cephalexin is dissolved in 10 mL of methanol to yield 500 mg/L stock solutions. Each standard is then serially diluted tenfold. Working standards for the other drugs are prepared similarly, dissolving 5 mg of each compound (cefadroxil, cefaclor, and cephradine) in 10 mL of methanol to give 500 mg/L stock solutions, which are diluted by tenfold serial dilutions to yield 50 mg/L and 5 mg/L working standards.

Aliquots of the working standard solutions are added to polyethylene microcentrifuge tubes to give the desired drug concentrations. The solvent is then evaporated under a stream of nitrogen. The residue is reconstituted with 0.1 mL of serum, a known volume of internal standard (cefixime for the other four compounds, cephalexin for cefixime), and 0.1 mL of acetonitrile to precipitate serum proteins. Samples are vortex-mixed for 15 seconds and centrifuged at 14,000 × g for 2 minutes. The clear supernatant is evaporated under a stream of nitrogen. The residue is reconstituted with 0.1 mL of the mobile phase, and 50 to 80 μL is delivered by a WISP autoinjector (Waters) into the chromatograph.

Performance

The peak height ratio is linear over the concentration ranges studied (0.1 to 10 mg/L for cefixime and 1 to 100 mg/L for the others). The range for the coefficients of variation for intra- and interday measurements is less than 15%. With the exception of cefaclor, the recovery of each cephalosporin is greater than 81.4% over these concentration ranges. The lower recovery of cefaclor is probably because of its limited solubility in the mobile phase. This becomes a problem only at concentrations of more than 50 mg/L. These drug levels are not normally observed clinically. Other than salicylic acid, which absorbs UV light at 240 nm, commonly administered drugs do not generally interfere with the assay. Moreover, salicyclic acid is eluted at 22.1 minutes, not in the same time frame as any of the cephalosporins. The performance data for the cephalosporin assays are shown in Table 8.17.

By using a single system for all five cephalosporins, this HPLC method allows for monitoring without delays due to changes in equipment (222).

Penicillins

Because new semisynthetic penicillins continue to be developed and require pharmaceutical, pharmacokinetic, and clinical assessment, HPLC has much to offer for this antibiotic group. Additionally, because of possible side effects, particularly those that are dose-related, selected therapeutic monitoring seems reasonable. Table 8.16 summarizes HPLC methods available for the penicillins. Note that some methods are designed

TABLE 8.17

Performance Data for the Antibiotics Studied (222)

Drug	Concentration Range (μg/mL)	Mean Coefficient of Variation (%)		Mean Net Recovery (%)
		Within-Day	Between-Day	
Cefixime	0.1–1	5.8	8.3	81.4
	1–10	4.7	4.2	
Cefaclor	1–20	5.7	6.0	72.6
	10–100	5.2	9.8	
Cefadroxil	1–20	8.8	7.1	90.1
	10–100	11.4	14.2	
Cephalexin	1–20	7.6	7.2	82.3
	10–100	4.0	5.6	
Cephradine	1–20	6.9	7.7	84.2
	10–100	7.3	8.6	

for the assessment of pharmaceutical dosage forms but can probably be modified for use with biologic fluids (1,30,33,63,101,112,122,136,144,145,161,164,172, 256,335). Assays for some major clinically useful penicillin and penicillin derivative antibiotics are presented in this chapter.

Aztreonam

Aztreonam is a totally synthetic, monocyclic, β-lactam antibiotic with low toxicity that exhibits specific activity against aerobic Gram-negative bacteria and aminoglycoside and cephalosporin-resistant Gram-negative organisms. Assays performed by microbiologic methods are lengthy and do not separate metabolites. The following assay describes an ion-pair HPLC method for the quantitative analysis of aztreonam and its metabolites in human and animal serum and urine.

Equipment

Two HPLC systems may be used interchangeably and yield equivalent results. One consists of the following components: two M-6000A solvent delivery pumps, a model 660 solvent gradient programmer and a model U6K injector (all from Waters Associates), a model LC75 variable-wavelength UV detector set at 293 nm, an autocontroller (Perkin-Elmer, Inc., Welleshey, MA), and a model 3390A printer/plotter/integrator (Hewlett-Packard, Avondale, PA). The other HPLC system is a Hewlett-Packard model 1084B HPLC, which is equipped with a built-in variable-wavelength UV detector also set at 293 nm, an autosampler, and a printer/integrator. With both systems, the analysis is performed using the same column system, i.e., a Bondapak C_{18} column (inside diameter, 3.9 mm; length, 3.0 cm) and a guard column (inside diameter, 3.9 mm; length, 3.0 cm). The guard column is packed with Bondapak C_{18} on Corasil (Waters).

Chromatographic Conditions

The mobile phase consists of 0.005 mol/L tetrabutylammonium hydrogen sulfate/0.005 mol/L $(NH_4)_2SO_4$ and acetonitrile (80:20 by volume), adjusted to pH 3.0. The solution is filtered and degassed before HPLC use and is pumped at a flow rate of 2.0 mL/minute.

Procedure

Serum is diluted with an equal volume of acetonitrile and centrifuged for 2 minutes at ambient temperature at 15,000 × g. Supernatants are removed, and 50 μL is used for HPLC analysis. Urine samples are diluted tenfold with 0.005 mol/L tetrabutylammonium hydrogen sulfate, pH 3.0. Fifty microliters of sample is used for analysis.

Standards of aztreonam for serum and urine are dissolved in the mobile phase and prepared at concentrations of 1,000, 500, 200, 100, 50, 20, 10, 5, 1, and 0.5 μg/mL. A standard curve is constructed using peak area versus concentration. Serum standards are prepared over the same concentration ranges as the mobile-phase standards, but are diluted with an equal volume of acetonitrile and centrifuged. Supernatants are then used for HPLC analysis. Aztreonam urine standards are made in the same concentration ranges as described. Urine samples are diluted tenfold with 0.005 mol/L tetrabutylammonium hydrogen sulfate and are analyzed by HPLC under the same conditions as the standards that are dissolved in the mobile phase. Peak areas for aztreonam obtained from the serum standards are plotted on the previously constructed standard curve of aztreonam standards dissolved in the HPLC mobile phase.

Performance

It is possible to analyze urine and serum from all species for aztreonam without encountering interfering peaks. The results are linear for serum and urine over the concentration range of 0.1 mg/mL to 0.5 μg/mL. Recovery of samples is between 96% and 102%, and total analysis time for either specimen type is less than 10.0 minutes per sample. Use of tetrabutylammonium hydrogen sulfate with acetonitrile and $(NH_4)_2SO_4$ to ion-pair the SO_3 group of aztreonam to the reverse-phase column gives a good retention time, a symmetrical peak shape for aztreonam, and also allows the drug to be separated from biologic fluid components. HPLC agrees well with a microbiologic assay for both sample types. The HPLC method offers the advantages of speed and the ability to separate chemical entities. Only a small sample is required for HPLC analysis (256).

Mezlocillin

Mezlocillin, an acylureidopenicillin, is a semisynthetic penicillin with a broad spectrum of antimicrobial activity against Gram-positive and Gram-negative organisms, including *Enterobacteriaceae*, *P. aeruginosa*, and *Bacteroides* spp. Previous assay methods, including HPLC, that have been developed to measure the drug's concentrations have not used internal standards. The following is a description of a reverse-phase, ion-pair, extraction HPLC assay that uses piperacillin as the internal standard.

Chromatographic Conditions

The mobile phase consists of 5 mmol/L of a phosphate buffer, pH 7.0, that contains 5 mmol/L tetrabutylammonium phosphate/acetonitrile (75:25). Fifteen microliters of the reconstituted eluate is injected onto a 250 × 4.5 mm Econosphere C_{18} column (5 μm particle size). Column effluent products are eluted at ambient temperature with the mobile phase at a flow rate of 1.0 mL/minute and are monitored at 220 nm.

Procedure

Solid-phase preparation is used for samples in the following manner: 0.5 mL of serum sample that contains 100 μL of tetrabutylammonium phosphate and 15 μL of piperacillin internal standard (1.0 g/L) are applied to solid-phase extraction columns that have been previously activated by washing with methanol and 5 mmol/L tetrabutylammonium phosphate. The column is then washed with water and dried by aspiration. The drug is eluted with 600 μL of an equivolume solution of chloroform/acetone. The eluate is then evaporated and reconstituted with 100 μL of the mobile phase. The assay is calibrated with drug-free serum spiked with mezlocillin (10 to 300 mg/L).

Performance

The peak-area ratio of mezlocillin to the internal standard is linearly related to the mezlocillin concentration. The run-to-run coefficient of variation is less than 5%. Analytical recovery is 67%. There are no known interferences with other antibiotics that have been tested. The use of a solid-phase preparation and an internal standard had made this method unique compared with other HPLC assays for mezlocillin (172).

Carbapenems

(5*R*,6*S*)-2-Aminomethyl-6-[(1*R*)-hydroxyethyl]-2-penem-3-carboxylic acid (Ciba-Geigy, Corp., Ardsley, NY) belongs to a class of β-lactam antibiotics, the carbapenems, of which imipenem, meropenem, and ertapenem are now used clinically in the United States. It combines, in a single structure, the antimicrobial properties of penicillin and the cephalosporins. The drug is broadly active against Gram-positive and Gram-negative aerobic and anaerobic organisms. These drugs have excellent effectiveness against *P. aeruginosa* and methicillin-resistant *S. aureus*. The following method is an HPLC assay for the determination of (5*R*,6*S*)-2-aminomethyl-6-[(1*R*)-hydroxyethyl]-2-penem-3-carboxylic acid in plasma and urine. It uses the closely related aminoethyl derivative of (5*R*,6*S*)-2-aminomethyl-6-[(1*R*)-hydroxyethyl]-2-penem-3-carboxylic acid as the internal standard.

Equipment

A reverse-phase HPLC system consisting of a Hewlett-Packard (Palo Alto, CA) model 1084B instrument equipped with a variable-volume injector and a variable-wavelength detector that is set at 320 nm may be used. Analysis is performed using a prepacked column (20 cm × 4.6 mm, internal diameter) filled with LiChrosorb RP-8 (10 μM Hewlett-Packard) and a precolumn (1 cm × 4.6 mm, internal diameter) filled with Nucleosil C_{18} (30 μm). For the plasma assay, both columns must be replaced after 120 to 150 injections to prevent a decrease in separation efficiency. Peak areas are given by the integrator/recorder (79 850 A LC terminal), while peak heights are measured manually.

Chromatographic Conditions

The mobile phase consists of a phosphate buffer (8×10^{-3} mol/L Na_2HPO_4/5.9×10^{-3} mol/L KH_2PO_4), pH 6, and is degassed and filtered before use. The mobile phase is delivered at a flow rate of 1 mL/minute at room temperature.

Procedure

Plasma samples are prepared by adding 50 μL of internal standard solution (116.2 mol/L prepared in phosphate buffer, pH 6), 50 μL of phosphate buffer, pH 6, and 250 μL of a saturated solution of ammonium sulfate (53 μg of ammonium sulfate in 72 mL of water) to 250 μL of plasma in a glass tube. The solution is vortex-mixed for 30 seconds and centrifuged at 1400 × g for 10 minutes. One hundred microliters of supernatant is used for analysis. For urine samples, a 1 mL volume of urine is diluted to 25 mL with phosphate buffer, pH 6. One milliliter of the diluted sample is added to 100 μL of the internal standard solution and 100 μL of phosphate buffer, pH 6, in a glass tube and vortex-mixed for 15 seconds. Thirty microliters of the mixture is used for analysis. For reasons of chemical stability, both samples needed to be injected as soon as possible after preparation.

Solutions of internal standards (116.2 μmol/L) as well as (5*R*,6*S*)-2-aminomethyl-6-[(1*R*)-hydroxyethyl]-2-penem-3-carboxylic acid stock solutions (2.05 mmol/L) are prepared in phosphate buffer, pH 6. Reference solutions are prepared by dilution with the same buffer. Plasma-calibrated samples are prepared by adding 50 μL of reference solution of (5*R*,6*S*)-2-aminomethyl-6-[(1*R*)-hydroxyethyl]-2-penem-3-carboxylic acid to 250 μL of drug-free plasma, and correspond to concentrations ranging from 1.64 to 410 μmol/L. Urine-calibrated samples are prepared by adding 100 μL of reference solutions of (5*R*,6*S*)-2-aminomethyl-6-[(1*R*)-hydroxyethyl]-2-penem-3-carboxylic acid to 1 mL of 25-fold diluted urine. Resulting concentrations range from 41 μmol/L to 1.025 mmol/L.

Performance

(5*R*,6*S*)-2-Aminomethyl-6-[(1*R*)-hydroxyethyl]-2-penem-3-carboxylic acid and the internal standard are well separated from plasma and urine components without any interferences. Calibration graphs for plasma and urine are obtained by plotting the (5*R*,6*S*)-2-aminomethyl-6-[(1*R*)-hydroxyethyl]-2-penem-3-carboxylic acid/internal standard peak-area ratio against the concentration of (5*R*,6*S*)-2-aminomethyl-6-[(1*R*)-hydroxyethyl]-2-penem-3-carboxylic acid. Their equations are calculated using weighted linear regression. The coefficients of variation are 3% to 8.6% and recoveries are close to 100%. The method described is suitable for the determination of (5*R*,6*S*)-2-aminomethyl-6-[(1*R*)-hydroxyethyl]-2-penem-3-carboxylic acid in plasma and urine (136).

Sulbactam

Sulbactam, a penicillanic acid sulfone and a competitive and noncompetitive β-lactamase inhibitor, is administered with cefoperazone to expand the drug's antimicrobial spectrum to include β-lactam-resistant organisms. Assays that were described before the following method showed interference from metabolic products and lacked the sensitivity to determine sulbactam concentrations in tissue. The assay next presented is an HPLC method that is able to determine sulbactam and cefoperazone concentrations in plasma, urine, and prostate tissue.

Equipment

A reverse-phase HPLC system that consists of a model 510B pump to deliver the mobile phase and a model 481 variable-wavelength detector (Waters Associates) may be used. The detector settings include a wavelength of 313 nm, 0.05 absorbance units full-scale for plasma, and 0.01 absorbance units full-scale for tissues. The analysis is performed with a Beckman ODS-5 stainless steel column (Beckman Instruments, Fullerton, CA).

Chromatographic Conditions

The mobile phase consists of 89% of a 0.1 mol/L phosphate buffer, pH 6.1/11% acetonitrile. Tetrabutylammonium hydroxide (40%, 2 mL) is added to 1 liter of buffer. The buffer is degassed and filtered before use. The mobile phase is delivered at a flow rate of 2.21 mL/minute. The retention time of the sulbactam imidazole derivative is 6.0 minutes.

Procedure

Sample preparation involves a two-step procedure: derivatization and extraction. The derivatization procedure for all three specimen types consists of adding 0.5 mL of an imidazole reagent to 1.0 mL of each specimen and standard. The specimens and standards are then vortex-mixed and stored at 4°C to allow the derivatization process to be completed. Imidazole reagent is prepared by dissolving 8.5 g of imidazole in water, adding 5 N HCl to bring the solution to pH 6.8, and adjusting the volume to 40 mL with water. Specimens are then extracted by using an acetonitrile/dichloromethane procedure. The procedure includes the addition of 2.0 mL of acetonitrile to the specimen test tube to precipitate the plasma proteins, centrifugation at 3000 × g for 5 minutes, and the decanting of the supernatant into 3.0 mL of dichloromethane. The test tube is mixed and centrifuged. A WISP automated sample processor is used to deliver 15 μL of the upper aqueous layer that contains the sulbactam imidazole derivative.

Prostate tissue is blotted, weighed, diluted with phosphate buffer, pH 6.1, and homogenized. A standard curve for the determination of sulbactam concentrations in pooled plasma is prepared with concentrations ranging from 0 to 100 μg/mL. A standard curve for determination of sulbactam concentrations in prostate tissue is prepared by the addition of 2 to 25 μg of sulbactam per gram to a tissue supernatant. A standard curve for the determination of sulbactam concentrations in normal urine is prepared with concentrations of 0 to 100 μg/mL. No internal standard is added to any sample.

Chromatograms do not contain interfering peaks from body metabolites in plasma, urine, or prostate tissue, or show interference with cefoperazone or other antimicrobial agents (34). The two-step procedure is linear from 100 to 1.0 μg/mL. Extraction efficiency of the sulbactam imidazole derivative is more than 90% for all specimen types. The coefficient of variation for inter- and intrabatch studies for all specimens is generally less than 11.4%. The recovery of sulbactam from urine is more than 50%.

Aminoglycosides

A number of different methods are available for therapeutic monitoring of aminoglycoside levels. Most frequently, aminoglycoside levels in human specimens are obtained with nonisotopic immunoassays. Microbiologic assays, RIA, EMIT, HPLC, and several other assays have been compared for the monitoring of gentamicin concentrations (87). RIA, EMIT, FPIA, and HPLC are advantageous in that their results are available within a few hours, compared with 4 to 10 hours for microbiologic assays, depending on the method employed. However, interference from other aminoglycosides should be anticipated when using RIA or EMIT to quantify one of the members of this group. HPLC, although more complex and time-consuming than EMIT and, to a lesser extent, RIA, offers greater specificity than either method. Additionally, it is the only one of these methods that separates the components of gentamicin and other aminoglycosides. Table 8.16 provides information on several HPLC methods that are available to therapeutically monitor the aminoglycosides. If the decision is made to monitor an aminoglycoside by HPLC, the specific method selected will probably depend on the nature of the available equipment and the level of technical expertise within the laboratory (25,271). It has been the authors' opinion that the HPLC method of Marples and Oates (215) deserves initial consideration.

Examples of the major clinically useful aminoglycoside/aminocyclitol antibiotics are presented here. Gentamicin was the first major aminoglycoside to be analyzed by HPLC. Its assay serves as a model for the assay of the other aminoglycosides.

Reagents

A potassium borate buffer (0.4 mol/L) is prepared by the titration of 24.7 g of boric acid into 900 mL of distilled water. The pH is brought to 10.40 with concentrated potassium hydroxide solution. The solution is then diluted to 1 liter.

o-Phthaldehyde (OPA) is prepared by dissolving 60 mg of OPA in 1 mL of methanol, followed by the addition of 2-mercaptoethanol (0.2 mL). The solution is gently stirred until complete decolorization occurs. Potassium borate buffer (100 mL) is added, and the mixture is vigorously stirred. The solution is placed in the supply vessel for OPA and flushed several times with nitrogen. It must be used within 2 days of preparation.

Stock gentamicin is prepared at a concentration of 1,000 μg/mL in 0.1 mol/L phosphate buffer, pH 8.0, and stored at −20°C until use. Appropriate dilutions of the stock solutions are made with water. A serum solution that contains 10 μg/mL gentamicin is prepared by the addition of gentamicin standard at 100 μg/mL to serum. Further dilutions from this serum standard are made in normal human serum.

Equipment

A Tracor model 990 pump (Tracor Instruments, Austin, TX) is used to deliver mobile phase. A Schoeffel model 970 fluorometer (Schoeffel Instrument Corp., Westwood, NJ) is used to detect the fluorescence product that is formed by continuous flow, postcolumn derivation with OPA. Fluorescence excitation is at 340 nm and a KV418 filter is used for emission. The photomultiplier voltage is varied between 1,000 and 1,100 V, depending on the sensitivity required. OPA is supplied to a mixing tee from a pressurized glass vessel. A Cheminer fitting (CJ-303 1; Laboratory Data Control, Riviera Beach, FL) is used for the mixing tee, and a delay coil consisting of a Teflon tube (2.0 × 0.6 mm, inner diameter) is used between the mixing tee and detector. Analysis is performed by using a Bondapak C_8 column (30 cm × 3.9 mm, inner diameter; Water Associates), with a precolumn (4.3 cm × 4.2 mm, inner diameter) packed with Micropart C_{18} phase-bonded silica gel (5 μm; Applied Science Laboratories). The detector signal is processed and recorded by using a CDS 101 computing integrator (Varian) and a model 7123A recorder (Hewlett-Packard). Samples are injected using a Valco CV-6-VHPa-C20 injection valve with a 15 μL injection loop modified for variable-volume injection (Glenco Scientific, Houston, TX).

Chromatographic Conditions

Mobile-phase compositions are expressed as the ratio of components, by volume, that are added to produce the final solution. No corrections need to be made for volume changes that occur as a result of mixing. Predominantly aqueous mobile phases are degassed before use by vacuum filtration through a Millipore type HA membrane filter (0.45 μm; Millipore Corp., Bedford, MA). Solutions that contain predominantly methanol are filtered through a solvent-resistant type of FH filter (0.5 μm). The mobile phase that is used for analysis contains 0.2 mol/L Na_2SO_4, 0.02 mol/L sodium pentasulfonate, and 0.1% (v/v) acetic acid in a water/methanol (97:3) mixture. The column flow rate is 2 mL/minute at 184 atm. The OPA flow rate is approximately 0.5 mL/minute.

Gentamicin is separated from interfering compounds in serum by ion-exchange gel chromatography. A 1.5-cm column with a bed volume of 1 mL is prepared with CM-Sephadex C-25 using 0.2 mol/L Na_2SO_4 as the

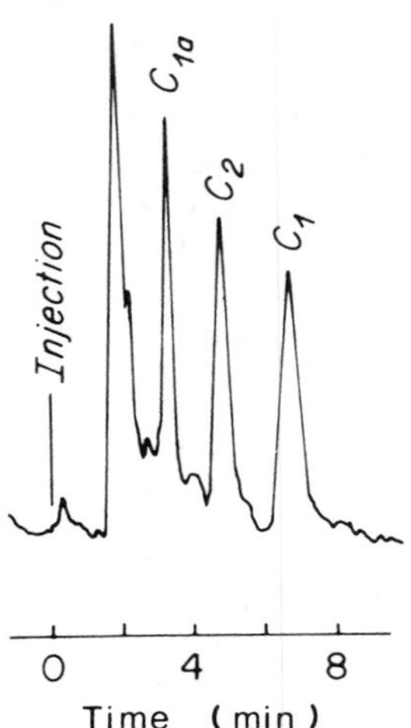

FIGURE 8.20 ● HPLC assay of gentamicin compounds. The serum contained 1.0 μg/mL. Each gentamicin compound is distinctly separated and can be assayed. (From Anhalt [11], with permission.)

initial buffer. Four hundred microliters of serum is applied to this column and eluted with 1 mL and 4 mL of the initial buffer in succession. The eluting buffer is changed to 0.01 mol/L NaOH in 0.2 mol/L Na_2SO_4, and 600 μL of this buffer is added to the column. After the column has drained completely, a second volume of alkaline buffer (400 μL) is added and the eluate is collected. Fifteen microliters of this fraction are injected for chromatographic analysis. Figure 8.20 presents the results of a typical assay. The chromatogram of a mixture of C_{1a}, C_2, and C_1 gentamicin, all at 2.5 μg/mL, is pictured.

Teicoplanin

Equipment

The liquid chromatography system is from Kontron with a Uvikon photometric detector. The LiChrosorb columns are connected by an Eco-tube cartridge system.

Chromatographic Conditions

The mobile phase is methanol/water (5:95, v/v) containing 0.01 mol/L disodium *n*-heptanesulfonate adjusted to pH 14.0 with sodium acetate and acetic acid. The HPLC system is operated at a flow rate of 0.8 mL/minute, a pressure of 59 bar, and a temperature of 30°C.

Procedure

A 1.0-mL plasma sample is extracted by dilution with *n*-heptanesulfonic acid and forced through a SAX Bond-Elut sample clean-up cartridge by vacuum. Plasma constituents are eluted from the cartridge with *n*-heptanesulfonic acid and teicoplanin is eluted with methanol. Detection is performed by measurement of the absorbance at 240 nm.

Performance

The calibration graph is linear in the range of 3 to 50 μg/mL. The detection limit is 0.2 to 0.4 μg/mL (131).

Clindamycin

CLD, synthesized from microbially fermented lincomycin, is an antibiotic that is often used to treat infections with Gram-positive and Gram-negative anaerobes, as well as Gram-positive aerobes. Other analytical procedures, including GC and microbiologic assays, exist for the detection of CLD in biologic fluids. However, the GC assay requires lengthy extraction and derivatization procedures, while the microbiologic assay lacks specificity and is less accurate than HPLC. Both of these assays are time-consuming and labor-intensive. Previously used HPLC assays have been applied only to the analysis of CLD concentrations in sterile fluids or water and have not been used with biologic fluids. The following assay is an excellent HPLC assay for the quantification of CLD in biologic fluids, serum, and plasma.

Equipment

A reverse-phase HPLC system is used that includes a model 510 pump (Waters Associates) to deliver the mobile phase. A model 783 variable wavelength UV detector (Spectros, Ramsey, NJ) with a detector wavelength of 198 nm and a filter response time of 0.1 second provides a reproducible, quantifiable peak that corresponds to 0.17 μg/mL. The monochromator of the detector is continuously purged with purified nitrogen to help decrease oxygen quenching and temperature-drift instability. Analysis is performed by using a Nova-Pak C_{18} octadecylsilane column (5 μm, 15 cm × 3.8 mm; Waters) that has been wrapped in styrofoam to help stabilize the temperature. The detector signal is processed and recorded by using a Pro-840 computer printer (Waters) for data collection, system operation, and data storage/retrieval.

Chromatographic Conditions

The mobile phase consists of acetonitrile/water/phosphoric acid/7.6 mmol/L trimethylammonium chloride (30:70:0.2:0.75), with a final pH of 6.7. The mobile phase is prepared in 2-liter quantities in the following manner. A 600-mL volume of acetonitrile is transferred to a 2-liter graduated cylinder. Nanopure (Millipore, Milford, MA) water is then poured into the cylinder until the fluid level reaches the 1900 mL mark. Four milliliters of phosphoric acid is added along with 15 mL of a previously prepared 10% trimethylammonium chloride solution. Water is added to the 2-liter mark and the contents are filtered under vacuum with a 0.45-μm membrane filter. The pH is adjusted to 6.7 with 1 mol/L sodium hydroxide and pumped through the column at a flow rate of 1.0 mL/minute and a pressure of 130 bar. A constant slow bubbling of helium through the mobile phase during operation is required to minimize the amount of oxygen in the system. Retention times for CLD and triazolam average 8 and 11.8 minutes, respectively.

Procedure

Heparinized plasma and serum samples (200 μL) are prepared by protein precipitation with 0.5 mL of acetonitrile that contains the internal standard triazolam (44 ng/100 mL). Samples are vortex-mixed for 20 seconds and centrifuged at 3000 × g for 10 minutes. The resulting supernatant is poured off the protein pellet and evaporated under nitrogen to a volume of 250 μL. A WISP autoinjector is used to deliver 15 to 30 μL of the concentrated supernatant into the HPLC system. Standards are human plasma samples with the addition of the internal standard triazolam and CLD, at 1.5 and 12 μg/mL, respectively.

Performance

Standard curves are constructed using an unweighted least squares ($y = mx + b$) method with the origin as a data point and a floating intercept. All chromatograms must be recalculated with forced baselines, as provided in a special chromatographic software package (Waters Associates). The use of peak height provides better linearity than peak area, when applied over the entire standard curve. Replicate standard curves run over a 36-hour period show no loss of integrity. The ranges for the coefficients of variation for intraday and interday measurement are 2.4% to 5.7%. The recovery range is 96% to 118%, and there is no degradation of CLD in human plasma stored at −20°C for up to 56 days.

The use of a low wavelength setting combined with the simple removal of oxygen from critical areas of the system allows for precise measurement of CLD concentrations in human plasma. This HPLC method also has the ability to measure CLD in other biologic fluids. It is fast, simple, and requires no extraction (193).

Roxithromycin

Roxithromycin is a macrolide antibiotic with an antibacterial spectrum of activity similar to that of erythromycin that exhibits enhanced, clinically desirable pharmacokinetic properties. Specifically, plasma levels are more sustained and are higher than for erythromycin, allowing for lower doses and less frequent administration. Previous assays for the macrolides have included microbiologic assays and HPLC using UV absorption fluorescence and electrochemical detection methods. Bioassays are lengthy and are not selective in the presence of active metabolites. HPLC that uses UV detection is limited because of weak macrolide absorbance in the low UV wavelength range (less than 235 nm). Thus, large volumes of patient specimens (2 to 3 mL) are required to attain sufficient sensitivity and the weak macrolide absorbance results in increased background noise and large interferences from coextracted samples. The following HPLC assay uses electrochemical detection of roxithromycin in plasma and urine.

Equipment

A reverse-phase HPLC system is used and consists of a solvent delivery pump (type 364.000; Knauer, Berlin, Germany), a manual injector (model U6K; Waters Associates), and a dual electrode electrochemical detector (ESA model 5100A; Coulochem Environmental Sciences, Bedford, MA). The electrochemical detector is equipped with a guard cell that has been placed in-line before the injector to electrolyze components of the mobile phase. The model 5010 dual-electrode cell is operated in the oxidative screen mode. The applied cell potential of the screen electrode E1 is set at +0.7 V and the sample electrode E2 at +0.9 V. This allows irreversible oxidation of many compounds in plasma and urine at the first electrode (E1) without a decrease in the response for roxithromycin and the internal standard. Analysis is performed using a Bondapak C_{18} reverse-phase column (30 cm × 3.9 mm, internal diameter; 10 μm particle size; Waters). The detector signal is recorded by an Omniscribe recorder (Houston Instruments, Houston, TX).

Chromatographic Conditions

The mobile phase consists of acetonitrile/83 mmol/L ammonium acetate/methanol (55:23:22, by volume), with the pH adjusted to 7.5 with acetic acid. The pH affects the retention times and oxidation of the macrolides. A pH of 7.5 is optimal. The low ionic strength of the buffer also helps provide adequate conductivity and minimizes background current. Before use, the mobile phase is filtered and pumped at ambient temperature through the column at a flow rate of 1.0 mL/minute. The retention times of roxithromycin and erythromycin base are 9.8 and 7.0 minutes, respectively.

Procedure

Two hundred-microliter aliquots of plasma or diluted urine (diluted 1:2 with isotonic NaCl solution), 100 μL of internal standard (10 μg/mL erythromycin), 600 μL of phosphate buffer, pH 9, and 3 mL of dichloromethane are pipetted into 10-mL glass extraction tubes, which are stoppered and mixed by shaking for 10 minutes. Following centrifugation at 2000 × g for 5 minutes, the upper layer is discarded and the organic phase (2.5 mL) is evaporated at ambient temperature under a stream of nitrogen. The residue is reconstituted with 50 μL of methanol and vortex-mixed for 10 seconds. A 15-mL aliquot is injected into the HPLC system. Standards are human plasma and urine samples with roxithromycin at concentrations of 1 to 20 μg/mL. The internal standard erythromycin concentration is 10 μg/mL in doubly distilled water.

Chromatograms are recorded at a chart speed of 0.25 cm/minute and peaks are well resolved from endogenous plasma or urine compounds. Peak height ratios of roxithromycin to erythromycin are measured.

Performance

There is a linear relationship between concentration and response up to 25 μg/mL in plasma samples and diluted urine samples. Instrument precision as determined by repeated injection of 500 mg of roxithromycin is 2.3%. The ranges for the coefficients of variation for intraday and interday variation are 1.6% to 5.5% and 2.2% to 7.0%, respectively. The recovery ranges for roxithromycin and erythromycin are 6.82 ± 1.0% and 78.8 ± 2.4%, respectively, with no interfering peaks. Roxithromycin does not degrade upon storage at 37°C, 4°C, or −20°C. The use of dual coulometric electrodes that are operated in the oxidative screen mode allow for the rapid and sensitive detection of roxithromycin in small patient samples (88).

Pyrazinamide

Pyrazinamide, an analog of nicotinamide, exhibits antimycobacterial activity when it is administered with other drugs. The drug is well absorbed after oral administration and hydrolyzed and hydroxylated to the following metabolites: 5-hydroxypyrazinamide, pyrazinoic acid, and 5-hydroxypyrazinoic acid. All of these may be important in drug-level monitoring to avoid the dose-related adverse effects of hyperuricemia and hepatotoxicity. Earlier assays, including an HPLC method that measures pyrazinamide and its three major metabolites, are time-consuming, tedious, and involve difficult extractions. The following method is rapid and allows simultaneous determination of pyrazinamide and its metabolites.

Equipment

The chromatographic system consists of an LC-6A chromatograph (Shimadzu, Kyoto, Japan) with an RF 530 HPLC fluorescence monitor (Shimadzu) set at 410/365 nm. Analysis is performed using a 10-μm Bondapak C_{18} column (30 cm × 3.9 mm, internal diameter; Waters Associates) at a column temperature of 25°C. The signal is recorded using a C-R3A Chromatopac recorder (Shimadzu).

Chromatographic Conditions

The mobile phase consists of 0.02 mol/L KH_2PO_4, pH 2.56, and is delivered at a flow rate of 2.0 mL/minute. Peaks elute between 2 and 8 minutes in the following order: 2,3-pyrazinedicarboxamide, pyrazinoic acid, and pyrazinamide.

Procedure

A 100-μL aliquot of 2 mol/L perchloric acid is placed in a 5-mL glass tube that contains 0.5 mL of plasma, 0.3 mL of distilled water, and 100 μL of 10 mmol/L 2,3-pyrazinedicarboxamide (as the internal standard) and is thoroughly mixed for 10 seconds. After centrifugation at 1500 × g for 10 minutes, a 200-μL aliquot of supernatant is neutralized with 48 μL of 1 mol/L sodium hydroxide solution. Sixty microliters of the supernatant is loaded onto the column.

The calibration graph is constructed by using 0.5 mL of drug-free plasma and adding 0.1 mL of a standard solution that contains pyrazinamide, its metabolites, and the internal standard plus 0.3 mL of distilled water, to obtain a calibration between 5 and 80 μg/mL for pyrazinamide, between 2.5 and 50 μg/mL for pyrazinoic acid, between 1 and 10 μg/mL for 5-hydroxypyrazinamide, and between 2.5 and 0.25 μg/mL for 5-hydroxypyrazinoic acid. This allows creation of a calibration graph because a small peak of an endogenous compound in plasma overlaps the peak of 5-hydroxypyrazinamide under these chromatographic conditions.

Performance

Peak area versus concentration is linear with standards in aqueous solutions up to 100, 50, 10, 2.5, and 150 μg/mL for pyrazinamide, pyrazinoic acid, 5-hydroxypyrazinamide, 5-hydroxypyrazinoic acid, and 2,3-pyrazinedicarboxamide, respectively. Detection limits for 5-hydroxypyrazinoic acid, 5-hydroxypyrazinamide, pyrazinoic acid, and pyrazinamide are 3, 3, 30, and 30 ng, respectively, with an apparatus detection limit of 0.45 ng/12 μL cell (353).

Linezolid

Linezolid, a new oxazolidinone antibiotic has broad activity against Gram-positive organisms, including methicillin-resistant *Staphylococcus aureus* (MRSA), vancomycin-resistant enterococci, and penicillin-resistant pneumococci. HPLC protocols for the measurement of Linezolid levels in serum and other body fluids have been published. (355–360) The following is a representative example of an HPLC assay for the measurement of Linezolid concentrations in human serum. (355)

Equipment

The stationary phase consists of Hypersil 5ODS, 10 cm × 4.6 mm (Waters Corporation, Milford, MA). A Ginà 50 autosampler (Dionex, Macclesfield, UK) for UV absorbance detection (λ_{max} 254), and the intergrator is a Trilab 2000 (Trivector, Sandy, UK).

Chromatographic Conditions

The mobile phase consists of 1% *ortho*-phosphoric acid (BDH, Analar grade, Poole, UK), 30% methanol (Prolabs Fontenay, France), 2 g/L, heptane sulphonic acid (Sigma-Aldrich, St. Louis, MO), adjusted to pH 5 by the addition of 10M sodium hydroxide. The flow rate is 1.0 mL/min. Retention time for Linezolid is 384 seconds.

Procedure

Samples are prepared by mixing aliquots (50:50) of the specimen with acetonitrile (Prolabs Fontenay, France). After mixing, the samples are incubated at room temperate for 10 minutes, then centrifuged at 5000g for 5 minutes. Twenty microliters of the supernant is injected.

Performance

The assay has been demonstrated to be reproducible, accurate, and linear at a concentration range from 0.0 mg/L to 30 mg/L. Intra-day and inter-day reproducibility was $<6\%$ and $<12.5\%$, with good correlation between drug concentration and peak for both aqueous and serum samples ($r = 0.9999$ for both). Linezolid recovery from serum approached 100% for concentrations tested. Accuracy of the assay expressed as percentage error was 4.0 for a 2.5 mg/L sample, 1.3 for an 8 mg/L sample, and 0.0 for an 18 mg/L sample. The lowest limit of quantification was 0.1 mg/L. No interference from 23 commonly used antimicrobial agents or unknown compounds in linezolid-free patient sera was found. Linezolid was shown to be stable in serum after sample preparation with acetonitrile for 24 hours at room temperature, and was stable in serum alone for at least 7 days at room temperature and at 4°C.

GAS-LIQUID CHROMATOGRAPHY

GLC has been used successfully in the past to assay for antibiotics that could be volatilized. With the application of HPLC to virtually all antibiotic classes, the need for GLC analyses has become significantly reduced. The general principle of GLC analysis of antibiotics and an abbreviated assay of one drug, CAM, are presented. The method often has includes a step that involves the conversion material to be assayed into a compound of high volatility so that it may be passed through a column in the gaseous phase. The general steps involved in GLC are:

1. Extraction of the drug from the serum sample
2. Conversion of the drug to a highly volatile form
3. Separation by GLC
4. Detection by flame-ionization electron capture, and so on
5. Quantitation of the drug by peak height or peak area

The finding that compounds can be rapidly converted to trimethylsilyl derivatives caused the gas chromatograph to become a tool for clinical laboratories. However, HPLC is the chromatographic technology of choice for the analysis of most antibiotics. The measurement of the concentrations of cephalosporin and (228) spectinomycin (52) antibiotics, CAM (266,295) and its chemically modified analogs (195,235), and the aminoglycosides have been determined using GLC.

Chloramphenicol

Equipment

A model 571 OA gas chromatograph equipped with dual flame ionization detector and a 1 mV model 7123A recorder (Hewlett-Packard), or the equivalent, is used. Glass columns are 122 cm × 2 mm (inner diameter) (configuration 5) for on-column injection (Hewlett-Packard), packed with 3% OV-I on 100/120 Gas Chrom Q (Applied Science Laboratory Alltech Associates, Inc. (Deerfield, IL)). Septa are type HT-9 (high temperature, low speed; Applied Science Laboratory).

The instrument conditions are as follows: injector temperature, 250°C; detector temperature, 300°C; oven temperature, programmed from 190°C to 270°C at 16°C per minute; gas flow rate, 40 mL/minute nitrogen, 250 mL/minute air, and 40 mL/minute hydrogen; and recorder chart speed, 13 mm/minute (Fig. 8.19).

Procedure

Serum (500 μL) is combined in 16 × 125 mm test tubes (Teflon-lined, screw cap) with 500 μL of a phosphate buffer (1 mol/L, pH 6.8) and 7 mL of ethyl acetate (Nanograde; Mallinckrodt Baker, Phillipsburg, NJ) that contains 21 μg of the internal standard. The tubes are mixed by shaking for 10 minutes in an Eberbach shaker at 350 oscillations/minute and centrifuged at 2,000 rpm in a desktop centrifuge for 10 minutes. The upper (organic) phase is transferred to fresh 16 × 125 mm tubes and is evaporated under a stream of nitrogen in a water bath at 40°C. Four milliliters of HCl (0.5 mol/L) are added and the tubes are held in an ultrasonic bath for 10 seconds to ensure that the residue completely dissolves. Seven milliliters of hexane is added and the tubes are mixed by shaking for 10 minutes in the Eberbach shaker (Eberbach Corporation, Ann Arbor, MI) and centrifuged for 3 minutes at 2,000 rpm. The upper (organic) phase is transferred into 7-mL screw-capped septum vials and evaporated under a stream of nitrogen in a 40°C water bath. Fifty microliters of Trisil (Pierce Chemical Co., Rockford, IL) is added to the residue and each vial is immediately capped. The vial contents are mixed on a vortex-type mixer and are allowed to stand for 8 minutes at room temperature. Two microliters of sample is injected into the gas chromatograph. One may silylate the next sample immediately after injection to save time. The results are calculated by the peak height ratio method, using CAM and the acetyl analog of CAM as internal standards.

Standard curves are prepared by analyzing samples of normal serum containing known amounts of CAM. It is convenient to run 10, 20, 40, 60, and 80 μg/mL in normal serum as standards.

THIN-LAYER CHROMATOGRAPHY

TLC has been used in the clinical laboratory for many years to separate high molecular weight, biologically active compounds. Like all forms of chromatography, the unknown may be identified based on a comparison of the mobility of the unknown compound in a defined matrix with the mobility of standards. A TLC method has been developed that first separates antibiotics from a mixture based on their mobilities in the chromatograph and then, using a test strain of indicator organism, quantitates them by their biologic activities.

Tobramycin (Nebramycin Complex)

Apparatus

Thin-layer plates (20 × 20 cm) are prepared from silica gel G. Glass plates of sizes 20 × 2 × 0.03 cm and 16 × 2 × 0.3 cm are used for framing the chromatograms.

Reagents

All standard antibiotic solutions are dissolved in distilled water. Two developing solvents are employed: methylethyl ketone (96%)/ethanol (25%)/ammonium hydroxide (1:1:1) and chloroform/methanol (25%)/ammonium hydroxide (1:7:4). Solvent systems are made fresh before use (Table 8.18). Bioautograms are stained with 1% tetrazolium blue and 0.02% tetrazolium violet.

TABLE 8.18

R_F Values of Closely Related Antibiotics in a Chloroform/Methanol/Ammonium Hydroxide Solvent System (250)

Antibiotic	$R_F \times 100$
Amikacin	6
Gentamicin (C_{1a}, C_1, C_2)	63
Kanamycin A	30
Neamine	37
Neomycin	12
Paromomycin	23
Sisomicin	60
Tobramycin (nebramycin) (2,5; 4,5; 5′)	32, 42, 51

Bacteria

The test organism used is *B. subtilis* ATCC strain 6633.

Procedure

Silica plates with a Camag or Desaga coater are made 0.25-mm thick, dried at room temperature for 2 days, and used without further pretreatment. Lines are drawn before use to ensure separate, 1.5-cm wide tracks. Tobramycin standard solutions are each diluted to a final content of 0.1 to 0.5 μg of the analyte. Patient specimens are dissolved in distilled water to also cover this range. Chromatography is allowed to proceed for a distance of 15 cm at room temperature. The plate is subsequently air-dried.

For the detection of microbiologic activity, nutrient agar is melted and the *B. subtilis* test organism is added to a final organism concentration of 1×10^8/mL. A 25-mL volume of this medium is poured onto the glass frame in order to cover the silica gel surface uniformly. The agar is covered with a 20 × 20 cm glass chromatographic plate and incubated for 10 to 16 hours at 37°C.

Interpretation

Quantitative determinations are performed using a calibration graph. The zones of inhibition of the *B. subtilis* test organism are measured with the standards and unknowns, and the concentration of tobramycin is calculated in the same manner as for the analogous electrophoresis/bioautography procedure.

Performance

The TLC/bioautography method is able to measure as little as 0.1 to 0.3 μg of tobramycin (nebramycin complex). It is able to separate tobramycin into nebramycin 2, 4, 5′, 5, and 6. Furthermore, the TLC/bioautography method is able to differentiate between closely related aminoglycoside antibiotics by their gel mobilities.

The tetrazolium blue solution gives a colorless spot on a deep red background in order to measure the zones of inhibition more efficiently. In addition to tobramycin, the method is able to detect 0.2 μg of gentamicin and 0.1 μg of neomycin, paromomycin, and kanamycin (250). TLC is a useful method for the detection of tetracyclines (246,247).

ION-EXCHANGE CHROMATOGRAPHY OF AMINOGLYCOSIDES

A procedure based on the ion-exchange chromatographic separation of aminoglycosides from human body specimens has been developed for the spectrofluorometric assay of aminoglycosides/aminocyclitol antibiotics. The aminoglycosides are separated by elution from the column with sulfuric acid, followed by fluorometric analysis after derivatization.

Ion-Exchange Assay

Reagents

Reagents for ion-exchange chromatography include 0.1 mol/L sulfuric acid and 0.5 mol/L sulfuric acid. Reagents for the analysis of aminoglycoside concentrations include acetylacetone, formaldehyde (30%), and Britton-Robinson buffer, made by mixing 100 mL of solution 1 (0.2 mol/L phosphoric acid, 0.2 mol/L acetic acid, and 0.2 mol/L boric acid) with 15 mL of 1.0 mol/L sodium hydroxide (15). To 10 mL of the final buffer, which is at pH 2.6, 0.8 mL of acetylacetone and 2.0 mL of formaldehyde are added.

Procedure

The aminoglycosides are analyzed spectrophotometrically with a fluorescent dihydrolutidine derivative that is developed by the condensation of the primary amino group with acetylacetone and formaldehyde under acidic conditions. A 13.9 × 290 mm glass column is packed with 3 mL of Amberlite IRC 50 resin (sodium form). Either human urine (2 mL) or human serum (5 mL) is diluted to 10 mL with distilled water and applied to the column. Twenty milliliters of distilled water are applied to the column and impurities are diluted with 20 mL of 0.1 mol/L sulfuric acid. The aminoglycoside antibiotics are eluted from the column with 20 mL of 0.5 mol/L sulfuric acid. Two milliliters of this eluent is analyzed for the aminoglycoside concentration. The elution rate is approximately 0.5 mL/minute.

Two milliliters of the eluent is added to 2 mL of the analysis reagent and heated at 100°C for 10 minutes. After heating, the aminoglycoside is quantitated by determining its absorbance at an excitation wavelength of 421 nm and an emission wavelength of 488 nm, in a 1-cm light path.

Performance

The method should be able to analyze any of the aminoglycoside antibiotics. Tobramycin, neomycin, sisomicin, kanamycin, and amikacin have been quantitated. The method is sensitive to 0.5 μg/mL.

MICELLAR ELECTROKINETIC CHROMATOGRAPHY OF ASPOXICILLIN

Micellar electrokinetic chromatography is a type of capillary zone electrophoresis in which a detergent forms micelles with electrically neutral substances, allowing their separation and detection by UV absorption (238). This method permits the quantitation of penicillin in plasma. Plasma proteins are solubilized by the detergent and thus do not interfere with the assay.

Micellar Method

Reagents

Sodium dodecyl sulfate is dissolved in a buffer of 0.02 mol/L sodium dihydrogen phosphate with 0.02 mol/L sodium tetraborate, passed through a 0.45-μm membrane filter, and degassed by sonication. Standards are dissolved in water to a concentration of 1 mg/mL.

Apparatus

A fused silica capillary tube with dimensions of 650 mm × 50 μm is used as a separation tube. Detection of antibiotic is achieved by on-column UV absorption measurement at 210 nm, using a Uvidec 100-V1 detector (Jasco, Tokyo, Japan) with a time constant of 0.05 second.

Performance

The calibration graph for aspoxicillin is linear in the range of 25 to 300 μg/mL. The detection limit is 1.3 μg/mL. The average recovery is 94% to 104%.

NUCLEAR MAGNETIC RESONANCE SPECTROSCOPY

Nuclear magnetic resonance techniques, while not widely available in the clinical setting, have been investigated for the measurement of antibiotic concentrations. When spinning nuclei in a magnetic field are irradiated by a second, perpendicular field, they change their alignment to the new field. The amount of energy required for the transformation is characteristic of the molecule and depends on factors such as electronic configuration and intermolecular interactions. Nuclear magnetic resonance spectroscopy can provide information about the kinetic and structural aspects of the interactions between ligands and macromolecules, such as drugs and receptors. It offers both sensitivity and specific simultaneous identification and quantification of drugs and their metabolites in plasma, serum, and urine. Antibiotics that have been assayed include tetracyclines, penicillins, cephalosporins, and erythromycin (48).

POLAROGRAPHY OF CLAVULANIC ACID

Gonzalez Perez et al. (138) have described a method for the determination of levels of clavulanic acid in the presence of amoxicillin by differential pulse polarography. Clavulanic acid is hydrolyzed in a sulfuric medium to obtain an electroactive product with a reduction peak at 0.75 V. The procedure can detect clavulanic acid in the range of 8 to 2 mol/L.

REFERENCES

1. Abuirejeie MA, Abdel-Hamid ME. Simultaneous high-pressure liquid chromatographic analysis of ampicillin

and cloxacillin in serum and urine. *J Clin Pharmacol* 1988;13:101–108.

2. Ace LN, Jaffe JM. Modified fluorometric assay for minocycline. *Biochem Med* 1975;12:401–402.
3. Ackerman BH, Berg HG, Strate RG, et al. Comparison of radioimmunoassay and fluorescent polarization immunoassay for quantitative determination of vancomycin concentrations in serum. *J Clin Microbiol* 1983;18:994–995.
4. Ackers IM, Myers CM, Blumer JL. Determination of cefsulodin in biological fluids by high-pressure liquid chromatography. *Ther Drug Monit* 1984;6:91–95.
5. Adamovics J. Rapid determination of metronidazole in human serum and urine using a normal-phase high-performance liquid chromatographic column with aqueous solvents. *J Chromatogr* 1984;309:436–440.
6. Alture-Werber E, Lowe L. A method for the routine determination of streptomycin levels in body fluids. *Proc Soc Exp Biol Med* 1946;63:277–280.
7. Amicon Corp. Amicon micropartition system. Lexington, MA: Amicon Corp., 1977.
8. Amina Watson RA, Landon J, Shaw EJ, et al. Polarization fluoroimmunoassay of gentamicin. *Clin Chim Acta* 1976;73:51–55.
9. Anders RJ, Lau A, Sharifi R, et al. Comparison of EMIT versus bioassay to evaluate inactivation of tobramycin by piperacillin. *Ther Drug Monit* 1987;9:472–477.
10. Andrews JM, Wise R. A comparison of the homogeneous enzyme immunoassay and polarization fluoroimmunoassay of gentamicin. *J Antimicrob Chemother* 1984;14:509–520.
11. Anhalt JP. Assay of gentamicin in serum by high-pressure liquid chromatography. *Antimicrob Agents Chemother* 1977;11:651–655.
12. Annesley T, Wilkerson K, Matz K, et al. Simultaneous determination of penicillin and cephalosporin antibiotics in serum by gradient liquid chromatography. *Clin Chem* 1984;30:908–910.
13. Araj GF, Khattar MA, Thulesius O, et al. Measurements of serum gentamicin concentrations by a biological method, fluorescence polarization immunoassay and enzyme multiplied immunoassay. *Int J Clin Pharmacol Ther Toxicol* 1986;24:542–555.
14. Aravind MD, Miceli JN, Kauffman RE, et al. Simultaneous measurement of chloramphenicol and chloramphenicol succinate by high-performance liquid chromatography. *J Chromatogr* 1980;221:176–181.
15. Aravind MK, Miceli JN, Kauffman RE. Determination of moxalactam by high-performance liquid chromatography. *J Chromatogr* 1982;228:418–422.
16. Arret B, Eckert J. New developments in antibiotic interference. *J Pharm Sci* 1968;57:871–878.
17. Arret B, Johnson DP, Kirshbarum A. Outline of details for microbiological assays of antibiotics: second revision. *J Pharm Sci* 1971;60:1689–1694.
18. Ascalone V, Dal-Bo L. Determination of ceftriaxone, a novel cephalosporin, in plasma, urine and saliva by high-performance liquid chromatography on an NH_2 bonded-phase column. *J Chromatogr* 1983;273:357–366.
19. Assenza SP, Brown PR. Evaluation of reversed-phase, radially-compressed, flexible-walled columns for the separation of low molecular weight, UV-absorbing compounds in serum. *J Liquid Chromatogr* 1980;3:41–59.
20. Asukabe H, Sasaki T, Harada KI, et al. Improvement of chemical analysis of antibiotics. IV. Fluorodensitometric determination of polyether antibiotics. *J Chromatogr* 1984;295:453–461.
21. Baer DM, Paulson RA. The effect of hyperlipidemia on therapeutic drug assays. *Ther Drug Monit* 1987;9:72–77.
22. Bakerman S. Fluorescence polarization immunoassay. *Lab Manage* 1983;July:16–18.
23. Barbhaiya RH, Forgue ST, Shyu WC, et al. High-pressure liquid chromatographic analysis of BMY-28142 in plasma and urine. *Antimicrob Agents Chemother* 1987;31:55–59.
24. Barbhaiya RH, Turner P, Shaw E. A simple rapid fluorimetric assay of amoxicillin in plasma. *Clin Chim Acta* 1977;77:373–377.
25. Barends DM, Blauw JS, Smits MH, et al. Determination of amikacin in serum by high-performance liquid chromatography with ultraviolet detection. *J Chromatogr* 1983;276:385–394.
26. Barry AL, Packer RR. Roxithromycin bioassay procedures for human plasma, urine and milk specimens [corrected and issued with original pagination in *Eur J Clin Microbiol* 1986;5(6)]. *Eur J Clin Microbiol* 1986;5:536–540.
27. Barry AL, Sabath LD. Special tests: bactericidal activity and activity of antimicrobics in combination. In: Lenette EH, Spaulding EH, Truant JP, eds. *Manual of clinical microbiology.* 2nd ed. Washington DC: American Society for Microbiology, 1974;431–435.
28. Bartlett JG, Chang TW, Gurwith M, et al. Antibiotic-associated pseudomembranous colitis due to toxin-producing clostridia. *N Engl J Med* 1978;298:534.
29. Barza M, Brusch J, Bergeron MG, et al. Penetration of antibiotics into fibrin loci in vivo. *J Infect Dis* 1974;129:73–78.
30. Baskerville AJ, Flemingham D, Gruneberg RN. A high performance liquid chromatography method for the determination of FCE 22101, a novel penem antimicrobial, in serum. *Drugs Exp Clin Res* 1988;14:645–648.
31. Bastiani RJ. The EMIT system: a commercially successful innovation. *Antibiot Chemother* 1979;26:89–97.
32. Bauchet J, Pussard E, Garaud JJ. Determination of vancomycin in serum and tissues by column liquid chromatography using solid-phase extraction. *J Chromatogr* 1987;414:472–476.
33. Bawdon RE, Madsen PO. High-pressure liquid chromatographic assay of sulbactam in plasma, urine, and tissue. *Antimicrob Agents Chemother* 1986;30:231–233.
34. Beezer AE, Miles RJ, Shaw EJ, et al. Antibiotic bioassay by flow microcalorimetry. *Experientia* 1980;36:1051–1052.
35. Bennett JV, Brodie JL, Benner EJ, et al. Simplified, accurate method for antibiotic assay of clinical specimens. *Appl Microbiol* 1966;14:170–177.
36. Benveniste R, Davies J. R-factor mediated gentamicin resistance: a new enzyme which modifies aminoglycoside antibiotics. *FEBS Lett* 1971;14:293–296.
37. Berry DJ. Chloramphenicol assay by EMIT [letter]. *Antimicrob Chemother* 1988;21:684–685.
38. Berti MA, Maccari M. Stability of frozen plasma containing different antibiotics. *Antimicrob Agents Chemother* 1975;8:633–637.
39. Black RE, Lau WK, Weinstein RJ, et al. Ototoxicity of amikacin. *Antimicrob Agents Chemother* 1976;9:956–961.
40. Black SB, Levine P, Shinefield HR. The necessity for monitoring chloramphenicol levels when treating neonatal meningitis. *J Pediatr* 1978;92:235–236.
41. Blecka LJ. Fluorescence polarization immunoassay: a review of methodology and applications. *Ther Drug Monit* 1983;March:16.
42. Bliss M, Mayersohn M. Liquid-chromatographic assay of

cefamandole in serum, urine, and dialysis fluid. *Clin Chem* 1986;32:197–200.

43. Bolton AE, Hunter WM. The labelling of proteins to high specific radioactivities by conjugation to a ^{125}I-containing acylating agent. *Biochem J* 1973;133:529–539.
44. Bowman DB, Aravind MK, Miceli JN, et al. Reversed-phase high-performance liquid chromatographic method to determine ceftriaxone in biological fluids. *J Chromatogr* 1984;309:209–213.
45. Boyce EG, Lawson LA, Gibson GA, et al. Comparison of gentamicin immunoassays using univariate and multivariate analyses. *Ther Drug Monit* 1989;11:97–104.
46. Boylon JC, Simmons JL, Winchly GL. Stability of frozen solutions of sodium cephalothin and cephaloridine. *Am J Hosp Pharm* 1972;29:687–689.
47. Brajtburg J, Elberg S, Bolard J, et al. Interaction of plasma proteins and lipoproteins with amphotericin B. *J Infect Dis* 1984;149:986–989.
48. Branch SK, Casy AF. Applications of modern high-field NMR spectroscopy in medicinal chemistry. *Prog Med Chem* 1989;26:355–436.
49. Brendel E, Zschunke M, Meineke I. High-performance liquid chromatographic determination of cefonicid in human plasma and urine. *J Chromatogr* 1985;339:359–365.
50. Brisson AM, Fourtillan JB. High-performance liquid chromatographic determination of piperacillin in plasma. *Antimicrob Agents Chemother* 1982;21:664–665.
51. Brisson AM, Fourtillan JB. Determination of cephalosporins in biological material by reversed-phase liquid column chromatography. *J Chromatogr* 1981;223:393–399.
52. Bronson LW, Bowman PB. Gas chromatographic assay for the antibiotic spectinomycin. *J Chromatogr Sci* 1974;12:373–376.
53. Broughall JM, Pugsley DJ, Reeves DS. Potential pitfall in bioassay of serum-gentamicin. *Lancet* 1975;2:1095.
54. Broughall JM, Reeves DS. The acetyltransferase enzyme method for the assay of serum gentamicin concentrations and a comparison with other methods. *J Clin Pathol* 1975;28:140–145.
55. Broughton A. Monitoring antibiotic levels in body fluids. *Lab Manage* 1977;12:10–12.
56. Broughton A, Strong JE. Radioimmunoassay of antibiotics and chemotherapeutic agents. *Clin Chem* 1976;22:726–732.
57. Broughton A, Strong JE, Pickering LK, et al. Radioimmunoassay of iodinated tobramycin. *Antimicrob Agents Chemother* 1976;10:652–656.
58. Buchs RP, Maxim TE, Allen N, et al. Analysis of cefoxitin, cephalothin and their deacylated metabolites in human urine by high-performance liquid chromatography. *J Chromatogr* 1974;99:609–618.
59. Butcher RH. Rapid serum gentamicin assay by enzymatic adenylation. *Am J Clin Pathol* 1977;68:566–569.
60. Butterfield AG, Hughes DW, Pound NJ, et al. Separation and detection of tetracycline by high-speed liquid chromatography. *Antimicrob Agents Chemother* 1973;4:11–15.
61. Campbell GW, Mageau RP, Schwab B, et al. Detection and quantitation of chloramphenicol by competitive enzyme-linked immunoassay. *Antimicrob Agents Chemother* 1984;25:205–211.
62. Carling DC, Idelson BA, Casano AA, et al. Nephrotoxicity associated with cephalothin administration. *Arch Intern Med* 1975;135:797–801.
63. Carlqvist J, Westerlund D. Automated determination of amoxycillin in biological fluids by column switching in ion-pair reversed-phase liquid chromatographic systems with post-column derivatization. *J Chromatogr* 1985;344:285–296.
64. Carroll MA, White ER, Jancsik Z, et al. The determination of cephradine and cephalexin by reverse phase high-performance liquid chromatography. *J Antibiot* 1977;30:397–403.
65. Cavenaghi L, Corti A, Cassani G. Comparison of the solid phase enzyme receptor assay (SPERA) and the microbiological assay for teicoplanin. *J Hosp Infect* 1986; 7(Suppl A):85–89.
66. Chan CY, Chan K, French GL. Rapid high performance liquid chromatographic assay of cephalosporins in biological fluids. *J Antimicrob Chemother* 1986;18:537–545.
67. Chen ML, Chiou WL. Analysis of erythromycin in biological fluids by high-performance liquid chromatography with electrochemical detection. *J Chromatogr* 1983;278:91–100.
68. Cheng AF, Lam AW, French GL. Comparative evaluation of the Abbott TDX, the Abbott ABA200, and the Syva LAB5000 for assay of serum gentamicin. *J Antimicrob Chemother* 1987;19:127–133.
69. Chow AW, Montgomerie JZ, Guze LB. Parenteral clindamycin therapy for severe anaerobic infections. *Arch Intern Med* 1974;134:7882.
70. Cooper MJ, Anders MW, Mirkin BL. Ion-pair extraction and high-speed liquid chromatography of cephalothin and diacetylcephalothin in human serum and urine. *Drug Metab Dispos* 1973;1:659–662.
71. Corti A, Cavenaghi L, Giani E, et al. A receptor-antibody sandwich assay for teicoplanin. *Clin Chem* 1987;33:1615–1618.
72. Corti A, Rurali C, Borghi A, et al. Solid-phase enzyme-receptor assay (SPERA): a competitive-binding assay for glycopeptide antibiotics of the vancomycin class. *Clin Chem* 1985;31:1606–1610.
73. Cosgrove RF. Rapid microbiological assay for chlorhydroxyquinoline that uses a cryogenically stored inoculum. *Antimicrob Agents Chemother* 1977;11:848–851.
74. Cowlishaw MG, Sharman JR. Liquid-chromatographic assay of cefoperazone from plasma and bile. *Clin Chem* 1986;32:894.
75. Croteau D, Vallee F, Bergeron MG, et al. High-performance liquid chromatographic assay of erythromycin and its esters using electrochemical detection. *J Chromatogr* 1987;419:205–212.
76. Cummings KC, Jatlow PI. Sample preparation by ultrafiltration for direct gas chromatographic analysis of ethylene glycol in plasma. *J Anal Toxicol* 1982;6:324–326.
77. Cummings KC, Torres AR, Edberg SC. The analysis of antimicrobial agents in biological fluids by high-performance liquid chromatography. II. Applications. *J Clin Lab Autom* 1984;4:244–255.
78. Dahlgren JC, Anderson ET, Hewitt WL. Gentamicin blood levels: a guide to nephrotoxicity. *Antimicrob Agents Chemother* 1975;8:58–62.
79. Daigneault R, Gagne M, Brazeau M. A comparison of two methods of gentamicin assay: an enzymatic procedure and an agar diffusion technique. *J Infect Dis* 1974;130:642–645.
80. Dalbey M, Gano C, Izutsu A, et al. Quantitative chloramphenicol determination by homogeneous enzyme-immunoassay. *Clin Chem* 1985;31:933.
81. Dandliker WB, Kelly RJ, Dandliker J. Fluorescence polarization immunoassay: theory and experimental method. *Immunochemistry* 1973;10:219–227.
82. Davidson AG, Stenlake JB. The spectrophotometric

determination of ampicillin and cloxacillin in combined injections. *Analyst* 1974;99:476–481.
83. Davidson DF. A simple chemical method for the assay of amoxycillin in serum and urine. *Clin Chim Acta* 1976;69:67–71.
84. Davies J, Brzezinska M, Benveniste R. R factors: biochemical mechanisms of resistance to aminoglycoside antibiotics. *Ann NY Acad Sci* 1971;182:226–233.
85. De Louvois J. A rapid method of assaying gentamicin and kanamycin concentrations in serum. *J Med Microbiol* 1974;7:11–16.
86. Deacon S. Assay of gentamicin in cerebrospinal fluid. *J Clin Pathol* 1976;29:749–751.
87. Delaney CJ, Opheim KE, Smith AL, et al. Performance characteristics of bioassay, radioenzymatic assay, homogeneous enzyme immunoassay, and high-performance liquid chromatographic determination of serum gentamicin. *Antimicrob Agents Chemother* 1982;21:19–25.
88. Demotes-Mainaird FM, Vincon GA, Jarry CH, et al. Micro-method for the determination of roxithromycin in human plasma and urine by high-performance liquid chromatography using electrochemical detection. *J Chromatogr* 1989;490:115–123.
89. Dipiro JT, Taylor AT, Steele JCH Jr. Lack of influence of commonly used drugs on bioassay indicator organisms. *Antimicrob Agents Chemother* 1983;23:703–705.
90. Dow J, Lemar M, Frydman A, et al. Automated high-performance liquid chromatographic determination of spiramycin by direct injection of plasma, using column-switching for sample clean-up. *J Chromatogr* 1985;344:275–283.
91. Duda E, Marton L, Kiss G. Modification of the thiobarbituric acid assay of streptomycin. *Biochem Med* 1976;15:330–332.
92. Durr A, Schatzmann HJ. A simple fluorometric assay for ampicillin in serum. *Experientia* 1975;31:503–504.
93. Edberg SC. Pharmacokinetics. In: Edberg SC, Berger SA, eds. *Antibiotics and infection.* New York: Churchill-Livingstone, 1983;1–15.
94. Edberg SC, Bottenbley CJ, Gam K. Use of sodium polyanethol sulfonate to selectively inhibit aminoglycoside and polymyxin antibiotics in a rapid blood level antibiotic assay. *Antimicrob Agents Chemother* 1976;9:414–417.
95. Edberg SC, Bottenbley CJ, Singer JM. The mechanism of inhibition of aminoglycoside and polymyxin class antibiotics by polyanionic detergents. *Proc Soc Exp Biol Med* 1976;153:49–51.
96. Edberg SC, Chu A. Determining antibiotic levels in the blood. *Am J Med Technol* 1975;41:99–105.
97. Edberg SC, Chu A, Melnick G. Preparation of organisms for determining antibiotic concentrations from the blood. *Lab Med* 1973;4:36–37.
98. Edberg SC, Mishkin A. Turbidimetric determination of blood aminoglycoside levels by growth curve analysis. *J Pharm Sci* 1981;69:1442–1443.
99. Edberg SC, Sabath LD. Determination of antibiotic levels in body fluids: techniques and significance. In: Lorian V, ed. *Antibiotics in laboratory medicine.* Baltimore: Williams & Wilkins, 1980;206–264.
100. Edberg SC, Young LS, Barry AL. Therapeutic drug monitoring: antimicrobial agents. In: *Cumitech 20.* Washington DC: American Society for Microbiology, 1984;120.
101. Egger HJ, Fischer G. Determination of the monocyclic-lactam antibiotic carumonam in plasma and urine by ion-pair and ion-suppression reversed-phase high-performance liquid chromatography. *J Chromatogr* 1987;420:357–372.
102. Ehret W, Probst H, Ruckdeschel G. Determination of aztreonam in faeces of human volunteers: comparison of reversed-phase high pressure liquid chromatography and bioassay. *J Antimicrob Chemother* 1987;19:541–549.
103. el-Yazigi A, Yusuf A, Al-Humaidan A. Direct, simultaneous measurement of chloramphenicol and its monosuccinate ester in micro-samples of plasma by radial-compression liquid chromatography. *Clin Chem* 1987;33:1814–1816.
104. Emm TA, Leslie J, Chai M, et al. High-performance liquid chromatographic assay of cephalexin in serum and urine. *J Chromatogr* 1988;427:162–165.
105. Engvall E, Perlman P. Enzyme-linked immunosorbent assay, ELISA. *J Immunol* 1972;109:129–135.
106. Engvall E, Perlmann P. Enzyme-linked immunosorbent assay (ELISA): quantitative assay of immunoglobulin G. *Immunochemistry* 1971;8:871–874.
107. Erni F. Liquid chromatography-mass spectrometry in the pharmaceutical industry: objectives and needs. *J Chromatogr* 1982;251:141–151.
107a. Evenson M. Spectrophotmetric techniques. In: Burtis C, Ashwood E, eds. *Teitz textbook of clinical chemistry,* 3rd ed. Philadelphia: WB Saunders, 1999;96–98.
108. Evrin FR, Bullock WE. Simple assay for clindamycin in the presence of aminoglycosides. *Antimicrob Agents Chemother* 1974;6:831–835.
109. Faine S, Knight DC. Rapid microbiological assay of antibiotic in blood and other body fluids. *Lancet* 1968;2:375–378.
110. Falkowski AJ, Greger RJ. Hydroxylamine technique for in vitro prevention of penicillin inactivation of tobramycin. *Antimicrob Agents Chemother* 1984;26:643–646.
111. Falkowski AJ, Look ZM, Noguchi H, et al. Determination of cefixime in biological samples by reversed-phase high-performance liquid chromatography. *J Chromatogr* 1987;422:145–152.
112. Fan-Havard P, Nahata MC. A rapid analysis of nafcillin using high-performance liquid chromatography. *Ther Drug Monit* 1989;11:105–108.
113. Fasching CE, Hughes CE, Hector RF, et al. High-pressure liquid chromatographic assay of Bay N 7133 in human serum. *Antimicrob Agents Chemother* 1984;25:596–598.
114. Fekety R. Vancomycin (Symposium on Antimicrobial Therapy). *Med Clin North Am* 1982;66:175–181.
115. Fernandes PB, Ramer N, Rode RA, et al. Bioassay for A-56268 (TE-031) and identification of its major metabolite, 14-hydroxy-6-O-methyl erythromycin. *Eur J Clin Microbiol Infect Dis* 1988;7:73–76.
116. Filburn BH, Shull VH, Tempera YM, et al. Evaluation of an automated fluorescence polarization immunoassay for vancomycin. *Antimicrob Agents Chemother* 1983;24:216–220.
117. Fiore D, Auger FA, Drusano GL, et al. Improved micromethod for mezlocillin quantitation in serum and urine by high-pressure liquid chromatography. *Antimicrob Agents Chemother* 1984;26:775–777.
118. Fisher AM. A method for the determination of antibacterial potency of serum during therapy of acute infections: a preliminary report. *Bull Johns Hopkins Hosp* 1952;90:313–320.
119. Fleming A. On a remarkable bacteriolytic element found in tissues and secretions. *Proc R Soc Lond [Biol]* 1922;93:306–317.
120. Foglesong A, Kavanagh F, Dietz JV. Possibility for error in FDA diffusion assays. *J Pharm Sci* 1978;68:797–798.
121. Forchetti C. High-performance liquid chromatographic procedure for the quantitation of norfloxacin in urine, serum and tissues. *J Chromatogr* 1984;309:177–182.

122. Forgue ST, Pittman KA, Barbhaiya RH. High-performance liquid chromatographic analysis of a novel carbapenem antibiotic in human plasma and urine. *J Chromatogr* 1987;414:343–353.
123. Forrey AW, Blair A, O'Neill M, et al. Enzymatic assay for gentamicin. *N Engl J Med* 1973;288:108.
124. Foulds G, Gans DJ, Girard D, et al. Assays of sulbactam in the presence of ampicillin. *Ther Drug Monit* 1986;8:223–227.
125. Fowler W, Khan MH. Mezlocillin in gonorrhea: a pilot study. *Curr Med Res Opin* 1979;5:790–792.
126. Friis JM, Lakings DB. High-performance liquid chromatographic method for the determination of cefpimizole in tissue. *J Chromatogr* 1986;382:399–404.
127. Fujimoto T, Tsuda Y, Tawa R, et al. Fluorescence polarization immunoassay of gentamicin or netilmicin in blood spotted on filter paper. *Clin Chem* 1989;35:867–869.
128. Garrod LP, Lambert HP, O'Grady F. *Antibiotics and chemotherapy.* Edinburgh: Churchill Livingstone, 1973.
129. Gentamicin radioimmunoassay. Newport Beach, CA: Monitor Science Corp., 1976.
130. Gentry LO, Jemsek JG, Natelson EA. Effects of sodium piperacillin on platelet function in normal volunteers. *Antimicrob Agents Chemother* 1981;19:532–533.
131. Georgopoulos A, Czejka MJ, Starzengruber N, et al. High-performance liquid chromatographic determination of teicoplanin in plasma: comparison with a microbiological assay. *J Chromatogr* 1989;494:340–346.
132. Giamerellou H, Zimelis VM, Matulionis DO, et al. Assay of aminoglycoside antibiotics in clinical specimens. *J Infect Dis* 1975;132:399–406.
133. Giddings JC. Theory of chromatography. In: Heftman E, ed. *Chromatography.* New York: Reinhold, 1967.
134. Giese RW. Technical considerations in the use of high-performance liquid chromatography in therapeutic drug monitoring. *Clin Chem* 1983;29:1331–1343.
135. Gochin R, Kanfer I, Haigh JM. Simultaneous determination of trimethoprim, sulphamethoxazole and N^4-acetylsulphamethoxazole in serum and urine by high-performance liquid chromatography. *J Chromatogr* 1981;223:139–145.
136. Godbillon J, Duval M, Gauron S, et al. High-performance liquid chromatographic determination of the penem antibiotic (5R,6S)-2-aminomethyl-6-[(1R)-hydroxyethyl]-2-penem-3-carboxylic acid in human plasma and urine. *J Chromatogr* 1988;427:269–276.
137. Golas CL, Prober CG, MacLeod SM, et al. Measurement of amphotericin B in serum or plasma by high-performance liquid chromatography. *J Chromatogr* 1983;278:387–395.
138. Gonzalez Perez C, Gonzalez Martin I, et al. Polarographic determination of clavulanic acid. *J Pharm Biomed Anal* 1991;9:383–386.
139. Granich GG, Krogstad DJ. Ion pair high-performance liquid chromatographic assay for ceftriaxone. *Antimicrob Agents Chemother* 1987;31:385–388.
140. Gravallese DA, Musson DG, Pauliukonis LT, et al. Determination of imipenem (N-formimidoyl thienamycin) in human plasma and urine by high-performance liquid chromatography: comparison with microbiological methodology and stability. *J Chromatogr* 1984;310:71–84.
141. Grove DC, Randall WA. *Assay methods of antibiotics: a laboratory manual.* New York: Medical Encyclopedia, 1955.
142. Guiochon G. Optimization in liquid chromatography. In: Horvath C, ed. *High-performance liquid chromatography:* advances and perspections. New York: Academic Press, 1980;2:1–56.
143. Haataja H, Kokkonen P. Determination of 2-acetyl erythromycin and erythromycin in human tonsil tissue by HPLC with coulometric detection. *J Antimicrob Chemother* 1988;21(Suppl D):67–72.
144. Haginaka J, Wakai J. Liquid chromatographic determination of penicillins by postcolumn alkaline degradation using a hollow-fiber membrane reactor. *Anal Biochem* 1988;168:132–140.
145. Haginaka J, Yasuda H, Uno T, et al. High-performance liquid chromatographic assay of clavulanate in human plasma and urine by fluorimetric detection. *J Chromatogr* 1986;377:269–277.
146. Hall D. Fluorimetric assay of tetracycline mixtures in plasma. In: Williams JD, Geddes AM, eds. *Chemotherapy,* vol. 2. New York: Plenum Press, 1975;111–114.
147. Hanka LJ, Barnett MS. Microbiological assays and bioautography of maytansine and its homologues. *Antimicrob Agents Chemother* 1974,6:651–652.
148. Hanka LJ, Gerpheide SA, Spieles PR, et al. Improved methods for production, isolation, and assay of two new chloroisoxazoline amino acid antitumor antimetabolites: U-42,126 and U-43,795. *Antimicrob Agents Chemother* 1975;7:807–810.
149. Harber MJ, Asscher AW. A new assay technique for antibiotics. In: Williams JD, Geddes AM, eds. *Chemotherapy,* vol. 2. New York: Plenum Press, 1975;125–131.
150. Harrison LI, Schuppan D, Rohlfing SR, et al. Determination of flumequine and a hydroxy metabolite in biological fluids by high-pressure liquid chromatographic, fluorometric, and microbiologial methods. *Antimicrob Agents Chemother* 1984;25:301–305.
151. Heimdahl A, Cars O, Hedberg M, et al. A micromethod for determination of antimicrobial agents in bone. *Drugs Exp Clin Res* 1988;14:649–654.
152. Hendrickx L, Roets E, Hoogmartens J, et al. Identification of penicillins by thin-layer chromatography. *J Chromatogr* 1984;291:211–218.
153. Henlon JD, Thomson BA, Dawson PH. Determination of sulfa drugs in biological fluids by liquid chromatography/mass spectrometry/mass spectrometry. *Anal Chem* 1982;54:451–456.
154. Heppel LA. Selective release of enzymes from bacteria. *Science* 1967;156:1541–1555.
155. Hildebrandt R, Gundert-Remy U. Improved procedures for the determination of the ureidopenicillins azlocillin and mezlocillin in plasma by high-performance liquid chromatography. *J Chromatogr* 1982;228:409–412.
156. Holdiness MR. Chromatographic analysis of antituberculosis drugsin biological samples [review]. *J Chromatogr* 1985;340:321–359.
157. Holmes RK, Sanford JP. Enzymatic assay for gentamicin and related aminoglycoside antibiotics. *J Infect Dis* 1974;129:519–527.
158. Holt DE, de Louvois J, Hurley R, et al. A high performance liquid chromatography system for the simultaneous assay of some antibiotics commonly found in combination in clinical samples. *J Antimicrob Chemother* 1990;26:107–115.
159. Horvath CS, Lipsky S. Use of liquid ion exchange chromatography for the separation of organic compounds. *Nature* 1966;211:748–749.
160. Hosotsubo H, Takezawa J, Taenaka N, et al. Rapid determination of amphotericin B levels in serum by high-performance liquid chromatography without interference by bilirubin. *Antimicrob Agents Chemother* 1988;32:1103–1105.
161. Hung CT, Lim JK, Zoest AR, et al. Optimization of high-performance liquid chromatographic analysis for

isoxazolyl penicillins using factorial design. *J Chromatogr* 1988;425:331–341.

162. Irwin WJ, Hempenstall JM, Li Wan Po A. Controlled-release pencillin complexes: high-performance liquid chromatography and assay. *J Chromatogr* 1984;278:85–96.
163. Issell BF, Bodey GP. Mezlocillin for treatment of infections in cancer patients. *Antimicrob Agents Chemother* 1980;17:1008–1013.
164. Jamaluddin AB, Sarwar G, Rahim MA, et al. Assay for cloxacillin in human serum utilising high-performance liquid chromatography with ultraviolet detection. *J Chromatogr* 1989;490:243–246.
165. Jarvis JD, Leung TWC. Some factors influencing the assay of gentamicin. In: Williams JD, Geddes AM, eds. *Chemotherapy,* vol. 2. New York: Plenum Press, 1975;143–146.
166. Jehl F, Gallion C, Monteil H. High-performance chromatography of antibiotics. *J Chromatogr* 1990;531:509–548.
167. Jehl F, Gallion C, Thierry RC, et al. Determination of vancomycin in human serum by high-pressure liquid chromatography. *Antimicrob Agents Chemother* 1985;27:503–507.
168. Jehl F, Monteil H, Tarral A. HPLC quantitation of the six main components of teicoplanin in biological fluids. *J Antimicrob Chemother* 1988;21(Suppl A):53–59.
169. Johnson GJ, Rao GHR, White JG. Platelet dysfunction induced by parenteral carbenicillin and ticarcillin. *Am J Pathol* 1978;91:85–106.
170. Jolley ME. Fluorescence polarization immunoassay for determination of therapeutic drug levels in human plasma. *J Anal Toxicol* 1981;5:236–240.
171. Jolley ME, Stroupe SD, Schwenzer KS, et al. Fluorescence polarization immunoassay. III. An automated system for therapeutic drug determination. *Clin Chem* 1981;27:1575–1579.
172. Jones CW, Chmel H. Solid-phase ion-pair extraction and liquid chromatography of mezlocillin in serum. *Clin Chem* 1988;34:2155–2156.
173. Jones SM, Blazevic DJ, Balfour HH. Stability of gentamicin in serum. *Antimicrob Agents Chemother* 1976;10:866–867.
174. Jonsson S. Immunochemical study of the structural specificity of an antigentamicin antiserum, useful also for radioimmunoassay of sisomycin. In: Williams JD, Geddes AM, eds. *Chemotherapy,* vol. 2. New York: Plenum Press, 1975;165–168.
175. Joos B, Luthy R. Determination of teicoplanin concentrations in serum by high-pressure liquid chromatography. *Antimicrob Agents Chemother* 1987;31:1222–1224.
176. Jorgensen JH, Lee JC. Rapid bioassay for clindamycin alone in the presence of aminoglycoside antibiotics. *J Infect Dis* 1977;136:422–427.
177. Joslyn DA, Galbraith M. A turbidimetric method for the assay of antibiotics. *J Bacteriol* 1950;59:711–716.
178. Jusko WJ. Fluorometric analysis of ampicillin in biological fluids. *J Pharm Sci* 1971;60:728–732.
179. Kabay A. Rapid quantitative microbiological assay of antibiotics and chemical preservatives of nonantibiotic nature. *Appl Microbiol* 1971;22:752–755.
180. Kalina M, Plapinger RE, Hoshino Y, et al. Nonosmiophilic tetrazolium salts that yield osmiophilic, lipophobic formazans for ultrastructural localization of dehydrogenase activity. *J Histochem Cytochem* 1972;20:685–695.
181. Kallner A, Tryding N. Laboratory tests to evaluate drug administration. *Scand J Clin Lab Invest Suppl* 1989;195: 19–21.
182. Kavanaugh F. *Analytical microbiology.* New York: Academic Press, 1972;11.
183. Kaye D, Levinson ME, Lebovitz ED. The unpredictability of serum concentrations of gentamicin: pharmacokinetics of gentamicin in patients with normal and abnormal renal function. *J Infect Dis* 1974;130:150–154.
184. Khabbaz RF, Standiford HC, Bernstein D, et al. Measurement of amikacin in serum by a latex agglutination inhibition test. *J Clin Microbiol* 1985;22:669–701.
185. Kim H, Lin C. High-pressure liquid chromatographic method for determination of SCH 28191 in biological fluids. *Antimicrob Agents Chemother* 1984;25:45–48.
186. Kirkland KM, McCombs DA, Kirkland JJ. Rapid high-resolution high performance liquid chromatographic analysis of antibiotics. *J Chromatogr* 1994;A660:327–337.
187. Kitagawa T, Kanamaru T, Wakamatsu H, et al. A new method for preparation of an antiserum to pencillin and its application for novel enzyme immunoassay of pencillin. *J Biochem* 1978;84:491–494.
188. Knoller J, Konig W, Schonfeld W, et al. Application of high-performance liquid chromatography of some antibiotics in clinical microbiology. *J Chromatogr* 1988;427:257–267.
189. Kohlstaedt KG. Propionyl erythromycin ester lauryl sulfate and jaundice. *JAMA* 1961;178:89–90.
190. Kondo S. Punch hole method, a new technique of antibiotic concentration bio-assay: a preliminary report. *Bull Osaka Med Sch* 1973;19:132–135.
191. Kramer WG, Pickering LK, Culbert S, et al. Mezlocillin pharmacokinetics in pediatric oncology patients. *Antimicrob Agents Chemother* 1984;25:62–64.
192. Kurta MJ, Billings M, Koh T, et al. Inexpensive double-antibody fluoroimmunoassay for aminoglycoside antibiotics, phenytoin, and theophylline in serum. *Clin Chem* 1983;29:1015–1019.
193. LaFollette G, Gambertoglio J, White JA, et al. Determination of clindamycin in plasma or serum by high-performance liquid chromatography with ultraviolet detection. *J Chromatogr* 1988;431:379–388.
194. Lauriault A, Awang DVX, Kindack D. High-performance liquid chromatographic determination of dicloxacillin in the presence of its degradation products. *J Chromatogr* 1984;283:449–452.
195. Least CJ Jr, Wiegand NJ, Johnson GF, et al. Quantitative gas-chromatographic flame-ionization method for chloramphenicol in human serum. *Clin Chem* 1977;23:220–222.
196. Lecaillon JB, Rouan MC, Souppart C, et al. Determination of cefsulodin, cefotiam, cefalexin, cefotaxime, desacetyl-cefotaxime, cefuroxime and cefroxadin in plasma and urine by high-performance liquid chromatography. *J Chromatogr* 1982;228:257–267.
197. Leeder JS, Spino M, Tesoro AM, et al. High-pressure liquid chromatographic analysis of ceftazidime in serum and urine. *Antimicrob Agents Chemother* 1983;24:720–724.
198. LeFrock JL, Molavi A, Prince RA. Clindamycin (Symposium on Antimicrobial Therapy). *Med Clin North Am* 1982;66:103–120.
199. Lever M. Improved fluorometric determination of tetracyclines. *Biochem Med* 1972;6:216–222.
200. Levison ME. Microbiological agar diffusion assay for metronidazole concentrations in serum. *Antimicrob Agents Chemother* 1974;5:466–468.
201. Levy J, Truong BL, Goignau H, et al. High-pressure liquid chromatographic quantitation of teicoplanin in human serum. *J Antimicrob Chemother* 1987;19:533–539.
202. Lewis AS, Taylor G, Rowe HN, et al. Modified enzyme

immunoassays for tobramycin using reduced sample and reagent volumes. *Am J Hosp Pharm* 1987;44:568–571.

203. Liberman DF, Fitzgerald J, Robertson RG. Rapid disk test for determining clindamycin serum levels. *Antimicrob Agents Chemother* 1974;5:458–461.
204. Lightbrown JW. Assay of individual antibiotics in drug combinations. In: PJ Watt, ed. *The control of chemotherapy*. London: E & S Livingstone, 1970;19.
205. Lindberg RLP, Huupponene RK, Huovinen P. Rapid high-pressure chromatographic method for analysis of phenoxymethylenicillin in human serum. *Antimicrob Agents Chemother* 1984;26:300–302.
206. Line DH, Poole GW, Waterworth PM. Serum streptomycin levels and dizziness. *Tubercle* 1970;51:7681.
207. Little JR, Little KD, Plut E, et al. Induction of amphotericin B-specific antibodies for use in immunoassays. *Antimicrob Agents Chemother* 1984;26:824–828.
208. Lovering AM, White LO, Reeves DS. Identification of aminoglycoside-acetylating enzymes by high-pressure liquid chromatographic determination of their reaction products. *Antimicrob Agents Chemother* 1984;26:10–12.
209. Lund ME, Blazevic DJ, Matsen JM. Rapid gentamicin bioassay using a multiple-antibiotic resistant strain of *Klebsiella pneumoniae*. *Antimicrob Agents Chemother* 1973;4:569–573.
210. Lu-Steffes M, Pittluck GW, Jolley ME, et al. Fluorescence polarization immunoassay. IV. Determination of phenytoin and phenobarbital in human serum and plasma. *Clin Chem* 1982;28:2278–2282.
211. Mahon WA, Ezer J, Wilson TW. Radioimmunoassay for measurement of gentamicin in blood. *Antimicrob Agents Chemother* 1973;3:585–589.
212. Mahon WA, Feldman RI, Scherr GH. Hemagglutination inhibition assay of gentamicin. *Antimicrob Agents Chemother* 1977;11:359–361.
213. Maitra SK, Yoshikawa TT, Hansen JL, et al. Serum gentamicin assay by high-performance liquid chromatography. *Clin Chem* 1977;23:2273–2278.
214. Marengo PB, Wilkins J, Overturf GD. Rapid specific microbiological assay for amikacin (BB-KB). *Antimicrob Agents Chemother* 1974;6:498–500.
215. Marples J, Oates MDG. Serum gentamicin, netilmicin and tobramycin assays by high-performance liquid chromatography. *J Antimicrob Chemother* 1982;10:311–318.
216. Martin AJP, Synge RLM. A new form of chromatogram employing two liquid phases. *Biochem J* 1941;35:1358–1368.
217. Marunaka T, Maniwa M, Matsushima E, et al. High-performance liquid chromatographic determination of a new β-lactamase inhibitor and its metabolite in combination therapy with piperacillin in biological materials. *J Chromatogr* 1988;431:87–101.
218. Marunaka T, Matsushima E, Maniwa M. Determination of cefodizime in biological materials by high-performance liquid chromatography. *J Chromatogr* 1987;420:329–339.
219. Mattiasson B, Svensson K, Borrebaeck C, et al. Non-equilibrium enzyme immunoassay of gentamicin. *Clin Chem* 1978;24:1770–1773.
220. Mattila J, Mannisto PT, Mantyla R, et al. Comparative pharmacokinetics of metronidazole and tinidazole as influenced by administration route. *Antimicrob Agents Chemother* 1983;23:721–725.
221. Mayhew JW, Fiore C, Murray T, et al. An internally-standardized assay for amphotericin B in tissues and plasma. *J Chromatogr* 1983;274:271–279.
222. McAteer JA, Hiltke MF, Silber BM, et al. Liquid-chromatographic determination of five orally active cephalosporinscefixime, cefaclor, cefadroxil, cephalexin, and cephradinein human serum. *Clin Chem* 1987;33: 1788–1790.
223. McClain JBL. Vancomycin quantitation by high-performance liquid chromatography in human serum. *J Chromatogr* 1982;231:463–466.
224. McCormick EM, Echols RM, Rosano TG. Liquid chromatographic assay of ceftizoxime in sera of normal and uremic patients. *Antimicrob Agents Chemother* 1984;25:336–338.
225. Melikian V, Wise R, Allum WH. Mezlocillin and gentamicin in the treatment of infections in seriously ill and immunosuppressed patients. *J Antimicrob Chemother* 1981;7:657–663.
226. Morris HC, Miller J, Campbell RS, et al. A rapid enzymatic method for the determination of chloramphenicol in serum. *J Antimicrob Chemother* 1988;22:935–944.
227. Morse GC, Nairn DK, Bertino JS Jr, et al. Overestimation of vancomycin concentrations utilizing fluorescence polarization immunoassay in patients on peritoneal dialysis. *Ther Drug Monit* 1987;9:212–215.
228. Mullen PW, Mawer GE, Tooth JA. An indirect method for the determination of cephaloridine in serum by gas chromatography. *Res Commun Chem Pathol Pharmacol* 1974;7:85–94.
229. Munro AJ, Landon J, Shaw EJ. The basis of immunoassays for antibiotics. *J Antimicrob Chemother* 1982;9:423–432.
230. Murachi T. Knowledge reactions. In: Ishikawa E, Kawai T, Miyai K, eds. *Enzyme immunology*. New York: Igaku-Shoin, 1981;513.
231. Murthy VV, Goswami SL. A modified fluorimetric procedure for the rapid estimation of oxytetracycline in blood. *J Clin Pathol* 1973;22:548–550.
232. Musson DG, Maglietto SM, Hwang SS, et al. Simultaneous quantification of cycloserine and its prodrug acetylacetonylcycloserine in plasma and urine by high-performance liquid chromatography using ultraviolet absorbence and fluorescence after post-column derivatization. *J Chromatogr* 1987;414:121–129.
233. Myers CM, Blumer JL. Determination of imipenem and cilastin in serum by high-pressure liquid chromatography. *Antimicrob Agents Chemother* 1984;26:78–81.
234. Najib NM, Suleiman MS, el-Sayed YM, et al. High-performance liquid chromatographic analysis of cephalexin in serum and urine. *J Clin Pharmacol Ther* 1987;12:419–426.
235. Nakagawa T, Masada M, Uno T. Gas chromatographic mass spectrometric analysis of chloramphenicol, thiamphenicol and their metabolites. *J Chromatogr* 1975;111:355–364.
236. Nilsson-Ehle I. High-pressure liquid chromatography as a tool for the determination of antibiotics in biological fluids. *Acta Pathol Microbiol Scand Suppl* 1977;259:61–66.
237. Nilsson-Ehle I, Yoshikawa TI, Schotz MC, et al. Quantitation of antibiotics using high-pressure liquid chromatography: tetracycline. *Antimicrob Agents Chemother* 1976;9:754–760.
238. Nishi H, Fukuyama T, Matsuo M. Separation and determination of aspoxicillin in human plasma by micellar electrokinetic chromatography with direct sample injection. *J Chromatogr* 1990;515:245–255.
239. Noone P, Parson TMC, Pattison JR, et al. Experience in monitoring gentamicin therapy during treatment of serious Gram-negative sepsis. *Br Med J* 1974;1:477–481.
240. Noone P, Pattison JR, Slack RCB. Rapid antibiotic assay. *Lancet* 1973;2:315–316.

241. Noone P, Pattison JR, Slack RB. Assay of gentamicin. *Lancet* 1973;1:49–50.
242. Norrby SR, Alestig K, Ferber F, et al. Pharmacokinetics and tolerance of N-formimidoyl-thienamycin (MK0787) in humans. *Antimicrob Agents Chemother* 1983;23:293–299.
243. Nossel NG, Heppel LA. The release of enzymes by osmotic shock from *Escherichia coli* in exponential phase. *J Biol Chem* 1966;241:3055–3062.
244. Oden EM, Stander H, Weinstein MJ. Microbiological assay of gentamicin. *Antimicrob Agents Chemother* 1963;8:13–19.
245. O'Gorman Hughes DW, Diamond LK. Chloramphenicol: simple chemical estimations in patients receiving multiple antibiotics. *Science* 1964;144:296–297.
246. Oka H, Uno K. Improvement of chemical analysis of antibiotics. VI. Detection reagents for tetracyclines in thin-layer chromatography. *J Chromatogr* 1984;295:129–139.
247. Oka H, Uno K. Improvement of chemical analysis of antibiotics. VII. Simple method for the analysis of tetracyclines on reversed-phase thin-layer plates. *J Chromatogr* 1984;284:227–234.
248. Oldfield N, Chang D, Garland W, et al. Quantitation of ceftetrame in human plasma and urine by high-performance liquid chromatography. *J Chromatogr* 1987;422:135–143.
249. Patton KR, Beg A, Felmingham D, et al. Determination of teicoplanin concentration in serum using a bioassay technique. *Drugs Exp Clin Res* 1987;13:547–550.
250. Pauncz JK, Harsanyi I. Aminoglycoside antibiotics: thin-layer chromatography, bioautographic detection and quantitative assay. *J Chromatogr* 1980;195:251–256.
251. Peng GW, Gadella MAF, Peng A, et al. High-pressure liquid-chromatographic method for determination of gentamicin in plasma. *Clin Chem* 1977;23:1838–1844.
252. Peng GW, Jackson GG, Chiou WL. High-pressure liquid chromatographic assay of netilmicin in plasma. *Antimicrob Agents Chemother* 1977;12:707–709.
253. Peromet M, Schoutens E, Vanderlinden MP, et al. Specific assay of gentamicin in the presence of penicillins and cephalosporins. *Chemotherapy* 1974;20:15.
254. Perrin F. Polarization de la lumiere de fluorescence: vie moyenne des molecules dans l'etat excite. *J Phys Radium* 1926;7:390–401.
255. Phillips I, Warren C, Smith SE. Serum gentamicin assay: a comparison and assessment of different methods. *J Clin Pathol* 1974;27:447–451.
256. Pilkiewicz FG, Remsburg BJ, Fisher SM, et al. High-pressure liquid chromatographic analysis of aztreonam in sera and urine. *Antimicrob Agents Chemother* 1983;23:852–856.
257. Place JD, Thompson SG, Clements HM, et al. Gentamicin substrate-labeled fluorescent immunoassay containing monoclonal antibody. *Antimicrob Agents Chemother* 1983;24:246–251.
258. Popelko SR, Miller DM, Holen JT, et al. Fluorescence polarization immunoassay. II. Analyzer for rapid, precise measurement of fluorescence polarization with use of disposable cuvettes. *Clin Chem* 1981;27:1198–1201.
259. Provoost AP, Schalkwijk WP, Olusanya A, et al. Determination of aminoglycosides in rat renal tissue by enzyme immunoassay. *Antimicrob Agents Chemother* 1984;25:497–498.
260. Raahave D. Paper disc-agar diffusion assay of penicillin in the presence of streptomycin. *Antimicrob Agents Chemother* 1974;6:603–635.
261. Raeburn JA. A method for studying antibiotic concentration in inflammatory exudate. *J Clin Pathol* 1972;24:633–635.
262. Rahal JJ Jr, Chan YK, Johnson G. Relationship of staphylococcal tolerance, teichoic acid antibody, and serum bactericidal activity to therapeutic outcome in *Staphylococcus aureus* bacteremia. *Am J Med* 1986;81:43–52.
263. Rake G, McKree CM, Jones H. A rapid test for the activity of certain antibiotic substances. *Proc Soc Exp Biol Med* 1942;51:273–274.
264. Ralph ED, Clarke JT, Libke RD, et al. Pharmacokinetics of metronidazole as determined by bioassay. *Antimicrob Agents Chemother* 1974;6:691–696.
265. Reeves DS, Bywater MJ. Quality control of serum gentamicin assays: experience of national surveys. *J Antimicrob Chemother* 1975;1:103–116.
266. Resnick GL, Corbin D, Sandberg DH. Determination of serum chloramphenicol utilizing gas-liquid chromatography and electron capture spectrometry. *Anal Chem* 1966;38:582–585.
267. Riva E, Ferry N, Cometti A, et al. Determination of teicoplanin in human plasma and urine by affinity and reversed-phase high-performance liquid chromatography. *J Chromatogr* 1987;421:99–110.
268. Robard D, Bridson W, Rayford PL. Rapid calculation of radioimmunoassay results. *J Lab Clin Med* 1969;74:770–781.
269. Robison LR, Seligsohn R, Lerner SA. Simplified radioenzymatic assay for chloramphenicol. *Antimicrob Agents Chemother* 1978;13:25–29.
270. Rouan MC. Antibiotic monitoring in body fluids [review]. *J Chromatogr* 1985;340:361–400.
271. Rumble RH, Roberts MS. High-performance liquid chromatographic assay of the major components of gentamicin in serum. *J Chromatogr* 1987;419:408–413.
272. Rybak MJ, Bailey EM, Reddy VN. Clinical evaluation of teicoplanin fluorescence polarization immunoassay. *Antimicrob Agents Chemother* 1991;35:1586–1590.
274. Sabath LD, Casey JI, Ruch PA, et al. Rapid microassay of gentamicin, kanamycin, neomycin, streptomycin, and vancomycin in serum or plasma. *J Lab Clin Med* 1971;78:457–463.
275. Sabath LD, Casey JI, Ruch PA, et al. Rapid microassay for circulating nephrotoxic antibiotics. *Antimicrob Agents Chemother* 1970;1969:83–89.
276. Sabath LD, Toftegaard I. Rapid microassays for clindamycin and gentamicin when present together and the effect of pH and of each on the antibacterial activity of the other. *Antimicrob Agents Chemother* 1974;6:54–59.
277. Sande MA, Kaye D. Evaluation of methods for determining antibacterial activity of serum and urine after colistimethate injection. *Clin Pharmacol Ther* 1970;11:873–882.
278. Sanders S, Bergan T, Fossberg E. Piperacillin in the treatment of urinary tract infections. *Chemotherapy* 1980;26:141–144.
279. Schlichter JG, McLean H. Method of determining effective therapeutic level in treatment of subacute bacterial endocarditis with penicillin: preliminary report. *Am Heart J* 1947;34:209–211.
280. Schlichter JG, MacLean H, Milzer A. Effective penicillin therapy in subacute bacterial endocarditis and other chronic infections. *Am J Med Sci* 1949;217:600–608.
281. Schwartz DW, Koechlin BA, Weinfeld RE. Spectrofluorimetric method for the determination of trimethoprim in body fluids. *Chemotherapy* 1969;14(Suppl):22–29.
282. Schwartz JG, Casto DT, Ayo S, et al. A commercial

enzyme immunoassay method (EMIT) compared with liquid chromatography and bioassay methods for measurement of chloramphenicol. *Clin Chem* 1988;34:1872–1875.

283. Schwertschlag U, Nakata LM, Gal J. Improved procedure for determination of flucytosine in human blood plasma by high-pressure liquid chromatography. *Antimicrob Agents Chemother* 1984;26:303–305.
284. Sears SD, Standiford HC, Bernstein D, et al. Comparison of the latex agglutination inhibition assay for tobramycin with radioimmunoassay. *Eur J Clin Microbiol* 1986;5:347–350.
285. Shaikah K, Talati PG, Gang DM. Spectrophotometric method for the estimation of 6-aminopenicillinic acid. *Antimicrob Agents Chemother* 1973;3:194–197.
286. Shannon KP, Philips I. The use of aminoglycoside 2-N-acetyltransferase for the assay of gentamicin in serum, plasma and urine. *J Antimicrob Chemother* 1977;3:25–33.
287. Shanson DC, Hince CD. Serum gentamicin assays of 100 clinical serum samples by a rapid 40°C Klebsiella method compared with overnight plate diffusion and acetyltransferase assays. *J Clin Pathol* 1977;30:521–525.
288. Shanson DC, Hince CJ, Daniels JV. Rapid microbiological assay of tobramycin. *J Infect Dis* 1976;134(Suppl):104–109.
289. Shanson DC, Hince C, Daniels JV. Assay of gentamicin and tobramycin by a reliable 2 1/2-hour Klebsiella plate method. In: Williams JD, Geddes AM, eds. *Chemotherapy*, vol. 2. New York: Plenum Press, 1975;147–153.
290. Sharma JP, Berill RF. Improved high-performance liquid chromatographic procedure for the determination of tetracyclines in plasma, urine and tissues. *J Chromatogr* 1978;166:213–220.
291. Shaw EJ. Immunoassays for antibiotics. *J Antimicrob Chemother* 1979;5:625–634.
292. Shaw EJ, Amina-Watson RA, Landon J, et al. Estimation of serum gentamicin by quenching fluoroimmunoassay. *J Clin Pathol* 1977;30:526–531.
293. Shaw EJ, Watson RAA, Smith DS. Continuous flow fluoroimmunoassay of serum gentamicin, with automatic sample blank correction. *Clin Chem* 1979;75:322–324.
294. Shaw FN, Sivner AL, Aarons L, et al. A rapid method for the simultaneous determination of the major metabolites of sulphasalazine in plasma. *J Chromatogr* 1983;274:393–397.
295. Shaw PD. Gas chromatography of trimethylsilyl derivatives of compounds related to chloramphenicol. *Anal Chem* 1963;35:1580–1582.
296. Shaw WV. Comparative enzymology of chloramphenicol resistance. *Ann NY Acad Sci* 1971;182:234–242.
297. Signs SA, File TM, Tan JS. High-pressure liquid chromatographic method for analysis of cephalosporins. *Antimicrob Agents Chemother* 1984;26:652–655.
298. Skinner M, Kanfer I. High-performance liquid chromatographic analysis of josamycin in serum and urine. *J Chromatogr* 1988;459:261–267.
299. Smith AL, Smith DH. Improved enzymatic assay of chloramphenicol. *Clin Chem* 1978;24:1452–1457.
300. Smith AL, Smith DH. Gentamicin:adenine mononucleotide transferase: partial purification, characterization and use in the clinical quantitation of gentamicin. *J Infect Dis* 1974;129:391–401.
301. Smith AL, Waitz JA, Smith DH, et al. Comparison of enzymatic microbiological gentamicin assays. *Antimicrob Agents Chemother* 1974;6:316–319.
302. Smith DH, Van Otto B, Smith AL. A rapid chemical assay for gentamicin. *N Engl J Med* 1972;286:583–586.
303. Snyder LR, Kirkland JJ. *Introduction to modern liquid chromatography*. New York: John Wiley & Sons, 1979;246–268.
304. Snyder LR, Kirkland JJ. *Introduction to modern liquid chromatography*. New York: John Wiley & Sons, 1979;552–556.
305. Sood SP, Green VI, Bailey CL. Routine methods in toxicology and therapeutic drug monitoring by high performance liquid chromatography. II. A rapid microscale method for determination of chloramphenicol in blood and cerebrospinal fluid. *Ther Drug Monit* 1987;9:347–352.
306. Spencer RD, Toledo FB, William BT, et al. Design, construction, and two applications for an automated flow-cell polarization fluorometer with digital readout. *Clin Chem* 1973;19:838–844.
307. Spreauz-Varoquaux O, Chapalain JP, Cordonnier P, et al. Determination of trimethoprim, sulphamethoxazole and its N^4-acetyl metabolite in biological fluids by high-performance liquid chromatography. *J Chromatogr* 1983;274:187–199.
308. Standiford HC, Tatem BA. Technical aspects and clinical correlations of the serum bactericidal test [review]. *Eur J Clin Microbiol* 1986;5:79–87.
309. Stevens P, Young LS. Simple method for elimination of aminoglycosides from serum to permit bioassay of other antimicrobial agents. *Antimicrob Agents Chemother* 1977;12:286–287.
310. Stevens P, Young LS, Hewitt WL. Radioimmunoassay, acetylating radioenzymatic assay, and microbiological assay of gentamicin: a comparative study. *J Lab Clin Med* 1975;86:349–359.
311. Stobberingh EE, Hourben AW, Van Boven CP. Comparison of different tobramycin assays. *Clin Microbiol* 1982;15:797–801.
312. Stratton CW, Reller LB. Serum dilution test for bactericidal activity: selection of a physiologic diluent. *J Infect Dis* 1977;136:187–195.
313. Stroy SA. Modified microbiological assay for rapid estimation of antibiotic concentration in human sera. *Appl Microbiol* 1969;18:31–34.
314. Svinarov DA, Dotchev DC. Simultaneous liquid-chromatographic determination of some bronchodilators, anticonvulsants, chloramphenicol, and hypnotic agents, with Chromosorb P columns used for sample preparation. *Clin Chem* 1989;35:1615–1618.
315. Thadepalli H, Rao B. Clinical evaluation of mezlocillin. *Antimicrob Agents Chemother* 1979;16:605–610.
316. Thompson SG, Burd JF. Substrate-labeled fluorescent immunoassay for amikacin in human serum. *Antimicrob Agents Chemother* 1980;18:264–268.
317. Tilton RC, Murphy JR, Mallet E. Assay for gentamicin. *N Engl J Med* 1972;287:1100.
318. Toothaker RD, Wright DS, Pachla LA. Recent analytical methods for cephalosporins in biological fluids [review]. *Antimicrob Agents Chemother* 1987;31:1157–1163.
319. Turley CP, Kearns GL, Jacobs RF. Microanalytical high-performance liquid chromatography assay for cefpirome (HR 810) in serum. *Antimicrob Agents Chemother* 1988;32:1481–1483.
320. Ueda Y, Saita A, Fukuoka Y, et al. Interactions of β-lactam antibiotics and antineoplastic agents. *Antimicrob Agents Chemother* 1983;23:374–378.
321. Uematsu T, Mizuno A, Suzuki Y, et al. Evaluation of a fluorescence polarization immunoassay procedure for quantitation of isepamicin, a new aminoglycoside antibiotic. *Ther Drug Monit* 1988;10:459–462.

322. Uematsu T, Sato R, Mizuno A, et al. A fluorescence polarization immunoassay evaluated for quantifying astromicin, a new aminoglycoside antibiotic. *Clin Chem* 1988;34:1880–1882.
323. Ueno H, Nishikawa M. Chromatographic separation and chemical analysis of polymers formed by penicillin G. *J Chromatogr* 1984;288:117–126.
324. Ulitzur S. Determination of antibiotic activities with the aid of luminous bacteria. *Methods Enzymol* 1986;133: 275–284.
325. Ulitzur S, Goldberg I. Sensitive, rapid and specific bioassay for the determination of antilipogenic compounds. *Antimicrob Agents Chemother* 1977;12:308–313.
326. Undenfriend S. *Fluorescence assay in biology and medicine*. New York: Academic Press, 1962.
327. Velagapudi R, Smith RV, Ludden TM, et al. Simultaneous determination of chloramphenicol and chloramphenicol succinate in plasma using high-performance liquid chromatography. *J Chromatogr* 1982;228:423–428.
328. Voller A, Bidwell DE, Bartlett A. Enzyme immunoassays in diagnostic medicine. *Bull WHO* 1976;53:55–65.
329. Wade JD, Schimpff SC, Newman KA, et al. Potential of mezlocillin as empiric single-agent therapy in febrile granulocytopenic cancer patients. *Antimicrob Agents Chemother* 1980;18:299–306.
330. Wagner JG. *Fundamentals of clinical pharmacokinetics*. Hamilton, IL: Drug Intelligence Publications, 1975.
331. Wagner JC, Novak E, Patel NC, et al. Absorption, excretion and half-life of clindamycin in normal adult males. *Am J Med Sci* 1968;256:25–37.
332. Warren C, Phillips I. A comparison of the homogeneous enzyme immunoassay (EMIT) autocarousel and quantitative single test (QST) systems with the radioenzymatic assay. *J Antimicrob Chemother* 1986;17:255–262.
333. Warren E, Snyder RJ, Washington JA. Four-hour microbiological assay of gentamicin in serum. *Antimicrob Agents Chemother* 1972;1:46–48.
334. Waterworth PM. Which gentamicin assay method is the most practicable? *J Antimicrob Chemother* 1977;3:18.
335. Watson ID. Clavulanate-potentiated ticarcillin: high-performance liquid chromatographic assays for clavulanic acid and ticarcillin isomers in serum and urine. *J Chromatogr* 1985;337:301–309.
336. Watson RA, Landon J, Shaw EJ, et al. Polarisation fluoroimmunoassay of gentamicin. *Clin Chim Acta* 1976;73:51–55.
337. Weber A, Opheim KE, Wong K, et al. High-pressure liquid chromatographic quantitation of azlocillin. *Antimicrob Agents Chemother* 1983;24:750–753.
338. Weber AF, Opheim KE, Koup JR, et al. Comparison of enzymatic and liquid chromatographic chloramphenicol assays. *Antimicrob Agents Chemother* 1981;19:323–325.
339. Weber G. Rotational Brownian motion and polarization of the fluorescence of solutions. *Adv Protein Chem* 1953;8:415–459.
340. Wells P, Robbins E, Cowley R, et al. Comparative analysis of two rapid automated methods and a semiautomated version of the urease method for determining aminoglycoside concentrations in serum. *J Clin Microbiol* 1987;25:1583–1586.
341. Wheals BB, Jane I. Analysis of drugs and their metabolites by high-performance liquid chromatography. *Analyst* 1977;102:625–644.
342. White LO, Edwards R, Holt HA, et al. The in vitro degradation at 37°C of vancomycin in serum, CAPD fluid and phosphate-buffered saline. *J Antimicrob Chemother* 1988;22:739–745.
343. Williams JW, Langer JS, Northrop DB. A spectrophotometric assay for gentamicin. *J Antibiot* 1975;27:982–987.
344. Williamson J, Russel F, Doig WM, et al. Estimation of sodium fusidate levels in human serum, aqueous humor, and vitreous body. *Br J Ophthalmol* 1970;54:126–130.
345. Wilson C, Greenhood G, Remmington JS, et al. Neutropenia after consecutive treatment courses with nafcillin and piperacillin. *Lancet* 1979;1:1150.
346. Winston DJ, Murphy W, Young LW. Pipercillin therapy for serious bacterial infections. *Am J Med* 1980;69:225–261.
347. Winters RE, Litwack KD, Hewitt WL. Relation between dose and levels of gentamicin in blood. *J Infect Dis* 1971;124:S90–S95.
348. Witebsky FG, Selepak ST. Feasibility of gentamicin measurement in icteric sera by the Syva EMIT system. *Antimicrob Agents Chemother* 1983;23:172–174.
349. Wold JS. Rapid analysis of cefazolin in serum by high-pressure liquid chromatography. *Antimicrob Agents Chemother* 1977;11:105–109.
350. Woo J, Wong CL, Teoh R, et al. Liquid chromatographic assay for the simultaneous determination of pyrazinamide and rifampicin in serum samples from patients with tuberculous meningitis. *J Chromatogr* 1987;420:73–80.
351. Wyss R, Bucheli F. Determination of cefetamet and its orally active ester, cefetamet pivoxyl, in biological fluids by high-performance liquid chromatography. *J Chromatogr* 1988;430:81–92.
352. Yamada Y, Sasaki J, Matsuzaki T, et al. Influence of medium and diluent pH and diffusion time on antibiotic bioassay. *Exp Clin Med* 1981;6:23–33.
353. Yamamoto T, Moriwaki Y, Takahashi S, et al. Rapid and simultaneous determination of pyrazinamide and its major metabolites in human plasma by high-performance liquid chromatography. *J Chromatogr* 1987;413:342–346.
354. Yeo KT, Traverse W, Horowitz GL. Clinical performance of the EMIT vancomycin assay. *Clin Chem* 1989;35:1504–1507.
355. Tobin CM, Sunderland J, White LO, MacGowan AP. A simple isocratic high-performance liquid chromatography assay for linezolid in human serum. *J Antimicrob Chemother* 2001;48:605–608.
356. Rana B, Butcher I, Grigoris P, Murnaghan C, Seaton RA, Tobin CM. Linezolid penetration into osteo-articular tissues. *J Antimicrob Chemother* 2002;50:747–750.
357. Conte JE, Golden JA, Kipps J, Zurlinden E. Intrapulmonary Pharmacokinetics of Linezolid. *Antimicrob Agents Chemother* 2002;46:1475–1480.
358. Tobin CM, Sunderland J, Lovering AM, MacGowan AP. A high performance liquid chromatography (HPLC) assay for linezolid in continuous ambulatory peritoneal dialysis fluid (CAPDF). *J Antimicrob Chemother* 2003;51:1041–1042.
359. Saralaya D, Peckham DG, Hulme G, Tobin CM, Denton M, Conway S, Etherington C. Serum and sputum concentrations following the oral administration of linezolid in adult patients with cystic fibrosis. *J Antimicrob Chemother* 2004;53:325–328.
360. Fiscella RG, Lai WW, Buerk B, Khan M, Rodvold K, Pulido JS, Labib S, Shapiro MJ, Blair NP. Aqueous and Vitreous Penetration of Linezolid (Zyvox) after Oral Administration. *Ophtalmology* 2004;111:1191–1195.

Antimicrobial Combinations

Satish K. Pillai and Robert C. Moellering, Jr.,
George M. Eliopoulos

Antimicrobial combinations are used most frequently to provide broad-spectrum empiric coverage in treatment of patients who are seriously ill and who may be septicemic. Less frequently, combinations of antimicrobials are chosen because an identified pathogen is resistant to inhibition and/or killing by conventional doses of single antimicrobials, but more susceptible to inhibition or killing by the combination. In both instances, the clinical outcome may depend on the interactions of these antimicrobial agents against individual microorganisms. In this chapter, we examine the effects of antimicrobial combinations against single microorganisms *in vitro*, presented according to their presumed mechanisms of interaction. Data on the activities of various combinations against specific pathogens are summarized in the Appendix at the end of the chapter, organized by the genus and species of the pathogen.

Two types of antimicrobial interactions have been excluded from consideration and are not discussed. The first is enhanced effectiveness of an antimicrobial due to another drug that interferes with the elimination or metabolism of the first drug, but is not itself an antimicrobial, e.g., the increased penicillin activity produced *in vivo* by probenecid, which interferes with excretion of penicillin by the kidney (292). The second is the inactivation of one antimicrobial by another, unrelated to the presence of a microorganism, e.g., the inactivation of aminoglycosides by penicillins by a mechanism involving nucleophilic substitution (384,636). Such reactions may proceed readily *in vitro* (226,384), but are probably insignificant *in vivo* unless the usually rapid excretion of both drugs by the kidney is markedly reduced. For this reason, it is important to measure serum aminoglycoside levels in patients with renal failure who are receiving β-lactam/aminoglycoside combinations (137) to ensure that the desired serum aminoglycoside concentrations are attained. We begin by examining the reasons for the use of antimicrobials in combination.

RATIONALES FOR THE USE OF ANTIMICROBIAL COMBINATIONS

Decreased Emergence of Resistant Strains

Antibiotics are sometimes used in combination in an attempt to prevent or delay the *in vivo* emergence of drug-resistant subpopulations of the pathogenic organism. With the simultaneous use of two or more agents against which bacteria develop resistance by different mechanisms, the probability that colonies will emerge resistant to all of the antimicrobials employed is theoretically very low. This is best illustrated in the treatment of tuberculosis, where simultaneous treatment with multiple drugs clearly reduces the risk of resistance during therapy (563,567). This rationale is often discussed for other combinations and may be relevant for combinations containing rifampin, an agent to which many bacteria readily develop resistance if it is used alone. For example, combinations of rifampin with vancomycin and/or other antibiotics have been used successfully in the treatment of prosthetic valve endocarditis due to coagulase-negative staphylococci. Although use of such combinations does appear to suppress the emergence of rifampin resistance in the infecting pathogen, some clinical failures associated with the development of resistant strains have been described (102,303). This may be due to the emergence of resistant clones in deep foci of infection into which there may be differential penetration of rifampin. Similarly, the combination of oxacillin with rifampin suppresses the emergence of *Staphylococcus aureus* populations resistant to the latter, despite the fact that rifampin can antagonize the bactericidal activity of β-lactams *in vitro* (220,368, 625).

There are also data to support this rationale for the use of antimicrobial combinations in the treatment of *Pseudomonas aeruginosa* pneumonia. Data from several studies indicated that administration a β-lactam alone was associated with the emergence of *P. aeruginosa* resistant to β-lactams (178,240,271,513,561,570,628). Although several experimental and clinical studies have produced evidence that combination therapy of *P. aeruginosa* infections with a β-lactam plus an aminoglycoside might reduce the incidence of resistance to either component of the combination (209,291,383,493), results of other studies have not supported this conclusion (46,55,104). Nevertheless, in addition to any benefit that may arise from suppression of drug-resistant colonies when infections due to Gram-negative bacteria are treated with combinations of antimicrobials, such combinations may also exhibit synergistic inhibitory or bactericidal activity, as will be discussed in the next section.

Decreased Dose-Related Toxicity as a Result of Reduced Dosage

Several important antimicrobials have significant dose-related toxicities that seriously limit their use, e.g., chloramphenicol, 5-fluorocytosine (marrow suppression), aminoglycosides, and sulfonamides (nephrotoxicity). Therefore, there are theoretical grounds on which to attempt reduction in the dose of a potentially toxic antimicrobial while using an additional agent to ensure a successful clinical outcome. This approach is exemplified by the former use of sulfonamide combinations (triple sulfonamides) to reduce the incidence of crystalluria with stone formation (350,351). The success of such regimens—now of historical interest only—was based on the fact that the solubilities of the three sulfonamides (sulfadiazine, sulfamerazine, and sulfamethiazine) are independent of one another, although their antibacterial effects are cumulative (350,652). At present, there are no antimicrobial combinations specifically designed to permit a significant reduction in the dose of the toxic antimicrobial without compromising antimicrobial activity. The more recent approach has been to develop antimicrobials with intrinsically superior safety profiles, which may, in many cases, be substituted for older, more toxic agents. For example, it may be possible to substitute a β-lactam (or a fluoroquinolone) for an aminoglycoside (for Gram-negative bacillary coverage) in some antibiotic regimens (529).

Polymicrobial Infection

Another important use of antimicrobial combinations is in the treatment of documented or suspected mixed (polymicrobial) infections. In some polymicrobial infections, it may be necessary to target each of several major pathogens for antimicrobial therapy. A classic example of this is the rat peritonitis model, in which treatment with agents active against both *Enterobacteriaceae* and anaerobes is necessary. Drugs active against the former (e.g., a cephalosporin or aminoglycoside) protect against early death from peritonitis, while agents active against anaerobes (e.g., clindamycin) prevent late abscess formation (372). Although such combinations are still frequently employed, the development of newer agents such as carbapenems or β-lactam–β-lactamase inhibitor antibiotics, which are broadly active against both components of mixed infections, now permits successful monotherapy of many polymicrobial infections.

Antimicrobial combinations (or equivalent broad-spectrum single agents) may not always be essential for the treatment of polymicrobial infections. Earlier studies indicated that penicillin alone was effective for the treatment of lung abscess, even when both penicillin-susceptible Gram-positive cocci and penicillin-resistant *B. fragilis* were present (40). However, later work did suggest that clindamycin (which is usually active against both groups of organisms) may be more effective than penicillin for the treatment of lung abscess (356).

Antimicrobial Synergism

Antimicrobial combinations were first used to treat patients early in the antibiotic era when it became apparent that not all infections responded to treatment with sulfonamides, penicillin, or streptomycin used alone. Despite its obvious empiricism, some of this early experience was remarkably successful, as illustrated by the discovery and study of the synergistic bactericidal activity of penicillin and streptomycin against enterococci by Hunter (278,279) and Jawetz et al. (287–289). This use of antimicrobial combinations to achieve *in vitro* activity and clinical efficacy against organisms resistant to inhibition and/or killing by acceptable (i.e., nontoxic) concentrations of single agents continues to be of great clinical relevance.

There is now a considerable body of literature pertaining to the role of antimicrobial synergism in the treatment of infections due to a wide variety of Gram-positive and Gram-negative organisms. However, in addition to the well-documented value of synergistic bactericidal combinations of penicillin (or ampicillin or vancomycin) plus an aminoglycoside (streptomycin or gentamicin) for the treatment of enterococcal endocarditis (425,426,650) and the obvious merit of fixed combinations such as trimethoprim (TMP)/sulfamethoxazole (SMZ) in selected situations, there are surprisingly few circumstances in which *in vitro* documentation of antimicrobial synergism has been highly predictive of superior clinical efficacy. Potential advantages of synergistic combinations in the treatment of infections due to Gram-negative bacilli (particularly *P. aeruginosa)* have been observed primarily in neutropenic patients (10,105,144,343). Even among this group, however, it remains uncertain whether such apparent benefits accrue from synergistic interactions per se or arise instead from the superior serum bactericidal activity of certain combinations, relative to those attainable with individual agents. The significance of this admittedly subtle distinction lies in the fact that serum bactericidal titers against various Gram-negative pathogens that can be attained with several of the newer β-lactam antibiotics may actually exceed those achieved using combinations of aminoglycosides with older β-lactams (627). (These issues are discussed further elsewhere [163].)

Further stimulus for study of antimicrobial interactions derives from the increasing awareness that certain combinations of agents may yield antagonistic effects. A classic example of such effects emerges from studies by Lepper and Dowling (355), who found that the addition of chlortetracycline markedly reduced the survival rate of children treated with penicillin for pneumococcal meningitis from 79% to 21%. More recent observations document the potential for antagonistic interactions between two β-lactam antibiotics used in combination against Gram-negative bacteria possessing inducible (derepressible), chromosomally mediated β-lactamases (228,550,552,555). Based on the preceding comments, it should be apparent that situations may arise in which it would be useful to confirm synergistic interactions between two antimicrobials against an infecting microorganism, or to exclude antagonistic interactions between antibiotics when these cannot be accurately anticipated from general knowledge of drug characteristics. Several methods have been developed to assess such potential drug interactions either quantitatively or qualitatively.

Definitions of Antimicrobial Interactions *In Vitro*

Despite differences in experimental methods and the criteria used to define quantitatively the results of antimicrobial combinations, there is general agreement on qualitative definitions of synergism and antagonism. Synergism is a positive interaction; the combined effect of the drugs being examined is significantly greater than the expected result, based on their independent effects when the drugs are used separately. Antagonism is a negative interaction; the combined effect of the drugs being examined is significantly less than their independent effects when they are tested separately. Many of the problems involved in assessing antimicrobial combinations result from uncertainty about the expected result with combinations in which there is no significant interaction between the antimicrobials being tested, whether that result should be described as additivity, indifference, or autonomy. Additivity is the basis of the checkerboard system and assumes that the result observed with more than one drug should be the sum of the separate effects of the drugs being tested if those drugs do not interact with one another. Autonomy (or indifference) is based on the idea that only one metabolic pathway can be growth rate-limiting for an organism at a time (312). Based on this observation, autonomy suggests that the combined effect of drugs that do not interact with one another should be simply the effect of the more (most) active drug alone (311,312).

LABORATORY METHODS USED TO ASSESS THE ACTIVITY OF ANTIMICROBIAL COMBINATIONS

Checkerboard Arrays

The checkerboard method is the technique that has been used most frequently to assess antimicrobial combinations *in vitro* (207,536), presumably because (a) its rationale is easy to understand, (b) the mathematics necessary to calculate and interpret the results are simple, (c) it can be performed in microbiology laboratories using equipment that is readily available, and (d) it has been the technique most frequently used in studies that have suggested an advantage of synergistic therapy in the treatment of neutropenic patients with Gram-negative septicemia (315, 343). The term "checkerboard" refers to the pattern (of tubes or microtiter wells or agar plates) formed by multiple dilutions of the two antimicrobials being tested, in concentrations equal to, above, and below their minimal inhibitory concentrations (MICs) against the organisms being tested (Fig. 9.1).

The concentrations tested for each antimicrobial typically range from four or five dilutions below the expected MIC to twice the anticipated MIC (or higher if antagonism is suspected), using twofold dilutions of each antimicrobial. Also included is a row (or column) of tubes or wells for each drug alone without any amount of the second antimicrobial. Thus, the checkerboard consists of columns in which each tube (or well or plate) contains the same amount of the drug (drug A) being diluted along the x axis and rows in which each tube (or well or plate) contains the same amount of the drug (drug B) being diluted on the y axis (Fig. 9.1). The result is that each square in the checkerboard (which represents one tube or well) contains a unique combination of the two drugs being tested. The dilutions of the antimicrobials being tested are usually performed in Mueller-Hinton broth or another suitable broth for bacterial studies, so that the drug-containing solutions can be mixed with drug-free medium to produce the final concentrations designated on the diagram. As noted later (see "Modifications of the Checkerboard Technique"), this technique may be performed with other liquid or semisolid (agar) media, with microtiter trays rather than racks of test tubes, using other than twofold dilutions, using more than two drugs, and with organisms other than bacteria.

Broth Method

With test tubes, it is convenient to use a final volume of 1.0 mL in each tube: 0.5 mL of broth containing antimicrobials (0.25 mL of broth for each drug if two

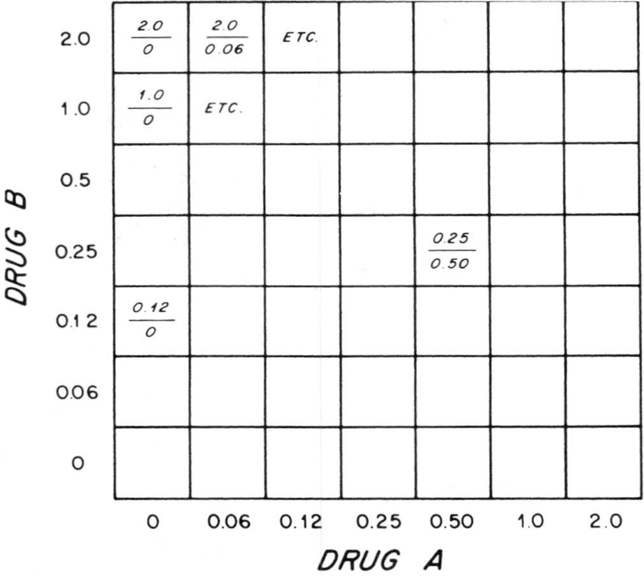

FIGURE 9.1 ● Checkerboard technique. In the checkerboard, serial dilutions of two drugs are performed using drug concentrations proportional to MICs of the drugs being tested. (Although usually expressed in micrograms per milliliter, the concentrations of drugs A and B are expressed here as multiples of the MIC.)

drugs are being tested) and 0.5 mL of broth containing a suspension of the organism to be tested. Because the final volume (1.0 mL) is four times as great as the volume of broth for each antimicrobial (0.25 mL) with this method, the antimicrobial concentrations used in the initial (stock) solutions should be fourfold greater than the desired final concentrations. For example, if the MIC of drug A (Fig. 9.1) is 1.0 μg/mL, the concentration of drug A in the solution added to the tubes in the far right column of the figure should be 8 μg/mL to produce a final concentration of 2 μg/mL, which is twice the MIC of the organism being tested. Similarly, the inoculum of the bacterial suspension added to each tube (in 0.5 mL of broth) should be approximately 2×10^5 colony-forming units (CFU)/mL after the addition of an equal volume of the antimicrobial solutions. If broth dilution studies are being performed to assess bactericidal activity by culturing a 10-μL sample for more than 99.9% killing, a final inoculum between 3 and 10×10^5 CFU/mL ensures greater accuracy of test results (492).

With a series of antimicrobial solutions containing four times the desired final concentrations, one can then produce the desired range of drug concentrations. Instead of making a separate set of dilutions for each tube, most workers find it more convenient to prepare larger volumes of the working (four times) antimicrobial solutions and to add an aliquot of those solutions to each tube in the appropriate row or column (as noted in Table 9.1). Cation-adjusted Mueller-Hinton broth works well for many bacteria, but other liquid media can be used as appropriate. This dilution scheme can be readily modified when it is desirable to work with different final or transfer volumes of antimicrobials or bacteria.

Although the dilutions used in the checkerboard are exponential (by powers of two) (Fig. 9.1), the results of checkerboard testing are interpreted by the pattern they form on the isobologram (which converts those data from an exponential [logarithmic] scale to an arithmetic one) (Fig. 9.2) (312). In Figure 9.2 A to C, experimental results are shown (shading indicates observable growth) that

TABLE 9.1

Dilution of an Antimicrobial for Checkerboard Testing in Broth[a]

Desired final concentration of drug	0	0.06	0.12	0.25	0.50	1.0	2.0
Concentration of drug in stock solution	0	0.25	0.50	1.0	2.0	4.0	8.0
Volume of stock solution per tube (mL)	0.25	0.25	0.25	0.25	0.25	0.25	0.25

[a] For the purpose of this table, concentrations of drug are expressed in multiples of the MIC. Each tube contains a total volume of 1.0 mL: 0.25 mL of drug A, 0.25 mL of drug B, and 0.5 mL of bacterial inoculum.

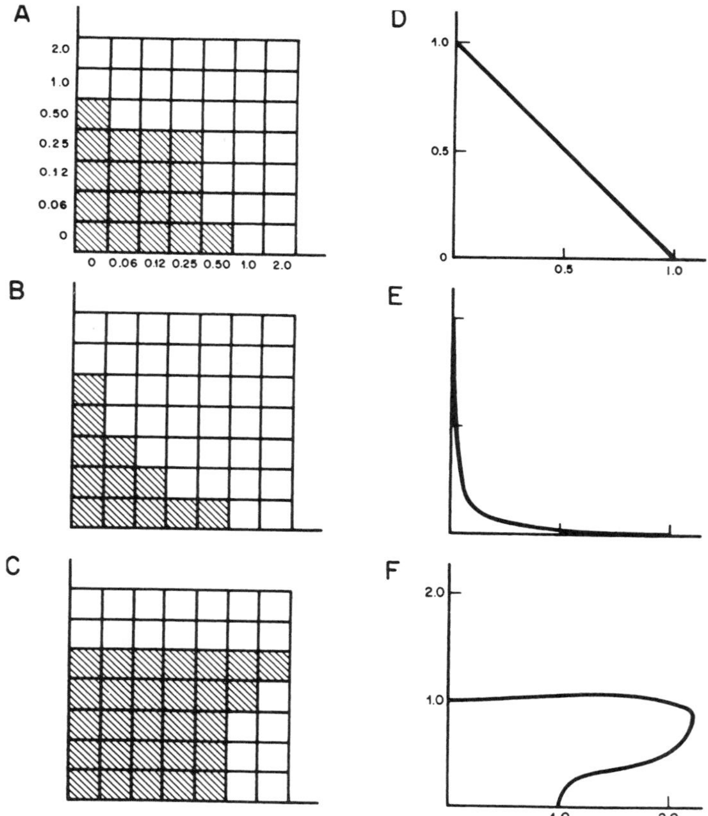

FIGURE 9.2 • Assessment of antimicrobial combinations with the checkerboard method. **A, B,** and **C:** results of testing combinations of two drugs (diluted in geometric twofold increments along the *x* and *y* axes, as in Fig. 9.1). *Shading,* visible growth. Concentrations are expressed as multiples of the MIC. **D, E,** and **F:** isobolograms (plotted on an arithmetic scale) that represent the results of checkerboards shown in **A, B,** and **C,** respectively. **A** and **D,** additive effect; **B** and **E,** synergism; **C** and **F,** antagonism.

corresponds to additive (Fig. 9.2A), synergistic (Fig. 9.2B), and antagonistic (Fig. 9.2C) interactions, as diagrammed in the isobologram in Figure 9.2 D, E, and F, respectively. The isobologram is constructed as follows. For each concentration of drug along the [*x*-] axis (plotted as the [*x*-] coordinate), the lowest concentration of the drug diluted along the [*y*-] axis that inhibits growth in the column of tubes is taken as the [*y*-] coordinate of this plot. An isobologram is constructed by connecting the series of coordinate points generated for each drug combination forming the "step" boundary between inhibition and growth on the checkerboard.

Agar Dilution Method

The principles of the techniques outlined for the broth method can also be adapted for use in an agar dilution system. This method may be advantageous when a large number of strains are to be tested against a limited number of antibiotic combinations. The volume of the bacterial inoculum does not enter into the calculations used to determine the dilution of the initial antimicrobial stock solutions with this method because the inoculum is applied to the surface of the agar plate. Therefore, some workers have mixed equal parts of molten agar medium containing each of the drugs being tested, using stock concentrations twice the desired final concentrations. If antimicrobials are added to the agar after it has been autoclaved, the agar should first be allowed to cool to 50°C to 55°C in a water-bath to prevent loss of activity with antimicrobials susceptible to heat (614). As discussed for broth testing, serial twofold dilutions can then be performed with plain agar to obtain the desired range of drug concentrations. However, serial dilutions in agar are tedious and difficult to perform accurately. Therefore, it is often more convenient and more accurate first to dilute the antimicrobials in broth and then to add that broth (containing antimicrobials) to the molten agar. In order to maintain the desired concentrations of both agar and antimicrobials, the volume of broth (containing antimicrobial) added to the agar should be small (i.e., 5% of the total volume). Thus, the concentration of the antimicrobial in the broth added to the molten agar medium should be 20 times the desired final antimicrobial concentration in the agar (Table 9.2). Mueller-Hinton agar permits satisfactory growth of most bacteria of interest, but other media or supplements can be used as appropriate.

After the agar plates have been poured and allowed to cool and dry, the bacteria to be tested can be applied to

TABLE 9.2

Dilution of an Antimicrobial for Checkerboard Testing in Agar[a]

Final concentration of antimicrobial desired	0	0.06	0.12	0.25	0.50	1.0	2.0
Concentration of antimicrobial stock solution	0	1.25	2.5	5.0	10.0	20.0	40.0
Volume of stock solution added to 19.0 mL of agar (mL)	1.0	1.0	1.0	1.0	1.0	1.0	1.0

[a] Concentrations of drug are expressed in multiples of the MIC. For testing two drugs, each 20-mL aliquot for a 100-mm agar plate contains 1.0 mL of the appropriate stock solution of drug A, 1.0 mL of drug B, and 18.0 mL of agar

the agar surface with a replicating device (589) designed to deliver a standard inoculum (usually approximately 10^4 CFU). The surface of the agar plate must be dry before the inoculum is applied because a watery film may permit one or two resistant organisms to spread over the entire agar surface. Condensation on the agar surface is often a concern because agar plates are frequently kept refrigerated after their initial preparation (because some antimicrobial agents remain stable in agar for at least 1 week at 4°C) (534). Therefore, agar plates should be removed from the refrigerator several hours before their expected use to permit them to reach room temperature. Plates with persistent condensation should be dried, with their lids ajar, at 35°C to 37°C for 1 to 2 hours before they are inoculated.

Inoculum

Use of the correct inoculum is critical for the accuracy and reproducibility of checkerboard testing, as it is for other susceptibility testing. An excessively large inoculum may result in a falsely high estimate of the MIC due to the inoculum effect, which usually reflects either the inactivation of β-lactams by β-lactamase or the selection of resistant mutants, although in many cases the mechanisms of this effect are poorly understood. Conversely, an excessively small inoculum may lead to a falsely low estimate of the MIC.

For most bacterial studies, the inoculum can be standardized by matching the turbidity of the culture to the 0.5 McFarland standard (448). This produces a suspension of approximately 10^8 CFU/mL for most bacteria, which is then further diluted in fresh broth to achieve final inocula of approximately 10^5 CFU/mL for broth dilution studies using MIC endpoints or to achieve larger final inocula if minimal bactericidal concentration (MBC) endpoints are to be assessed (492). For agar dilution studies the initial 0.5 McFarland inoculum is diluted approximately 1:10 in fresh broth, and 1 to 2 μL of that suspension are applied to the surface of an agar plate with a calibrated wire loop or a multiprong replicator (589), for an inoculum of approximately 10^4 CFU/spot. The National Committee for Clinical Laboratory Standards has recommended that susceptibility tests with anaerobic bacteria be performed at an inoculum tenfold greater than that for aerobes (447). Other inocula may be appropriate for testing specific microorganisms (448). In any case, it is prudent to verify the actual inoculum density by determining colony counts for representative strains of the species to be tested.

Modifications of the Checkerboard Technique

Use of Microtiter Trays. Large amounts of antimicrobials and media are required for standard checkerboard testing with racks of test tubes containing mixtures of both drugs being tested. Therefore, many workers prefer to use microtiter trays because they require smaller quantities of antibiotics and broth. In addition, automated equipment can be used to prepare and dispense the antimicrobial dilutions and to deliver the inoculum.

Dilutions may be made with handheld or automated microdiluters. Similarly, the transfer plate technique may be used (either manually or with automated microdiluters) to prepare dilutions of a second drug (153). The contents of the transfer plate are then transferred to a standard microdilution plate containing appropriate concentrations of the first antimicrobial, thus creating the desired two-dimensional matrix of drug concentrations. Although smaller volumes are used with this technique than with the standard test tube (macro) checkerboard technique, the conceptual aspects of the test and the nature of the information produced are basically similar. However, there are several potential problems with microtiter checkerboard testing that are not encountered when using the macro (test tube) method.

The first problem is evaporation. Because the volumes in each microtiter well are small (100 to 200 μL), modest amounts of evaporation may significantly increase the concentrations of the antimicrobials being tested and thus produce artifactually low MICs (and/or MBCs). This can be prevented best by using plastic adhesive sheets or lids available through the manufacturers of these plates.

The second problem is anaerobiosis. The experience of many investigators suggests that these plastic sheets or lids (previously mentioned) do not inhibit the growth of strict aerobes. However, the best control to exclude this possibility is luxuriant growth of the test organism in the well(s) without antimicrobial. (It is also possible to punch small holes in the plastic sheets over each microtiter well with a pin. This allows equilibration with the ambient atmosphere of the incubator and also decreases the condensation on the undersurface of the plastic sheet, but does increase the likelihood of contamination.)

The third problem is surface electricity. Static electricity may accumulate under certain conditions and may interfere with effective dilution of the antimicrobials. Wiping the bottom of the plate with a moist cloth is usually sufficient to resolve this problem.

Variable Dilutions. Although twofold dilutions have been used traditionally with this method (in both its macro- and microtiter versions), they may be insufficiently sensitive for some organisms, especially if the breakpoint is at the upper end of the clinically acceptable range of concentrations for a toxic antimicrobial, such as an aminoglycoside. For this reason, it is often helpful to use less than twofold dilutions (for the whole series of dilutions or at least for those of greatest interest) (311). From a mathematical point of view, the smallest dilution increments provide the greatest precision for subsequent evaluation of the results. Giant checkerboards can be created by combining a series of smaller matrices, each using different dilutions of the two drugs in an attempt to increase precision of endpoint determinations (276). This technique involves considerable work and does not fully circumvent limitations inherent in the standard twofold dilution method.

Testing More than Two Drugs. Using the same dilution scheme, it is also possible to create a three-dimensional (or *n*-dimensional) lattice to study combinations of three (or *n*-) drugs against a single pathogen. This strategy was developed by Berenbaum (48–50), who also used it to quantitate the results with the fractional inhibitory concentration (FIC) index (see following discussion).

Testing Organisms Other than Bacteria. The same approach has also been used to examine the activity of other antimicrobial combinations against nonbacterial pathogens such as parasites and fungi (145,380,468,591). (For a review of antimicrobial combinations against fungi, see reference Johnson et al. [293].) Measures of antimicrobial action used in these studies have included morphologic criteria (e.g., reductions in parasite counts as measured by Giemsa-stained smears, isotope uptake (the reduction of [^{3}H]-hypoxanthine or [^{3}H]-thymidine uptake for antiparasitic and antiviral agents) (95,275,502,594), and quantitative cultures (of fungi and viruses) (148,275,595). From a conceptual point of view, the nature of the testing scheme is the central issue, not the specific microorganism being tested.

Definition of the Endpoint. Most checkerboard tests are read by examining the tubes (or wells or plates) for evidence of visible growth after 16 to 20 hours of incubation at 35°C to 37°C. Occasionally, endpoints may be determined earlier for rapidly growing organisms, or may require longer incubation for slowly growing isolates. Bactericidal data may be obtained if the tubes (or wells) without visible evidence of bacterial growth are sampled to determine the concentrations of the combination producing 99.9% killing (the MBC). Similarly, some investigators have modified the determination (and the definition) of the MIC by using 50% reduction in the optical density produced by bacterial growth to replace visual inspection. They believe that this measure (the 50% inhibitory concentration), when assessed with a spectrophotometer, may be more accurate than the traditional MIC (2,486).

Interpretation of the Results

In interpreting the results of checkerboard studies, the critical question is usually whether an apparently synergistic combination is significantly below the additive line of the isobologram. Because the margin of error in these studies is plus or minus one dilution, a combination should inhibit growth (or achieve killing) at least two dilutions below the additive line of the isobologram to be considered synergistic or at least two dilutions above the additive line to be considered antagonistic. Because the determination of synergism often depends on the tubes (wells) near the midpoint of the isobologram, many workers have examined only the MIC (or MBC) and one lower concentration of each drug alone, in addition to a group of comparably increasing concentrations of both drugs (in a ratio of their MICs or MBCs), beginning from the control (without drug A or B) and progressing toward the point with x = one half the MIC of drug A and y = one half the MIC of drug B. This scheme substantially reduces the number of tubes and dilutions necessary to perform the test, while retaining sufficient discrimination at the midpoint to define synergism in most cases (Fig. 9.3). The FIC index of Elion et al. (161) can be viewed as a mathematical restatement of the isobologram (Table 9.3) and is the method most commonly used in the literature to report the results of studies with antimicrobial combinations. In this method, the FIC for each drug is derived by dividing the concentration of that drug necessary to inhibit growth in a given row or column by the MIC of the test organism for that drug alone. The FIC index is then calculated by summing the separate FICs for each of the drugs present in that tube (or well) (Table 9.3).

Although each antimicrobial checkerboard produces a series of FIC index values if one calculates separate FIC indexes for each row or column in the isobologram, most investigators use the value obtained for equally effective concentrations of the two drugs being tested (i.e., the result obtained by examining combinations in which the ratios of the concentrations of the two antimicrobials are equal to the ratios of their MICs, as in the 45 degree line in Fig. 9.3) as representative of that combination. Although this approach simplifies the calculations, it may be misleading because the ratios of the two drugs may not remain constant *in vivo*, even if they are administered

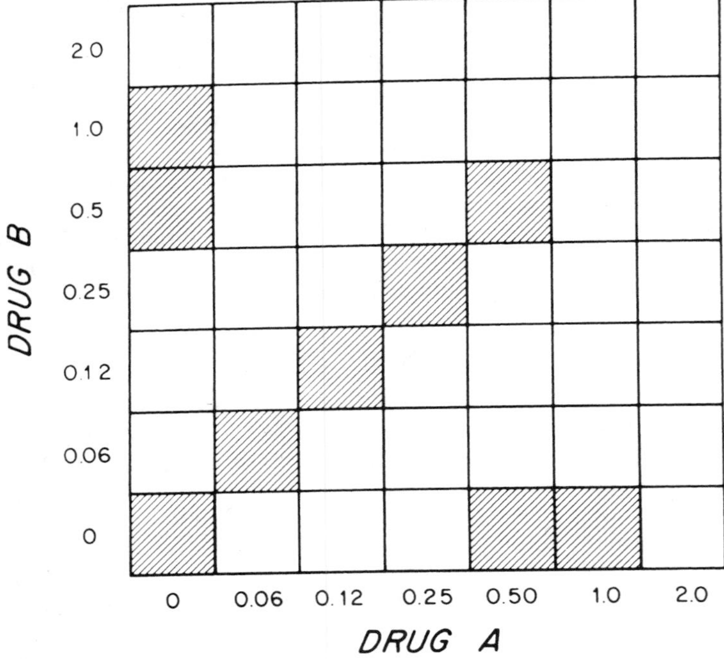

FIGURE 9.3 ● Simplified checkerboard testing of antimicrobial combinations. With this approach, the number of combinations tested may be substantially reduced (e.g., in this case to only 7 of 49 combinations). *Hatching,* combinations tested.

in doses proportional to their MICs. Also, it may be important to detect significant synergism or antagonism that occur at drug concentrations off of the 45 degree line, if such concentrations are clinical relevant.

With this method, synergism has traditionally been defined as an FIC index of 0.5 or less and additivity as a FIC index of 1.0; antagonism has been often defined as a FIC index of 2.0 (207,536). More recent criteria suggest that a FIC index of more than 4 should be applied to definitions of antagonism to account for inherent imprecision of the technique when twofold dilutions are used and because of FIC index of 2.0 is probably indicative of an indifferent, rather than a true antagonistic, effect (15). In some cases it may be appropriate to use a more rigorous definition of synergism (e.g., a FIC index of less than 0.5) to discriminate more completely between synergistic and additive effects (379,557). Although most investigators use the FIC index calculation only for two-drug combinations, this approach can be applied to combinations of three or more drugs (50).

Because of the inherent variability in results derived from the traditional twofold dilution scheme described, it is usually not possible to distinguish between "additivity" and "indifference" with confidence, when FIC indices lie between 0.5 and 4. Although such distinctions may be useful in assessing mechanisms of drug interactions, they may be misleading when used to describe potentially beneficial clinical interactions (e.g., "partial synergy" or "additivity"). For this reason, use of such terms (for conditions other than strictly defined synergism or antagonism) is discouraged, in favor of more neutral terms such as "no interaction" or "indifferent" (15,293,469).

TABLE 9.3

Calculation of the Fractional Inhibitory Concentration (FIC) Index for Combinations of Two Antimicrobials[a]

$$\frac{(A)}{(MIC_A)} + \frac{(B)}{(MIC_B)} = FIC_A + FIC_B = \text{FIC index}$$

[a] (A) is the concentration of drug A in a tube that is the lowest inhibitory concentration in its row. (MIC_A) is the MIC of the organism to drug A alone. FIC_A is the fractional inhibitory concentration of drug A. (B) is the concentration of drug B in a tube that is the lowest inhibitory concentration in its column. (MIC_B) and FIC_B are defined in the same fashion for drug B.

Limitations of the Technique

As practiced by most laboratories, the checkerboard method has several significant limitations. First, unless each of the tubes (or wells) without obvious macroscopic evidence of growth is sampled to determine microbicidal activity, it yields only inhibitory data. This lack of microbicidal data can be a serious limitation because the organisms most frequently submitted for such testing are from patients with infections that most clinicians believe should be treated with microbicidal therapy when possible (e.g., endocarditis, meningitis, or osteomyelitis).

Second, both the FIC index calculation and the usual interpretation of the isobologram assume incorrectly that all antimicrobials have linear dosage-response curves (311). Although checkerboard results are often used to characterize the dose-response relationship between an antimicrobial and microorganism, the checkerboard method as usually performed provides only all-or-none responses (i.e., growth or no growth) and is thus incapable of measuring the graded responses necessary to define dose-response curves. Finally, because the results are usually examined only at one point in time, the checkerboard method typically provides a static, rather than a dynamic, view of antimicrobial interaction. Despite these limitations, the checkerboard technique is simple to perform and remains a widely used technique to assess antimicrobial combinations.

Killing Curves (Time-Kill Curves or Time-Kill Plots)

In contrast to the checkerboard technique, which typically provides only inhibitory data, the killing-curve technique measures the microbicidal activity of the combination being tested. For this reason, it is often more relevant for clinical situations in which bactericidal therapy is desirable. The other major advantage of killing curves over the checkerboard technique is that they provide a dynamic picture of antimicrobial action and interaction over time (based on serial colony counts), as opposed to the checkerboard technique, which is usually examined only once (after 16 to 24 hours of incubation).

However, the repetitive colony counts that this technique requires are tedious and seriously limit the number of antimicrobial concentrations and combinations that can be tested with any one isolate. Therefore, if the laboratory results are to be useful in guiding therapy, it is essential that the antimicrobial concentrations tested be chosen carefully and that they represent concentrations that are achievable at the presumed site of infection. Because the medium is sampled repetitively for colony counts, killing-curve studies must be performed in liquid media and care is required to avoid contamination. Most experiments are performed with a final inoculum of 10^5 to 10^7 CFU/mL, which is produced by diluting an overnight culture of the pathogen in cation-adjusted Mueller-Hinton broth or another suitable broth. It is usually convenient first to adjust the overnight culture (or logarithmic-phase culture if desired) to match the 0.5 McFarland standard (448) and then to dilute a second time with fresh broth and the appropriate amounts of antimicrobials in the tube or flask in which the study is to be performed. The initial sampling for colony counts should take place as soon as the inoculum is added (within 5 minutes). Assuming that the volume of the culture is at least 10 mL, it is usually convenient to take 0.5-mL samples for colony counts, which may be performed by one of several methods. Especially if short sampling intervals are being used, the culture flasks should be returned to the incubator immediately after the aliquots have been removed.

Saline Dilution

As usually performed, this method uses a series of tubes containing 4.5 mL of sterile saline (0.9% NaCl) or another appropriate sterile diluent. One pipettes a 0.5-mL sample from the culture into the first tube (producing a 10^1 dilution) and then, after thorough mixing, transfers 0.5 mL from that tube (with a new sterile pipette) to the next tube (which becomes the 10^2 dilution), repeating the procedure until a series of tubes have been prepared (usually from 10^1 to 10^8). Precise aliquots from these tubes are then plated on an agar plate without antimicrobials and incubated overnight (or longer, for slowly growing organisms or when there is a prolonged postantibiotic effect (e.g., Caron et al. [91]). If aliquots of 0.1 mL are used, they should be spread on the surface of a whole agar plate. However, if smaller volumes are used (e.g., drops of 0.025 mL), it is often feasible to use a single plate for the results of all dilutions from one colony count (Fig. 9.4). In either case, it should be possible to use a single sterile

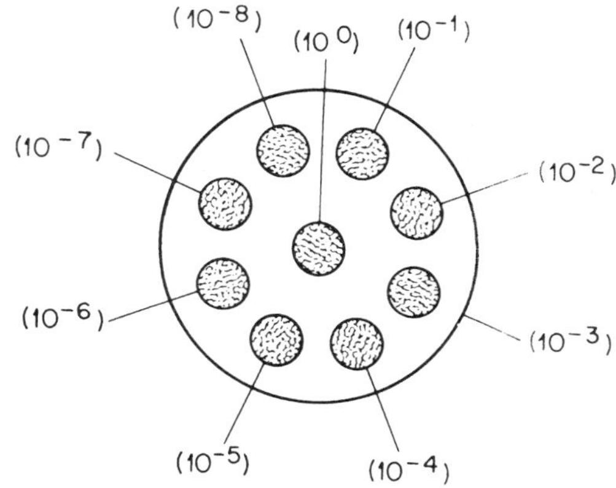

FIGURE 9.4 ● Arrangement of drops of culture broth on an agar plate for counting colony-forming units per milliliter. *Shading,* area of the plate typically covered by single 0.025-mL drops from each tenfold dilution.

pipette to apply all dilutions for a single colony count by beginning with the most diluted tubes (i.e., working from the 10^8 dilution to the 10^1 dilution) after the dilutions have been performed. Replicate colony counts obtained in this fashion should agree within $\pm 10\%$. In contrast, significant differences among antimicrobials and antimicrobial combinations are usually defined as tenfold to 100-fold changes in the number of CFU per milliliter after 4 to 24 hours of incubation. If one expects that the colony count will be close to zero, it is helpful to place an aliquot of the undiluted sample in the center of the plate (with the micropipette method) or to use an extra agar plate with 0.1 mL of undiluted material (with the macro 0.1-mL pipette method).

In many cases, it is also necessary to ascertain that carryover of antimicrobials from the dilution tubes is not of sufficient magnitude to lower falsely the resulting colony counts. This is usually not a problem when counting is performed on drops derived from the fourth or fifth dilution tube or beyond because the process of dilution usually reduces residual antimicrobial concentrations to negligible levels. It is important to note, however, that, for antibiotics demonstrating marked inoculum effects against the test microorganism, drug concentrations significantly below the MIC (derived at standard inocula) may inhibit the growth of the few colonies present in that given dilution. When there is doubt about the possible effects of antibiotic carryover, control experiments should be performed in which small inocula of the test strain are suspended in saline, with or without antimicrobial at concentrations of interest, and then plated immediately on drug-free agar. Resulting colony counts should be in close agreement in the absence of significant carryover effects.

Another approach is to inactiviate the antibiotic(s) prior to plating, if this can be accomplished without affecting the organism. This is generally feasible only for β-lactam antibiotics, which can be inactiviated in many cases by addition of commercially available β-lactamase. When significant carryover of a potent antimicrobial is anticipated, it may be necessary to employ alternative methods to remove residual antibiotic in order to obtain accurate colony counts. One method is to collect bacteria by filtering aliquots through a 0.45-μm filter, washing the filter with sterile saline, and finally eluting organisms from the filter by vigorous agitation in a volume of saline equal to that of the original aliquot. Alternatively, samples may be spun to pellet the bacteria, discarding the supernatant containing the carried-over antibiotic, and resuspending in fresh medium. The resulting bacterial suspension is then plated for colony counts. Whatever method is used, all specimens (including an antibiotic-free growth control) should be handled in an identical fashion because of the possibility that some colonies will be retained on the filter or will not be completely resuspended, even after vigorous agitation.

Another pitfall, which is somewhat less obvious, is the handling of the tubes with 4.5 mL of sterile saline. If these tubes are autoclaved after (rather than before) the saline has been added, the autoclaving process inevitable produces enough evaporation after the tubes are removed from the autoclave to significantly reduce the volume (usually to 4.0 mL). The only certain way to control this source of error is to dispense the sterile saline into the tubes after the saline and the tubes have been sterilized.

The agar plates used for the colony counts must not contain any antimicrobials. Although Mueller-Hinton agar is quite sufficient for most bacteria, we have used blood, brain-heart, and nutrient agars for work with enterococci, and other media (e.g., chocolate agar) would clearly be necessary if one were to work with more fastidious organisms such as *Neisseria*. It is important not to tilt (and preferably not to move) the plates onto which drops have been applied until the drops have had time to dry thoroughly. This is less of a problem with 0.1-mL aliquots spread on individual agar plates because the relatively small volume (in relation to the surface area) dries much more rapidly.

Agar Dilution

Colony counts may also be determined by agar dilution. Typically, a 1.0-mL aliquot is removed from the culture and diluted in sterile saline. Aliquots of this suspension are added to 19 mL of molten agar medium that has been allowed to cool to 50°C to 55°C after autoclaving and the mixture is poured into agar plates (100 mm in diameter), allowed to harden, and then incubated overnight at 35° to 37° prior to colony counting. Penicillinase or sodium polyanetholsulfonate can be used to inactivate penicillin or aminoglycosides, respectively, with the agar dilution method because it requires the pouring of fresh agar plates. If penicillinase is added, 1.0 to 1.3 mL of penicillinase/20-mL plate equivalent to 10^6 kinetic units of penicillinase/mL is sufficient to inactivate several hundred micrograms of penicillin per milliliter in the sample. Sodium polyanetholsulfonate concentrations of 0.025 to 0.050 g/100 mL (or 5% NaC1) should inactivate clinically relevant concentrations of aminoglycosides and polymyxin (335).

After incubation of the agar plates at 35°C to 37°C for 16 to 18 hours (or less with some rapidly growing organisms), colony counts may be performed. In some cases, it may be necessary to incubate plates 48 to 72 hours in order for surviving colonies to be visualized for counting (91). When using the saline tube dilution method, we customarily place drops from each dilution tube onto duplicate antibiotic-free plates for counting and then average the results at each dilution. A colony counter with a magnifying glass is ofen helpful because up to several hundred colonies may be clustered in the approximately 1.5-cm diameter circles produced by the drops on the agar plate (Fig. 9.4). Although there are usually fewer colonies per unit surface area with the macro technique (in which 0.1-mL aliquots of culture or diluted specimen are spread over the surface of a 100-mm agar plate), colony-counting devices are also helpful with that method.

Interpretation of Results

When the colony counts have been determined, the easiest way to visualize the results is to plot them on semilogarithmic paper (using the abscissa for time and the ordinate [the logarithmic sale] for the colony counts, as in Fig. 9.5). If arithmetic paper is used, colony counts between powers of 10 should be plotted (on the ordinate) as their logarithms, rather than arithmetically, i.e., 3.1×10^7 (not 5×10^7) CFU/mL should be midway between 10^7 and 10^8 CFU/mL. The definitions of antimicrobial interaction with this technique are based on studies with enterococci, against which clinically acceptable concentrations of the aminoglycosides alone are generally inactive and penicillin is only bacteriostatic. The results are interpreted by the effect of the combination in comparison with the most active single drug alone. Synergism is defined at a 100-fold increase in killing at 24 hours (as measured by colony counts) with the combination, in comparison with the most active single drug. Antagonism is defined as a 100-fold decrease in killing at 24 hours with the combination, compared with the most active single drug alone (424,425).

These definitions assume that at least one of the drugs being tested produces no significant inhibition or killing alone. Although this assumption is true for enterococci (against which clinically acceptable concentrations of aminoglycosides are inactive), it is not true for most other organisms (especially Gram-negative bacilli), against which clinically acceptable concentrations of aminoglycosides are often quite active. There are no established criteria with which to evaluate the results obtained (with the killing curve technique) using two or more drugs, each of which has significant activity alone, to determine whether those drugs are synergistic. One approach has been to examine antimicrobials alone and then in combination at some fraction of the MIC or MBC (e.g., one-fourth of the MIC or MBC). Typically, however, this results in some degree of killing with one or both of the agents used alone at an early time point, followed by regrowth at 24 hours. In such cases, the combination may result in sustained bactericidal activity over the entire sampling period, but it is difficult, if not impossible, to differentiate a true synergistic interaction from merely additive effects or from the phenomenon of mutual suppression of resistance to the single agents. Especially when penicillins are tested by time-kill methods against Gram-negative bacilli, late regrowth of microorganisms is often associated with loss of antimicrobial activity in the culture medium over time because of slow inactivation of drugs. In such cases, determination of bactericidal activity of the single agents and combinations at earlier time points (e.g., 6 to 8 hours) may be more relevant (225).

Some authors have used statistical techniques to evaluate microbicidal interactions measured by killing curves (148,245). In this method, survival probabilities at various time points for each drug and their combinations are examined for evidence of statistically significant differences.

Limitations of the Technique

The major disadvantage of the killing-curve technique is that the repetitive sampling necessary for each of the flasks being tested and the multiple colony counts required seriously limit the number of antimicrobial combinations that can be tested. For this reason, it is essential that the

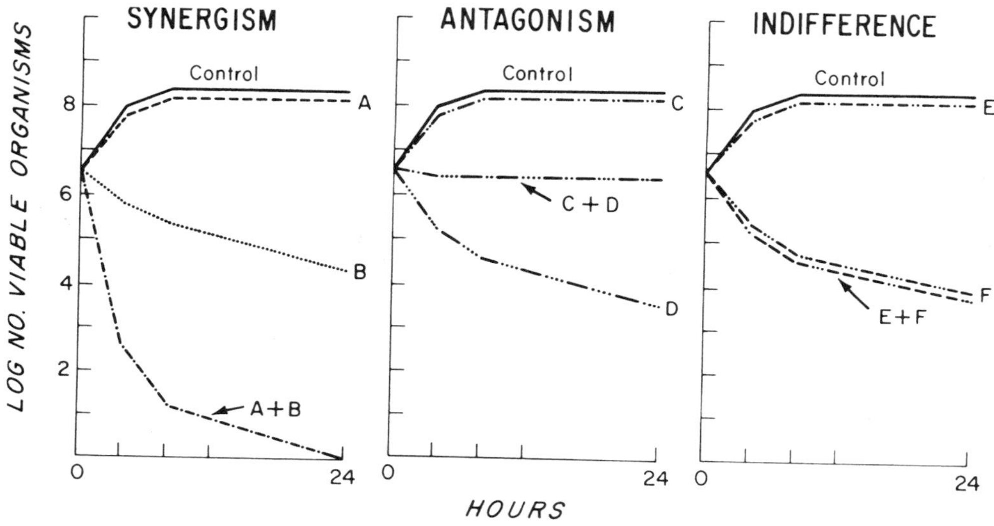

FIGURE 9.5 ● Effects of antimicrobial combinations as measured with the killing-curve method. *A + B*, synergism; *C + D*, antagonism; *E + F*, autonomy (or indifference).

concentrations that are tested be chosen with knowledge of the antimicrobial concentrations that are achievable at the site(s) of the infection. Furthermore, only fixed concentrations of drugs can be studied with traditional methods. One modification of the time-kill curve technique employs programmable pumps to deliver antibiotics into a central culture chamber at variable concentrations over time, simulating drug concentrations achieved in man (679). Although this method is subject to the same difficulties in interpretation of results as in the static time-kill curve model, it does provide useful insights into the net effect of drugs employed in combination in their relevant clinical doses. The model may be further modified to permit simulation of multiple dosing regimens.

Serum Bactericidal Testing

Rationale

As already noted, one limitation of the killing-curve technique is that the few antimicrobial concentrations tested must represent concentrations achievable *in vivo*. To ensure that the antimicrobial concentrations tested are relevant clinically, several groups have employed the serum bactericidal titer to estimate the activity of antimicrobials in combination (121,154). The advantage of this approach is obviously that it measures the activity of antimicrobial concentrations that are achievable *in vivo*. Its disadvantages include the fact that serum may include inhibitory substances other than antibiotics, and the added precautions needed to process patient serum specimens in the laboratory.

Interpretation of the Results

One practical approach is to measure serum bactericidal activity while the patient is receiving one antimicrobial, and then to repeat the test after addition of a second agent to see if the combination results in enhanced activity. However, the use of serum bactericidal titers in this fashion does not exclude the possibility that the increment in activity observed results from the last agent added (alone), rather than from antimicrobial interaction. For this reason, the results obtained with this method should be described qualitatively and not as synergism or antagonism, unless several serum samples are also available that contain similar concentrations of each drug alone.

Diffusion Methods

A variety of methods have been explored to assess, primarily in a qualitative fashion, interactions of antimicrobials as they diffuse through agar plates seeded with a test organism. One major advantage of the diffusion method is that commercially produced antimicrobial-impregnated disks and Mueller-Hinton agar plates may be employed. Paper strips soaked in antimicrobial solutions are used in some modifications of this method.

Disk Technique

This technique uses the same standard inoculum and Mueller-Hinton agar as a routine Bauer-Kirby susceptibility test (43). To assess possible interactions between two drugs (e.g., drugs A and B), disks containing drugs A and B are placed on a plate that has been inoculated in the usual fashion with the organisms to be tested. The distance by which the disks are separated may be varied, but it should generally be equal to or slightly greater than the sum of the radii of the zones of inhibition of the drugs when examined alone. After overnight (16- to 18-hour) incubation at 35°C to 37°C, the plates are ready for examination.

The pattern observed with additive or indifferent combinations is that of two independent circles (Fig. 9.6A). With synergistic combinations, enhancement or bridging is observed at or near the junction of the two zones of inhibition (Fig. 9.6B). With antagonistic combinations, truncation is observed near the junction of the two zones of inhibition (Fig. 9.6C). A special instance in which this technique can be very persuasive is when neither drug A nor drug B alone inhibits the test organism. In this

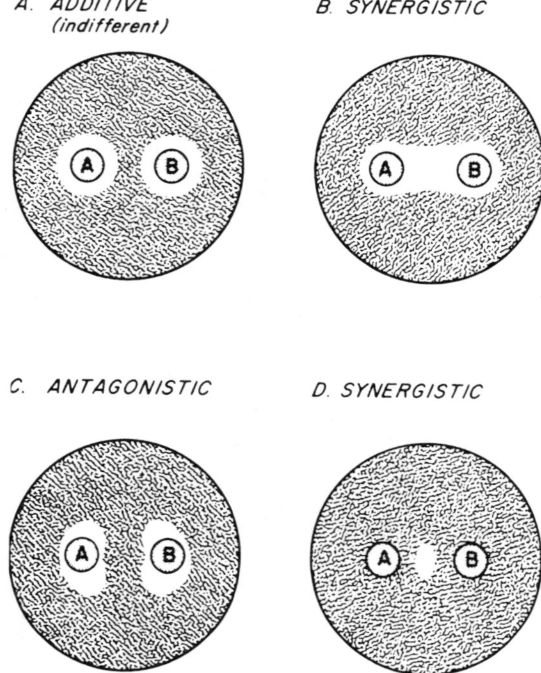

FIGURE 9.6 ● Assessment of antimicrobial combinations with the disk diffusion technique, using disks containing only one antimicrobial. **A:** additive or autonomous result. **B** and **D:** synergism. **C:** antagonism. *Shading,* bacterial growth; *clear areas,* zones of growth inhibition.

situation, inhibition of growth can only be due to the combined effects of drugs A and B (Fig. 9.6D) (419). An example of an actual experiment showing synergism and antagonism is shown in Figure 9.7. An example of how this test is used in clinical practice is the approximation of clindamycin and erythromycin disks onto an agar plate seeded with an erythromycin-resistant, clindamycin-susceptible strain of *S. aureus* to determine whether resistance to clindamycin might be inducible (i.e, MLS_B resistance mechanisms present) or not (i.e., macrolide resistance most likely due to efflux). In the former case, induction by erythromycin results in blunting of the inhibition zone around the clindamycin disk.

Another modification of this technique is the comparison of zones of inhibition produced by drugs A and B alone with the zone produced by a single disk containing both A and B. Although a larger zone of inhibition around A plus B than around either drug alone excludes significant antagonism, it may be impossible to distinguish between additive and synergistic interactions unless disks containing two times A and two times B are also tested. (The simplest instance is that found when zones of inhibition for A and B are equal, in which case the zone of inhibition for A plus B must be significantly greater than that of disks containing two times A or two times B to satisfy the criteria for synergism.)

Although the advantages of this technique as described are its simplicity and the use of readily available materials, it yields only qualitative information about antimicrobial interactions. Moreover, the results of this test may differ from results obtained when the same agents and organisms are tested in liquid media. Information about bacterial killing may be obtained by adding an agent to inactivate one or both of the drugs employed, thus permitting the detection of organisms that have been inhibited but not killed (e.g., the addition of β-lactamase to a penicillin-containing plate) (348,666). A less specific method that provides similar information is the use of a velvet impression from the test plate, which may then be replica-plated onto an agar plate without antimicrobials (347).

Paper Strip Diffusion with Cellophane or Membrane Filter Transfer

This method has been described by a number of investigators (58,98–100,158,371), but is now only of historical interest. Filter paper strips (0.5 to 0.9, 4 to 5 cm) are soaked in antimicrobial solution and placed at right angles to one another on an agar plate (Fig. 9.8). After overnight incubation at 35°C to 37°C, the filter paper strips are removed, leaving behind drug that has diffused into the agar medium. After removal of the filter paper strips, a transferable material (cellophane [99] or a filter membrane [371]) that permits diffusion of the two drugs now contained on the agar plate is placed on the agar surface and inoculated with a suspension

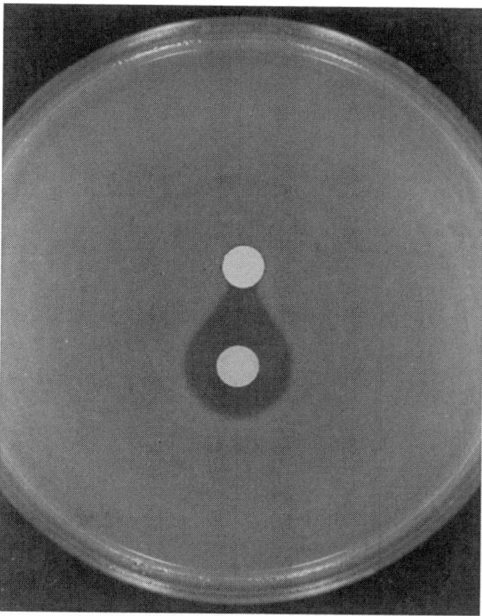

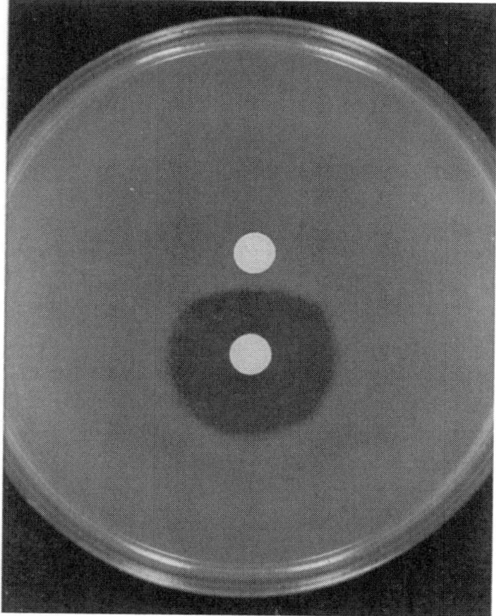

FIGURE 9.7 ● Assessment of antimicrobial combinations with the disk approximation technique. Combinations of β-lactams were tested against one strain of *E. cloacae*. *Left,* synergism between the two drugs. *Right,* activity of one drug is antagonized by the second, at concentrations below those that inhibit growth of the organism.

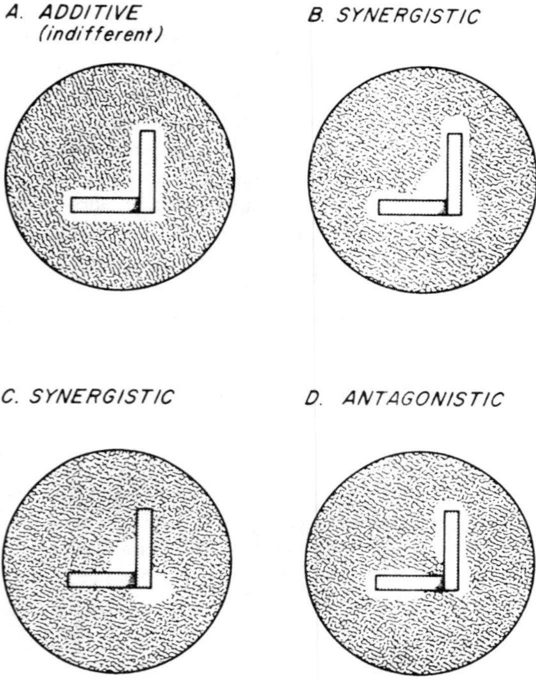

FIGURE 9.8 ● Assessment of antimicrobial combinations with the paper strip diffusion technique, using paper strips containing only one antimicrobial. **A:** additive or indifferent result. **B** and **C:** synergistic results. **D:** antagonistic result. *Shading* and *clear areas,* as in Figure 9.6.

of the organism to be tested. After 16 to 18 hours of incubation, the transferable material is removed from the agar plate containing drugs A and B and transferred to another agar plate without antimicrobials. After an additional 18 hours of incubation at 35°C to 37°C, the growth pattern is examined.

The filter paper test may be modified by streaking culture plates with enough organisms to produce confluent growth. Filter paper strips soaked in different antimicrobials (in concentrations equal to or greater than the MIC for the organisms to be tested) are then placed on the plate at right angles. After several hours at room temperature (to allow the antibiotics to diffuse into the agar), the filter paper strips are removed and the plates are incubated for 18 to 24 hours at 35°C to 37°C. The patterns of growth inhibition that result with both methods are interpreted as described in Figure 9.8 (371,574).

More recently, commercially prepared antimicrobial gradient diffusion strips (Epsilometer Etest strips, AB Biodisk, Solna, Sweden) have been used to increase the utility this type of testing and to provide quantitive determination of the potential synergistic activity of antibiotic combinations (57,388,656).

Other Methods of Assessing Antibacterial Combinations

Some workers have used regression lines derived from least-squares analysis of MIC (x axis) versus zone diameter (y axis) to quantitate the effectiveness of combination therapy *in vitro* (152). They have suggested that synergism is indicated by a steeper negative slope (i.e., a more negative value of "m" in the equation "$y = mx+b$" of the regression line for the combination of the two drugs, compared with each drug alone. Because the data on which each line has been based span only a short distance on the abscissa, their validity outside this range remains unclear. In addition, multiple MIC and zone size determinations with different organisms are required to determine a single line. Therefore, this method is of limited value when examining a single isolate for the presence of synergism with a given drug combination.

Sanders et al. (557) have described a technique using graphic and statistical analysis of inhibition zone sizes using disks impregnated with various concentrations of each study drug. Concentrations were selected to represent decimal fractions of a biological equivalence factor equivalent to the amount of each agent producing identical zone sizes. Results from the combinations were compared with expected additive effects (each drug combined with itself). This method (decimal assay for additivity) requires preliminary steps to establish biological equivalence factors and appropriate zone size ranges. However, it may be useful for detailed study of interactions for research purposes.

Mathematical Models to Assess Interactions

Various authors have applied mathematical methods in an effort to enhance the validity of conclusions regarding drug interactions when dose-response relationships are nonlinear or to display concentration-effect relationships three-dimensionally. Li et al. (360) described a method using initial bactericidal rate constants at various drug concentrations. Pharmacodynamic models are tested to describe appropriate concentration-response curves, and results are expressed with isobolograms on two-dimensional plots where axes represent fractional maximal effects for each drug (on a scale of zero to one). A method of exploring drug interactions derived from nonlinear enzyme kinetic equations described by Chou and Talalay (110) has been applied in studies of antiviral drugs against human immunodeficiency virus (120,328). In these examples, measurements of p24 antigen production, reverse transcriptase activity, and so on are taken at various concentrations of the drugs alone and combined.

Both activities and toxicities of antimicrobial combinations have been examined using a three-dimensional graphic method described by Pritchard and Shipman

(143,514,515). Concentrations of the two drugs (in this case antivirals) tested are plotted along x and y axes forming a horizontal plane, and the effect being measured (e.g., p24 antigen) is plotted on the *z* axis perpendicular to the plane. Plotting of experimental data points (with the aid of a microcomputer) yields a three-dimensional surface. A second surface representing the additive interactions generated from dose-response curves of individual agents is subtracted from this, leaving a series of peaks and valleys corresponding to areas of significant deviation from additivity (515). Assumptions inherent to each of these models have been discussed elsewhere (360,515).

Summary of Methods for the Study of Synergism

The salient features, advantages, and disadvantages of several methods have been tabulated (Table 9.4). Before selecting a specific technique, it is useful to consider both the laboratory's capabilities and the type of information that would potentially be most helpful. For situations in which simplicity is important and qualitative results adequate, diffusion testing might be a reasonable choice. However, it must be noted that these methods have generally not been validated by comparison with more quantitative methods. If many different combinations of the drugs must be examined or for reference work, a checkerboard method may be optimal. If the MIC and MBC are close to one another, the results of checkerboard testing using agar and broth dilution techniques may be in good agreement with killing-curve data. When assessment of bactericidal activity is paramount, killing curve techniques are usually most appropriate.

Inoculum

For clinical purposes, four or five colonies of the same morphology should be used to inoculate broth cultures. For research purposes, single-colony isolates that have been purified (streaked to single colonies) at least twice should be employed. Clearly, a mixed culture cannot produce a satisfactory result.

Standardization of the Inoculum

As previously noted, an excessively heavy inoculum tends to produce falsely high MIC and MBC values with all methods described, and an excessively light inoculum tends to produce a falsely low value. This tendency is typically accentuated with organisms capable of inactivating the antimicrobials being tested (e.g., in the testing of β-lactamase-producing organisms with penicillins). When determining the MBC, it is important to use a large enough inoculum (3 to 10 $\times$ 10^5 CFU/mL) so that 99.9% killing can be measured accurately (492).

Media

Mueller-Hinton agar and (cation-adjusted) broth are recommended for susceptibility testing because they permit growth of the most common pathogens and contain few substances that interfere with antimicrobial activity. Exceptions to this generalization include the use of specialized media for fastidious organisms and the study of antimicrobials subject to antagonism by certain medium components, e.g., chocolate agar for *Neisseria* and the addition of lysed horse blood for TMP/SMZ testing (256).

Because the action of several antimicrobials is pH-dependent, another cause of difficulty is failure to adjust the pH of the medium to between 7.2 and 7.4. For example, pH levels below 7.0 begin to adversely affect activities of most aminoglycosides (35). Activities of some antibiotics such as fluoroquinolones and polymyxins, as well as daptomycin, are sensitive to variations in the concentrations of Mg^{2+} and/or Ca^{2+} (133,165,172,218,523). In these situations, it is appropriate to ensure that media are supplemented approximately (448).

ANTIMICROBIAL INTERACTIONS RESULTING IN ANTAGONISM

From a clinical viewpoint, antagonism is the most disadvantageous outcome possible with an antimicrobial combination because the effect of the combination may be less than that of either drug alone. However, there are few reports in which clinically significant antagonism has been documented (355,472,648) despite the large number of reports of *in vitro* antagonism in the literature. It is possible that clinically significant antagonism unrecognized in patients with complex disease states or under-reported. It is also possible that antagonism defined under relatively controlled conditions *in vitro* may not be significant *in vivo*, especially in the presence of intact host defenses. For whatever reasons, documented reports of clinically significant antagonism are uncommon.

Combinations of Bacteriostatic Agents with β-Lactam Antibiotics

Older Protein-Synthesis Inhibitors and β-Lactams

The clearest example of clinically significant antagonism was reported in a study of pneumococcal meningitis (355). In that study, patients who were treated with penicillin/chlortetracycline had a mortality rate of 79%, versus a mortality rate of only 21% for patients who were treated with penicillin alone. Those results presumably reflected antimicrobial antagonism *in vivo* because tetracycline also prevents the bactericidal action of penicillin against the pneumococcus *in vitro*. Although the exact

TABLE 9.4

Comparison of Different Techniques Used to Assess Antimicrobial Combinations

Technique	Medium	Antibacterial Effect	Modifications	Advantages/Disadvantages
Checkerboard	Broth dilution, Microdilution in broth	Bacteriostatic	Killing can be assessed by sampling clear tubes/wells	Many different combinations and concentrations can be tested; bactericidal data require extra sampling steps; does not assess killing rates. Microtiter plate preparation can be automated.
	Agar dilution	Bacteriostatic		Useful for testing many organisms against a few antimicrobials.
Killing curve	Broth	Bactericidal	Can adapt to pharmacodynamic models simulating human pharmacokinetics	Few combinations can be tested, but killing effect over time can be determined
Disk diffusion	Agar	Bacteriostatic		Gradient produced by drug diffusion does not necessarily have a clear relationship with achievable concentrations; qualitative information may be useful for screening
Paper strip diffusion	Agar	Bacteriostatic	Can use commercial gradient diffusion strips	Traditional paper strip method produces only qualitative results, difficult to relate to achievable concentrations
Kinetic spectrophoto-metric	Broth	Bacteriostatic	Killing can be assessed by performing colony counts at selected time points	Provides a potentially helpful kinetic view of antimicrobial action and interaction; bactericidal data can be obtained only with addition of colony counts

mechanism responsible for this effect is unknown, it is known that a bacterium must be growing for penicillin to express its bactericidal activity and that the bacteriostatic action of tetracycline on the ribosome inhibits bacterial growth. An additional potential mechanism is inhibition (by tetracycline) of the production of autolysin by the pneumococcus (607).

Like tetracycline, chloramphenicol (a reversible inhibitor of protein synthesis that binds to the 50S subunit of the ribosome) has also been shown to antagonize bacterial killing by penicillin *in vitro* (289,516) and to reduce the activity of β-lactams such as cefotaxime and aztreonam against *Klebsiella pneumoniae* (66). Although such studies would raise serious questions about the use of chloramphenicol/β-lactam combinations (especially for meningitis), attempts to reproduce this phenomenon *in vivo* met with mixed success. For example, antagonism was demonstrated in a dog model of pneumococcal meningitis only when chloramphenicol was administered before penicillin. When the drugs were given simultaneously or when penicillin was given first, antagonism was less marked or absent. Regardless of the initial protocol, continued administration of both drugs produced complete killing of the organism in this model (638). Other studies failed to demonstrate antagonism with penicillin/chloramphenicol combinations in the rabbit model of meningitis with *Haemophilus influenzae* or *Streptococcus pneumoniae* (56). The fact that penicillin does not inhibit the antibacterial activity of chloramphenicol against these organisms (even though chloramphenicol is less effective than penicillin against both) may account for the lack of significant *in vivo* antagonism in these studies. Studies of the autolytic enzyme system indicate that chloramphenicol inhibits the activity of the autolysin responsible for the penicillin-induced lysis and killing of pneumococci (607). Chloramphenicol inhibits bacterial growth and protein synthesis, which may account in part for its ability to inhibit the bactericidal action of penicillin *in vitro*.

Linezolid Plus β-Lactams or Vancomycin

Several studies employing time-kill methods have shown that the bacteriostatic oxazolidinone agent, linezolid, exerts an antagonistic effect on the killing of *S. aureus* by vancomycin (242,286). However, against clinical staphylococcal isolates, Mulazimoglu et al. (432) reported that the combination of the linezolid with vancomycin, both at one-fourth of their respective MICs, demonstrated indifference by time-kill methods. It may be relevant that the studies demonstrating antagonism between linezolid and vancomycin used higher concentrations of linezolid than those used by Mulazimoglu et al. (432). Several other studies have failed to demonstrate antagonism between linezolid and either β-lactams or vancomycin. Using the checkerboard technique, Sweeney and Zurenko (599) found that the combination of the linezolid with a variety of β-lactams or vancomycin yielded predominantly indifferent effects against several Gram-positive organisms (*S. aureus*, enterococci, and pneumococci). A mouse intraperitoneal infection model demonstrated indifference or additivity when oxazolidinones were combined with either vancomycin or imipenem/cilastatin against methicillin-resistant *S. aureus* (197). However, Chiang and Climo (108), while finding the combination of linezolid plus vancomycin indifferent by checkerboard methods (average FIC index = 2), demonstrated in a rabbit model of endocarditis that both linezolid alone and linezolid combined with vancomycin resulted in less killing of *S. aureus* in cardiac vegetations than was seen with vancomycin alone. On the other hand, in an *in vitro* pharmacodynamic system intended to model human pharmaockinetics, the combination of linezolid with either vancomycin or cefepime resulted in modestly improved killing of methicillin-resistant *S. aureus* and *Stapylococcus epidermidis,* methicillin-susceptible *S. aureus,* and glycopeptide-intermediate *S. aureus* (linezolid+cefepime only) (from 0.37 to 2.28 log CFU/ml greater, compared with the most active single agent) (5). Indifference and additivity were the predominant findings for the combination of linezolid and amoxicillin against *Helicobacter pylori* (262).

Combinations of 50S Subunit Ribosomal Inhibitors

Many antimicrobials (e.g., erythromycin, clindamycin, spiramycin, linezolid, chloramphenicol) inhibit bacterial protein synthesis by binding to the 50S subunit of ribosome. Because a number of these agents bind to the same (or very similar) sites on the ribosome, the use of more than one of these antimicrobials may result in competition for target sites, with resultant loss of activity of the most active compound. For example, lincomycin, erythromycin, oleadomycin, and spiramycin have been shown to inhibit the binding of chloramphenicol to intact *Bacillus megaterium* and to ribosomes isolated from them (630). Incubation of staphylococci with erythromycin, a good inducer of ribosomal methylases, may result in resistance to agents such as clindamycin or spiramycin, which are themselves poor inducers of, but susceptible to, this resistance mechanism (34,367, 418).

It has been noted that some clinical isolates of *S. aureus* that have developed resistance to linezolid remain susceptible to erythromycin (615,660). Furthermore, Howe et al. (274) demonstrated that *in vitro* selection for linezolid resistance in *S. aureus* could result in loss of erythromycin resistance. These observations raised the possibility that since both agents act on the same region of the bacterial ribosome (the 50S subunit), mutations causing resistance to linezolid might be incompatible with expression of macrolide resistance. However, Sakoulas et al. (543) were unable to demonstrate the restoration of linezolid susceptibility following the transformation of the *erm*(C) gene (conferring erythromycin resistance) into a linezolid-resistant *S. aureus*.

For other strains of *S. aureus* and for pneumococci, checkerboard assays have shown predominantly indifferent effects for linezolid combined with various other 50S ribosomal subunit inhibitors (including erythromycin, clindamycin, chloramphenicol) (599). Similarly, the combination of linezolid and clarithromycin yielded mostly additive/indifferent effects against *H. pylori* (262).

It also appears that the physical state of the ribosome may be an important determinant of the interactions of drugs acting on the ribosome. For example, the macrolide antibiotics (erythromycin, oleandomycin, and spiramycin) prevent the binding of chloramphenicol to individual 70S ribosomes, but not to polysomes (ribosomes on messenger RNA), raising questions about the validity of observations made with these agents in cell-free systems (499).

Although there is convincing evidence that antagonism can occur *in vitro* with agents that both bind to the 50S subunt of the ribosome, there have been no clinical reports (of which we are aware) to establish that these observations are relevant *in vivo*. The lack of such reports is particularly interesting because the combination of erythromycin plus chloramphenicol was used to provide broad-spectrum coverage for many years before the advent of the newer aminoglycosides and cephalosporins (516).

Combinations of Aminoglycosides with Bacteriostatic Agents

Bactericidal activity of the aminoglycosidic aminocyclitols (such as gentamicin, tobramycin, amikacin, netilmicin, kanamycin, and streptomycin) is potentially antagonized *in vitro* by bacteriostatic agents such as tetracycline or chloramphenicol (288,516). Although the exact mechanism responsible for this antagonism remains unknown, it is possible that chloramphenicol and tetracycline inhibit the active transport mechanisms necessary for the energy-dependent uptake of aminoglycosides into bacterial cells (68) or that they prevent the movement of the ribosome along messenger RNA so that it cannot return to form the initiation complex that may be a critical site for the bactericidal action of aminoglycosides (516).

Jacqueline et al. (286) have shown that linezolid antagonizes the early bactericidal activity of gentamicin against methicillin-resistant *S. aureus* in time-kill assays. They speculated that the antagonism of aminoglycoside activity may be due to either linezolid preventing the formation of the initiation complex for protein synthesis or by inhibition of the active transport mechanisms necessary for aminoglycoside uptake into cells (286). However, other investigators, using checkerboard tests of linezolid combined with gentamicin against several Gram-positive organisms, have documented predominantly indifferent effects (599); studies with a mouse intraperitoneal *S. aureus* infection model concluded that combinations of an oxazolidinone with gentamicin are indifferent or additive (197). Grohs et al. (242) demonstrated that combining linezolid with gentamicin prevented the emergence of gentamicin-resistant colonies of *S. aureus in vitro*.

Several studies have demonstrated *in vivo* antagonism of aminoglycoside action by chloramphenicol in experimental animal models. Combinations of gentamicin plus chloramphenicol were antagonistic in the treatment of meningitis due to *Proteus mirabilis* in rabbits (592) and for *P. mirabilis* peritonitis in neutropenic mice (549); effects were less clear in studies of *Serratia marcescens* peritonitis in normal mice (516). Although there are no published reports (of which we are aware) of antagonism in humans with these combinations (and tetracycline/aminoglycoside combinations have been commonly used in the treatment of brucellosis), the animal studies cited here suggest that combinations of aminoglycosides with chloramphenicol or tetracycline should be used with caution, if at all, in the treatment of immunosuppressed patients or in the treatment of meningitis.

Several reports have suggested that the combination of erythromycin (or clindamycin) plus gentamicin may be synergistic by the checkerboard method (188,189,354). However, time-kill curve studies with these same combinations suggest that clindamycin may antagonize the early bactericidal activity of gentamicin (687).

Combinations of β-Lactams

A number of troublesome Gram-negative pathogens, such as *P. aeruginosa, Enterobacter, Citrobacter,* and *Serratia,* possess chromosomally mediated β-lactamases that are inducible on exposure of the organisms to β-lactam antibiotics (231). Some β-lactamase-resistant cephalosporins not only are potent inducters of these enzymes, but also may allow selection of stably derepressed (i.e., fully induced) mutant strains of these organisms (232,550,552,554). Against strains possessing such enzymes, the combination of a potent inducer of chromosomal β-lactamase (e.g., cefoxitin) with an intrinsically more potent agent that is not fully resistant to hydrolysis (e.g., a ureidopenicillin) may result in significant loss of activity of the latter. This is illustrated in Figure 9.7 (right panel), where such a combination was employed against a strain of *Enterobacter cloacae*.

Even drugs that appear to be relatively resistant to β-lactamase hydrolysis, such as the third-generation cephalosporins, suffer loss of activity against fully depressed mutant strains. Although alternative hypotheses have been proposed (550), this phenomenon is best explained by the combined roles of the permeability barrier created by the outer cell membrane of Gram-negative organisms and of the previously underestimated hydrolytic capacity of periplasmic β-lactamases. Vu and Nikaido (634) have demonstrated that, in the presence of intact outer-cell envelope barriers to the penetration of β-lactams, the periplasmic β-lactamases of induced cells are capable of hydrolyzing the low concentrations of (even relatively stable) cephalosporins or penicilllins that can be achieved in this space.

Several animal models have been used to demonstrate that β-lactam/β-lactam antagonism also occurs *in vivo* (218,337). Although the clinical significance of these observations was not clear initially (553,646), several investigators demonstrated rapid development of resistance to cephalosporins used for treatment of bacteremias and other serious infections caused by Gram-negative organisms with inducible β-lactamases (441,552). During treatment of *Enterobacter* bacteremias with cephalosporins to which the organisms appear susceptible by standard laboratory tests, a substantial breakthrough rate of stably derepressed mutants has been documented (113). Sanders (551) described such Gram-negative organisms with inducible chromosomal β-lactamases as not truly susceptible to the second- and third-generation cephalosporins because the resistance genes are present but not activated during routine susceptibility testing.

Combinations of Quinolones with Other Agents

Because of widespread clinical use of fluoroquinolone antimicrobials, several studies have explored combinations of these drugs with a variety of other antibiotics. Fortunately, such combinations have demonstrated antagonism relatively infrequently (164). *In vitro,* chloramphenicol antagonized the bactericidal activity of ciprofloxacin against some strains of *S. aureus, Escherichia coli,* and *P. aeruginosa* (521,678). By checkerboard methods, the combination of various quinolone antimicrobials with linezolid was predominantly indifferent against a variety of Gram-positive and Gram-negative organisms (599). However, by time-kill methods, the bactericidal rate of ciprofloxacin against staphylococci can be reduced in the presence of other agents demonstrating weaker bactericidal activity, including vancomycin (485), rifampin (26,624), or linezolid (242). The bactericidal activity of levofloxacin against pneumococci (220) and *Listeria monocytogenes* (413) could also be reduced in the presence of rifampin.

Combinations of quinolones with quinupristin/dalfopristin have demonstrated antagonism against vancomycin-resistant *Enterococcus faecium* (300,402). However, because such combinations (a) do not inevitably result in decreased serum bactericidal activities (relative to the most active drug alone), (b) demonstrate antagonism against exponentially growing organisms (staphylococci), but additivity toward stationary-phase staphylococci (26), and (c) may result in the mutual suppression of resistant subpopulations (26), it is not certain that such potential antagonism discerned by *in vitro* testing would be clinically relevant. Antagonistic effects *in vitro* between fluoroqinolones and novobiocin, an older antibiotic that also inhibits DNA gyrase, have been reported against staphylococci (359).

ANTIMICROBIAL INTERACTIONS RESULTING IN SYNERGISM

Having introduced the most frequent justifications for the use of combination therapy and the techniques commonly used to assess antimicrobial interaction, we now consider the major mechanisms responsible for antimicrobial synergism against bacteria.

There are four generally accepted mechanisms of antibacterial synergism: (a) serial (sequential) inhibition of a common biochemical pathway (e.g., TMP/SMZ), (b) inhibition of protective bacterial enzymes (e.g., β-lactamases) or efflux systems, (c) use of combinations of cell wall-active agents (e.g., amdinocillin (mecillinam) plus ampicillin), and (d) use of cell wall-active agents to enhance the uptake of other antimicrobials (e.g., penicillin plus streptomycin). In addition, there are other instances in which the criteria for synergism are fulfilled but the mechanism of drug interaction is either unique (e.g., quinupristin/dalfopristin) or unclear (e.g., SMZ plus colistin).

In this section we consider each of these groups of interactions, beginning with the known mechanisms of action and resistance (citing examples from both laboratory and clinical studies) and concluding with a discussion of the laboratory results and their clinical application, as well as simple tests that may be used to predict resistance to combination therapy.

Sequential (Serial) Inhibition of a Common Biochemical Pathway

The best known example of antimicrobial synergism by sequential inhibition of a common biochemical pathway is the combination of TMP and SMZ. Two additional combinations that most likely also involve sequential inhibition of a common pathway are those containing amdinocillin (mecillinam) or vancomycin plus penicillins or cephalosporins (30,151). For the purposes of this chapter, the latter interactions are considered as combinations of agents acting on the cell wall, although they can also be considered to act in sequence on biochemical pathways involved in cell wall synthesis.

Mechanism of Action

SMZ and other sulfonamides are thought to exert their antibacterial effect by competing with *p*-aminobenzoic acid to prevent the formation of 7,8-dihydropteroate (Fig. 9.9) (65). This compound, 7,8-dihydropteroate, is combined with L-glutamate to form dihydrofolic acid and is then reduced (in the presence of dihydrofolate reductase) to tetrahydrofolic acid, which is an essential donor of one-carbon fragments for the synthesis of thymidine, methionine, glycine, adenine, and guanine in both bacterial and mammalian cells (161,263). TMP, pyrimethamine, and other antifolate agents inhibit dihydrofolate reductase and thus inhibit the production of tetrahydrofolic acid from dihydrofolic acid (264). Because the effects of TMP plus SMZ, including cell death, can be reversed by thymidine, thymineless death is thought to be the mechanism by which TMP/SMZ exerts its bactericidal effect (326,605). Bacterial cells generally cannot take up exogenous folates; thus, they are unable to bypass the block created by TMP plus SMZ (263). Mammalian cells, which can absorb exogenous folate, are also protected because they contain a different dihydrofolate reductase. TMP is more than 10,000 times more active against bacterial dihydrofolate reductase than it is against the mammalian enzyme (72,254,298).

Although the TMP/SMZ combination acts at least two points in the folate pathway, there has been some uncertainty, on theoretical grounds, whether sequential inhibition of a linear pathway could produce a truly

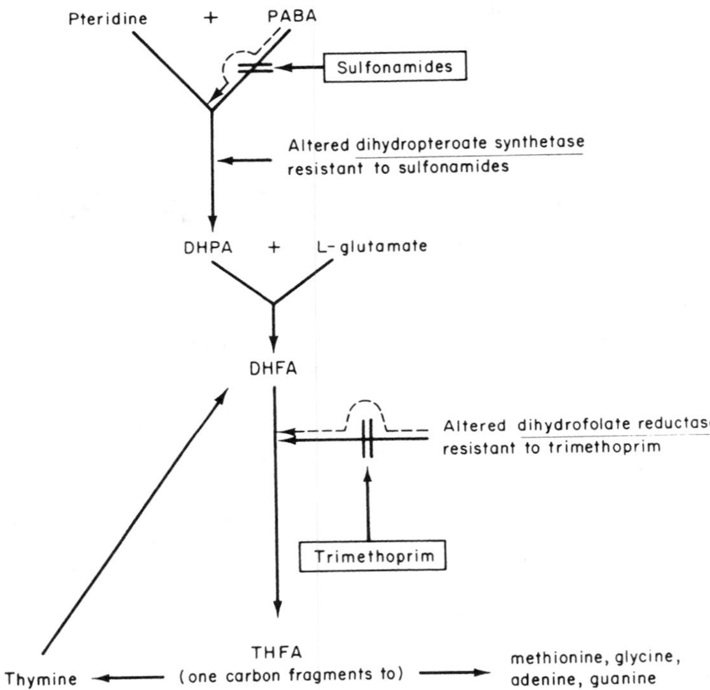

FIGURE 9.9 ● Mechanisms of resistance to sulfonamides and TMP *in vitro*. The more prevalent mechanisms of resistance are altered dihydropteroate synthetase and dihydrofolate reductase enzymes with decreased affinities for sulfonamides and TMP, respectively. See text for details. *PABA*, *p*-aminobenzoic acid; *DHPA*, 7, 8-dihydropteroate; *DHFA*, dihydrofolic acid; *THFA*, tetrahydrofolic acid.

synergistic effect (647). Therefore, it had been proposed that sulfonamides may act synergistically with TMP on the same enzyme, dihydrofolate reductase (510). In support of this concept, a variety of sulfonamides synergize with TMP against an *E. coli* dihydrofolate reductase *in vitro* (510), but only at concentrations several orders of magnitude greater than those achievable *in vivo*; this mechanism would therefore require that the organism concentrate sulfonamide for synergism to occur either *in vitro* or *in vivo* (71,604). Because there is no evidence for such high intracellular concentrations of sulfonamides, this possibility seems unlikely. Other workers have pointed out that dihydrofolate reductase may be in a cyclic rather than a linear pathway (considering the recycling of tetrahydrofolate after it has been oxidized to dihydrofolate) and that sequential inhibition in such a system should therefore be capable of producing synergism if the sulfonamides reduce the quantity of intermediates available (71,647). Another objection to the aforementioned hypothesis was that several dihydrofolate reductase inhibitors with structure quite different from that of TMP were all capable of synergizing with sulfonamides, which would not have been expected if both compounds were acting together on the same enzyme (604).

In summary, although sulfonamides and TMP have been shown to synergistically inhibit dihydrofolate reductase activity *in vitro*, the concentrations of sulfonamide at which this occurs are significantly higher than those achievable *in vivo*, where synergism has been demonstrated (71,79). Thus, it seems reasonable to regard sequential inhibition of a common pathway as the most likely basis for the synergism observed with TMP plus SMZ.

Laboratory Studies of TMP Plus SMZ

Laboratory studies have been performed on a wide variety of organisms, using many different methods. The drugs are most frequently employed in a 1:20 ratio of TMP to SMZ (the usual ratio of serum concentrations achieved with oral administration of the commercially available 1:5 combination). The optimal ratio of two drugs for the production of synergism is thought to be the ratio of their MICs for the organism being tested (79), and TMP is 20 to 100 times as active as SMZ against most bacteria. Therefore, using this fixed 1:20 ratio is usually appropriate. Nevertheless, this ratio may not be optimal for all organisms, because at least three general—*Neisseria, Brucella,* and *Nocardia*—are more susceptible to SMZ than to TMP and should presumably be studied with a different TMP/SMZ mixture (79).

Many Gram-negative organisms are often reported as susceptible to TMZ plus SMZ *in vitro*, including *E. coli* and other *Enterobacteriaceae* (2,79), *H. influenzae* (382) and *Bordetella pertussis* (79). Although resistant isolates are recognized, TMP/SMZ is one of a few antimicrobials with substantial activity against some strains of *Burkholderia cepacia* and *Stenotrophomonas maltophilia* (358,394). *P. aeruginosa,* which is generally resistant to both TMP and SMZ separately, is characteristically also resistant to TMP/SMZ synergism. Similarly,

Mycobacterium tuberculosis, which is usually resistant to both drugs, has also been resistant to the TMP/SMZ combination (79).

In spite of their relative TMP resistance, a number of *Neisseria gonorrhoeae* strains are synergistically inhibited by TMP plus SMZ. This is most noticeable using a 3:1 combination (rather than the usual 1:20 combination) (24), which more closely approximates the ratios of the MICs of these two drugs for *N. gonorrhoeae*. Among Gram-positive organisms, many streptococci and pneumococci are susceptible to TMP plus SMZ, as are some strains of *S. aureus*. Enterococci *(Enterococcus faecalis)* are typically resistant to TMP/SMZ synergism *in vivo* because they are able to absorb exogenous folate and thus bypass the metabolic block produced by the drug combination (79,263,264). Among the actinomycetes, synergism has been shown *in vitro* for *Nocardia asteroides* (385). Thus, the *in vitro* laboratory data suggest a wide range of bacteria against which the TMP/SMZ combination might be effective *in vivo*.

Mechanism of Resistance *in Vitro*

There are several mechanisms by which bacteria may be resistant to TMP/SMZ synergism *in vitro* (Fig. 9.9): (a) an altered dihydropteroate synthetase with a decreased affinity for sulfonamides, (b) an altered dihydrofolate reductase with a decreased affinity for TMP, and (c) resistance based on poor drug penetration or enhanced drug efflux by transmembrane pumps (280,327).

Sulfonamide resistance was noted shortly after sulfa drugs were first introduced for clinical use. In 1952, it was postulated that the basis of this resistance might be an enzyme with decreased affinity for sulfonamides (138). Subsequently, in 1963, it was demonstrated that the dihydropteroate synthetase activity of sulfonamide-resistant *E. coli* mutants was resistant to sulfonamide inhibition (484). These findings were later corroborated by kinetic studies of dihydropteroate synthetase activity in sulfonamide-resistant *Neisseria meningitidis* and *N. gonorrhoeae* (267). It is now clear that the basis of resistance in some clinical isolates of sulfonamide-resistant *E. coli* are plasmid-encoded dihydropteroate synthetases with decreased affinity for sulfonamides. It was demonstrated in 1945 that some sulfonamide-resistant strains produced increased quantities of *p*-aminobenzoic acid (341). However, the clinical importance of this observation remains unclear, even though it was subsequently confirmed by other workers (283,655).

TMP resistance was not a problem in early studies. TMP had been chosen from a group of several antifolates after examination of their activities against the dihydrofolate reductases of several species (72,263,264). The concentration of TMP necessary for 50% inhibition of human dihydrofolate reductase activity in these studies was 60,000 times that required for a similar effect on bacterial dihydrofolate reductase (72,263,264). Thus, the choice of TMP as a therapeutic agent took advantage of naturally occurring species differences in enzyme specificity. However, several bacterial dihydrofolate reductases that are resistant to TMP were soon described (9,489,572). Since that time, several additional distinct and transferable TMP-resistant dihydrofolate reductases have been recognized (280).

Mechanisms of Resistance to TMP Plus SMZ *in Vivo*

As mentioned, enterococci are generally resistant to the TMP/SMZ combination *in vivo* because they are able to absorb the exogenous folates preset in human plasma (50,79,263,264). Two animal studies demonstrated lack of activity of TMP plus SMZ against enterococcal infections *in vivo*, despite activity *in vitro* (107,237). In the rat endocarditis model, numbers of residual bacteria in cardiac vegetations of TMP/SMZ-treated animals were identical to those of untreated controls (237).

Clinical Studies of TMP Plus SMZ

Most clinical trials of TMP/SMZ synergism have used a fixed combination with five times as much SMZ as TMP (by weight). This combination usually produces serum levels of SMZ in humans approximately 20 times those of TMP (in micrograms per milliliter) (126,187), which is close to the most frequent ratio of their MICs against common pathogens.

Problems associated with the use of TMZ/SMZ combination include decreased intestinal absorption of oral drug in critically ill patients with ileus and fluid overload with intravenous administration in patients with renal and/or cardiac failure (because both drugs are only sparingly soluble in water). TMP/SMZ toxicity is most frequently due to hypersensitivity reactions to one of the two components (especially SMZ). Although neutropenia and thrombocytopenia do occur with TMP plus SMZ, particularly in children (20), marrow depression secondary to the antifolate effect of TMP alone has not commonly been reported under ordinary circumstances when the drug has been used as an antibacterial agent (198). Higher frequencies of adverse effects, including hypersensitivity reactions and hematologic effects, however, have been observed in patients with human immunodeficiency virus infection (116). On theoretical grounds, it should be possible to reverse marrow toxicity (when it occurs) with folinic acid, which mammalian cells (but not bacteria other than enterococci) can absorb from their external environment. The primary route of excretion for both drugs is through the kidneys, with an elimination half-life of 11 to 14 hours (302,463). Although the dose should therefore be reduced in patients with renal failure (653), TMP/SMZ has been successfully used for the treatment of urinary tract infections in these patients (47).

Substantial experience has been accumulated with the use of TMP plus SMZ for meningitis and brain abscess. The available data suggest that SMZ readily crosses the blood–brain barrier into the cerebrospinal fluid and that

TMP penetrates well across mildly inflamed meninges. Levels of TMP and SMZ in brain tissue of a patient being treated for *N. asteroides* brain abscess were reported to be 5.1 and 36.0 μg/g of tissue, respectively, 6 hours after the last TMP/SMZ dose, using only 160/800 mg twice daily (385).

TMP/SMZ demonstrated activity against *Salmonella typhi* and *Shigella* spp resistant to earlier agents including ampicillin and chloramphenicol and was used successfully to treat infections caused by these organisms (84,106,219,449,471). Unfortunately, TMP/SMZ resistant strains of *S. typhi* and *Shigella* are now recognized (363,635). *H. influenzae* type b organisms resistant to ampicillin were first noted in the United States in 1974 (310,608). Soon thereafter, such strains appeared widely in the United States (562). Although both erythromycin/SMZ (562) and streptomycin/SMZ (406) combinations have also been used, TMP/SMZ has continued to play an important role in the treatment of ampicillin-resistant *H. influenzae* infection.

Other infections in which TMP/SMZ has been efficacious include gonorrhea (24) (although many strains are now resistant) and infections due to *Enterobacter* spp, multiply resistant *Acinetobacter, Stenotrophomonas* and *N. asteroides* (385,394,462). This combination has also proven useful in the treatment of serious infections due to methicillin-resistant but TMP/SMZ-susceptible strains of *S. aureus* in patients who cannot tolerate vancomycin (517). TMP/SMZ has been employed successfully in the treatment of infections due to *L. monocytogenes* (582).

TMP/SMZ is widely used for the treatment of urinary tract infections due to Gram-negative organisms, especially the *Enterobacteriaceae*. Its effectiveness is enhanced by attainment of high urinary levels of the components. Unfortunately, resistance to TMP/SMZ is now increasing among urinary tract isolates of *E. coli* (305).

Additional uses for TMP/SMZ include the prevention of recurrent urinary tract infection (255,586) and the treatment of chronic prostatitis because TMP penetrates especially well into prostatic fluid (407). (TMP is concentrated in prostatic secretions to levels three times plasma levels, but SMZ levels in prostatic secretions are only one-tenth those found in plasma [663]). TMP/SMZ has also been established as effective for the prophylaxis and treatment of *Pneumocystis (jiroveci) carinii* pneumonia (79,80,99).

Predicting Resistance to Therapy

Problems with TMP/SMZ susceptibility testing were most frequently related to the thymidine content of the testing media, i.e., the TMP MIC has been shown to rise with the thymidine content (326). Similar problems occurred earlier in sulfonamide testing, and in 1945 it was demonstrated that lysed horse blood could improve otherwise unsuitable media (256). Lysed horse red blood cells contain thymidine phosphorylase, which converts thymidine to thymine, thus decreasing its ability to antagonize the TMP/SMZ blockade by approximately 100-fold (79).

For this reason, Bushy (79) recommended the addition of lysed horse blood to media used for TMP/SMZ testing, unless the thymidine content is known to be less than 0.3 μg/mL. Unsupplemented Mueller-Hinton agar is now usually satisfactory (39). Agar lots can be screened for the absence of significant amounts of thymidine or thymine by demonstrating inhibition of control strains of *E. faecalis* by TMP/SMZ disks (39). For susceptibility testing with TMP/SMZ in broth, supplementation of the medium with lysed horse blood or addition of commercially available thymidine phosphorylase usually results in satisfactory performance (448).

Inhibition of Enzymes That Render Antimicrobial Agents Inactive

This section describes antimicrobial combinations in which one drug interferes with either the production or the action of a bacterial enzyme, thus permitting another drug (which would otherwise have been ineffective) to be active.

Mechanism of Action

Bacterial enzymes may exert a protective effect by hydrolyzing a substrate such as penicillin, thus rendering it inactive against the bacterial cell. Two approaches to antimicrobial synergism have attempted to circumvent this mechanism, by (a) using another drug to prevent the production of β-lactamase or (b) binding the enzyme so tightly that it is not free to act on the susceptible (hydrolyzable) penicillin, thus allowing that penicillin to remain intact and to exert its bactericidal effect on the β-lactamase-producing organism. Inhibitors of an aminoglycoside-modifying enzyme (aminoglycoside-2-*O*-adenylyltransferase) have been described that potentiate aminoglycoside activities against enzyme-producing Gram-negative bacilli (6). A third example has been the use of a urease inhibitor (acetohydroxamic acid) (443) to prevent the rise in urinary pH associated with urease activity (e.g., *Proteus* infections), so that drugs that require acidic urine (methenamine mandelate) (442) might be effective. This urease inhibitor also inhibits growth of *H. pylori* at high concentrations and appears to augment activities of various antimicrobials against some isolates (505). However, neither the aminoglycoside-modifying enzyme inhibitors nor inhibitors of urease activity have been developed to a level of clinical utility.

Laboratory Studies of Synergism by Inhibition of Enzymes That Render Antimicrobial Agents Inactive

Penicillin Combinations Using an Inhibitor β-Lactam to Bind β-Lactamase. A substantial body of literature describes the use of penicillin combinations against β-lactamase-producing strains *in vitro*. In early

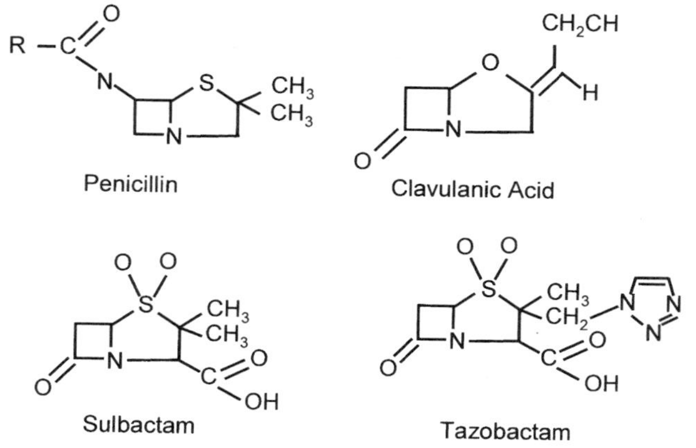

FIGURE 9.10 ● Structures of penicillin, clavulanic acid, tazobactam and sulbactam. The β-lactamase inhibitors (clavulanic acid sulbactam and tazobactam) share a double-ring structure and the β-lactam bond in common with penicillin.

studies, these combinations usually involved an inhibitor (less hydrolyzable) penicillin (e.g., cloxacillin) to bind the β-lactamase and a hydrolyzable penicillin (e.g., penicillin G), which would ordinarily have been inactivated by β-lactamase. It has been suggested that four criteria must be met for such combinations to successfully produce synergism (537): (a) β-lactamase must be a major factor in the resistance of the organism to penicillin, (b) the inhibitor β-lactam must be resistant to the β-lactamase of the organism, (c) the inhibitor β-lactam must have a greater affinity for the β-lactamase than does the hydrolyzable penicillin, and (d) the inhibitor β-lactam must be relatively ineffective as an antimicrobial against the test strain at the concentration employed (otherwise, it would inhibit and kill the test organism alone).

The failure to demonstrate synergism in early studies with *S. aureus* (540) was attributed to a low affinity of the inhibitor penicllin for staphylococcal penicillinase (537). The affinity of methicillin (the inhibitor penicillin) for staphylococcal β-lactamase is less than 10^{-4} that of benzylpenicllin (466). However, study of Gram-negative organisms, particularly *Pseudomonas,* revealed that their β-lactamases have a much greater affinity for methicillin and cloxacillin than for penicillin or ampicillin, thus opening the way for consideration of synergistic penicillin combinations (538). This type of synergism has been reported *in vitro* against *P. aeruginosa* (539), *E. coli* (598), *Proteus* spp (467), *Klebsiella* spp (539), *Enterobacter* spp (184), and a number of other Gram-negative organisms. Because it requires very high concentrations of methicillin or cloxacillin to produce synergism with penicillins against Gram-negative bacilli, such combinations were useful only in the treatment of urinary tract infections.

Clavulanic acid, a β-lactam isolated from *Streptomyces clavuligerus,* has also been shown to inhibit the penicillinases produced by a numer of bacteria (77,520). Although it shares a common β-lactam ring with penicillin, it differs structurally in several aspects (Fig. 9.10) (520): (a) the sulfur atom of the thiazolidine ring is replaced by an oxygen, producing an oxazolidine ring; (b) there is no side chain connected by an amide linkage at position 6 of the β-lactam ring; and (c) the two methyl groups at position 2 of the thiazolidine ring are replaced by a β-hydroxylethylidine group. Also shown in Figure 9.10 is the chemical structure of the sulfone sulbactam (175), another β-lactamase inhibitor that has been developed for clinical use. *In vitro* studies have shown that clavulanic acid, sulbactam, and another penicillinic acid sulfone β-lactamase inhibitor, tazobactam (16), inhibit the plasmid-mediated β-lactamases of *S. aureus* and many *Enterobacteriaceae* but are usually ineffective against the chromosomal β-lactamases of *P. aeruginosa* and *E. cloacae* and a chromosomally mediated enzyme from *E. coli* (77,520).

Although none of these inhibitors demonstrates significant antimicrobial activity against most commonly encountered organisms (except that sulbactam does have activity against *Acinetobacter*) (78,455,666), all three drugs considerably extend the spectrum of hydrolyzable penicillins and cephalosphorins against a broad range of Gram-negative and Gram-positive organisms possessing β-lactamases susceptible to inhibition by these drugs (16,175,336,349,501,507,520,668). Synergism between amoxicillin and clavulanate, ticarcillin and clavulanate, ampicillin and sulbactam, or piperacillin and tazobactam, the four fixed-dose β-lactam/β-lactamase inhibitor combinations currently available in the United States, yields useful antimicrobial activity against many strains of *S. aureus, Bacteroides fragilis, H. influenzae, K. pneumoniae,* and other *Enterobacteriaceae,* among others (38,233,336,629). These inhibitors also restore activities of several third-generation cephalosporins against *Enterobacteriaceae* producing several extended-spectrum β-lactamases, most of which are related to TEM or SHV enzymes (285,477). These combinations offer little advantage against most *P. aeruginosa* or *E. cloacae* strains, whose chromosomal β-lactamases are poorly inhibited by these agents. In fact, at high concentrations, clavulanic acid may function as an inducer of these β-lactamases, hence antagonizing the activities of the intrinsically more active penicillins against some strains (162). Compounds that inhibit chromosomal β-lactamases of Gram-negative bacteria have been described, e.g., BRL 42715 (117,682), but none has been developed for clinical use.

Inhibition of β-Lactamase Production. Because β-lactamases are proteins, the use of drugs that inhibit protein synthesis might theoretically inhibit their production enough to render β-lactamase-producing organisms susceptible to β-lactams. Therefore, several investigators have examined antimicrobial combinations of inhibitors of protein synthesis (e.g., chloramphenicol) with penicillin *in vitro* against strains that produce β-lactamase and are thus characteristically penicillin-resistant.

It was demonstrated in 1973 that chloramphenicol could synergize with β-lactam antibiotics against *Klebsiella, Enterobacter,* and *Serratia* (375). Because these combinations were more frequently synergistic against strains resistant to β-lactams, it seemed possible that chloramphenicol might exert its effect through inhibition of the protein synthesis required for β-lactamase production. This hypothesis was later supported by a study of *Enterobacteriaceae* in which the killing-curve technique was used to demonstrate synergism between cephaloridine (12.5 to 500 μg/mL) and chloramphenicol (6 μg/mL) against 10 of 10 β-lactamase-producing strains (411). Although chloramphenicol reduced the loss of cephaloridine activity in the medium (measured by bioassay) in that study, β-lactamase was not directly determined, so chloramphenicol-induced inhibition of β-lactamase production was implied but not proven. The same group of investigators later reported penicillin/chloramphenicol synergism against 17 of 20 β-lactamase-producing strains of *S. aureus* (412). Although high concentrations of chloramphenicol antagonized the inhibitory effect of penicillin, lower concentrations (4 μg/mL) prevented measurable β-lactamase production and produced synergism (99). More recently, clindamycin was shown to inhibit derepression of the inducible β-lactamases of *E. cloacae* and *P. aeruginosa* (555). Combined with cefamandole (an agent susceptible to hydrolysis by the *E. cloacae* enzyme), clindamycin augmented the *in vitro* bactericidal activity and *in vivo* efficacy of the cephalosporin.

Resistance to Synergism by Inhibition of Bacterial Enzymes That Render Antimicrobial Agents Inactive

Combinations Using an Inhibitor β-Lactam to Bind β-Lactamase. As mentioned, a β-lactam inhibitor that is bound more tightly to β-lactamase than is a hydrolyzable penicillin or cephalosporin may produce synergism against certain organisms when combined with that penicillin or cephalosporin. Inadequate binding of cloxacillin to staphylococcal β-lactamase was a major reason for failure to demonstrate penicillin/cloxacillin synergism against *S. aureus* (540). Such combinations (ampicillin/cloxacillin) also synergistically inhibit Gram-negative organisms, but poor penetration of the latter drug into these organisms severely limits the usefulness of such combinations (60). Obviously, addition of clavulanic acid, sulbactam, or tazobactam to penicillins or cephalosporins offers no advantage against strains resistant to the latter, based on production of enzymes (primarily chromosomal) against which the inhibitors are inactive (77). Several novel, plasmid-mediated β-lactamases that are resistant to inhibition by the currently available inhibitors have been reported (285,478,504). Resistance to β-lactam/β-lactamase combinations (e.g., amoxicillin/clavualanate) among some strains of *E. coli* has been attributed to hyperproduction of TEM-type β-lactamases (against which clavulanate is usually active) encoded by small multicopy plasmids (396).

Inhibition of β-Lactamase Production. The use of inhibitors of protein synthesis to inhibit β-lactamase synthesis and thereby potentiate activity of an otherwise hydrolyzable β-lactam has not proven feasible for general use. Therefore, resistance mechanisms are largely theoretical and would include: (a) emergence of resistance to the inhibitor of protein synthesis, rendering it ineffective in inhibiting β-lactamase synthesis; and (b) manifestation of antagonistic interations arising from interference with β-lactam-induced lysis, either by direct inhibition (e.g., by chloramphenicol) of cellular autolysins or by generation of population of nongrowing cells that are less susceptible to penicillin-induced lysis (607).

Clinical Studies of Synergism by Inhibition of Bacterial Enzymes That Render Antimicrobial Agents Inactive

Penicillin Combinations Using an Inhibitory β-Lactam to Bind β-Lactamase. The use of older β-lactamase-resistant penicillins (e.g., cloxacillin) to synergistically enhance the activities of hydrolyzable penicillins (e.g., ampicilllin) against Gram-negative bacilli was severely constrained by the fact that effective concentrations of the former often exceeded levels readily achievable in serum (184). Therefore, use of such combinations was limited to treatment of urinary tract infections (537,539). In contrast, combinations of clavulanic acid with amoxicillin or ticarcillin, of sulbactam with ampicillin, and of tazobactam with piperacillin have proven efficacious against infections caused by a wide variety of susceptible pathogens and are currently approved for clinical use in the Untied States (16,233,666). Such combinations not only provide greater potency than the penicillin alone against some organisms (e.g., *B. fragilis*), but also extend the antibacterial spectrum to bacteria usually resistant to clinically achievable concentrations of these penicillins alone (e.g., *K. pneumoniae* and *S. aureus*). One novel approach was to combine ampicillin with sulbactam through an ester linkage to create a new compound (sultamicillin) that, after *in vivo* hydrolysis to the parent drugs, produced higher serum levels after oral administration than observed with either of the single agents alone.

Inhibition of β-Lactamase Production. Clinical trials have not been performed to test the use of inhibitors of protein synthesis to block penicillinase production and thus render β-lactamase-producing organisms penicillin-sensitive. The major theoretical reason for the lack of such trials is probably the narrow range of chlorampehnicol concentrations over which synergism has been observed *in vitro*, with documented antagonism at slightly higher levels (412).

Inhibition of Efflux Systems That Render Antimicrobial Agents Inactive. It has recently been appreciated that active efflux of antimicrobials contributes significantly to antimicrobial resistance in both Gram-positive and Gram-negative bacteria. Numerous efflux systems have been described (366). Efflux mechanisms contribute to resistance to a broad range of antimicrobial agents including β-lactams, aminoglycosides, fluoroquinolones, oxazolidinones, macrolides, tetracyclines, trimethoprim, antiseptics, and others. Several investigational efflux inhibitors have been studied. One of these was shown to enhance the potency of levofloxacin against a susceptible strain of *P. aeruginosa,* restore susceptibility to levofloxacin of a resistant strain, and reduce the frequency at which resistant subpopulations emerged following exposure to the quinolone (365). At the present time, no efflux inhibitor has been developed for clinical use.

Combinations of Agents That Act on the Bacterial Cell Wall

Although the β-lactam/β-lactamase inhibitor combinations described earlier are combinations of agents that, in principle, have activity against bacterial cell wall synthesis, the inhibitor in those combinations is primarily functioning to bind β-lactamase and probably does not affect cell wall synthesis of most organisms at clinically relevant concentrations. In this section, we consider combinations in which both antimicrobials appear to act on the bacterial cell wall. It has been known for many years that penicillin inhibits bacterial cell wall synthesis, particularly at the cross-linking step (52). There has been interest in combinations of penicillins with drugs that act at earlier steps of cell wall synthesis (e.g., β-chloro-D-alanine, phosphonic acid derivatives, or vancomycin) or with other β-lactams (e.g., amdinocillin, formerly known as mecillinam) that target different penicillin-binding proteins (PBPs) (479) than those that are the primary targets of penicillin. Examples of such combinations, few of which are clinically important, are given in this section.

Mechanism of Action

β-Chloro-D-Alanine Plus Penicillin. β-Chloro-D-alanine (an analog of D-alanine) probably acts by competitively inhibiting the synthesis and/or attachment of the terminal D-alanine dipeptide to generate the pentapeptide necessary for production of the bacterial cell wall (387). The enzymes that have been implicated as the sites of this inhibition are alanine racemase (which converts L-alanine to D-alanine) and D-glutamate-D-alanine transaminase (which transfers the D-alanine dipeptide to the *N*-acetyl-uridine diphosphate peptide) (579). Thus, the synergism observed with β-chloro-D-alanine plus penicillin is presumably the result of activity exerted at two points in the sequence of cell wall synthesis: (a) decreased production and attachment of the D-alanine dipeptide due to β-chloro-D-alanine and (b) inhibition of the later cross-linking step due to penicillin.

Phosphonic Acid Derivatives Plus β-Lactams. Phosphonic acid derivatives, such as fosmidomycin, alafosfalin, and fosfomycin, also inhibit the early steps of cell wall synthesis. Thus, mechanisms of synergy with β-lactams are presumabaly analogous to those of β-chloro-D-alanine. These drugs have been shown to inhibit alanine racemase and uridine 5-diphosphate *N*-acetylmuramyl-L-alanine synthetase (alafosfalin) (21) and UDP-*N*-acetylglucosamine enolpyruvyl transferase (fosmidomycin and fosfomycin) (44,297,458,459). Fosfomycin may also affect the synthesis of PBPs (243,623), providing yet another possible mechanism of interaction with β-lactams.

Amdinocillin Plus Other β-Lactams. Amdinocillin is a β-lactam antibiotic that differs in structure from penicillin in one major respect: it has an amidino side chain at the 6-position, in contrast to the acylamino side chain at the 6-position of the more traditional penicillins (376). Exposure of bacteria to amdinocillin results in the formation of large spherical cells that lyse without formation of spheroplasts (239,376,479). These observations suggest a different mode of action for amdinocillin than for penicillin, which typically produces filamentous forms of *E. coli* at low concentrations, bulges in bacilli at intermediate concentrations, and finally spheroplasts (which lyse unless maintained in a hypertonic medium) at high concentrations (584). Binding of amdinocillin to its primary target, PBP-2 in *E. coli,* accounts for the morphologic changes mentioned here (583,585,606). Because most of the other penicillins and cephalosporins used clinically bind preferentially to other PBPs (606), combination of amdinocillin with β-lactams acting at complementary target sites could result in synergistic antibacterial interactions.

Vancomycin Combined with Penicillins and Cephalosporins. Although amdinocillin/penicillin combinations are probably the best example of synergism due to combinations of agents that act on the bacterial cell wall, combinations of vancomycin with penicillins and cephalosporins could act by a similar mechanism (151). Because vancomycin acts earlier than the cross-linking step of cell wall synthesis (it inhibits the synthesis of peptidoglycan) (400), its interaction with penicillins or cephalosporins could be classified either as sequential inhibition of a common biochemical pathway or (as we have done) as synergism due to a combination of agents that act on the bacterial cell wall.

Laboratory Studies Using Combinations of Agents That Act on the Bacterial Cell Wall

β-Chloro-D-alanine Plus Penicillin. Using a *Salmonella typhimurium* strain resistant to penicillin, synergism has been demonstrated with penicillin and concentrations of β-chloro-D-alanine that are ineffective when used alone (4 to 8 μg/mL) (579).

Phosphonic Acid Derivatives Plus β-Lactams. Alafosfalin plus amdinocillin or ampicillin act synergistically against a variety of *Enterobacteriaceae* (21). Similarly, fosmidomycin plus penicillin or cephalosporin combinations demonstrated synergism against many *E. coli, K. pneumoniae,* and *S. marcescens* (458). Combinations of fosfomycin with a variety of β-lactams have yielded synergistic inhibition of a wide range of organisms, including *Enterobacteriaceae* (495), *Pseudomonas* (600), and staphylococci (8,241). However, because bacterial strains resistant to fosfomycin can be selected easily, both *in vitro* and *in vivo* (603), it is not clear in most cases whether a beneficial interaction of two drugs results primarily from true synergism or from the suppression of resistant clones. Combination of fosfomycin with daptomycin, a cyclic lipopeptide antibiotic (included here for convenience, although it is not a β-lactam) active at the level of cell wall synthesis, has resulted in synergism against *E. faecalis,* including strains demonstrating high-level resistance to gentamicin (527). Against *S. aureus,* the combination of fosfomycin and vancomycin has resulted in antagonistic effects by the checkerboard technique; however, time-kill studies failed to demonstrate antagonism with this combination (241).

Fosfomycin induces alterations in PBP patterns in *S. aureus* resulting in variable, concentration-dependent interactions with oxacillin (445). Alterations in PBP patterns on incubation in fosfomycin have also been demonstrated with enterococci; this has been suggested as a mechanism for enhanced activity when this drug is combined with penicillin *in vitro* (243).

Amdinocillin Plus Other β-Lactams. A number of reports have described the action of amdinocillin on bacterial cells. Susceptibility studies indicate that amdinocillin alone is active *in vitro* (MIC of less than 6.3 μg/mL) against many *Enterobacteriaceae* (including *E. coli, Klebsiella, Enterobacter, Salmonella,* and *Shigella).* Resistant organisms include *P. aeruginosa, Acinetobacter, Serratia, Proteus, Providencia, H. influenzae,* most Gram-positive cocci and bacilli, and the Gram-negative anaerobes. *In vitro* combinations of amdinocillin with other β-lactams have demonstrated synergism against *E. coli* (450,620), *Klebsiella* (30,450), *Enterobacter* (450), *Citrobacter* (451), indole-negative *Proteus* (30,450), *Shigella* (451), *Salmonella* (451), and other Gram-negative aerobes, especially *Enterobacteriaceae,* which are typically susceptible to amdinocillin. Synergism is usually not seen against Gram-positive cocci (streptococci or staphylococci), Gram-positive bacilli (*Clostridia* or *Listeria),* indole-positive *Proteus,* or Gram-negative anaerobes (450), which are generally resistant to amdinocillin alone. Although studies of amdinocillin/β-lactam synergism have usually employed amdinocillin/ampicillin combinations, the use of cloxacillin (48), amoxicillin (450), carbenicillin (30), cepahlothin (451), cephradine (309), and other β-lactams with amdinocillin has yielded similar results.

Gutmann et al. (247) demonstrated rapid bactericidal effects against *E. coli* with combinations of amdinocillin (PBP-2-specific) plus aztreonam (PBP-3-specific) at drug concentrations that were only bacteriostatic individually. The relevance of PBP binding in these observations was further clarified by studies with temperature-sensitivie PBP-2 or PBP-3 mutants. Under conditions in which one or the other of these was not expressed, addition of the drug specifically binding the complementary PBP resulted in cell lysis comparable with that seen when the two antibiotics were combined.

Studies by Sanders et al. (556) have revealed another possible mechanism by which amdinocillin may potentiate the activities of other β-lactams. Exposure of Gram-negative bacilli to amdinocillin caused leakage of β-lactamase into the culture medium. It can be postulated that defects in the cell envelope leading to leakage may also facilitate penetration of other β-lactams or may render the cell more vulnerable to β-lactams by virtue of diminished inactivity enzyme in the periplasmic space.

Other β-Lactam Combinations. Several authors have reported synergism between different β-lactams against various organisms. These include imipenem or meropenem with other β-lactams against methicillin-resistant *S. aureus* (399,470,518,597) and imipenem plus ampicillin (63) or amoxicillin plus cefotaxime (386) against enterococci. Sader et al. (541) reported instances of synergism between aztreonam with other β-lactams against *P. aeruginosa* (ceftazidime or cefepime) and various *Enterobacteriaceae* (imipenem, ceftazidime or cefepime), although the predominant effect was additivity. A special case of double β-lactam interaction arises with the use of cefotaxime. The desacetyl metabolite of this drug is biologically active and its combination with the parent compound sometimes results in apparently synergistic interactions against staphylococci and *S. pneumoniae* (87,290), anaerobes (87,290,392,428), and Gram-negative bacilli (290,392,428).

Vancomycin in Combination with Penicillins or Cephalosporins. Synergistic results have been observed with high concentrations of vancomycin plus β-lactams (carbenicillin or cephalothin) against some Gram-negative organisms in early checkerboard studies (151). Against *S. aureus,* synergistic interactions have been recorded for combinations of vancomycin with cefpirome

(566) or cefepime (374), and for teicoplanin or vancomycin combined with imipenem (37,613); the latter interaction was also documented with *in vivo* experiments. Likewise, combinations of vancomycin with antistaphylococcal penicillins have resulted in synergistic inhibitory activity against vancomycin-intermediate *Staphylococcus aureus* strains *in vitro*, and have exhibited enhanced effects in animal models (115). Synergistic interactions between vancomycin and cefepime have been demonstrated against methicillin-susceptible and -resistant *S. epidermidis* (374). In an *in vitro* pharmacodynamic model designed to mimic human pharmacokinetics, the combination of vancomycin and cefepime increased the killing of methicillin-susceptible and -resistant *S. aureus*, methicillin-resistant *S. epidermidis*, and glycopeptide-intermediate *S. aureus*, compared with either agent alone (5).

Combinations of glycopeptides with β-lactams can result in bacteriostatic synergism against vancomycin-resistant enterococci (51,345). Such interactions do not occur predictably nor are they necessarily seen at clinically achievable drug concentrations (96). It has been hypothesized that the novel peptidoglycan synthesized following induction of the vancomycin resistance system cannot be adequately processed by enterococcal PBPs with low affinity for penicillin, rendering the cells hypersusceptible to the β-lactam (7). In animal models of infection with vancomycin- and penicillin-resistant *E. faecium*, combinations of vancomycin or teicoplanin with penicillin or ceftriaxone have demonstrated synergistic inhibitory activity, which in turn results in synergistic bactericidal activity when gentamicin is added (90,92,93).

Resistance to Synergism by Combinations of Agents That Act on the Bacterial Cell Wall

Resistance to Phosphonic Acid Derivative Plus β-Lactam Synergism. The presently available studies suggest that Gram-negative bacilli susceptible to phosphonic acid compounds alone are less susceptible to phosphonic acid derivative/β-lactam synergism (458). Our studies with the fosfomycin/daptomycin combination against enterococci revealed bactericidal synergism only when a low daptomycin concentration employed yielded a relatively weak bactericidal effect as a single agent (527). Otherwise, the magnitude of killing by daptomycin was so great that further improvement by drug combinations could not be demonstrated.

Resistance to Amdinocillin Plus β-Lactam Synergism. Data from a number of laboratories suggest that strains that are resistant to amdinocillin *in vitro* are usually also resistant to amdinocillin/β-lactam synergism. Mechanisms of such resistance may include alterations in PBP-2 targets, alterations at the level of the outer bacterial cell membrane resulting in diminished penetration of drug, or elaboration of β-lactamases capable of hydrolyzing the drug. In the laboratory, exposure of bacteria to amdinocillin in culture medium or urine can also permit the selection of phenotypically resistant variants that revert to normal morphology, antibiotic susceptibility, and generation time when returned to antibiotic-free medium (11,401).

Resistance to Synergism by Vancomycin in Combination with Penicillins or Cephalosporins. The mechanism by which some strains of Gram-negative bacteria are resistant to vancomycin/β-lactam synergism *in vitro* is not known. However, isolates that are synergistically inhibited (by the checkerboard technique) tend to have higher vancomycin MICs (5000 μg/mL or more) than do isolates that are resistant to synergism (MICs of 1250 to 2500 μg/mL) (151).

In animal experiments with vancomycin-resistant enterococci that demonstrate susceptibility to glycopeptide/β-lactam inhibitory synergism, colonies resistant to the synergistic interaction can be recovered among surviving bacteria at the completion of treatment (93). Studies of mutant colonies resistant to synergism sometimes demonstrate alterations in PBPs, but for other strains mechanisms of resistance remain obscure (246).

Clinical Studies of Synergism by Combinations of Agents That Act on the Bacterial Cell Wall

β-Chloro-D-alanine or Phosphonic Acid Derivatives Plus Penicillin. This approach to antimicrobial synergism has not achieved clinical application for β-chloro-D-alanine. In the United States, fosfomycin (trometamol) is used only for treatment of urinary tract infections. Elsewhere, fosfomycin has been used in combination antimicrobial regimens (461), but the exact role of synergism in outcomes observed is not clear. Fosmidomycin is currently under study as an antimalarial agent because it inhibits an enzymatic pathway that is essential in *P. falciparum* but not in humans (60a,353).

Amdinocillin Plus β-Lactam Synergism. Several controlled trials of amdinocillin/β-lactam combined therapy have been reported. An early study suggested that a combination of pivmecillinam (the pivaloyloxymethyl ester of amdinocillin) plus amoxicillin was superior to amoxicillin alone when given three times daily for 10 days to patients with purulent exacerbations of chronic bronchitis (507). The authors suggested that the mechanism of the more rapid general improvement and more rapid conversion of purulent mucoid sputum might be antimicrobial synergism against *H. influenzae* (244,665), which is normally resistant to amdinocillin alone. File and Tan (193) studied amdinocillin plus cefoxitin versus cefoxitin alone in the treatment of mixed soft-tissue infections, including diabetic foot infections. Although a higher percentage of patients responded satisfactorily to combined therapy (90% versus 71%), the number of patients studied was too small for the differences to reach statistical significance. Sattler et al.

(558) compared amdinocillin plus β-lactam therapy with amdinocillin plus aminoglycoside treatment for serious Gram-negative infections. The therapetic responses were similar in the two groups. Amdinocillin plus cefoxitin combinations have also been used successfully in the treatment of urinary tract infections due to multiply resistant *S. marcescens* (639).

Although amdinocillin was approved for clinical use in the United States, its application was limited by the relatively narrow spectrum of the drug itself, by the inability to predict definitively, without actual testing *in vitro*, whether synergism would occur against a given isolate and by the availability of highly effective alternative agents (163).

Vancomycin Combined with Penicillins or Cephalosporins. The levels of vancomycin required to produce synergism with β-lactams against Gram-negative bacilli *in vitro* (78 to 2500 μg/mL) (151) are equal to or greater than those that have been related to ototoxicity (80 to 100 μg/mL) (208). Therefore, such interactions are not clinically relevant. Synergism between vancomycin and β-lactams against vancomycin-resistant enterococci can occur at clinically attainable concentrations of both drugs. However, the survival of mutant clones resistant to synergism after treatment in animal models sheds doubt on the applicability of such regimens (93). Human studies with such regimens have not been reported.

Use of Agents Active on the Cell Wall to Enhance the Uptake of Aminoglycosides

Although resistance to antimicrobials may be the result of drug-inactivating enzymes (136) or an insensitive target site (e.g., a ribosome resistant to aminoglycosides) (685,686), it may also be due to permeability barriers. In such situations, a given drug could be active if another agent enhanced its entry to the site of action. It has been postulated that agents that act on the cell wall may enhance the entry of aminoglycosides in this manner in a number of bacterial species. Amphotericin B similarly facilitates the entry of 5-fluorocytosine and other agents into fungi (409). In this section, we consider combinations of agents active on the bacterial cell wall with aminoglycoside antibiotics.

Mechanism

Studies with enterococci (*E. faecalis*) have shown that the uptake of ^{14}C-labeled streptomycin is significantly increased in the presence of penicillin (Fig. 9.11) (423). Furthermore, this effect is not specific for penicillin and is also seen with other agents acting on the cell wall (cycloserine, bacitracin, and vancomycin), all of which presumably act similarly to permit increased entry of aminoglycosides (423). To the extent that the aminoglycoside is active intracellularly—that is, unless the drug is rendered ineffective by aminoglycoside-modifying enzymes or unless the organism is resistant at the ribosomal level (163,166)—such combinations usually exert a synergistic effect. Enhancement of intracellular uptake of aminoglycosides in the presence of cell wall-active agents, with resulting bactericidal synergism, has also been documented in viridans streptococci (671) and *S. aureus* (681). As early as 1962, Plotz and Davis (509) demonstrated enhanced bactericidal activity against Gram-negative bacilli, with augmented uptake of ^{14}C-streptomycin, in the presence of penicillin. Similar mechanisms have also been demonstrated to be operative in *P. aeruginosa* (414). Mechanisms of interaction are potentially more complicated in Gram-negative organisms, however. For example, in Gram-negative bacilli, exposure to aminoglycosides may produce relative permeabilization of the outer cell envelope to some β-lactam antibiotics (253,254).

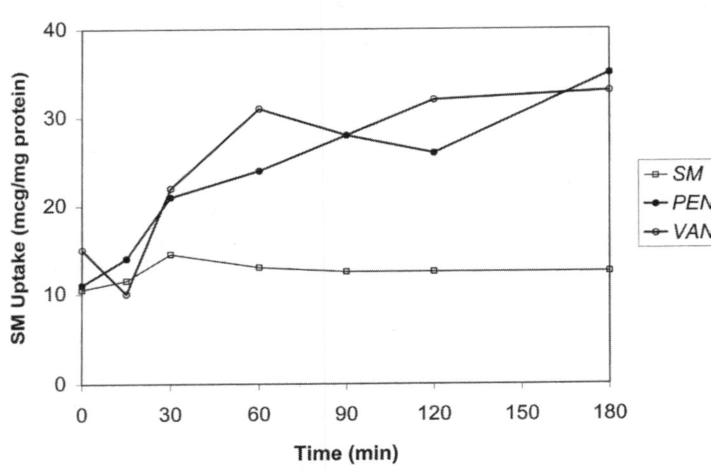

FIGURE 9.11 ● Effect of penicillin (*PEN*) 6.25 μg/mL or vancomycin (*VAN*) 10 μg/mL on the uptake of ^{14}C-streptomycin (*SM*) 200 μg/mL by *E. faecalis.* (Data from Moellering and Weinberg [423]; *SM* only results are an average value from two experiments.)

In both *E. faecalis* and *E. coli,* sequential exposure to ampicillin followed by an aminoglycoside (amikacin) results in a greater bactericidal effect than when the drugs are applied in the reverse order (369), providing support for the primary effect of the cell wall-active agent in the initiation of bactericidal synergism when the agents are administered simultaneously.

Laboratory Studies Using Agents Active on the Cell Wall to Enhance the Uptake of Aminoglycosides

Because many different inhibitors of cell wall synthesis have been combined with aminoglycosides against a variety of bacteria, discussion of laboratory studies has been organized by the bacteria examined.

Enterococci. The original observation of penicillin/aminoglycoside synergism was probably made in 1947 (278). Subsequently, many other investigators have demonstrated a synergistic effect of penicillin plus various aminoglycosides against enterococci, including streptomycin, kanamycin, gentamicin, tobramycin, netilmicin, sisomicin, and amikacin (85,231,287,332,424,426,427).

The cell wall-active agents that enhance the uptake of ^{14}C-labeled streptomycin by enterococci (e.g., penicillin, cycloserine, bacitracin, vancomycin, and ethylenediaminetetraacetic acid) (423) also produce synergism against enterococci when combined with streptomycin (Fig. 9.12) (425). Thus, the present model of penicillin/aminoglycoside synergism in enterococci assumes that the role of agents active on the cell wall is to facilitate the entry of the aminoglycoside (Fig. 9.13). A number of penicillins, including ampicillin, carbenicillin, and penicillin G, have been shown to produce synergism with aminoglycosides against enterococci (231,361). Among the semisynthetic β-lactamase-resistant penicillins, the available data suggest that the ability to produce bactericidal synergy *in vitro* with aminoglycosides correlates with the effectiveness (as judged by the MIC) of the semisynthetic penicillin alone against enterococci. Thus, nafcillin is more effective than oxacillin, which is more effective than methicillin (224,642). In addition to these killing-curve studies, oxacillin/gentamicin synergism against enterococci has been shown by the checkerboard technique (389). (The latter technique, however, is not recommended for documentation of bactericidal synergism against enterococci [535].)

Streptococci. Combinations of penicillin and streptomycin have been shown to be synergistic against many strains of viridans streptococci *in vitro* by the killing-curve technique (279,667) and by the checkerboard method (156). Group B streptococci are likewise killed more rapidly *in vitro* by penicillin (or ampicillin) plus gentamicin than by either drug alone (25,154,559).

Staphylococci. Enhanced activity was demonstrated by the time-kill method when nafcillin or oxacillin was combined with gentamicin, tobramycin, netilmicin, or sisomicin against clinical isolates of methicillin-susceptible *S. aureus* (546,641,643). One group reported that the enhanced activity against *S. aureus* observed with the addition of a β-lactam to an aminoglycoside fulfilled criteria for synergism (by the killing-curve technique) most frequently for nafcillin plus tobramycin (29%) and slightly less frequently for other combinations, including oxacillin plus sisomicin (23%), nafcillin plus gentamicin (20%), nafcillin plus netilmicin (20%), oxacillin plus netilmicin (20%), and nafcillin plus sisomicin (11%) (641,643). A synergistic effect by the killing-curve method was found against eight of eight penicillinase-producing *S. aureus* strains with the combination of nafcillin (5 μg/mL) plus gentamicin (2 or 0.5 μg/mL) (546). Using the checkerboard technique and a criterion of FIC index 0.5 or less, synergism was demonstrated with penicillin plus gentamicin against five of six penicillin-susceptible *S. aureus* strains (590). A synergistic effect against methicillin-resistant *S. aureus* (determined by the killing-curve technique) was shown for combinations of cephalothin (10 μg/mL) plus kanamycin (20 μg/mL) (70) and for high concentrations (50 μg/mL) of either oxacillin or cephalothin plus gentamicin (5 μg/mL) (314). By time-kill techniques, combinations of vancomycin with gentamicin failed to achieve synergistic killing of methicillin-resistant *S. aureus* with high-level resistance to the aminoglycoside; against other isolates, synergism or indifference could not be predicted by the level of resistance to gentamicin (431).

It is worth noting, however, that beneficial interactions between β-lactams and aminoglycosides against *S. aureus* may also be attributable to other mechanisms. Specifically, such combinations may suppress the late regrowth of colonies seen in time-kill studies when aminoglycosides are tested as single agents (163), which has been associated with decreased susceptibility to bactericidal effects of the aminoglycoside among surviving colonies (357).

Other Gram-Positive Organisms. Bactericidal synergism between β-lactam antibiotics and aminoglycosides against *L. monocytogenes* has been recognized for years (421). Such interactions can be demonstrated by time-kill methods using subinhibitory concentrations of aminoglycosides and inhibitory concentrations of the β-lactams, which are typically bacteriostatic against *Listeria* (168,378).

Combinations of β-lactams with aminoglycosides have also produced bactericidal synergism against some strains of pathogenic *Corynebacteria* spp (434). Synergism generally cannot be demonstrated against strains of JK corynebacteria that are resistant to aminoglycosides (MIC more than 128 μg/mL), but resistance to penicillin only may not always preclude synergism (434). Against this group of organisms, bactericidal synergism can also be shown between aminoglycosides and the cell wall-active drugs vancomycin or daptomycin (580).

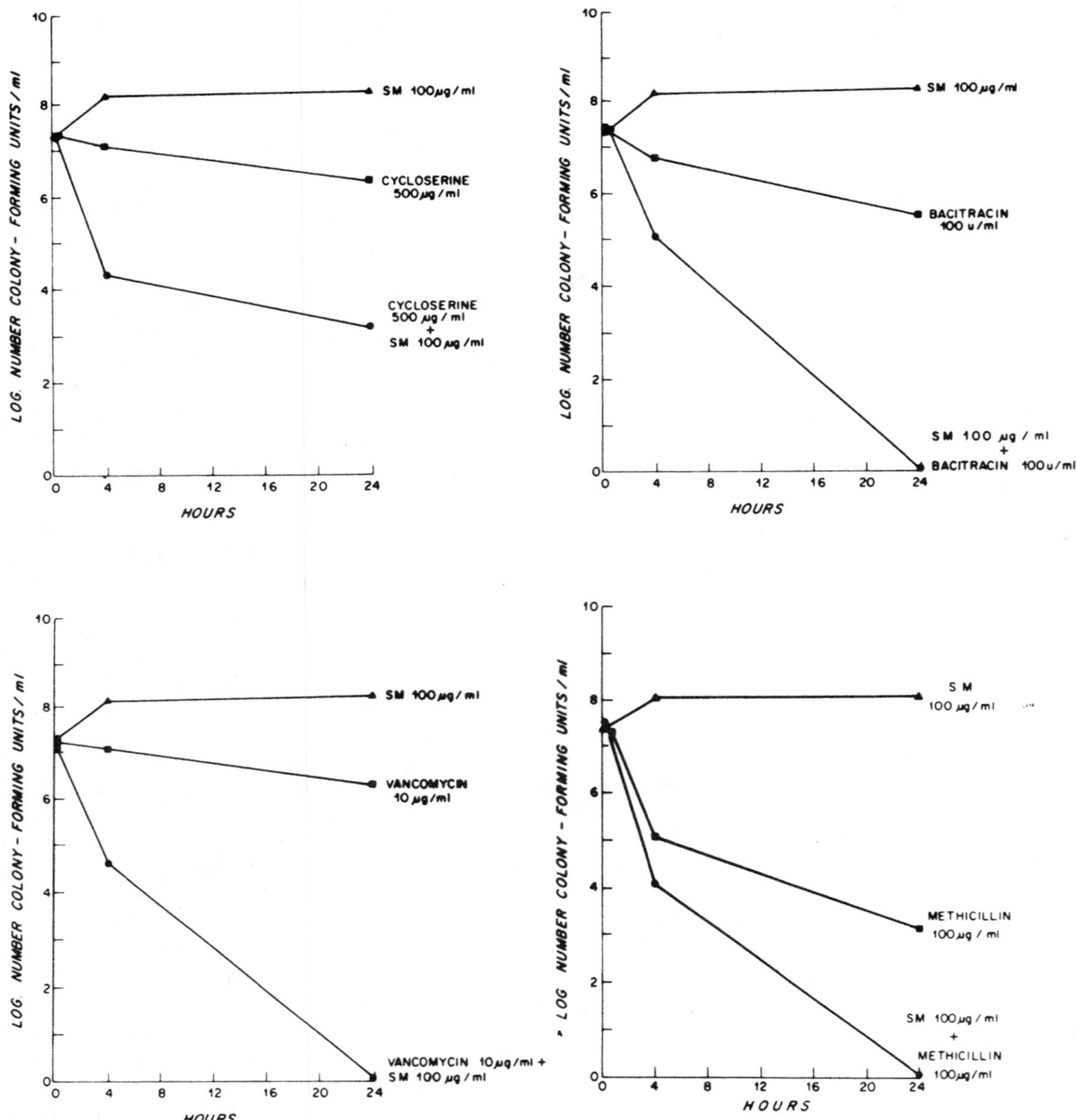

FIGURE 9.12 ● Effect of cycloserine, bacitracin, vancomycin, or methicillin plus streptomycin (*SM*) against *E. faecalis*. (RC Moellering, Jr., unpublished observations, 1969; see ref 425.)

Pseudomonas. Pseudomonads not uncommonly cause life-threatening infection in immunocompromised hosts and other seriously ill patients (54). In addition, they are frequently resistant to multiple drugs (3). Thus, when gentamicin and carbenicillin became available, a number of investigators examined the activity of this combination against clinical isolates of *Pseudomonas in vitro*. Following the initial description of gentamicin/carbenicillin synergism in 1967 (67), several laboratories reported a synergistic effect of this combination against *P. aeruginosa* by checkerboard or agar diffusion techniques (159,322,574,578,588,674). Killing-curve studies have also shown synergism of this combination against a number of *P. aeruginosa* strains (578,588).

Subsequently, ticarcillin, ticarcillin/clavulanate, piperacillin, piperacillin/tazobactam, azlocillin, aztreonam, ceftriaxone, ceftazidime, cefepime, meropenem, imipenem, and mezlocillin were also found to enhance the activity of gentamicin and other aminoglycosides against *P. aeruginosa*, including isolates that were

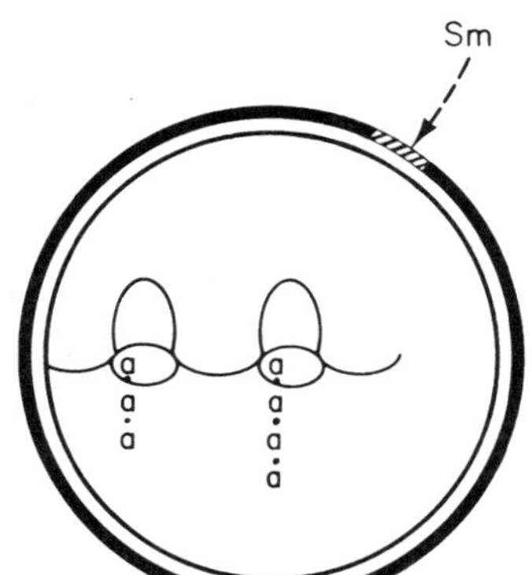

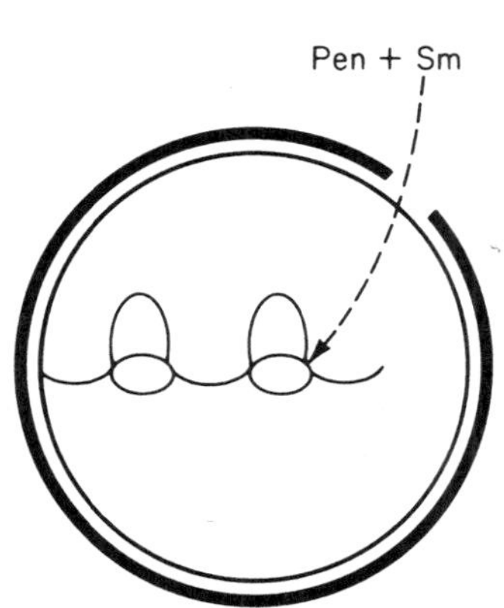

FIGURE 9.13 ● Mechanisms of penicillin plus aminoglycoside synergism against enterococci. Based on studies of the uptake ^{14}C-streptomycin (*Sm*) (see Fig. 9.11), aminoglycosides appear to be unable to enter the enterococcal cell or to reach its ribosomes in the absence of penicillin (*Pen*) (or other agents that act on the bacterial cell wall).

resistant to either one or both drugs in the combination (12,75,118,163,212,446,476,637). Some investigators have noted that penicillin-derivatives (such as ticarcillin or piperacillin) combined with a β-lactamase inhibitor, provide greater synergism when combined with an aminoglycoside, than cephalosporin-aminoglycoside combinations against *P. aeruginosa* (476).

As judged by their MICs, ticarcillin is approximately twice as active as carbenicillin against *P. aeruginosa,* mezlocilllin is approximately as active as ticarcillin, and piperacillin is two to four times more active than mezlocillin (160,169,480,601,637). Similarly, aminoglycosides other than gentamicin, including tobramycin, amikacin, sisomicin, and netilmicin, are synergistic with β-lactams against pseudomonads by the checkerboard technique (118,318,321,324,391,404). Rand et al. (519) have called attention to the lack of reproducibility of the microdilution checkerboard method for determining β-lactam/aminoglycoside interactions against *P. aeruginosa* and recommended establishing consistency of test results in replicate determinations if that method is used. Furthermore, results derived from checkerboard methods of determining synergism between β-lactams and aminoglycosides against *Pseudomonas* spp may not correlate with those based on time-kill curve techniques (88,404).

Similarly, a variety of β-lactams have also been shown to enhance the activity of aminoglycosides against *Acinetobacter baumannii* by time-kill or checkerboard assays (222,393,437,438,476). However, the combination of imipenem and amikacin was not synergistic in a mouse pneumonia model (530).

Klebsiella. Using the checkerboard technique, one study found synergism between cephalothin plus gentamicin against 73% of 61 strains of *Klebsiella* (316). Cefazolin plus amikacin was synergistic, by both killing-curve and checkerboard techniques, against 11 of 20 *Klebsiella* strains studied (320). Another study using the checkerboard technique demonstrated synergism with cephalothin plus gentamicin, kanamycin, or amikacin against most (69% to 95%) of the 38 *Klebsiella* isolates tested (132). In other studies against *Klebsiella* spp, amikacin plus imipenem (230), ceftazidime (230), or cefotaxime (225) resulted in synergism against 5% to 83% of strains tested. This wide range in outcome undoubtedly reflects differences in strain collections and/or methods used (checkerboard versus time-kill). The aforementioned studies were performed before the widespread occurrence of extended-spectrum β-lactamases in *Klebsiella* spp.

Other *Enterobacteriaceae*. Numerous studies have documented the synergistic potential of older β-lactams (e.g., ampicillin, carbenicillin, cephalothin, etc.) plus aminoglycosides against many strains of *E. coli* (195,316), *Proteus* spp (160,195,316,318,575), and *Enterobacter* spp (194,316). Several more recent studies using similar techniques have noted synergism between several extended-spectrum acylaminopenicillins or third-generation cephalosporins and aminoglycosides (often amikacin or gentamicin) against 52% to 90% of *Enterobacteriaceae* tested (163). Similar results have also been seen for various β-lactam/β-lactamase inhibitor plus aminoglycoside as well as cephalosporin plus aminoglycoside combinations using checkerboard techniques (476) and in animal models (415,416).

Mechanism of Resistance

Enterococci. Following the original descriptions of penicillin/streptomycin synergism, it became apparent that not all enterococci were synergistically killed by this combination. The explanation for this discrepant behavior among clinical isolates of enterococci (610) was not clear until 1970, when two groups of investigators pointed out that isolates with high-level streptomycin resistance (MIC of more than 2000 μg/ml) were resistant to penicillin/streptomycin synergism and that strains without high-level streptomycin resistance (MIC of 2000 μg/mL or less) were susceptible to penicillin/streptomycin synergism (424,587). Although the correlation between high-level streptomycin resistance and resistance to synergism seemed clear, the mechanism of this resistance was unknown.

Subsequent work showed that penicillin enhances the uptake of radiolabeled ^{14}C-streptomycin in strains with or without high-level streptomycin resistance (423). Therefore, it seemed unlikely that the resistance to synergism observed in strains with high-level streptomycin resistance was due to a permeability barrier. It was later demonstrated that an enterococcal strain that was highly resistant to streptomycin and resistant to penicillin/streptomycin synergism contained ribosomes that were insensitive to the *in vitro* effects of streptomycin on protein synthesis (i.e., streptomycin failed to inhibit the incorporation of radiolabeled phenylalanine into trichloroacetic acid-precipitable material and also failed to cause misreading) (685,686). Thus, it seemed reasonable to postulate that the resistance to penicillin/aminoglycoside synergism observed in clinical isolates of enterococci might be due to the same mechanism. This hypothesis was consistent with the observation that all clinical enterococcal isolates examined at that time were susceptible to high levels of gentamicin (2000 μg/mL) and to penicillin/gentamicin synergism (426).

However, the strain used in these ribosome studies of streptomycin activity was a laboratory mutant derived from a clinical isolate that had been susceptible to penicillin/streptomycin synergism and to high levels of streptomycin (MIC of 400 μg/mL) (686). Continued study of enterococci *(E. faecalis)* showed that 40% to 50% of clinical isolates in Boston had high-level resistance to both streptomycin and kanamycin and were likewise resistant to both penicillin/streptomycin and penicillin/kanamycin synergism (85). None of 203 isolates examined was found to harbor high-level resistance (MIC of more than 2000 μg/mL) to gentamicin, sisomicin, or tobramycin, and all ten strains tested by the killing-curve technique were synergistically killed by penicillin plus gentamicin, sisomicin, or tobramycin (85). The findings with amikacin were at variance with those obtained with other aminoglycosides. Although only one of ten strains tested for synergism had high-level amikacin resistance (amikacin MIC of more than 2000 μg/mL), six of those ten strains were resistant to synergistic killing by the penicillin/amikacin combination (the same six strains also exhibited high-level resistance to kanamycin [MIC of more than 2000 μg/mL]). Resistance to penicillin/amikacin synergism in enterococci was simultaneously reported by another group (41).

Additional study of clinical isolates with high-level streptomycin and kanamycin resistance revealed an explanation for these findings. The strains with high-level streptomycin and kanamycin resistance contained a 45-MDa plasmid that was transferable by conjugation and produced high-level resistance to both streptomycin and kanamycin and resistance to penicillin/streptomycin and penicillin/kanamycin synergism in a recipient strain that was previously susceptible (334). Curing with novobiocin produced simultaneous loss of the plasmid, of high-level aminoglycoside resistance, and of resistance to penicillin/aminoglycoside synergism (334). Thus, it seemed clear that, at least in some clinical isolates of enterococci, a conjugative plasmid was responsible for the observed resistance to penicillin/aminoglycoside synergism.

The mechanism of this plasmid-mediated resistance is not an altered ribosome. *In vitro* studies revealed no difference in the aminoglycoside susceptibility of ribosomes from the susceptible recipient strain and the resistant donor strain (a clinical isolate with high-level resistance) when studied with varying concentrations of streptomycin, kanamycin, and amikacin (0.1 to 100 μg/mL) (333). Subsequently, aminoglycoside-modifying enzymes, which explain the observed resistance to synergism, were found. A phosphotransferase in resistant strains inactivates kanamycin and amikacin by phosphorylating the 3′-hydroxyl group, and an adenylyltransferase inactivates streptomycin (333). The absence of 3′-hydroxyl group in gentamicin, tobramycin, netilmicin, and sisomicin protects them from phosphorylation by this enzyme. The adenylyltransferase that inactivates streptomycin has no activity against 2-deoxystreptamine-containing aminoglycosides, such as kanamycin, amikacin, gentamicin, tobramycin, netilmicin, and sisomicin.

Studies of the relative activities of these modifying enzymes against various aminoglycoside substrates also explain the apparent discrepancy between the infrequent occurrence of high-level amikacin resistance and the frequency of resistance to penicillin/amikacin synergism. Amikacin has a 3′-hydroxyl group that is phosphorylated by the *E. faecalis* phosphotransferase. However, this enzyme is less active against amikacin than kanamycin (333). This finding presumably explains why MICs of amikacin were generally lower than those observed against kanamycin (41,85). Nevertheless, the activity of this enzyme is sufficient to confer resistance to penicillin/amikacin (as well as penicillin/kanamycin) synergism in strains with high-level kanamycin resistance.

Among the strains of *E. faecalis* producing the 3′-phosphotransferase enzyme, combinations of penicillin or ampicillin with amikacin frequently are less bactericidal (slight-to-moderate degrees of antagonism by time-kill curves) than the β-lactam alone (602). Against such isolates, even concentrations of amikacin well above the MIC exert primarily a bacteriostatic effect, thus presumably antagonizing the lethal effect of penicillin, which is greatest among growing cells (602). The presence of a 3′-phosphotransferase in strains of enterococci with high-level resistance to streptomycin and kanamycin has also been reported in the absence of streptomycin-modifying enzymes (573). Some strains with high-level resistance to streptomycin do not have enzymes that inactivate streptomycin (by acetylation, phosphorylation, or adenylylation). The mechanism of their resistance has been elucidated and involves an altered ribosome (166), as noted in the laboratory mutant of *E. faecalis* studied earlier (686).

E. faecium strains are usually resistant to penicillin/tobramycin synergism (427), even though most *E. faecalis* strains that have been examined are susceptible to penicillin/tobramycin. Elaboration of low levels of a 6′-acetyltransferase enzyme (which inactivates tobramycin as well a sisomicin and netilmicin) by *E. faecium* explains resistance to penicillin/tobramycin synergism (122,654). In contrast to the other aminoglycoside-inactivating enzymes described in enterococci, this activity is not transferable by conjugation and is chromosomally mediated (122,654). As noted for *E. faecalis,* plasmid-mediated resistance to streptomycin and kanamycin has also been described in *E. faecium* (344). A more recently described 4′, 4″-nucleotidyltransferase confers high-level resistance to kanamycin and tobramycin, with resistance to synergism by amikacin combinations as well (89).

High-level resistance to gentamicin was unknown among enterococci prior to 1978, when it was first encountered in *E. faecalis* isolated in France (273). High-level resistance to gentamicin, with failure of penicillin/gentamicin synergism, can be attributed principally to the elaboration of a bifunctional enzyme with 6′-acetyltransferase and 2″-phosphotransferase activity to which the aminoglycoside is susceptible. Such isolates typically produce multiple aminoglycoside-modifying enzymes with adenylylating, acetylating, and phosphorylating activities (119). These enzymes are plasmid- or transposon-mediated and transmissible by conjugation to recipient strains *in vitro* (125,268,408). A single isolate of *E. faecalis* was described that resisted penicillin/gentamicin but not penicillin/tobramycin synergism (422). The mechanism involved in resistance to synergism appeared to be a specific defect in the transport of gentamicin (but not tobramycin). High-level gentamicin-resistant *E. faecalis* strains have now been isolated from centers around the world and they comprise a significant fraction of clinical enterococcal isolates at many institutions (269). Characterization of the first reported clinical isolates of high-level gentamicin-resistant *E. faecium* revealed enzymatically mediated resistance mechanisms completely analogous to those described among *E. faecalis* (171). A few enterococcal isolates that have moderate levels of gentamicin resistance (MICs of 256 to 1000 μg/mL) and that are resistant to penicillin/gentamicin synergism have been encountered (32). These strains produce the bifunctional enzyme, but at levels that may be insufficient to yield MICs of more than 2000 μg/mL, at least in some media. Subsequently, additional phosphotransferases have been described which inactivate gentamicin, but which have various effects on synergism with combinations using other aminoglycosides (112).

Resistance to the β-lactam component of β-lactam/aminoglycoside combinations has also been studied. Although combinations of cephalosporins and aminoglycosides are synergistic against enterococci *in vitro* (173,191,649,651), experience with clinical use of cephalosporin/aminoglycoside combinations has been unsatisfactory (516). It has been suggested that the high MICs of cephalothin (16 to 32 μg/mL) and other cephalosporins against most enterococci may be a major factor in their lack of efficacy because β-lactams typically do not produce synergism with aminoglycosides against enterococci unless they are present in concentrations near or greater than their MICs (612,651).

Other studies have suggested that combinations of semisynthetic penicillinase-resistant penicillins (nafcillin, oxacillin, or methicillin) plus gentamicin are significantly less effective *in vivo* than penicillin/gentamicin, although their activities are similar to that of penicillin/gentamicin *in vitro* (362). The reason for this discrepancy is almost certainly related to the high levels of protein binding (80% to 92%) of nafcillin and oxacillin because these drugs are much less effective *in vitro* (even with gentamicin) against enterococci when serum is added to the culture media (221).

In 1983, Murray and Mederski-Samoraj (435) described β-lactamase production in a clinical isolate of *E. faecalis*. Genetic determinants mediating production of this enzyme, which derive from staphylococcal penicillinase genes (436), were found to be transferable to recipient enterococcal strains by conjugation *in vitro* (435). Since that time, additional β-lactamase-producing isolates have been recovered in Philadelphia, New Haven, Boston, and elsewhere (433,439,488,526). Such isolates demonstrate a marked resistance to penicillin or ampicillin at high inocula. Most isolates described to date have also been highly resistant to gentamicin. Elaboration of β-lactamase has been described in an *E. faecium* isolate (124). Resistance to penicillin (and other β-lactams), which is characteristic of the majority of clinical isolates of this species, is usually due, however, to the presence of a low-affinity PBP (PBP-5) (659).

There has been increasing resistance to β-lactams among *E. faecium* since the late 1980s. The concentration of penicillin required to inhibit 90% of isolates from one Boston hospital rose from 64 μg/mL in the 20-year period up to 1988 to 512 μg/mL for strains collected in 1989 and 1990 (236). Strains with very high levels of resistance to penicillin may fail to exhibit bactericidal synergism when combined at clinically achievable concentrations with an aminoglycoside (612).

Vancomycin resistance has now emerged in both *E. faecium* (346,460,658) and *E. faecalis* (568) (as well as other species) (301,542). The genetic determinants of vancomycin resistance can be found on transposons and are often transferable to recipient strains by conjugation (19,346,568). The net effect of activation of these genes is production of altered peptidoglycan precursors, most often terminating in D-alanine-D-lactate, to which vancomycin binds with much less affinity than it does to its normal target, D-alanine-D-alanine. In some enterococci, altered peptidoglycan terminating D-alanine-D-serine is produced (405).

The present model of resistance to synergism in enterococci relies primarily on the association between high-level resistance to an aminoglycoside and resistance to synergism with a cell wall-active agent plus that aminoglycoside. The mechanism of high-level aminoglycoside resistance in clinical isolates of *E. faecalis* studied to date is usually synthesis of aminoglycoside-inactivating enzymes, but ribosomal resistance and other mechanisms play a role in some *E. faecalis* strains, especially those with high-level resistance to streptomycin alone. Resistance to achievable concentrations of the cell wall-active agent (e.g., ampicillin or vancomycin) also results in resistance to synergism. Mechanisms of resistance to synergism *in vivo* (to combinations that are synergistic *in vitro*) are probably multiple. At present, the most important factors appear to be protein binding and the relationship of the MIC of the β-lactam or glycopeptide to achievable serum and tissue levels *in vivo*.

Viridans Streptococci. Although these organisms have been typically susceptible to penicillin/streptomycin synergism (156,667), both high-level streptomycin resistance (180) and penicillin resistance (150,181) are now found among clinical isolates. Both ribosomal (180) and enzyme-mediated (182) resistance mechanisms have been described that produce resistance to penicillin/streptomycin synergism. The penicillin resistance observed is associated with alterations in PBPs (181), similar to the alterations observed in penicillin-resistant pneumococci (249,683). High-level gentamicin resistance has now also been detected in viridans group streptococci (306).

Other Genera. Resistance to penicillin/aminoglycoside synergism in other bacteria is presumably due to similar mechanisms, although studies to clarify the relative importance of aminoglycoside-resistant ribosomes, aminoglycoside-inactivating enzymes, permeability barriers, altered PBPs, and β-lactamases have rarely been performed. The limited data that are available suggest that, as the MIC of one of the drugs rises, the combination tends to become less effective. For example, with increasing resistance (MIC) to gentamicin, fewer strains of *Enterobacteriaceae* are susceptible to ampicillin/gentamicin and cephalothin/gentamicin synergism by the checkerboard technique (316). Similarly, the addition of antipseudomonal penicillins to gentamicin was ineffective against *P. aeruginosa* highly resistant to gentamicin (MIC of 80 μg/mL or more) (638). Likewise, a major factor in resistance to carbenicillin/aminoglycoside synergism in *A. baumannii* is the aminoglycoside MIC; strains resistant to β-lactam/aminoglycoside synergism had MICs of 31 μg/mL or more for tobramycin (two of two strains) or 62.5 μg/mL or more for gentamicin (two of four strains) (222). The mechanism of aminoglycoside resistance in these strains is the production of aminoglycoside-modifying enzymes (437,438).

However, resistance to either the β-lactam or the aminoglycoside component of a given regimen does not completely preclude the possibility of a synergistic interaction. For example, in one study imipenem/amikacin inhibitory synergism was observed against 45% of imipenem-resistant *P. aeruginosa* (81), while another study noted piperacillin/amikacin synergism against 55% of amikacin-susceptible and 88% of amikacin-resistant strains of this species (339).

Animal and Human Studies of Penicillin/Aminoglycoside Synergism

Enterococci. Use of the penicillin plus streptomycin combination for the treatment of enterococcal endocarditis began with the observation that this combination cured patients who had failed to respond to penicillin alone (278,287). The effectiveness of penicillin plus streptomycin combinations was subsequently documented in the rabbit endocarditis model (94,332). Since the discovery of enterococcal strains with high-level streptomycin and kanamycin resistance (MICs more than 2000 μg/mL) that are resistant to penicillin plus streptomycin and penicillin plus kanamycin synergism *in vitro* (424,588), penicillin plus gentamicin has been used widely for the treatment of patients with enterococcal endocarditis. Although there have been no controlled clinical trials, penicillin plus gentamicin has been clearly shown to be effective for the treatment of enterococcal endocarditis due to strains with high-level streptomycin (and/or kanamycin) resistance in patients (650) and in the rabbit model (332). In addition, using the rabbit model, penicillin plus streptomycin is no more effective than penicillin alone (and is significantly less effective than penicillin plus gentamicin or penicillin plus sisomicin) in the treatment of enterococcal endocarditis due to strains with high-level streptomycin resistance (94). The emergence of enterococci demonstrating high-level resistance to gentamicin (and other deoxystreptamine aminoglycosides) has posed a major therapeutic challenge. Although a minority of such isolates may prove not to be highly streptomycin-resistant (444), thus presumably permitting penicillin/streptomycin synergism, there are no known combinations of cell wall-active agents with clinically available aminoglycosides that would be synergistic for the majority of such organisms that are highly resistant to both streptomycin and gentamicin. Some patients with documented or presumed endocarditis due to highly gentamicin-resistant organisms have responded to a cell wall-active agent alone or as an adjunct to surgery (192,364,420,487).

As discussed, there is no role for currently available cephalosporins or antistaphylococcal penicillins, alone or in combination with any aminoglycoside, in the treatment of serious enterococcal infections. There is no evidence that imipenem (22) or any of the acylaminopenicillins (169) is superior to penicillin or ampicillin in combination regimens for the treatment of enterococcal infections. Imipenem, vancomycin, or ampicillin plus sulbactam may play a role in the treatment of infections due to β-lactamase-producing strains (261), but such regimens are limited by the fact that most β-lactamase-producing strains have also been highly gentamicin resistant, as noted earlier.

Streptococci. Animal studies have suggested that penicillin/aminoglycoside combinations might also be useful in the treatment of streptococcal infections. Penicillin plus streptomycin was more effective than either drug alone against viridans group streptococcal endocarditis in the rabbit model (i.e., it produced more rapid sterilization of vegetations) (547), and ampicillin plus gentamicin produced increased survival, compared with either drug alone, in a group B streptococcal mouse peritonitis model (146). Penicillin plus streptomycin has also been shown to be more effective than penicillin alone in the prevention of viridans group streptococcal endocarditis in the rabbit model (157). In another animal model of endocarditis due to *Streptococcus sanguinis,* superiority of the penicillin/streptomycin combination over penicillin alone was demonstrable only against penicillin-tolerant or relatively resistant (penicillin MIC of 1 μg/mL) strains; no advantage was noted against a fully penicillin-susceptible strain, against which the single β-lactam was highly effective (662).

In the treatment of viridans streptococcal endocarditis in humans, relapse rates of 6% to 15% were initially reported after 2 weeks of treatment with penicillin alone (252). However, when penicillin therapy is extended to 4 weeks (for penicillin-susceptible isolates), it has not been convincingly demonstrated that penicillin/streptomycin therapy (252,609,611,667) is more effective than treatment with penicillin alone (272,304). Nonetheless, combination therapy may allow a shorter duration of treatment (i.e., 2 weeks) for patients with uncomplicated endocarditis due to fully penicillin-susceptible organisms (661).

Staphylococci. Animal studies using penicillin-susceptible stains have shown penicillin plus gentamicin to be more effective than penicillin alone in the treatment of *S. aureus* peritoneal infection in mice (590) and endocarditis in rabbits (548). Nafcillin plus gentamicin has been found to be more effective than nafcillin alone in the treatment of endocarditis due to penicillinase-producing *S. aureus* in the rabbit model (546). Retrospective studies and a large, controlled, clinical trial of nafcillin plus gentamicin versus nafcillin alone in *S. aureus* endocarditis have failed to provide evidence for superior efficacy of nafcillin/gentamicin combinations in the therapy of human *S. aureus* endocarditis (1,331). However, combination therapy may allow shorter treatment courses in injection drug uses with *S. aureus* right-sided endocarditis due to methicillin-susceptible strains (149).

Pseudomonas. Animal studies have shown that combinations of carbenicillin or ticarcillin plus gentamicin or tobramycin are more effective than the individual drugs alone in the treatment of *Pseudomonas* peritonitis in normal rats (13,14), in the treatment of *Pseudomonas* peritonitis and bacteremia in neutropenic rats (564), and in the therapy of *Pseudomonas* peritonitis in mice (118). Several clinical studies on the use of antibiotic combinations for the therapy of Gram-negative infections, especially in neutropenic or immunosuppressed patients, have demonstrated that the results of treatment with synergistic combinations (defined by reduction of the MIC to one-fourth or less of its original value for each of the two drugs in the combination, i.e., a FIC index of 0.5 or less) are superior to those in which synergism did not occur (315,319,343). Each of these studies included infections due to *P. aeruginosa* that responded well to synergistic therapy, but none contained enough patients with *Pseudomonas* infections alone to determine whether synergistic combinations significantly increased the survival of patients with *Pseudomonas* infection. In the study by Anderson et al. (10), ten of 12 patients with *P. aeruginosa* bacteremia who received synergistic antimicrobial therapy responded, whereas none of six responded to nonsynergistic regimens. However, in a retrospective analysis of more than 400 cases of *P. aeruginosa* bacteremia (in both neutropenic and nonneutropenic patients), no differences in response were noted among patients treated with an appropriate antipseudomonas β-lactam plus an aminoglycoside compared with a β-lactam alone (55).

Chamot et al. (101) reviewed 30-day survival in 115 episodes of *P. aeruginosa* bacteremia encountered from 1988 to1998. In that study, adequate empirical combination antipseudomonas therapy (β-lactam plus aminoglycoside or ciprofloxacin, or ciprofloxacin plus aminoglycoside) resulted in improved 30-day survival compared with adequate monotherapy (an aminoglycoside alone was not considered adequate monotherapy) or inadequate therapy. However, the use of adequate combination therapy was not superior to adequate monotherapy for definitive treatment (based on availability of antibiogram results).

These and other studies stress the importance of treatment with a β-lactam active against the pathogen, at the very least (163). If high-serum bactericidal titers can be achieved with such an agent alone (which may not always be the case), the added benefit of synergistic therapy becomes less clear. Reyes et al. (525) studied, *in vitro*, strains of *P. aeruginosa* isolated from patients with endocarditis and they concluded that synergism between drugs used for treatment (carbenicillin plus gentamicin or tobramycin) was necessary for, but not a guarantee of, cure with medical therapy. In a prospective study of 200 patients with *P. aeruginosa* bacteremia, the mortality rate was significantly lower in patients receiving combination therapy (antipseudomonal β-lactam plus aminoglycoside in all but one case), compared with those receiving monotherapy (27% versus 47%) (259). Whether the combination used was synergistic against the infecting organism (FIC of 0.5 or less or FIC of 1.0 or less or by killing curves at one-fourth the MIC of each) did not significantly influence outcome, although there was a trend toward improved survival in combinations demonstrating bactericidal synergism. Notably, there was incomplete correlation between results of *in vitro* studies using different methods. In another study, addition of rifampin to antipseudomonal β-lactam/aminoglycoside combinations resulted in increased bacteriologic eradication rates, but not in survival, of patients with *P. aeruginosa* bacteremia (330).

Other Gram-Negative Bacteria. Animal studies have shown that ticarcillin and carbenicillin enhance the activity of gentamicin or tobramycin against *E. coli* or *E. cloacae* in the mouse peritonitis model (118). Confirmatory evidence from human studies is restricted to the studies of Gram-negative septicemia cited here, which involve many *Enterobacteriaceae*, including *E. coli, Citrobacter, Klebsiella, Enterobacter,* and *Proteus,* as well as *P. aeruginosa* (315,319,343). Several studies have also supported the value of combination therapy for Gram-negative rod bacteremia in neutropenic patients. One older study noted a 75% response among patients receiving two drugs active against the pathogen, but only a 44% response rate for organisms susceptible to only one drug (323). A large multicenter trial comparing two-drug regimens of amikacin plus ticarcillin, azlocillin, or cefotaxime noted a 66% response when organisms were susceptible to both components but only a 21% response when the strain was resistant to the β-lactam (317). DeJongh et al. (144) observed that synergism (by MIC checkerboard) was important for patients with persistent, profound (less than 100 cells/μL) neutropenia. On the other hand, other trials have found little benefit in adding an aminoglycoside to cefoperazone (506) or aztreonam (294) for the treatment of Gram-negative rod bacteremia (including patients who were neutropenic). The apparent success of such single-drug regimens employing more potent β-lactams may relate to the higher serum bactericidal titers against many pathogens that can be attained using these agents (627).

Nevertheless, because of high mortality rates associated with Gram-negative sepsis, particularly in neutropenic patients, and because of the necessity to start empirical antibiotic therapy early (often before susceptibility results are known, and certainly before synergy studies can be done or serum bactericidal titers established), many clinicians still prefer to use β-lactam/aminoglycoside combinations in this setting. A multicenter trial comparing ceftazidime plus 3 days of amikacin versus ceftazidime plus 9 days of amikacin for the treatment of Gram-negative bacteremia in neutropenic cancer patients found improved response with the longer course of combination therapy (81% versus 48%) (177). In a prospective observational study of *Klebsiella* spp bacteremia in 230 patients, outcome was similar for patients receiving monotherapy with an active agent and for those receiving combination therapy (almost always β-lactam plus aminoglycoside) (329). However, mortality rates were significantly lower for combination-treated patients with hypotension (24% versus 50%). In that study, antibiotic interactions *in vitro* were not reported.

Leibovici et al. (352) prospectively observed 2,124 patients with Gram-negative rod bacteremia treated at one medical center from 1988 to 1995. Mortality rates were not different for patients who received a single, active β-lactam or for those receiving active-combination therapy with a β-lactam and (for the great majority) an aminoglycoside, either for empirical or definitive therapy. Although there was a trend in favor of empirical combination therapy for subsets of patients with neutropenia or *P. aeruginosa* bacteremia, and in favor of combinations for definitive therapy in neutropenic patients, these differences did not reach statistical significance. However, in that study, patients receiving an active β-lactam plus an aminoglycoside to which the organism was resistant were classified as having received monotherapy. Because the possibility of a synergistic interaction cannot be excluded, even when an organism is resistant to the aminoglycoside, it is possible that any differences between monotherapy and combination therapy may have been blunted in this analysis. Although the possible role of synergistic therapy in treatment of *A. baumannii* infection has been raised (223), there have been no controlled animal or human trials to study the question *in vivo.*

Combinations of Antimicrobial Agents That Act by Other or Unknown Mechanisms

This section considers combinations of antimicrobials that synergize against bacteria by other or unknown mechanisms. Therefore, the discussion of some of these is restricted to available laboratory and clinical studies because both the mechanisms of synergistic activity and the mechanisms of resistance to synergism are unknown.

Laboratory Studies of Antimicrobial Combinations That Act by Other or Unknown Mechanisms

Trimethoprim/sulfamethoxazole Plus β-Lactams. TMP/SMZ has been shown to synergize with ticarcillin/clavulanate against ticarcillin-, ticarcillin/clavulante-, and TMP/SMZ-resistant *S. maltophilia,* by checkerboard assay and in a time-kill assay using clinically achievable peak levels of each drug (512). Synergy was also seen with piperacillin/tazobactam (557a).

Quinupristin/Dalfopristin Plus Vancomycin or β-Lactams. Quinupristin/dalfopristin is a combination of two semisynthetic pristinamycin derivatives derived from pristinamycin I_A (quinupristin) and pristinamycin II_A (dalfopristin) (23). This combination results both in inhibitory synergism against various Gram-positive organisms (62,453) and in bactericidal activity lacking in the individual components. It has been proposed that binding of dalfopristin to the ribosome induces a conformational change that increases binding of the I_A component, resulting in a very stable ternary complex that blocks protein synthesis (23). Several studies have evaluated the activity of quinupristin/dalfopristin combined with another antimicrobial against a variety of organisms.

Enterococci

Studies of quinupristin/dalfopristin plus cell wall-active agents have yielded conflicting results. In one study, the combination of ampicillin/sulbactam with quinupristin/dalfopristin was synergistic by checkerboard assay against vancomycin-resistant *E. faecium* (VREF); however, time-kill studies documented synergism against only 25% of these VREF isolates (402). Bonilla et al. (59) also could not document synergism between quinupristin/dalfopristin and ampicillin against VREF by time-kill methods. However, in an *in vitro* pharmacodynamic model simulating human pharmacokinetics, enhanced killing of a vancomycin-resistant *E. faecalis* isolate was noted when quinupristin/dalfopristin was combined with ampicillin (5).

Quinupristin/dalfoprisin modal MICs were reduced against VREF when the streptogramin was combined with teicoplanin, but not with vancomycin (260). We found predominantly indifference by checkerboard MIC testing when quinupristin/dalfopristin was combined with glycopeptides (or β-lactams) against VREF, and only minor enhancement in killing by time-kill methods (170). Kang and Rybak (300) demonstrated synergy between quinupristin/dalfopristin and vancomycin against VREF using checkerboard assays, but found only additivity by time-kill assays. Lorian and Fernandes (370) reported that subinhibitory concentrations of quinupristin/dalfopristin and vancomycin produced synergisitic killing of VREF, whereas against vancomycin-susceptible *E. faecium* synergism was less evident. Vancomycin concentrations required to show this effect against VREF strains ($0.5 \times$ MIC was 200 to 250 μg/mL) exceeded concentrations achievable in serum.

Staphylococci

The report of a patient with MRSA bacteremia and polyarticular joint infections failing vancomycin, rifampin and gentamicin combination therapy, who demonstrated rapid blood culture sterilization and clinical improvement following the institution of quinupristin/dalfopristin plus vancomycin (430) stimulates interest in exploring results of combination studies against *S. aureus in vitro*. Here, too, reported effects have been somewhat inconsistent. Studies using checkerboard methods have shown predominantly additivity between quinupristin/dalfopristin and vancomycin (299,633), with some instances of synergy (FIC index 0.5 or less) between quinupristin/dalfopristin and β-lactams (633) against both MLS_B-susceptible and -resistant *S. aureus*. Time-kill assays have revealed bactericidal synergism against MRSA when quinupristin/dalfopristin and vancomycin were combined (299,300,490), but others have documented antagonism against a significant minority of MLS_B-resistant isolates (202). Results may also depend on the concentrations of antimicrobials studied. Time-kill experiments using MRSA isolates with constitutive MLS_B resistance found that the combination of quinupristin/dalfopristin plus cefepime, at concentrations approximating trough serum levels, resulted in 1 to 2 $\log_{10}$ CFU/mL greater killing than seen with each antibiotic alone (633). However, using peak antibiotic concentrations, this beneficial effect was lost and a trend toward antagonism was noted. Fuchs et al. (202) also found instances of antagonism when quinupristin/dalfopristin was combined with various β-lactams against 10 MLS_B-resistant *S. aureus* (ranging between 1 to 3 isolates for individual agents).

In general, though, models using infected fibrin clots (299), pharmacodynamic modeling (5), or experimental endocarditis (490,633) to study combinations of quinupristin/dalfopristin with either vancomycin or cephems against *S. aureus* have shown trends toward greater killing activity with combinations than with any drug alone.

Quinupristin/Dalfopristin and Other Antimicrobials. Additional studies have examined the effects of this streptogramin antibiotic with other antimicrobial classes. As in the preceeding discussion, the results are sometimes inconsistent, the mechanisms of potential interactions are unknown, and the practical significance of the observations remains unclear.

Enterococci

Some authors have found favorable interactions between quinupristin/dalfopristin and tetracyclines (170,260,402). Our own studies revealed inhibitory synergism between quinupristin/dalfopristin and doxycycline against 36% to 40% of vancomycin-resistant enterococci (both *E. faecium* and *E. faecalis*) by checkerboard assays (170). We reported that such interactions did not result in bactericidal synergism by time-kill experiments. Aeschilimann et al. (4) also could not demonstrate synergism between quinupristin/dalfopristin and doxycycline against VREF by time-kill curves or in an *in vitro* simulated endocarditis vegetation model; however, they did find that the combination either prevented or delayed the emergence of resistance to quinupristin/dalfopristin in the test isolates. Patel et al. (483) did not find synergistic interactions between quinupristin/dalfopristin and the minocycline derivative, tigecycline (GAR-936), against vancomycin-resistant enterococci.

Studies of other combinations with quinupristin/dalfopristin against VREF have generally found little evidence of synegistic interactions. Against vancomycin-resistant *E. faecalis* and *E. faecium*, combinations of quinupristin/dalfopristin with chloramphenicol have yielded mostly additive/indifferent inhibitory effects by checkerboard assays (170,410). Combinations of quinupristin/dalfopristin plus ciprofloxacin, rifampin, or novobiocin are not predictably synergistic against VREF by time-kill methods (59). Although some data suggest the potential for synergism between quinupristin/dalfopristin and gentamicin (300), most reports do not (54,170,260,300). The combination of quinupristin/dalfopristin with linezolid improved killing of a vancomycin-resistant *E. faecalis* by approximately 1-$\log_{10}$ CFU/mL compared with the most active single agent in an *in vitro* pharmacodynamic model (5).

Staphylococci

Bactericidal synergism can occasionally be seen when quinupristin/dalfopristin is combined with rifampin (202,545). Enhanced killing of MLS_B-susceptible MRSA using quinupristin/dalfopristin plus rifampin has been shown in animal models (544,677). In a rabbit prosthetic-joint infection model, all animals treated with quinupristin/dalfopristin plus rifampin had sterilization of bone (compared with five of 11 treated with vancomycin plus rifampin) and there was no emergence of rifampin resistance (versus detection of rifampin resistance in five of 11 animals treated with vancomycin plus rifampin) (544). In an endocarditis model, quinupristin resistance (constitutive MLS_B phenotype) was associated with loss of synergy between quinupristin/dalfopristin and rifampin and the permitted the emergence of rifampin resistance during combination therapy (677).

Combinations of quinupristin/dalfopristin with gentamicin have generally been indifferent by checkerboard testing, time-kill, or experimental models (42,202). Bactericidal synergism against *S. aureus* is sometimes reported with quinupristin/dalfopristin plus ciprofloxacin (545), but antagonism has also been encountered (202). Also, studies using an *in vitro* pharmacodynamic system demonstrated that the combination of quinupristin/dalfopristin plus linezolid increased the killing of a clinical MRSA isolate, compared with activity of each antimicrobial individually (5).

Fosfomycin and Other Antimicrobials. Against staphylococci, combinations of fosfomycin with rifampin, linezolid, quinupristin/dalfopristin, or moxifloxacin have shown synergism by checkerboard techniques, but not in time-kill assays (241).

Clindamycin Plus Gentamicin. Utilizing the checkerboard technique, clindamycin/gentamicin was shown to be synergistic against 33 of 62 Enterobacteriaceae and *P. aeruginosa* strains that were susceptible to 6.2 μg/mL or less gentamicin (188). However, the concentrations of clindamycin required for synergism were frequently 50 to 100 μg/mL, which is significantly greater than clinically achievable levels (5 to 25 μg/mL) (189). Other studies also suggested that the clindamycin plus gentamicin combination was synergistic against *E. coli* and certain other *Enterobacteriaceae* when tested by a modified checkerboard technique (354). However, the use of techniques that measure the early bactericidal activity of amikacin and gentamicin has demonstrated antagonism between clindamycin and the aminoglycoside (687). Our own data support the latter observations. We have noted decreased early killing of a number of Gram-negative bacilli, including *S. marcescens,* with the combination of clindamycin plus gentamicin versus gentamicin alone. With gentamicin alone there was often overgrowth of gentamicin-resistant colonies after 24 hours of incubation. With clindamycin plus gentamicin such colonies did not emerge, and at 24 hours the colony counts in tubes containing clindamycin plus gentamicin were often lower than those in tubes that contained gentamicin alone (RC Moellering, Jr., and CBG Wennersten, unpublished observations, 1976). Thus, the net effect of the combination (at 24 hours) is increased killing (presumably due to the decreased emergence of resistant mutants), despite early antagonism (in the first few hours). This effect may account for the synergism noted by investigators who used an overnight incubation for the checkerboard determination (354).

Clindamycin/gentamicin synergism has also been reported against some strains of viridans streptococci (156). However, this combination has produced antagonism against other streptococci (577) and the clinical significance of these observations remains to be established. *In vitro* synergism, of uncertain mechanism and clinical significance, has been reported between clindamycin and gentamicin against *Chlamydia trachomatis* (491).

Polymyxins Plus Sulfonamides or TMP. Polymyxins are effective *in vitro* against most aerobic and facultative Gram-negative bacilli, except *Proteus* and *Serratia* spp (238). However, when combined with a sulfonamide or TMP, which are also ineffective alone, polymyxins synergistically inhibit both *Proteus* and *Serratia* spp. Synergism of colistin (polymyxin E) and a sulfonamide against *Proteus* spp was first noted in 1959 (258) and was later confirmed by other investigators (474,619). Others have also demonstrated synergism between colistin and TMP/SMZ or rifampin against nonfermenting Gram-negative rods (213,214). Strains that were resistant to polymyxin B/sulfonamide synergism have been killed by polymyxin B plus TMP (238). TMP, SMZ, and polymyxin B have been studied alone and in combination against a number of Gram-negative bacilli (531). Successful *in vitro* combinations included SMZ plus polymyxin B against *Klebsiella-Enterobacter-Serratia* spp (21 of 26 strains demonstrated either synergism or an additive effect), TMP plus polymyxin B against *Proteus-Providencia* spp (14 of 14 strains), and all three drugs together against nine of 12 strains studied by the killing-curve technique (531).

Although the mechanism of this interaction has not been established, the ability of TMP to synergize with polymyxins against strains resistant to sulfonamide/polymyxin synergism suggests that the folate pathway is involved. In addition, two lines of evidence imply that the function of the sulfonamide may be to allow polymyxin to reach the cell membrane. (a) There is a lag of four generation times for the synergistic bacterial effect of the combination after the addition of sulfonamide. The same lag occurs if both drugs are added together or if the sulfonamide is added first, followed by colistin four generations later, in which case the effect occurs immediately after the addition of colistin (473). (b) Artificial lipid membranes prepared from *Proteus* spp resistant to polymyxins *in vitro* are as susceptible to disruption by polymyxin B in the laboratory as are those prepared from sensitive strains (238). Thus, the available information suggests that sulfonamides and/or TMP may act on the cell through the folate pathway to increase the access of polymyxin to the cell membrane. The mechanism by which these effects occur remains unknown. Polymyxin combinations with sulfonamides and/or TMP have received very little clinical attention in recent years because of polymyxin toxicity. However, the emergence of multidrug-resistant, Gram-negative bacteria as a cause of serious infections has rekindled an interest in the use of polymyxins.

Linezolid Plus Rifampin. Checkerboard broth microdilution tests of linezolid plus rifampin reveal predominantly indifferent activity against a variety of Gram-positive organisms, including *E. faecalis, E. faecium,* and *S. aureus* (599). The combination is also indifferent against staphylococci by time-kill methods (432). The absence of synergistic interactions between oxazolidinones and rifampin is also supported by results from studies of experimental *S. aureus* infection (134,197).

In contrast to these studies with staphylococci and enterococci, pharmacodynamic simulation of human-achievable antibiotic peak concentrations and elimination half-lives demonstrated rifampin to augment the bactericidal activity of linezolid against a pencillin-intermediate, vancomycin-tolerant *S. pneumoniae* (97).

Several lines of evidence suggest that linezolid may prevent the emergence of resistance to rifampin. With both methicillin-susceptible (242) and methicillin-resistant *S. aureus* (242,286), linezolid inhibited the development of rifampin resistance *in vitro*. In the previously described rabbit endocarditis model (134), resistance to rifampin did not occur in animals achieving therapeutic levels of linezolid. Given the rapidity with which rifampin resistance can develop in the clinical setting, the combination of linezolid and rifampin could prove useful, despite the lack of data for important synergistic interactions between linezolid and rifampin.

TMP Plus Aminoglycosides. Limited study has shown that TMP plus amikacin may produce synergism against *Enterobacteriaceae* that are susceptible to TMP (MIC of 1.6 μg/mL or less) and amikacin (MIC of 6.4 μg/mL or less) alone (481). Although most strains studied were examined by the checkerboard technique, killing curves also showed that some strains were synergistically killed by this combination.

Doxycycline and Other Antimicrobials. Against a clinical isolate of *A. baumannii,* the combination of amikacin with doxycycline, each at 4 × MIC, was found to be synergistic by time-kill methods (530). In a mouse pneumonia model employing this isolate, combination therapy was more effective in sterilizing lung tissue than either antibiotic alone (530). The combination of doxycycline with linezolid led to greater killing of vancomycin-resistant enterococci than observed with the most active single agent in an *in vitro* pharmacodynamic model (5).

Metronidazole Plus Clindamycin. Metronidazole and clindamycin exhibited synergistic activity at clinically achievable concentrations (0.125 to 1.0 μg/mL and 2.0 μg/mL, respectively) against a majority of *B. fragilis* strains tested in one early study (76).

Quinolones and Other Antimicrobials

Gram-Negative Organisms

Synergism between ciprofloxacin and aminoglycosides (250) or various β-lactams (251) is infrequently demonstrable against *Enterobacteriaceae* and antagonism seems quite rare. Against *P. aeruginosa,* combinations of ciprofloxacin with aminoglycosides demonstrated synergism against less than one-third of isolates (109,135,210,215), whereas combination with various β-lactams (e.g., azlocillin, cefpiramide, or imipenem) resulted in synergism more frequently (up to 70% of interactions) (74,75,135,199,215,532). Differences in rates of synergism for quinolone-aminoglycoside combinations compared with quinolone-β-lactam combinations are also seen with quinolones other than ciprofloxacin and against nonfermenting Gram-negative bacilli other than *P. aeruginosa* (139,631,632). Although reported rates of quinolone/β-lactam synergism for combinations of various quinolones (e.g., ciprofloxacin, ofloxacin, moxifloxacin, gatifloxacin, levofloxacin, and trovafloxacin) and β-lactams (e.g., cephalosporins, monobactams, and carbapenems) against a range of bacteria (including *Enterobacteriaceae, P. aeruginosa, S. matophilia, A. baumanii* and *B. cepacia*) vary widely, antagonism is rarely encountered (128,217,282, 296a,475,541,632).

Demonstration of synergism can depend on the activities of the individual agents, concentrations tested, and methods used. In many studies, time-kill studies demonstrate synergism more often than checkerboard tests for a variety of quinolone-β-lactam combinations against *Enterobacteriaceae* (114,234) and nonfermenters including *P. aeruginosa* (27,114,234,235,632). Pohlman et al. (511) assessed the activity of ciprofloxacin combined with β-lactams against *Enterobacteriaceae* and *P. aeruginosa*. They found synergism most often at later sampling points (7 hours) and with antibiotic concentrations equal to 0.5 × to 1 × MIC, while antagonism was seen predominantly at lower antibiotic concentrations (0.25 × MIC) and at earlier sampling points. Burgess and colleagues (73) found bactericidal synergism more often with a low concentration (2 μg/mL) of levofloxacin than with a higher concentration (4 μg/mL) when combined with various β-lactams against *P. aeruginosa*. However, used alone, the higher concentration of levofloxacin had greater bactericidal activity over 24 hours than did the lower concentration; also, the higher concentration combined with a β-lactam more often achieved a bactericidal endpoint over 24-hours incubation. The effects of quinolone susceptibility on quinolone/β-lactam synergism against *P. aeruginosa* have been inconsistent. Some have reported synergism even against quinolone-resistant organisms (82,196), while others have shown predominantly additive effects irrespective of susceptibities to either the quinolone or β-lactam agent (494). One group found ciprofloxacin plus β-lactam synergy against *S. maltophilia* only in the absence of high-level ciprofloxacin resistance (512).

Against *Legionella pneumophila,* checkerboard analysis of macrolide (erythromycin, clarithromycin, or azithromycin) plus quinolone (levofloxacin or ciprofloxacin) combinations revealed predominantly additive/indifferent results (FIC indices from 0.5 to 2). In that study, only two of 34 isolates were synergistically inhibited (FIC index 0.375), and both instances occurred with combinations of azithromycin plus ciprofloxacin (395). Other investigators, using time-kill methods found the combination of levofloxacin plus rifampin to produce synergistic bactericidal activity against *L. pneumophila* (29).

Pneumococci

In vitro, combinations of quinolones with glycopeptides or β-lactams can result in synergistic killing of pneumococci (325,497) and may reduce the emergence of resistance to the quinolone (123,338). Animal models also provide evidence of enhanced killing of penicillin-resistant *S. pneumoniae* by combinations of levofloxacin with meropenem or cefotaxime (123,338) and by gatifloxacin combined with cefepime (497).

Staphylococci

Combinations of enoxacin, ofloxacin, or norfloxacin with coumermycin (which inhibits the B-subunit of DNA gyrase) were synergistic against *S. aureus* isolates (454). However, in a rat *S. aureus* endocarditis model, ciprofloxacin/coumermycin was less effective than the fluoroquinolone alone (498). Novobiocin, another agent that acts at the level of DNA gyrase, inhibited the bactericidal activities of ciprofloxacin and ofloxacin against *S. aureus* and *Staphylococcus warneri in vitro* (359). Addition of rifampin to ciprofloxacin tended to decrease the bactericidal activity of the latter against *S. aureus,* but the combination did appear to suppress the emergence of rifampin-resistant colonies (248,624). Combination of quinolones with β-lactams or aminoglycosides can result in synergistic killing of *S. aureus,* but reported frequencies vary widely (139,234).

Enterococci

Against vancomycin-resistant enterococci, combinations of ciprofloxacin with vancomycin sometimes yield inhibitory synergism, but at concentrations of the former too high to be of likely importance (622). Such interactions may be due to diminished induction of proteins mediating glycopeptide resistance (622). By checkerboard methods, the combination of gatifloxacin plus a β-lactam (including cefepime, meropenem, piperacillin) or gentamicin demonstrated predominantly indifferent effects against VREF (139). Combinations of sparfloxacin or clinafloxacin with either streptomycin or gentamicin resulted in bactericidal synergism against some enterococcal isolates studied by time-kill methods (496). High concentrations of ampicillin combined with ciprofloxacin have produced a bactericidal effect against some strains of enterococci resistant to both classes of agents (340). Mechanisms of such interactions have not been determined. Subinhibitory concentrations of ampicillin combined with levofloxacin also resulted in synergistic activity against ampicillin-resistant, levofloxacin-susceptible *E. faecium* by time-kill assays (576); however, such combinations do not necessarily meet criteria for bactericidal activity. No evidence of synergy for this combination was detected against either levofloxacin-intermediate or -resistant *E. faecium* isolates that were ampicillin-resistant (576).

Antineoplastic Agents Plus Antimicrobials. Several investigators have shown that antineoplastic agents such as bleomycin, mitomycin C, and 5-fluorouracil, some of which demonstrate antimicrobial activity at attainable serum concentrations (53), can synergize with known antibiotics (such as aminoglycosides and β-lactams) against *S. aureus* (284) and Gram-negative bacilli (621,670). Although some of these interactions are bactericidal, their clinical significance is not defined.

SUMMARY

Mechanisms of Antimicrobial Interactions Resulting in Synergism

There are several well-established general mechanisms of antimicrobial interaction that produce synergism. Synergism may result from sequential inhibition of a common biochemical pathway (e.g., TMP plus SMZ) or from inhibition of complementary targets (e.g., amdinocillin plus a second β-lactam). Protection of an antibiotic susceptible to degrading enzymes (e.g., β-lactamases) or elimination mechanisms (e.g., efflux pumps) by the use of enzyme inhibitors (e.g., β-lactamase inhibitors), inhibitors of protein synthesis, or efflux pump inhibitors may enhance activities of the antimicrobial agents, resulting in synergistic inhibitory or bactericidal effects. Combination of cell wall-active agents (e.g., penicillins or glycopeptides) with otherwise poorly penetrating antibiotics (e.g., aminoglycosides) can enhance the access of the latter to their intracellular targets, resulting in bactericidal synergism.

Other mechanisms of synergism are possible, as exemplified by the interactions that occur at the level of the bacterial ribosome between quinupristin and dalfopristin, which can result both in enhanced inhibitory activity and in bactericidal activity absent in the individual components.

Mechanisms Resulting in Antimicrobial Antagonism

Combining a bacteriostatic agent (e.g., tetracycline or chloramphenicol) with bactericidal agents (e.g., penicillins) can result in demonstrably less killing than seen with the latter agent alone. The clinical signficance of such antagonism was illustrated only once by the adverse experience with combinations of penicillin with chlortetracycline in the treatment of bacterial meningitis. Drugs that act at the same target (e.g., 50S ribosomal subunit) may also exhibit antagonistic interactions *in vitro*, but the clinical importance of such interactions is not usually as well defined. Combinations of agents, one of which induces a resistance mechanism to which the second agent is susceptible, can result in antagonistic interactions. Examples of this include the induction by one β-lactam of chromosomal β-lactamase that hydrolyzes a second β-lactam, and induction of ribosomal methylases by erythromycin, conferring resistance to clindamycin. Fortunately, there would usually be little reason to consider using such combinations in clinical practice.

Significance of *In Vitro* Antimicrobial Interactions

In spite of the large body of literature describing antibiotic interactions *in vitro* and in animal models, there are few clinical scenarios in which synergism has been shown unequivocally to be an important factor in response of infections to therapy with antimicrobial combinations (e.g., enterococcal endocarditis). Obviously, drug combinations that are specifically formulated for enhanced activity are an exception (e.g., β-lactam/β-lactamase inhibitor combinations, TMP/SMZ, quinupristin/dalfopristin). Synergistic interactions may be but one means to achieve an end (e.g., enhanced bactericidal activity). In many cases, other ways of achieving this end (e.g., selection of a highly potent single agent) might result in equivalent outcomes. In other cases, even where the potential for antagonism has been demonstrated *in vitro* (e.g., rifampin with a bactericidal agent), the potential benefits of such combinations (e.g., suppression of rifampin-resistant mutants to allow therapy of a biofilm-associated infection) may well outweigh the theoretical risks of combined therapy.

REFERENCES

1. Abrams B, Sklaver A, Hoffman T, et al. Single or combination therapy of staphylococcal endocarditis in intravenous drug abusers. *Ann Intern Med* 1979;90:789–791.
2. Acar JF, Goldstein F, Chabbert YA. Synergistic activity of trimethoprim-sulfamethoxazole on Gram-negative bacilli: observations in vitro and in vivo. *J Infect Dis* 1973;128 (Suppl):S470–S477.
3. Acar JF, Witchitz JL, Goldstein F, et al. Susceptibility of aminoglycoside-resistant Gram-negative bacilli to amikacin: delineation of individual resistance patterns. *J Infect Dis* 1976;134(Suppl 1):S280–S285.
4. Aeschlimann JR, Zervos MJ, Rybak MJ. Treatment of vancomycin-resistant *Enterococcus faecium* with RP 59500 (quinupristin-dalfopristin) administered by intermittent or continuous infusion, alone or in combination with doxycycline, in an in vitro pharmacodynamic infection model with simulated endocardial vegetations. *Antimicrob Agents Chemother* 1998;42:2710–2717.
5. Allen GP, Cha R, Rybak MJ. In vitro activities of quinupristin-dalfopristin and cefepime, alone and in combination with various antimicrobials, against multidrug-resistant staphylococci and enterococci in an in vitro pharmacodynamic model. *Antimicrob Agents Chemother* 2002;46:2606–2612.
6. Allen NE, Alborn WE Jr, Hobbs JN Jr, et al. 7-Hydroxytropolone: an inhibitor of aminoglycoside-2-*O*-adenylyltransferase. *Antimicrob Agents Chemother* 1982;22:824–831.
7. Al-Obeid S, Billot-Klein D, van Heijenoort J, et al. Replacement of the essential penicillin-binding protein 5 by high-molecular mass PBPs may explain vancomycin—β-lactam synergy in low-level vancomycin-resistant *Enterococcus faecium* D366. *FEMS Microbiol Lett* 1992;91:79–84.
8. Alvarez S, Jones M, Berk SL. In vivo activity of fosfomycin, alone and in combination, against methicillin-resistant *Staphylococcus aureus*. *Antimicrob Agents Chemother* 1985;28:689–690.
9. Amyes SGB, Smith JT. R-factor trimethoprim resistance mechanism: an insusceptible target site. *Biochem Biophys Res Commun* 1974;58:412–418.
10. Anderson ET, Young LS, Hewitt WL. Antimicrobial synergism in the therapy of Gram-negative rod bacteremia. *Chemotherapy* 1978;24:45–54.
11. Anderson JD, Adams MA, Webster HM, et al. Growth properties of mecillinam-resistant bacterial variants in urine. *Antimicrob Agents Chemother* 1977;12:559–562.
12. Andrews R, Fasoli R, Scoggins WG, et al. Combined aztreonam and gentamicin therapy for pseudomonal lower respiratory tract infections. *Clin Ther* 1994;16:236–252.
13. Andriole VT. Synergy of carbenicillin and gentamicin in experimental infection with *Pseudomonas*. *J Infect Dis* 1971;124(Suppl):S46–S55.
14. Andriole VT. Antibiotic synergy in experimental infection with *Pseudomonas*. II. The effect of carbenicillin, cephalothin or cephanone combined with tobramycin or gentamicin. *J Infect Dis* 1974;129:124–133.
15. Anonymous. Instructions to authors. *Antimicrob Agents Chemother* 2004;48:i–xxi.
16. Anonymous. Piperacillin/tazobactam. *Med Lett Drugs Ther* 1994;36:79.
17. Arain TM, Goldstein BP, Scotti R, et al. Synergic activity of teicoplanin with ethambutol against *Mycobacterium tuberculosis*. *J Antimicrob Chemother* 1994;33:359–360.
18. Aronoff SC, Klinger JD. In vitro activities of aztreonam, piperacillin, and ticarcillin combined with amikacin

against amikacin-resistant *Pseudomonas aeruginosa* and *P. cepacia* isolates from children with cystic fibrosis. *Antimicrob Agents Chemother* 1984;25:279–280.
19. Arthur M, Molinas C, Depardieu F, et al. Characterization of Tn*1546*, a Tn*3*-related transposon conferring glycopeptide resistance, by synthesis of depsipeptide peptidoglycan precursors in *Enterococcus faecium* BM4147. *J Bacteriol* 1993;175:117–127.
20. Asmar BI, Maqbool S, Dajani AS. Hematologic abnormalities after oral trimethoprim-sulfamethoxazole therapy in children. *Am J Dis Child* 1981;135:1100–1103.
21. Atherton FR, Hall MJ, Hassall CH, et al. Antibacterial properties of alafosfalin combined with cephalexin. *Antimicrob Agents Chemother* 1981;20:470–476.
22. Auckenthaler R, Wilson WR, Wright AJ, et al. Lack of an in vivo and in vitro bactericidal activity of *N*-formimidoyl thienamycin against enterococci. *Antimicrob Agents Chemother* 1982;22:448–452.
23. Aumercier M, Bouhallab S, Capman M-L, et al. RP 59500: a proposed mechanism for its bactericidal activity. *J Antimicrob Chemother* 1992;30(Suppl 4):914.
24. Austin TW, Brooks CF, Bethel M, et al. Trimethoprim-sulfamethoxazole in the treatment of gonococcal urethritis: clinical and laboratory correlates. *J Infect Dis* 1973;128 (Suppl):S666–672.
25. Backes RJ, Rouse MS, Henry NK, et al. Activity of penicillin combined with an aminoglycoside against group B streptococci in vitro and in experimental endocarditis. *J Antimicrob Chemother* 1986;18:491–498.
26. Bahl D, Miller DA, Leviton I, et al. In vitro activities of ciprofloxacin and rifampin alone and in combination against growing and nongrowing strains of methicillin-susceptible and methicillin-resistant *Staphylococcus aureus*. *Antimicrob Agents Chemother* 1997;41:1293–1297.
27. Bajaksouzian S, Visalli MA, Jacobs MR, et al. Activities of levofloxacin, ofloxacin, and ciprofloxacin, alone and in combination with amikacin, against acinetobacters as determined by checkerboard and time-kill studies. *Antimicrob Agents Chemother* 1997;41:1073–1076.
28. Baker CN, Thornsberry C, Facklam RR. Synergism, killing, and antimicrobial susceptibility of group A and B streptococci. *Antimicrob Agents Chemother* 1981;19:716–725.
29. Baltch AL, Smith RP, Ritz W. Inhibitory and bactericidal activities of levofloxacin, ofloxacin, erythromycin, and rifampin used singly and in combination against *Legionella pneumophila*. *Antimicrob Agents Chemother* 1995;39:1661–1666.
30. Baltimore RS, Klein JO, Wilcox C, et al. Synergy of mecillinam (FL 1060) with penicillins and cephalosporins against *Proteus* and *Klebsiella*, with observations on combinations with other antibiotics and against other bacterial species. *Antimicrob Agents Chemother* 1976;9:701–705.
31. Bansal MB, Thadepalli H. Antimicrobial effect of β-lactam antibiotic combinations against *Bacteroides fragilis* in vitro. *Antimicrob Agents Chemother* 1983;23:166–168.
32. Bantar CE, Micucci M, Fernandez Canigia L, et al. Synergy characterization for *Enterococcus faecalis* strains displaying moderately high-level gentamicin and streptomycin resistance. *J Clin Microbiol* 1993;32:1921–1923.
33. Barakett V, Lesage D, Delisle F, et al. Synergy of cefotaxime and fosfomycin against penicillin-resistant pneumococci. *J Antimicrob Chemother* 1993;31:105–109.
34. Barber M, Waterworth PM. Antibacterial activity of lincomycin and pristinamycin: a comparison with erythromycin. *Br Med J* 1964;2:603–606.
35. Barber M, Waterworth PM. Activity of gentamicin against pseudomonas and hospital staphylococci. *Br Med J* 1966;1:203–205.
36. Baron EJ, Young LS. Amikacin, ethambutol, and rifampin for treatment of disseminated *Mycobacterium avium-intracellulare* infections in patients with acquired immune deficiency syndrome. *Diag Microbiol Infect Dis* 1986;5:215–220.
37. Barr JG, Smyth ET, Hogg GM. In vitro antimicrobial activity of imipenem in combination with vancomycin or teicoplanin against *Staphylococcus aureus* and *Staphylococcus epidermidis*. *Eur J Clin Microbiol Infect Dis* 1990;9:804–809.
38. Barry AL, Ayers LW, Gavan TL, et al. In vitro activity of ticarcillin plus clavulanic acid against bacteria isolated in three centers. *Eur J Clin Microbiol* 1984;3:203–206.
39. Barry AL, Thornsberry C. Susceptibility testing: diffusion test procedures. In: Lennette EH, Balows A, Hausler WJ Jr., et al., eds. *Manual of clinical microbiology,* 4th ed. Washington, DC: American Society for Microbiology, 1985;978–987.
40. Bartlett JG, Gorbach SL. Treatment of aspiration pneumonia and primary lung abscess: penicillin G vs. clindamycin. *JAMA* 1975;234:935–937.
41. Basker MJ, Slocombe B, Sutherland R. Aminoglycoside-resistant enterococci. *J Clin Pathol* 1977;30:375–380.
42. Batard E, Jacqueline C, Boutoille D, et al. Combination of quinupristin-dalfopristin and gentamicin against methicillin-resistant *Staphylococcus aureus*: experimental rabbit endocarditis study. *Antimicrob Agents Chemother* 2002;46:2174–2178.
43. Bauer AW, Kirby WMM, Sherris JC, et al. Antibiotic susceptibility testing by a standardized single disk method. *Am J Clin Pathol* 1966;45:493–496.
44. Baum EZ, Montenegro DA, Licata L, et al. Identification and characterization of new inhibitors of the *Escherichia coli* MurA enzyme. *Antimicrob Agents Chemother* 2001;45:3182–3188.
45. Bayer AS, Chow AW, Morrison JO, et al. Bactericidal synergy between penicillin or ampicillin and aminoglycosides against antibiotic-tolerant lactobacilli. *Antimicrob Agents Chemother* 1980;17:359–363.
46. Bayer AS, Norman D, Kim KS. Efficacy of amikacin and ceftazidime in experimental aortic valve endocarditis due to *Pseudomonas aeruginosa*. *Antimicrob Agents Chemother* 1985;28:781–785.
47. Bennett WM, Craven R. Urinary tract infections in patients with severe renal disease: treatment with ampicillin and trimethoprim-sulfamethoxazole. *JAMA* 1976;236:946–948.
48. Berenbaum MC. A method for testing for synergy with any number of agents. *J Infect Dis* 1978;137:122–130.
49. Berenbaum MC. Correlations between methods for measurement of synergy. *J Infect Dis* 1980;142:476–478.
50. Berenbaum MC, Yu VL, Felegie TP. Synergy with double and triple combinations compared. *J Antimicrob Chemother* 1983;12:555–563.
51. Bingen E, Lambert-Zechovsky N, Leclercq R, et al. Bactericidal activity of vancomycin, daptomycin, ampicillin and aminoglycosides against vancomycin-resistant *Enterococcus faecium*. *J Antimicrob Chemother* 1990;26:619–626.
52. Blumberg PM, Strominger JL. Interaction of penicillin with the bacterial cell: penicilllin-binding proteins and penicillin-sensitive enzymes. *Bacteriol Rev* 1974;38:291–335.
53. Bodet CA, Jorgensen JH, Drutz DJ. Antibacterial activities of antineoplastic agents. *Antimicrob Agents Chemother* 1985;28:437–439.

54. Bodey GP. Epidemiological studies of *Pseudomonas* species in patients with leukemia. *Am J Med Sci* 1970;260: 82–89.
55. Bodey GP, Jadeja L, Elting L. *Pseudomonas* bacteremia. Retrospective analysis of 410 episodes. *Arch Intern Med* 1985;145:1621–1629.
56. Bodine J, Murray T, Sande MA. Combination therapy of experimental *Haemophilus influenzae* and *Streptococcus pneumoniae* meningitis. *Clin Res* 1977;25:27A.
57. Bonapace CR, White RL, Friedrich LV, et al. Evaluation of antibiotic synergy against *Acinetobacter baumannii*: a comparison with Etest, time-kill, and checkerboard methods. *Diagn Microbiol Infect Dis* 2000;38:43–50.
58. Bonifas V. Determination de l'association synergique binaire d'antibiotes et de sulfamides. *Experientia* 1952; 8:234–235.
59. Bonilla HF, Perri MB, Kauffman CA, et al. Comparative in vitro activity of quinupristin/dalfopristin against multidrug resistant *Enterococcus faecium. Diagn Microbiol Infect Dis* 1996;25:127–131.
60. Bornside GH. Synergistic antibacterial activity of ampicillin-cloxacillin mixtures against *Proteus morganii. Appl Microbiol* 1968;16:1507–1511.

60a. Borrmann S, Issifou S, Esser G. Fosmidomycin-Clindamycin for the treatment of *Plasmodium falciparum* malaria. *J Infect Dis* 2004;190:1534–1540.

61. Bosso JA, Saxon BA, Matsen JM. In vitro activity of aztreonam combined with tobramycin and gentamicin against clinical isolates of *Pseudomonas aeruginosa* and *Pseudomonas cepacia* from patients with cystic fibrosis. *Antimicrob Agents Chemother* 1987;31:1403–1405.
62. Bouanchaud DH. In-vitro and in-vivo synergic activity and fractional inhibitory concentration (FIC) of the components of a semisynthetic streptogramin, RP 59500. *J Antimicrob Chemother* 1992;30(Suppl A):95–99.
63. Brandt CM, Rouse MS, Laue NW, et al. Effective treatment of multidrug resistant enterococcal experimental endocarditis with combinations of cell-wall active agents. *J Infect Dis* 1996;173:909–913.
64. Brook I, Coolbaugh JC, Walker RI, et al. Synergism between penicillin, clindamycin, or metronidazole and gentamicin against species of the *Bacteroides melaninogenicus* and *Bacteroides fragilis* groups. *Antimicrob Agents Chemother* 1984;25:71–77.
65. Brown GM. The biosynthesis of folic acid. II. Inhibition by sulfonamides. *J Biol Chem* 1962;237:536–540.
66. Brown TH, Alford RH. Antagonism by chloramphenicol of broad-spectrum β-lactam antibiotics against *Klebsiella pneumoniae. Antimicrob Agents Chemother* 1984;25:405–407.
67. Brumfitt W, Percival A, Leigh DA. Clinical and laboratory studies with carbenicillin: a new penicillin active against *Pseudomonas pyocyanea. Lancet* 1967;1:1289–1293.
68. Bryan LE, Van den Elzen HM. Streptomycin accumulation in susceptible and resistant strains of *Escherichia coli* and *Pseudomonas aeruginosa. Antimicrob Agents Chemother* 1976;9:928–938.
69. Buesing MA, Jorgensen JH. *In vitro* activity of aztreonam in combination with newer β-lactams and amikacin against multiply-resistant Gram-negative bacilli. *Antimicrob Agents Chemother* 1984;25:283–285.
70. Bulger RJ. In vitro activity of cephalothin/kanamycin and methicillin/kanamycin combinations against methicillin-resistant *Staphylococcus aureus. Lancet* 1967;1:17–19.
71. Burchall JJ. Synergism between trimethoprim and sulfamethoxazole. *Science* 1977;197:1300–1301.
72. Burchall JJ, Hitchings GH. Inhibitor binding analysis of dihydrofolate reductases from various species. *Mol Pharmacol* 1965;1:126–136.
73. Burgess DS, Hall RG, Hardin TC. In vitro evaluation of the activity of two doses of levofloxacin alone and in combination with other agents against *Pseudomonas aeruginosa. Diagn Microbiol Infect Dis* 2003;46:131–137.
74. Burgess DS, Hastings RW. Activity of piperacillin /tazobactam in combination with amikacin, ciprofloxacin, and trovafloxacin against *Pseudomonas aeruginosa* by time-kill. *Diagn Microbiol Infect Dis* 2000;38:37–41.
75. Burgess DS, Nathisuwan S. Cefepime, piperacillin /tazobactam, gentamicin, ciprofloxacin, and levofloxacin alone and in combination against *Pseudomonas aeruginosa. Diagn Microbiol Infect Dis* 2002;44:35–41.
76. Busch DF, Sutter VL, Finegold SM. Activity of combinations of antimicrobial agents against *Bacteroides fragilis. J Infect Dis* 1976;133:321–328.
77. Bush K. Characterization of β-lactamases. *Antimicrob Agents Chemother* 1989;33:259–263.
78. Bush K, Sykes RB. β-Lactamase inhibitors in perspective. *J Antimicrob Chemother* 1983;11:97–107.
79. Bushby SRM. Trimethoprim-sulfamethoxazole: in vitro microbiological aspects. *J Infect Dis* 1973;128(Suppl): S442–S462.
80. Bushby SRM, Hitchings GH. Trimethoprim: a sulfonamide potentiator. *Br J Pharmacol Chemother* 1968;33: 72–90.
81. Bustamante CI, Drusano GL, Wharton RC, et al. Synergism of the combinations of imipenem plus ciprofloxacin and imipenem plus amikacin against *Pseudomonas aeruginosa* and other bacterial pathogens. *Antimicrob Agents Chemother* 1987;31:632–634.
82. Bustamante CI, Wharton RC, Wade JC. In vitro activity of ciprofloxacin in combination with ceftazidime, aztreonam, an azlocillin against multiresistant isolates of *Pseudomonas aeruginosa. Antimicrob Agents Chemother* 1990;34:1814–1815.
83. Butler T, Linh NN, Arnold K, et al. Therapy of antimicrobial-resistant typhoid fever. *Antimicrob Agents Chemother* 1977;11:645–650.
84. Butler T, Linh NN, Arnold K, et al. Chloramphenicol-resistant typhoid fever in Vietnam associated with R factor. *Lancet* 1973;2:983–985.
85. Calderwood SA, Wennersten CBG, Moellering RC Jr, et al. Resistance to six aminoglycosidic aminocyclitol antibiotics among enterococci: prevalence, evolution, and relationship to synergism with penicillin. *Antimicrob Agents Chemother* 1977;12:401–405.
86. Calderwood SB, Gardella A, Philippon AM, et al. Effects of azlocillin in combination with clavulanic acid, sulbactam, and *N*-formimidoyl-thienamycin against β-lactamase-producing, carbenicillin-resistant *Pseudomonas aeruginosa. Antimicrob Agents Chemother* 1982;22:266–271.
87. Canawati HN. A reassessement of the activity of the third-generation cephalosporins against anaerobes and *Staphylococcus aureus. Am J Surg* 1992;164(Suppl 4A):24S–27S.
88. Cappelletty DM, Rybak MJ. Comparison of methodologies for synergism testing of drug combinations against resistant strains of *Pseudomonas aeruginosa. Antimicrob Agents Chemother* 1996;40:677–683.
89. Carlier C, Courvalin P. Emergence of 4′,4″-aminoglycoside nucleotidyltransferase in enterococci. *Antimicrob Agents Chemother* 1990;34:1565–1569.
90. Caron F, Carbon C, Gutmann L. Triple-combination penicillin-vancomycin-gentamicin for experimental endocarditis caused by a moderately penicillin- and highly glycopeptide-resistant isolate of *Enterococcus faecium. J Infect Dis* 1991;164:888–893.

91. Caron F, Gold HS, Wennersten CB, et al. Influence of erythromycin resistance, inoculum growth phase, and incubation time on assessment of the bactericidal activity of RP 59500 (quinupristin-dalfopristin) against vancomycin-resistant *Enterococcus faecium*. *Antimicrob Agents Chemother* 1997;41:2749–2753.
92. Caron F, Lemeland J-F, Humbert G, et al. Triple combination penicillin-vancomycin-gentamicin for experimental endocarditis caused by a highly penicillin- and glycopeptide-resistant isolate of *Enterococcus faecium*. *J Infect Dis* 1993;168:681–686.
93. Caron F, Pestel M, Kitzis M-D, et al. Comparison of different β-lactam-glycopeptide-gentamicin combinations for an experimental endocarditis caused by a highly β-lactam resistant and highly glycopeptide-resistant isolate of *Enterococcus faecium*. *J Infect Dis* 1995;171:106–112.
94. Carrizosa J, Kaye D. Antibiotic synergism in enterococcal endocarditis. *J Lab Clin Med* 1976;88:132–141.
95. Cedeno JR, Krogstad DJ. Susceptibility testing of *Entamoeba histolytica*. *J Infect Dis* 1983;148:1090–1095.
96. Cercenado E, Eliopoulos GM, Wennersten CB, et al. Absence of synergistic activity between ampicillin and vancomycin against highly vancomycin-resistant enterococci. *Antimicrob Agents Chemother* 1992;36:2201–2203.
97. Cha R, Rybak MJ. Linezolid and vancomycin, alone and in combination with rifampin, compared with moxifloxacin against a multidrug-resistant and a vancomycin-tolerant *Streptococcus pneumoniae* strain in an in vitro pharmacodynamic model. *Antimicrob Agents Chemother* 2003;47:1984–1987.
98. Chabbert YA. Une technique nouvelle d'etude de l'action bactericide des associations d'antibiotiques: le transfert sur cellophane. *Ann Inst Pasteur* 1957;93:289–299.
99. Chabbert YA, Patte JC. Cellophane transfer application to the study of combinations of antibiotics. *Appl Microbiol* 1960;8:193–199.
100. Chabbert YA, Waterworth PM. Studies on the carry over of antibiotic using of the cellophane transfer technique. *J Clin Pathol* 1965;18:314–316.
101. Chamot E, Boffi El Amari E, et al. Effectiveness of combination antimicrobial therapy for *Pseudomonas aeruginosa* bacteremia. *Antimicrob Agents Chemother* 2003;47:2756–2764.
102. Chamovitz B, Bryant RE, Gilbert DN, et al. Prosthetic valve endocarditis caused by *Staphylococcus epidermidis*: development of rifampin resistance during vancomycin and rifampin therapy. *JAMA* 1985;253:2867–2868.
103. Chan EL, Zabransky R. Determination of synergy by two methods with eight antimicrobial combinations against tobramycin-susceptible and tobramycin-resistant strains of *Pseudomonas*. *Diagn Microbiol Infect Dis* 1987;6:157–164.
104. Chandrasekar PH, Crane LR, Bailey EJ. Comparison of the activity of antibiotic combinations in vitro with clinical outcome and resistance emergence in serious infection by *Pseudomonas aeruginosa* in non-neutropenic patients. *J Antimicrob Chemother* 1987;19:321–329.
105. Chang HY, Rodriguez V, Narboni G, et al. Causes of death in adults with acute leukemia. *Medicine* 1976;55:259–268.
106. Chang MJ, Dunkle LM, Van Reken D, et al. Trimethoprim-sulfamethoxazole compared to ampicillin in the treatment of shigellosis. *Pediatrics* 1977;59:726–729.
107. Chenoweth CE, Robinson KA, Schaberg DR. Efficacy of ampicillin versus trimethoprim-sulfamethoxazole in a mouse model of lethal enterococcal peritonitis. *Antimicrob Agents Chemother* 1990;34:1800–1802.
108. Chiang FY, Climo M. Efficacy of linezolid alone or in combination with vancomycin for treatment of experimental endocarditis due to methicillin-resistant *Staphylococcus aureus*. *Antimicrob Agents Chemother* 2003;47:3002–3004.
109. Chin NX, Jules K, Neu HC. Synergy of ciprofloxacin and azlocillin in vitro and in a neutropenic mouse model of infection. *Eur J Clin Microbiol* 1986;5:23–28.
110. Chou T-C, Talalay P. Quantitative analysis of dose-effect relationships: the combined effects of multiple drugs or enzyme inhibitors. *Adv Enzyme Regul* 1984;22:27–55.
111. Chow AW, Wong J, Bartlett KH. Synergisitc interactions of ciprofloxacin and extended-spectrum β-lactams or aminoglycosides against multiply drug-resistant *Pseudomonas maltophilia*. *Antimicrob Agents Chemother* 1988;32:782–784.
112. Chow JW. Aminoglycoside resistance in enterococci. *Clin Infect Dis* 2000;31:586–589.
113. Chow JW, Fine MJ, Shlaes DM, et al. *Enterobacter* bacteremia: clinical features and emergence of antibiotic resistance during therapy. *Ann Inern Med* 1991;115:585–590.
114. Clark CL, Jacobs MR, Appelbaum PC. Activities of clinafloxacin, alone and in combination with other compounds, against 45 gram-positive and -negative organisms for which clinafloxacin MICs are high. *Antimicrob Agents Chemother* 1999;43:2295–2298.
115. Climo MW, Patron RL, Archer GL. Combinations of vancomycin and beta-lactams are synergistic against staphylococci with reduced susceptibilities to vancomycin. *Antimicrob Agents Chemother* 1999;43:1747–1753.
116. Cockerill FR III, Edson RS. Trimethoprim-sulfamethoxazole. *Mayo Clin Proc* 1991;66:1260–1269.
117. Coleman K, Griffin DRJ, Page JWJ, et al. In vivo evaluation of BRL42715, a novel β-lactamase inhibitor. *Antimicrob Agents Chemother* 1989;33:1580–1587.
118. Comber KR, Basker MJ, Osborne CD, et al. Synergy between ticarcillin and tobramycin against *Pseudomonas aeruginosa* and Enterobacteriaceae in vitro and in vivo. *Antimicrob Agents Chemother* 1977;11:956–964.
119. Combes T, Carlier C, Courvalin P. Aminoglycoside-modifying enzyme content of multiply-resistant strains of *Streptococcus faecalis*. *J Antimicrob Chemother* 1983; 11:41–47.
120. Connell EV, Hsu M-C, Richman DD. Combinative interactions of a human immunodeficiency virus (HIV) Tat antagonist with HIV reverse transcriptase inhibitors and an HIV protease inhibitor. *Antimicrob Agents Chemother* 1994;38:348–352.
121. Coppens L, Hansen B, Klastersky J. Therapy of staphylococcal infections with cefamandole or vancomycin alone or with a combination of cefamandole and tobramycin. *Antimicrob Agents Chemother* 1983;23:36–41.
122. Costa Y, Galimand M, Leclercq R, et al. Characterization of the chromosomal *aac-Ii* gene specific for *Enterococcus faecium*. *Antimicrob Agents Chemother* 1993;37:1896–1903.
123. Cottagnoud P, Cottagnoud M, Acosta F, et al. Meropenem prevents levofloxacin-induced resistance in penicillin-resistant pneumococci and acts synergistically with levofloxacin in experimental meningitis. *Eur J Clin Microbiol Infect Dis* 2003;22:656–662.
124. Coudron PE, Markowitz SM, Wong ES. Isolation of a β-lactamase-producing, aminoglycoside-resistant strain of *Enterococcus faecium*. *Antimicrob Agents Chemother* 1992;36:1125–1126.
125. Courvalin P, Carlier C, Collatz E. Plasmid-mediated resistance to aminocyclitol antibiotics in group D streptococci. *J Bacteriol* 1980;143:541–551.
126. Craig WA, Kunin CM. Trimethoprim-sulfamethoxazole:

pharmacodynamic effects of urinary pH and impaired renal function. *Ann Intern Med* 1973;78:491–497.

127. Credito KL, Jacobs MR, Appelbaum PC. Anti-anaerobic activity of levofloxacin alone and combined with clindamycin and metronidazole. *Diagn Microbiol Infect Dis* 2000;38:181–183.
128. Critchley IA, Sahm DF, Kelly LJ, et al. In vitro synergy studies using aztreonam and fluoroquinolone combinations against six species of Gram-negative bacilli. *Chemotherapy* 2003;49:44–48.
129. Crosby MA, Gump DW. Activity of cefoperazone and two β-lactamase inhibitors, sulbactam and clavulanic acid, against *Bacteroides* spp. correlated with β-lactamase production. *Antimicrob Agents Chemother* 1982;22:398:405.
130. Cynamon MH, Palmer GS. In vitro susceptibility of *Mycobacterium fortunitum* to amoxicillin or cepahlothin in combination with clavulanic acid. *Antimicrob Agents Chemother* 1983;23:935–937.
131. Cynamon MH, Palmer GS. In vitro activity of amoxicillin in combination with clavulanic acid against *Mycobacterium tuberculosis*. *Antimicrob Agents Chemother* 1983;24:429–431.
132. D'Alessandri RM, McNeeley DJ, Kluge RM. Antibiotic synergy and antagonism against clinical isolates of *Klebsiella* species. *Antimicrob Agents Chemother* 1976;10:889–892.
133. D'Amato RF, Thornsberry C, Baker CN, et al. Effect of calcium and magnesium ions on the susceptibility of *Pseudomonas* species to tetracycline, gentamicin, polymyxin B, and carbenicillin. *Antimicrob Agents Chemother* 1975;7:596–600.
134. Dailey CF, Pagano PJ, Buchanan LV, et al. Efficacy of linezolid plus rifampin in an experimental model of methicillin-susceptible *Staphylococcus aureus* endocarditis. *Antimicrob Agents Chemother* 2003;47:2655–2658.
135. Davies GSR, Cohen J. In vitro study of the activity of ciprofloxacin alone and in combination against strains of *Pseudomonas aeruginosa* with multiple antibiotic resistance. *J Antimicrob Chemother* 1985;16:713–717.
136. Davies JE, Benveniste RE. Enzymes that inactivate antibiotics in transit to their targets. *Ann NY Acad Sci* 1974;235:130–136.
137. Davies M, Morgan JR, Anand CR. Interactions of carbenicillin and ticarcillin with gentamicin. *Antimicrob Agents Chemother* 1975;7:431–434.
138. Davis BD, Maas WK. Analysis of the biochemical mechanism of drug resistance in certain bacterial mutants. *Proc Natl Acad Sci USA* 1952;38:775–785.
139. Dawis MA, Isenberg HD, France KA, et al. In vitro activity of gatifloxacin alone and in combination with cefepime, meropenem, piperacillin and gentamicin against multidrug-resistant organisms. *J Antimicrob Chemother* 2003;51:1203–1211.
140. Day CA, Marceau-Day ML, Day DF. Increased susceptibility of *Pseudomonas aeruginosa* to ciprofloxacin in the presence of vancomycin. *Antimicrob Agents Chemother* 1993;37:2506–2508.
141. Debbia E, Pesce A, Schito GC. In vitro activity of LY 146032 alone and in combination with other antibiotics against Gram-positive bacteria. *Antimicrob Agents Chemother* 1988;32:279–281.
142. Debbia E, Varaldo PE, Schito GC. In vitro activity of imipenem against enterococci and staphylococci and evidence for high rates of synergism with teicoplanin, fosfomycin, and rifampin. *Antimicrob Agents Chemother* 1986;30:813–815.
143. Declercq E, Yamamoto N, Pauwels R, et al. Highly potent and selective inhibitions of human immunodeficiency virus by the bicyclam derivative JM3100. *Antimicrob Agents Chemother* 1994;38:668–674.
144. DeJongh CA, Joshi JH, Thompson BW, et al. A double β-lactam combination versus an aminoglycoside-containing regimen as empiric antibiotic therapy for febrile granulocytopenic cancer patients. *Am J Med* 1986;80(Suppl 5C):101–111.
145. Denning DW, Hanson LH, Perlman AM, et al. In vitro susceptibility and synergy studies of *Aspergillus* species to conventional and new agents. *Diagn Microbiol Infect Dis* 1992;15:21–34.
146. Deveikis A, Schauf V, Mizen M, et al. Antimicrobial therapy of experimental Group B streptococcal infection in mice. *Antimicrob Agents Chemother* 1977;11:817–820.
147. Dhople AM, Ibanez MA. In-vitro activity of three new fluoroquinolones and synergy with ansamycins against *Mycobacterium leprae*. *J Antimicrob Chemother* 1993;32:445–451.
148. Diamond DM, Bauer M, Daniel BE, et al. Amphotericin B colloidal dispersion combined with flucytosine with or without fluconazole for treatment of murine cryptococcal meningitis. *Antimicrob Agents Chemother* 1998;42:528–533.
149. DiNubile MJ. Short-course antibiotic therapy for right-sided endocarditis caused by *Staphylococcus aureus* in injection drug users. *Ann Intern Med* 1994;121:873–876.
150. Doern GV, Ferraro MJ, Brueggemann AB, et al. Emergence of high rates of antimicrobial resistance among viridans group streptococci in the United States. *Antimicrob Agents Chemother* 1996;40:891–894.
151. Donabedian H, Andriole VT. Synergy of vancomycin with penicillins and cephalosporins against *Pseudomonas, Klebsiella,* and *Serratia*. *Yale J Biol Med* 1977;50:165–176.
152. Dornbusch K. Regression line analysis of the synergistic effect for the combination of trimethoprim-sulfamethoxazole. *Chemotherapy* 1971;16:229–238.
153. Dougherty PF, Yotter DW, Matthews TR. Microdilution transfer plate technique for determining in vitro synergy of antimicrobial agents. *Antimicrob Agents Chemother* 1977;11:225–228.
154. Drake TA, Hackbarth CJ, Sande MA. Value of serum tests in combined drug therapy of endocarditis. *Antimicrob Agents Chemother* 1983;24:653–657.
155. Dumon L, Adriens P, Anne J, et al. Effect of clavulanic acid on the minimum inhibitory concentration of benzylpenicillin, ampicillin, carbenicillin, or cephalothin against clinical isolates resistant to β-lactam antibiotics. *Antimicrob Agents Chemother* 1979;15:315–317.
156. Duperval R, Bill NJ, Geraci JE, et al. Bactericidal activity of combinations of penicillin or clindamycin with gentamicin or streptomycin against species of viridans streptococci. *Antimicrob Agents Chemother* 1975;8:673–676.
157. Durack DT, Petersdorf RG. Chemotherapy of experimental streptococcal endocarditis. I. Comparison of commonly recommended prophylactic regimens. *J Clin Invest* 1973;52:592–598.
158. Dye WE. An agar diffusion method for studying the bacteriostatic action of combinations of antimicrobial agents. *Antibiot Annu* 1955–1956;374–382.
159. Eickhoff TC. In vitro effects of carbenicillin combined with gentamicin or polymyxin B against *Pseudomonas aeruginosa*. *Appl Microbiol* 1969;18:469–473.
160. Eickhoff TC, Ehret JM. Comparative activity in vitro of ticarcillin, BL-P1654, and carbenicillin. *Antimicrob Agents Chemother* 1976;10:241–244.
161. Elion GB, Singer S, Hitchings CH. Antagonists of

nucleic acid derivatives. VIII. Synergism in combinations of biochemically related antimetabolites. *J Biol Chem* 1954;208:477–488.
162. Eliopoulos GM. Induction of β-lactamases. *J Antimicrob Chemother* 1988;22(Suppl A):37–44.
163. Eliopoulos GM, Eliopoulos CT. Antibiotic combinations: should they be tested? *Clin Microbiol Rev* 1988;1:139–156.
164. Eliopoulos GM, Eliopoulos CT. Ciprofloxacin in combination with other antimicrobials. *Am J Med* 1989;87(Suppl 5A):17S–22S.
165. Eliopoulos GM, Eliopoulos CT. Activity in vitro of the quinolones. In: Hooper DC, Wolfson JS, eds. *Quinolone antimicrobial agents,* 2nd ed. Washington DC: American Society for Microbiology, 1993;161–193.
166. Eliopoulos GM, Farber BF, Murray BE, et al. Ribosomal resistance of clinical enterococcal isolates to streptomycin. *Antimicrob Agents Chemother* 1984;25:398–399.
167. Eliopoulos GM, Gardella A, DeGirolami P, et al. In vitro activity of U-63196E, a new cephalosporin, against clinical bacterial isolates. *Antimicrob Agents Chemother* 1984;25:401–404.
168. Eliopoulos GM, Moellering RC Jr. Susceptibility of enterococci and *Listeria monocytogenes* to *N*-formimidoyl-thienamycin alone and in combination with an aminoglycoside. *Antimicrob Agents Chemother* 1981;19:789–793.
169. Eliopoulos GM, Moellering RC Jr. Azlocillin,mezlocillin, and piperacillin: new broad-spectrum penicillins. *Ann Intern Med* 1982;97:755–760.
170. Eliopoulos GM, Wennersten CB. Antimicrobial activity of quinupristin-dalfopristin combined with other antibiotics against vancomycin-resistant enterococci. *Antimicrob Agents Chemother* 2002;46:1319–1324.
171. Eliopoulos GM, Wennersten C, Zighelboim-Daum S, et al. High-level resistance to gentamicin in clinical isolates of *Streptococcus faecium. Antimicrob Agents Chemother* 1988;32:1528–1532.
172. Eliopoulos GM, Willey S, Reiszner E, et al. In vitro and in vivo activity of LY146032, a new cyclic lipopeptide antibiotic. *Antimicrob Agents Chemother* 1986;30:532–535.
173. Elliot AM, Karam GH, Cobbs CG. Interaction of cefotaxime and aminoglycosides against enterococci in vitro. *Antimicrob Agents Chemother* 1983;24:847–850.
174. Enciso MD, Lindemann MLM, Altes AG. In vitro evaluation of *N*-formimidoyl-thienamycin (MK0787) combined with amikacin against Gram-negative bacilli and *Staphylococus aureus. Antimicrob Agents Chemother* 1982;22:1064–1066.
175. English AR, Retsema JA, Girard AE, et al. CP 45,899, a β-lactamase inhibitor that extends the antibacterial spectrum of β-lactams: initial bacteriological characterization. *Antimicrob Agents Chemother* 1978;14:414–419.
176. Ermertcan S, Hosgor M, Tunger O, et al. Investigation of synergism of meropenem and ciprofloxacin against *Pseudomonas aeruginosa* and *Acinetobacter* strains isolated from intensive care unit infections. *Scand J Infect Dis* 2001;33:818–821.
177. European Organization for Research on Treatment of Cancer International Antimicrobial Therapy Cooperative Group. Ceftazidime combined with a short or long course of amikacin for empirical therapy of Gram-negative bacteremia in cancer patients with granulocytopenia. *N Engl J Med* 1987;317:1692–1698.
178. Ervin FR, Bullock WE. Clinical and pharmacologic studies of ticarcilllin in Gram-negative infections. *Antimicrob Agents Chemother* 1976;9:94–101.
179. Esposito S, Gupta A, Thadepalli H. In vitro synergy of ciprofloxacin and three other antibiotics against *Bacteroids fragilis. Drugs Exp Clin Res* 1987;13:489–492.
180. Farber BF, Eliopoulos GM, Ward JI, et al. Resistance to penicillin-streptomycin synergy among clinical isolates of viridans streptococci. *Antimicrob Agents Chemother* 1983;24:871–875.
181. Farber BF, Eliopoulos GM, Ward JI, et al. Multiply resistant viridans streptococci: susceptibility to β-lactam antibiotics and comparison of penicillin-binding protein patterns. *Antimicrob Agents Chemother* 1983;24:702–705.
182. Farber BF, Yee Y. High-level aminoglycoside resistance mediated by aminoglycoside-modifying enzymes among viridans streptococci: implications for the therapy for endocarditis. *J Infect Dis* 1987;155:948–953.
183. Farber BF, Yee YC, Karchmer AW. Interaction between rifampin and fusidic acid against methicillin-resistant coagulase positive and negative staphylococci. *Antimicrob Agents Chemother* 1986;30:174–175.
184. Farrar WE Jr, O'Dell NM, Krause JM. Use of penicillinase-resistant penicillins to increase the susceptibility of Gram-negative bacteria to antibiotics. *Ann Intern Med* 1967;67:733–743.
185. Fass RJ. Inconsistency of synergy between the β-lactamase inhibitor CP-45,899 and β-lactam antibiotics against multiply drug-resistant Enterobacteriaceae and *Pseudomonas* species. *Antimicrob Agents Chemother* 1981;19:361–363.
186. Fass RJ. Comparative in vitro activities of β-lactam-tobramycin combinations against *Pseudomonas aeruginosa* and multidrug-resistant Gram-negative enteric bacilli. *Antimicrob Agents Chemother* 1982;21:1003–1006.
187. Fass RJ, Prior RB, Perkins RL. Pharmacokinetics and tolerance of a single twelve tablet dose of trimethoprim (960 mg) and sulfamethoxazole (4800 mg). *Antimicrob Agents Chemother* 1977;12:102–106.
188. Fass RJ, Rotilie VA, Prior RB. Interaction of clindamycin and gentamicin in vitro. *Antimicrob Agents Chemother* 1974;6:582–587.
189. Fass RJ, Scholand JF, Hodges GR, et al. Clindamycin in the treatment of serious anaerobic infections. *Ann Intern Med* 1973;78:853–859.
190. Fass RJ, Wright CA. Comparative efficacies of mezlocillin and ampicillin alone or in combination with gentamicin in the treatment of *Streptococcus faecalis* endocarditis in rabbits. *Antimicrob Agents Chemother* 1984;25:408–410.
191. Fekety FR Jr, Weiss P. Antibiotic synergism: enhanced susceptibility of enterococci to combinations of streptomycin and penicillins or cephalosporins. *Antimicrob Agents Chemother* 1966;6:156–164.
192. Fernandez-Guerrero ML, Barros C, Rodriguez et al. Aortic endocarditis caused by gentamicin-resistant *Enterococcus faecalis. Eur J Clin Microbiol* 1988;7:525–527.
193. File TM Jr, Tan JS. Amdinocillin plus cefoxitin versus cefoxitin alone in therapy of mixed soft tissue infections (including diabetic foot infections). *Am J Med* 1983;75(Suppl):100–105.
194. Finland M, Garner C, Wilcox C, et al. Susceptibility of Enterobacteria to aminoglycoside antibiotics: comparisons with tetracycline, polymyxins, chloramphenicol, and spectinomycin. *J Infect Dis* 1976;134(Suppl):S57–S74.
195. Finland M, Garner C, Wilcox C, et al. Susceptibility of Enterobacteria to penicillins, cepahalosporins, lincomycins, erythromycin, and rifampin. *J Infect Dis* 1976;134(Suppl):S75–S96.
196. Fish DN, Choi MK, Jung R. Synergic activity of

cephalosporins plus fluoroquinolones against *Pseudomonas aeruginosa* with resistance to one or both drugs. *J Antimicrob Chemother* 2002;50:1045–1049.

197. Ford CW, Hamel JC, Wilson DM, et al. In vivo activities of U-100592 and U-100766, novel oxazolidinone antimicrobial agents, against experimental bacterial infections. *Antimicrob Agents Chemother* 1996;40:1508–1513.
198. Frisch MJ. Clinical experience with adverse reactions to trimethoprim-sulfamethoxazole. *J Infect Dis* 1973;128(Suppl):S607–S611.
199. Fu KP, Hetzel N, Gregory FJ, et al. Therapeutic efficacy of cefpiramide-ciprofloxacin combination in experimental *Pseudomonas* infections in neutropenic mice. *Antimicrob Agents Chemother* 1987;20:541–546.
200. Fu KP, Kimble EF, Zoganas H, et al. Synergistic activity of cefsulodin combined with cefoxitin and sulbactam against *Bacteroides* species. *J Antimicrob Chemother* 1984;13:257–265.
201. Fu KP, Neu HC. Comparative inhibition of β-lactamases by novel β-lactam compounds. *Antimicrob Agents Chemother* 1979;15:171–176.
202. Fuchs PC, Barry AL, Brown SD. Interactions of quinupristin-dalfopristin with eight other antibiotics as measured by time-kill studies with 10 strains of *Staphylococcus aureus* for which quinupristin-dalfopristin alone was not bactericidal. *Antimicrob Agents Chemother* 2001;45:2662–2665.
203. Fuchs PC, Barry AL, Thornsberry C, et al. In vitro activity of ticarcillin plus clavulanic acid against 632 clinical isolates. *Antimicorb Agents Chemother* 1984;25:392–394.
204. Fuchs PC, Barry AL, Thornsbery C, et al. In vitro evaluation of Augmentin by broth microbilution and disk diffusion susceptibility testing: regression analysis, tentative interpretive criteria, and quality control limits. *Antimicrob Agents Chemother* 1983;24:31–38.
205. Fuchs PC, Jones RN, Barry AL, et al. Effect of clavulanic acid on the susceptibility of clinical anaerobic bacteria to ticarcillin. *Diagn Microbiol Infect Dis* 1988;9:47–50.
206. Fung-Tomc J, Huczko E, Kolek B, et al. In vitro activities of cefepime alone and with amikacin against aminoglycoside-resistant Gram-negative bacteria. *Antimicrob Agents Chemother* 1991;35:2652–2654.
207. Garrod LP, Waterworth PM. Methods of testing combined antibiotic bactericidal action and the significance of the results. *J Clin Pathol* 1962;15:328–338.
208. Geraci JE, Nichols DR, Wellman WE. Vancomycin in serious staphylococcal infections. *Arch Intern Med* 1962;109:507–515.
209. Gerber AU, Vastola AP, Brandel J, et al. Selection of aminoglycoside-resistant variants of *Pseudomonas aeruginosa* in an in vivo model. *J Infect Dis* 1982;146:691–697.
210. Gerceker AA, Gurler B. In-vitro activities of various antibiotics, alone and in combination with amikacin against *Pseudomonas aeruginosa*. *J Antimicrob Chemother* 1995;36:707–711.
211. Gevaudan MJ, Mallet MN, Gulian C, et al. Etude de la sensibilite de sept especes de mycobacteries aux nouvelles quinolones. *Pathol Biol* 1988;36:477–481.
212. Giamarellos-Bourboulis EJ, Grecka P, Giamarellou H. In-vitro interactions of DX-8739, a new carbapenem, meropenem and imipenem with amikacin against multiresistant *Pseudomonas aeruginosa*. *J Antimicrob Chemother* 1996;38:287–291.
213. Giamarellos-Bourboulis EJ, Karnesis L, Giamarellou H. Synergy of colistin with rifampin and trimethoprim/sulfamethoxazole on multidrug-resistant *Stenotrophomonas maltophilia*. *Diagn Microbiol Infect Dis* 2002;44:259–263.
214. Giamarellos-Bourboulis EJ, Xirouchaki E, Giamarellou H. Interactions of colistin and rifampin on multidrug-resistant *Acinetobacter baumannii*. *Diagn Microbiol Infect Dis* 2001;40:117–120.
215. Giamarellou H, Petrikkos G. Ciprofloxacin interactions with imipenem and amikacin against multiresistant *Pseudomonas aeruginosa*. *Antimicrob Agents Chemother* 1987;31:959–961.
216. Giamarellou H, Zissis NP, Tagari G, et al. In vitro synergistic activities of aminoglycosides and new β-lactams against multiresistant *Pseudomonas aeruginosa*. *Antimicrob Agents Chemother* 1984;25:534–536.
217. Gimeno C, Borja J, Navarro D, et al. In vitro interaction between ofloxacin and cefotaxime against gram-positive and gram-negative bacteria involved in serious infections. *Chemotherapy* 1998;44:94–98.
218. Gilbert DN, Kutscher E, Ireland P, et al. Effect of the concentrations of magnesium and calcium on the in vitro susceptibility of *Pseudomonas aeruginosa* to gentamicin. *J Infect Dis* 1971;124(Suppl):S37–S45.
219. Gilman RH, Terminel M, Levine MM, et al. Comparison of trimethoprim-sulfamethoxazole and amoxicillin in therapy of chloramphenicol-resistant and chloramphenicol-sensitive typhoid fever. *J Infect Dis* 1975;132:630–636.
220. Giron KP, Gross ME, Musher DM, et al. In vitro antimicrobial effect against *Streptococcus pneumoniae* of adding rifampin to penicillin, ceftriaxone, or 1-ofloxacin. *Antimicrob Agents Chemother* 1995;39:2798–800.
221. Glew RH, Moellering RC Jr. Effect of protein binding on the activity of penicillins in combination with gentamicin against enterococci. *Antimicrob Agents Chemother* 1979;15:87–92.
222. Glew RH, Moellering RC Jr, Buettner KR. In vitro synergism between carbenicillin and aminoglycoside aminocyclitols against *Acinetobacter calcoaceticus* var. *anitratus*. *Antimicrob Agents Chemother* 1977;11:1036–1041.
223. Glew RH, Moellering RC Jr, Kunz LJ. Infections with *Acinetobacter calcoaceticus* (*Herellea vaginicola*): clinical and laboratory studies. *Medicine* 1977;56:79–97.
224. Glew RH, Moellering RC Jr, Wennersten CBG. Comparative synergistic activity of nafcillin, oxacillin, and methicillin in combination with gentamicin against enterococci. *Antimicrob Agents Chemother* 1975;7:828–832.
225. Glew RH, Pavuk RA. Early synergistic interaction between semisynthetic penicillins and aminoglycosidic aminocyclitols against Enterobacteriaceae. *Antimicrob Agents Chemother* 1983;23:902–906.
226. Glew RH, Pavuk RA. Stability of gentamicin, tobramycin, and amikacin in combination with four β-lactam antibiotics. *Antimicrob Agents Chemother* 1983;24:474–477.
227. Glew RH, Pavuk RA. Early synergistic interactions between amikacin and six β-lactam antibiotics against multiply resistant members of the family Enterobacteriaceae. *Antimicrob Agents Chemother* 1984;26:378–381.
228. Goering RV, Sanders CC, Sanders WE Jr. Antagonism of carbenicillin and cefamandole by cefoxitin in treatment of experimental infections in mice. *Antimicrob Agents Chemother* 1982;21:963–967.
229. Gombert ME, Aulicino TM. Synergism of imipenem and amikacin in combination with other antibiotics against *Nocardia asteroides*. *Antimicrob Agents Chemother* 1983;24:810–811.
230. Gombert ME, Aulicino TM. Amikacin synergism with

β-lactam antibiotics against selected nosocomial pathogens. *J Antimicrob Chemother* 1986;17:323–326.

231. Gootz TD, Jackson DB, Sherris JC. Development of resistance to cephalosporins in clinical strains of *Citrobacter* spp. *Antimicrob Agents Chemother* 1984;25:591–595.
232. Gootz TD, Sanders CC, Goering RV. Resistance to cefamandole: derepression of β-lactamases by cefoxitin and mutation in *Enterobacter cloacae*. *J Infect Dis* 1982;146:34–42.
233. Gordin FM, Sande MA. Amdinocillin therapy of experimental animal infections. *Am J Med* 1983;75(Suppl 2A):48–53.
234. Gould IM, Milne K. In-vitro pharmacodynamic studies of piperacillin/tazobactam with gentamicin and ciprofloxacin. *J Antimicrob Chemother* 1997;39:53–61.
235. Gradelski E, Valera L, Bonner D, et al. Synergistic activities of gatifloxacin in combination with other antimicrobial agents against *Pseudomonas aeruginosa* and related species. *Antimicrob Agents Chemother* 2001;45:3220–3222.
236. Grayson ML, Eliopoulos GM, Wennersten CB, et al. Increasing resistance to β-lactam antibiotics among clinical isolates of *Enterococcus faecium*: a 22-year review at one institution. *Antimicrob Agents Chemother* 1991;35:2180–2184.
237. Grayson ML, Thauvin-Eliopoulos C, Eliopoulos GM, et al. Failure of trimethoprim-sulfamethoxazole therapy in experimental enterococcal endocarditis. *Antimicrob Agents Chemother* 1990;34:1792–1794.
238. Greenfield S, Feingold DS. The synergistic action of the sulfonamides and the polymyxins against *Serratia marcescens*. *J Infect Dis* 1970;121:555–558.
239. Greenwood D, O'Grady F. FL 1060: a new β-lactam antibiotic with novel properties. *J Clin Pathol* 1973;26:1–6.
240. Gribble MJ, Chow AW, Naiman SC, et al. Prospective randomized trial of piperacillin monotherapy versus carboxypenicilllin-aminoglycoside combination regimens in the empirical treatment of serious bacterial infections. *Antimicrob Agents Chemother* 1983;24:388–393.
241. Grif K, Dierich MP, Pfaller K, et al. In vitro activity of fosfomycin in combination with various antistaphylococcal substances. *J Antimicrob Chemother* 2001;48:209–217.
242. Grohs P, Kitzis MD, Gutmann L. In vitro bactericidal activities of linezolid in combination with vancomycin, gentamicin, ciprofloxacin, fusidic acid, and rifampin against *Staphylococcus aureus*. *Antimicrob Agents Chemother* 2003;47:418–420.
243. Grossato A, Sartori R, Fontana, R. Effect of non-β-lactam antibiotics on penicillin-binding protein synthesis of *Enterococcus hirae* ATCC 9790. *J Antimicrob Chemother* 1991;27:263–271.
244. Grunberg E, Cleeland R, Beskid G, et al. In vivo synergy between 6-amidinopenicillanic acid derivatives and other antibiotics. *Antimicrob Agents Chemother* 1976;9:589–595.
245. Guerillot F, Carret G, Flandrois JP. A statistical evaluation of the bactericidal effects of ceftibutin in combination with aminoglycosides and ciprofloxacin. *J Antimicrob Chemother* 1993;32:685–694.
246. Gutmann L, Al-Obeid S, Billot-Klein D, et al. Synergy and resistance to synergy between β-lactam antibiotics and glycopeptides against glycopeptide-resistant strains of *Enterococcus faecium*. *Antimicrob Agents Chemother* 1994;38:824–829.
247. Gutmann L, Vincent S, Billot-Klein D, et al. Involvement of penicillin-binding protein 2 with other penicillin-binding proteins in lysis of *Escherichia coli* by some β-lactam antibiotics alone and in synergistic lytic effect of amdinocillin (mecillinam). *Antimicrob Agents Chemother* 1986;30:906–912.
248. Hackbarth CJ, Chambers HF, Sande MA. Serum bactericidal activity of rifampin in combination with other antimicrobial agents against *Staphylococcus aureus*. *Antimicrob Agents Chemother* 1986;29:611–613.
249. Hakenbeck R, Tarpay M, Tomasz A. Multiple changes of penicillin-binding proteins in penicillin-resistant clinical isolates of *Streptococcus pneumoniae*. *Antimicrob Agents Chemother* 1980;17:364–371.
250. Haller I. Comprehensive evaluation of ciprofloxacin-aminoglycoside combinations against Enterobacteriaceae and *Pseudomonas aeruginosa* strains. *Antimicrob Agents Chemother* 1985;28:663–666.
251. Haller I. Comprehensive evaluation of ciprofloxacin in combination with β-lactam antibiotics against Enterobacteriaceae and *Pseudomonas aeruginosa*. *Arzneimittelforschung* 1986;36:226–229.
252. Hamburger M, Stein L. *Streptococcus viridans* subacute bacterial endocarditis: two week treatment schedule with penicillin. *JAMA* 1952;149:542–545.
253. Hancock REW, Wong PGW. Compounds which increase the permeability of the *Pseudomonas aeruginosa* outer membrane. *Antimicrob Agents Chemother* 1984;26:48–52.
254. Handwerger S, Tomasz A. Antibiotic tolerance among clinical isolates of bacteria. *Rev Infect Dis* 1985;7:368–386.
255. Harding GKM, Ronald AR. A controlled study of antimicrobial prophylaxis of recurrent urinary tract infection in women. *N Engl J Med* 1974;291:597–601.
256. Harper GJ, Cawston WC. The in vitro determination of the sulphonamide sensitivity of bacteria. *J Pathol Bacteriol* 1945;57:59–66.
257. Heineman HS, Lofton WM. Unpredictable response of *Pseudomonas aeruginosa* to synergistic antibiotic combinations in vitro. *Antimicrob Agents Chemother* 1978;13:827–831.
258. Herman LG. Antibiotic sensitivity using pretreated plates. II. A demonstration of inhibitory activity with a low level combination of a sulfonamide and polymyxin B against *Proteus* species. *Antibiot Annu* 1959;836–839.
259. Hilf M, Yu VL, Sharp J, et al. Antibiotic therapy for *Pseudomonas aeruginosa* bacteremia: outcome correlations in a prospective study of 200 patients. *Am J Med* 1989;87:540–546.
260. Hill RL, Smith CT, Seyed-Akhavani M, et al. Bactericidal and inhibitory activity of quinupristin/dalfopristin against vancomycin- and gentamicin-resistant *Enterococcus faecium*. *J Antimicrob Chemother* 1997;39 Suppl A:23–28.
261. Hindes RG, Willey SH, Eliopoulos GM, et al. Treatment of experimental endocarditis caused by β-lactamase-producing strain of *Enterococcus faecalis* with high-level resistance to gentamicin. *Antimicrob Agents Chemother* 1989;33:1019–1022.
262. Hirschl AM, Apfalter P, Makristathis A, et al. In vitro activities of linezolid alone and in combination with amoxicillin, clarithromycin, and metronidazole against *Helicobacter pylori*. *Antimicrob Agents Chemother* 2000;44:1977–1979.
263. Hitchings GH. Chemotherapy and comparative biochemistry. *Cancer Res* 1969;29:1895–1903.
264. Hitchings GH. Species differences among dihydrofolate reductases as a basis for chemotherapy. *Postgrad Med J* 1969;45(Suppl):7–10.
265. Hjelm U, Kaustova J, Kubin M, et al. Susceptibility of *Mycobacterium kansasii* to ethambutol and its combination with rifamycins, ciprofloxacin and isoniazid. *Eur J Clin Microbiol Infect Dis* 1992;11:51–54.

266. Ho JL, Klempner MS. In vitro evaluation of clindamycin in combination with oxacillin, rifampin or vancomycin against *Staphylococcus aureus*. *Diagn Microbiol Infect Dis* 1986;4:133–138.
267. Ho RI, Corman L, Morse SA, et al. Alterations in dihydropteroate synthetase in cell-free extracts of sulfanilamide-resistant *Neisseria meningitidis* and *Neisseria gonorrhoeae*. *Antimicrob Agents Chemother* 1974;5: 388–392.
268. Hodel-Christian SL, Murray BE. Characterization of the gentamicin resistance transposon Tn*538* from *Enterococcus faecalis* and comparison to staphylococcal transposons Tn*4001* and Tn*4031*. *Antimicrob Agents Chemother* 1991;35:1147–1152.
269. Hoffmann SA, Moellering RC Jr. The enterococcus: putting the bug in our ear. *Ann Intern Med* 1987;106:757–761.
270. Hoffner SE, Svenson SB, Kallenius G. Synergistic effects of antimycobacterial drug combinations on *Mycobacterium avium* complex determined radiometrically in liquid medium. *Eur J Clin Microbiol* 1987;6:530–535.
271. Holmes KK, Clark H, Silverblatt F, et al. Emergence of resistance in *Pseudomonas* during carbenicillin therapy. *Antimicrob Agents Chemother* 1970;1969:391–397.
272. Hoppes WL. Treatment of bacterial endocarditis caused by penicillin-sensitive streptococci. *Arch Intern Med* 1977;137:1122–1123.
273. Horodniceanu T, Bougueleret L, El-Solh N, et al. High-level, plasmid-borne resistance to gentamicin in *Streptococcus faecalis* subsp. *zygomeses*. *Antimicrob Agents Chemother* 1979;16:686–689.
274. Howe RA, Noel A, Bowker KE, et al. Emergence of linezolid (LIN) resistance in *Staphylococcus aureus* can be associated with loss of erythromycin (ERY) resistance. In: *Program and Abstracts of the Forty-second Interscience Conference on Antimicrobial Agents and Chemotherapy,* Abstract C1–1608, San Diego, CA. Washington, DC: American Society for Microbiology, 2002;75.
275. Hruska JF, Bernstein JM, Douglas RG Jr, et al. Effects of ribavirin on respiratory syncytial virus in vitro. *Antimicrob Agents Chemother* 1980;17:770–775.
276. Hsieh MH, Yu CM, Yu VL, et al. Synergy assessed by checkerboard: a critical analysis. *Diagn Microbiol Infect Dis* 1993;16:343–349.
277. Hunter PA, Coleman K, Fisher J, et al. In vitro synergistic properties of clavulanic acid, with ampicillin, amoxycillin and ticarcillin. *J Antimicrob Chemother* 1980;6:455–470.
278. Hunter TH. Use of streptomycin in treatment of bacterial endocarditis. *Am J Med* 1947;2:436–442.
279. Hunter TH. The treatment of some bacterial infections of the heart and pericardium. *Bull NY Acad Med* 1952;28:213–228.
280. Huovinen P. Resistance to trimethoprim-sulfamethoxazole. *Clin Infect Dis* 2001;32:1608–1614.
281. Iannini PB, Ehret J, Eickhoff TC. Effects of ampicillin-amikacin and ampicillin-rafampin on enterococci. *Antimicrob Agents Chemother* 1976;9:448–451.
282. Isenberg HD, Alperstein P, France K. In vitro activity of ciprofloxacin, levofloxacin, and trovafloxacin, alone and in combination with beta-lactams, against clinical isolates of *Pseudomonas aeruginosa, Stenotrophomonas maltophilia,* and *Burkholderia cepacia*. *Diagn Microbiol Infect Dis* 1999;33:81–86.
283. Ivler D, Leedom JM, Thrupp LD, et al. Naturally occurring sulfadiazine-resistant meningococci. *Antimcrob Agents Chemother* 1965;1964:444–450.
284. Jacobs JY, Michael J, Sacks T. Bactericidal effect of combinations of antimicrobial drugs and antineoplastic agents against *Staphylococcus aureus*. *Antimicrob Agents Chemother* 1979;15:580–586.
285. Jacoby GA, Medeiros AA. More extended-spectrum β-lactamases. *Antimicrob Agents Chemother* 1991;35: 1697–1704.
286. Jacqueline C, Caillon J, Le Mabecque V, et al. In vitro activity of linezolid alone and in combination with gentamicin, vancomycin or rifampicin against methicillin-resistant *Staphylococcus aureus* by time-kill curve methods. *J Antimicrob Chemother* 2003;51:857–864.
287. Jawetz E, Gunnison JB, Colman VR. The combined action of penicillin with streptomycin or chloromycetin on enterococci in vitro. *Science* 1950;111:254–256.
288. Jawetz E, Gunnison JB, Speck RS. Studies on antibiotic synergism and antagonism: the interference of aureomycin, chloramphenicol, and terramycin with the action of streptomycin. *Am J Med Sci* 1951;222:404–412.
289. Jawetz E, Gunnison JB, Speck RS, et al. Studies on antibiotic synergism and antagonism: the interference of chloramphenicol with the action of penicillin. *Arch Intern Med* 1951;87:349–359.
290. Jenkins SG, Lewis JW. Synergistic interaction between ofloxacin and cefotaxime against common clinical pathogens. *Infection* 1995;23:154–161.
291. Johnson DE, Thompson B. Efficacy of single-agent therapy with azlocillin, ticarcillin, and amikacin and beta-lactam/amikacin combinations for treatment of *Pseudomonas aeruginosa* bacteremia in granulocytopenic rats. *Am J Med* 1986;80(Suppl 5C):53–58.
292. Johnson DW, Kvale PA, Afable VL, et al. Single-dose antibiotic treatment of asymptomatic gonorrhea in hospitalized women. *N Engl J Med* 1970;283:16.
293. Johnson MD, MacDougall C, MacDougall Ostrosky-Zeichner L, et al. Combination antifungal therapy. *Antimicrob Agents Chemother* 2004;48:693–715.
294. Jones PG, Rolston KVI, Fainstein V, et al. Aztreonam therapy in neutropenic patients with cancer. *Am J Med* 1986;81:243–248.
295. Jones RN, Barry AL, Packer RB, et al. In vitro antimicrobial spectrum, occurrence of synergy, and recommendations for dilution susceptibility testing concentrations of the cefoperazone-sulbactam combination. *J Clin Microbiol* 1987;25:1725–1729.
296. Jones RN, Packer RR. Antimicrobial activity of amikacin combinations against Enterobacteriaceae moderately susceptible to third-generation cephalosporins. *Antimcirob Agents Chemother* 1982;22:985–989.
296a. Jung R, Husain M, Choi MK, Fish DN. Synergistic activities of moxifloxacin combined with piperacillin-tazobactam or cefepime against *Klebsiella pneumoniae, Enterobacter cloacae,* and *Acinetobacter baumannii* clinical isolates. *Antimicrob Agents Chemother* 2004;48:1055–1057.
297. Kahan FM, Kahan JS, Cassidy PJ, et al. The mechanism of action of fosfomycin (phosphomycin). *Ann NY Acad Sci* 1974;235:364–286.
298. Kahn SB, Fein SA, Brodsky I. Effects of trimethoprim on folate metabolism in man. *Clin Pharmacol Ther* 1968;9:550–560.
299. Kang SL, Rybak MJ. Pharmacodynamics of RP 59500 alone and in combination with vancomycin against *Staphylococcus aureus* in an in vitro-infected fibrin clot model. *Antimicrob Agents Chemother* 1995;39:1505–1511.
300. Kang SL, Rybak MJ. In-vitro bactericidal activity of quinupristin/dalfopristin alone and in combination against resistant strains of *Enterococcus species* and *Staphylococcus aureus*. *J Antimicrob Chemother* 1997;39(Suppl A):33–39.

301. Kaplan AH, Gilligan PH, Facklam RR. Recovery of resistant enterococci during vancomycin prophylaxis. *Antimicrob Agents Chemother* 1988;26:1216–1218.
302. Kaplan SA, Weinfeld RE, Abruzzo CW, et al. Pharmacokinetic profile of trimethoprim-sulamethoxazole in man. *J Infect Dis* 1973;128(Suppl):S547–S555.
303. Karchmer AW, Archer GL, Dismukes WE. Rifampin treatment of prosthetic valve endocarditis due to *Staphylococcus epidermidis*. *Rev Infect Dis* 1983;5(Suppl 3):S543–S548.
304. Karchmer AW, Moellering RC Jr, Maki DG, et al. Single antibiotic treatment of streptococcal endocarditis. *JAMA* 1978;241:1801–1806.
305. Karlowsky JA, Kelly LJ, Thornsberry C, et al. Trends in antimicrobial resistance among urinary tract infection isolates of *Escherichia coli* from female outpatients in the United States. *Antimicrob Agents Chemother* 2002;46:2540–2545.
306. Kaufhold A, Potgieter E. Chromosomally mediated high-level gentamicin resistance in *Streptococcus mitis*. *Antimicrob Agents Chemother* 1993;37:2740–2742.
307. Kelly MT, Matsen JM. In vitro activity, synergism, and testing parameters of amikacin, with comparisons to other aminoglycoside antibiotics. *Antimicrob Agents Chemother* 1976;9:440–447.
308. Kent RJ, Bakhtiar M, Shanson DC. The in-vitro bactericidal activities of combinations of antimicrobial agents against clinical isolates of *Mycobacterium-avium-intracellulare*. *J Antimicrob Chemother* 1992;30:643–650.
309. Kerry DW, Hamilton-Miller JMT, Brumfitt W. Laboratory studies on mecillinam; activity alone and in combination with cephradine. *J Antimicrob Chemother* 1977;3(Suppl B):53–58.
310. Khan W, Ross S, Rodriguez W, et al. *Haemophilus influenzae* type B resistant to penicillin: a report of two cases. *JAMA* 1974;229:298–301.
311. King TC, Krogstad DJ. Spectrophotometric assessment of dose-response curves for single antimicrobials and antimicrobial combinations. *J Infect Dis* 1983;147:758–764.
312. King TC, Schlessinger D, Krogstad DJ. The assessment of drug combinations. *Rev Infect Dis* 1981;3:627–633.
313. Kitzis MD, Gutmann L, Acar JF. In vitro susceptibility of *Nocardia asteroides* to 21 β-lactam antibiotics, in combination with β-lactamase inhibitors, and its relationship to the β-lactamase content. *J Antimicrob Chemother* 1985;15:23–30.
314. Klastersky J. Antibiotic susceptibility of oxacillin-resistant staphylococci. *Antimcirob Agents Chemother* 1972;1:441–446.
315. Klastersky J, Cappel R, Daneau D. Clinical significance of in vitro synergism between antibiotics in Gram-negative infections. *Antimicrob Agents Chemother* 1972;2:470–475.
316. Klastersky J, Cappel R, Swings G, et al. Bacteriological and clinical activity of the ampicillin/gentamicin and cephalothin/gentamicin combinations. *Am J Med Sci* 1971;262:283–290.
317. Klastersky J, Glauser MP, Schimpff SC, et al. Prospective randomized comparison of three antibiotic regimens for empirical therapy of suspected bacteremic infection in febrile granulocytopenic patients. *Antimicrob Agents Chemother* 1986;29:263–270.
318. Klastersky J, Henri A, Vandenborre L. Antimicrobial activity of tobramycin and gentamicin used in combination with cephalothin and carbenicillin. *Am J Med Sci* 1973;266:13–21.
319. Klastersky J, Hensgens C, Meunier-Carpentier F. Comparative effectiveness of combinations of amikacin with penicillin G and amikacin with carbenicillin in Gram-negative septicemia: a double-blind clinical trial. *J Infect Dis* 1976;134(Suppl):S433–S440.
320. Klastersky J, Meunier-Carpentier F, Prevost JM, et al. Synergism between amikacin and cefazolin against *Klebsiella:* in vitro studies and effect on the bactericidal activity of serum. *J Infect Dis* 1976;134:271–276.
321. Klatersky J, Nyamubeya B, Vandenborre L. Antimicrobial effectiveness of kanamycin, aminosidin, BBK-8, sisomicin, gentamicin, and tobramycin combined with carbenicillin or cephalothin against Gram-negative rods. *J Med Microbiol* 1974;7:465–472.
322. Klastersky J, Swings G, Daneau D. Antimicrobial activity of the carbenicillin/gentamicin combination against Gram-negative bacilli. *Am J Med Sci* 1970;260:373–380.
323. Klastersky J, Zinner SH. Synergistic combinations of antibiotics in Gram-negative bacillary infections. *Rev Infect Dis* 1982;4:294–301.
324. Kluge RM, Standiford HC, Tatem B, et al. Comparative activity of tobramycin, amikacin, and gentamicin alone and with carbenicillin against *Pseudomonas aeruginosa*. *Antimicrob Agents Chemother* 1974;6:442–446.
325. Klugman KP, Capper T, Bryskier A. In vitro susceptibility of penicillin-resistant *Streptococcus pneumoniae* to levofloxacin, selection of resistant mutants, and time-kill synergy studies of levofloxacin combined with vancomycin, teicoplanin, fusidic acid, and rifampin. *Antimicrob Agents Chemother* 1996;40:2802–2804.
326. Koch AE, Burchall JJ. Reversal of the antimicrobial activity of trimethoprim by thymidine in commercially prepared media. *Appl Microbiol* 1971;22:812–817.
327. Kohler T, Kok M, Michea-Hamzehpour M, et al. Multidrug efflux in intrinsic resistance to trimethoprim and sulfamethoxazole in *Pseudomonas aeruginosa*. *Antimicrob Agents Chemother* 1996;40:2288–2290.
328. Kong X-B, Zhu Q-Y, Ruprecht R, et al. Synergistic inhibition of human immunodeficiency virus type 1 replication in vitro by two-drug and three-drug combinations of 3-azido-3-deoxythymidine, phosphonoformate, and 2,3-dideoxythymidine. *Antimicrob Agents Chemother* 1991;35:2003–2011.
329. Korvick JA, Bryan CS, Farber B, et al. Observational study of *Klebsiella* bacteremia in 230 patients: outcome for antibiotic combinations versus monotherapy. *Antimicrob Agents Chemother* 1992;36:2639–2644.
330. Korvick JA, Peacock JE Jr, Muder RR, et al. Addition to rifampin to combination antibiotic therapy for *Pseudomonas aeruginosa* bacteremia: prospective trial using the Zelen protocol. *Antimicrob Agents Chemother* 1992;36:620–625.
331. Korzeniowski O, Sande MA, National Collaborative Endocarditis Study Group. Combination antimicrobial therapy for *Staphylococcus aureus* endocarditis in patients addicted to parenteral drugs and in nonaddicts. *Ann Intern Med* 1982;97:496–503.
332. Korzeniowski O, Wennersten CBG, Moellering RC Jr, et al. Penicillin-netilmicin synergism against *Streptococcus faecalis*. *Antimicrob Agents Chemother* 1978;13:430–434.
333. Krogstad DJ, Korfhagen TR, Moellering RC Jr, et al. Aminoglycoside-inactivating enzymes: an explanation for resistance to penicillin-aminoglycoside synergism in enterococci. *J Clin Invest* 1978;62:480–486.
334. Krogstad DJ, Korfhagen TR, Moellering RC Jr, et al. Plasmid-mediated resistance to antibiotic synergism in enterococci. *J Clin Invest* 1978;61:1645–1653.
335. Krogstad DJ, Murray PR, Granich GG, et al. Sodium polyanethol sulfonate inactivation of aminoglycosdes. *Antimicrob Agents Chemother* 1981;20:272–274.

336. Kuck NA, Jacobus NV, Petersen PJ, et al. Comparative in vitro and in vivo activities of piperacillin combined with the β-lactamase inhibitors tazobactam, clavulanic acid and sulbactam. *Antimicrob Agents Chemother* 1989;33:1964–1969.
337. Kuck NA, Testa RT, Forbes M. In vitro and in vivo antibacterial effects of combinations of β-lactam antibiotics. *Antimicrob Agents Chemother* 1981;19:634–638.
338. Kuhn F, Cottagnoud M, Acosta F, et al. Cefotaxime acts synergistically with levofloxacin in experimental meningitis due to penicillin-resistant pneumococci and prevents selection of levofloxacin-resistant mutants in vitro. *Antimicrob Agents Chemother* 2003;47:2487–2491.
339. Kurtz TO, Winston DJ, Bruckner DA, et al. Comparative in vitro synergistic activity of new β-lactam antimicrobial agents and amikacin against *Pseudomonas aeruginosa* and *Serratia marcescens*. *Antimicrob Agents Chemother* 1981;20:239–243.
340. Landman D, Mobarakai NK, Quale JM. Novel antibiotic regimens against *Enterococcus faecium* resistant to ampicillin, vancomycin, and gentamicin. *Antimicrob Agents Chemother* 1993;37:1904–1908.
341. Landy M, Gerstung RB. *P*-Aminobenzoic acid synthesis by *Neisseria gonorrhoeae* in relation to clinical and cultural sulfonamide resistance. *J Immunol* 1945;51:269–277.
342. Lapointe J-R, Lavallee C, Meilleur R, et al. Roxithromycin alone and in combination with sulphamethoxazole against *Haemophilus influenzae*. *J Antimicrob Chemother* 1987;20(Suppl B):21–29.
343. Lau WK, Young LS, Black RE, et al. Comparative efficacy and toxicity of amikacin/carbenicillin versus gentamicin/carbenicillin in leukopenic patients: a randomized prospective trial. *Am J Med* 1977;62:959–966.
344. LeBouguenec C, Horodniceanu T. Conjugative R plasmids in *Streptococcus faecalis* (group D). *Antimicrob Agents Chemother* 1982;21:698–705.
345. Leclercq R, Bingen E, Su QH, et al. Effects of combinations of β-lactams, daptomycin, gentamicin and glycopeptides against glycopeptide-resistant enterococci. *Antimicrob Agents Chemother* 1991;35:92–98.
346. Leclercq R, Derlot E, Duval J, et al. Plasmid-mediated resistance to vancomycin and teicoplanin in *Enterococcus faecium*. *N Engl J Med* 1988;319:157–161.
347. Lederberg J, Lederberg EM. Replica plating and indirect selection of bacterial mutants. *J Bacteriol* 1952;63:399–406.
348. Lee WS, Komarmy L. Simple technique for the assay of antibiotic synergism against enterococci. *Antimicrob Agents Chemother* 1975;7:82–84.
349. Lees L, Milson JA, Knirsch AK, et al. Sulbactam plus ampicillin: interim review of efficacy and safety for therapeutic and prophylactic use. *Rev Infect Dis* 1986;8(Suppl 5):S644–S650.
350. Lehr D. Inhibition of drug precipitation in the urinary tract by the use of sulfonamide mixtures. I. Sulfathiazole-sulfadiazine mixture. *Proc Soc Exp Biol Med* 1945;58:11–14.
351. Lehr D. Prevention of renal damage by use of mixtures of sulfonamides: animal-experimental and clinical studies. *Br Med J* 1947;2:943–946.
352. Leibovici L, Paul M, Poznanski O, et al. Monotherapy versus beta-lactam-aminoglycoside combination treatment for gram-negative bacteremia: a prospective, observational study. *Antimicrob Agents Chemother* 1997;41:1127–1133.
353. Lell B, Ruangweerayut, Wiesner J, et al. Fosmidomycin, a novel chemotherapeutic agent for malaria. *Antimicrob Agents Chemother* 2003;47:735–738.
354. Leng B, Meyers BR, Hirschman SZ, et al. Susceptibilities of Gram-negative bacteria to combinations of antimicrobial agents in vitro. *Antimicrob Agents Chemother* 1975;8:164–171.
355. Lepper MH, Dowling HF. Treatment of pneumococcic meningitis with penicillin compared with penicillin plus aureomycin: studies including observations on an apparent antagonism between penicillin and aureomycin. *Arch Intern Med* 1951;88:489–494.
356. Levison ME, Mangura CT, Lorber B, et al. Clindamycin compared with penicillin for the treatment of anaerobic lung abscess. *Ann Intern Med* 1983;98:466–471.
357. Levy J, Klastersky J. Synergism between amikacin and cefazolin against *Staphylococcus aureus:* a comparative study of oxacillin-sensitive and oxacillin-resistant strains. *J Antimicrob Chemother* 1979;5:365–373.
358. Lewin C, Doherty C, Govan J. In vitro activities of meropenem, PD 127391, PD 131628, ceftazidime, chloramphenicol, co-trimoxazole, and ciprofloxacin against *Pseudomonas cepacia*. *Antimicrob Agents Chemother* 1993;37:123–125.
359. Lewis CS, Howard BM, Smith JT. 4-Quinolone interactions with gyrase subunit B inhibitors. *J Med Microbiol* 1991;35:358–362.
360. Li RC, Schentag JJ, Nix DE. The fractional maximal effect method: a new way to characterize the effect of antibiotic combinations and other nonlinear pharmacodynamic interactions. *Antimicrob Agents Chemother* 1993;37:523–531.
361. Libke RD, Regamey C, Clarke JT, et al. Synergism of carbenicillin and gentamicin against enterococci. *Antimicrob Agents Chemther* 1973;4:564–568.
362. Lincoln LJ, Weinstein AJ, Gallagher M, et al. Penicillinase-resistant penicillins plus gentamicin in experimental enterococcal endocarditis. *Antimicrob Agents Chemother* 1977;12:484–489.
363. Ling J, Kam KM, Lam AW, et al. Susceptibilities of Hong Kong isolates of multiply resistant *Shigella* spp. to 25 antimicrobial agents, including ampicillin plus sulbactam and new 4-quinolones. *Antimicrob Agents Chemother* 1988;32:20–23.
364. Lipman ML, Silva J Jr. Endocarditis due to *Streptococcus faecalis* with high-level resistance to gentamicin. *Rev Infect Dis* 1989;11:325–328.
365. Lomovskaya O, Warren MS, Lee A, et al. Identification and characterization of inhibitors of multidrug resistance efflux pumps in *Pseudomonas aeruginosa:* novel agents for combination therapy. *Antimicrob Agents Chemother* 2001;45:105–116.
366. Lomovskaya O, Watkins W. Inhibition of efflux pumps as a novel approach to combat drug resistance in bacteria. *J Mol Microbiol Biotechnol* 2001;3:225–236.
367. Lorian V. Some effects of subinhibitory concentrations of antibiotics on bacteria. *Bull NY Acad Med* 1975;51:1046–1055.
368. Lorian V, Atkinson B, Kim Y. Effect of rifampin and oxacillin on the ultrastructure and growth of *Staphylococcus aureus*. *Rev Infect Dis* 1983;5(Suppl 3):S418–S427.
369. Lorian V, Ernst J. Activity of amikacin and ampicillin in succession and in combination. *Diagn Microbiol Infect Dis* 1988;11:163–169.
370. Lorian V, Fernandes F. Synergic activity of vancomycin-quinupristin/dalfopristin combination against *Enterococcus faecium*. *J Antimicrob Chemother* 1997;39(Suppl A):63–66.
371. Lorian V, Fodor G. Technique for determining the bactericidal effect of drug combinations. *Antimicrob Agents Chemother* 1974;5:630–633.
372. Louie TJ, Onderdonk AB, Gorbach SL, et al. Therapy for

experimental intraabdominal sepsis: comparison of four cephalosporins with clindamycin plus gentamicin. *J Infect Dis* 1977;135(Suppl):S18–S22.

373. Lowy FD, Chang DS, Lash PR. Synergy of combinations of vancomycin, gentamicin, and rifampin against methicillin-resistant, coagulase-negative staphylococci. *Antimicrob Agents Chemother* 1983;23:932–934.
374. Lozniewski A, Lion C, Mory F, et al. In vitro synergy between cefepime and vancomycin against methicillin-susceptible and -resistant *Staphylococcus aureus* and *Staphylococcus epidermidis*. *J Antimicrob Chemother* 2001;47:83–86.
375. Luboshitzky R, Sacks T, Michael J. Bactericidal effect of combinations of antibiotics on *Klebsiella-Enterobacter-Serratia*. *Chemotherapy* 1973;19:354–366.
376. Lund F, Tybring L. 6-β-Amidinopenicillinanic acids: a new group of antibiotics. *Nature New Biol* 1972;236:135–137.
377. Lyon MD, Smith KR, Saag MS, et al. In vitro activity of piperacillin, ticarcillin and mezlocillin alone and in combination with aminoglycosides against *Pseudomonas aeruginosa*. *Antimicrob Agents Chemother* 1986;30:25–30.
378. MacGowan AP, Holt HA, Reeves. In-vitro synergy testing of nine antimicrobial combinations against *Listeria monocytogenes*. *J Antimicrob Chemother* 1990;25:561–566.
379. MacGowan AR, Bowker K, Bedford KA, et al. Synergy testing of macrolide combinations using the chequerboard technique. *J Antimicrob Chemother* 1993;32:913–915.
380. McCormick GJ, Canfield CJ. In vitro evaluation of antimalarial drug combinations. *Proc Helminthol Soc Wash* 1972;39(Suppl):292–297.
381. McDougal LK, Thornsberry C. In vitro bacterial synergism of rifampin and trimethoprim and implications for treatment of carriers of *Haemophilus influenzae*. *J Antimicrob Chemother* 1982;9:369–378.
382. McGowan JE, Terry PM, Nahmias AJ. Susceptibility of *Haemophilus influenze* isolates from blood and cerebrospinal fluid to ampicillin, chloramphenicol and trimethoprim-sulfamethoxazole. *Antimicrob Agents Chemother* 1976;9:137–139.
383. McLaughlin FJ, Matthews WJ Jr, Strieder DJ, et al. Clinical and bacteriological responses to three antibiotic regimens for acute exacerbations of cystic fibrosis: ticarcillin-tobramycin, azlocillin-tobramycin, and azlocillin-placebo. *J Infect Dis* 1983;147:559–567.
384. McLaughlin JE, Reeves DS. Clinical and laboratory evidence for inactivation of gentamicin by carbenicillin. *Lancet* 1971;1:261–264.
385. Maderazo EG, Quintiliani R. Treatment of norcardial infection with trimethoprim and sulfamethoxazole. *Am J Med* 1974;57:671–675.
386. Mainardi JL, Gutmann L, Acar JF, et al. Synergistic effect of amoxicillin and cefotaxime against *E. faecalis*. *Antimicrob Agents Chemother* 1995;39:1984–1987.
387. Manning JM, Merrifield NE, Jones WM, et al. Inhibition of bacterial growth by β-chloro-D-alanine. *Proc Natl Acad Sci USA* 1974;71:417–421.
388. Manno G, Ugolotti E, Belli ML, et al. Use of the E test to assess synergy of antibiotic combinations against isolates of *Burkholderia cepacia*-complex from patients with cystic fibrosis. *Eur J Clin Microbiol Infect Dis* 2003;22:28–34.
389. Marier RL, Joyce N, Andriole VT. Synergism of oxacillin and gentamicin against enterococci. *Antimicrob Agents Chemother* 1975;8:571–573.
390. Markowitz SM, Sibilla DJ. Comparative susceptibilities of clinical isolates of *Serratia marcescens* to newer cephalosporins, alone and in combination with various aminoglycosides. *Antimicrob Agents Chemother* 1980;18:651–655.
391. Marks MI, Hammerberg S, Greenstone G, et al. Activity of the newer aminoglycosides and carbenicillin, alone in combination, against gentamicin-resistant *Pseudomonas aeruginosa*. *Antimicrob Agents Chemother* 1976;10:399–401.
392. Marone P, Navarra A, Monzillo V, et al. Antibacterial activity of combined cefotaxime and desacetyl-cefotaxime against aerobic and anaerobic Gram-negative bacilli. *Drugs Exp Clin Res* 1990;16:629–633.
393. Marques MB, Brookings ES, Moser SA, et al. Comparative in vitro antimicrobial susceptibilities of nosocomial isolates of *Acinetobacter baumannii* and synergistic activities of nine antimicrobial combinations. *Antimicrob Agents Chemother* 1997;41:881–885.
394. Marshall WF, Keating MR, Anhalt JP, et al. *Xanthomonas maltophilia*: an emerging nosocomial pathogen. *Mayo Clin Proc* 1989;64:1097–1104.
395. Martin SJ, Pendland SL, Chen C, et al. In vitro synergy testing of macrolide-quinolone combinations against 41 clinical isolates of *Legionella*. *Antimicrob Agents Chemother* 1996;40:1419–1421.
396. Martinez JL, Vincente MF, Delgado-Iribarren A, et al. Small plasmids are involved in amoxicillin-clavulanate resistance in *Escherichia coli*. *Antimicrob Agents Chemother* 1989;33:595.
397. Maslow MJ, Simberkoff MS, Rahal JJ. Clinical efficacy of a synergistic combination of cefotaxime and amikacin against multiresistant *Pseudomonas* and *Serratia* infections. *J Antimicrob Chemother* 1985;16:227–234.
398. Masuda G, Nakamura K, Yajima T, et al. Bacteriostatic and bactericidal activities of β-lactam antibiotics enhanced by the addition of low concentration of gentamicin. *Antimicrob Agents Chemother* 1980;17:334–336.
399. Matsuda K, Asahi Y, Sanada M, et al. In-vitro activity of imipenem combined with β-lactam antibiotics for methicillin-resistant *Staphylococcus aureus*. *J Antimicrob Chemother* 1991;27:809–815.
400. Matsuhashi M, Dietrich CP, Strominger JL. Biosynthesis of the peptidoglycan of bacterial cell walls. III. The role of soluble ribonucleic acid of lipid intermediates in glycine incorporation in *Staphylococcus aureus*. *J Biol Chem* 1967;242:3191–3206.
401. Matsuhashi T, Kamiryo T, Blumberg PM, et al. Mechanisms of action and development of resistance to a new amidino penicillin. *J Bacteriol* 1974;117:578–587.
402. Matsumura SO, Louie L, Louie M, et al. Synergy testing of vancomycin-resistant *Enterococcus faecium* against quinupristin-dalfopristin in combination with other antimicrobial agents. *Antimicrob Agents Chemother* 1999;43:2776–2779.
403. Matsuura M, Nakazawa H, Hashimoto T, et al. Combined antibacterial activity of amoxicillin with clavulanic acid against ampicillin-resistant strains. *Antimicrob Agents Chemother* 1980;17:908–911.
404. Mayer I, Nagy E. Investigation of the synergic effects of aminoglycoside-fluoroquinolone and third-generation cephalosporin combinations against clinical isolates of *Pseudomonas* spp. *J Antimicrob Chemother* 1999;43:651–657.
405. McKessar SJ, Berry AM, Bell JM, et al. Genetic characterization of vanG, a novel vancomycin resistance locus of *Enterococcus faecalis*. *Antimicrob Agents Chemother* 2000;44:3224–3228.
406. Meade RH III. Streptomycin and sulfisoxazole for treatment of *Haemophilus influenzae* meningitis. *JAMA* 1978;239:324–327.

407. Meares EM Jr. Observations on activity of trimethoprim-sulfamethoxazole in the prostate. *J Infect Dis* 1973; 128(Suppl):S679–S685.
408. Mederski-Samoraj BD, Murray BE. High-level resistance to gentamicin in clinical isolates of enterococci. *J Infect Dis* 1983;147:751–757.
409. Medoff G, Comfort M, Kobayashi GS. Synergistic action of amphotericin B and 5-fluorocytosine against yeast-like organisms. *Proc Soc Exp Biol Med* 1971;138:571–574.
410. Messick CR, Pendland SL. In vitro activity of chloramphenicol alone and in combination with vancomycin, ampicillin, or RP 59500 (quinupristin/dalfopristin) against vancomycin-resistant enterococci. *Diagn Microbiol Infect Dis* 1997;29:203–205.
411. Michel J, Bornstein H, Luboshitzky R, et al. Mechanisms of chloramphenicol-cephaloridine synergism on Enterobacteriaceae. *Antimicrob Agents Chemother* 1975;7:845–849.
412. Michel J, Jacobs J, Sacks T. Bactericidal synergistic effect due to chloramphenicol-induced inhibition of staphylococcal penicillinase. *Chemotherapy* 1977;23:32–36.
413. Michelet C, Avril JL, Arvieux C, et al. Comparative activities of new fluoroquinolones, alone or in combination with amoxicillin, trimethoprim-sulfamethoxazole, or rifampin, against intracellular *Listeria monocytogenes*. *Antimicrob Agents Chemother* 1997;41:60–65.
414. Miller MH, Feinstein SA, Chow RT. Early effects of β-lactams on aminoglycoside uptake, bactericidal rates, and turbidimetrically measured growth inhibition in *Pseudomonas aeruginosa*. *Antimicrob Agents Chemother* 1987;31:108–110.
415. Mimoz O, Jacolot A, Leotard S, et al. Efficacies of cefepime, ceftazidime, and imipenem alone or in combination with amikacin in rats with experimental pneumonia due to ceftazidime-susceptible or -resistant *Enterobacter cloacae* strains. *Antimicrob Agents Chemother* 1998;42:3304–3308.
416. Mimoz O, Jacolot A, Padoin C, et al. Cefepime and amikacin synergy in vitro and in vivo against a ceftazidime-resistant strain of *Enterobacter cloacae*. *J Antimicrob Chemother* 1998;41:367–372.
417. Mintz L, Drew WL. Comparative synergistic activity of cefoperazone, cefotaxime, moxalactam, and carbenicillin, combined with tobramycin, against *Pseudomonas aeruginosa*. *Antimicrob Agents Chemother* 1981;19:332–334.
418. Mitsuhashi S, Inoue M. Resistance to macrolides and lincomycins. In: Bryan LE, ed. *Antimicrobial drug resistance*. Orlando, FL: Academic Press, 1984;279–281.
419. Moeller O, Holmgren J. A paper disc technique for studying antibacterial synergism. *Acta Pathol Microbiol Scan* 1969;76:141–145.
420. Moellering RC Jr. The enterococcus: a classic example of the impact of antimicrobial resistance on therapeutic options. *J Antimicrob Chemother* 1991;28:1–12.
421. Moellering RC Jr, Medoff G, Leech I, et al. Antibiotic synergism against *Listeria monocytogenes*. *Antimicrob Agents Chemother* 1972;1:30–34.
422. Moellering RC Jr, Murray BE, Schoenbaum SC, et al. A novel mechanism of resistance to penicillin-gentamicin synergism in *Streptococcus faecalis*. *J Infect Dis* 1980; 141:71–86.
423. Moellering RC Jr, Weinberg AN. Studies on antibiotic synergism against enterococci. II. Effect of various antibiotics on the uptake of ^{14}C-labeled streptomycin by enterococci. *J Clin Invest* 1971;50:2580–2584.
424. Moellering RC Jr, Wennersten CB, Medrek T, et al. Prevalence of high-level resistance to aminoglycosides in clinical isolates of enterococci. *Antimicrob Agents Chemother* 1971;1970:335–340.
425. Moellering RC Jr, Wennersten CB, Weinberg AN. Studies on antibiotic synergism against enterococci. I. Bacteriologic studies. *J Lab Clin Med* 1971;77:821–828.
426. Moellering RC Jr, Wennersten CB, Weinberg AN. Synergy of penicillin and gentamicin against enterococci. *J Infect Dis* 1971;124 (Suppl):S207–S209.
427. Moellering RC Jr, Wennersten CB, Weinberg AN. Penicillin-tobramycin synergism against enterococci: a comparison with penicillin and gentamicin. *Antimicrob Agents Chemother* 1973;3:526–529.
428. Molinari G, Saverino D, Paglia P, et al. Synergistic antibacterial interaction of cefotaxime and desacetylecefotaxime. *J Chemother* 1991;3:6–12.
429. Moody JA, Peterson LR, Gerding DN. In vitro activity of ciprofloxacin combined with azlocillin. *Antimicrob Agents Chemother* 1985;28:849–850.
430. Moyenuddin M, Ohl CA, Williamson JC, et al. Disseminated oxacillin-resistant *Staphylococcus aureus* infection responsive to vancomycin and quinupristin-dalfopristin combination therapy. *J Antimicrob Chemother* 2003;51:202–203.
431. Mulazimoglu L, Drenning SD, Muder RR. Vancomycin-gentamicin synergism revisited: effect of gentamicin susceptibility of methicillin-resistant *Staphylococcus aureus*. *Antimicrob Agents Chemother* 1996;40:1534–1535.
432. Mulazimoglu L, Drenning SD, Yu VL. In vitro activities of two novel oxazolidinones (U100592 and U100766), a new fluoroquinolone (trovafloxacin), and dalfopristin-quinupristin against *Staphylococcus aureus* and *Staphylococcus epidermidis*. *Antimicrob Agents Chemother* 1996;40:2428–2430.
433. Murray BE, Church DA, Wanger A, et al. Comparison of two β-lactamase-producing strains of *Streptococcus faecalis*. *Antimicrob Agents Chemother* 1986;30:861–864.
434. Murray BE, Karchmer AW, Moellering RC Jr. Diphtheroid prosthetic valve endocarditis: a study of clinical features and infecting organisms. *Am J Med* 1980;69:838–848.
435. Murray BE, Mederski-Samoraj B. Transferable β-lactamase: a new mechanism for in vitro penicillin resistance in *Streptococcus faecalis*. *J Clin Invest* 1983;72:1168–1171.
436. Murray BE, Mederski-Samoraj B, Foster SK, et al. In vitro studies of plasmid-mediated penicillinase from *Streptococcus faecalis* suggest a staphylococcal origin. *J Clin Invest* 1986;77:289–293.
437. Murray BE, Moellering RC Jr. Aminoglycoside-modifying enzymes among clinical isolates of *Acinetobacter calcoaceticus* subsp. *anitratus (Herellea vaginicola)*: explanation for high-level aminoglycoside resistance. *Antimicrob Agents Chemother* 1979;15:190–199.
438. Murray BE, Moellering RC Jr. Evidence of plasmid-mediated production of aminoglycoside-modifying enzymes not previously described in *Acinetobacter calcoaceticus*. *Antimicrob Agents Chemother* 1980; 17:30–36.
439. Murray BE, Singh KV, Markowitz SM, et al. Evidence for clonal spread of a single strain of β-lactamase-producing *Enterococcus (Streptococcus) faecalis* to six hospitals in five states. *J Infect Dis* 1991;163:780–785.
440. Murray PR. Activity of cefotaxime-aminoglycoside combinations against aminoglycoside-resistant *Pseudomonas*. *Antimicrob Agents Chemother* 1980;17:474–476.
441. Murray PR, Granich GG, Krogstad DJ, et al. In vivo selection of resistance to multiple cephalosporins. *J Infect Dis* 1983;147:590.
442. Musher DM, Griffith DP. Generation of formaldehyde

from methenamine: effect of pH and concentration, and antibacterial effect. *Antimicrob Agents Chemother* 1974;6:708–711.

443. Musher DM, Griffith DP, Tyler M, et al. Potentiation of the antibacterial effect of methenamine by acetohydroxamic acid. *Antimicrob Agents Chemother* 1974;5:101–105.
444. Nachamkin I, Axelrod P, Talbot GH, et al. Multiply high-level aminoglycoside-resistant enterococci isolated from patients in a university hospital. *J Clin Microbiol* 1988;26:1287–1291.
445. Najioullah F, Pellon G, Freney J, et al. Fosfomycin enhances the expression of penicillin-binding protein 2 in methicillin-sensitive and methicillin-resistant *Staphylococcus aureus* strains. *FEMS Microbiol Lett* 1992;76:221–226.
446. Nakamura A, Hosoda M, Kato T, et al. Combined effects of meropenem and aminoglycosides on *Pseudomonas aeruginosa* in vitro. *J Antimicrob Chemother* 2000;46:901–904.
447. National Committee for Clinical Laboratory Standards. *Methods for antimicrobial susceptibility testing of anaerobic bacteria: approved standard,* 4th ed. National Committee for Clinical Laboratory Standards document M11-A4. Villanova, PA: National Committee for Clinical Laboratory Standards, 1997.
448. National Committee for Clinical Laboratory Standards. *Methods for dilution antimicrobial susceptibility tests for bacteria that grow aerobically: approved standard,* 6th ed. National Committee for Clinical Laboratory Standards document M7-A6. Villanova, PA: National Committee for Clinical Laboratory Standards, 2003.
449. Nelson JD, Kusmiesz H, Jackson LH, et al. Trimethoprim-sulfamethoxazole therapy for shigellosis. *JAMA* 1976; 235:1239–1243.
450. Neu HC. Synergy of mecillinam, a β-amidinopenicillanic acid derivative, combined with β-lactam antibiotics. *Antimicrob Agents Chemother* 1976;10:535–542.
451. Neu HC. Mecillinam: an amidino penicillin which acts synergistically with other β-lactam compounds. *J Antimicrob Chemother* 1977;3(Suppl B):43–52.
452. Neu HC. Synergistic activity of mecillinam in combination with the β-lactamase inhibitors clavulanic acid and sulbactam. *Antimicrob Agents Chemother* 1982;22:518–519.
453. Neu HC, Chin N-X, Gu J-W. The in-vitro activity of new streptogramins, RP 59500, RP 57669, and RP 54476, alone and in combination. *J Antimicrob Chemother* 1992;30(Suppl A):83–94.
454. Neu HC, Chin N-X, Labthavikul P. Antibacterial activity of coumermycin alone and in combination with other antibiotics. *Antimicrob Agents Chemother* 1984;25:687–689.
455. Neu HC, Fu KP. Clavulanic acid, a novel inhibitor of β-lactamase. *Antimicrob Agents Chemother* 1978;14:650–655.
456. Neu HC, Fu KP. Synergy of azlocillin and mezlocillin combined with aminoglycoside antibiotics and cephalosporins. *Antimicrob Agents Chemother* 1978;13:813–819.
457. Neu HC, Fu KP. Synergistic activity of piperacillin in combination with β-lactamase inhibitors. *Antimicrob Agents Chemother* 1980;18:582–585.
458. Neu HC, Kamimura T. Synergy of fosmidomycin (FR-31564) and other antimicrobial agents. *Antimicrob Agents Chemother* 1982;22:560–563.
459. Neuman M. Recent developments in the field of phosphonic acid antibiotics. *J Antimicrob Chemother* 1984;14:309–311.
460. Nicas TI, Yu CYE, Hobbs JN Jr, et al. Characterization of vancomycin resistance in *Enterococcus faecium* and *Enterococcus faecalis*. *Antimicrob Agents Chemother* 1989;33:1121–1124.
461. Nissen LR, Jacobsen J, Ravn TJ, et al. Fosfomycin-ampicillin versus gentamicin-ampicillin in the treatment of critically ill patients with pneumonia. *Infection* 1986;14:246–249.
462. Nitidandhaprabhas P, Sittapairochan D. Treatment of nocardial mycetoma with trimethoprim and sulfamethoxazole. *Arch Dermatol* 1975;111:1345–1348.
463. Nolte H, Buettner H. Pharmacokinetics of trimethoprim and its combination with sulfamethoxazole in man after single and chronic oral administration. *Chemotherapy* 1973;18:274–284.
464. Norden CW, Shaffer MA. Activities of tobramycin and azlocillin alone and in combination against experimental oteomyelitis caused by *Pseudomonas aeruginosa*. *Antimicrob Agents Chemother* 1982;21:62–65.
465. Norden CW, Shafer M. In vitro synergism between mezlocillin and isoxazolyl penicillins against β-lactamase-producing Gram-negative organisms. *J Antimicrob Chemother* 1983;11:377–380.
466. Novick RP. Staphylococcal penicillinase and the new penicillins. *Biochem J* 1962;83:229–235.
467. O'Callaghan CH, Muggleton PW, Kirby SM, et al. Inhibition of β-lactamase decomposition of cephaloridine and cephalothin by other cephalosporins. *Antimicrob Agents Chemother* 1967;1966:337–343.
468. Odds FC. Interactions among amphotericin B, 5-fluorocytosine, and miconazole against pathogenic fungi in vitro. *Antimicrob Agents Chemother* 1982;22:763–770.
469. Odds FC. Synergy, antagonism, and what the chequerboard puts between them. *J Antimicrob Chemother* 2003;52:1.
470. Oka S, Goto M, Kaji Y, et al. Synergistic activity of imipenem/cilastin combined with cefotiam against methicillin-resistant *Staphylococcus aureus*. *J Antimicrob Chemother* 1993;31:533–541.
471. Olarte J, Galindo E. *Salmonella typhi* resistant to chloramphenicol, ampicillin, and other antimicrobial agents: strains isolated during an extensive typhoid fever epidemic in Mexico. *Antimicrob Agents Chemother* 1973;4:597–601.
472. Olsson RA, Kirby JC, Romansky MJ. Pneumococcal meningitis in the adult: clinical therapeutic and prognostic aspects in forty-three patients. *Ann Intern Med* 1961;55:545–549.
473. Onozawa Y, Kumagi K, Ishida N. Mode of synergism between colistin and sulfisomezole in inhibiting the growth of *Proteus* organisms. *Jpn J Microbiol* 1967;11:221–227.
474. Onozawa Y, Sato S, Kumagai K, et al. The combination effect of colistin sulfate and sulfixomezole-Na against *Proteus* species. I. *J Antibiot(B)* 1964;17:61–64.
475. Otsuki M, Nishino T. The synergic effects of quinolones and oral cephem antibiotics on *Serratia marcescens*. *J Antimicrob Chemother* 1996;38:771–776.
476. Owens RC Jr, Banevicius MA, Nicolau DP, et al. In vitro synergistic activities of tobramycin and selected beta-lactams against 75 gram-negative clinical isolates. *Antimicrob Agents Chemother* 1997;41:2586–2588.
477. Papanicolaou GA, Medeiros AA. Discrimination of extended-spectrum β-lactamase by a novel nitrocefin competition assay. *Antimicrob Agents Chemother* 1990;34:2184–2192.
478. Papanicolaou GA, Medeiros AA, Jacoby GA. Novel plasmid-mediated β-lactamase (MIR-1) conferring

resistance to oxyimino and α-methoxy β-lactams in clinical isolates of *Klebsiella pneumoniae*. *Antimicrob Agents Chemother* 1990;34:2200–2209.

479. Park JT, Burman L. FL-1060: a new penicillin with a unique mode of action. *Biochem Biophys Res Commun* 1973;51:863–868.
480. Parry MF, Neu HC. Comparison and evaluation of ticarcillin and carbenicillin using disk diffusion methods. *Antimicrob Agents Chemother* 1976;9:625–632.
481. Parsley TL, Provonchee RB, Clickman C, et al. Synergistic activity of trimethoprim and amikacin against Gram-negative bacilli. *Antimicrob Agents Chemother* 1977;12:349–352.
482. Patel JA, Pachucki CT, Lentino JR. Synergy of levofloxacin (L-ofloxacin) and oxacillin against quinolone-resistant *Staphylococcus aureus* measured by the time-kill method. *Antimicrob Agents Chemother* 1993;37:339–341.
483. Patel R, Rouse MS, Piper KE, et al. In vitro activity of GAR-936 against vancomycin-resistant enterococci, methicillin-resistant *Staphylococcus aureus* and penicillin-resistant *Streptococcus pneumoniae*. *Diagn Microbiol Infect Dis* 2000;38:177–179.
484. Pato ML, Brown GM. Mechanisms of resistance of *Escherichia coli* to sulfonamides. *Arch Biochm Biophys* 1963;103:443–448.
485. Paton JH, Williams EW. Interaction between ciprofloxacin and vancomycin against staphylococci. *J Antimicrob Agents Chemother* 1987;20:251–254.
486. Patte JC, Hirsch H, Chabbert YA. Etude des courbes d'effet bacteriostatique des associations d'antibiotiques. *Ann Inst Pasteur* 1958;94:621–635.
487. Patterson JE, Colodny, JE, Zervos MJ. Serious infection due to β-lactamase-producing *Streptococcus faecalis* with high-level resistance to gentamicin. *J Infect Dis* 1988;158:1144–1145.
488. Patterson JE, Masecar BL, Zervos MJ. Characterization and comparison of two penicillinase-producing strains of *Streptococcus (Enterococcus) faecalis*. *Antimicrob Agents Chemother* 1988;32:122–124.
489. Pattishal KH, Acar J, Burchall JJ, et al. Two distinct types of trimethoprim resistant dihydrofolate reductase specified by R-plasmids of different compatibility groups. *J Biol Chem* 1977;252:2319–2323.
490. Pavie J, Lefort A, Zarrouk V, et al. Efficacies of quinupristin-dalfopristin combined with vancomycin in vitro and in experimental endocarditis due to methicillin-resistant *Staphylococcus aureus* in relation to cross-resistance to macrolides, lincosamides, and streptogramin B-type antibiotics. *Antimicrob Agents Chemother* 2002;46:3061–3064.
491. Pearlman MD, Faro S, Riddle GD, et al. In vitro synergy of clindamycin and aminoglycosides against *Chlamydia trachomatis*. *Antimicrob Agents Chemother* 1990;34:1399–1401.
492. Pearson RD, Steigbigel RT, Davis HT, et al. Method of reliable determination of minimal lethal antibiotic concentrations. *Antimicrob Agents Chemother* 1980;18:699–708.
493. Pechere JC, Marchou B, Michea-Hamzehpour M, et al. Emergence of resistance after therapy with antibiotics used alone or combined in a murine model. *J Antimicrob Chemother* 1986;17(SupplA):11–18.
494. Pendland SL, Messick CR, Jung R. In vitro synergy testing of levofloxacin, ofloxacin, and ciprofloxacin in combination with aztreonam, ceftazidime, or piperacillin against *Pseudomonas aeruginosa*. *Diagn Microbiol Infect Dis* 2002;42:75–78.
495. Perea EJ, Torres MA, Borobio MV. Synergism of fosfomycin-ampicillin and fosfomycin-chloramphenicol against *Salmonella* and *Shigella*. *Antimicrob Agents Chemother* 1978;13:705–709.
496. Perri MB, Chow JW, Zervos MJ. In vitro activity of sparfloxacin and clinafloxacin against multidrug-resistant enterococci. *Diagn Microbiol Infect Dis* 1993;17:151–155.
497. Perrig M, Acosta F, Cottagnoud M, et al. Efficacy of gatifloxacin alone and in combination with cefepime against penicillin-resistant *Streptococcus pneumoniae* in a rabbit meningitis model and in vitro. *J Antimicrob Chemother* 2001;47:701–704.
498. Perronne CM, Malinverni R, Glauser MP. Treatment of *Staphylococcus aureus* endocarditis in rats with coumermycin A1 and ciprofloxacin, alone or in combination. *Antimicrob Agents Chemother* 1987;31:539–543.
499. Pestka S. Antibiotics as probes of ribosomal structure: binding of chloramphenicol and erythromycin to polyribosomes: effect of other antibiotics. *Antimicrob Agents Chemother* 1974;5:255–267.
500. Pfaller M, Bale M, Preston T, et al. In vitro inhibitory and bacterial activity of cefiramide and seven antipseudomonal agents against *Pseudomonas aeruginosa*. *Diagn Microbiol Infect Dis* 1986;5:17–23.
501. Pfaller M, Barry A, Fuchs P, et al. Relative efficacy of tazobactam, sulbactam and clavulanic acid in enhancing the potency of ampicillin against clinical isolates of *Enterobacteriaceae*. *Eur J Clin Microbiol Infect Dis* 1993;12:200–205.
502. Pfaller MA, Segal JJ, Krogstad DJ. Activity of ketoconazole and its deacyl derivative against *Plasmodium falciparum* and *Candida* isolates. *Antimicrob Agents Chemother* 1982;22:917–919.
503. Phair JP, Watanakunakorn C, Bannister T. In vitro susceptibility of *Pseudomonas aeruginosa* to carbenicillin and the combination of carbenicillin and gentamicin. *Appl Microbiol* 1969;18:303–306.
504. Philippon A, Arlet G, Jacoby GA. Plasmid-determined AmpC-type beta-lactamases. *Antimicrob Agents Chemother* 2002;46:1–11.
505. Phillips K, Munster DJ, Allardyce RA, et al. Antibacterial action of the urease inhibitor acetohydroxamic acid on *Helicobacter pylori*. *J Clin Pathol* 1993;46:372–373.
506. Piccart M, Klastersky J, Meunier F, et al. Single-drug versus combination empirical therapy for Gram-negative bacillary infections in febrile cancer patients with and without granulocytopenia. *Antimicrob Agents Chemother* 1984;26:870–875.
507. Pines A, Nandi AR, Raafat H, et al. Pivmecillinam and amoxycillin as combined treatment in purulent exacerbations of chronic bronchitis. *J Antimicrob Chemother* 1977;3(Suppl B):141–148.
508. Piot P, van Dyke E. In vitro activity of BRL 17421 against *Haemophilus influenzae, Neisseria gonorrhoeae,* and *Branhamella catarrhalis*. *Antimicrob Agents Chemother* 1982;21:166–167.
509. Plotz PH, Davis BD. Synergism between streptomycin and penicillin: a proposed mechanism. *Science* 1962;135:1067–1068.
510. Poe M. Antibacterial synergism: a proposal for chemotherapeutic potentiation between trimethoprim and sulfamethoxazole. *Science* 1976;194:533–535.
511. Pohlman JK, Knapp CC, Ludwig MD, et al. Timed killing kinetic studies of the interaction between ciprofloxacin and beta-lactams against gram-negative bacilli. *Diagn Microbiol Infect Dis* 1996;26:29–33.
512. Poulos CD, Matsumura SO, Willey BM, et al. In

vitro activities of antimicrobial combinations against *Stenotrophomonas (Xanthomonas) maltophilia*. *Antimicrob Agents Chemother* 1995;39:2220–2223.
513. Preheim LC, Penn RG, Sanders CC, et al. Emergence of resistance to β-lactam and aminoglycoside antibiotics during moxalactam therapy of *Pseudomonas aeruginosa* infections. *Antimicrob Agents Chemother* 1982;22:1037–1041.
514. Prichard MN, Prichard LE, Baguley WA, et al. Three-dimensional analysis of the synergistic cytotoxicity of ganciclovir and zidovudine. *Antimicrob Agents Chemother* 1991;35:1060–1065.
515. Prichard MN, Shipman C Jr. A three-dimensional model to analyze drug-drug interactions. *Antiviral Res* 1990;24:181–206.
516. Rahal JJ. Antibiotic combinations: the clinical relevance of synergy and antagonism. *Medicine* 1978;57:179–195.
517. Rahal JJ. Treatment of methicillin-resistant staphylococci infections. In: Peterson PK, Verhoef J, eds. *Antimicrobial agents annual*, vol. 1. Amsterdam: Elsevier, 1986;489–514.
518. Rand KH, Brown P. Concentration-dependent synergy and antagonism between cefoperazone and imipenem against methicillin-resistant *Staphylococcus aureus*. *Antimicrob Agents Chemother* 1995;39:1173–1177.
518a. Rand KH, Houck HJ. Synergy of daptomycin with oxacillin and other β-Lactams against methicillin-resistant *Staphylococcus aureus*. *Antimicrob Agents Chemother* 2004;48:2871–2875.
519. Rand KH, Houck HJ, Brown P, et al. Reproducibility of the microdilution checkerboard method for antibiotic synergy. *Antimicrob Agents Chemother* 1993;37:613–615.
520. Reading C, Cole M. Clavulanic acid: a β-lactamase inhibiting β-lactam from *Streptomyces clavuligerus*. *Antimicrob Agents Chemother* 1977;11:852–857.
521. Reeves DS, Bywater MJ, Holt HA, et al. In vitro studies with ciprofloxacin, a new 4-quinolone compound. *J Antimicrob Chemother* 1984;13:333–336.
522. Rein MF, Elliott WC, Swenson JM, et al. Sulfamethoxaxole-trimethoprim synergism for *Neisseria gonorrhoeae*. *Antimicrob Agents Chemother* 1980;17:247–250.
523. Reller LB, Schoenknecht FD, Kenny MA, et al. Antibiotic susceptibility testing of *Pseudomonas aeruginosa:* selection of a control stain and criteria for magnesium and calcium content in media. *J Infect Dis* 1974;130:454–463.
524. Retsema JA, English AR, Girard AE. CP-45,899 in combination with penicillin or ampicillin against penicillin-resistant *Staphylococcus, Haemophilus influenzae* and *Bacteroides*. *Antimicrob Agents Chemother* 1980;17:615–622.
525. Reyes MP, El-Khatib MR, Brown WJ, et al. Synergy between carbenicillin and an aminoglycoside (gentamicin or tobramycin) against *Pseudomonas aeruginosa* isolated from patients with endocarditis and sensitivity of isolates to normal human serum. *J Infect Dis* 1979;140:192–202.
526. Rhinehart E, Smith NE, Wennersten C, et al. Rapid dissemination of β-lactamase-producing, aminoglycoside-resistant *Enterococcus faecalis* among patients and staff on an infant-toddler surgical ward. *N Engl J Med* 1990;323:1814–1818.
527. Rice LB, Eliopoulos GM, Moellering RC Jr. In vitro synergism between daptomycin and fosfomycin against *Enterococcus faecalis* isolates with high-level gentamicin resistance. *Antimcirob Agents Chemother* 1989;33:470–473.
528. Riley TV, Digiovanni C, Hoyne GF. Susceptibility of *Branhamella catarrhalis* to sulphamethoxazole and trimethoprim. *J Antimicrob Chemother* 1987;19:39–43.
529. Rodriguez JR, Ramirez-Ronda CH, Nevarez M. Efficacy and safety of aztreonam-clindamycin versus tobramycin-clindamycin in the treatment of lower respiratory tract infections caused by aerobic Gram-negative bacilli. *Antimicrob Agents Chemother* 1985;27:246–251.
530. Rodriguez-Hernandez MJ, Pachon J, Pichardo C, et al. Imipenem, doxycycline and amikacin in monotherapy and in combination in *Acinetobacter baumannii* experimental pneumonia. *J Antimicrob Chemother* 2000;45:493–501.
531. Rosenblatt JE, Steward PR. Combined activity of sulfamethoxazole, trimethoprim and polymyxin B against Gram-negative bacilli. *Antimicrob Agents Chemother* 1974;6:84–92.
532. Rudin JE, Norden CW, Shinners EM. In vitro activity of ciprofloxacin against aerobic Gram-negative bacteria. *Antimicrob Agents Chemother* 1984;26:597–598.
533. Rudoy RC, Nelson JD, Haltalin KC. In vitro susceptibility of *Shigella* strains to trimethoprim and sulfamethoxazole. *Antimicrob Agents Chemother* 1974;5:439–443.
534. Ryan KJ, Neeham GM, Dunsmoor CL, et al. Stability of antibiotics and chemotherapeutics in agar plates. *Appl Microbiol* 1970;20:447–451.
535. Ryan RW, Kwasnik I, Tilton RC. Methodological variation in antibiotic synergy tests against enterococci. *J Clin Microbiol* 1981;13:73–75.
536. Sabath LD. Synergy of antibacterial substances by apparently known mechanisms. *Antimicrob Agents Chemother* 1968;1967:210–217.
537. Sabath LD, Elder HA, McCall CE, et al. Synergistic combinations of penicillins in the treatment of bacteriuria. *N Engl J Med* 1967;277:232–238.
538. Sabah LD, Jago M, Abraham EP. Cephalosporinase and penicillinase activities of β-lactamase from *Pseudomonas pyocyanea*. *Biochm J* 1965;96:739–752.
539. Sabath LD, McCall CE, Steigbigel NH, et al. Synergistic penicillin combinations for treatment of human urinary tract infections. *Antimicrob Agents Chemother* 1967;1966:149–155.
540. Sabath LD, Steinhauser BW, Finland M. Combined action of penicillin G with methicillin or oxacillin against *Staphylococcus aureus*. *N Engl J Med* 1963;268:284–286.
541. Sader HS, Huynh HK, Jones RN. Contemporary in vitro synergy rates for aztreonam combined with newer fluoroquinolones and beta-lactams tested against gram-negative bacilli. *Diagn Microbiol Infect Dis* 2003;47:547–550.
542. Sahm DF, Kissinger J, Gilmore MS, et al. In vitro susceptibility studies of vancomycin-resistant *Enterococcus faecalis*. *Antimicrob Agents Chemother* 1989;33:1588–1591.
543. Sakoulas G, Gold HS, Venkataraman L, et al. Introduction of erm(C) into a linezolid- and methicillin-resistant *Staphylococcus aureus* does not restore linezolid susceptibility. *J Antimicrob Chemother* 2003;51:1039–1041.
544. Saleh-Mghir A, Ameur N, Muller-Serieys C, et al. Combination of quinupristin-dalfopristin (Synercid) and rifampin is highly synergistic in experimental *Staphylococcus aureus* joint prosthesis infection. *Antimicrob Agents Chemother* 2002;46:1122–1124.
545. Sambatakou H, Giamarellos-Bourboulis EJ, Grecka P, et al. In-vitro activity and killing effect of quinupristin/dalfopristin (RP59500) on nosocomial *Staphylococcus aureus* and interactions with rifampicin and ciprofloxacin against methicillin-resistant isolates. *J Antimicrob Chemother* 1998;41:349–55.
546. Sande MA, Courtney KB. Nafcillin-gentamicin synergism in experimental staphylococcal endocarditis. *J Lab Clin Med* 1976;88:118–124.
547. Sande MA, Irvin RG. Penicillin-aminoglycoside synergy

in experimental *Streptococcus viridans* endocarditis. *J Infect Dis* 1974;129:572–576.

548. Sande MA, Johnson ML. Antimicrobial therapy of experimental endocarditis caused by *Staphylococcus aureus*. *J Infect Dis* 1975;131:367–375.
549. Sande MA, Overton JW. In vivo antagonism between gentamicin and chloramphenicol in neutropenic mice. *J Infect Dis* 1973;128:247–250.
550. Sanders CC. Inducible β-lactamases and non-hydrolytic resistance mechanisms. *J Antimicrob Chemother* 1984; 13:13.
551. Sanders CC. New β-lactams: new problems for the internist. *Ann Intern Med* 1991;115:650–651.
552. Sanders CC, Moellering RC Jr, Martin RR, et al. Resistance to cefamandole: a collaborative study of emerging clinical problems. *J Infect Dis* 1982;145:118–125.
553. Sanders CC, Sanders WE Jr. Emergence of resistance to cefamandole: possible role of cefoxitin-inducible β-lactamases. *Antimicrob Agents Chemother* 1979;15:792–797.
554. Sanders CC, Sanders WE Jr, Goering RV. In vitro antagonism of β-lactam antibiotics by cefoxitin. *Antimicrob Agents Chemother* 1982;21:968–975.
555. Sanders CC, Sanders WE Jr, Goering RV. Influence of clindamycin on derepression of β-lactamases in *Enterobacter* spp. and *Pseudomonas aeruginosa*. *Antimicrob Agents Chemother* 1983;24:48–53.
556. Sanders CC, Sanders WE Jr, Goering RV, et al. Leakage of β-lactamase: a second mechanism for antibiotic potentiation by amdinocillin. *Antimicrob Agents Chemother* 1987;31:1164–1168.
557. Sanders CC, Sanders WE Jr, Moland ES. Decimal assay for additivity of drugs permits delineation of synergy and antagonism. *Antimicrob Agents Chemother* 1993;37:260–264.

557a. San Gabriel P, Zhou J, Tabibi S, Chen Y, et al. Antimicrobial susceptibility and synergy studies of *Stenotrophomonas maltophilia* isolates from patients with cystic fibrosis. *Antimicrob Agents Chemother* 2004;48:168–171.

558. Sattler FR, Hall S, Hanna CE, et al. Efficacy of amdinocillin and lack of nephrotoxicity when combined with a second β-lactam antibiotic for therapy of serious Gram-negative bacillary infections. *Am J Med* 1983;75(Suppl):106–112.
559. Schauf V, Deveikis A, Riff L, et al. Antibiotic-killing kinetics of group B streptococci. *J Pediatr* 1976;89:194–198.
560. Scheld WM, Alliegro GM, Field MR, et al. Synergy between ampicillin and gentamicin in experimental meningitis due to group B streptococci. *J Infect Dis* 1982;146:100.
561. Schleupner CJ, Engle JC. Clinical evaluation of cefotaxime for therapy of lower respiratory tract infections. *Antimicrob Agents Chemother* 1982;21:327–333.
562. Schwartz R, Rodriguez W, Khan W, et al. The increasing incidence of ampicillin-resistant *Haemophilus influenzae*: a cause of otitis media. *JAMA* 1978;239:320–323.
563. Schwartz WS. Isoniazid alone compared with isoniazid and PAS in the treatment of minimal and noncavitary, moderately advanced, previously untreated pulmonary tuberculosis. XI. A report of the Veterans Administration-Armed Forces Cooperative Study. *Am Rev Respir Dis* 1963;87:424–428.
564. Scott RE, Robson HG. Synergistic activity of carbenicillin and gentamicin in experimental *Pseudomonas* bacteremia in neutropenic rats. *Antimicrob Agents Chemother* 1976;10:646–651.
565. Scribner RK, Marks MI, Weber AH, et al. Activities of various β-lactams and aminoglycosides, alone and in combination, against isolates of *Pseudomonas aeruginosa* from patients with cystic fibrosis. *Antimicrob Agents Chemother* 1982;21:939–943.
566. Seibert G, Isert D, Klesel N, et al. The in-vitro antibacterial activity of a combination of cefpirome or cefoperazone with vancomycin against enterococci and *Staphylococcus aureus*. *J Antimicrob Chemother* 1992;29(Suppl A):25–30.
567. Selkon JB, Devadatta S, Kulkarnia KG, et al. The emergence of isoniazid-resistant cultures in patients with pulmonary tuberculosis during treatment with isoniazid alone or isoniazid plus PAS. *Bull WHO* 1964;31:273–294.
568. Shlaes DM, Bouvet A, Devine C, et al. Inducible, transferable resistance to vancomycin in *Enterococcus faecalis* A256. *Antimicrob Agents Chemother* 1989;33:198–203.
569. Silva M, Jacobus NV, Gorbach SL. In vitro activity of LY 146032 against Gram-positive bacteria. *Diagn Microbiol Infect Dis* 1988;9:79–85.
570. Simon GL, Snydman DR, Tally FP, et al. Clinical trials of piperacillin with acquisition of resistance by *Pseudomonas* and clinical relapse. *Antimicrob Agents Chemother* 1980;18:167–170.
571. Sirisanthana T, Lerner SA. Effect of clavulanic acid on the in vitro synergism between carbenicillin and gentamicin against *Serratia marcescens*. *Antimicrob Agents Chemother* 1979;15:630–632.
572. Skold O, Widh A. A new dihydrofolate reductase with low trimethoprim sensitivity induced by an R factor mediating high resistance to trimethoprim. *J Biol Chem* 1974;249:4324–4325.
573. Slocombe B. Transmissible aminoglycoside resistance in strains of *Streptococcus faecalis*. In: Siegenthaler W, Leuthy R, eds. *Current chemotherapy,* vol. 2 *(Proceedings of the 10th International Congress of Chemotherapy).* Washington, DC: American Society for Microbiology, 1978;891–893.
574. Smith CB, Dans PE, Wilfert JN, et al. Use of gentamicin in combination with other antibiotics. *J Infect Dis* 1969;119:370–377.
575. Smith CB, Wilfert JN, Dans PE, et al. In vitro activity of carbenicillin and results of treatment of infections due to *Pseudomonas* with carbenicillin singly and in combination with gentamicin. *J Infect Dis* 1970;122(Suppl):S14–S25.
576. Smith CE, Foleno BE, Barrett JF, et al. Assessment of the synergistic interactions of levofloxacin and ampicillin against *Enterococcus faecium* by the checkerboard agar dilution and time-kill methods. *Diagn Microbiol Infect Dis* 1997;27:85–92.
577. Snyder RJ, Wikowski CJ, Washington JA II. Bactericidal activity of combinations of gentamicin with penicillin or clindamycin against *Streptococcus mutans*. *Antimicrob Agents Chemother* 1975;7:333–335.
578. Sonne M, Jawetz E. Combined action of carbenicillin and gentamicin on *Pseudomonas aeruginosa* in vitro. *Appl Microbiol* 1969;17:893–896.
579. Soper TS, Manning JM. Synergy in the antimicrobial action of penicillin and β-chloro-D-alanine *in vitro*. *Antimicrob Agents Chemother* 1976;9:347–349.
580. Spitzer PG, Eliopoulos GM, Karchmer AW, et al. Comparative in vitro activity of the new cyclic lipopeptide LY 146032 against *Corynebacterium* species. *Eur J Clin Microbiol* 1987;6:183–185.
581. Spitzer PG, Eliopoulos GM, Karchmer AW, et al. Synergistic activity between vancomycin or teicoplanin and gentamicin or tobramycin against pathogenic diphtheroids. *Antimicrob Agents Chemother* 1988;32:434–437.
582. Spitzer PG, Hammer SM, Karchmer AW. Treatment

of *Listeria monocytogenes* infection with trimethoprim-sulfamethoxazole: case report and review of the literature. *Rev Infect Dis* 1986;8:427–430.
583. Spratt BG. Distinct penicillin binding proteins involved in the division, elongation, and shape of *Escherichia coli* K12. *Proc Natl Acad Sci USA* 1975;72:2999–3003.
584. Spratt BG. The mechanism of action of mecillinam. *J Antimicrob Chemother* 1977;3(Suppl B):13–19.
585. Spratt BG, Pardee AB. Penicillin-binding proteins and cell shape in *E. coli*. *Nature* 1975;254:516–517.
586. Stamey TA, Condy M, Mihara G. Prophylactic efficacy of nitrofurantoin macrocrystals and trimethorim-sulfamethoxazole in urinary tract infections. *N Engl J Med* 1977;296:780–783.
587. Standiford HC, deMaine JB, Kirby WMM. Antibiotic synergism of enterococci: relation to inhibitory concentration. *Arch Intern Med* 1970;126:255–259.
588. Standiford HC, Kind AC, Kirby WMM. Laboratory and clinical studies of carbenicillin against Gram-negative bacilli. *Antimicrob Agents Chemother* 1969;1968:286–291.
589. Steers E, Foltz El, Graves BS, et al. An inocula replicating apparatus for routine testing of bacterial susceptibility to antibiotics. *Antibiot Chemother* 1959;9:307–311.
590. Steigbigel RT, Greenman RL, Remington JS. Antibiotic combinations in the treatment of experimental *Staphylococcus aureus* infection. *J Infect Dis* 1975;131:245–251.
591. Stevens DA, Vo PT. Synergistic interaction of trimethoprim and sulfamethoxazole on *Paracoccidioides brasiliensis*. *Antimicrob Agents Chemother* 1982;21:852–854.
592. Strausbaugh LJ, Sande MA. Factors influencing the therapy of experimental *Proteus mirabilis* meningitis in rabbits. *J Infect Dis* 1978;137:251–260.
593. Stutman HR, Welch DF, Scribner RK, et al. In vitro antimicrobial activity of aztreonam alone and in combination against bacterial isolates from pediatric patients. *Antimicrob Agents Chemother* 1984;25:212–215.
594. Sud IJ, Feingold DS. Heterogeneity of action mechanisms among antimycotic imidazoles. *Antimicrob Agents Chemother* 1981;20:71–74.
595. Sud IJ, Feingold DS. Effect of ketoconazole on the fungicidal action of amphotericin B in *Candida albicans*. *Antimicrob Agents Chemother* 1983;23:185–187.
596. Sugiura A, Jono K, Kono T, et al. The effect of combinations of cefotiam and other antibiotics on methicilin-resistant *Staphylococcus aureus*. *J Antimicrob Chemother* 1991;28:707–717.
597. Sumita Y, Mitsuhashi S. In vitro synergistic activity between meopenem and the β-lactams against methicillin-resistant *Staphylococcus aureus*. *Eur J Clin Microbiol Infect Dis* 1991;10:77–84.
598. Sutherland R, Batchelor FR. Synergistic activity of penicillins against penicillinase-producing Gram negative bacilli. *Nature* 1964;201:868–869.
599. Sweeney MT, Zurenko GE. In vitro activities of linezolid combined with other antimicrobial agents against staphylococci, enterococci, pneumococci, and selected gram-negative organisms. *Antimicrob Agents Chemother* 2003;47:1902–1906.
600. Takahashi K, Kanno H. Synergistic activities of combinations of β-lactams, fosfomycin, and tobramycin against *Pseudomonas aeruginosa*. *Antimicrob Agents Chemother* 1984;26:789–791.
601. Thadepalli H, Roy I, Bach VT, et al. In vitro activity of mezlocillin and its related compounds against aerobic and anaerobic bacteria. *Antimicrob Agents Chemother* 1979;15:487–490.
602. Thauvin C, Eliopoulos GM, Wennersten C, et al. Antagonistic effect of penicillin-amikacin combinations against enterococci. *Antimicrob Agents Chemother* 1985;28:78–83.
603. Thauvin C, Lemeland J-F, Humbert G, et al. Efficacy of pefloxacin-fosfomycin in experimental endocarditis caused by methicillin-resistant *Staphylococcus aureus*. *Antimicrob Agents Chemother* 1988;32:919–921.
604. Then R. Synergism between trimethoprim and sulfamethoxazole. *Science* 1977;197:1301.
605. Then R, Angehrn P. Nature of the bactericidal action of sulfonamides and trimethoprim, alone and in combination. *J Infect Dis* 1973;128(Suppl):S498–S501.
606. Tomasz A. From penicillin-binding proteins to the lysis and death of bacteria: a 1979 view. *Rev Infect Dis* 1979;1:434–467.
607. Tomasz A, Waks S. Mechanism of action of penicillin: triggering of the pneumococcal autolytic enzyme by inhibitors of cell wall synthesis. *Proc Natl Acad Sci USA* 1975;72:4162–4166.
608. Tomeh MO, Starr SE, McGowan JE Jr, et al. Ampicillin-resistant *Haemophilus influenzae* type b infection. *JAMA* 1974;229:295–297.
609. Tompsett R, Hurst ML. Bacterial endocarditis: selected aspects of treatment. *Trans Am Clin Climatol Assoc* 1972;83:95–103.
610. Tompsett R, Pizette M. Enterococcal endocarditis: lack of correlation between therapeutic results and antibiotic sensitivity tests. *Arch Intern Med* 1962;109:146–150.
611. Tompsett R, Robbins WC, Berntsen C Jr. Short-term penicillin and dihydrostreptomycin therapy of streptococcal endocarditis. *Am J Med* 1958;24:57–67.
612. Torres C, Tenorio C, Lantero M, et al. High-level penicillin resistance and penicillin-gentamicin synergism in *Enterococcus faecium*. *Antimicrob Agents Chemother* 1993;37:2427–2431.
613. Totsuka K, Shiseki M, Kikuchi K, et al. Combined effects of vancomycin and imipenem against methicillin-resistant *Staphylococcus aureus* (MRSA) in vitro and in vivo. *J Antimicrob Chemother* 1999;44:455–460.
614. Traub WH, Leonard B. Heat stability of the antimicrobial activity of sixty-two antibacterial agents. *J Antimicrob Chemother* 1995;35:149–154.
615. Tsiodras S, Gold HS, Sakoulas G, et al. Linezolid resistance in a clinical isolate of *Staphylococcus aureus*. *Lancet* 2001;358:207–208.
616. Tuazon CA, Miller H. Comparative in vitro activity of teichomycin and vancomycin alone and in combination with rifampin and aminoglycosides against staphylococci and enterococci. *Antimicrob Agents Chemother* 1984;25:411–412.
617. Tuazon CU, Shamsuddin D, Miller H. Antibiotic susceptibility and synergy of clinical isolates of *Listeria monocytogenes*. *Antimicrob Agents Chemother* 1982;21:525–527.
618. Tuomanen E, Gilbert K, Tomasz A. Modulation of bacteriolysis by cooperative effects of penicillin-binding proteins 1a and 3 in *Escherichia coli*. *Antimicrob Agents Chemother* 1986;30:659–663.
619. Turner FJ, Lindo FL, Storino PJ, et al. Sulfonamide potentiation of the inhibitory activity of colistin on *Proteus vulgaris*. *Antimicrob Agents Chemother* 1963;1962:815–826.
620. Tybring L, Melchoir NH. Mecillinam (FL 1060), a 6-amidinopenicillanic acid derivative: bactericidal action and synergy in vitro. *Antimicrob Agents Chemother* 1975;8:271–276.
621. Ueda Y, Saito A, Fukuoka Y, et al. Interactions of β-lactam antibiotics and antineoplastic agents. *Antimicrob Agents Chemother* 1983;23:374–378.
622. Unal S, Flokowitsch J, Mullen DL, et al. In-vitro synergy and mechanism of interaction between vancomycin and

ciprofloxacin against enterococcal isolates. *J Antimicrob Chemother* 1993;31:711–723.

623. Utsui Y, Ohya S, Magaribuchi T, et al. Antibacterial activity of cefmetazole alone and in combination with fosfomycin against methicillin- and cephem-resistant *Staphylococcus aureus*. *Antimicrob Agents Chemother* 1986;30:917–922.
624. Van der Auwera P, Joly P. Comparative in vitro activities of teicoplanin, vancomycin, coumermycin, and ciprofloxacin, alone and in combination with rifampin or LM 427, against *Staphylococcus aureus*. *J Antimicrob Chemother* 1987;19:313–320.
625. Van der Auwera P, Klastersky J. In vitro study of the combination of rifampin with oxacillin against *Staphylococcus aureus*. *Rev Infect Dis* 1983;5(Suppl 3):S509–S514.
626. Van der Auwera P, Vandermies A, Lieppe S, et al. Ceftazidime combined with mecillinam: serum bactericidal titers compared with in vitro synergy against Gram-negative bacilli. *J Antimicrob Chemother* 1988;21:745–753.
627. Van Laethem Y, Klastersky J. Serum bactericidal activity of mezlocillin, ceftazidime, mezlocillin/ceftazidime and mezlocillin/amikacin against *Klebsiella pneumoniae* and *Pseudomonas aeruginosa*. *Eur J Clin Microbiol* 1986;5:110–114.
628. Van Laethem Y, Lagast H, Klastersky J. Serum bactericidal activity of ceftazidime and cefoperazone alone or in combination with amikacin against *Pseudomonas aeruginosa* and *Klebsiella pneumoniae*. *Antimicrob Agents Chemother* 1983;23:435–439.
629. Van Landuyt HW, Pyckavet M, Lambert AM. Comparative activity of BRL 25,000 with amoxycillin against resistant clinical isolates. *J Antimicrob Chemother* 1981;7:65–70.
630. Vasquez D. Binding of chloramphenicol to ribosomes: the effect of a number of antibiotics. *Biochem Biophys Acta* 1965;114:277–288.
631. Visalli MA, Jacobs MR, Appelbaum PC. Determination of activities of levofloxacin, alone and combined with gentamicin, ceftazidime, cefpirome, and meropenem, against 124 strains of *Pseudomonas aeruginosa* by checkerboard and time-kill methodology. *Antimicrob Agents Chemother* 1998;42:953–955.
632. Visalli MA, Jacobs MR, Appelbaum PC. Activities of three quinolones, alone and in combination with extended-spectrum cephalosporins or gentamicin, against *Stenotrophomonas maltophilia*. *Antimicrob Agents Chemother* 1998;42:2002–2005.
633. Vouillamoz J, Entenza JM, Feger C, et al. Quinupristin-dalfopristin combined with beta-lactams for treatment of experimental endocarditis due to *Staphylococcus aureus* constitutively resistant to macrolide-lincosamide-streptogramin B antibiotics. *Antimicrob Agents Chemother* 2000;44:1789–1795.
634. Vu H, Nikaido H. Role of beta-lactam hydrolysis in the mechanism of resistance of a beta-lactamase-constitutive *Enterobacter cloacae* strain to expanded spectrum beta-lactams. *Antimicrob Agents Chemother* 1985;27:393–398.
635. Wain J, Diem Nga LT, Kidgell C, et al. Molecular analysis of incHI1 antimicrobial resistance plasmids from Salmonella serovar Typhi strains associated with typhoid fever. *Antimicrob Agents Chemother* 2003;47:2732–2739.
636. Waitz AJ, Drube CG, Moss EL Jr, et al. Biological aspects of the interaction between gentamicin and carbenicillin. *J Antibiot* 1972;25:219–255.
637. Wald ER, Standiford HC, Tatem BA, et al. BL-P1654, ticarcillin and carbenicillin: in vitro comparison alone and in combination with gentamicin against *Pseudomonas aeruginosa*. *Antimicrob Agents Chemother* 1975;7:336–340.
638. Wallace JF, Smith RH, Garia M, et al. Studies on the pathogenesis of meningitis. VI. Antagonism between penicillin and chloramphenicol in experimental pneumococcal meningitis. *J Lab Clin Med* 1967;70:408–418.
639. Ward TT, Amon MB, Krause LK. Combination of adminocillin and cefoxitin therapy of multiply-resistant *Serratia marcescens* urinary tract infections. *Am J Med* 1983;75(Suppl):85–89.
640. Watanakunakorn C. Effects of inoculum size on the activity of carboxy- and ureido-penicillins and effects of combinations of ureido-penicillins with aminoglycosides against resistant *Pseudomonas aeruginosa*. *J Antimicrob Chemother* 1986;17:91–95.
641. Watanakunakorn C, Glotzbecker C. Enhancement of the effects of anti-staphylococcal antibiotics by aminoglycosides. *Antimicrob Agents Chemother* 1974;6:802–806.
642. Watanakunakorn C, Glotzbecker C. Comparative in vitro activity of nafcillin, oxacillin and methicillin in combination with gentamicin and tobramycin against enterococci. *Antimicrob Agents Chemother* 1977;11:88–91.
643. Watanakunakorn C, Glotzbecker C. Enhancement of anti-staphylococcal activity of nafcillin and oxacillin by sisomicin and netilmicin. *Antimicrob Agents Chemother* 1977;12:346–348.
644. Watanakunakorn C, Tisone JAC. Synergism between vancomycin and gentamicin or tobramycin for methicillin-susceptible and methicillin-resistant *Staphylococcus aureus* strains. *Antimicrob Agents Chemother* 1982;22:903–905.
645. Watanakunakorn C, Tisone JAC. Synergism between *N*-formimidoyl-thienamycin and gentamicin or tobramycin against enterococci. *Antimicrob Agents Chemother* 1982;22:1082–1083.
646. Waterworth PM, Emmerson AM. Dissociated resistance among cephalosporins. *Antimicrob Agents Chemother* 1979;15:497–503.
647. Webb JL. *Enzyme and metabolic inhibitors*. New York: Academic Press, 1963;498–500.
648. Wehrle PF, Mathies AW, Leedom JM, et al. Bacterial meningitis. *Ann NY Acad Sci* 1967;145:488–498.
649. Weinstein AJ, Lentnek AL. Cephalosporin-aminoglycoisde synergism in experimental enterococcal endocarditis. *Antimicrob Agents Chemother* 1976;9:983–987.
650. Weinstein AJ, Moellering RC Jr. Penicillin and gentamicin therapy for enterococcal infections. *JAMA* 1973;223:1030–1032.
651. Weinstein AJ, Moellering RC Jr. Studies of cephalothin-aminoglycoside synergism against enterococci. *Antimicrob Agents Chemother* 1975;7:522–529.
652. Weinstein L. Antimicrobial agents: sulfonamides and trimethoprim-sulfamethoxazole. In: Goodman LS, Gilman A, eds. *The pharmacological basis of therapeutics*, 5th ed. New York: Macmillan, 1975;1113–1119.
653. Welling PG, Craig WA, Amidon GL, et al. Pharmacokinetics of trimethoprim and sulfamethoxazole in normal subjects and in patients with renal failure. *J Infect Dis* 1973;128(Suppl):S556–S566.
654. Wennersten CB, Moellering RC Jr. Mechanisms of resistance to penicillin-aminoglycoside synergism in *Streptococcus faecium*. In: *Current chemotherapy and infectious disease*, vol. 1 *(Proceedings of the 11th International Congress of Chemotherapy)*. Washington DC: American Society for Microbiology, 1980;710–712.
655. White PJ, Woods DD. The synthesis of *p*-aminobenzoic acid and folic acid by staphylococci sensitive and resistant to sulfonamides. *J Gen Microbiol* 1965;40:243–253.

656. White RL, Burgess DS, Manduru M, et al. Comparison of three different in vitro methods of detecting synergy: time-kill, checkerboard, and E test. *Antimicrob Agents Chemother* 1996;40:1914–1918.
657. Whiting JL, Cheng N, Chow AW. Interactions of ciprofloxacin with clindamycin, metronidazole, cefoxitin, cefotaxime, and mezlocillin against Gram-positive and Gram-negative anaerobic bacteria. *Antimicrob Agents Chemother* 1987;31:1379–1382.
658. Williamson R, Al-Obeid S, Shlaes JH, et al. Inducible resistance to vancomycin in *Enterococcus faecium* D366. *J Infect Dis* 1989;159:1095–1104.
659. Williamson R, LeBouguenec C, Gutmann L, et al. One or two low affinity penicillin-binding proteins may be responsible for the range of susceptibility of *Enterococcus faecium* to benzylpenicillin. *J Gen Microbiol* 1985;131:1933–1940.
660. Wilson P, Andrews JA, Charlesworth R, et al. Linezolid resistance in clinical isolates of *Staphylococcus aureus*. *J Antimicrob Chemother* 2003;51:186–188.
661. Wilson WR, Thompson RL, Wilkowski CJ, et al. Short-term therapy for streptococcal infective endocarditis: combined intramuscular administration of penicillin and streptomycin. *JAMA* 1981;254:360–363.
662. Wilson WR, Zak O, Sande MA. Penicillin therapy for treatment of experimental endocarditis caused by viridans streptococci in animals. *J Infect Dis* 1985;151:1028–1033.
663. Winningham DG, Stamey TA. Diffusion of sulfonamides from plasma into prostatic fluid. *J Urol* 1970;104:559–563.
664. Wise R, Andrews JM, Bedford KA. In vitro study of clavulanic acid in combination with penicillin, amoxycillin, and carbenicillin. *Antimicrob Agents Chemother* 1978;1:389–393.
665. Wise R, Ayliffe GAJ, Andrews JM, et al. The activity of mecillinam (FL-1060), in combination with other antibiotics, against *H.influenzae* and *Streptococcus faecalis*, vol. 5. In: Williams JD, Geddes AM, eds. *Chemotherapy*. New York: Plenum Press, 1976;191–198.
666. Wise RW. β-lactamase inhibitors. *J Antimicrob Chemother* 1982;9(Suppl B):31–40.
667. Wolfe JC, Johnson WD Jr. Penicillin-sensitive streptococcal endocarditis: in vitro and clinical observations on penicillin-streptomycin therapy. *Ann Intern Med* 1974;81:178–181.
668. Wust J, Hardegger U. In vitro activity of ceftriaxone combined with tazobactam against anaerobic bacteria. *Eur J Clin Microbiol Infect Dis* 1994;13:177–181.
669. Yajko DM, Sanders CA, Nassos PS, et al. In vitro susceptibility of *Mycobacterium avium* complex to the new fluoroquinolone sparfloacin (CI-978;AT-4140) and comparison with ciprofloxacin. *Antimicrob Agents Chemother* 1990;34:2442–2444.
670. Yamashiro Y, Fukuoka Y, Yotsuji A, et al. Interactions of antimicrobial agents and antineoplastic agents. *J Infect Dis* 1986;154:531–534.
671. Yee Y, Farber B, Mates S. Mechanism of penicillin-streptomycin synergy for clinical isolates of viridans streptococci. *J Infect Dis* 1986;154:531–534.
672. Yogev R, Kabat WJ. Synergistic action of nafcillin and ampicillin against ampicillin-resistant *Haemophilus influenzae* type b bacteremia and meningitis in infant rats. *Antimicrob Agents Chemother* 1980;18:122–124.
673. Yogev R, Melick C, Kabat WJ. In vitro and in vivo synergism between amoxicillin and clavulanic acid against ampicillin-resistant *Haemophilus influenzae* type b. *Antimicrob Agents Chemother* 1981;19:993–996.
674. Young LS. Gentamicin: clinical use with carbenicillin and in vitro studies with recent isolates of *Pseudomonas aeruginosa*. *J Infect Dis* 1971;124(Suppl):S202–S206.
675. Yu PKW, Edson RS, Washington JA II, et al. Bactericidal and synergistic activity of moxalactam alone and in combination with gentamicin against *Pseudomonas aeruginosa*. *Antimicrob Agents Chemother* 1983;23:179–181.
676. Yu VL, Felegie TP, Yee RB, et al. Synergistic interaction in vitro with use of three antibiotics simultaneously against *Pseudomonas maltophilia*. *J Infect Dis* 1980;142:602–607.
677. Zarrouk V, Bozdogan B, Leclercq R, et al. Activities of the combination of quinupristin-dalfopristin with rifampin in vitro and in experimental endocarditis due to *Staphylococcus aureus* strains with various phenotypes of resistance to macrolide-lincosamide-streptogramin antibiotics. *Antimicrob Agents Chemother* 2001;45:1244–1248.
678. Zeiler HJ. Evaluation of the in vitro bactericidal action of ciprofloxacin on cells of *Escherichia coli* in the logarithmic and stationary phases of growth. *Antimicrob Agents Chemother* 1985;28:524–527.
679. Zelenitsky SA, Booker B, Laing N, et al. Synergy of an investigational glycopeptide, LY333328, with once-daily gentamicin against vancomycin-resistant *Enterococcus faecium* in a multiple-dose, in vitro pharmacodynamic model. *Antimcirob Agents Chemother* 1999;43:592–597.
680. Zemelman R, Bello H, Dominguez M, et al. Activity of imipenem, third-generation cephalosporins, aztreonam, and ciprofloxacin against multi-resistant Gram-negative bacilli isolated form Chilean hospitals. *J Antimicrob Chemother* 1993;32:413–419.
681. Zenilman JM, Miller MH, Mandel LJ. In vitro studies simultaneously examining effect of oxacillin on uptake of radiolabeled streptomycin and on associated bacterial lethality in *Staphylococcus aureus*. *Antimicrob Agents Chemother* 1986;30:877–882.
682. Zhou XY, Kitzis MD, Acar JF, et al. Activity of the β-lactamase inhibitor BRL 42715 against cephalosporinases produced by Enterobacteriaceae. *J Antimicrob Chemother* 1993;31:473–480.
683. Zighelboim S, Tomasz A. Penicillin-binding proteins of multiply-resistant South African strains of *Streptococcus pneumoniae*. *Antimicrob Agents Chemother* 1980;17:434–442.
684. Zimmer BL, DeYoung DR, Roberts GD. In vitro synergistic activity of ethambutol, isoniazid, kanamycin, rifampin, and streptomycin against *Mycobacterium avium-intracellulare* complex. *Antimicrobial Agents Chemother* 1982;22:148–150.
685. Zimmerman RA, Moellering RC Jr, Weinberg AN. Enterococcal resistance to antibiotic synergism. *Antimicrob Agents Chemother* 1971;1970:517–521.
686. Zimmerman RA, Moellering RC Jr, Weinberg AN. Mechanism of resistance to antibiotic synergism in enterococci. *J Bacteriol* 1971;105:873–879.
687. Zinner SH, Provonchee RB, Elias KS, et al. Effect of clindamycin on the in vitro activity of amikacin and gentamicin against Gram-negative bacilli. *Antimicrob Agents Chemother* 1976;9:661–664.
688. Zuravleff JJ, Yu VL, Yee RB, et al. Effect of calcium, magnesium, and zinc on ticarcillin and tobramycin alone and in combination against *Pseudomonas aeruginosa*. *Antimicrob Agents Chemother* 1982;22:839–843.

APPENDIX 9.1

Examples of Synergistic Antimicrobial Combinations *in Vitro*[a]

Organism	Mechanism of Synergism	Antimicrobial Combination	Techniques and Modifications	Effect Measured	References
Gram-negative Bacilli					
Acinetobacter spp	β-Lactam + aminoglycoside	Carbenicillin + kanamycin, tobramycin or gentamicin	Killing curve	Bactericidal	222
		Imipenem, ceftazidime, ceftriaxone, ampicillin/sulbactam, ticarcillin/clavulante or piperacillin/tazobactam + amikacin or tobramycin	Checkerboard-broth microtiter	Bacteriostatic	230, 393, 476
	Unknown	Doxycycline + amikacin	Killing curve	Bactericidal	530
		Colistin + rifampin	Killing curve	Bactericidal	214
		Gatifloxacin or ciprofloxacin + ceftazidime, aztreonam, ticarcillin/clavulanate or meropenem	Killing curve	Bactericidal	176, 235
		Ciprofloxacin + azlocillin	Checkerboard-broth	Bacteriostatic	429
	β-Lactam + aminoglycoside or unknown	Piperacillin/tazobactam + gentamicin or ciprofloxacin	Checkerboard-broth microtiter with sampling	Bactericidal	234
Citrobacter spp	Sequential enzyme inhibition	TMP + SMZ	Checkerboard-agar dilution (fractional inhibitory concentration [FIC] index)	Bacteriostatic	79
	Inhibition of protective enzymes	Clavulanic acid or sulbactam + ampicillin or amoxicillin	Checkerboard-broth	Bacteriostatic	175, 204
		Chloramphenicol + ampicillin, cephaloridine or carbenicillin	Cellophane transfer	Bacteriostatic	411
	Inhibition of cell wall synthesis	Amdinocillin + ampicillin, cefoxitin, or cefamandole	Checkerboard-agar	Bacteriostatic	451
	β-Lactam + aminoglycoside	Amikacin or tobramycin + apalcillin, azlocillin, ceftazidime, ceftriaxone, piperacillin/tazobactam, or ticarcillin/clavulanate	Checkerboard-broth microtiter	Bacteriostatic	230, 476
	β-Lactam + aminoglycoside or unknown	Piperacillin/tazobactam + gentamicin or ciprofloxacin	Checkerboard-broth microtiter with sampling	Bactericidal	234

(continued)

APPENDIX 9.1 (Continued)

Examples of Synergistic Antimicrobial Combinations *in Vitro*[a]

Organism	Mechanism of Synergism	Antimicrobial Combination	Techniques and Modifications	Effect Measured	References
Enterobacter spp	Sequential enzyme inhibition	TMP + SMZ	Checkerboard-agar dilution (FIC index)	Bacteriostatic	79
	Inhibition of protective enzymes	Nafcillin + penicillin, ampicillin or cephalothin	Checkerboard-broth dilution	Bacteriostatic	184
		Clavulanic acid or sulbactam + ampicillin	Checkerboard-broth microtiter and agar dilution	Bacteriostatic	201, 520
		Chloramphenicol + ampicillin, cephaloridine, or carbenicillin	Cellophane transfer	Bacteriostatic	411
		Chloramphenicol + cephaloridine	Killing curve	Bactericidal	411
		Clindamycin + cefamandole	Killing curve	Bactericidal	555
	Inhibition of cell wall synthesis	Amdinocillin + amoxicillin	Checkerboard-broth and agar dilution	Bacteriostatic	450
		Amdinocillin + ceftazidime	Checkerboard-broth microtiter with sampling	Bacteriostatic and bactericidal	626
	β-Lactam and aminoglycoside	Ampicillin or cephalothin + gentamicin	Checkerboard-agar dilution	Bacteriostatic	316
		Amikacin + piperacillin, cepthalothin, moxalactam, cefepime, cefotaxime, or cefoxitin	Killing curve	Bactericidal	225, 227, 416
		Amikacin or tobramycin + imipenem, aztreonam, cefmenoxime, ceftazidime, ceftriaxone, ticarcillin/clavulante, or piperacillin/tazobactam	Checkerboard-broth microtiter	Bacteriostatic	230, 476
	Unknown	Ciprofloxacin + aztreonam, ceftazidime, piperacillin/tazobactam, or ticarcillin/clavulanate	Killing curve	Bactericidal	511
	β-Lactam + aminoglycoside or unknown	Piperacillin/tazobactam + gentamicin or ciprofloxacin	Checkerboard-broth microtiter with sampling	Bactericidal	234
Enterobacteriaceae (misc)	Inhibition of protective enzymes	Cefoperazone + sulbactam	Checkerboard-broth microtiter	Bacteriostatic	295
		Ampicilliin + sulbactam, clavulanate, or tazobactam	Broth microdilution	Bacteriostatic	501

	β-Lactam + aminoglycoside	Moxalactam, cefoperazone, cefotaxime, or ceftazidime + amikacin	Checkerboard-broth microtiter	Bacteriostatic	296
	Inhibition of cell wall synthesis	Aztreonam + imipenem, cefepime, or ceftazidime	Checkerboard-broth microdilution	Bacteriostatic	541
	Unknown	Aztreonam + ciprofloxacin, gatifloxacin or levofloxacin	Checkerboard-broth microdilution	Bacteriostatic	541
Escherichia coli	Sequential enzyme inhibition	TMP + SMZ	Checkerboard-broth and agar dilution, paper strip diffusion	Bacteriostatic	2
	Inhibition of protective enzymes	Cloxacillin or dicloxacillin + ampicillin, penicillin, mezlocillin, or cephalothin	Checkerboard-broth agar dilution	Bacteriostatic	465, 539, 598
		Clavulanic acid or sulbactam + ampicillin, amoxicillin, piperacillin or cephaloridine	Checkerboard-broth microtiter and agar dilution	Bacteriostatic	155, 175, 201, 403, 457, 520, 664
		Clavulanic acid or sulbactam + amdinocillin (amdinocillin-resistant isolates)	Checkerboard-agar dilution	Bacteriostatic	452
		Sulbactam + cefoperazone	Checkerboard-broth	Bacteriostatic	295
		Chloramphenicol + ampicillin, cephaloridine, or carbenicillin	Cellophane transfer	Bacteriostatic	411
	Inhibition of cell wall synthesis	β-Chloro-D-alanine + penicillin	Killing curve	Bactericidal	579
		Amdinocillin + amoxicillin or ampicillin	Checkerboard-broth and agar dilution	Bacteriostatic	450, 620
			Killing curve	Bactericidal	450
		Fosmidomycin + cefazolin, cephalexin, ampicillin, or ticarcillin	Checkerboard-agar dilution	Bacteriostatic	458
	β-Lactam + aminoglycoside	Ampicillin or cephalothin + gentamicin	Checkerboard-agar	Bacteriostatic	316, 398
		Piperacillin, cefotaxime, or cefamandole + amikacin or gentamicin	Killing curve	Bactericidal	225, 227
	Unknown	Clindamycin + gentamicin	Checkerboard-broth dilution	Bacteriostatic	354
		Cefotaxime + ofloxacin	Checkerboard	Bacteriostatic	217
Klebsiella spp	Sequential enzyme inhibition	TMP + SMZ	Checkerboard-agar dilution	Bacteriostatic	79

(continued)

APPENDIX 9.1 (Continued)

Examples of Synergistic Antimicrobial Combinations *in Vitro*[a]

Organism	Mechanism of Synergism	Antimicrobial Combination	Techniques and Modifications	Effect Measured	References
	Inhibition of protective enzymes	Cloxacillin + ampicillin or cephalothin	Checkerboard-broth and agar dilution	Bacteriostatic	539
		Clavulanic acid or sulbactam + ampicillin, amoxicillin, cefotaxime, ceftriaxone, aztreonam, or piperacillin	Checkerboard-broth microtiter and agar	Bacteriostatic	155, 175, 201, 204, 457, 664, 680
		Chloramphenicol + ampicillin, cephaloridine, or carbenicillin	Cellophane transfer	Bacteriostatic	411
		Clavulanic acid + amdinocillin (against amdinocillin-resistant isolates)	Checkerboard-agar dilution	Bacteriostatic	452
	Inhibition of cell wall synthesis	Fosmidomycin + cefazolin, cephalexin, or ticarcillin	Checkerboard-agar	Bacteriostatic	458
		Amdinocillin + cephalothin, cefazolin, amoxicillin, ampicillin, or ceftazidime	Checkerboard-broth and agar	Bacteriostatic	30, 450, 626
			Killing curve	Bactericidal	451
		Vancomycin + cephalothin or carbenicillin	Checkerboard-broth microtiter	Bacteriostatic	151
	β-Lactam + aminoglycoside	Cephalothin + gentamicin	Checkerboard-agar dilution and broth microtiter	Bacteriostatic	316, 398
		Cefazolin + amikacin	Checkerboard-agar dilution and broth microtiter with sampling	Bacteriostatic and bactericidal	320
		Apalcillin, cefmenoxime, or ceftazidime + amikacin	Checkerboard-broth microtiter	Bacteriostatic	230
		Piperacillin, cefotaxime, cefamanadole, cefoxtin, cephalothin, or moxalactam + amikacin	Killing curve	Bactericidal	225, 227
	Unknown	Ciprofloxacin + aztreonam, ceftazidime, piperacillin/tazobactam, or ticarcillin/clavulanate	Killing curve	Bactericidal	511
		Gatifloxacin + gentamicin or cefepime	Checkerboard-agar dilution	Bacteriostatic	139
		Gatifloxacin + gentamicin or meropenem	Killing curve	Bactericidal	139
Legionella pneumophila	Unknown	Ciprofloxacin or levofloxacin + azithromycin	Checkerboard-agar dilution	Bacteriostatic	395
		Rifampin + levofloxacin, ofloxacin, or erythromycin	Killing curve	Bactericidal	29

Morganella morganii	β-Lactam + aminoglycoside	Imipenem + amikacin	Checkerboard-agar dilution	Bacteriostatic	174
Proteus spp	Inhibition of protective enzymes	Nafcillin, oxacillin, or methicillin + ampicillin	Checkerboard-broth dilution	Bacteriostatic	539
		Clavulanic acid or sulbactam + ampicillin, amoxicillin, cephalodrine, carbenicillin, or ticarcillin	Checkerboard-broth microtiter and agar dilution	Bacteriostatic	155, 175, 203, 204, 520, 664
		Chloramphenicol + ampicillin, cephaloridine, or carbenicillin	Cellophane transfer	Bacteriostatic	411
		Acetohydroxaminic acid + methenamine (in urine)	Killing curve	Bactericidal	443
	Inhibition of cell wall synthesis	Amdinocillin + ampicillin, cephalothin, cephradine, cefazolin, or carbenicillin	Checkerboard-broth and agar	Bacteriostatic	30, 309, 450
	β-Lactam + aminoglycoside	Cephalothin, carbenicillin, or ampicillin + gentamicin	Checkerboard-agar	Bacteriostatic	316, 318
		Azlocillin, aztreonam, ceftazidime, or ceftriaxone + amikacin	Checkerboard-broth microtiter	Bacteriostatic	230
		Piperacillin, cefotaxime, or moxalactam + amikacin	Killing curve	Bactericidal	225, 227
Providencia spp	Inhibition of protective enzymes	Chloramphenicol + ampicillin, cephaloridine, or carbenicillin	Cellophane transfer	Bacteriostatic	411
		Sulbactam + ampicillin	Checkerboard-broth microtiter	Bacteriostatic	175
Pseudomonas aeruginosa	Inhibition of protective enzymes	Methicillin, cloxacillin, or nafcillin + penicillin or ampicillin	Checkerboard-broth	Bacteriostatic	539
		Clavulanic acid or sulbactam + azlocillin or ampicillin	Checkerboard-broth	Bacteriostatic	86, 175
	Inhibition of cell wall synthesis	Vancomycin + cephalothin or carbenicillin	Checkerboard-broth microtiter	Bacteriostatic	151
		Aztreonam + cefepime or ceftazidime	Checkerboard-broth microtiter	Bacteriostatic	541
	β-Lactam + aminoglycoside	Carbenicillin, ticarcillin, piperacillin, moxalactam ceftriaxone, ceftazidime, cefotaxime, azlocillin, cefsulodin, imipenem, cefpiramide, mezlocillin, cefpimizole, cefepime, meropenem or aztreonam + gentamicin, tobramycin, amikacin, netilmicin, or sisomicin	Checkerboard-agar dilution, broth microtiter, or broth dilution with sampling	Bacteriostatic	12, 18, 61, 81, 103, 118, 167, 186, 206, 210, 216, 230, 257, 307, 322, 324, 339, 377, 391, 397, 417, 440, 446, 464, 565, 593, 674, 688

(continued)

APPENDIX 9.1 (Continued)

Examples of Synergistic Antimicrobial Combinations *in Vitro*[a]

Organism	Mechanism of Synergism	Antimicrobial Combination	Techniques and Modifications	Effect Measured	References
			Killing curve	Bactericidal	69, 75, 103, 118, 212, 318, 456, 464, 500, 503, 578, 588, 593, 640, 675
		Ceftazidime, piperacillin/tazobactam, or ticarcillin/clavulanate + tobramycin	Checkerboard-broth microtiter	Bacteriostatic	476
	Unknown	Clindamycin + gentamicin	Checkerboard-broth microtiter	Bacteriostatic	188
		Ciprofloxacin + imipenem, azlocillin, cefoperazone, aztreonam, ceftazidime, or vancomycin	Checkerboard-broth dilution	Bacteriostatic	81, 82, 135, 140, 429, 532
		Ciprofloxacin + imipenem or amikacin	Killing curve	Bactericidal	215
		Ciprofloxacin + aztreonam or ceftazidime	Killing curve	Bactericidal	511
		Ciprofloxacin, levofloxacin or trovafloxacin + cefepime, meropenem, or piperacillin/tazobactam	Killing curve	Bactericidal	73, 74, 75, 176
		Gatifloxacin + cefepime, meropenem, piperacillin, or gentamicin	Checkerboard-agar dilution	Bacteriostatic	139
		Gatifloxacin + piperacillin, cefepime, cefoperazone, ceftazidime, imipenem, aztreonam, or amikacin	Killing curve	Bactericidal	139, 235
		Levofloxacin + ceftazidime, cefpirome, cefepime, imipenem, meropenem, piperacillin/tazobactam, or gentamicin	Killing curve	Bactericidal	74, 631
		Levofloxacin or ofloxacin + ceftazidime, cefpirome, cefotaxime, meropenem, or gentamicin	Checkerboard	Bacteriostatic	217, 631
		Aztreonam + ciprofloxacin, gatifloxacin, or levofloxacin	Checkerboard-broth microdilution	Bacteriostatic	541
	β-Lactam + aminoglycoside or unknown	Piperacillin/tazobactam + gentamicin or ciprofloxacin	Checkerboard-broth microtiter with sampling	Bactericidal	234
Burkholderia cepacia	β-Lactam + aminoglycoside	Piperacillin or aztreonam + amikacin	Checkerboard-agar dilution	Bacteriostatic	18

		Aztreonam + gentamicin or tobramycin	Checkerboard-broth microtiter with sampling	Bacteriostatic	61
				Bactericidal	61
	Unknown	Gatifloxacin + gentamicin, ceftazidime, or aztreonam	Killing curve	Bactericidal	139, 235
		Levofloxacin + cefoperazone or imipenem	Checkerboard-agar dilution	Bacteriostatic	282
Stenotrophomonas maltophilia	Unknown	Rifampin + gentamicin + carbenicillin	Checkerboard-broth microtiter	Bacteriostatic	676
		Rifampin + TMP + SMZ + carbenicillin	Checkerboard-broth microtiter	Bacteriostatic	676
		Ciprofloxacin + mezlocillin, piperacillin, imipenem, meropenem, aztreonam, ceftriaxone, ceftazidime, cefoperazone, or gentamicin	Checkerboard-agar dilution	Bacteriostatic	111, 282
		Gatifloxacin + cefepime, or piperacillin	Checkerboard-agar dilution	Bacteriostatic	139
		Gatifloxacin + ceftazidime, ticarcillin/clavulanate, or aztreonam	Killing curve	Bactericidal	235
		Ciprofloxacin, levofloxacin, or trovafloxacin + cefpirome, cefoperazone, ceftazidime, piperacillin/tazobactam, ticarcillin/clavulanate, or gentamicin	Checkerboard-broth microtiter	Bacteriostatic	512, 632
			Killing curve	Bactericidal	632
		Colistin + rifampin or TMP/SMZ	Killing curve	Bactericidal	213
	β-Lactam + aminoglycoside	Ceftazidime + tobramycin	Checkerboard-broth microtiter	Bacteriostatic	103
	β-Lactam + aminoglycoside or unknown	Piperacillin/tazobactam + gentamicin or ciprofloxacin	Checkerboard-broth microtiter with sampling	Bactericidal	234
Salmonella typhi	Sequential enzyme inhibition	TMP + SMZ	Checkerboard-agar dilution	Bacteriostatic	83
Salmonella typhimurium	Inhibition of protective enzymes	Chloramphenicol + ampicillin cephaloridine, or carbenicillin	Cellophane transfer	Bacteriostatic	411
	Inhibition of cell wall synthesis	β-Chloro-D-alanine + penicillin	Killing curve	Bactericidal	579
		Amdinocillin + ampicillin	Killing curve	Bactericidal	451
Salmonella spp	Inhibition of protective enzymes	Sulbactam + ampicillin	Checkerboard-broth microtiter	Bacteriostatic	175

(continued)

APPENDIX 9.1 (Continued)

Examples of Synergistic Antimicrobial Combinations *in Vitro*[a]

Organism	Mechanism of Synergism	Antimicrobial Combination	Techniques and Modifications	Effect Measured	References
Serratia marcescens	Inhibition of protective enzymes	Sulbactam + ampicillin	Checkerboard-broth	Bacteriostatic	175
		Clavulanic acid or sulbactam + amdinocillin (versus amdinocillin-resistant isolates)	Checkerboard-agar dilution	Bacteriostatic	452
		Chloramphenicol + ampicillin, cephaloridine, or carbenicillin	Cellophane transfer	Bacteriostatic	411
	Inhibition of cell wall synthesis	Fosmidomycin + cefazolin, cephalexin, ampicillin, or ticarcillin	Checkerboard-agar	Bacteriostatic	458
		Amdinocillin + cephradine	Checkerboard-broth dilution	Bacteriostatic	309
		Amdinocillin + ceftazidime	Checkerboard-broth microtiter dilution with sampling	Bacteriostatic Bactericidal	626 626
		Vancomycin + cephalothin or carbenicillin	Checkerboard-broth microtiter	Bacteriostatic	151
	β-Lactam + aminoglycoside	Piperacillin, moxalactam, cefotaxime, or cefoperazone + amikacin	Checkerboard-agar dilution	Bacteriostatic	339
		Azlocillin, aztreonam, ceftazidime, ceftriaxone, cefmenoxime, imipenem, piperacillin/tazobactam, ticarcillin/clavulanate, or moxalactam + amikacin tobramycin or netilmicin	Checkerboard-broth microtiter	Bacteriostatic	230, 390, 476
	Unknown	Ciprofloxacin + aztreonam, ceftazidime, piperacillin/tazobactam, ticarcillin/clavulanate, cefcamate, or cefpodoxime	Killing curve	Bactericidal	475, 511
		Ciprofloxacin or ofloxacin + cefcamate or cefpodoxime	Checkerboard-agar dilution	Bacteriostatic	475
		Sulfadiazine + polymyxin B	Checkerboard-broth dilution	Bacteriostatic	238
Serratia spp	β-Lactam + aminoglycoside or unknown	Piperacillin/tazobactam + gentamicin or ciprofloxacin	Checkerboard-broth microtiter with sampling	Bactericidal	234

Shigella spp	Sequential enzyme inhibition	TMP + SMZ	Checkerboard-broth and agar dilution	Bacteriostatic	533
	Inhibition of protective enzymes	Sulbactam + ampicillin	Checkerboard-agar dilution	Bacteriostatic	201
		Chloramphenicol + ampicillin, cephaloridine, or carbenicillin	Cellophane transfer	Bacteriostatic	411
	Inhibition of cell wall synthesis	Amdinocillin + ampicillin	Killing curve	Bactericidal	451
Gram-negative Coccobacilli					
Haemohilus influenzae	Sequential enzyme	TMP + SMZ	Checkerboard-agar dilution	Bacteriostatic	79
	Inhibition of cell wall synthesis	Amdinocillin + ampicillin	Checkerboard-agar dilution	Bacteriostatic	665
	Inhibition of protective enzymes	Nafcillin + ampicillin	Checkerboard-broth dilution	Bacteriostatic	672
		Clavulanic acid or sulbactam + ampicillin, amoxicillin or ticarcillin	Checkerboard-agar dilution, broth microtiter, and broth microtiter with sampling	Bacteriostatic	175, 185, 203, 508, 524, 664, 673
				Bactericidal	185, 524, 673
	Unknown	Rifampin + TMP	Checkerboard-broth	Bactericidal	381
		Roxithromycin + sulfamethoxazole	Checkerboard-broth microtiter with sampling	Bacteriostatic and bactericidal	342
Moraxella catarrhalis	Inhibition of protective enzymes	Clavulanic acid + amoxicillin	Checkerboard-agar dilution	Bacteriostatic	277
	Sequential enzyme inhibition	TMP + SMZ	Checkerboard-agar dilution	Bacteriostatic	528
Neisseria gonorrhoeae	Sequential enzyme inhibition	TMP + SMZ (1:1)	Checkerboard-agar dilution	Bacteriostatic	522
	Inhibition of protective enzymes	Clavulanic acid or sulbactam + ampicillin, amoxicillin, or ticarcillin	Checkerboard-broth microtiter	Bacteriostatic	175, 203, 277, 508
Bordetella pertussis	Sequential enzyme inhibition	TMP + SMZ	Checkerboard-agar dilution	Bacteriostatic	79

(continued)

APPENDIX 9.1 (Continued)

Examples of Synergistic Antimicrobial Combinations *in Vitro*[a]

Organism	Mechanism of Synergism	Antimicrobial Combination	Techniques and Modifications	Effect Measured	References
Gram-negative Anaerobes					
Bacteroides fragilis group	Inhibition of protective enzymes	Cefoxitin + carbenicillin, piperacillin, or mezlocillin	Checkerboard-agar dilution	Bacteriostatic	31
		Clavulanic acid or sulbactam + cefoperazone, cefulodin, ampicillin, amoxicillin, ticarcillin, piperacillin, or penicillin G	Checkerboard-agar dilution and microtiter broth dilution with sampling	Bacteriostatic	129, 175, 185, 200, 203, 205, 277, 295, 457, 524, 664
				Bactericidal	185, 200, 524
		Tazobactam + ceftriaxone or piperacillin	Agar dilution	Bacteriostatic	668
	Unknown	Metronidazole + clindamycin	Checkerboard-agar dilution and broth dilution microtiter with sampling	Bacteriostatic and Bactericidal	76
		Ciprofloxacin + clindamycin, mezlocillin, cefoxitin, or cefotaxime	Checkerboard-broth microtiter or agar	Bacteriostatic	179, 657
		Levofloxacin + clindamycin or metronidazole	Killing curve	Bactericidal	127
Prevotella melaninogenica	β-Lactam + aminoglycoside	Penicillin + gentamicin	Checkerboard-agar dilution	Bacteriostatic	64
	Inhibition of protective enzymes	Clavulanic acid + ticarcillin	Checkerboard-broth microdilution	Bacteriostatic	205
		Tazobactam + ceftriaxone or piperacillin	Agar dilution	Bacteriostatic	668
P. disiens	Unknown	Levofloxacin + metronidazole	Killing curve	Bactericidal	127
P. intermedia	Unknown	Levofloxacin + metronidazole	Killing curve	Bactericidal	127
Gram-positive Cocci					
Viridans streptococci	β-Lactam + aminoglycoside	Penicillin + streptomycin	Checkerboard-broth dilution with sampling	Bactericidal	156
			Killing curve	Bactericidal	667
Diphtheroids	Cell wall-active agent + aminoglycoside	Vancomycin or teicoplanin + gentamicin or tobramycin	Killing curve	Bactericidal	434, 581
		Daptomycin + gentamicin or tobramycin	Killing curve	Bactericidal	580

Group A streptococci	β-Lactam + aminoglycoside	Penicillin + gentamicin	Checkerboard-broth microdilution with sampling at 3 and 6 hr	Bactericidal	28
			Killing curve		28
	β-Lactam + aminoglycoside or unknown	Piperacillin/tazobactam + gentamicin or ciprofloxacin	Checkerboard-broth microtiter with sampling	Bactericidal	234
Group B streptococci	β-Lactam + aminoglycoside	Ampicillin or penicillin + gentamicin	Checkerboard-broth microdilution with sampling at 3 and 6 hr	Bactericidal	28, 559, 560
			Killing curve	Bactericidal	28, 559, 560
Pneumococci	Inhibition of cell wall synthesis	Cefotaxime + fosfomycin	Killing curve	Bactericidal	33
	Unknown	Levofloxacin + vancomycin or teicoplanin	Killing curve	Bactericidal	325
		Levofloxacin or gatifloxacin + cefepime, cefotaxime, or meropenem	Killing curve	Bactericidal	123, 338, 497
			Checkerboard-microdilution	Bacteriostatic	338, 497
		Ofloxacin + cefotaxime or desacetylcefotaxime	Checkerboard-agar dilution	Bacteriostatic	290
Enterococci	β-Lactam (or other agent acting on the cell wall) + aminoglycoside	Penicillin, ampicillin, carbenicillin, nafcillin, oxacillin, or vancomycin + streptomycin, kanamycin, gentamicin, tobramycin, amikacin, netilmicin, or sisomicin	Killing curve or checkerboard-broth dilution with sampling	Bactericidal	85, 190, 224, 281, 332, 361, 389, 425, 427
		Imipenem + gentamicin, tobramycin, or amikacin	Killing curve	Bactericidal	168, 230, 645
	Inhibition of cell wall synthesis	Daptomycin + imipenem or fosfomycin	Checkerboard-broth microdilution	Bacteriostatic	141
			Killing curve	Bactericidal	141
		Imipenem + fosfomycin or teicoplanin	Checkerboard-broth microdilution	Bacteriostatic	142
			Killing curve	Bactericidal	142
	β-Lactam + aminoglycoside or unknown	Piperacillin/tazobactam + gentamicin or ciprofloxacin	Checkerboard-broth microtiter with sampling	Bactericidal	234
		Levofloxacin + ampicillin	Killing curve	Bactericidal	576
	Inhibition of cell wall synthesis	Glycopeptides + various β-lactams	Checkerboard-microdilution	Bacteriostatic	96
	(Vanco-R strains)		Checkerboard-microdilution	Bacteriostatic	345

(continued)

APPENDIX 9.1 (Continued)

Examples of Synergistic Antimicrobial Combinations *in Vitro*[a]

Organism	Mechanism of Synergism	Antimicrobial Combination	Techniques and Modifications	Effect Measured	References
		Amoxicillin + cefotaxime	Checkerboard-agar dilution	Bacteriostatic	386
	Unknown	Imipenem + rifampin	Checkerboard-microdilution	Bacteriostatic	142
			Killing curve	Bactericidal	142
	Unknown (Vanco-R strains)	Ciprofloxacin + vancomycin	Checkerboard-microdilution	Bacteriostatic	622
		Ciprofloxacin + ampicillin	Killing curve	Bactericidal	340
		Sparfloxacin or clinafloxacin + gentamicin	Killing curve	Bactericidal	496
	Unknown	Quinupristin/dalfopristin + doxycycline	Killing curve	Bactericidal	402
		Quinupristin/dalfopristin + ampicillin/sulbactam	Checkerboard	Bacteriostatic	402
			Killing curve	Bactericidal	402
		Quinupristin/dalfopristin + vancomycin	Killing curve	Bactericidal	370
		Quinupristin/dalfopristin + vancomycin or gentamicin	Checkerboard-microdilution	Bacteriostatic	300
Staphylococcus aureus	Inhibition of protective enzymes	Clavulanic acid or sulbactam + ticarcillin, piperacillin, ampicillin, amoxicillin, or penicillin G	Checkerboard-broth microtiter and agar	Bacteriostatic	155, 175, 277, 457, 520, 524, 664
		Chloramphenicol + penicillin G	Cellophane transfer	Bacteriostatic	412
	Inhibition of cell wall synthesis	Daptomycin + aztreonam or ceftriaxone	Checkerboard-broth microdilution	Bacteriostatic	569
		Imipenem + teicoplanin or fosfomycin	Checkerboard-broth microdilution	Bacteriostatic	142
			Killing curve	Bactericidal	142
		Imipenem + vancomycin or teicoplanin	Checkerboard-broth microdilution with sampling	Bacteriostatic Bactericidal	37
		Cefepime + vancomycin	Checkerboard-agar dilution	Bacteriostatic	374
			Killing curve	Bactericidal	374
		Fosfomycin + cefazolin or meropenem	Checkerboard microdilution	Bacteriostatic	241
	β-Lactam (cell wall agent) + aminoglycoside	Nafcillin, oxacillin, cephalothin, or vancomycin + kanamycin, gentamicin, tobramycin, netilmicin, or sisomicin	Killing curve	Bactericidal	70, 314, 641, 643, 644

	Unknown	Daptomycin + tobramycin	Checkerboard-broth microdilution	Bacteriostatic	569
		Teicoplanin + rifampin	Checkerboard-broth microtiter	Bacteriostatic and bactericidal	616
		Vancomycin + rifampin	Killing curve	Bactericidal	544
		Clindamycin or imipenem + rifampin	Killing curve	Bactericidal	142, 266
		Ciprofloxacin + azlocillin	Checkerboard-broth microdilution	Bacteriostatic	429
		Levofloxacin + oxacillin	Killing curve	Bactericidal	482
		Fosfomycin + rifampin, linezolid, quinupristin/dalfopristin, or moxifloxacin	Checkerboard microdilution	Bacteriostatic	241
	β-Lactam + aminoglycoside or unknown	Piperacillin/tazobactam + gentamicin or ciprofloxacin	Checkerboard-broth microtiter with sampling	Bactericidal	234
S. aureus (penicillin-susceptible)	β-Lactam + aminoglycoside	Penicillin + gentamicin	Checkerboard-broth dilution	Bacteriostatic	590
S. aureus (methicillin-resistant)	Inhibition of protective enzymes	Sulbactam + ampicillin or penicillin G	Checkerboard-broth dilution	Bacteriostatic	524
	Inhibition of cell wall synthesis	Fosfomycin + methicillin or cefamandole	Checkerboard-broth microdilution	Bacteriostatic	8
		Daptomycin + oxacillin or ampicillin-sulbactam	Killing curve	Bactericidal	518a
		Imipenem + cefotiam, cefpiramide, or piperacillin	Checkerboard-agar	Bacteriostatic	399
			Killing curve	Bactericidal	
		Vancomycin + cefoperazone, cefpirome, or imipenem	Checkerboard methods	Bacteriostatic	566, 613
		Meropenem + various β-lactams	Checkerboard-agar	Bacteriostatic	597
		Cefotiam or cefoperazone + cefmetazole, imipenem, vancomycin, and others	Checkerboard-agar	Bacteriostatic	518, 596
		Cefepime + vancomycin	Checkerboard-agar dilution	Bacteriostatic	374
			Killing curve	Bactericidal	374
	Unknown	Quinupristin/dalfopristin + ciprofloxacin or rifampin	Killing curve	Bactericidal	545
		Teicoplanin + rifampin	Checkerboard-broth	Bacteriostatic and bactericidal	616
S. aureus (MSSA and/or MRSA)	Unknown	Fusidic acid + rifampin	Killing curve	Bactericidal	183
		Quinupristin/dalfopristin + vancomycin	Killing curve	Bactericidal	299, 490

(continued)

APPENDIX 9.1 (Continued)

Examples of Synergistic Antimicrobial Combinations *in Vitro*[a]

Organism	Mechanism of Synergism	Antimicrobial Combination	Techniques and Modifications	Effect Measured	References
		Quinupristin/dalfopristin + amoxicillin, flucloxacillin, cefuroxime, cefamandole, cefepime, imipenem, or tetracycline	Checkerboard microdilution	Bacteriostatic	633
		Ofloxacin + cefotaxime or desacetylcefotaxime	Checkerboard	Bacteriostatic	217, 290
Coagulase-negative staphylococci	Inhibition of protective enzymes	Sulbactam + ampicillin	Checkerboard-broth	Bacteriostatic	524
	β-Lactam (or other agent acting on the cell wall) + aminoglycoside	Vancomycin + gentamicin or tobramycin	Killing curve	Bactericidal	373
	Inhibition of cell wall synthesis	Daptomycin + tobramycin	Checkerboard-broth microdilution	Bacteriostatic	569
		Daptomycin + aztreonam or ceftriaxone	Checkerboard-broth microdilution	Bacteriostatic	569
		Imipenem + fosfomycin or teicoplanin	Checkerboard-broth microdilution	Bacteriostatic	142
			Killing curve	Bactericidal	142
		Imipenem + vancomycin or teicoplanin	Checkerboard-broth microdilution with sampling	Bacteriostatic Bactericidal	37
		Cefepime + vancomycin	Checkerboard-agar dilution	Bacteriostatic	374
			Killing curve	Bactericidal	374
	β-Lactam + aminoglycoside or unknown	Piperacillin/tazobactam + gentamicin or ciprofloxacin	Checkerboard-broth microtiter with sampling	Bactericidal	234
	Unknown	Vancomycin + rifampin	Killing curve	Bactericidal	373
		Gentamicin + rifampin	Killing curve	Bactericidal	373
		Ofloxacin + cefotaxime or desacetylcefotaxime	Checkerboard	Bacteriostatic	290
		Fosfomycin + rifampin, linezolid, quinupristin/dalfopristin, or moxifloxacin	Checkerboard microdilution	Bacteriostatic	241
		Imipenem + rifampin	Checkerboard-broth microtiter	Bacteriostatic	142
			Killing curve	Bactericidal	142

Gram-positive Bacilli					
Lactobacilli	β-Lactam + aminoglycoside	Penicillin or ampicilin + streptomycin, or gentamicin	Checkerboard-broth dilution with sampling	Bactericidal	45
Listeria monocytogenes	β-Lactam + aminoglycoside	Ampicillin or penicillin + streptomycin or gentamicin	Killing curve	Bactericidal	378, 421
		Imipenem + gentamicin	Killing curve	Bactericidal	168
	Unknown	Rifampin + penicillin G, ampicillin, or cefamandole	Checkerboard-broth microtiter with sampling	Bactericidal	617
		Rifampin + erythomycin	Checkerboard-broth microtiter	Bacteriostatic	617
		Trimethoprim +gentamicin	Killing curve	Bactericidal	378
Gram-positive Anaerobes[b]					
Peptostreptococcus asaccharolyticus	Unknown	Levofloxacin + metronidazole	Killing curve	Bactericidal	127
Clostridium perfrigens	Unknown	Levofloxacin + clindamycin or metronidazole	Killing curve	Bactericidal	127
Other Organisms					
Nocardia asteroides	Sequential enzyme inhibition	TMP + SMZ	Checkerboard	Bacteriostatic	385
	Inhibition of protective enzymes	Clavulanic acid + penicillin, ampicillin, carbenicillin, mezlocillin, piperacillin, or amdinocillin	Checkerboard-agar dilution	Bacteriostatic	313
			Paper strip	Bacteriostatic	313
	Inhibition of cell wall synthesis	Imipenem + cefotaxime	Checkerboard-agar dilution	Bacteriostatic	229
	Unknown	TMP + SMZ + imipenem	Checkerboard-agar dilution	Bacteriostatic	229
		TMP +SMZ + amikacin	Checkerboard-agar dilution	Bacteriostatic	229
Mycobacterium[c] *avium complex*	Unknown	Ethambutol + rifampin, streptomycin, kanamycin, amikacin, clarithromycin, or ciprofloxacin	Checkerboard-agar dilution	Bacteriostatic	36, 308, 684
		Rifampin + streptomycin, kanamycin, isonazid, or clarithromycin			
		Isonazid + streptomycin or kanamycin			

(continued)

APPENDIX 9.1 (Continued)

Examples of Synergistic Antimicrobial Combinations *in Vitro*[a]

Organism	Mechanism of Synergism	Antimicrobial Combination	Techniques and Modifications	Effect Measured	References
		Streptomycin + ethambutol, rifampin + ethambutol, or INH-isoniazid, rifampin + ethambutol	Growth rate broth	Bacteriostatic	270
		Ethambutol + sparfloxacin ± rifampin	Broth dilution	Bacteriostatic Bactericidal	669
Mycobacterium fortuitum	Inhibition of protective enzymes	Clavulanic acid + amoxicillin or cephalothin	Checkerboard-agar dilution	Bacteriostatic	130
	Unknown	Ciprofloxacin + amikacin or TMP + SMZ	Checkerboard-agar	Bacteriostatic	211
M. tuberculosis	Inhibition of protective Enzymes	Clavulanic acid + amoxicillin	Broth dilution with sampling	Bactericidal	131
	Unknown	Teicoplanin + ethambutol	Checkerboard-broth dilution	Bacteriostatic	17
M. kansasii	Unknown	Ethambutol + ciprofloxacin, rifampin, or isoniazid	Growth rate broth	Bacteriostatic	265
M. leprae	Unknown	Rifabutin + clinafloxacin or sparfloxacin	Checkerboard measurement of metabolic activity	Bacteriostatic Bactericidal	147

[a] Demonstration of synergism is often strain- and concentration-dependent. Other effects, including antagonism, can result from some combinations described as showing synergism against some isolates at some antimicrobial concentrations. Effects noted are presented as examples of interactions which have been described, but may not always occur at clinically achievable concentrations. *In vitro* activity does not necessarily predict enhanced efficacy *in vivo*. Grouping of similar antimicrobials in each component of a combination regimen does not necessarily imply that all possible combinations result in the effect noted.

[b] See also Chapter 4, "Antimicrobial Susceptibilty Testing of Anaerobic Bacteria."

[c] See also Chapter 5, "Antimycobacterial Agents."

CHAPTER 10

Genetic and Biochemical Mechanisms of Bacterial Resistance to Antimicrobial Agents

Louis B. Rice, Robert A. Bonomo

The emergence and spread of antimicrobial resistance determinants continues to challenge our abilities to treat serious infections. Over the past decade, we have witnessed growing challenges of antimicrobial resistance in both the nosocomial and the community setting. While new antimicrobial agents designed to treat multiresistant pathogens have been introduced in the past few years, resistance has continued to emerge and spread. Roughly 25% of clinical enterococcal isolates (now the fourth most common cause of nosocomial infection) are now resistant to both ampicillin and vancomycin, for years the two most reliable antienterococcal drugs (www.cdc.gov/ncidod/hip/SURVEILL/NNIS.HTM). Many of these strains are resistant to multiple additional antibiotics. The clinical availability of linezolid, daptomycin, and quinupristin-dalfopristin has offered therapeutic alternatives for such strains, but resistance to these newer compounds is also emerging. Methicillin-resistant *Staphylococcus aureus* (MRSA) now represent more than 50% of isolates recovered from patients in intensive care units (www.cdc.gov/ncidod/hip/SURVEILL/NNIS.HTM), and new strains of MRSA are causing soft tissue infections in the community at an alarming rate. Gram-negative bacterial pathogens have kept pace, especially *Acinetobacter baumannii* and *Pseudomonas aeruginosa,* in which multiresistance is frequently recognized (271). We have learned much over the past decade about the mechanisms by which these bacteria become resistant to multiple antimicrobial agents. It is hoped that this knowledge will better inform future strategies for drug development and at the same time allow us to limit the morbidity and mortality associated with bacterial infections more effectively and efficiently.

Several factors influence increases in bacterial resistance. The increased use of a variety of antimicrobials and the clinical introduction of numerous closely related compounds in the 1980s and 1990s are clearly associated with the emergence and dissemination of resistant strains. Increasing numbers of immunocompromised patients, including patients undergoing intensive cancer chemotherapy or organ or bone marrow transplantation and those suffering from acquired immunodeficiency syndrome, have created environments where host immune response is diminished (320). Cost-containment requirements in modern hospitals have led to increased patient-to-staff ratios, which have been associated with reduced adherence to strict infection control measures (263). Finally, the flourishing of intensive care units, with the prolonged stays and close proximity of many patients whose physical and immunologic defenses are compromised, has created settings in which the emergence and spread of resistant bacteria have accelerated (181,283).

The development of antimicrobial resistance is an entirely predictable consequence of our use of potent antimicrobial agents. Compared to humans, whose evolution is relatively slow, bacteria multiply and evolve rapidly. A 24-hour period allows 1 million or more opportunities for the development of mutations for many bacteria. Mutations that provide a selective advantage in a given environment are rapidly propagated. Moreover, bacteria have been faced with antimicrobial challenges for a considerably longer time than these agents have been used to treat clinical infections. Most antibiotics in current use are natural products (or derivatives of natural products) of fungi or bacteria. It stands to reason that bacteria able to produce an antibiotic must have developed mechanisms by which its lethal action could be avoided. In addition, because, pure cultures are rarely found in nature, it also stands to reason that bacteria that share an environment with antibiotic-producing organisms must develop mechanisms by which they can survive in this environment. Therefore many, if not all of the acquired resistance genes now arising in clinically important bacteria were likely in existence long before the human discovery of antibiotics. Their appearance in modern times merely reflects the scavenging ability of clinically important bacteria and the significant selective advantage these determinants confer in antimicrobial-rich environments.

Although antimicrobial resistance is likely to result in improved bacterial survival in an antimicrobial-rich milieu, there is little evidence to date to support a role for antimicrobial resistance determinants as virulence factors themselves. Nevertheless, because both true virulence factors and antimicrobial resistance determinants may be found as transferable genetic elements, coselection for both resistance and virulence determinants remains a significant concern (115,210,259). The explosion in genomic data that has occurred during the past decade has dramatically improved our understanding of the relationships that exist between antimicrobial resistance and virulence determinants, especially within large genomic regions designated "pathogenicity islands." Moreover, our increasing knowledge of the complex regulatory networks employed by bacteria makes it clear that global regulators may activate virulence determinants and resistance determinants at the same time.

The past two decades have produced substantial research into the mechanisms by which bacteria develop and disseminate resistance determinants. Although there is much yet to be learned, it is clear from work already accomplished that bacteria are highly evolved in their abilities to share advantageous genes. In this chapter, we review what is known about the genetic mechanisms by which bacteria develop and disseminate antibiotic resistance determinants. We also review how our knowledge of bacterial genetic systems has furthered our ability to understand the spread of resistant bacteria in the human population. Finally, we summarize current knowledge of the biochemical mechanisms of bacterial antimicrobial resistance.

GENETIC BASIS OF ANTIMICROBIAL RESISTANCE

Intrinsic Resistance

When discussing bacterial resistance to antibiotics, we normally restrict our comments to the emergence of resistance in previously susceptible species. This is not to imply that intrinsic resistance is unimportant—it is not—but merely reflects the fact that intrinsic resistance is normally discovered in the early stages of drug development and does not present therapeutic dilemmas for well-informed physicians (assuming, of course, that therapeutic alternatives exist). The study of intrinsic resistance characteristics of different species can help us predict potential problems that may emerge under selective pressure. For example, the emergence of *Stenotropomonas maltophilia* as a significant nosocomial pathogen corresponded with the clinical introduction of imipenem, to which *S. maltophilia* is intrinsically resistant (329). The study of intrinsic resistance may also help in choosing effective treatment strategies. It is essential, for example, to understand that the intrinsic resistance of enterococci to all clinically available cephalosporins is due to a decreased binding affinity of the penicillin-binding proteins (PBPs) rather than to the production of β-lactamase (375). Combining a cephalosporin with an inhibitor of β-lactamase would have little chance of producing a clinical cure of an enterococcal infection. A complete explication of intrinsic resistance mechanisms is beyond the scope of this chapter and can be found elsewhere in this volume.

Resistance Due to Structural Mutations in Preexisting Genetic Determinants

It has been recognized since early in the antibiotic era that resistance to certain antimicrobial agents can be elicited either by inoculating a large number of bacteria onto an agar plate containing the antibiotic or by exposing a bacterial strain to ever increasing concentrations of the antimicrobial over time (47). Antibiotics for which one-step mutation to resistance occurs at a high enough frequency to be detectable in the laboratory include streptomycin, rifampin, and the fluoroquinolones (74,146,172). Resistance in these instances generally results from point mutations (addition, deletion, or substitution of a nucleotide or nucleotides, resulting in an alteration of the protein sequence of the translated gene product) somewhere in the gene encoding the proteins that are targeted by the antibiotic. Point mutations presumably occur at random. Those that are not recognized and repaired by host repair systems are passed on to successive generations of bacteria, assuming that they do not result in a change that is lethal or seriously deleterious to the organism.

Not all mutations are clinically significant. In many cases, single nucleotide changes do not result in an alteration in the amino acid sequence of the protein product. These are referred to as silent mutations. Other nucleotide changes may result in amino acid changes that do not detectably alter the physical or functional characteristics of the protein product. Such mutations are insignificant phenotypically but may be of value in tracing the evolution or epidemiology of certain resistance determinants. In the case of streptomycin, one-step resistance occurs via point mutations in the genes encoding ribosomal proteins, resulting in an inability of streptomycin to bind to its target, the ribosome. In *Mycobacterium tuberculosis,* the majority of streptomycin-resistant (Sm^r) clinical isolates have a nucleotide change from adenine to guanine in codon 43 of the *rpsL* gene, which encodes the ribosomal protein S12

(74). Mycobacteria are somewhat unusual in this regard, because the streptomycin resistance seen in most other bacterial species commonly results from the acquisition of exogenous genes encoding enzymes that modify the antibiotic (316). The reliance of *M. tuberculosis* on ribosomal mechanisms for streptomycin resistance may simply be a necessary consequence of what appears to be an undeveloped system for acquiring exogenous genes, although there are data that suggest that at least some mycobacterial species are capable of acquiring exogenous DNA (251). Resistance to rifampin, which targets the cellular DNA-dependent RNA polymerase, occurs at a high frequency in most bacteria. In *Escherichia coli*, resistance results from amino acid changes in one of six highly conserved regions of *rpoB*, which encodes the β-subunit of the RNA polymerase (172). Most of the resistant *E. coli* that have been examined have had point mutations in a short conserved region of this gene and in well-defined clusters within this region. Mutations in the RNA polymerase genes have now been identified in rifampin-resistant (Rif^r) isolates of a number of species, among these *Mycobacterium leprae, M. tuberculosis, Neisseria meningitides, Rhodococcus equi, and Chlamydia trachomatis* (55,155,337). In all cases, rifampin resistance appears to result from mutations in regions corresponding to the conserved regions of the *E. coli* protein.

Fluoroquinolones such as ciprofloxacin target the host topoisomerases, DNA gyrase and topoisomerase IV. These enzymes are essential for cellular maintenance and replication through their involvement in the coiling and uncoiling of chromosomal DNA and the segregation of daughter molecules (156). The DNA gyrase enzyme has two A and B subunits; the A subunits are the primary targets for fluoroquinolone action. Fluoroquinolones vary in their specificity for gyrase or topoisomerase IV in different genera, and strains that emerge resistant to these antibiotics will generally contain mutations in locations that reflect these specificities (156). High-level ciprofloxacin-resistant isolates frequently employ several resistance mechanisms, including one or more topoisomerase mutations along with active efflux from the cell. Efflux, in fact, may be a critically important first step to resistance. Although efflux of fluoroquinolones does not by itself confer very high levels of resistance, the activation of efflux mechanisms may amplify levels of resistance associated with point mutations in the topoisomerase genes. Mutations that might not normally survive the challenge of clinical concentrations of fluoroquinolones may, under these circumstances, allow propagation of the mutation and the eventual emergence of high-level resistance.

One-step mutations can have significant clinical impact. The initial excitement over the efficacy of streptomycin as a treatment for tuberculosis was rapidly diminished by the recurrence of resistant organisms during streptomycin therapy (223). Rifampin remains one of our most broadly active antimicrobials but is seldom if ever used as a single agent because resistance emerges rapidly during therapy, although this drug has proven effective in combination with other antibiotics against several important pathogens (230). Ciprofloxacin remains an excellent and highly effective antibiotic, but its usefulness has rapidly diminished against methicillin-resistant staphylococci due to the widespread isolation of fluoroquinolone-resistant strains (34), and its activity against nosocomial strains of *P. aeruginosa* is rapidly diminishing (www.cdc.gov/ncidod/hip/SURVEILL/NNIS.HTM). In general, the mechanisms by which rifampin and fluoroquinolone resistance occurs in clinical isolates closely parallel those that have been observed in laboratory mutants. As noted, due to the widespread presence of aminoglycoside-modifying enzyme genes, the same is not true for streptomycin (316).

In the laboratory, the occurrence of stable, one-step resistant mutants has been used to great advantage in several areas. The ability to create such mutants allows the study of the resistance mutations in isogenic susceptible and resistant strains, eliminating the question of whether undetectable additional genetic events have resulted in levels of resistance seen in clinical isolates. The ability to create stable resistant mutants has also greatly aided the study of transferable resistance determinants. Laboratory-derived resistant mutants serve as excellent plasmid recipients in mating experiments, as long as the plasmid transfer frequency exceeds by a significant degree the frequency of spontaneous donor resistance to the counter-selecting antibiotic. Rif^r and Sm^r mutants of different bacterial species remain the most commonly used recipient strains (72,163). If the transfer event being studied is very rare (i.e., less than 10^{-9}/recipient colony-forming unit [CFU]), additional resistance markers may be necessary. In *E. coli*, the second marker is frequently resistance to nalidixic acid (a precursor of the fluoroquinolones that is also a DNA gyrase inhibitor), resistance to which occurs spontaneously in *E. coli* at a rate of approximately 2×10^{-8}/CFU (286). In Gram-positive bacteria, recipients expressing resistance to fusidic acid in addition to rifampin are frequently used (167). The rationale for the second resistance determinant is simple. If resistance to the two antibiotics occurs by independent events, then the chance of the two mutations occurring in a single organism is the product of each mutation occurring alone. Therefore, if the rate of rifampin resistance in enterococci is 1×10^{-7} and the rate of spontaneous resistance to fusidic acid is 1×10^{-8}, then the rate of spontaneous resistance to both antibiotics at the same time will be 1×10^{-15}. Protocols for the isolation of resistant mutants using antibiotic selection are included in the appendices at the end of this chapter.

Important recently introduced antimicrobial agents have proved susceptible to point mutations as a cause of resistance. Linezolid, the first clinically available member of the oxazolidinone class, acts by inhibiting protein synthesis through its binding to the initiation complex (319). A single point mutation in the 23S rRNA gene can confer resistance (269). Since there are 4–6 23S rRNA genes present in most of the bacteria that linezolid is used against, a single point mutation confers little or no resistance. However, when several of the genes possess the mutation, high-level resistance can result (211). In recombination-proficient cells, mutation of additional 23S rRNA genes occurs relatively rapidly through the process of gene conversion (202). As a result, linezolid-resistant isolates of multiresistant *E. faecium* have been frequently isolated and have caused outbreaks in areas where patients are significantly immunocompromised (122,149).

Resistance Due to Regulatory Mutations in Preexisting Genetic Determinants

One-step mutation to antibiotic resistance can also result from changes in the regulation of preexisting genes. All Gram-negative bacteria thus far examined (with the exception of *Salmonella*) have been found to possess a chromosomal β-lactamase gene whose product in most instances is primarily a cephalosporinase that results in resistance to all cephalosporins and penicillins when produced in large amounts (29). In particular genera, notably *Citrobacter, Enterobacter, Pseudomonas,* and *Serratia,* the production of this enzyme can be induced by exposure to antibiotics that are good inducers, among them cefoxitin and imipenem (26). The *Enterobacter ampC* is under the regulatory control of several other genes, designated *ampR, ampD, ampE,* and *ampG,* via an interaction that involves normal cellular processes for the uptake and reprocessing of cell wall breakdown products (Fig. 10.1) (26). AmpR serves two functions. Under normal circumstances, cellular concentrations of the peptidoglycan precursor *N*-acetyl-muramic acid pentapeptide (MurNAc-penta) are sufficient to bind to AmpR and maintain it as a repressor of *ampC* transcription. MurNAc-penta can be displaced from its site on AmpR by the cell wall breakdown product anhydro-*N*-acetyl muramic acid tripeptide (anhydro-murNAc-tri), resulting in conversion of AmpR to a potent activator of *ampC* transcription. Entry of anhydro-MurNAc-tri into the cell is facilitated by AmpG, a permease that transports it across the cell membrane. Concentrations of anhydro-MurNAc-tri are normally modulated by AmpD, a cytosolic *N*-acetylmuramyl-L-alanine amidase that converts anhydro-murNAc-tri to murNAc-tri, which can then be processed into precursors for the growing peptidoglycan. Importantly, murNAC-tri does not bind to AmpR. Therefore, conditions in which excesses of anhydro-murNAc-tri are present will be associated with excessive production of AmpC β-lactamase. When AmpD is absent or nonfunctional or when an excess of cell wall breakdown products overwhelms its capabilities (e.g., in the presence of a β-lactam that is a good inducer), the excess of anhydro-MurNAc-tri displaces MurNAc-penta from its binding site on AmpR, increasing *ampC* expression (168). AmpE contributes to the activity of the AmpD but is not essential for activity. Overexpression of *ampC* yields clinical resistance to virtually all β-lactam agents, with the possible exception of imipenem and meropenem, resistance to which requires associated decreases in the expression of specific outer membrane proteins or the activation of specific efflux pumps (344,379). Derepressed mutants occur frequently enough (approximately 10^{-8}/CFU) to be significant problems in the treatment of clinical *Enterobacter* and *Pseudomonas* infections (8,199).

In many instances, regulatory mutants either decrease the expression of outer membrane porins or increase the expression of multidrug efflux pumps. The importance of efflux pumps for the expression of resistance is understood in most detail for *P. aeruginosa.* A very important class of efflux pumps is the "resistance-nodulation-cell division" (RND) class. RND pumps are found in a wide variety of Gram-negative bacteria. The structure of one such pump, the AcrAB-TolC pump of *E. coli,* has been elucidated in the greatest detail (Fig. 10.2) (233). It is presumed that other RND pumps are similar in their structure. RND pumps have three components. The pump itself spans the cytoplasmic membrane, connecting the cytoplasm to the periplasmic space. The periplasmic portion of the pump is connected to an outer membrane protein by a periplasmic connector. The specificity of the pump is contributed primarily by two large periplasmic loops located in the cytoplasmic membrane portion (380), which also contains channels that can allow entry (and efflux) of β-lactam antibiotics from the periplasmic space (233). A scan of the *P. aeruginosa* genome reveals roughly a dozen potential RND-type efflux pumps, at least six of which have now been characterized as antibiotic efflux pumps (332). Most of these pumps are not expressed under normal conditions, but they can be activated under antimicrobial selective pressure (Table 10.1). Most pumps thus far described in *P. aeruginosa* efflux fluoroquinolone antibiotics, explaining in part the rapid increase in fluoroquinolone resistance in this species and offering insight into the frequency of multiresistance as well.

The complexity and interplay of the different pumps are best exemplified by the emergence of carbapenem resistance in strains of *P. aeruginosa*. Under normal circumstances, the only RND-type pump expressed in *P. aeruginosa* is the MexAB-OprM pump. This pump effluxes a variety of different antimicrobial agents, including many β-lactams. Meropenem serves as a substrate for this pump, but imipenem does not. The MexEF-OprN pump, expression of which is normally repressed, was originally thought to efflux meropenem, but that is no longer considered to be true. There is no pump yet identified that efficiently effluxes imipenem. Resistance to imipenem, however, can be achieved relatively easily by reducing the quantity of outer membrane protein D2 (OMP D2). Reductions in this outer membrane protein impede imipenem entry into the periplasmic space, making the *P. aeruginosa* AmpC β-lactamase more effective and conferring

(*text continues on page 447*)

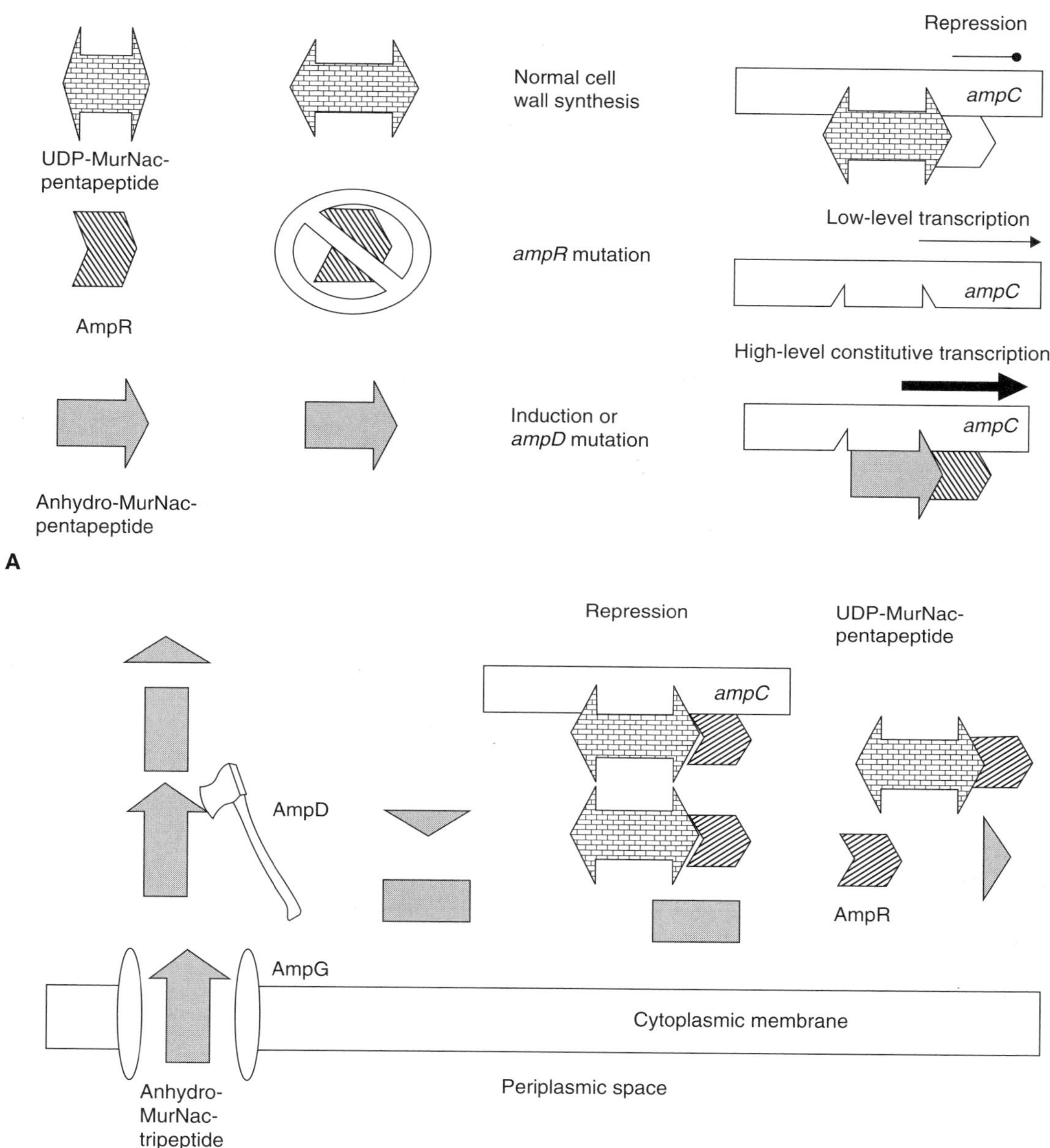

FIGURE 10.1 ● **A**. Schematic representation of the different states of β-lactamase expression in *Enterobacter* spp. UDP-MurNAc, when complexed with AmpR, represses *ampC* transcription. Loss of AmpR results in low-level *ampC* transcription; anhydro-MurNAc-tripeptide, when complexed with AmpR, activates high-level *ampC* transcription. **B**. Mechanism for maintaining repression of *ampC* transcription under baseline circumstances. AmpG is a permease that allows reentry of anhydro-MurNAC-tripeptide into the cytoplasm. Under normal circumstances, the amidase encoded by *ampD* removes the anhydro moiety, preventing interaction with AmpR as an activator. Under inducing conditions, the amount of anhydro-MurNAc-tripeptide entering the cell overwhelms the activity of AmpD. Under "stably derepressed" conditions, null mutations in *ampD* result in constitutive activation.

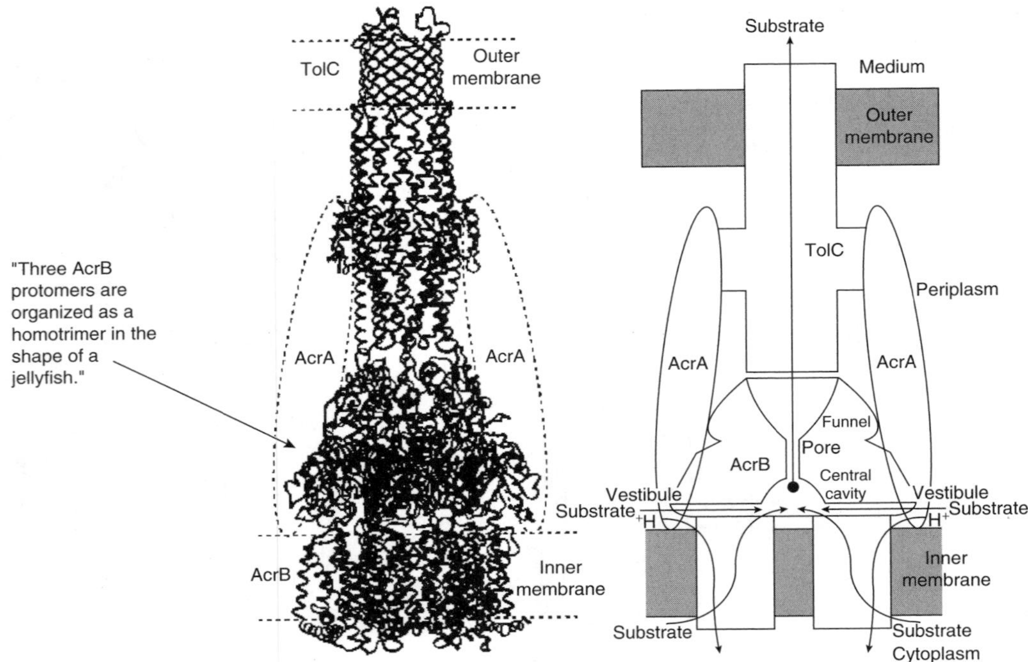

FIGURE 10.2 ● Representation of the crystal structure of the RND pump AcrAB-TolC. There are three components to this pump. The AcrB portion, which spans the cytoplasmic membrane, defines the substrate specificity. It also contains channels that allow extrusion of β-lactam antibiotics from the periplasmic space. Reprinted with permission from Murakami et al. (233).

TABLE 10.1

Pseudomonas aeruginosa RND-type Efflux Pumps and Their Substrates

RND Efflux Pump	Expression in Wild-type *Pseudomonas aeruginosa*	Substrates
MexAB-OprM	+	Quinolones, macrolides, tetracyclines, lincomycin, chloramphenicol, novobiocin, β-lactams except imipenem, triclosan (216)
MexCD-OprJ	−	Quinolones, macrolides, tetracyclines, lincomycin, chloramphenicol, novobiocin, penicillins except carbenicillin and sulbenicillin, cephems except ceftazidime, flomoxef, meropenem, triclosan (216)
MexEF-OprN	−	Quinolones, chloramphenicol, trimethoprim, tetracycline (213)
MexGHI-OpmD	+	Vanadium (2)
Mex JK-OprM	−	Erythromycin, tetracycline, triclosan (67)
MexWV-OprM	−	Quinolones, tetracycline, chloramphenicol, erythromycin, ethidium bromide, acriflavine (198)
MexXY-OprM	−	Aminoglycosides, quinolones, macrolides, tetracyclines, lincomycin, chloramphenicol, novobiocin, penicillins except carbenicillin and sulbenicillin, cephems except cefsulodin and ceftazidime, flomoxef, meropenem (3,216,226)

clinically significant levels of resistance. Entry of meropenem into the periplasmic space is not as dependent on OMP D2, so OMP D2 mutants generated by exposure to imipenem generally remain susceptible to meropenem. Activation of the MexEF-OprN pump has been linked to mutations in an upstream regulatory gene designated *mexT*. *mexT* expression is associated with increased expression of MexEF-OprN and decreased expression of OprD2 (248). Clinical strains have been reported that exhibit resistance to both imipenem and meropenem. These strains have expressed high levels of both MexAB-OprM and MexEF-OprN, along with decreased expression of OprD (99). Although it was originally thought that meropenem resistance was conferred by overexpression of the MexEF-OprN pump, it is probably more likely that meropenem resistance results from combined MexAB-OprM overexpression and increased expression of the *P. aeruginosa* AmpC. Imipenem resistance is the result of the combination of AmpC expression and OprD2 reduction, since neither reduction of OprD2 alone nor expression of AmpC alone confers significant levels of resistance (199). Such strains remain modestly susceptible to cefepime (a good substrate only for the MexCD-OprJ pump) and amikacin, and patients infected with such strains have responded to these combinations (99).

Insertion sequences, small segments of mobile bacterial DNA, may also play a role in apparent one-step mutations to resistance. It has been noted that certain strains of *Bacteroides fragilis* mutate to resistance to imipenem in a single step (265). The resistant strains produce a β-lactamase that is able to hydrolyze carbapenems. Cloning and sequencing of the segments of *B. fragilis* chromosome that confer this resistance phenotype have revealed that the production of the β-lactamase within these strains correlates with the placement of an insertion sequence, IS*1186*, upstream of the structural gene (266). Located within the end of IS*1186* is a region that promotes transcription of the β-lactamase gene. Without the promoter supplied by the IS element, the β-lactamase gene is unexpressed (266). A similar insertion sequence has been identified upstream of genes that confer resistance to 5-nitroimidazoles in *B. fragilis* (132). Insertion sequence-supplied promoter sequences may also be involved in the increased expression of β-lactamase genes responsible for resistance to ceftazidime in *Klebsiella pneumoniae* (264,287). Many of the insertion sequences described in Gram-negative bacilli possess potential promoter sequences in their terminal inverted repeats, suggesting that regulatory mutations resulting from the mobility of IS elements may be relatively common (119).

Point Mutations in Acquired Resistance Genes

The mushrooming number of new antimicrobial agents has led to the isolation of some classes of mutants that would have been unlikely to become clinically important in the absence of an antimicrobial-rich environment. These mutations result in the so-called extended-spectrum β-lactamases (ESBLs) most commonly found in clinical *K. pneumoniae* isolates (40). The development of the extended-spectrum cephalosporins was fueled in part by the need for antibiotics that were resistant to hydrolysis by the plasmid-mediated β-lactamases of Gram-negative bacilli, the most common of which were the TEM-1 and SHV-1 enzymes (40). These enzymes were acquired by and became prevalent within *E. coli* and other enterobacteria after the clinical introduction of ampicillin, the first penicillin with clinically important activity against enteric Gram-negative bacilli. The cephalosporins avoided hydrolysis by these enzymes via relatively minor alterations in the β-lactam molecular structure that precluded effective interaction with the β-lactamase molecule but did not preclude interaction with their target molecules, the PBPs. Because the extended activity of the newer cephalosporins is due to relatively minor modifications of the β-lactam molecule, it stands to reason that relatively minor modifications of the β-lactamase enzyme would be able to restore some degree of activity. Such minor modifications in the enzymes were identified with astonishing rapidity, with ceftazidime-hydrolyzing ability frequently resulting from a change of just one or two nucleotides (and resulting amino acids) in the roughly 1000–base pair gene (40). The emergence and spread of organisms producing these enzymes have threatened to significantly decrease the utility of the entire cephalosporin class of antibiotics (180,254,256). Moreover, newer classes of ESBLs, including the increasingly widespread CTX-M class, continue to be described (37). In contrast, the staphylococcal β-lactamases have remained remarkably stable, despite the fact that the β-lactamase–resistant semisynthetic penicillins (methicillin, nafcillin, and oxacillin) have been in clinical use for over 40 years (387). The reasons for this wide variation in the evolution frequencies of the enterobacterial and staphylococcal plasmid-mediated enzymes are unknown.

RESISTANCE VIA ACQUISITION OF FOREIGN DNA

Mechanisms of Acquiring Foreign DNA

Resistance to the majority of currently used antimicrobial agents has been accomplished via the acquisition of exogenous DNA. Resistance mediated by β-lactamase is most frequently exogenously acquired, as is resistance to aminoglycosides, chloramphenicol, erythromycin, sulfonamides, tetracyclines, trimethoprim, and vancomycin. Genes encoding low-affinity PBPs may also be exogenously acquired. It is generally accepted that there are three primary mechanisms by which bacteria share DNA: transduction, transformation, and conjugation.

Transduction is the process of DNA transfer mediated by bacteriophages (87). Bacteriophages invade and replicate within bacterial cells. Replicated phage genome is packaged into phage heads, which are released after lysis of the host cell. Packaged phage genomes then invade other cells, and the process repeats itself. Many bacteriophages integrate into the bacterial chromosome after invasion. In some instances, the phage genome is excised from the chromosome along with a neighboring segment of DNA. The neighboring segment of DNA then gets packaged into the phage head along with the phage genome. This process is known as specialized transduction, because it results in the transfer of only relatively small segments of chromosomal DNA adjacent to the integrated phage genome (100). If the phage genome is integrated next to an antimicrobial resistance determinant, then specialized transduction is a potential mechanism by which resistance genes can be transferred. Generalized transduction is a process whereby a segment of bacterial DNA unrelated to the phage genome becomes packaged within a phage head (100). This unrelated DNA can then be injected into a new cell. If the packaged DNA is a piece of chromosome, it may integrate into the new cell's chromosome via homologous recombination. If it is a plasmid, it will be able to replicate within the recipient cell as long as the host is permissive of plasmid replication and there are no incompatible plasmids already present. If the transduced DNA contains transposons, some segments of the transferred DNA can be integrated into the recipient genome via mechanisms mediated by transposon-encoded genes.

The extent to which transduction mechanisms have been responsible for the spread of antimicrobial resistance genes is not known. It is thought that generalized transduction has been responsible for the rapid and nearly complete spread of β-lactamase and heavy metal resistance plasmids in *Staphylococcus aureus,* since the plasmids that commonly encode these determinants approximate the size of an average phage genome (roughly 40 kb) (203). The rapid spread and genomic diversity of the recently described community-acquired methicillin-resistant *S. aureus* strains raise concern that the spread may be bacteriophage-mediated, since the methicillin-resistance chromosomal cassette in these strains is small enough to be packaged into a bacteriophage head (83,205,249). Bacteriophages have proven to be important tools for genetic manipulation of bacteria in the laboratory (100). They also serve as useful, although by no means foolproof, methods of typing bacteria for the study of the epidemiology of many infectious diseases (214).

Transformation is the process by which bacteria are able to absorb naked DNA from the surrounding environment. This is a process characteristic of a variety of bacteria. Those that have used it to acquire resistance to antimicrobial agents include *Streptococcus pneumoniae,* viridans streptococci, *Haemophilus influenzae, Neisseria gonorrhoeae,* and *Neisseria meningitidis,* among others (95,96). The genetic basis for the creation of the low-affinity PBPs in *S. pneumoniae* and *N. meningitidis,* for example, is the formation of mosaic PBP genes (95,96). Mutations of PBP2b and PBP2x of *S. pneumoniae* are responsible for different resistance phenotypes observed in clinical isolates (126). Mosaic genes contain segments of normal pneumococcal, meningococcal, or gonococcal PBP genes, but regions of the gene have been replaced by segments that are derived from relatively penicillin resistant viridans streptococci (for pneumococci) or commensual *Neisseria* spp. (for gonococci and meningococci) (Fig. 10.3) (4). In the case of pneumococci, these genes are transmitted vertically, and the spread of resistance is accomplished, to a significant degree, by the human spread of resistant clones (although horizontal transfer of altered pneumococcal PBPs may also occur) (96). Chromosomally resistant strains of *N. gonorrhoeae* have been responsible for outbreaks of penicillin-resistant gonococcal infection and represent a considerable percentage of penicillin-resistant gonococcal strains (111).

Transformation techniques have proven useful in the genetic manipulation of bacterial species. In nonnaturally transformable species, successful transformation requires manipulation of the recipient cells, generally with

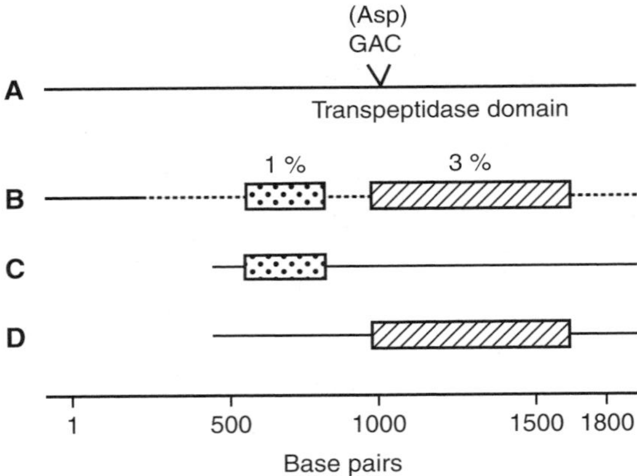

FIGURE 10.3 ● Schematic representation of mosaiclike *penA* genes of *Neisseria* strains. The *penA* gene of *N. gonorrhoeae* and the coding region for PBP2 are represented. The *penA* genes of cefixime-susceptible *N. gonorrhoeae* strain NG-12 (A), an *N. gonorrhoeae* strain with reduced susceptibility to cefixime (strain NG-3) (B), *N. cinerea* strain LPN3173 (C), and *N. perflava* (*N. sicca*) strain 1654/1659 (D) are shown. The nucleotide sequence divergences (in percentages) between regions of the *N. gonorrhoeae* NG-3 *penA* genes and the corresponding regions in the *penA* genes of *N. cinerea* LPN3173 and *N. perflava* (*N. sicca*) 1654/1659 are shown. Reprinted with permission from Ameyama et al. (4).

chemical reagents or with electrical current, to make them transformation-competent (102). Transformation protocols are detailed in Appendix V. These techniques range in complexity from relatively simple and highly efficient (for *E. coli*) to difficult and inefficient (for *Enterococcus faecalis*). More recently, mosaic genes and natural transformation have been implicated as mechanisms for acquired resistance to ampicillin in *Helicobacter pylori* (183).

Conjugation is the process by which different bacterial cells come into contact to exchange genetic material (87). It is generally presumed that conjugation represents the primary mechanism by which resistance genes spread between related, and in some cases unrelated, bacteria. In most cases, the sequence of events that makes conjugation possible is encoded on plasmids within the donor strain. In these instances, transfer of the plasmid to the recipient strain is the result. In other instances, however, chromosomally integrated elements are able to induce conjugation events, with resulting exchange of the integrated elements, either with or without the concomitant exchange of other regions of the donor genome.

Plasmids are extrachromosomal replicating elements that range widely in size and encoded functions. Some plasmids exceed 180 kb and encode a wide variety of antimicrobial resistance genes (293). Others may be quite small (less than 3 kb) and encode a single resistance gene or no resistance genes at all (77). Plasmids that do not encode detectable resistance or metabolic genes are termed cryptic. It appears likely that most plasmids, even those that do not encode antimicrobial resistance genes, must encode some genes that are beneficial to the host cell, because studies have shown that plasmid transfer within a bacterial population does not occur with a great enough frequency to explain their persistence without an associated selective advantage (123). Plasmids may encode many different types of genes, including those for carbohydrate fermentation enzymes, bacteriocins, toxins, adhesive and colonization factors, and conjugation, in addition to antimicrobial resistance determinants. Plasmids may reside in cells either as a single copy or as multiple copies. Large plasmids tend to have a lower copy number, whereas smaller plasmids may be present in dozens of copies per cell. Small, high–copy number plasmids tend to be fairly stable within a bacterial strain because the chance of segregating all of the resident copies in one descendent following replication is rather small (373). For single-copy plasmids, the chance of plasmid loss is considerably greater, if loss occurs merely by chance. Hence, many larger, low–copy number plasmids encode partitioning genes whose purpose is to ensure that a single copy of the plasmid ends up in each offspring after replication (373).

Among the best-studied plasmids in Gram-negative bacteria are the F (fertility) factor from *E. coli* and plasmid RP4 from *P. aeruginosa*. These plasmids conjugate at extremely high frequencies, with the result that most recipient cells contain a copy of the plasmid within 2 hours of the initiation of the mating event. The F factor encodes genes for the production of the F pilus, a proteinaceous strand that connects donor and recipient cells, drawing them close together so that DNA can be exchanged (372). The conjugation genes of the F factor are encoded over a 33-kb region, implying that the conjugative plasmids must be at least this size. The RP4 transfer system is encoded over two regions (Tra1 and Tra2) that encode 30 transfer functions (128). The plasmids are led into the recipient cell as a single-stranded molecule by a nucleic acid–protein complex (the relaxosome) formed at the plasmid origin of transfer (*oriT*) (128). Plasmids pass into the recipient cell through a channel whose structure and genetics bear significant similarity to Type IV secretion systems, which are virulence factors in several pathogenic bacteria (187). Complementary strand synthesis and relegation of the plasmid then occur in the recipient strain using recipient host cell enzymes (372).

In some strains, the F factor becomes integrated into the bacterial chromosome. The integration event occurs via homologous recombination between insertion sequences located on the F factor and similar elements in the chromosome (372). From these strains the F factor may transfer to recipients, followed by large segments of the *E. coli* chromosome. Strains in which the F factor is integrated into the bacterial chromosome are referred to as Hfr (high-frequency recombinant) strains. This characteristic of the F factor has proven highly useful in mapping the *E. coli* chromosome. Genetic determinants are mapped according to the number of minutes of conjugation required to cotransfer with the F factor from a known F integration site. Hence, the mar (multiple antibiotic resistance) locus is described as mapping to 34 minutes in the *E. coli* chromosome (73).

Although clinical strains may harbor multiple plasmids, some plasmids are unable to coexist within the same cell. In other words, they are incompatible. Investigators have used this characteristic of some plasmids to form a classification scheme known as incompatibility grouping (77). RP4, for example, is a member of the IncP incompatibility group. Simply put, plasmids that employ the same genetic mechanism for replication are generally incompatible. The incompatibility group within which a given plasmid falls is determined by introducing (by either conjugation, transduction, or transformation) a plasmid of known incompatibility group into a strain harboring the plasmid in question. Selection is generally for the resistance determinants present on the introduced plasmid. After several generations of growth, colonies are scored for the presence of resistances encoded by each of the plasmids. If transconjugants expressing resistances encoded by both the known plasmid and the plasmid in question cannot be isolated, then the plasmids are considered to fall into the same incompatibility group. If colonies expressing both sets of resistances are present, then the presumption is that the plasmids occupy different incompatibility groups, as long as a recombination event between the two plasmids has not occurred. Recombination between the two plasmids can be ruled out either by secondary mating experiments (in which transfer of resistance determinants specific to each plasmid is looked for) or by direct physical characterization of the plasmids.

Among the most extensively studied plasmids from Gram-positive bacteria are the pheromone-responsive plasmids from *E. faecalis*. Many enterococci possess large (more than 50 kb) pheromone-responsive plasmids (69). These elements encode their own intercellular transfer via a series of regulatory and structural genes (128). Three pheromone-responsive plasmids, pAD1, pCF10 and pPD1, have been studied in the greatest detail (70). These plasmids possess similar genes responsible for the production of an aggregation protein (in response to exposure to pheromone produced by potential recipient cells) and a surface exclusion protein, involved in cellular resistance to entry by plasmids with similar pheromone response genes (70,103). Recipient cells produce an extracellular material known as binding substance. Production of aggregation substance results in the visible clumping of donor and recipient cells in liquid media. Expression of mating proteins is under both positive and negative regulatory control encoded by the plasmids themselves. Pheromones are internalized through an oligopeptide permease encoded by the plasmids (194), where they interact with a regulatory cytoplasmic target molecule (TraA in pAD1 and pPD1), inhibiting the repression of the mating genes (70). Exposure to pheromone may result in the transfer of these plasmids to 1% to 10% of recipient cells in broth matings. Scanning electron micrographs of enterococcal cells expressing these proteins are shown in Figure 10.4 (151). The host range of most pheromone-responsive plasmids is restricted to *E. faecalis*, so the contribution of these elements to interspecies or intergeneric transfer of antimicrobial resistance determinants is likely negligible.

There is some restriction on the host range of most plasmids from clinical isolates, although in some instances this restriction appears to be fairly mild. Plasmid RP4, originally isolated from *P. aeruginosa*, is transferable to a wide variety of enterobacteria, among other bacteria. Host species also differ in their ability to support a wide range of plasmids. In general, *E. coli* is a permissive host and therefore serves as a common background for the investigation of plasmids from many different sources (41). In addition to the narrow-range, pheromone-responsive plasmids, enterococci also harbor conjugative plasmids with broad host ranges. These broad–host range plasmids, which are able to transfer to and replicate within a wide variety of species, transfer at a lower frequency than the pheromone-responsive plasmids and require conjugation on solid media (128). Genera into which these plasmids, typified by pAMβ1 and pIP501, can transfer include the staphylococci, streptococci, lactobacilli, *Bacillus* spp., and *Clostridium* spp. (43,335). Enterococcal broad–host range plasmids have been found to harbor resistance determinants for erythromycin and chloramphenicol, among others, and have been implicated in the transfer of important antimicrobial resistance determinants between enterococci and staphylococci (116, 285).

In practice, most plasmid analyses performed today use techniques designed to determine the physical, rather than functional, characteristics of the replicons. Most techniques for isolating plasmids take advantage of the fact that plasmids are present within cells in a covalently closed, supercoiled state, making them more resistant to denaturation in alkaline solutions. The ability to separate plasmids from the chromosome allows determination of their size (generally measured in kilobases) by separation on agarose gels. Plasmids may be further characterized by digestion with restriction enzymes, proteins that cleave double-stranded DNA at highly specific sequences that are usually palindromes. *Hind*III, for example, cleaves the sequence A!AGCTT in a manner that leaves a four-base single-stranded overhang. By measuring the size of the fragments (restriction fragments) resulting from digestion, maps of plasmids can be constructed to look for similarities with previously characterized replicons. Further differentiation can be made by hybridizing plasmids to one another, although the frequent presence of insertion sequences on plasmids makes this technique somewhat treacherous unless one is certain of the sequence being used as a probe. With the widespread and relatively inexpensive availability of nucleotide sequencing in recent years, restriction mapping and hybridization studies have sometimes given way to determining the complete nucleotide sequence of plasmids as a mechanism for characterization.

Mobile DNA Elements

There are many mobile elements found in bacterial cells that do not encode their own replication functions and hence must "hitch a ride" on other replicative elements (such as the chromosome or a plasmid) in order to replicate. These transposable elements come in many sizes. Insertion sequences are small segments of DNA (generally less than 2 kb) that translocate from one replicon to another independently of the host cell recombination machinery (119). By definition, they encode only genes responsible for their own transposition. Mobile elements that encode additional genes, such as antimicrobial resistance determinants, are referred to as transposons. Many insertion sequences have been described in Gram-negative species and have been implicated in a wide variety of genetic events, including insertional inactivation of genes, increases in expression via the placement of promoter sequences upstream of structural genes,

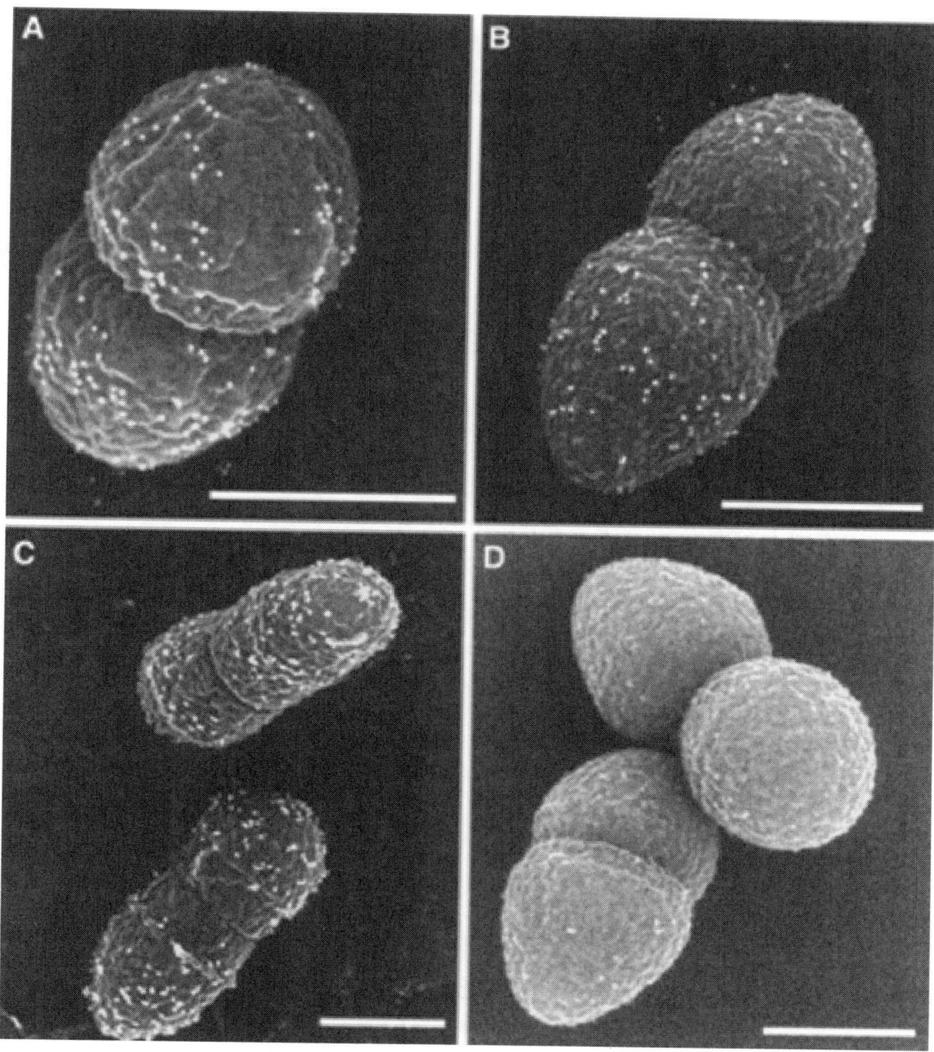

FIGURE 10.4 ● Electron microscopy of *Enterococcus faecalis* or *Lactococcus lactis* cells expressing aggregation substance. Aggregation substance is detected using a primary mouse monoclonal antibody, followed by a 12-nm-diameter gold particle-labeled secondary antibody. (**A**) *E. faecalis* (pCF10), cCF10 induced. (**B**) *E. faecalis* (pMSP7517) induced with nisin at 25 ng/mL. (**C**) *L. lactis* (pMSP7517) induced with nisin at 25 ng/mL. (**D**) *E. faecalis* (pMSP7517), no nisin induction. Scale bars, 0.5 μm. Reprinted with permission from Hirt et al. (151).

duplication and deletion of genes and surrounding segments, and, most important from a resistance point of view, formation of transposons by flanking an otherwise nonmobile resistance gene or group of genes (119). Although largely unappreciated until the past 10 years, the contribution of insertion elements to genetic variability in Gram-positive species has also been substantial (82,285).

Transposons are mobile elements with genes encoding functions other than those necessary for the translocation of the element. In most cases, because of the ease of detection, transposons have been found to encode antimicrobial resistance determinants, but they may encode other determinants as well (276). Most, but not all, transposons are flanked by inverted repeat DNA sequences of varying lengths that are important for transposition, presumably as recognition sites for the transposases that catalyze movement. Several classes of transposable elements have been described. The present discussion focuses on three of these classes: (a) the Tn*3* family elements, (b) the conjugative transposons, and (c) composite transposons.

Several Tn*3* family elements have been described in Gram-negative bacilli. Tn*3* family transposons are generally medium-sized elements (5 to 12 kb) flanked by approximately 35– to 48–base pair inverted repeats that demonstrate significant conservation across the family (318). Another Tn*3* family characteristic is that transposition is replicative (i.e., the final transposition products include copies of the transposon on both the donor and recipient molecules). Structurally, Tn*3* family transposons are characterized by the presence of two genes responsible for encoding transposition functions. The transposase is responsible for the initial transposition and replication of the element, resulting in a cointegrate in which donor and target replicons are joined at each end by copies of the transposon. The resolvase is responsible for the resolution of this cointegrate, resulting in the final product. In some Tn*3* family elements (Tn*3*, Tn*1000*, Tn*2501*, and Tn*1546*), the transposase and resolvase are transcribed in opposite directions. In others (Tn*501*, Tn*21*, and Tn*917*), the transposase and resolvase are adjacent to one another and transcribed in the same direction (318).

Tn*3* family elements have been described in Gram-positive species as well. Tn*917*, an enterococcal element that encodes inducible resistance to the macrolide/lincosamide/streptogramin B (MLS_B) group of antibiotics, is a Tn*3* family element, as is Tn*552*, a staphylococcal β-lactamase putative transposon (302,315). A particularly important Tn*3* family transposon is Tn*1546*, the transposon encoding VanA-type high-level resistance to the glycopeptide antibiotics vancomycin and teicoplanin in enterococci (12). Tn*1546* is a complex element that encodes, in addition to a transposase and resolvase, six genes responsible for the regulation and expression of glycopeptide resistance. A diagram of the functions of the various resistance genes is presented in Fig. 10.5 (121). Glycopeptide resistance in enterococci results from the formation of an abnormal pentapeptide peptidoglycan precursor in which the normal vancomycin-binding site has been changed in a manner that prevents binding but does not prevent the formation of a normal cell wall (15). Tn*1546* encodes not only the structural gene responsible for the production of the abnormal ligase that is the heart of vancomycin resistance but also two additional genes, *vanX* and *vanY*, whose purpose is to decrease the amount of normal peptidoglycan precursor, thereby favoring the incorporation of the abnormal precursor and amplifying the expression of vancomycin resistance. The *vanZ* gene of Tn*1546* contributes to teicoplanin resistance by an unknown mechanism but does not appear to affect the level of resistance to vancomycin (10). Tn*1546*-like elements appear to be widespread in vancomycin-resistant enterococci (82,175,312).

The availability of large-scale genomic analysis over the past decade has led to a significant evolution in the

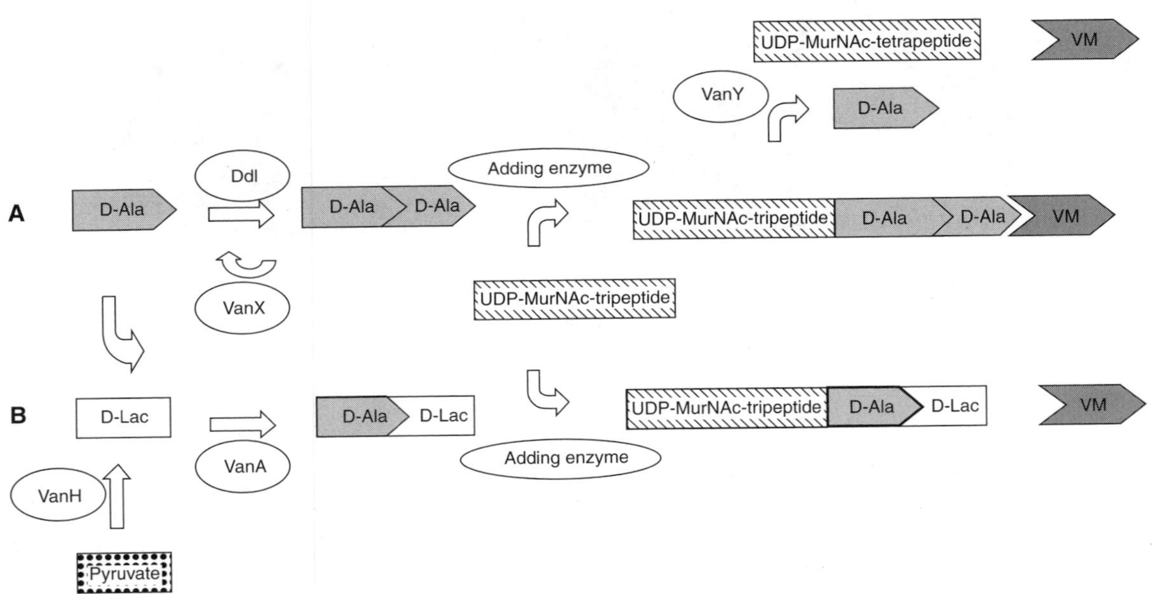

FIGURE 10.5 ● Schematic representation of the peptidoglycan synthesis pathways in vancomycin-susceptible and vancomycin-resistant cells. The upper pathway (**A**) produces the native peptidoglycan precursor that is the target for vancomycin. The altered peptidoglycan precursor produced by the lower pathway (**B**) binds vancomycin with roughly 1000-fold lower affinity than the wild-type peptidoglycan precursor. VanY, encoded by the *vanA* gene cluster, modifies the finished native peptidoglycan precursor. D-Ala, D-alanine; D-Ala D-Ala, D-alanyl D-alanine; D-Ala D-Lac, D-alanyl D-lactate; Ddl, D-Ala:D-Ala ligase; D-Lac, D-lactate; UDP-MurNAc, uridine diphosphate-*N*-acetyl muramyl; VM, vancomycin. Reprinted with permission from Gold (121).

understanding of elements known as conjugative transposons. We now recognize that there are a variety of large integrative, conjugative elements found in a number of Gram-positive, Gram-negative, facultative, and anaerobic species (1,22,232,282,314,371). The prototype conjugative transposon, *E. faecalis* 18-kb element Tn*916,* still serves as a paradigm for these elements, but it is now recognized that there is considerable variation between them (117,280). Common to all of these elements is that they encode their own integration, excision, and transfer functions but are nonreplicative. Some, like Tn*916,* exhibit a broad host range and a relative lack of specificity (in most species) for integration sites. Others are restricted in their host range and are site-specific in their integration (22). Many are composite elements that encode different resistance determinants that have been integrated through the activity of flanking IS elements (152,285). One transposon, Tn*5397* from *Clostridium difficile,* is essentially identical to Tn*916,* except that it has acquired different ends and a different integration apparatus (295). Most of the integrases found on conjugative transposons are tyrosine recombinases similar to the integrase found on bacteriophage lambda (232). The size range of these elements is large, from less than 20 kb to greater than 100 kb. The variety and internal heterogeneity of these elements force us to rethink the artificial distinctions we have made between transposons, plasmids, and bacteriophages and highlight the fact that bacterial evolution occurs along many paths. In the same way that bacteria use the same basic mechanisms to transfer DNA as they use to inject toxins into host cells, they also employ common mechanisms to integrate and mobilize plasmids, transposons, and bacteriophages. It has recently been suggested that the conjugative transposons epitomized by Tn*916* be consigned to a subgroup of a larger group of integrative conjugative elements (ICEs) (50). There is little reason to doubt that the range of elements known to transfer resistance and other determinants between bacterial species will only broaden as the database of genomic information expands and our ability to analyze this information develops.

Composite transposons are elements whose mobility functions are supplied by insertion sequences present at both ends. Many different composite elements have been described in Gram-negative species, including Tn*A,* which confers ampicillin resistance; Tn*5,* which confers resistance to kanamycin, bleomycin, and streptomycin; and Tn*10,* which confers resistance to tetracycline. Flanking IS elements may be present as either direct or inverted repeats, and in some cases only one need be a functional insertion sequence (179). In general, the mechanism of movement of composite elements reflects the mechanism of movement of the flanking elements. Because most insertion sequences appear to transpose via a replicative mechanism, most composite transposons appear to transpose via replicative mechanisms as well. Resolution functions are not usually encoded by composite transposons. Resolution of cointegrates after the movement of composite elements generally requires the host cell recombination machinery. One composite transposon that moves via a conservative cut-and-paste-type mechanism is Tn*10,* a tetracycline resistance transposon flanked by inverted copies of the IS element IS*10*. IS*10* excises from its donor molecule prior to transposition. Interestingly, it appears as though the donor molecule is lost (not rejoined) in this process, in contrast to the excision method for conjugative transposons, where the junction fragments are rejoined in the donor replicon (179,284).

Multiple antimicrobial resistance determinants have also been discovered integrated into plasmids or transposons at specific sites known as integrons (25,134, 136). Integrons serve as sinks for the accumulation of resistance determinants. The integron contains a gene, *int,* encoding a site-specific recombinase adjacent to an integration site. Many plasmid-determined resistance genes are located inserted into integrons, and all are in the same orientation. This orientation specificity has been attributed to characteristics of the integration event and appears to be affected by changes in a 59-base element found 3′ to the antimicrobial resistance gene in each integration (75,135). Expression of genes integrated into integrons, which do not generally arrive with their own promoter sequences, is directed from promoters within the 5-region of the integron. The level of expression of the genes within the integrons is related to the proximity of the inserted gene to the 5-promoter sequences (76). In integrons with multiple resistance inserts, this distance may be substantial. Integrons appear to be a powerful mechanism by which plasmids can accumulate multiple antimicrobial resistance determinants (25). Integrons appear to be very ancient structures that have had a significant impact on many aspects of microbial evolution (301).

MOLECULAR GENETICS IN THE STUDY OF ANTIMICROBIAL RESISTANCE

Among the more important advances in understanding the molecular genetics of bacterial resistance was the discovery of plasmids and the ability to separate these elements from the bacterial chromosome. Plasmids, because they are significantly smaller than the chromosome, are much more amenable to study. In addition, plasmids exist in a supercoiled state, making them more resistant to denaturation by alkali than the more loosely coiled chromosome. This relative resistance to alkaline denaturation forms the basis for most plasmid extraction protocols used today. The supercoiled state of plasmid DNA also forms the basis for the separation of plasmid and chromosomal DNA using the technique of cesium chloride/ethidium bromide equilibrium density gradients, in which the intercalation of ethidium bromide into the plasmid and chromosome results in differential density, allowing separation of the two types of molecules in cesium chloride by ultracentrifugation. In practice, cesium chloride/ethidium bromide gradient separations of plasmid and chromosomal DNA are infrequently used these days because more rapid techniques for the purification of plasmid DNA have been developed. These newer technologies allow purification of large amounts of plasmid DNA without exposure to ethidium bromide, a well-known mutagen.

A recounting of the history of molecular biology exceeds the reach of this chapter, but a few important advances deserve mention. These include the discovery and purification of numerous restriction enzymes; the development of *E. coli* strains with well-characterized genetic backgrounds; the discovery and purification of T4 DNA ligase, which allowed the ligation of different DNA molecules with compatible ends; the development of well-characterized cloning vectors with multiple restriction sites and antibiotic resistance genes; the development of transformation techniques by which plasmids could be introduced into bacteria without employing conjugation or transduction systems; the isolation of thermoresistant DNA polymerases that allow amplification of specific DNA sequences; the discovery of reverse transcriptase, which allows complementary DNA to be synthesized from mRNA; and the development of rapid and reliable sequencing methods, along with the computer power and databases required to perform sophisticated analysis.

Use of Conjugation, Hybridization, Cloning, and Sequencing to Identify Mechanisms of Ceftazidime Resistance in *K. pneumoniae*

Ceftazidime resistance mediated by the production of ESBLs has been a problem of importance in this country and around the world (40). This problem has been primarily seen in strains of *K. pneumoniae,* although extended-spectrum enzymes have been identified in a wide variety of Gram-negative bacilli. In 1988, the authors of this chapter were alerted to the isolation of an increasing number of ceftazidime-resistant *K. pneumoniae* isolates at a chronic care facility in Cambridge, Massachusetts (293). Ceftazidime resistance in these strains was reversible by combining this agent with the β-lactamase inhibitor sulbactam, confirming the presence of an extended-spectrum enzyme. The evaluation of the mechanism of resistance of these strains proceeded in the following manner:

1. Determine the plasmid content of the donor strains.
2. Determine whether the resistance determinant was transferable to an *E. coli* recipient.
3. Select ceftazidime-resistant transconjugants possessing only a single plasmid.
4. Characterize the transferred plasmid by susceptibility testing.
5. Characterize the transferred plasmid by restriction enzyme analysis.
6. Characterize the ESBL biochemically by isoelectric focusing (IEF).
7. Characterize the ESBL genetically by hybridization with known β-lactamase genes or by amplification using specific primers.
8. Conclusively characterize the ESBL by cloning and sequencing the β-lactamase gene.

Plasmid profiles of a sampling of the ceftazidime-resistant clinical isolates are shown in Fig. 10.6A. Based on plasmid analysis, many of the strains isolated during the outbreak appeared to be distinct. Common to all of the isolates was an extremely large plasmid (more than 180 kb) that transferred to *E. coli* J53–2 (Rif^r) from 9 of 15 strains examined. When minimal inhibitory concentrations (MICs) for the transconjugants were determined, the strains were all found to express resistance to ceftazidime, chloramphenicol, gentamicin, kanamycin, streptomycin, sulfonamide, tetracycline, trimethoprim, mercuric chloride, and potassium tellurite. Despite the overall similarities in resistance profiles, the levels of resistance to ceftazidime differed in some of the strains. Some strains exhibited very high MICs for ceftazidime (256 μg/mL), whereas others exhibited somewhat lower MICs (64 μg/mL) (293).

The presumably different β-lactamases were then characterized by isoelectric point (pI) determination, wherein the cellular proteins are separated along a pH gradient and the pI of the β-lactamases is determined using filter paper impregnated with the chromogenic cephalosporin nitrocefin (362). IEF of the plasmids conferring different levels of resistance to ceftazidime confirmed that two distinct β-lactamases were expressed, one with a pI of 5.57 and the other with a pI of 5.2 (293). Restriction digests of the plasmids expressing the different β-lactamases revealed that they were different plasmids, although the large number of similarly sized bands suggested that they were related to one another (Fig. 10.6B). Probing with a TEM-1 gene revealed hybridization to bands of both plasmids, although the sizes of the bands differed (Fig. 10.6B). Incompatibility experiments suggested that both plasmids were of the same incompatibility group, IncH12 (293).

The natural conclusion to be drawn from the data is that the two ceftazidimase genes occupied plasmids that were ancestrally related but had evolved differently. In addition, it would be reasonable to assume that the two ceftazidimase genes were closely related and had developed either separate or sequential mutations that resulted in different levels of resistance to ceftazidime and different IEF points. The final piece of the puzzle was supplied by cloning and sequencing the two ceftazidimase

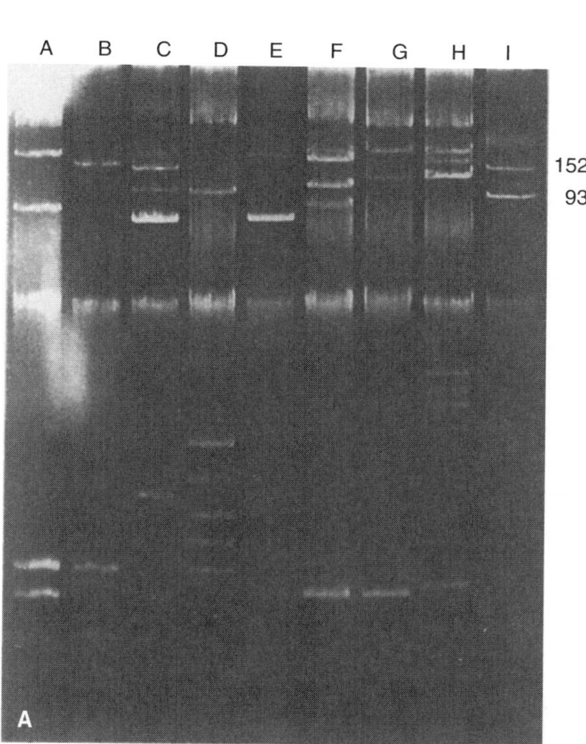

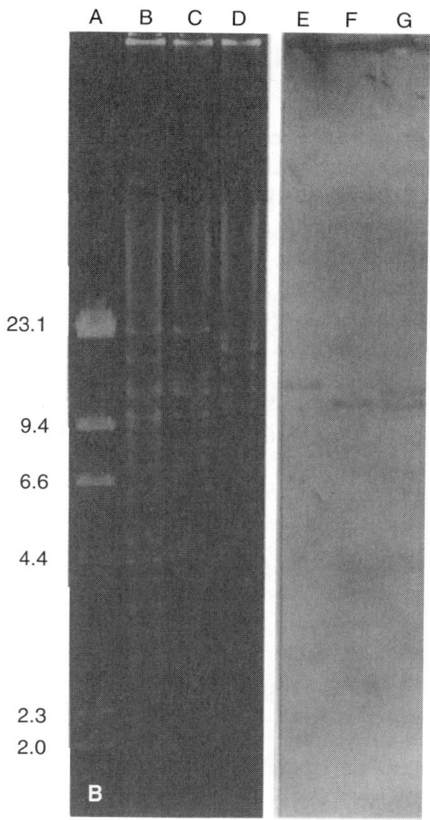

FIGURE 10.6 ● **A**. *Klebsiella pneumoniae* plasmids from an outbreak of ESBL-producing *K. pneumoniae* organisms in Cambridge, MA. Note the different plasmid patterns. The ESBL-producing plasmids are very large and barely visible at the top of the gel. *Hind*III restriction digestion of plasmids from two of the outbreak strains are shown (lanes A, B, E, F). The additional plasmid was an ESBL-producing isolate from another hospital in town. Note the large number of similar bands between the plasmids, despite the fact that they produced different ESBLs (TEM-12, TEM-26). **B.** Hybridization with a TEM-probe reveals that the TEM ESBL genes are also on different sized *Hind*III fragments in the two plasmids. Note that the third strain has two TEM-type genes present. Reprinted with permission from Rice et al. (293).

genes (292). Nucleotide sequence analysis revealed that the gene conferring the lower level of resistance to ceftazidime had a single mutation that resulted in an amino acid change consistent with that previously described for the extended-spectrum enzyme TEM-12 (285). The gene conferring the higher level of ceftazidime resistance had the identical change seen in TEM-12 plus an additional mutation, and the consequent enzyme was consistent with the previously described TEM-26 (292).

These investigations suggested that the outbreak of ceftazidime resistance was fueled more by the spread of a related group of resistance plasmids between different organisms than by the dissemination of a single resistant clone throughout the facility. The plasmids responsible for the dissemination of the resistance determinants diverged from one another both in their restriction maps and in the sequences of their ceftazidimases. TEM-12 and TEM-26, along with TEM-10, are among the most commonly encountered ESBLs in the United States (40). In practice, modern laboratories would short-cut the analysis by amplifying suspected genes from the clinical strains and sequencing the amplification products to determine which of the many already characterized ESBLs was present. Although such a strategy is no doubt efficient, it should be recognized that the resulting data are necessarily incomplete. The presence of a gene does not entail that it is expressed, and even if expressed, it does not conclusively prove that the gene is the cause of resistance. Moreover, many ESBL-producing *K. pneumoniae* produce three or more β-lactamases (256), sometimes combining expression of an extended-spectrum enzyme with expression of its narrow-spectrum parent. The cumbersome process of transfer, cloning, and then characterization offers the potential for greater certainty that the conclusions drawn are valid. In addition, it is a more effective (and efficient) method of identifying previously unidentified resistance determinants.

Use of Molecular Techniques to Isolate and Characterize Mobile DNA Elements

The presence of a resistance determinant on a plasmid greatly facilitates its analysis. The same is true for discrete, relatively small mobile elements. The most commonly employed strategies for isolating and purifying mobile elements involve mobilization onto well-characterized plasmids. In general, a well-characterized transferable plasmid is introduced, usually by conjugation, into a strain harboring a mobile element on a nontransferable replicon. Mating experiments are then performed with a plasmid-free recipient strain to detect transfer of the resistance determinant(s) carried on the mobile element in addition to those present on the transferable plasmid. Many different transferable plasmids have been employed for this purpose. In Gram-negative bacilli, derivatives of the F factor (i.e., pOX38Km) have proven especially useful for this purpose (225). In enterococci, the pheromone-responsive plasmid pAD1 has been frequently used (164).

We used pAD1 to mobilize tetracycline resistance from *E. faecalis* CH116, which encodes multiple antimicrobial resistance determinants (β-lactamase production, erythromycin resistance, gentamicin resistance, streptomycin resistance, and tetracycline resistance) on the chromosome (290). pAD1 was first introduced into CH116 by mating this strain with *E. faecalis* OG1X (pAD1) (Sm^r) on sterile nitrocellulose filters and selecting for transconjugants on brain-heart infusion (BHI) agar containing 4% horse blood and gentamicin (500 μg/mL). CH116 (pAD1) was then mated with *E. faecalis* JH2–7 (fusidic acid-resistant [Fus^r], Rif^r, and thymine-deficient [Thy^-]), and transconjugants were selected on BHI agar plates containing 4% horse blood, tetracycline, rifampin, and fusidic acid. Tetracycline-resistant, hemolytic colonies were subjected to secondary matings with OG1X (Sm^r), with selection on agar containing horse blood, tetracycline, and streptomycin. Donors for all transconjugants in secondary matings that were both tetracycline-resistant and hemolytic were presumed to have the transposon integrated into pAD1. Restriction digestions (using *Eco*RI) and Southern hybridizations of these transposon-containing plasmids, using the *tetM* gene from Tn*916* as a probe, are shown in Figure 10.7. In three of the instances shown in Figure 10.7, integration has occurred into the *Eco*RI B fragment (the second largest) of

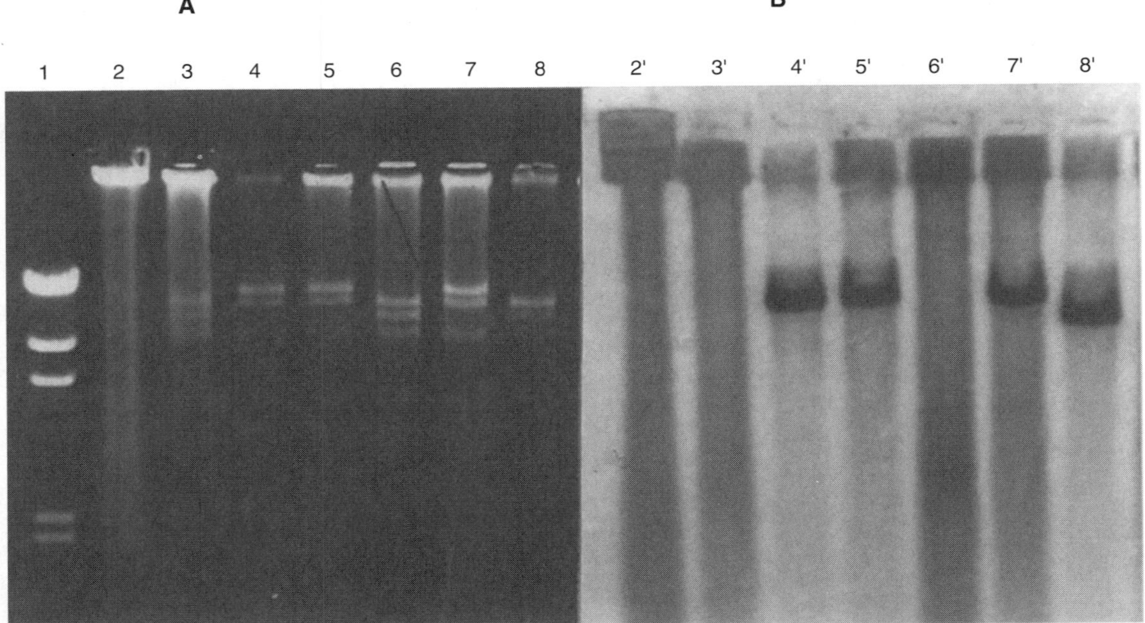

FIGURE 10.7 ● Restriction digestion of donor and transconjugant enterococcal strains in which pheromone-responsive plasmid pAD1 has been used to capture tetracycline-resistant transposon Tn*5383*. Lanes 2 and 2′: CH116, a plasmid-free *E. faecalis* strain in which Tn*5383* is present in the chromosome. Lanes 3 and 3′: CH116 with pAD1. Lanes 4, 5, 7, 4,′ 5,′ 7′: Transconjugants in which Tn*5383* has inserted into the *Eco*RI B fragment of pAD1. Lanes 6 and 6′: Transconjugant in which Tn*5383* has inserted into the chromosome. Lanes 8 and 8′: Transconjugant in which Tn*5383* has inserted elsewhere within pAD1. Hybridization at the right is with a *tet*(M) probe. Reprinted with permission from Rice et al. (291).

pAD1, with a resulting loss of that fragment on restriction digestion and the appearance of two additional fragments. The appearance of two new fragments (lower fragment not visible in Figure 10.7) after an integration event suggests the presence of an *Eco*RI site within the transposon itself. Subsequent comparison of restriction digestions of this transposon, designated Tn*5381*, and Tn*916* revealed an extensive amount of restriction similarity and DNA homology.

Transposons have also been employed as mutagens for inactivation of a variety of cellular genes in many species. A complete discussion of the variety of transposon delivery vectors is beyond the scope of this chapter but can be found in a recent review (137,173). Many transposon constructs have been developed that offer specific advantages over natural transposons. Among the most useful of these constructs have been the mini-Tn*5* transposon delivery vectors (90). Tn*5* is a composite transposon with kanamycin, bleomycin, and streptomycin resistance genes flanked by copies of IS*50* (28). Mini-Tn*5* elements contain only the terminal sequences of the insertion elements flanking one or more of several resistance determinants. They also contain an internal *Not*I restriction site for cloning genes of interest. Mini-Tn*5* elements are integrated into a suicide vector, pUT::miniTn*5*, which can be introduced into clinical strains by mating *E. coli* S17.1 pir/pUT::miniTn*5* with the clinical strain. Encoded on this plasmid, independently of the mobile element, is the transposase responsible for transposition of IS*50*. Hence, in selecting for transfer of the resistance encoded by the mini-Tn*5*, one selects for insertion of the mobile element into the bacterial chromosome or a resident plasmid of the recipient strain. Once inserted into the chromosome, the mini-Tn*5* is locked in position, because the transposase responsible for its movement stays behind with the plasmid (90). Because insertion is essentially random, transformants can be analyzed for the phenotypic characteristics associated with the regulatory or structural gene being examined. Mini-Tn*5* delivery vectors have been used with success in the investigation of several regulatory genes in Gram-negative bacilli (274,275).

Transposon insertion mutagenesis has also been employed in the analysis of genes in Gram-positive bacteria, although the choice of transposons is considerably less extensive (27). The most common transposon to be used in the setting is Tn*917*, an enterococcal erythromycin resistance transposon (315,341). Tn*917* is generally delivered on temperature-sensitive plasmids. Using this strategy, strains are transformed with the Tn*917*-carrying vector. Transformants in which the plasmid is stably maintained are then grown overnight at a restrictive temperature, generally 42°C or higher, and cells are plated onto erythromycin-containing agar. Erythromycin-resistant colonies emerging in this setting have the transposon integrated into the chromosome or resident plasmid. Insertions conferring phenotypes of interest can then be identified, and the flanking sequence can be cloned for use in sequencing and to identify the native gene by Southern hybridization. The native gene can then be cloned and used for complementation studies and confirmatory sequence analysis. Genetic regions of Gram-positive replicons or operons analyzed with Tn*917* mutagenesis include the pheromone-response genes of the enterococcal plasmid pAD1, the staphylococcal β-lactamase regulatory region, and the enterococcal vancomycin resistance operon, among many others (140,162,386). Other transposons that have been used for insertional mutagenesis in Gram-positive species are Tn*916* and the related Tn*1545* as well as Tn*4001* (207,313,345).

Genome Analysis in the Study of the Epidemiology of Infectious Diseases

Among the most important questions asked in the analysis of outbreaks of infection with resistant bacteria is the following: are all of the infections caused by the same strain or are multiple strains involved? Phenotypic techniques—biochemical profiling, serogrouping, and antimicrobial resistance profiling—were employed to answer this question before the advent of molecular analysis. Each of these techniques has substantial shortcomings. Biochemical profiles are poorly discriminatory beyond the species level. Serogrouping is applicable to only certain species of bacteria and cannot discriminate between strains of the same serotype. In addition, serogroup can be a transferable characteristic (20). Antimicrobial resistance profiling is fraught with the hazards imposed by the frequent transfer of resistance determinants between different strains on transferable plasmids or transposons.

The ability to extract and manipulate bacterial genomic DNA proved an important advance in the analysis of the molecular epidemiology of infection. Initial efforts focused on the analysis of plasmid content as a marker for strain identity. Plasmid profiles have proven useful in the analysis of many outbreaks of infection. Plasmid analysis, however, has proven to have significant discriminatory limitations (268). For one thing, different plasmids may be the same size, and very closely related plasmids may differ in size following the addition or subtraction of a segment due to transposition or homologous recombination with another plasmid or the chromosome (see the earlier discussion of ESBL-producing *K. pneumoniae*). To address this problem, investigators began to digest plasmids with restriction enzymes prior to agarose gel separations. Restriction digestion provides an extra measure of discriminatory ability but is more reliable in the analysis of large plasmids, where there may be multiple bands to compare in size. Small plasmids, which may be digested to only one or two fragments, are less reliably distinguished using this technique. To add an additional measure of discrimination, plasmids can be labeled and hybridized to one another under conditions of high stringency. Plasmids that cross-hybridize to multiple bands are presumed to be related. The problem with this method is that, without knowing the precise content of the probe (plasmid), it is impossible to determine with certainty what is being hybridized. Hence, a common antimicrobial resistance gene or common insertion sequence may imply the identity of fragments of different sizes even though the majority of each targeted fragment bears no sequence homology with the probe.

The frequent transferability of plasmids limits their utility in identifying clonal relationships of bacterial strains. Identical plasmid profiles may simply reflect a recent transfer event, as clearly occurred with the ESBL-producing isolates described earlier (293). Plasmid profiling is most useful in the investigation of small localized outbreaks where a clinical pattern of transmission has been identified and the clinical isolates have seemingly been shown to be identical by biochemical and antimicrobial resistance profiling. The presence of identical plasmid restriction patterns in outbreak strains in such settings strongly suggests the spread of a single epidemic strain (382).

Optimal discriminatory ability in molecular epidemiology requires the analysis of restriction digestions of the bacterial chromosome. The most widely used of these techniques is restriction digestion of genomic DNA using enzymes that, by virtue of their specificity, digest DNA of a given species infrequently, followed by separation of the digested DNA on agarose gels using pulsed-field gel electrophoresis (PFGE) (214). PFGE allows reasonably accurate size estimations of DNA fragments as large as 1000 kb. An additional advantage of PFGE is that it is applicable to virtually any bacterial or fungal species as long as DNA can be extracted. The problems associated with the use of PFGE derive from the substantial startup cost of purchasing the equipment, the technical expertise required to obtain reproducibly clear gels, and the difficulty of determining precisely how many bands must differ in size before it can be concluded that two strains are not clonally related (214). Most investigators use the criteria that identical strains must have identical bands and clonally related strains must differ by less than 10% of bands. An example of the power of PFGE to determine the clonal relationship of different methicillin-resistant staphylococci is shown in Fig. 10.8 (234).

Digestion of genomic DNA with standard restriction enzymes frequently results in agarose separations that have the appearance of long smears, with the differentiation of individual bands being difficult, if not impossible. Standard enzyme genomic digestion patterns can be considerably simplified if the digested DNA is transferred onto a filter and hybridized with a probe that hybridizes to a limited number of bands. The resulting banding pattern observed on the Southern blot may then be used to distinguish clonally related and clonally unrelated strains. The most frequent sequences used as probes for these experiments are insertion sequences and ribosomal RNA (rRNA) gene probes (323,334). Another technique that is highly discriminatory is multilocus enzyme electrophoresis, in which a series of enzymes within different strains are separated on polyacrylamide gels (324). Point mutations in the genes encoding these enzymes are, in many cases, reflected as a difference in electrophoretic mobility. Although this technique appears to be highly accurate, it is cumbersome and time consuming. As a result, it is available only in a few reference laboratories. More recently, a variety of PCR-based techniques have been introduced (89). In general, these techniques measure the distances within the genome between repetitive sequences. They have the virtue of rapidity and ease of use.

In the final analysis, a truly reliable assessment of the clonal relationship of bacterial strains that do not have a clear epidemiological link will be achievable only by using more than one typing technique. Molecular epidemiological tools are obviously very powerful, but they all suffer from the fact that they are analyzing a chemical structure that replicates itself more than 1 million times a day (in growing bacteria). In addition, the increasingly obvious promiscuity of many bacterial genera provides a constant opportunity for the acquisition of foreign DNA, which, in many cases, alters the structural details of the resident DNA molecules. Thus, it is naive to assume that the chromosomal structure of bacteria would stay precisely the same over long periods of time. Fortunately, the true importance of these techniques is in the analysis of strains that have spread within a relatively narrow temporal and physical environment. In the hospital environment, for example, many of the techniques just described have proven highly valuable in the establishment of patterns of bacterial spread.

Mechanism-based Strategies for the Prevention and Control of Antimicrobial Resistance

The notable advances in our understanding of the molecular mechanisms of antimicrobial resistance and resistance transfer offer the tantalizing potential for the development of enlightened strategies for preventing the emergence and spread of resistant bacterial strains. Such strategies will require an understanding of the origins of the resistance genes, the mechanisms by which these determinants are exchanged between organisms, the environments that promote their spread, and the characteristics of the individual bacteria that promote survival in a given setting. Obviously, we have not advanced very far on many of these fronts for most bacteria. However, some important examples exist of scenarios in which molecular and biochemical knowledge has offered insight into the design of optimal prevention and eradication strategies. Three such examples are the emergence and spread of glycopeptide resistance in enterococci, of ESBLs in nosocomial

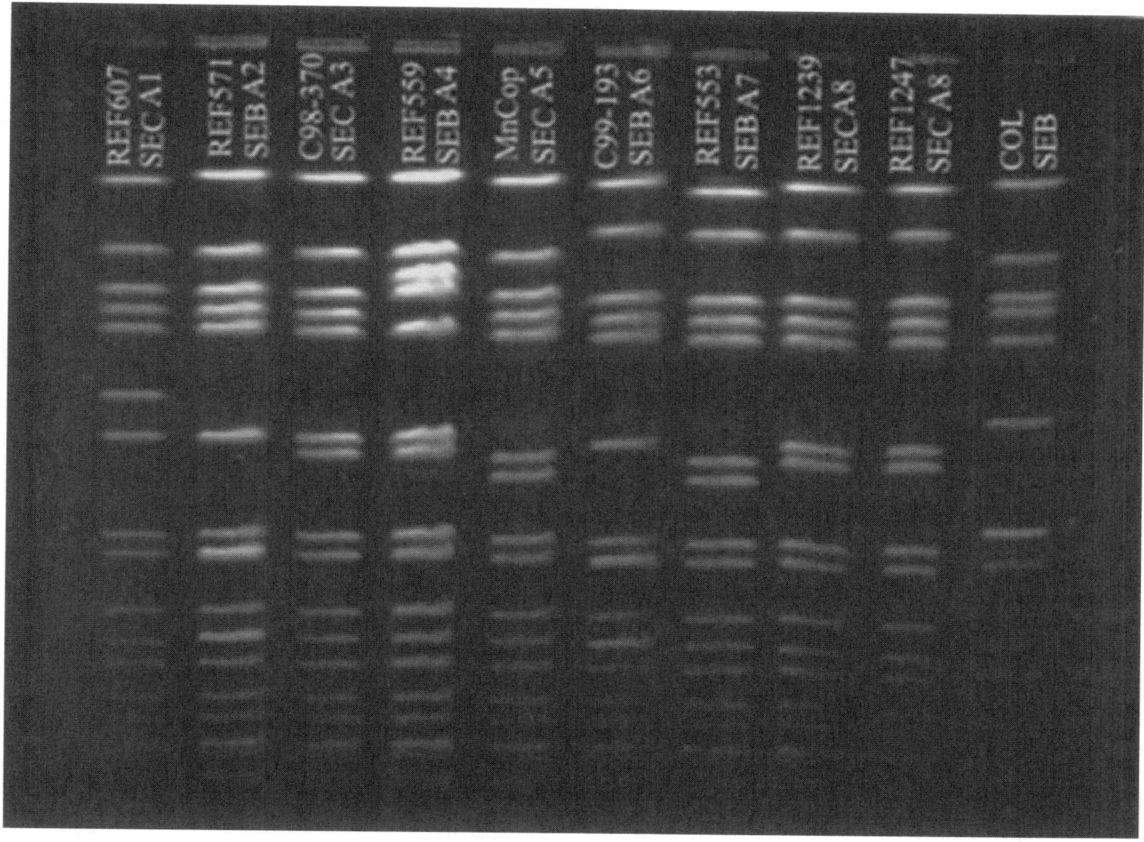

FIGURE 10.8 ● Pulsed-field gel electrophoresis of *Sma*I-digested genomic DNA from community-acquired MRSA strains (first nine lanes) and a typical hospital-acquired MRSA strain (lane 10). Results indicate clonal relationship between all of the community-acquired strains and a difference between them and the hospital-acquired strain. Reprinted with permission from Fey et al. (114).

isolates of *K. pneumoniae,* and of methicillin resistance in nosocomial and community-acquired strains of *S. aureus*.

One of the more intriguing questions surrounding the emergence of many strains of glycopeptide-resistant enterococci is why they appeared 30 years after the clinical introduction of vancomycin. Prior to the mid-1980s, acquired resistance to vancomycin in enterococci had not been described. Since that time, we have witnessed a multicentric explosion of different enterococcal strains exhibiting such this resistance (281). The first clue to the possible origin of these resistance determinants came from a description of VanA transposon Tn*1546* (12). Tn*1546* encodes six separate genes involved in the regulation and expression of vancomycin resistance. It represents a highly sophisticated system designed to promote the bypassing of normal peptidoglycan precursors in favor of a structure that does not efficiently bind glycopeptides. The complexity of this transposon argues against its de novo evolution in the past 10 or 20 years. Rather, it is probably an intrinsic genetic structure for some as yet unidentified species, perhaps one that evolved in an ecologic niche in close proximity to a vancomycin-producing species.

If the vancomycin resistance determinants were acquired, where were they acquired from? Genomic data from glycopeptide producers suggest that the vancomycin resistance determinants originated in these organisms. Studies from Europe suggest that animal feces may be the source for the emergence of vancomycin-resistant enterococci (VRE) in that region, because the glycopeptide avoparcin is used in animal feed in many European countries (178). In support of this scenario, vancomycin-resistant enterococci have been found in the feces of nonhospitalized individuals in some European countries (358). Moreover, reductions in the use of avoparcin in many European countries have been associated with significant reductions in the isolation of VRE from animal feces and food products (177).

Glycopeptides are not used as animal feed supplements in the United States, however, so animals appear to be an unlikely source for VRE in this country. It is more likely that human use of oral glycopeptides, first recommended with the discovery that antibiotic-associated diarrhea in hospitalized patients was caused by toxin-producing *Clostridium difficile* (21), led to the emergence of VRE in humans in the United States. Oral administration of vancomycin results in stool concentrations of 1000 to 5000 μg/g, providing strong motivation for vancomycin-susceptible organisms to acquire resistance determinants. Most Gram-positive gut species are likely to be killed by such high concentrations of vancomycin. Enterococci, however, are tolerant of the bactericidal action of all cell wall–active agents and simply lay dormant until the concentration of vancomycin decreases to the point where they again multiply. Under these conditions, enterococci are much more likely to come into contact with bacterial species that possess expressed vancomycin resistance genes. Transconjugants resulting from mating events between enterococci and vancomycin-resistant gut organisms would have a strong selective advantage in this environment.

Although the entry of vancomycin resistance determinants into enterococci was almost certainly facilitated by the use of oral vancomycin, the subsequent spread of these organisms within U.S. hospitals has been facilitated by a wide variety of factors. Several classes of antibiotics have been associated with VRE colonization and infection, including vancomycin, drugs with potent activity against anaerobic bacteria, and extended-spectrum cephalosporins (281). The vancomycin association is logical. The association with drugs with potent activity against anaerobic bacteria appears primarily to involve promoting the persistence of high-level excretion of VRE in the feces (thus facilitating environmental contamination and eventual transmission) (92,93,270). The association with extended-spectrum cephalosporins is almost certainly due to the virtually universal association in the United States between VRE strains of vancomycin resistance determinants and resistance to ampicillin (304). Resistance to ampicillin in *E. faecium* is associated with expression of the low-affinity penicillin-binding protein PBP5 and was associated with extended-spectrum cephalosporin exposure even in the pre-VRE era (54,61,288). In at least some VRE strains, VanB transposon Tn*5382* and low-affinity *pbp5* are located adjacent to each other in the genome and transfer together to recipient strains *in vitro* (54,142). The transferability of vancomycin resistance determinants, their association with other resistance phenotypes, and the fact that enterococci are gut colonizers all would predict a polyclonal outbreak associated with a range of antimicrobial exposures, which is precisely what has been observed.

Once VRE become endemic within a health care institution, their persistence and spread also correlate strongly with lapses in infection control. Only when strict isolation precautions (e.g., the use of gloves, gowns, and dedicated equipment) have been instituted have outbreaks of colonization by these strains been aborted (38,39). Enterococci are hardy organisms that survive on many hospital surfaces (39,174,201). Hospital personnel have been implicated in the nosocomial transmission of enterococci (39,281,382). Many hospital outbreaks of VRE have involved only a few different strains, supporting person-to-person spread (38,39,281,382). However, others have involved multiple strains, highlighting the importance of antimicrobial selective pressure (231). Clearly, these strategies are complementary and both are critical for successful control of these troublesome pathogens.

Extended-spectrum β-Lactamase-producing *K. pneumoniae*

The emergence of ESBLs-producing *K. pneumoniae* differs somewhat from the emergence of VRE. First, the raw materials for cephalosporin resistance (plasmid-mediated β-lactamase genes) are already highly prevalent in *Klebsiella* species. Because point mutations in these prevalent genes can confer an extended spectra of resistance, there is a theoretical opportunity for the emergence of resistance with every replication of a β-lactamase–producing strain (40). Because these genes are frequently encoded on large conjugative, multiresistance plasmids, they may disseminate rapidly within the hospital environment (293). Most outbreaks appear to involve the transfer of plasmids between different bacterial strains (293), although some evidence suggests that even strains exhibiting different plasmid and resistance profiles may be clonally related (7,124).

The clinical use of large amounts of extended-spectrum cephalosporins has been associated with all reported outbreaks of ESBL-producing *K. pneumoniae.* In areas where a significant amount of ceftazidime is used, these organisms may become entrenched as part of the typical nosocomial colonizing flora (311). Unlike enterococci, however, the modes of spread of ceftazidime-resistant *Klebsiella* species within the hospital environment have not been well established. Of particular interest is the fact that, unlike outbreaks of enterococci, outbreaks of these strains appear to dissipate in response to decreases in the use of ceftazidime, whether or not strict infection control techniques have been used (258,289). These findings may reflect a lesser ability of *Klebsiella* organisms to survive on hospital surfaces, in comparison with enterococci. Other factors may also be important. Some investigators have found that expression of ceftazidime resistance has declined after passage of ESBL-producing strains on antibiotic-free media, suggesting that some ESBL-encoding plasmids may be unstable (352). This has not been a universal finding. Enzymatic analysis suggests that extended-spectrum enzymes have decreased activity against older, less extended spectrum antimicrobials such as ampicillin (169). It is likely that this decreased activity results from changes in the structure of the active site that allow entry of extended-spectrum cephalosporins but reduce the efficiency of the reaction with penicillins. In a hospital environment awash in penicillins rather than cephalosporins, it is possible that these mutations confer a selective disadvantage, explaining their disappearance when cephalosporins are replaced with, for example, β-lactam–β-lactamase inhibitor combinations (258,289).

Methicillin-resistant *S. aureus*

Detailed genetic information has provided significant insight into the evolution and spread of methicillin-resistant *S. aureus* (MRSA). Originally described in the early 1960s, MRSA first became a significant problem in Europe (298). Some countries, through extensive infection control efforts, managed to reverse the trend of *S. aureus* resistance (298). Others, such as the United States, saw MRSA emerge in hospitals slowly but inexorably, leading to the present situation, where more that 50% of *S. aureus* strains isolated from infections in ICU patients are resistant to methicillin (www.cdc.gov/ncidod/hip/SURVEILL/NNIS.HTM). Early molecular analysis of the *mec* (methicillin-resistance) determinant indicated that it was chromosomally encoded and located at a specific site within the *S. aureus* chromosome (6). Although it was logical that this was an acquired determinant, efforts to transfer the determinant *in vitro* were unsuccessful. Originally described *mec* regions were large (ca. 65 kb) and contained a variety of integrated plasmids and transposons, some of which encoded determinants for resistance to other antibiotics, thus explaining the frequency with which MRSA were resistant to multiple antibiotics (166).

Initial molecular epidemiological investigations using a variety of genetic typing tools indicated that the spread of MRSA was essentially clonal, with single clones spreading within hospitals and cities and even between continents (182,297). With the *mec* region essentially fixed in the genome, the spread of MRSA was mediated by the spread of resistant strains rather than by the transfer of determinants between unrelated strains. Moreover, primary sites of *S. aureus* colonization, such as the skin, were not heavily exposed to most antimicrobial agents that were administered systemically (this may change with the increased use of fluoroquinolone antimicrobial agents). In this sense, the molecular epidemiology of MRSA was quite different from that of VRE or ESBL-producing *K. pneumoniae*. In essence, the molecular data explain why control of MRSA was achievable with strict infection control measures.

The availability of rapid genome analysis has greatly facilitated the analysis of the more recent outbreaks of community-acquired MRSA (83,227,236). These strains have appeared around the world virtually simultaneously and have caused serious soft tissue infections and death. Genomic analyses of these strains indicate that the *mec* region is considerably smaller than the regions found in hospital strains and contains no additional resistance determinants beyond the pbp2a gene (205). Moreover, the entire region spans less that 20 kb, making it small enough to be readily transferred by generalized transduction. Finally, most of these strains express a variety of toxins that make them particularly likely to be associated with serious soft tissue infections (83,227,235). Hence, molecular analyses offer plausible explanations for the polyclonal, pauciresistant, and invasive nature of these isolates.

In sum, an understanding of the mechanisms of acquisition and persistence of resistance determinants has aided in the development of strategies designed to control the emergence and spread of these determinants in enterococci, *Klebsiella* species, and *S. aureus*. There remains much to be learned about the processes by which different species acquire and disseminate resistance determinants. Continued basic research into these processes will provide many important and clinically useful data to aid in the development and implementation of future strategies.

BIOCHEMICAL MECHANISMS OF ANTIMICROBIAL RESISTANCE

Bacteria have evolved sophisticated biochemical mechanisms to evade the lethal effects of antibiotics. These mechanisms include target overproduction or modification, permeability barriers (reduced uptake or active efflux), enzymatic inactivation, and sequestration (86). Antibiotic resistance can be primary (associated with a biosynthetic pathway naturally present in the organism) or secondary (associated with the acquisition of a resistance gene) (85). Resistance mechanisms can exist singly or in combination. Enzymatic inactivation is highly specific, because a precise stereochemical fit must be present for enzymes to efficiently inactivate antibiotics. Target alterations can affect the binding of either single or multiple antimicrobials, because some sites serve as targets for several different classes of antibiotics. In a similar manner, permeability barriers can be either general or specific, depending on the number of antimicrobials that traverse the altered pathway (241).

Bacterial Cell Membrane as a Permeability Barrier

The Gram-negative bacterial cell wall is a relatively thin structure sandwiched between two lipid-rich membranes, the cytoplasmic and outer membranes. The outer membrane is composed largely of a lipid bilayer that is largely impermeable to most antimicrobial agents and other hydrophilic compounds. The molecular basis of this permeability barrier was the subject of a comprehensive recent review by Hiroshi Nikaido (241). The space between the cytoplasmic and outer membrane is referred to as the periplasmic space. Entry into and exit from the periplasmic space is facilitated by a series of protein channels and pumps. Protein channels that are relatively nonspecific as regards the substrates they transport are generally referred to as *porins*. Entry of hydrophilic substances, such as most antimicrobial agents, into the periplasmic space can be facilitated or inhibited by increases or decreases in the quantities of various porins (243). When lipopolysaccharide is modified by the attachment of polycationic molecules, by mutation, or by removal, resistance to hydrophobic antibiotics increases (244). Penetration of antibiotics through the outer membrane can occur by passive diffusion through porin channels, by facilitated diffusion using siderophore receptors (normally involved in iron transport), or by self-promoted uptake (aminoglycosides) (64). The outer membrane can serve an important barrier function in the other direction as well, helping to concentrate protective enzymes such as β-lactamases in the periplasmic space (199). A significant permeability barrier can tip the balance in favor of even a relatively weak β-lactamase. Gram-positive bacteria lack an outer membrane. The peptidoglycan layer of Gram-positive bacteria, although considerably thicker than those found in Gram-negative bacteria, is permeable to most antibiotics, so defects in the uptake of antibiotics in Gram-positive bacteria normally result from changes involving the cytoplasmic membrane.

Porins exclude antibiotics mostly by their size. The porin designated OmpD2 in *P. aeruginosa* is a transporter of basic amino acids and also serves as the pathway for imipenem entry into the periplasmic space. The absence of OmpD2, combined with the presence of significant concentrations of periplasmic, chromosomally encoded β-lactamase, results in imipenem resistance (199). Resistance to cephalosporins due to loss of the OmpC porin has been observed in *Salmonella typhimurium* (222,244). Examples of porin-deficient strains have also been reported in *E. coli, H. influenzae, K. pneumoniae,* and *Serratia marcescens* (16,48,129,130,252, 287,309).

Active Efflux

An important mechanism of antimicrobial resistance based on an energy-dependent system is active efflux of antibiotic (354). Efflux is due to the presence of specialized membrane proteins. A large number of pump variants have been described. Bacterial efflux pumps that efflux antimicrobial agents fall into five classes: (a) major facilitator family (MFS), (b) multidrug and toxic efflux (MATE), (c) resistance-nodulation-division family (RND), (d) small multidrug resistance (SMR), and (e) adenosine triphosphate (ATP)-binding cassette (ABC) transporters. MFS, MATE, RND, and SMR efflux proteins are simple proteins that extrude drugs by using the proton motive force. ATP-binding cassette transporters use ATP hydrolysis to drive export (354,366).

Both porins and pumps are critically involved in antimicrobial resistance, despite the fact that alterations in either rarely confer clinically significant levels of resistance by themselves. Their role in resistance is best understood as supportive: they assist the bacterium in achieving significant levels of resistance. Assistance can take the form of supporting the bacterial strains through times of antimicrobial threat until a self-sufficient mechanism of resistance can be achieved. This supportive but transitory role may be the primary importance of porin mutations in the evolution of ESBLs. The ability of β-lactamases to confer resistance is ultimately dependent on the numbers of β-lactamase molecules in the periplasmic space relative to the number of β-lactam molecules, in combination with the specific activity of the β-lactamase against the β-lactam in question. Porin reductions can tilt the balance in favor of a relatively weak β-lactamase, allowing point mutants that confer little resistance when present in low-level inoculum to survive antibiotic challenge. Just such a progression in the clinical setting was suggested by a report by Rasheed and colleagues (273). According the report, an originally susceptible *E. coli* strain became resistant to ceftazidime when there was a reduction in the quantity of an outer membrane protein in combination with the expression of SHV-1 β-lactamase (which has weak activity against ceftazidime). Over time, the SHV-1 β-lactamase acquired a point mutation conferring an extended spectrum of activity (becoming SHV-8), permitting regeneration of the missing porin though the phenotype remained resistant.

The ESBL-producing *E. coli* described here exemplifies a circumstance wherein porin mutations are transition states that allow the emergence of independent mechanisms for high-level resistance. In other circumstances, however, porin mutations must persist for the continuation of high levels of resistance. An example of this persistence can be found in *Neisseria gonorrhoeae* strains expressing chromosomally mediated high levels of penicillin resistance (Fig. 10.9) (361). Penicillin resistance in *N. gonorrhoeae* is commonly associated with a reduced binding affinity of PBP2 resulting from insertion of an aspartate between positions 345 and 346 of the wild-type gene (*penA* mutation) (42). This mutation, acquired through horizontal transfer from other neisserial species, reduces susceptibility to penicillin approximately fourfold. Resistance to penicillin can also be associated with *mtr* mutations, which increase expression of the RND-type efflux pump (MtrC-MtrD-MtrE) and, when present alone, decrease the susceptibility of gonococci twofold (133). When these two mechanisms coexist within a strain, resistance is increased 8- to 10-fold. A third mutation, resulting in the replacement of the Por1A-encoding allele with

A

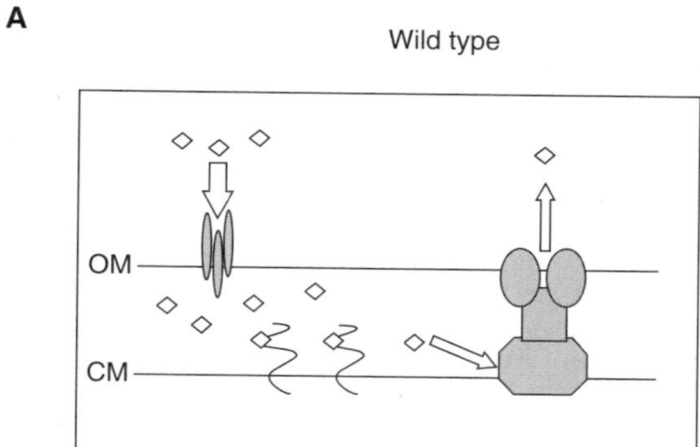

B

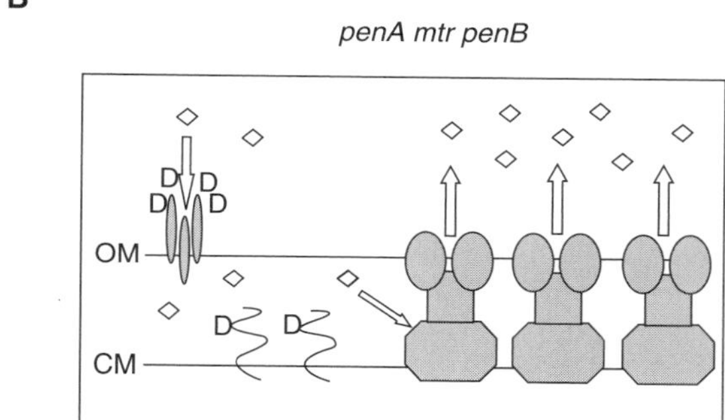

FIGURE 10.9 ● Model for the interaction of the MtrCDE efflux pump and other penicillin resistance determinants in conferring resistance to penicillin in *Neisseria gonorrhoeae.* **A.** Penicillin action in wild-type strains. Penicillin, represented by diamonds, crosses the outer membrane (OM) via the trimeric porin and reaches a concentration in the periplasmic space sufficient to bind to PBP2, the lethal target in gonococci. Some amount of penicillin is exported by the MtrCDE efflux system. **B.** Penicillin resistance due to *penA, mtrR,* and *penB* resistance determinants. In strains with the *penA, mtrR,* and *penB* mutations, influx of penicillin is reduced because of the replacement of two aspartate residues in loop 3 of the porin, binding of penicillin to PBP2 is reduced because of the additional aspartate residue present at codon 345A in PBP2, and efflux of penicillin is increased because of overexpression of MtrCDE as a result of the mutation affecting *mtrR*. CM, cytoplasmic membrane; D, aspartate. Reprinted with permission from Veal et al. (361).

the Por1B-encoding allele and subsequent amino acids replacements in loop 3 of Por1B, gives rise to the *penB* phenotype (120). When all three mutations are combined, there is a 66-fold reduction in penicillin susceptibility. Recent work (361) indicates that increased expression of the efflux pump is required for the *penB* mutation to have a significant impact on the MIC. Thus, in *N. gonorrhoeae*, the pump and porin mutations must both be present for resistance due to decreased PBP affinity to reach significant levels.

In considering the mechanisms of resistance (which we discuss in subsequent sections), it is worth remembering that many of the mechanisms will be amplified by the activity of different efflux pumps. Moreover, the combination of different efflux pumps can have a multiplicative effect on resistance. In the interests of space, however, we will not detail the specifics of pump or porin impact in each case.

Resistance to Aminoglycoside-Aminocyclitol Antibiotics

The aminoglycoside/aminocyclitol antibiotics as a class are characterized by two or more amino sugars linked by a glycosidic bond to the aminocyclitol (hexose) ring. The six-membered aminocyclitol ring is either streptidine (found in streptomycin) or 2-deoxystreptamine (found in other aminoglycosides). There are three classes of aminoglycoside-aminocyclitol antibiotics: 4,5-disubstituted deoxystreptamines, 4,6-disubstituted deoxystreptamines, and others (84). Select examples of the 4,5-disubstituted deoxystreptamines include neomycin and paromomycin. Kanamycin; tobramycin; amikacin; gentamicin C_{1a}, C_1, and C_2; and netilmicin are examples of 4,6-disubstituted deoxystreptamines. Streptomycin, spectinomycin, and kasugamycin are commonly used aminoglycoside/aminocyclitol antibiotics classified separately.

Resistance to aminoglycoside-aminocyclitol antibiotics is found in both Gram-positive and Gram-negative bacteria and occurs by three different mechanisms: target (ribosomal) alteration, aminoglycoside modification, and failure to transport drug into the cell. By far, enzymatic aminoglycoside modification is the most important mechanism. Aminoglycoside/aminocyclitol resistance determinants are encoded chromosomally and on plasmids and transposons.

Enzymatic Modification

Aminoglycosides are modified enzymatically by one of three mechanisms. These include *N*-acetylation, *O*-nucleotidylation, and *O*-phosphorylation (316). Specific enzymes attack certain amino or hydroxyl groups and add an acetyl, adenyl, or phosphate moiety (Fig. 10.10) (353). These enzymes are named after the molecular site where the modification occurs. The phosphorylating enzymes are designated APH; the acetylating enzymes, AAC; and the adenylating enzymes, ANT. By convention, the site the enzymes act upon is designated by an Arabic number; for example, the enzyme catalyzing adenylation of the 4-site is designated ANT(4). Roman numerals (I to V, etc.) are used for unique phenotypic resistance profiles. Lastly, a, b, and c are used for unique protein designations. Aminoglycoside-aminocyclitol–modifying enzymes often have broad substrate profiles. For example, the enzyme

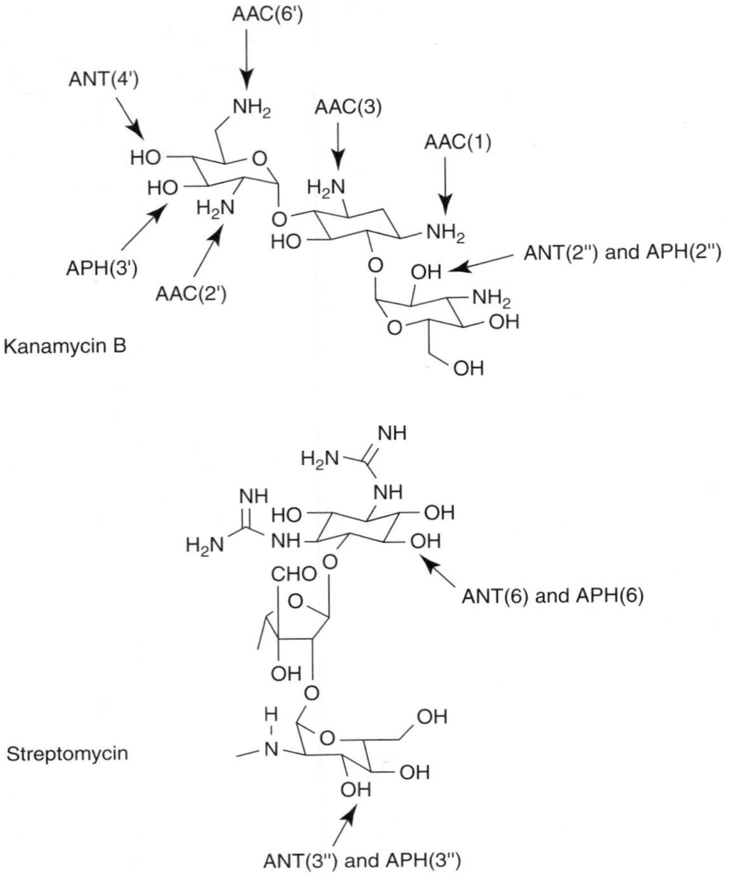

FIGURE 10.10 ● Sites of modification of aminoglycosides by aminoglycoside-modifying enzymes. Reprinted with permission from Vakulenko and Mobashery (354).

ANT(3/9) recognizes both the 9-hydroxyl group of spectinomycin and the 3-hydroxyl group of streptomycin. Certain aminoglycoside/aminocyclitol antibiotics can be modified by several enzymes. An excellent summary was recently published by Vakulenko and Mobashery (353), and its tables are summarized in Table 10.2. As is evident from Table 10.2, cross-resistance exists among many of the aminoglycoside-aminocyclitol–modifying enzymes. The fact that an antibiotic is a substrate for some forms of the enzyme does not mean that the strain containing the enzyme is resistant to the antibiotic. The molecular genetics of aminoglycoside resistance genes and the spectra of different aminoglycoside-modifying enzymes have been reviewed (316,353).

Aminoglycoside-modifying enzymes have several isozymic forms, forms that act on the same site of the compound but have different kinetic properties. Hence, the rate of modification of an aminoglycoside/aminocyclitol substrate can influence the clinical resistance observed. For example, AAC(3)-I has a greater affinity for gentamicin than tobramycin. This can be manifested in clinical isolates by gentamicin resistance and tobramycin susceptibility. The most common aminoglycoside-modifying enzymes in prokaryotes are the 3′-phosphotransferases.

Gentamicin-resistant staphylococci and high-level gentamicin-resistant enterococci most commonly express bifunctional aminoglycoside-modifying enzymes AAC(6′)/APH(2″) (113). This enzyme is a fused protein that possesses both phosphotransferase and acetyltransferase activities. Resistance to aminoglycosides in enterococci severely limits our ability to use synergistic therapy for serious enterococcal infections such as endocarditis. In enterobacteria, aminoglycoside-modifying enzymes are often plasmid-encoded and have been found in association with ESBLs, frequently on multiresistance plasmids (112,293).

Ribosomal Resistance

As a mechanism of resistance to aminoglycosides, ribosomal modification is less common. Streptomycin resistance can result from an alteration in ribosomal protein S12 of the 30S ribosome as well as a change in 16S rRNA

TABLE 10.2

Substrate Profiles of Different Aminoglycoside-modifying Enzymes[a]

Enzyme	Substrates
Phosphotransferase	
APH(3′)	
I	Kanamycin, neomycin, lividomycin, paromomycin, ribostamycin
II	Kanamycin, neomycin, butirosin, paromomycin, ribostamycin
III	Kanamycin, neomycin, lividomycin, paromomycin, ribostamycin, butirosin, amikacin, isepamicin
IV	Kanamycin, neomycin, butirosin, paromomycin, ribostamycin
V	Neomycin, paromomycin, ribostamycin
VI	Kanamycin, neomycin, paromomycin, ribostamycin, butirosin, amikacin, isepamicin
VII	Kanamycin, neomycin
APH(2″)	
Ia (bifunctional enzyme)	Kanamycin, gentamicin, tobramycin, sisomicin, dibekacin
Ib, Id	Kanamycin, gentamicin, tobramycin, netilmicin, dibekacin
Ic	Kanamycin, gentamicin, tobramycin
APH(3″)-Ia, -Ib	Streptomycin
APH(7″)-Ia	Hygromycin
APH(4)-Ia, -Ib	Hygromycin
APH(6)-Ia, -Ib, -Ic, -Id	Streptomycin
APH(9)-Ia, -Ib	Spectinomycin
Acetyltransferase	
AAC(6′)	
I (at least 24 different enzymes)	Tobramycin, amikacin, netilmicin, dibekacin, sisomicin, kanamycin, isepamicin
II	Tobramycin, gentamicin, netilmicin, dibekacin, sisomicin, kanamycin
AAC(3)	
Ia, Ib	Gentamicin, sisomicin, fortimicin
IIa, IIb, IIc	Tobramycin, gentamicin, netilmicin, dibekacin, sisomicin
IIIa, IIIb, IIIc	Tobramycin, gentamicin, dibekacin, sisomicin, kanamycin, neomycin, paromomycin, lividomycin
IV	Tobramycin, gentamicin, netilmicin, dibekacin, sisomicin, apramycin
VII	Gentamicin
AAC(1)	Paromomycin, lividomycin, ribostamycin, apramycin
AAC(2′)-Ia	Tobramycin, gentamicin, netilmicin, dibekacin, neomycin
Nucleotidyltransferase	
ANT(2″)-I	Tobramycin, gentamicin, dibekacin, sisomicin, kanamycin
ANT(3′)-I	Streptomycin, spectinomycin
ANT(4′)-Ia	Tobramycin, amikacin, dibekacin, kanamycin, isepamicin
ANT(4′)-IIa	Tobramycin, amikacin, kanamycin, isepamicin
ANT(6′)-I	Streptomycin
ANT(9)-I	Spectinomycin

[a] Reprinted with permission from Vakulenko and Mobashery (353).

(225). A mutation in S12 leads to high-level resistance. Ribosomal modification has been implicated as a cause of high-level streptomycin resistance in rare isolates of enterococci (109) and has also been implicated as a cause of streptomycin and spectinomycin resistance in *N. gonorrhoeae* (209). *M. tuberculosis* resistance to streptomycin is also associated with single 16S rRNA mutations as well as a mutation in ribosomal protein S12 (224). For other aminoglycosides, multiple ribosomal binding sites can be altered. Although ribosomally mediated resistance to streptomycin is reported in *E. coli* laboratory isolates, this mechanism of resistance appears to have little clinical importance.

Ineffective Transport

Aminoglycoside uptake is a complex process that is addressed in detail elsewhere in this volume. Ineffective aminocyclitol transport has been associated with bacterial proteins involved in electron transport or ATPase activity. This can be observed in *S. aureus* as well as in many Gram-negative organisms. Strict anaerobic bacteria are resistant to aminoglycosides because they lack an oxygen transport system (139,218,308). The essentially anaerobic metabolism of enterococci is thought to be responsible for the intrinsic resistance of these bacteria to the aminoglycosides (193).

Glycopeptide Resistance

The basic building block of cell wall peptidoglycan is the *N*-acetylmuramic acid pentapeptide. The terminal two amino acids of the pentapeptide in virtually all bacteria are D-alanines. The terminal D-alanine is cleaved from the pentapeptide, providing the energy required for the formation of the cross-link required for peptidoglycan formation. Glycopeptides bind to the terminal D-alanine-D-alanine and sterically inhibit the cross-linking reaction in Gram-positive bacteria. Gram-negative bacteria are intrinsically resistant to glycopeptides because these large molecules exceed the exclusion limit of the outer membrane porins of these species.

Lactobacilli, pediococci, and *Leuconostoc* species—Gram-positive bacteria that are intrinsically resistant to glycopeptides—produce a pentapeptide that terminates in D-alanine-D-lactate, to which glycopeptides bind poorly (30,140). The intrinsically resistant enterococcal species *Enterococcus gallinarum, E. casseliflavus,* and *E. flavescens* produce pentapeptides terminating in D-alanine-D-serine, which are responsible for resistance (30,238).

Acquired vancomycin resistance is a relatively recent phenomenon that has been described primarily in enterococci, especially *Enterococcus faecium* and *E. faecalis* (121). Glycopeptide-resistant enterococcal strains have acquired genes encoding ligases that incorporate D-lactate in place of D-alanine as the terminal amino acid of the peptide chain (141). This terminus has a reduced affinity for glycopeptide antibiotics.

Seven genotypic classes of glycopeptide resistance have been described. VanA-type strains predominate in most geographic regions. VanA strains express high-level resistance to both vancomycin and teicoplanin, resistance that is inducible by exposure to either antibiotic. VanB strains, which are less prevalent that VanA strains but have been associated with outbreaks in some cities, express moderate- to high-level resistance to vancomycin but appear susceptible to teicoplanin, a susceptibility that is misleading because it reflects only the fact that teicoplanin is a poor inducer of this group of enzymes. Constitutive VanB strains are resistant to teicoplanin. The VanC phenotype confers low-level resistance to vancomycin but not teicoplanin. This type of resistance, which is not inducible, is an intrinsic characteristic of *E. casseliflavus, E. flavescens,* and *E. gallinarum* and is of questionable clinical significance.

The Van operons are complex elements that at once synthesize and ligate low-affinity precursors while depleting the cells of precursors terminating in the native D-alanyl-D-alanine (Fig. 10.5). In VanA strains, VanH converts pyruvate to lactate, providing the substrate for the formation of the resistant depsipeptide (D-alanyl-D-lactate). VanA then ligates D-lactate to resident D-alanine. Meanwhile, VanX cleaves D-alanine-D-alanine, thereby decreasing the amount of normal precursor available for incorporation into the pentapeptide (13,279). An additional enzyme, VanY, is a carboxypeptidase that removes the terminal D-alanine from the normal pentapeptide precursor, rendering any normal pentapeptides present in the cell less efficient as acceptors of cross-links (11). The final gene within the VanA operon encodes VanZ, which contributes to teicoplanin resistance by an unknown mechanism. The combination of all of these actions results in high levels of resistance to the glycopeptides.

Regulation of glycopeptide resistance in VanA strains is encoded by a two-component system (VanR/VanS) in which both genes are transcribed from the same promoter (14). Transcription increases when cells are exposed to glycopeptide. Regulation of the VanB operon occurs through a similar system, although important differences exist in that the VanB regulation is not normally induced by teicoplanin (110). Mutations occur within the VanS sensor kinase that result either in constitutive expression of the VanB operon or in inducibility by exposure to teicoplanin (19). In the clinic, such mutants may emerge and cause treatment failure when VanB strains are treated with teicoplanin (145).

Enterococcal isolates have been reported that actually require vancomycin in the growth medium for survival (118,127). The mechanism for this vancomycin dependence is a malfunctioning normal cellular D-alanine-D-alanine ligase in a strain with inducible vancomycin resistance genes (355). In this situation, the only mechanism by which the organism can make peptidoglycan is via the abnormal depsipeptide pathway. Because this pathway is activated only in the presence of an inducer, vancomycin is required for bacterial replication.

Two types of glycopeptide resistance have appeared in staphylococci in recent years (59,68,321). Low-level glycopeptide resistance has appeared in strains of *S. aureus* isolated from patients given prolonged courses of vancomycin. This resistance is intrinsic and not transferable. The precise mechanisms underlying the resistance are not completely understood. However, strains that express the resistance (glycopeptide-intermediate *S. aureus* [GISA]) demonstrate abnormally thick cell walls that have large numbers of unlinked cell wall precursor molecules (79,80). It has been proposed that these unlinked monomers serve as "sponges" for vancomycin, siphoning off substantial amounts of the antibiotic before it reaches its true target precursors at the cytoplasmic membrane. It has also been noted that these strains have increased expression of PBP2, although the precise role of this PBP in resistance is not known (228). One study suggested that GISA strains are predominantly of a single lineage as determined by "*agr*" grouping (306,307). Since this resistance phenotype is not transferable, and since reversion to normal phenotype occurs at an appreciable frequency *in vitro* (and presumably *in vivo*), it is not clear whether these strains will emerge as a significant problem for anyone other than those patients exposed to prolonged vancomycin therapy.

The year 2002 saw the first two reports of high-level vancomycin resistance in *S. aureus* (59,357). In both cases, the *S. aureus* strains expressed VanA-type resistance. In one of these cases, the patient from whom the resistant strain was isolated was found to have a wound co-colonized by both a methicillin-resistant strain of *S. aureus* and a VanA-type vancomycin-resistant strain of *E. faecalis* (59). Compelling circumstantial evidence has emerged from the strains involved that transfer occurred from the vancomycin-resistant *E. faecalis* to the MRSA through the movement of a broad–host range plasmid (116). Once in the staphylococcal strain, Tn*1546* then transposed to a conjugative staphylococcal plasmid, where it was stably maintained (367). The occurrence of this transfer has been widely anticipated and has caused great concern for our continued ability to treat serious staphylococcal infections in the nosocomial setting.

Macrolide, Lincosamide, and Streptogramin B Resistance

MLS_B antibiotics are structurally distinct but have similar mechanisms of action. Macrolides are 14-, 15-, and 16-membered lactone rings that have one or more deoxysugars attached (strictly speaking, azithromycin is an azalide antibiotic). The 14-membered macrolides include roxithromycin, clarithromycin, erythromycin, oleandomycin, and dirithromycin. The 15-membered macrolide is azithromycin, and the 16-membered macrolides include midecamycin, josamycin, micocamycin, rokitamycin, and spiramycin. Lincosamides (lincomycin and clindamycin) are alkyl derivatives of proline (trans-L-4-*n*-propylhygrinic acid) attached to a sulfur-containing derivative of octose. Streptogramin antibiotics are made up of two components that act in synergy (193). The members of this group in clinical use include virginiamycin, pristinamycin, and the combination quinupristin-dalfopristin. Streptogramins are extremely potent and are bactericidal. Ketolides belong to a new class of semisynthetic 14-member-ring macrolides, which differ from erythromycin by having a 3-keto group instead of the neutral sugar L-cladinose. Ketolides bind to an additional site on the bacterial ribosome, increasing their binding affinity relative to other macrolides (94).

The prototypical MLS_B antibiotic is erythromycin. Erythromycin, clindamycin, and streptogramin B all inhibit bacterial protein synthesis by affecting ribosome function. MLS_B antibiotics bind to the 50S ribosome subunit. Bacterial resistance to erythromycin occurs by target site alterations, drug modification, and altered transport. The most common mechanisms of resistance to erythromycin are target site modification and active efflux (368,385). Resistance to erythromycin implies resistance to all macrolides and azalides though not necessarily to all lincosamides, streptogramins, or ketolides. MLS_B resistance may be plasmid-mediated or chromosomally mediated, inducible, or constitutive. A summary of erythromycin resistance mechanisms found in Gram-postive bacteria is presented in Table 10.3, which is taken from an excellent recent review by Roland Leclercq (189).

Target Site Alteration

Target site alteration of the ribosome occurs by posttranslational modification of the 23S rRNA by an adenine-specific *N*-methyltransferase (methylase). This enzyme is specified by a class of genes bearing the designation *erm* (erythromycin ribosome methylation). There are at least 30 *erm* genes that have been identified in diverse bacterial species (368). rRNA methylation leads to a conformational change in the ribosome that results in resistance to MLS_B-type antibiotics, because all of these antibiotics act at the same or overlapping sites (191,368). Ribosomal modification by *erm* methylases has been described in a wide variety of genera. In some strains that carry the *ermC* resistance gene, phenotypic resistance is inducible by exposure to erythromycin via a mechanism of translational attenuation. Bacteria with inducible MLS_B resistance normally contain inactive messenger RNA (mRNA) for the enzyme necessary to methylate the macrolide-binding site (MLS_B-type resistance is not expressed). In the presence of an inducer, induction of

TABLE 10.3

Phenotypes and Genotypes of Macrolide Resistance Due to Ribosomal Methylation, Drug Efflux, or Drug Inactivation in Gram-positive Cocci[a]

Species, Mechanism	Gene Class	Phenotype Designation	Phenotype of Resistance: 14- or 15-Md	16-Md	Cli
Staphylococcus species					
Ribosomal methylation	*erm*	MLS_B inducible	R	s	S
		MLS_B constitutive	R	R	R
Macrolide efflux	*msr*(A)	MS_B	R	S	S
Lincosamide inactivation	*lnu*(A)	L	S	S	S[b]
Streptococcus and *Enterococcus* species					
Ribosomal methylation	*erm*	MLS_B inducible	R or I	R, I, or s	R, I, or s
		MLS_B constitutive	R	R	R
Efflux	*mef*(A)	M	R or I	S	S
Enterococcus faecium					
Lincosamide inactivation	*lnu*(B)	L	S	S	S[b]

[a] Reprinted with permission from Leclercq (189).
[b] Diminished bactericidal activity.
Cli, clindamycin; 14-Md, 14-membered ring macrolides (clarithromycin, dirithromycin, erythromycin, and roxithromycin); 15-Md, 15-membered macrolide (azithromycin); I, intermediate resistance; L, lincosamides; M, 14- or 15-membered macrolides; MLS_B, macrolides, lincosamides, and streptogramins B; MS_B, macrolides and streptogramins B; R, resistant; S, susceptible; s, susceptible *in vitro* but risk of selection of constitutive mutants *in vivo*; 16-Md, 16-membered ring macrolides (josamycin and spiramycin).

mRNA leads to activation of the enzyme and expression of the methylase. Once induced, organisms are cross-resistant to all 14-, 15-, and 16-membered macrolides. Rokitamycin, josamycin, spiramycin, and miocamycin (16-membered macrolides) and clindamycin are poor inducers of the mRNA and do not induce the methylase. Binding of erythromycin to a susceptible ribosome results in an alteration of the conformation of the methylase mRNA in a manner that opens up the methylase ribosome–binding site, promoting translation of the methylase mRNA. The details of the molecular mechanisms of erythromycin induction of MLS_B resistance have been reviewed (368,369).

Telithromycin is a ketolide that is highly active against pneumococci (regardless of their susceptibility or resistance to erythromycin and/or penicillin), erythromycin-susceptible *S. pyogenes* strains, and erythromycin-resistant *S. pyogenes* strains of the M, $iMLS_B$, or $iMLS_c$ phenotype (in which resistance is mediated by a methylase encoded by the *ermTR* gene) (17). Ketolides are less active against erythromycin-resistant *S. pyogenes* strains with the cMLS phenotype or the iMLS-A subtype (where resistance is mediated by a methylase encoded by the *ermAM* gene), these strains ranging in phenotype from the upper limits of susceptibility to resistant. Methicillin-resistant staphylococci, which commonly express a $cMLS_B$ phenotype, are not susceptible to telithromycin (17).

erm-type genes have been described that do not confer resistance to erythromycin. These genes (*carB* and *tylA*) result in resistance to the action of the macrolides carbomycin and tylosin and are found in the organisms that naturally produce these antibiotics (109,381).

Active Efflux

An important mechanism of resistance to macrolides is by expression of efflux pumps encoded by *mef* genes (Mef in Gram-positive bacteria and Acr-AB-TolC in *H. influenzae* and *E. coli*) (385). The efflux pumps confer resistance to the macrolides but not to clindamycin, hence the phenotypic description of this resistance as "M" type. *Mef* genes have been studied most extensively in *S. pneumoniae* (*mef*(E)) and *S. pyogenes* (*mef*(A)), but similar genes have been described in a variety of Gram-positive genera. The prevalence of *mef*-mediated resistance versus resistance mediated by MLS_B-type mechanisms in *S. pneumoniae* varies in different parts of the world. Increases in macrolide resistance in *S. pyogenes* causing pediatric pharyngeal infections have been reported in some areas of the United States (212). Movement of *mef* genes in *S. pyogenes* may be facilitated by large mobile elements related to Tn*1207.3* (310).

Drug Modification

Unlike target site alteration, enzymatic modification of MLS_B antibiotics is highly specific. Macrolide-modifying enzymes have been detected in lactobacilli and enterobacteria (192). In enterobacteria, the lactone ring of the 14-membered macrolide is inactivated by erythromycin esterase or a macrolide 2-phosphotransferase. Erythromycin esterases appear to be restricted to Gram-negative bacilli (104). The macrolides with 16-membered rings are not as efficiently hydrolyzed as those with 14-membered rings. Two types of esterases have been described, type I (ereA) and type II (ereB) (9). Plasmid-mediated MLS_B antibiotic-inactivating enzymes that adenylate, acetylate, or hydrolyze macrolides have been described in *Staphylococcus haemolyticus* and *S. aureus*. Lincosamide resistance mediated by a 3-lincomycin 4-*O*-nucleotidyltransferase (2,3) has been detected in staphylococci (190). Enzymes inactivating streptogramin A and B have been also described in *S. aureus*. These enzymes, streptogramin A acetyltransferase and streptogramin B hydrolase, also confer resistance to low levels of lincosamides (192).

Quinupristin-dalfopristin is a mixture of semisynthetic streptogramins A and B. A related streptogramin A and B combination, virginiamycin, has been used as a growth promoter in animal feed. Resistance to quinupristin-dalfopristin can result from resistance to streptogramin A alone and was first described in staphylococci. In this case, it was conferred by genes encoding streptogramin A acetyltransferases [*vat*(A), *vat*(B), and *vat*(C)] or ATP-binding efflux genes [*vga*(A) and *vga*(B)]. Quinupristin-dalfopristin's excellent activity against *E. faecium* makes it an attractive alternative for the treatment of multiresistant *E. faecium* infections, especially since the combination retains good *in vitro* activity against streptogramin B–resistant strains. Two acetyltransferase-encoding resistance genes have now been described that confer resistance to quinupristin-dalfopristin in *E. faecium vat*(D) [previously *sat*(A)] and *vat*(E) [previously *sat*(G)] (325). In most cases, these resistance genes are found along with an *erm* resistance gene (325), suggesting that resistance to both streptogramin A and B may be necessary to confer clinically significant levels of resistance to quinupristin-dalfopristin in *E. faecium*. The presence of these resistance genes on transferable plasmids suggests that the potential for their spread within the genus is significant. Target site alterations and active efflux by ATP-binding cassette pumps have also been implicated in quinupristin-dalfopristin resistance (150).

Altered Transport and Decreased Permeability

An efflux mechanism that confers resistance to erythromycin and streptogramin but not to lincosamides has been described in *S. epidermidis* (104). This resistance is mediated by a 59.9-kDa protein that appears to function as an efflux pump. Decreased permeability has also been described in *Pseudomonas*, Enterobacteriaceae, and *Acinetobacter* organisms (191).

Quinolone Resistance

Resistance to fluoroquinolones most commonly involves mutations in the bacterial cellular type 2 topoisomerases (DNA gyrase and topoisomerase IV), impermeability, active efflux, or combinations of these mechanisms (156). DNA gyrase is an ATP-dependent, four-subunit enzyme that introduces negative supercoils into DNA, whereas topoisomerase IV plays an important role in partitioning daughter chromosomes (156). Fluoroquinolones interact with topoisomerase-DNA complexes and prevent movement of the replication fork, RNA polymerase and DNA helicase. The end result is cellular death by as yet undefined mechanisms.

The most extensively studied mechanisms of resistance to fluoroquinolones are point mutations within the GyrA and ParC subunits of the DNA gyrase and topoisomerase IV enzymes. Most GyrA mutations occur in a short region termed the quinolone resistance-determining region (QRDR). Examples include mutations at residues Ser-84, Ser-85, and Glu-88 in *S. aureus* and in codons 67, 81, 83, 84, 87, and 106 of *gyrA* in *E. coli* (147,237). Fluoroquinolones may exhibit different target specificities in different species. In general, GyrA is the primary target of fluoroquinolones in Gram-negative bacteria, whereas topoisomerase IV is often the primary target in Gram-positive species (33). The first point mutations that occur in response to fluoroquinolone exposure are usually in the primary target, conferring a lower level of resistance. Secondary mutations at other sites in the primary target or in the alternative enzyme will then occur and serve to amplify the level of resistance. The introduction of newer fluoroquinolones over the past 5 years has allowed a greater understanding of the role of mutations in resistance, and the discovered mutations have in turn informed our understanding of different target preferences for the newer agents.

Quinolone permeability changes and efflux have been demonstrated in many different bacteria. In

Gram-negative bacilli, efflux is most commonly mediated by RND-type pumps (see Table 10.1). Virtually all pumps thus far described efflux fluoroquinolones to some degree, explaining the ease with which some species become resistant to these agents. Efflux pumps are also important in Gram-positive bacteria. The two most thoroughly characterized of these pumps are NorA from *S. aureus* and PmrA from *S. pneumoniae* (45,238,360). As discussed earlier, the primary role of these pumps may be to amplify levels of resistance conferred by specific topoisomerase mutations, allowing them to survive and proliferate in the presence of selective concentrations of fluoroquinolones.

In rare instances, a plasmid-mediated and transferable mechanism of resistance to fluoroquinolones has been described in *K. pneumoniae*. The gene conferring this resistance, designated *qnr,* which encodes a 218-aa protein belonging to a pentapeptide repeat family that is thought to protect DNA gyrase from the action of microcin B17 (343). The prevalence and clinical importance of this mechanism of resistance remains uncertain. Finally, a recent report suggests that quinolone resistance can be achieved by decreasing the expression of the target enzyme (165). As this was an *in vitro* observation and there were growth rate disadvantages to the resistant phenotype, it is unclear that this will be an important mechanism in clinical isolates.

In general, fluoroquinolone resistance is class resistance, with demonstrable decreases in susceptibility to all agents for a bacterial strain expressing frank resistance to any fluoroquinolone. The increases in MIC for some fluoroquinolones may not exceed the breakpoints set for clinical resistance, however, so strains may be formally resistant to some fluoroquinolones and susceptible to others. The newer fluoroquinolones gatifloxacin and moxifloxacin, which were developed for their excellent activity against *S. pneumoniae,* will retain clinically significant activity against ciprofloxacin-resistant strains.

TABLE 10.4

Mechanisms of Resistance for Characterized *tet* and *otr* Genes[a]

Mechanism	Genes
Efflux	*tet*(A), *tet*(B), *tet*(C), *tet*(D), *tet*(E), *tet*(G), *tet*(H), *tet*(I), *tet*(J), *tet*(Z), *tet*(30)[b] *tet*(31)[b]
	tet(K), *tet*(L)
	otr(B), *tcr3*[c]
	*tet*P(A)
	tet(V)
	tet(Y)[d]
Ribosomal protection	*tet*(M), *tet*(O), *tet*(S), *tet*(W)
	tet(Q), *tet*(T)
	otr(A), *tet*P(B),[e] *tet*[c]
	Emzymatic, *tet*(X)
Unknown[f] genes	*tet*(U), *otr*(C)

[a] Reprinted with permission from Chopra et al. (65). grouped according to McMurry and Levy (221).
[b] First numbered genes (197).
[c] These genes have not been given new designations (197).
[d] Relatedness to groups 1 to 6 is unclear, since the gene has not been studied extensively.
[e] *tet*P(B) is not found alone, and *tet*P(A) and *tet*P(B) are counted as one gene (204,322).
[f] *tet*(U) has been sequenced but does not appear to be related to either efflux or ribosomal protection proteins; *otr*(C) has not been sequenced (251,294).

Resistance to Tetracyclines and Oxytetracyclines

Although nearly 1000 tetracycline derivatives exist, seven are in major clinical or veterinary use. These are chlortetracycline, demethylchlorotetracycline, doxycycline, minocyclin, methacycline, oxytetracycline, and tetracycline. Despite their differing pharmacokinetic properties, structural variations do not dramatically affect the antimicrobial activity of these agents, except for minocycline.

Bacteria develop resistance to tetracyclines by (a) energy-dependent efflux of tetracyclines by proteins inserted into the cytoplasmic membrane (196); (b) enzymatic alteration and inactivation of tetracycline by a reaction that requires oxygen, which renders the drug inactive as an inhibitor of protein synthesis (296,328); and (c) ribosomal protection proteins (48). The majority of tetracycline resistance determinants are located on plasmids or transposons. In general, resistance to one tetracycline indicates resistance to all tetracyclines. Resistance is primarily due to the acquisition of Tet determinants rather than mutations in existing genes (exceptions exist) (296).

Initial designations of tetracycline resistance determinants used the prefixes *tet* or *otr,* with letters (A, for example) designating the different determinants. Since the number of resistance determinants now exceeds the number of letters in the alphabet, a system using numbers has been devised (Table 10.4) (197).

Efflux of Tetracycline

Expulsion of tetracycline from the bacterial cell occurs via an energy-dependent efflux mechanism involving a 46-kDa membrane protein. This efflux protein consists of 12 hydrophobic membrane-spanning domains. Efflux of tetracyclines is driven by a proton motive force and involves an electrically neutral proton/tetracycline antiport system with exchange of a monocationic magnesium-tetracycline chelate complex for a proton. Tetracycline efflux proteins have amino acid and structural similarities to the multidrug efflux proteins implicated in the multiple-drug resistance phenotype (66).

Enzymatic Alteration

The TetX determinant in *Bacteroides* organisms is the only example of enzymatically mediated resistance to tetracycline. The presence of TetX is unusual in these hosts because it is not operational in the absence of oxygen. Hence, its clinical significance is questionable. Nevertheless, it does demonstrate that tetracycline can be modified enzymatically (327).

Ribosomal Protection

Cytosolic proteins exist with amino acid sequence similarity to elongation factor Tu and elongation factor G and protect the ribosome from the binding of tetracycline (48). TetM, TetO, TetS, TetB(P), TetQ, and OtrA encode for cytosolic proteins of 72.5 kDa. TetM has ribosome-dependent guanosine triphosphatase activity. It has been suggested that these proteins might modify ribosomal proteins or rRNA (208).

Glycylcyclines

Glycylcyclines inhibit ribosomal protein synthesis in tetracycline-sensitive and tetracycline-resistant TetM-protected ribosomes (383). These compounds (9-aminominocycline and 9-amino-6-demethyl-6-oxytetracycline) are active against strains resistant to tetracycline due to ribosomal protection (TetM) and the efflux pumps TetA, TetB, TetC, TetD, TetE, and TetK. Most promising is the activity of these agents against methicillin-resistant staphylococci, VRE, and penicillin-resistant pneumococci.

Bacitracin Resistance

Bacitracin is a polypeptide antibiotic made up of three individual compounds, bacitracin A, B, and C (342). Bacitracin A, the major component, contains a thiazolidine ring and peptide side chains. Bacitracin inhibits bacterial cell wall synthesis by forming a complex with C_{55}; *n*-prenol pyrophosphate. This complex prevents the incorporation of cell wall constituents into the growing cell wall. It also disrupts the bacterial cytoplasmic membrane. Resistance to bacitracin in *Bacillus licheniformis*, a producer of the antibiotic, is mediated by an ABC transporter (267). This has been identified in *E. coli*, an intergenic region disruption of which increases susceptibility to bacitracin and some other cell wall active agents (377). The mechanism by which this occurs is unknown. Resistance to bacitracin has been reported rarely in *S. aureus*.

β-Lactamase-mediated β-Lactam Resistance

β-Lactamase Classification

Two schemes are currently used to classify β-lactamases: the Ambler classification scheme and the Bush-Medeiros-Jacoby classification system (Table 10.5) (51). The Ambler scheme separates β-lactamases into four distinct classes based on similarities in amino acid sequence. Classes A, C, and D are serine β-lactamases, whereas class B enzymes are metallo-β-lactamases that require zinc for activity. The Bush-Medeiros-Jacoby system classifies β-lactamases according to functional similarities (substrate and inhibitor profiles). There are four categories and multiple subgroups in the Bush-Medeiros-Jacoby system (Groups 1, 2, 3, subgroups 2a, 2c, 3a, etc.). The two classification systems are compared in Table 10.5. Two comprehensive reviews have been recently written describing these systems and their highlights (40,148).

Class A β-Lactamases

Molecular class A β-lactamases are penicillinases and cephalosporinases. Among these are the clinically important β-lactamases usually found in *S. aureus* (PC1), *E. coli* (TEM-1), and *K. pneumoniae* (TEM-1 or SHV-1). In the Bush-Medeiros-Jacoby scheme, these enzymes are classified as Group 2b.

In staphylococci, β-lactamase production by *blaZ*, the structural β-lactamase gene, is inducible. The production of β-lactamase is under the control of three regulatory elements (*blaI*, *blaR1*, and *blaR2*). *BlaI* encodes a repressor protein that negatively regulates *blaZ*. *BlaR1* encodes a protein that spans the bacterial membrane and serves two roles: the extracellular domain senses the presence of

TABLE 10.5

β-Lactamase Classification Schemes

Bush-Jacoby-Medeiros Classification	Ambler Classification System
Group 1 cephalosporinases (clavulanic acid resistant)	Class A-penicillinases TEM, SHV, PC1, CTX-M
Group 2 penicillinases (clavulanic acid susceptible) 2a, 2b, 2be, 2br, 2c, 2d, 2e 2f-oxacillin hydrolyzing	Class B metallo-β-lactamases (zinc)
Group 3 metallo-β-lactamases 3a, 3b, 3c	Class C cephalosporinase (AmpC, P99)
Group 4 (miscellaneous)	Class D oxacillin-hydrolyzing enzymes

β-lactams and the intracellular domain produces a signal that derepresses *blaZ*. *BlaR2* down regulates β-lactamase production.

TEM-1 and SHV-1 are β-lactamases commonly found in *E. coli*. TEM-1, a plasmid-encoded β-lactamase, is by far the most prevalent β-lactam–inactivating enzyme found in enteric bacilli. SHV-1 (64% sequence identity with TEM-1) is the β-lactamase usually found in *K. pneumoniae*. In *Klebsiellae* species, SHV-1 can be plasmid or chromosomally encoded. As a rule, TEM-1 and SHV-1 β-lactamases confer higher levels of resistance to ampicillin, amoxicillin, and piperacillin than to cephalothin or other first-generation cephalosporins. Expressed in Gram-negative bacteria, TEM-1 and SHV-1 β-lactamases do not confer any significant resistance to cephamycins (cefoxitin and cefotetan), oxyimino-cephalosporins (ceftazidime, ceftriaxone, and cefotaxime), aztreonam, and carbapenems (imipenem and meropenem). Numerous variants of TEM and SHV have been found (www.lahey.org). Many of these mutants alter the substrate profile of the enzymes.

Extended-spectrum β-Lactamases

ESBLs are enzymes that have "expanded" or changed their substrate profile because of amino acid substitutions. Essentially, these novel TEM and SHV β-lactamases are able to hydrolyze oxyimino-cephalosporins (ceftazidime, ceftriaxone, and cefotaxime) and monobactams (aztreonam). ESBL detection methods were summarized previously. These novel enzymes have 1–4 amino acid substitutions (the most common amino acid substitutions that confer this phenotype are Gly238Ser, Ala237Thr, Arg164Ser or -His, Asp179Asn, -Gly, Gly240Lys, and Glu104Lys). The crystallography of these β-lactamases has been the focus of a great deal of attention.

Inhibitor Resistant β-Lactamases

Normally, bacteria that contain Class A β-lactamases and ESBLs (TEM and SHV) are susceptible to β-lactam–β-lactamase inhibitor combinations. The discovery of *E. coli* resistant to ampicillin/sulbactam and amoxicillin/clavulanic acid in 1993 in France undermined the sense of comfort that came from their susceptibility. The inhibitor-resistant TEMs (IRTs) have been described in *E. coli, Citrobacter freundii, K. pneumoniae, Klebsiella oxytoca, Proteus mirabilis, Shigella sonnei,* and *Enterobacter cloacae*. Unfortunately, the true frequency of IRTs in the United States is only now being investigated. Substitutions in TEM at positions Met69, Ser130, Arg244, Arg275, and Asn276 define the inhibitor-resistant phenotype.

Non-TEM and Non-SHV ESBLs

A large number of non-TEM and non-SHV Class A ESBLs are being described and have been reviewed. The most important families include the CTX-M family (Toho-1) and the PER family (PER-1 and PER-2). These β-lactamases have been found in *E. coli, Salmonella typhimurium, Citrobacter* spp, and *Enterobacter* spp.

Carbapenem-Hydrolyzing Class A β-Lactamases

A growing number of Class A β-lactamases that confer carbapenem resistance are known: Sme-1-3, NMC-A, IMI-1, and KPC-1 and KPC-2, and GES-2. These have been recently reviewed (40,148). In the main, NMC-A, IMI-1 and SME-1/2 hydrolyze aminopenicillin, carboxypenicillins, cephalothin, aztreonam and carbapenems. These β-lactamase posses a singular threat to β-lactam therapy (246b).

Class B β-Lactamases

Unlike the serine-dependent β-lactamases, Class B β-lactamases are metallo–β-enzymes. These enzymes are found in *Bacillus cereus* (Bc II), *Bacteroides fragilis* (CcrA), *P. aeruginosa* (IMP-1 and VIM-2), *Chryseobacterium meningosepticum* (Bla B), and *Legionella gormanii* (FEZ-1). Class B β-lactamases require zinc or another heavy metal for catalysis and are inhibited by chelating agents (EDTA). Class B β-lactamases are able to confer resistance to a wide range of β-lactam compounds, including cephamycins and carbapenems. These enzymes demonstrate resistance to inactivation by clavulanate, sulbactam, and tazobactam. Aztreonam, a monobactam, is neither hydrolyzed nor acts as an inhibitor. There are three broad subdivisions in this class. These are designated B1, B2 and B3. A standard numbering system has been applied that is based upon x-ray structures for B1 and B3 enzymes (119b,119c).

Class C β-Lactamases

Ambler Class C β-lactamases (Bush-Jacoby-Medeiros Group 1) are produced to some degree by virtually all Gram-negative bacteria (*Salmonella* spp. and *Klebsiella* spp. being the only known exceptions). Chromosomally encoded versions of these enzymes are particularly important in clinical isolates of *C. freundii, Enterobacter aerogenes, E. cloacae, Morganella morganii, P. aeruginosa,* and *Serratia marcescens*. They tend to hydrolyze cephalosporins (including extended-spectrum cephalosporins) more effectively than they do penicillins. These cephalosporinases have also been described on plasmids, making their spread to other bacteria a concern. β-Lactamases in this class are inducible. Most of plasmid mediated AmpC β-lactamases have been described in *K. pneumoniae*. These plasmid mediated AmpC β-lactamases have been described globally and CMY-2 β-lactamase is the most widely distributed (263b). Pathogen

---

**Nordmann P, Poirel L. Emerging carbapenemases in gram-negative aerobes.* Clin Microbiol Infect *2002;321–331.*

harboring AmpC β-lactamases are usually susceptible to cefepime and carbapenems–except when the host organism losses a porin. These enzymes may be divided into 6 distinct groups (263b). The conjugative plasmid mediated AmpC β-lactamases are disseminated thruout the US (3a).

Class D β-Lactamases

The OXA-type (oxacillin-hydrolysing) β-lactamase has been mostly described in enterobacteria, *Acinetobacter baumannii* and in *P. aeruginosa.* OXA enzymes impart resistance to penicillins, cloxacillin, oxacillin, and methicillin. In certain cases, they also confer resistance to cefepime and to carbapenems. They are weakly inhibited by clavulanic acid, but sodium chloride (NaCl) possesses a strong inhibition activity. Many of these β-lactamases demonstrate an ESBL phenotype (OXA-10 and OXA-14 to OXA-19). Like the situation with class A and B enzymes, OXA β-lactamases have their own unique numbering system—referred to as DBL (76a). At the time of this writing there have been more than 60 OXA enzymes described (120a,267a). Most of the oxacillinases are plasmid mediated, but few are chromasomally encoded. A recent report details the finding of a class D oxacillinase in *K. pneumoniae* in association with a porin loss (267a).

Chloramphenicol Resistance

Enzymatic Inactivation

Chloramphenicol contains a nitrobenzene ring and is a derivative of dichloroacetic acid. Chloramphenicol inhibits protein synthesis by binding to the 50S subunit of the 70S ribosome at a site that prevents the attachment of aminoacyl-transfer RNA (tRNA) to its binding site. Without this attachment, peptide bond formation cannot occur. Chloramphenicol attaches to the ribosome in proximity to the targets for erythromycin and clindamycin.

The most common mechanism of resistance to chloramphenicol is the enzymatic inactivation of the compound. In resistant strains, chloramphenicol is acetylated by a cytoplasmic enzyme, chloramphenicol acetyltransferase (CAT) (317). CAT acetylates chloramphenicol at the C3-hydroxyl. Acetylated forms of chloramphenicol cannot bind to the ribosome. Subsequent isomerization of the C3-acetylated molecule results in the formation of substrate for a second acetylation, resulting in 1,3-diacetyl-chloramphenicol. The ability of different CAT enzymes to catalyze this second acetylation varies, as do the conditions under which it occurs (317). In any case, the second acetylation is unlikely to be of substantial clinical significance, because the primary acetylation inactivates the molecule. There are at least a dozen different CAT enzymes. These enzymes may be plasmid encoded or chromosomally encoded.

Several variants of CAT have been described. Nucleotide sequence data suggest some conservation of the primary structure between the variants, but their spectra of activity are essentially the same (317). An interesting feature of type I CAT is its ability to bind (but not inactivate) fusidic acid, resulting in resistance to this unrelated antibiotic in addition to resistance to chloramphenicol (24). The nucleotide sequences of many CAT genes have been determined, and seven distinct classes have been defined (346).

Active Efflux

Chloramphenicol serves as a substrate for many of the multidrug efflux pumps that exist in Gram-positive and Gram-negative bacteria, including those found in *E. coli, P. aeruginosa, Bacillus subtilis,* and *S. aureus* (242). The first described chloramphenicol-specific efflux gene (as *cmlA* within the In*4* integron of Tn*1696* [32]) encodes a mechanism that effluxes chloramphenicol but not florfenicol. Subsequently, reports emerged of *E. coli* and *Salmonella* isolates expressing efflux genes (flo_{Pp}, flo_{St}) specific for both chloramphenicol and florfenicol (which is used exclusively in animals) (35,371). The chloramphenicol resistance expressed by multiresistant *S. typhimurium* DT104 is most commonly encoded by flo_{St} (35).

Colistin Resistance

Colistin is a polymyxin antibiotic (polymyxin E) structurally and pharmacologically related to polymyxin B (108). The sulfamethyl derivative of colistin, colistimethate sodium, is the major preparation available in the United States. This compound is hydrolyzed to colistin and acts like a cationic detergent, damaging cell membranes. Resistance is reversible and develops only rarely. Use of this agent has seen a resurgence in recent years, especially in regions experiencing high rates of multiresistant *P. aeruginosa* and *A. baumannii* infections (185).

Fosfomycin Resistance

Fosfomycin is a small molecule that inhibits the first step in cell wall synthesis by acting as an analog of phosphoenolpyruvate (235). It exhibits a broad spectrum of antimicrobial activity. Resistance occurs via inactivation by enzymes, with activity similar to that of glutathione *S*-transferases. Although readily obtained *in vitro*, resistance in clinical isolates is rare, perhaps because resistant mutants exhibit a slower growth rate than wild-type strains (245).

Fusidic Acid Resistance

Fusidic acid interferes with ribosome-associated elongation factor G, the 50S ribosome translocation protein. Mutant EF-Gs associated with fusidic acid resistance have been described in a number of species, and mutation of these genes has been associated with changes in accumulation of ppGpp in bacterial cells (186,206). The chromosomal mutation (*fusA*) lowers the affinity of the G factor for the antibiotic in *S. aureus* (63).

Resistance to Linezolid

Linezolid is the first representative of the oxazolidinone antibiotic class. It inhibits bacterial protein synthesis by interacting with the initiation complex, the *N*-formylmethionyl-tRNA-ribosome-mRNA ternary complex that starts the process of protein synthesis (321). Linezolid exerts potent bacteriostatic activity against a wide range of Gram-positive pathogens, including the vast majority of clinical methicillin-resistant staphylococci and multiresistant enterococci. Use of linezolid has been associated with resistance, particularly in VRE (122,250). One outbreak that involved several patients in a liver transplant unit has been reported (149). Analysis of linezolid-resistant enterococcal laboratory mutants suggests that resistance is most commonly associated with a G2576U (*E. coli* numbering scheme) point mutation in the 23S ribosomal RNA, although mutations at other positions may also contribute to resistance (269). A G2576U mutation has been described in resistant clinical isolates of *E. faecium* and in the analogous position of the 23S ribosomal subunit of a resistant *S. aureus* strain (122,349). Since the 23S subunit genes exist in multiple copies in different bacteria (four in *E. faecalis,* six in *E. faecium*), it has been suggested that more than one copy of the genes must be mutated to confer resistance. Several studies now have suggested that levels of linezolid resistance correlate with the number of 23S genes possessing the G2576U mutation (211,262). Increased numbers of these mutations are apparently easy to come by for most bacteria. Once the first 23S gene is mutated, subsequent mutations may result from recombination between homologous 23S genes, a process commonly referred to as *gene conversion* (202).

Metronidazole Resistance

The 5-nitroimidazoles are antimicrobial agents used extensively for the treatment of infections due to anaerobic bacteria. The 5-nitroimidazole molecule is a prodrug whose activation depends on reduction of the nitro group in the absence of oxygen. An exception to this rule occurs in *Helicobacter pylori,* where the *rdxA* gene is able to successfully reduce metronidazole in a microaerophilic environment (359). Metronidazole is a member of the nitroimidazole family of bactericidal antimicrobials. The hydroxy metabolite of metronidazole is also an active antibiotic. The nitro group of metronidazole accepts electrons from electron-transport proteins (ferredoxins) in bacteria. The activity of metronidazole appears to result in DNA damage and cell death (106). Resistance to metronidazole is rare but may be increasing. Decreased uptake and/or reduced rate of reduction are believed to be responsible for metronidazole resistance in some cases (105). In *H. pylori,* null mutations in the *rdxA* gene appear to be involved, although reduction may be accomplished by other cellular enzymes in this species (359). Four genes, *nimA–D,* that have been identified in *Bacteroides* organisms confer resistance to 5-nitroimidazole antibiotics. The polypeptides encoded by these genes do not appear to be membrane proteins and do not appear to involve modification of the penetration of the drug into cells. Expression of *nim* genes may vary, resulting in variable levels of resistance (131).

Mupirocin Resistance

Mupirocin (formerly pseudomonic acid A) is a unique antimicrobial that contains a short fatty acid side chain (9-hydroxy-nonanoic acid) linked to a monic acid by an ester linkage (253). Mupirocin inhibits bacterial RNA and protein synthesis by binding to isoleucyl-tRNA synthetase (158). Mupirocin contains an epoxide side chain structurally similar to isoleucine and competes with this amino acid for the binding site on isoleucyl-tRNA synthetase. As a result of this, no isoleucine is incorporated into the nascent peptide chain, and protein synthesis is aborted.

Resistance to mupirocin has been described in staphylococci (both methicillin-sensitive and -resistant *S. aureus* and *S. epidermis*) (261). Low-level resistance may be mediated by altered access to binding sites on isoleucyl-tRNA synthetase. High-level resistance is mediated by a transferable plasmid that codes for a modified isoleucyl-tRNA synthetase (153). Analysis of this gene product suggests it was acquired from another organism. *Pseudomonas fluorsecens,* the organism that produces mupirocin, is intrinsically resistant to this drug because its isoleucyl-tRNA synthetase is structurally distinct.

Nitrofurantoin Resistance

Nitrofurantoin is a synthetic nitrofuran antibiotic. As a class, nitrofuran antibiotics are reduced in bacterial cells and bind to a variety of proteins. They inhibit the synthesis of inducible enzymes by blocking translation, inhibit bacterial respiration, damage bacterial DNA, and induce an SOS-like response (349). Resistant bacteria are associated with reductions in the activity of nitrofuran reductase (the oxygen-insensitive, reduced nicotinamide adenine dinucleotide–linked form of the enzyme), thereby reducing the production of active derivatives (44).

Novobiocin Resistance

Novobiocin is an antimicrobial that holds some promise for use in combination with other agents against multiply resistant bacteria (5,184). It inhibits ATPase, resulting in a multitude of intracellular effects. The most well recognized of these effects is inhibition of DNA gyrase. Resistance emerges relatively rapidly during therapy, via unknown mechanisms. The use of this agent in combination with other agents may slow or prevent the emergence of resistance.

Polymyxin B Resistance

Polymyxin B is a rapidly bactericidal, cationic, cyclic decapeptide antibiotic that binds to phosphate groups in the lipids of bacterial cytoplasmic membranes and acts as a cationic detergent, altering the osmotic permeability of the bacterial membrane. Its activity is primarily limited to Gram-negative organisms. Organisms resistant to polymyxin B have cell walls that prevent access of the drug to the bacterial cell membrane. There is complete cross-resistance between colistin derivatives and polymyxin B. Cross-resistance to other antibiotics has not been reported. No activity against Gram-positive bacteria has been observed. Although *Pseudomonas* species are susceptible *in vitro* to polymyxin B, the concentration of divalent cations in body fluids usually nullifies its activity (108,154). *Proteus, Providencia, Serratia,* and *Neisseria* species are resistant. Polymyxin B can be considered for the treatment of multidrug resistant gram negative infections. There has been renewed interest in polymyxin B and colistin especially against A. baumannii and P. aeruginosa. There is evidence that colistin is effective in bacteremia, but not effective in experimental models of endocarditis (9–14).

Sulfonamide Resistance

Sulfonamides are synthetic bacteriostatic antimicrobials that interfere with bacterial folic acid synthesis. Sulfonamides competitively inhibit the incorporation of paraaminobenzoic acid into tetrahydropteroic acid by interfering with the action of dihydropteroic acid synthetase (46). This enzyme is not present in human cells. Decreasing folic acid synthesis results in a decrease in bacterial nucleotides, inhibiting bacterial growth.

Resistance to sulfonamides arises by bacterial mutations that result in overproduction of paraaminobenzoic acid or a change in the dihydropteroic acid synthetase enzyme. Dihydropteroate synthetase is competitively inhibited by sulfonamides. Clinically important bacteria in which chromosomal *dhps* mutations resulting in sulfonamide resistance have been described include *E. coli, S. pneumoniae, S. aureus, S. haemolyticus, Campylobacter jejuni,* and *H. pylori,* in which sequential point mutations are likely responsible for the resistant genotype. In contrast, *N. meningitides* and *Streptococcus pyogenes* chromosomal *dhps* appears to have acquired resistance mutations by transformation and recombination of foreign DNA. Plasmid-mediated resistance to sulfonamides is more common. To date, two plasmid-mediated mutant enzymes (SULI and SULII) have been described (193). Decreased cell permeability to sulfonamides may also contribute to resistance.

Organisms resistant to one sulfonamide are considered cross-resistant to all members of this class. Sulfones are very similar to sulfonamides in mechanism and activity. Resistance to sulfones has been a problem in *Mycobacterium leprae* infections.

Trimethoprim Resistance

Trimethoprim is a synthetic diaminopyrimidine antimicrobial 20-fold more potent than sulfamethoxazole. Trimethoprim competitively inhibits dihydrofolate reductase (DHFR), an essential cellular enzyme, and thereby interferes with the nicotinamide adenine dinucleotide phosphate–dependent reduction of dihydrofolate to tetrahydrofolate, the major precursor of purines. Eukaryotic DHFR is resistant to trimethoprim, hence the prokaryotic selectivity of this agent. Chromosomal trimethoprim resistance is usually due to mutations in the cellular *dhfr* gene, to promoter mutations yielding increased production of DHFR, or to a combination of these two mechanisms (159). Rarely, strains have been reported in which a separate mutation has resulted in a dependence on external thymine (thymine auxotrophy). In these instances, the cellular need for DHFR is largely bypassed.

Twenty or more plasmid-encoded DHFRs that confer resistance to trimethoprim have been identified (159). The different DHFRs have similar amino acid sequences, and the enzymes can be grouped (A to E) (161). Plasmid-borne enzymes may bear little structural resemblance to the host chromosomal enzyme. Trimethoprim resistance genes in Gram-negative bacilli are frequently found integrated into integrons, which themselves may be components of transposons. This mobility allows them to be located on plasmids or on the chromosome.

Trimethoprim resistance due to decreased cell permeability has been described in *K. pneumoniae, Enterobacter* species, and *S. marcescens* (130,160). Loss of a 37- to 41-kDa outer membrane protein (porin) is believed to be responsible.

ANTITUBERCULOUS AGENTS

See also Chapter 4.

Capreomycin Resistance

Capreomycin is a polypeptide antibiotic. Resistance is believed to occur in a stepwise manner. The mechanism of resistance to capreomycin is unknown.

Ethambutol Resistance

Ethambutol inhibits the incorporation of D-arabinase into arabinogalactan. It appears to do this by inhibiting arabinosyltransferases. Resistance to ethambutol has been linked to a missense mutation in *embB*, an arabinosyltransferase gene in *Mycobacterium smegmatis* and *M. tuberculosis* (195).

Ethionamide Resistance

Ethionamide is an isonicotinic acid derivative similar to isoniazid (see following section).

Isoniazid Resistance

Isoniazid is believed to be bactericidal against *M. tuberculosis* by inhibiting InhA, an enzyme involved in mycolic acid biosynthesis. Mycolic acids are long-chain, long-branched hydroxy-fatty acids found in mycobacterial cell walls. In order to be active, isoniazid requires catalase-peroxidase activation (a function performed by KATG). Resistance to isoniazid in *M. tuberculosis* has been most commonly attributed to mutations in *katG*, although mutations in *inhA* are not uncommon (229).

The *inhA* gene encodes a 32-kDa protein that serves as a target for isoniazid. This protein, InhA, is homologous to the *E. coli* enzyme EnvM and to the enoyl-acyl carrier protein reductase of *Brassica napus* (18). Either a single point mutation (Ser-94 to Ala-94 or Ile-16 to Thr-16) or target amplification of the wild-type gene confers resistance to isoniazid. This resistance is accompanied by resistance to ethionamide, an antimycobacterial drug related to isoniazid. Dessen et al. (91) demonstrated that InhA catalyzes the reduction of 2-trans-acetenoyl-acyl carrier protein, thus identifying the *inhA* gene product as an enoyl-acyl carrier protein reductase. This was consistent with the suggestion that InhA participates in mycolic acid biosynthesis. Crystals of the InhA protein were subsequently prepared; three-dimensional structural analyses of the InhA protein and mutant revealed that drug resistance is directly related to a perturbation in the hydrogen-bonding network that stabilizes reduced nicotinamide adenine dinucleotide binding (91).

Recently, a locus required for activation of ethionamide (structurally related to isoniazid) has been identified. Mutations within the *ethA* gene are frequently present in *M. tuberculosis* strains resistant to ethionamide. These mutations do not confer resistance to isoniazid. However, inhA mutations confer resistance to both antimicrobial agents (229).

Pyrazinamide Resistance

Pyrazinamide is a niacinamide derivative. The activity of the drug appears to be dependent on intracellular conversion. Pyrazinamide is converted by deamination to pyrazinoic acid by intracellular pyrazinamidase (a nicotinamidase). The primary mechanism of resistance to pyrazinamide appears to be mutations in the *pncA* gene, which encodes the pyrazinamidase that activates the molecule. Recent studies indicate that both a functional pyrazinamide uptake mechanism and pyrazinamidase activity are required for pyrazinamide antitubercular activity, as naturally resistant mycobacterial species with only one of these activities functional have been characterized (277).

Rifampin and Rifabutin Resistance

The prototypical drug for this class of antibiotics is rifamycin B. Rifampin, a zwitterionic derivative of rifamycin SV_1, is the most active and lipophilic drug of its class. Rifamycin inhibits DNA-dependent RNA polymerase at the a-subunit (330). Bacteria develop resistance to rifampin primarily via point mutations in the *rpoB* gene encoding the a-subunit of the polymerase (330). These mutations have been described in *M. leprae, E. coli,* and *M. tuberculosis*. Mutations occur at multiple sites in the RNA polymerase and occur with a very high frequency, making these drugs ineffective as monotherapy for clinical infections (although rifampin alone has been used effectively in the eradication of nasopharyngeal colonization with *N. meningitidis*).

Rifabutin, a derivative of rifamycin S, that has a similar mechanism of action, inhibiting DNA-dependent RNA polymerase. Resistance to rifabutin is similar to that to rifamycin.

In *Nocardia* species, resistance due to glycosylation of the 23-hydroxy group and phosphorylation of the 21-hydroxy group of rifampin has been recently described. Ribosylation of rifampin has also been described in *M. smegmatis* and several other mycobacterial species (81).

APPENDICES

The past decade has seen a virtual explosion in the availability of molecular biology techniques and tools for working with microbial genetics. There are now many commercial enterprises that offer easy-to-use kits to perform a variety of techniques, from cloning to hybridization to PCR amplification. DNA sequencing, once a tedious and arduous chore, is now readily available for very reasonable prices. For that reason, we have chosen to be selective in the techniques described in the appendices. In general, we describe older techniques for which modern commercial kits are not available or techniques that can be used for hard-to-work-with species (species for which commercial techniques may not be suited).

APPENDIX I: SELECTION OF ANTIBIOTIC-RESISTANT MUTANTS

In some cases, the first insight into the mechanism of action of a specific antibiotic, or the mechanisms of eventual resistance, is derived by the selection of antibiotic-resistant mutants in the laboratory. The selection of antibiotic-resistant mutants is therefore a useful tool for analyzing resistance mechanisms in bacteria. It can also be employed as technique for isolating bacteria with specific resistance characteristics that could play a role in future *in vitro* experiments. It should be kept in mind that there are many important resistance mechanisms that *in vitro* selection techniques would not predict, such as β-lactamase–mediated resistance in *E. coli* or *S. aureus* or vancomycin resistance in enterococci. In other instances, such as resistance to rifampin, streptomycin, or the fluoroquinolones, the *in vitro* experience has closely paralleled subsequent clinical findings.

Most mutation techniques are based on the inoculation of plates containing concentrations of antibiotic far in excess of the MIC of the organism and on the selection of colonies able to grow at higher than normal concentrations. Using concentrations far in excess of the MIC allows selection of single-step mutants. It is also possible to select for resistant mutants by progressively increasing the antibiotic concentration in which the organism is grown. Although this technique may lead to a higher yield of resistant organisms in some cases, it also has a higher risk of selecting mutants whose resistance is based on decreases in uptake of the antibiotic or on alterations of the bacterial growth rate (small-colony variant).

Single-step mutants are readily selectable if the rate of mutation is naturally between 10^{-8} and 10^{-7}/CFU. For mutations whose rate is below this limit, exposure to mutating agents may be necessary. It should be kept in mind that these techniques do not allow prediction of the nature of the mutation resulting in resistance. In some cases, the altered phenotype may simply involve the introduction of a point mutation in a specific gene or operon. In others, insertion sequences or transposons may inactivate, or activate, certain genes or operons, leading to resistance. Deletion events mediated by homologous recombination may also play a role. Determining the mechanism of resistance requires more detailed molecular studies. Following are two techniques for isolating resistant bacterial mutants.

A. Gradient Plate Method

1. Prepare two 30-mL aliquots of nutrient agar and autoclave.
2. Cool to 50°C to 55°C and pour 50 mL of molten agar into a tilted, 120 × 120 × 17 mm square Petri dish with one end propped up 0.25 inches. Allow the agar to solidify.
3. Add the desired concentration of antibiotic to another agar flask (the final concentration must be greater than the MIC).
4. Pour the antibiotic-containing agar over the solidified agar and allow it to solidify. The diffusion of the antibiotic through the solidified agar should provide a continuous concentration gradient across the plate. This process should be performed with several plates containing different starting antibiotic concentrations.
5. Inoculate the plates by spreading 100 μL of an overnight culture over the surface of the plate. Incubate overnight at 37°C.
6. The following day, confluent growth should be visible up to the point where the antibiotic concentration equals the MIC for that inoculum. Colonies growing at higher concentrations are antibiotic-resistant mutants.
7. Restreak mutant colonies on agar plates with high concentrations of antibiotic to determine the level of resistance.
8. Retest the MIC after several passages on antibiotic-free agar to test the stability of the resistant phenotype.

B. Nitrosoguanidine Method

This technique is derived from Prado et al. (261), who used it create a recombination-deficient strain of *E. faecalis*. Nitrosoguanidine is highly mutagenic, and this and similar techniques should be undertaken only with the utmost care and appropriate guidance from experienced individuals. Mutagenesis methods are generally used to induce mutations that fall below the detectable spontaneous mutation frequency.

1. Inoculate 250 mL of an overnight culture of *E. faecalis* JH2–2 into M9-YE broth and incubate at 37°C to midlogarithmic phase (80 Klett units, using a Klett-Summerson colorimeter with a no. 54 filter).
2. Pellet cells, resuspend them in 2.5 mL of M9-YE broth containing 100 μg/mL *N*-methyl-*N*-nitro-*N*-nitrosoguanidine, and incubate at 37°C for 30 minutes.
3. Wash cells thoroughly in broth and inoculate appropriate dilutions onto antibiotic plates with different concentrations or onto gradient plates, as described previously. Incubate at 37°C for 24 hours and examine for growth above the MIC for that antibiotic.
4. Confirm resistance level and stability of the phenotype using the same techniques as for the gradient plate method (steps 7 and 8).

APPENDIX II: CONJUGAL TRANSFER OF ANTIBIOTIC RESISTANCE

When examining resistance within a clinical strain, the first step is to attempt to transfer the determinant to a well-defined recipient strain. Many clinical isolates harbor multiple plasmids, making it difficult to pinpoint the location of a resistance determinant. Transfer of resistance to a recipient strain often allows one to implicate a specific plasmid as harboring the determinant. Placing a single plasmid in a defined genetic background also allows reasonable estimations regarding the entire complement of resistance determinants harbored by that plasmid and facilitates restriction digestion, hybridization studies, and cloning of plasmid fragments.

Mating experiments are designed to detect DNA transfer events that require cell-to-cell contact. More frequently, they result in the detection of the transfer of plasmids. Mating experiments can also detect the transfer of specific segments of chromosomal DNA, via transposition processes, mobilization of the chromosome by plasmids, or processes yet to be defined. Most mating experiments do not rule out the possibility that nonconjugative processes, such as transformation or transduction, are mediating the transfer event. Other experiments, such as mating experiments performed on DNase-containing media (to exclude transformation) or in environments designed to allow the passage of bacteriophages (to exclude transduction), are required to achieve certainly about the mechanism of transfer.

The mating experiment to be performed varies depending on the type of conjugation event that is anticipated. Some plasmids that mediate their own transfer pass into recipient cells quite readily during incubation in broth media. Examples of plasmids of this type are the F factor of *E. coli* and pAD1 of *E. faecalis* (162,372). Other plasmids transfer at a considerably lower frequency and require mating on solid media. Examples of plasmids that require solid media for transfer include broad–host range enterococcal plasmids such as pAM1 (335). Matings on solid media hold the donor and recipient strain in relatively fixed positions, thereby offering more stability and a greater period of time during which the cells can stay in contact. Transfers in which chromosomal determinants are exchanged almost always require solid media, except when the F factor is integrated into the *E. coli* chromosome.

The strategy guiding mating experiments is relatively simple. The goal is to mix two strains of bacteria with disparate resistance determinants and to search for bacterial strains (transconjugants) that express both types of resistance. The donor possesses the resistance determinant to be examined. The recipient must be susceptible to the antibiotic to which the transferable determinant confers resistance but resistant to one or more antibiotics to which the donor is susceptible. The resistance characteristics of the recipient should be chromosomally encoded and not transferable. It is also helpful if the recipient possesses other identifiable characteristics, such as auxotrophy for one or more amino acids, to allow positive identification. This arrangement allows the creation of plates that inhibit both the recipient and the donor, allowing growth of only those recipients that have acquired the transferable determinant.

One recipient commonly used for the transfer of resistance determinants from Gram-negative bacteria is *E. coli* J53–2 (71). This strain expresses chromosomal nontransferable resistance to rifampin and requires proline and methionine in the growth medium. We have used J53–2 extensively in the transfer of ceftazidime resistance from *K. pneumoniae*. In enterococci, strains that are frequently employed as recipients include *E. faecalis* JH2–2 (Fus^r and Rif^r), the closely related JH2–7 (Fus^r, Rif^r, and Thy$^-$), and *E. faecalis* OG1, which has several different resistant variants (OG1X [Sm^r];OG2RF [Fus^r and Rif^r]; and OG1SS; Sm^{r}and spectinomycin-resistant).

A. Broth Matings

Broth matings are generally used to detect transfer of determinants that are located on plasmids that encode their own transfer genes. These genes generally alter the surface of the cell (F pilus in *E. coli* and aggregation substance in enterococci) in a manner that allows close association of cells in liquid media, thereby increasing the frequency of DNA transfer.

1. Inoculate 5 mL of Luria-Bertani (LB) (Gram-negative) or BHI (Gram-positive) broth with a single colony from a recipient culture (e.g., *E. coli* J53–2). Inoculate 5 mL of broth with a single colony of donor culture and incubate both overnight at 37°C.
2. Set up three flasks with 4.5 mL of broth. Into one (mating flask), inoculate 50 μL of the donor overnight culture and 500 μL of the recipient culture. Into the second (recipient control flask), inoculate 500 μL of the recipient overnight culture. Into the third, inoculate 50 μL of the donor overnight culture.
3. Incubate at 37°C for 4 hours or overnight, without shaking.
4. Inoculate selective agar plates with 100 μL from the mating mixture and control flasks. In the case of matings between *K. pneumoniae* strain 5657 and *E. coli* J53–2, selection is on plates containing rifampin (100 μg/mL) and ceftazidime (5 μg/mL). Serial dilutions should also be performed on the mating mixtures to determine the number of donor and recipient CFU.

Transfer frequency is expressed as transconjugants/recipient CFU. LB broth contains 10 g/L Bacto-tryptone, 5 g/L yeast extract, and 10 g/L NaCl. The volume of the mating mixture is not critical to these experiments. It is important that the bacteria be well aerated and grown at a defined temperature. This broth protocol can be scaled down to allow for mating between a greater number of different mating pairs (e.g., in microtiter plates) as necessary.

B. Filter Matings

Filter matings are used to detect transfer events that require close cellular contact for a period of time.

1. Set up overnight cultures as in the preceding method.
2. Place three sterile nitrocellulose disks on a nonselective agar plate.
3. Inoculate tubes with mating mixtures as in the preceding method.
4. Place 100 μL of each mixture into a sterile 1.5-mL polypropylene tube, mix, transfer 100 μL to a sterile nitrocellulose filter, and allow the filter to dry at room temperature.
5. Place plates in an incubator overnight at 37°C.
6. Pick up filters with sterile forceps and place into test tubes with 1 to 2 mL of sterile 0.9% saline. Vortex-mix vigorously.
7. Inoculate 100-μL aliquots from each tube onto selective agar plates. Remember to inoculate plates selective for either donor or recipient CFU with serial dilutions of the mating mixture to allow for determination of the number of donors and transconjugants and calculation of the rate of transfer.

C. Mating Strategy for Very Low Frequency Events

Filter matings are adequate for detecting events that occur at a rate of at least 1×10^{-8} per recipient CFU. We have found that some transfer events in enterococci occur at rates as low as 10^{-10} to 10^{-9}. For example, the transfer of the chromosomally integrated gentamicin resistance gene of *E. faecalis* CH19 to recipient strain *E. faecalis* JH2–7 (Fus^r, Rif^r, and Thy$^-$) occurs at rates as low as 10^{-10} per recipient CFU (290). We have devised a strategy for detecting events of this frequency.

1. Grow donor and recipient strains as in the broth mating method.
2. Combine 500 μL of donor and 500 μL of recipient in a sterile test tube. Spread 100 μL of the mixture over a 20-mL BHI agar plate.
3. Allow the plate to dry and incubate it overnight at 37°C.
4. Harvest as many of the CFU on the mating plate as possible by scraping the plate with a sterile loop and transferring the cells to a tube with 1 mL of saline. Harvest the cells from the donor and recipient control plates in a similar fashion. Vortex-mix vigorously.
5. Perform serial dilutions of the mating mixture in sterile saline. Inoculate the serial dilutions onto plates containing either gentamicin (500 μg/mL) or fusidic acid (25 μg/mL) and rifampin (100 μg/mL).
6. Inoculate the entire mating mixture and control cells onto selective plates (BHI agar with 25 μg/mL fusidic acid, 100 μg/mL rifampin, and 500 μg/mL gentamicin) in 100- to 200-μL aliquots. Allow the plates to dry and incubate them overnight at 37°C. Perform serial dilutions on plates designed to detect donors or recipients as well.
7. Continue to check the plates while incubating at 37°C for 5 days before arriving at a final count of transconjugants.

A situation in which such high-inoculum experiments cannot be used is in the selection for transfer of ampicillin resistance in Gram-negative bacilli. With high inocula, even low levels of chromosomal β-lactamase production result in overgrowth on ampicillin-containing media.

APPENDIX III: EXTRACTION OF PLASMID AND GENOMIC DNA

Techniques for the extraction of plasmid DNA from *E. coli* have undergone significant advances over the past decade. Numerous biotechnology companies have developed reliable and rapid techniques for extracting and purifying large amounts of the high–copy number plasmids normally used as cloning vectors. These newer techniques largely avoid contact with toxic agents, such as phenol and ethidium bromide, commonly used in older techniques. We do not address these readily available protocols in this appendix. Instead, we detail several more complicated protocols that are designed to extract plasmid or genomic DNA from strains for which the newer techniques work poorly, either because of the nature of the host organism or because of the size of the plasmids to be extracted. Most of these protocols stop short of the final purification step using cesium chloride/ethidium bromide equilibrium density gradients, because this step is cumbersome, requires exposure to substantial amounts of ethidium bromide and phenol, and is not necessary for most purposes. Progression to the CsCl gradient is detailed for one protocol and can be applied to virtually all of the other protocols, although in some cases an increased amount of starting bacteria is required.

The protocols that follow separate plasmid from chromosomal DNA by taking advantage of the fact that most plasmids exist in the supercoiled state and hence are more resistant to denaturation in alkaline solution than is chromosomal DNA. Exposure of these DNA preparations to alkaline solutions denatures the chromosomal and nicked plasmid DNA, and this denatured DNA segregates with the cell wall pellet following neutralization. Supercoiled plasmid remains in solution and can be precipitated with salt and alcohol.

A. Isolation of Moderate-Size Plasmids (20–80 kb) from a Range of Bacteria

The following protocol, derived from Takahashi and Nagano (337), is ideal for the rapid isolation of moderate-size plasmid DNA (20–80 kb) from many species of Gram-negative bacilli, including *E. coli* and *K. pneumoniae*. With modification, it can also be used to isolate similar-sized plasmids from other species, such as *H. influenzae, P. aeruginosa,* and *S. aureus*. Buffers are as follows: buffer A (9), 400 mmol/L Tris-acetic acid and 20 mmol/L ethylenediaminetetraacetic acid (EDTA), pH 8.0; buffer B, 3 mol/L sodium acetate/acetic acid, pH 5.5; buffer C, 10 mmol/L Tris-acetic acid and 2 mmol/L disodium EDTA, pH 8.0; lysostaphin solution, 12 units/mL lysostaphin, 100 mmol/L NaCl, 40 mmol/L Tris-NaOH, and 50 mmol/L disodium EDTA, pH 6.9; lysing solution for enterobacteria and *S. aureus,* 4% sodium dodecyl sulfate (SDS)/100 mmol/L Tris mixed in equal volume with freshly prepared 0.4 N NaOH; lysing solution for *P. aeruginosa* and *H. influenzae*, 4% SDS/100 mmol/L tris mixed in equal volume with freshly prepared 0.16 N NaOH.

1. Culture as a broth culture overnight in 3 to 5 mL.
2. Harvest cells by centrifugation at room temperature at 2190 × g for 5 minutes.
3. Resuspend cells in 200 μL of either buffer A or lysostaphin solution with 100 mg/mL RNase. Transfer to a 1.5-mL polypropylene tube. For *S. aureus,* incubate further for 10 minutes at 37°C.
4. Add lysing solution (400 μL) and gently invert 5 to 10 times. Allow to stand at room temperature for 5 minutes.
5. Add 300 μL of cold (4°C) buffer B and gently invert 10 to 20 times.
6. Maintain at 0°C for 10 minutes, centrifuge at room temperature for 10 minutes, and then maintain at 0°C for 10 minutes.
7. Centrifuge for 10 minutes at 0°C and then transfer the supernatant to a fresh tube.
8. Extract with an equal volume of chloroform/isoamyl alcohol (24:1).
9. Transfer 500 μL of the aqueous phase to a fresh tube. Add 1 mL of cold 95% ethanol and mix by inversion. Place on ice for 5 minutes.
10. Centrifuge at 0°C for 30 minutes.
11. Wash pellet with 70% ethanol.
12. Resuspend in 125 μL of 50 mmol/L Tris, 10 mmol/L EDTA, pH 8 (TE buffer). Separate 25 μL on an agarose gel to determine plasmid content.

B. Isolation of Very Large Plasmids (More Than 100 kb) from Gram-Negative Bacilli

Very large plasmids are often difficult to isolate because they tend to break up and separate with the chromosomal DNA in most protocols. The following technique, from a protocol published by Hansen and Olsen (143), involves gentle and meticulous lysis steps as well as precipitation with polyethylene glycol, which is considerably gentler than precipitation with either ethanol or isopropanol.

1. After overnight growth on solid medium, inoculate 40 mL of broth and grow to an optical density at 425 nm of approximately 2.
2. Centrifuge cells for 10 minutes. Wash cells once in 0.1 mol/L sodium phosphate buffer, pH 7.0. Centrifuge again and resuspend in 1.35 mL of 25% sucrose/0.05 mol/L Tris, pH 8.0.
3. Add 0.1 mL of lysozyme solution (10 mg/mL in 0.25 mol/L Tris, pH 8.0) and mix by gentle inversion (20 times per minute). Place on ice for 5 minutes.
4. Add 0.5 mL of 0.25 mol/L EDTA, pH 8.0. Mix by five inversions. Place on ice for 5 minutes.
5. Add 0.5 mL of SDS (20%, w/v, in TE buffer), followed by eight cycles of a heat pulse at 55°C and five inversions at room temperature. A clear viscous solution of lysed cells should be produced.
6. Add 0.5 mL of 3 N NaOH (freshly prepared) and immediately begin 3 minutes of inversions.
7. Add 1 mL of 2 mol/L Tris, pH 7.0, in two 0.5-mL aliquots, followed by 30 seconds of inversion.
8. Add 0.65 mL of SDS (20%, w/v, in TE buffer), immediately followed by the addition of 1.25 mL of 5 mol/L NaCl and 20 inversions. This step is crucial for the removal of chromosomal DNA.
9. Chill tubes in an ice bath and then allow them to sit overnight at 4°C.
10. Centrifuge at 17,000 g at 4°C for 30 minutes.
11. Pour the supernatant into chilled plastic conical tubes. Remove any carried-over pieces of flocculent material with a Pasteur pipette. Measure the volume.
12. Decant the fluid into chilled polypropylene tubes. Add 0.313 volumes of polyethylene glycol 6000 (42%, w/v, in 0.1 mol/L sodium phosphate buffer). Mix gently by stirring with a plastic pipette. Refrigerate for 6 hours or overnight.

13. Centrifuge at 700 × g for 5 minutes at 4°C.
14. Resuspend the pellet in 150 μL of 50 mmol/L Tris, 5 mmol/L disodium EDTA, 50 mmol/L NaCl, pH 8.0. Crude plasmid preparation can be electrophoresed at this point. Ten to 40 μL should be used for electrophoresis. In our experience, restriction digestion of this crude preparation is generally unsuccessful.

C. Plasmid Isolation from Enterococci

This protocol, from C. Wennersten in the laboratory of R. C. Moellering Jr., represents a modification of the protocol of Birnboim (31). This protocol is useful for extracting plasmids from difficult-to-lyse organisms such as the enterococci but works with most Gram-negative organisms as well. It is primarily useful for the separation of undigested plasmids on agarose gels. Solutions are as follows: solution 1, 0.9 g of glucose, 0.346 g of EDTA, and 0.303 g of Tris (volume to 100 mL with water and pH to 8.0 with HCl); solution 2, 3% SDS in 0.3 mol/L NaOH, pH 13.03; solution 3, 29.4 g of potassium acetate and 5 mL of formic acid (volume to 100 mL with water).

1. Streak a single colony onto a blood agar plate and incubate overnight at 37°C.
2. Harvest colonies with a sterile cotton swab into dextrose phosphate broth to reach McFarland standards of 0.5 to 1 and incubate at 35°C for 2 hours.
3. Remove 15 mL, add to tubes with 0.75 g of glycine, and incubate at 35°C for 60 minutes.
4. Harvest 12 mL into a Falcon 2059 tube, centrifuge in a Sorvall RC-5B centrifuge at 6000 rpm for 10 minutes, and discard the supernatant.
5. Resuspend pellets in 1 mL of freshly made solution 1 with 5 mg/mL lysozyme, vortex-mix, and incubate on ice for 60 minutes.
6. Add 2 mL of solution 2, invert the tube six times, and incubate for 5 minutes on ice.
7. Add 1.5 mL of solution 3, invert the tube six times, and place on ice for 60 minutes.
8. Centrifuge at 10,000 rpm for 30 minutes and transfer the supernatant to a new Falcon tube.
9. Extract with an equal volume of chloroform/isoamyl alcohol (24:1) and transfer the aqueous phase to a new tube.
10. Add 9 mL of cold (20°C) 95% ethanol and place at 70°C overnight.
11. Centrifuge at 10,000 rpm for 30 minutes.
12. Wash the pellet with cold 70% ethanol, resuspend in 100 μL of TE buffer, and use 25 μL for separation on an agarose gel.

D. Small-Scale Isolation of Enterococcal Plasmids for Restriction Digestion Only

This rapid protocol, based on Ehrenfeld and Clewell (107), is designed to extract enough plasmid from an overnight 5-mL culture of enterococci to be visible on an agarose gel after digestion with restriction enzymes. It is primarily useful for screening transconjugants from mating experiments. It does not purify plasmids enough to be run on a gel without digestion. The solutions are as follows: solution 1, 50 mmol/L Tris-HCl, 10 mmol/L EDTA, 100 mmol/L glucose, and 10 mg/mL lysozyme; solution 2, 0.2 N NaOH and 1% SDS; solution 3, 30% potassium acetate, pH 5.0.

1. Grow the enterococcal strain overnight in 5 mL of BHI broth with selective antibiotics as necessary.
2. Centrifuge at 5000 rpm for 10 minutes and discard the supernatant.
3. Resuspend the pellet in 200 μL of solution 1, transfer to a 1.5-mL tube, and incubate for 30 minutes at 37°C.
4. Add 400 μL of solution 2 and invert until the solution clears. Incubate on ice for 5 minutes.
5. Add 300 μL of solution 3, invert, and incubate on ice for 5 minutes. Centrifuge.
6. Pour the supernatant into a new 1.5-mL tube, extract with an equal volume of phenol/chloroform/isoamyl alcohol (25:24:1), and centrifuge for 10 minutes.
7. Extract the aqueous phase with an equal volume of chloroform/isoamyl alcohol (24:1) and centrifuge for 10 minutes.
8. Add an equal volume of isopropanol, mix, and centrifuge for 30 minutes.
9. Resuspend the pellet in 200 μL of TE buffer, add 20 μL of 3 mol/L sodium acetate and 400 μL of cold 95% ethanol, mix, and centrifuge.
10. Resuspend the pellet in 20 μL of TE buffer. Digest the entire sample with a restriction enzyme and 1 mg/mL RNase.

E. Larger-Scale Isolation of Enterococcal Plasmid DNA

This protocol, from LeBlanc and Lee (188), is designed to extract moderately large amounts of plasmid from difficult-to-lyse organisms such as enterococci.

1. Grow the strain overnight in 20 mL of BHI broth with selective antibiotic as necessary.
2. Centrifuge overnight growth at 7000 rpm for 5 minutes.
3. Wash the pellet one time with sodium phosphate buffer, pH 7.0, and repeat the centrifugation.
4. Resuspend the washed cells in 730 μL of 50 mmol/L Tris-HCl, pH 8.0.

5. Add 720 μL of lysozyme solution (40 mg/mL in 50 mmol/L Tris-HCl, pH 8.0).
6. Incubate at 37°C for 20 minutes.
7. Add 500 μL of 0.25 mol/L EDTA and chill on ice for 5 minutes.
8. Add 500 μL of 20% SDS in 50 mmol/L Tris-HCl, 10 mmol/L EDTA.
9. Perform eight immersions at 55°C, each followed by five inversions of the tube at a rate of one inversion every 3 seconds.
10. Add 250 μL of 3 N NaOH. Invert 20 times per minute for 3 minutes.
11. Add 500 μL of water, mix, add 500 μL of 2 mol/L Tris-HCl, pH 7.0, and invert the tube 10 times.
12. Repeat step 11.
13. Add 650 μL of 20% SDS in TE buffer, mix, and incubate overnight at 4°C.
14. Centrifuge samples at 17,000 × g at 4°C for 30 minutes.
15. Add 6.1 mL of water, add RNase to a final concentration of 100 μg/mL, and incubate at 37°C for 60 minutes.
16. Extract with an equal volume of sodium-saturated phenol.
17. Extract with an equal volume of chloroform/isoamyl alcohol (24:1).
18. Add 1/20 volume of 3 mol/L sodium acetate and 2 volumes of 95% ethanol. Precipitate at 20°C for 4 hours or overnight.
19. Centrifuge at 17,000 × g for 30 minutes at 4°C.
20. Suspend the pellet in 100 μL of TE buffer.

F. Large-Scale Preparation of Genomic DNA from Gram-Negative Bacilli

In some situations, such as the investigation of resistance genes that are chromosomally encoded, it is desirable to extract chromosomal as well as plasmid DNA. It is not possible to obtain completely pure chromosomal DNA (i.e., without plasmid contamination) even with CsCl gradient centrifugation. This protocol, from Wilson (376), yields large amounts of genomic DNA from *E. coli*. For pure DNA, the CsCl step must be performed. However, the DNA extracted prior to the CsCl step is pure enough for most purposes.

1. Grow 100 mL of bacteria culture to saturation.
2. Centrifuge for 10 minutes at 4000 × g.
3. Resuspend the pellet in 9.5 mL of TE buffer, 0.5 mL of 10% SDS, and 50 L of 20 mg/mL proteinase K. Mix and incubate for 1 hour at 37°C.
4. Add 1.8 mL of 5 mol/L NaCl and mix thoroughly.
5. Add 1.5 mL of hexadecyltrimethyl ammonium bromide (CTAB)/NaCl solution (the solution is prepared by dissolving 4.1 g of NaCl in water and slowly adding 10 g of CTAB, with heating and stirring; the final volume is adjusted to 100 mL with water).
6. Extract with an equal volume of chloroform/isoamyl alcohol (24:1) and centrifuge for 10 minutes at 6000 × g at room temperature.
7. Transfer the aqueous phase to a fresh tube and extract with phenol/chloroform/isoamyl alcohol (25:24:1) if necessary.
8. Transfer the aqueous phase to a fresh tube. Precipitate DNA with 0.6 volumes of isopropanol. Remove the DNA clot with a glass rod and transfer it to a tube with 70% ethanol. Centrifuge and resuspend the pellet in 100 to 500 μL of TE buffer. DNA can be used directly at this point, after incubating for 30 minutes with RNase and repeating the extraction. Alternatively, it can be dissolved in 4 mL of TE buffer and purified by cesium chloride/ethidium bromide equilibrium density gradient centrifugation, as in the following steps.
9. Measure the DNA concentration. Adjust the concentration to give 50 to 100 μg/mL. Add 4.3 g of CsCl/4 mL of TE buffer. Add 200 mL of 10 μg/mL ethidium bromide. Transfer to sealable centrifuge tubes. Centrifuge for 4 hours at 70,000 rpm at 15°C.
10. Visualize the gradient with ultraviolet (UV) light and remove the chromosomal band.
11. Extract ethidium bromide with CsCl-saturated isopropanol.
12. Dialyze overnight against 2 L of TE buffer.
13. Precipitate with 1/10 volume of 3 mol/L sodium acetate and 2 volumes of 95% ethanol.

G. Small-Scale Miniprep for Genomic DNA from Gram-Positive Bacteria

This protocol, adapted from Storrs et al. (331), is useful for the isolation of genomic DNA from a large number of species of Gram-positive bacteria for screening purposes or for cloning of genomic fragments.

1. Culture cells overnight in 5 mL of BHI broth.
2. Centrifuge in a Sorvall RC-5B centrifuge at 5000 rpm for 5 minutes.
3. Resuspend the cell pellet in 400 μL of TE buffer with 25% sucrose and 20 mg/mL lysozyme (add lysostaphin for staphylococci).
4. Incubate at 37°C for 15 minutes.
5. Add 400 μL of TE buffer with 2% SDS and mix until clear.
6. Add 100 μL of proteinase K (5 mg/mL solution) and 100 μL of RNase (5 mg/mL solution).
7. Extract twice with phenol/chloroform/isoamyl alcohol (25:24:1).
8. Precipitate with an equal volume of isopropanol and transfer the DNA clot to a tube with cold 70% ethanol.
9. Centrifuge and resuspend pellet in 50 to 100 μL of TE buffer. Use 3 to 5 μL for genomic restriction digestion.

APPENDIX IV: TRANSFORMATION OF BACTERIA

Our understanding of gene structure and function has been dramatically increased by our ability to clone genes into high–copy number vectors in well-characterized strains of *E. coli*. The first step toward introduction of foreign DNA into cells is the preparation of competent cells. Following is a protocol for making competent cells using calcium chloride. Other chemical protocols exist that may yield an even higher frequency of transformation (138). The highest frequencies of transformation are reportedly obtained using electroporation, but this requires an expensive device and is generally not required for routine transformations.

A. Preparation of Competent *E. coli* using Calcium Chloride

1. Inoculate 1 mL of LB broth with an isolated colony from an appropriate *E. coli* strain (we prefer recombination-deficient strains such as HB101, DH5, and XL1-Blue).
2. Inoculate 100 mL of LB broth with 1 mL of overnight culture.
3. Incubate for 2 to 3 hours at 37°C with shaking.
4. Place the culture on ice for 5 to 10 minutes.
5. Pellet the culture at 7000 rpm for 5 minutes at 4°C.
6. Gently resuspend cells in 20 mL of sterile, ice-cold transformation buffer (50 mmol/L $CaCl_2$ and 10 mmol/L Tris-HCl, pH 8.0). Place on ice for 20 minutes.
7. Centrifuge for 5 minutes at 7000 rpm.
8. Carefully resuspend the pellet in 2 mL of ice-cold transformation buffer.
9. Allow cells to remain on ice for 1 to 2 hours. Store at 4°C for 12 to 24 hours.

Transformation efficiency should increase with increased time on ice. For long-term storage, cells should be immediately separated into 200-μL aliquots in 1.5-mL polypropylene tubes, snap frozen in dry ice/alcohol, and stored at 70°C. They can be thawed on ice prior to use.

APPENDIX V: MISCELLANEOUS PROCEDURES

A. Polymerase Chain Reaction Techniques

In the past 5 years, the technique of amplifying segments of DNA using PCR technology has seen countless new applications. PCR techniques are all based (a) on the activity of thermostable DNA polymerases, particularly the polymerase from *Thermus aquaticus,* to effectively polymerize DNA at high temperatures and (b) on the availability of computer-based water baths that can rapidly change temperatures between those required for denaturation, annealing, and extension. By subjecting even very small amounts of template to repeated reproduction, the target sequence can be amplified to more than 1 million copies in a few hours. In the microbiology laboratory, PCR techniques are useful both for documenting the presence of genes and for cloning and sequencing genes that would be otherwise difficult to clone (292). These techniques have also been used as epidemiological tools to assess the clonal relationship of clinical isolates (356). Following is just one example of a protocol in which PCR techniques were used with success to rapidly document the presence of the *mecA* gene in methicillin-resistant staphylococci (350,351). Primers (based on the published *mecA* sequence [326]) designed to yield an 1800-bp product are as follows: primer 1, 5-GTTGTAGTTGTCGGGTTTGG-3; primer 2, 5-CCACCCAATTTGTCTGCCAGTTTCTCC-3.

1. Harvest a 1-μL loopful of bacteria from an agar plate and resuspend in 50 μL of lysostaphin solution (100 g/mL in water).
2. Incubate for 10 minutes at 37°C.
3. Add 50 μL of proteinase K solution (100 μg/mL) and 150 μL of 0.1 mol/L Tris, pH 7.5.
4. Incubate at 37°C for 10 minutes.
5. Place in boiling water for 5 minutes.
6. Use 10 μL of the above mixture for PCRs. Follow the manufacturer's recommendations for the concentrations of various components. Calculate the amount of added primer based on the amount of primers in individual preparations. Reaction conditions for PCR amplification are as follows: denaturation at 94°C for 30 seconds, annealing at 55C for 30 seconds, and primer extension at 72°C for 2 minutes, for a total of 30 cycles. Run 10 μL of the reaction mixture on an agarose gel to demonstrate the expected 1.8-kb amplification product.

Several variations on PCR amplification techniques have been developed. Among these are inverse PCR, which allows amplification of sequences flanking regions of a known DNA sequence after a digested fragment has been ligated to itself (347), and anchor template PCR, which allows amplification between a known region and a restriction site when the sequence of only one specific primer is known (300). A full discussion of all of the uses of PCR techniques is beyond the scope of this appendix.

B. RNA Techniques

In instances in which decreased expression of a gene is being investigated, it is important to distinguish between processes that result in decreased transcription of the gene and processes that either decrease the half-life of the mRNA or posttranslationally modify the encoded protein. Northern blots are designed to detect the total amount of a specific mRNA produced by a bacterial strain. DNA probes are used to hybridize to total cellular RNA. When a region representing a gene between the transcriptional start site and the stop codon of the open reading frame for the protein is used, hybridization should be specific for the mRNA transcribed from that gene. Decreased expression of resistance in the presence of a detectable decrease in the mRNA for that resistance gene implies that the loss of the resistance characteristic involves a change in the regulation of the transcription of the gene. RNA can be readily extracted from *E. coli* using protocols that employ guanidine isothiocyanate/phenol/chloroform extraction techniques. Following is a rapid procedure by which RNA can be isolated from many different tissue sources or types of cells. It is based on Chomczynski and Sacchi (62). Next comes a protocol for the transfer and detection of RNA using a Northern blot.

RNA Extraction Protocol

Solution D (denaturing solution) contains 4 mol/L guanidine isothiocyanate, 25 mmol/L sodium citrate, pH 7.0, 0.5% sarkosyl, and 0.1 mol/L 2-mercaptoethanol (62).

1. Grow overnight the cells to be analyzed.
2. Pellet cells and resuspend them in 1 mL of solution D (or 100 μL/10^6 cells).
3. Add, in sequence, 0.1 mL of 2 mol/L sodium acetate, pH 4, 1 mL of water-saturated phenol, and 0.2 mL of chloroform/isoamyl alcohol mixture (49:1). Mix thoroughly by inversion after each addition.
4. Shake the final suspension vigorously for 10 seconds and place on ice for 15 minutes.
5. Centrifuge at 10,000 × g for 20 minutes at 4°C.
6. Transfer the aqueous phase to a fresh tube.
7. Mix with 1 mL of isopropanol and keep mixture at 20°C for 1 hour.
8. Centrifuge at 10,000 × g for 20 minutes at 4°C.
9. Redissolve the pellet in 300 μL of solution D and transfer to a 1.5-mL tube.
10. Precipitate with 1 volume of isopropanol at 20°C for 1 hour.
11. Centrifuge in an Eppendorf centrifuge for 10 minutes.
12. Wash the pellet in 75% ethanol.
13. Vacuum-dry the pellet and dissolve in 50 μL of 0.5% SDS at 65°C for 10 minutes; the preparation can then be used.

Northern Blot

1. Set up 2-mL cultures with or without antibiotics; incubate overnight at 37°C.
2. Extract RNA using Qiagen RNeasy kit, eluting with 60 μl DNase/RNase-free water.
3. Determine RNA quantity by checking OD 260 of a 1:10 dilution of sample.
4. Aliquot a 5-μL volume. If greater than 5 μL, precipitate using 2 volumes 100% ethanol and 10% 2M NaCl.
5. Resuspend in 5 μL DNase/RNase-free water.
6. Add 10 μL 1.5× RNA Sample Buffer.
7. Mix.
8. Heat at 65°C for 15 minutes.
9. Chill on ice.
10. Add 1 μL of 1 mg/mL ethidium bromide and 3 μL tracking dye.
11. Spin load on RNA/formaldehyde gel with 1× MOPS as running buffer in cold room overnight at a low voltage.
12. Set up the blot as follows (bottom to top): 20 SSC-soaked wick of three pieces of Whatman paper, upside-down gel, Magnagraph membrane, three pieces of Whatman paper, and paper towels.
13. Weigh down the blot with book weights, fill pyrex baking dishes with approximately 1 inch of 20 × SSC, and allow transfer to proceed overnight.
14. Mark ribosomal bands with a pencil under UV irradiation and bake the blot under vacuum for 2 hours.
15. Prehybridize at 42°C for at least 2 hours in 20 mL of Northern prehybridization solution (Northern prehybridization solution is 5 SSC, 50% formamide, 0.02% SDS, 0.1% *N*-laurylsarcosine, 2%, w/v, blocking reagent for nucleic acid hybridization, and 20 mmol/L sodium maleate, pH 7.5).
16. Boil digoxigenin-labeled probe for 10 minutes and quench on ice. Add the probe to 20 mL of fresh prehybridization solution and hybridize overnight at 42°C.
17. Wash the membrane once at room temperature in 2 SSC/0.1% SDS.
18. Wash the membrane twice at 65°C in 0.1 SSC/0.1% SDS.
19. Wash the membrane for 1 minute at room temperature in 50 mL of Northern blocking solution, with rocking (Northern blocking solution is 100 mmol/L sodium maleate, pH 7.5, 150 mmol/L NaCl, and 2% blocking reagent).
20. Incubate the membrane for 30 minutes in 50 mL of anti-digoxigenin-alkaline phosphatase conjugate (1:5000) in Northern blocking solution (see step 19).
21. Wash twice for 15 minutes in 200 mL of maleate buffer (maleate buffer is 100 mmol/L maleic acid, pH 7.5, and 150 mmol/L NaCl).

22. Equilibrate the membrane for 5 minutes in buffer 3 (see Southern blot protocol above).
23. Place the membrane in an envelope constructed from a clear overhead-transparency sheet. Add 500 μL of Lumi-Phos 530 and spread out the air bubbles. Tape shut and expose to film for varying periods of time until the optimal picture is obtained.

RT-PCR

In some cases, a more precise measure of RNA quantities is desired. Such a measure can be attained using cycling techniques and real-time PCR. A brief protocol is given here. More details are available from manufacturers of RT-PCR machines.

1. Prep RNA using Qiagen RNeasy mini kit as per the previous protocol.
2. Treat sample with DNase. We have used Promega's RQ1 RNase-free DNase and Ambion's DNA-free kit with equal success. We prefer Ambion's product because it cleans the sample of all buffer and ions without extraction and ethanol precipitation.
3. Perform PCR (should be negative) to confirm DNase treatment was successful.
4. Set up RT-PCR reaction for LightCycler using Roche LightCycler RNA master sybr green kit.
5. Follow recommendations of Roche to optimize reaction. Substantial differences exist between protocols because of differing primers, etc. Trial and error with different conditions is often necessary.

APPENDIX VI: β-LACTAMASE ANALYSIS

The major action of these bacterial hydrolytic enzymes is to inactivate β-lactam antibiotics. By destroying penicillins and cephalosporins, these enzymes are the major cause of resistance to β-lactam antibiotics. There are two general mechanisms by which β-lactamases hydrolyze β-lactams; a two-step serine ester mechanism and a zinc (Zn^{+2}) metallo-enzyme. In common with penicillin-binding proteins (PBPs), β-lactamases share amino acid sequence motifs that are conserved among all the penicillin-recognizing enzymes. The major catalytic difference between PBPs and β-lactamases rests in the rate of regeneration of the free enzyme. In β-lactamases, the rate of enzyme regeneration is rapid; in PBPs, the rate of regeneration is considerably slower (217).

Detection and Measurement of β-Lactamase Activity

Antimicrobial susceptibility data are usually very reliable indicators of β-lactamase activity. Much can be learned by the interpretation of resistance to classes of antibiotics. However, methods of greater sensitivity and specificity are often required. In the following sections, we summarize the general methods used to detect β-lactamases in the clinical and research laboratories. The following descriptions are based upon an earlier version of this text (Lorian, 4th Edition, 1996) written by David M. Livermore and J. David Williams. In many instances the original text and references were included. The clinician, clinical microbiologist, and researcher need to appreciate the limitations of each method. The detection of β-lactamases in certain clinical isolates is extremely important for therapy. For study purposes, it is often important to know the β-lactamase responsible for ceftazidime resistance in *E. coli* or *Klebsiella* spp because these genera are normally susceptible to extended-spectum β-lactams.

Types of β-Lactamase Tests

Three general methods are used to detect β-lactamases. One method incorporates the use of a chromogenic cephalosporin such as nitrocefin or CENTA, and the other two methods depend on the hydrolysis of penicillin linked to the decolorization of iodine (iodometric test) or linked to a pH indicator (acidimetric test). The former method is based on a very sensitive color change; the acidimetric and iodometric methods are less sensitive. The investigator should be mindful that high-level resistance observed *in vitro* by susceptibility tests (high β-lactam MICs) may not be easily measured.

Chromogenic Cephalosporins

Nitrocefin. This chromogenic cephalosporin undergoes a rapid yellow to red change after hydrolysis by β-lactamases (247). It is an extremely sensitive test, useful in most clinical situations, except for detecting the PC-1 β-lactamase of staphylococci and the ROB-1 β-lactamase of *H. influenzae* (299,303). A solution of the pure nitrocefin powder is made at 0.5 mmol/L concentration for applications in the laboratory. The nitrocefin powder (2.58 mg) is initially soluble in 0.5 mL of DMSO, and 9.5 mL of 0.1 mol/L phosphate buffer, pH 7, is added. The solution can be divided into 1-mL aliquots and frozen at −20°C or placed in a 4°C refrigerator wrapped in aluminum foil for immediate use (we do not keep nitrocefin more than a week at 4°C). To detect β-lactamase activity using this solution, colonies are scrapped from a plate and suspended in 20 μL of phosphate buffer, then 20 μL of nitrocefin test solution is added. If β-lactamases are present, the yellow to red changes should be readily observed in 1–3 minutes. Numerous commercial preparations based on this general method are available. Becton Dickinson, Unipath, and Difco all produce nitrocefin-impregnated paper disks for clinical applications. When β-lactamases are suspected and the organism identified is known to be impermeable to β-lactam antibiotics, a 0.1 mmol/L EDTA and 2 mg/mL lysozyme solution can be mixed with colonies when they are suspended in phosphate buffer before the addition of nitrocefin (23). By chelating Ca^{+2} in the outer membrane, the EDTA increases permeability, and the lysozyme acts to hydrolyze cell walls (257). If the investigator wishes to determine if more than one β-lactamase is present, solutions of 0.1 mmol/L cloxacillin (to inhibit AmpC cephalosporinases) and clavulanic acid (to inhibit the penicillinases) can be added as well (60,374).

PADAC. This cephalosporin (pyridinium 2 azo-p-dimethylaniline chromophore) undergoes a violet to yellow change upon hydrolysis by a β-lactamase. In the experience of one of the authors, it was very difficult to use this chromogenic cephalosporin in direct applications (e.g., on filter paper) due to the direction of color change. It is no longer commercially available.

CENTA. A third chromogenic cephalospoirin, CENTA, is also available for use. Although it not recommended for the direct detection of β-lactamase–producing colonies on agar plates, it is useful in kinetic analyses. A method for its preparation has been summarized (23) and been found useful for the characterization of all classes of enzymes except for the *Aeromonas hydrophila* metallo-enzyme. Unlike nitrocefin, it is highly soluble in aqueous buffers and does not require DMSO. This chromogenic cephalsosporin is prepared from cephalothin. Despite its low cost, CENTA has not been widely used.

Iodometric Tests

The hydrolysis of a β-lactam substrate results in the reduction of iodine to iodide, decolorizing the blue-black starch-iodine complex. Three iodometric tests are available (tube method, paper strip method, and agar overlay method). Of these tests, the most useful is the agar overlay method.

Agar Overlay Method. Herein, a 67-mL volume of 120% strength Mueller-Hinton agar at 55°C is supplemented with 33 mL of 0.6% iodine in 6% aqueous potassium iodide and with 600 mg of benzylpenicillin dissolved in 2 mL of 0.1 mol/L phosphate buffer, pH 7. After mixing, the agar is poured onto an overnight culture plate without disturbing the colonies. As the agar cools, a clear halo is seen around colonies with β-lactamases (36,378).

Paper Strip Method. Starch (0.2 g) is boiled in 100 mL of distilled water and slowly cooled. Upon cooling, 1 g of benzylpenicillin is added. Filter paper strips are then soaked with this solution and air-dried. When ready for use, the strips are moistened with 2% iodine in 53% aqueous potassium iodide, and colonies from an overnight plate are placed on the strips. The decolorization should take 5 minutes (378).

Tube Method. Bacterial colonies suspected of having β-lactamases are emulsified in benzylpenicillin-containing solution (6 mg/mL in 0.1 mol/L phosphate buffer), and 20 μL of 1% soluble starch is added, followed by 20 μL of iodine reagent (2% iodine in 53% aqueous potassium iodide). Decolorization of the iodine should occur in 5 minutes. Controls are absolutely required due to the nonspecific nature of these tests (57).

Acidimetric Tests

Like iodometric tests, acidimetric tests can done using a tube method, paper strip method, and an agar overlay method.

Tube Acidimetry. In this method, 2 mL of aqueous of phenol solution (0.5%) is diluted with 16.6 mL of distilled water, and 1.2 g of penicillin is added. The pH is adjusted to 8.5 with 1 mol/L NaOH. This violet solution is frozen till use. When required, the solution is thawed, 100 μL are aliquoted into a well or onto a glass slide, and bacterial colonies are added. The appearance of a yellow color in 5 minutes indicates β-lactamase activity. This method should not be used with liquid cultures since acid metabolites could interfere with the interpretation of results (101).

Paper Strip Method. This method works on the same principle as the tube method except that the chemistry occurs on a paper surface. In brief, filter paper is soaked in 125 mg/mL benzylpenicillin, 0.1% bromocresol purple, and 1.25 mmol/L NaOH, then dried and stored. Before use, the strips are moistened with distilled water. Bacteria are then smeared on them. The development of a yellow color indicates β-lactamase activity (101).

Agar Overlay Method. In this method, 10% benzylpenicillin, 0.25% *N*-phenyl-1-napthyl-amine-azo-*O*-carboxylbenzene, 6% NaOH, and 1.5% agar (55°C) are first prepared. The *N*-phenyl-1-napthyl-amine-azo-*O*-carboxylbenzene is rendered alkaline with NaOH, and 2 mL is mixed with 8 mL of agar. The molten agar is poured on an agar plate, with care taken not to disturb the colonies. Five milliliters of the penicillin solution is then poured on top, and the colonies possessing β-lactamase are identified by the purple color change (101). The above summarized iodometric and acidemetric tests are largely used when nitrocesin and CENTA are unavailable.

Interpretation of Antibiogram Data

Although prediction of β-lactamase content does not surpass definitive identification, interpretative reading of susceptibility results can be insightful. This approach requires the use of well-studied controls and reference standards obtained from the National Committee for Clinical Laboratory Standards and zone sizes or MIC data. Interpretative reading is not accurate when used with automated susceptibility testing methods (Vitek).

To perform this correctly, a wide range of β-lactams must be tested (e.g., penicillins, penicillin β-lactamase inhibitors, cefoxitin or cefotetan, ceftazidime, and carbapenems). It should be noted that these "marker antibiotics" might also reveal the resistance mechanism as well (cefoxitin can be used to induce a β-lactamase in *Enterobacter* spp. and *Citrobacter freundii* and to distinguish an ESBL [cefoxitin susceptible] from an AmpC [cefoxotin resistant]). There are certain caveats with interpretative reading. One must reserve confidence when interpreting antibiogram data from *Acinteobacter* spp and *Burkholderia cepacia*. It is the authors' experience that when multiple β-lactamases are present, this method is prone to serious error. We were recently challenged by the task of determining the β-lactamases present in a *Proteus mirabilis* clinical isolate that demonstrated resistance to ampicillin, amoxicillin clavulanate, cephalothin, ceftazidime, piperacillin/tazobactam, and ceftriaxone but was susceptible to imipenem and cefepime. Our investigations revealed the isolate contained a TEM-10 and a TEM-1 (unpublished observations). Similar experience has been gained interpreting the susceptibility data from a worldwide collection of *K. pneumoniae* isolates. The presence of a CTX-M TEM and SHV β-lactamases conferred resistance to all third-generation cephalosporins and β-lactamase inhibitors. Some clinical isolates can have up to five β-lactamase enzymes, confounding even the most insightful interpreters. The reader is referred to the 4th edition of this text for detailed listing of interpretative criteria.

Bioassays of β-Lactamase Activity

These highly sensitive methods can be used for detection as well as chemical screening purposes. The most widely used application of bioassays has been in the detection of ESBLs and qualitative β-lactamase induction.

Double-Disk Diffusion Assay and Etests for Gram-negative Bacteria

This test arose from the clinical observation that the susceptibility of ESBL-producing bacteria could be enhanced by the addition of a β-lactamase inhibitor. It is the authors' practice to take a standard suspension of bacteria in trypticase soy broth (0.5 MacFarland) and apply the suspension as a lawn to a standard agar plate (Mueller-Hinton agar). Antibiotic-containing disks (amoxicillin 20 μg/clavulanate 10 μg and cefotaxime or ceftazidme 30 μg) are placed 30 mm apart (center to center). Such disks are available from several suppliers (Becton Dickinson and Oxoid). After overnight incubation, an ESBL is inferred when the cephalosporin zone is expanded by the clavulanate. A difference of $\geq$5 mm between the zone diameters of either of the cephalosporin disks and the proximal β-lactam/clavulanate disk is taken to be phenotypic confirmation of ESBL production. Occassionally investigators will place multiple extended spectrum cephalosporin discs in a circular fashion around an amoxicillin/clavulanic acid disc to screen for the presence of an ESBL (e.g., cefotaxime, ceftazidime, cefpodoxime, ceftriaxone, and cefepime). This increases the sensitivity and specificity of the test. The reader is referred to the CDC web site: www.cdc.gov/NCIDOD/hip/Lab/FactSheet/esbl.htm and reference 15.

The purchase of Etest strips from AB Biodisk, which are fashioned with an extended-spectrum cephalosporin on one end and the extended-spectrum cephalosporin in combination with a β-lactamase inhibitor on the other, can also be reliably used. ESBL production is inferred when the ratio between the ceftazidime MIC and the ceftazidime clavulanate MIC equals or exceeds 16. It is common practice to regard *E. coli* and *Klebsiella* spp possessing an ESBL resistance to one extended-spectrum cephalosporin as resistant to *all* extended-spectrum cephalosporins. The standards for testing for ESBLs in genera other than *E. coli* and *Klebsiella* spp are still being investigated.

Three-Dimensional Test

The three-dimensional test (338) gives phenotypic evidence of ESBL-induced inactivation of extended-spectrum cephalosporins or aztreonam without relying on demonstration of inactivation of the β-lactamases by a β-lactamase inhibitor. In this test, developed by Thomson, the surface of the susceptibility plate is inoculated by using standard methods for disk diffusion testing, but additionally a circular slit is cut in the agar concentric with the margin of the plate. A heavy inoculum of organisms (10^9 to 10^{10} CFU) is pipetted into the slit. β-lactam–impregnated disks are then placed on the surface of the agar 3 mm outside of the inoculated circular slit. β-lactamase–induced inactivation of each test antibiotic is detected by inspection of the margin of the zone of inhibition in the vicinity of its intersection with the circular three-dimensional inoculation. The presence of β-lactamase–induced drug inactivation is visualized as a distortion or discontinuity in the usually circular inhibition zone or the production of discrete colonies in the vicinity of the inoculated slit.

A modification of the test involves removing a cylindrical plug of agar (diameter 4 mm), 2 mm from the antibiotic disks. The resulting cup is then filled with a milky suspension (McFarland no. 0.5 turbidity standard) of the test organism. Disadvantages of the test include the need for an additional indirect test if inhibition zones are small or absent. If the indirect test is used, the three-dimensional test is more sensitive than the double-disk diffusion test, but if the indirect test is not used, sensitivity declines.

Qualitative Induction Tests for Cephalosporinase Production in Gram-negative Bacteria

This test is performed to investigate if β-lactamase production can be induced. Generally, the presence or absence of induction can be readily shown for *Enterobacter* spp, *Citrobacter freundii,* and *Serratia* spp. As in the double-disk method, a lawn of bacteria is plated on Mueller-Hinton agar and a cefoxitin disk and a cefotaxime or cefuroxime disk are placed 15 and 20 mm apart. The plates are incubated overnight at 37°C, and the next day the blunting of the indicator zone adjacent to the cefoxitin disk is taken to mean the presence of induction. When the disks are placed at different distances, this method is very reliable.

Masuda Double-disk Assay

In the Masuda double-disk assay, an indicator organism (either the Oxford S. aureus strain, *Bacillus subtilis* or an ampicillin-susceptible *E. coli*) is grown overnight and added to 100 mL of agar. After mixing, the agar is poured into a Petri dish and allowed to set. Disks containing the antibiotic that the organism is susceptible to are placed on the plate. Adjacent to these disks are placed filter paper strips or disks containing the test organism or a concentrated cell extract containing the suspected bacterial β-lactamase from the test organism (the latter is preferred). The optimal distance is 15–18 mm (corresponding to MIC zones). After overnight incubation, the β-lactamase activity is determined by the qualitative indentation of the zone size of the susceptible bacteria around the test antibiotic. This is an extremely sensitive visual test and can be used when hydrolysis is not observed in the test tube yet MICs to the antibiotic are elevated. After overnight incubation, the zone size around the strip indicates hydrolysis (215).

Cloverleaf Method

In the cloverleaf method, an indicator organism is spread across an agar plate, as in the Masuda double-disk assay, and an antibiotic disk is placed in the center of the plate. Suspensions of the test organisms are streaked outward from the disk to the edge of the plate. Commonly, four isolates can be tested per plate. After overnight incubation, β-lactamase activity is noted where the test organism permits the indicator strain to grow closer to the disk than elsewhere on the plate. This method is preferred when testing staphylococcal isolates.

β-Lactamase Identification

aIEF

Currently, there are more than 470 unique β-lactamases described (51). Unlike the situation years ago, isoelectric point identification (pI) is no longer considered a reliable means of β-lactamase identification. Point mutations can drastically change pIs, and multiple enzymes share similar if not identical pIs. Although analytical isoelectric focusing (aIEF) remains an invaluable tool for detecting the numbers of β-lactamases in a clinical isolate, DNA sequencing is mandatory for definitive identification. Occasionally, the investigator can be tricked into thinking there are more β-lactamases than there really are owing the presence of satellite banding. In these instances, clarity can be achieved by reducing the quantity of β-lactamase solution loaded on the aIEF gel. The interested reader is referred to the following web site for an updated list of common pIs (www.lahey.org).

The charges carried by amino acid side chains of proteins and the presence of retained waters determine the migration of a protein in an electrically generated pH gradient. Whether the amino or carboxy side chains are charged or not depends on pH. In the electrically generated pH gradient established by the choice of buffers at the anode and cathode ends, a protein stops migrating at its pI. To perform aIEF correctly, a β-lactamase extract must be prepared (see below for methods). After β-lactamases are liberated, crude cell extracts are clarified by high-speed ultracentrifugation for 15–30 minutes. Our laboratory filter sterilizes crude cell extracts before they are stored at 4°C and applied to specially prepared gels.

In the past, numerous protocols existed for the design of aIEF gels with different pH ranges. Currently, aIEF gels can be purchased from Pharmacia. These commercial gels are convenient, made uniformly, and available in a variety of pH ranges. Although they are expensive, the safety and convenience far outweigh the cost. The reader may wish to consult earlier versions of this reference work on the preparation of individual gels. It is advisable to exercise caution using acrylamide stock solutions to make up aIEF gels since unpolymerized acrylamide is a neurotoxin.

Once in hand, 10 μL of clarified β-lactamase extract is loaded on an aIEF gel (aliquots are placed 0.5 cm apart) and located about 3 cm from the anode position. Usually 10 μL of sample will turn a nitrocefin solution pink in 1–3 minutes. If the coloration occurs faster, the investigator may wish to dilute the β-lactamase solution. Aliquots are applied to a gel surface, and commercially available standards (purchased from BioRad) with colored markers of various pI values are run simultaneously. The anode and cathode strips are usually made from a heavy chromatography paper (Munktel) and are soaked with acid and alkali to prevent migration of samples onto the electrodes. The gel is placed on a plate with electrodes on each end housed in the apparatus. Standard running conditions are 2000–3000 volts and 100–150 milliamps. A power of 10–15 watts allows focusing to occur within 2–3 hours. We usually run chromogenic standards (BioRad, aIEF standards) placed on opposite sides of the gel. These gels are run on a plate with a cold-water bath circulating through it. Various β-lactamases with known pIs are used as controls (257).

After the gel is run, the β-lactamase can be detected by overlying the gel with 0.5 mmol/L nitrocefin solution in the concentration as above. β-lactamase enzymes appear as red bands against a yellow background. In instances where β-lactamases do not hydrolyze nitrocefin (e.g., certain very high pI carbapenemases), investigators have used a 1% imipenem solution in a 0.9% agarose containing 0.5% bromthymol blue to detect high pI enzymes. These enzymes appear as yellow bands against a blue background. Occasionally, penicillin and iodine can be used as an overlay. It is also possible to overlay the isoelectric focusing gel with nutrient agar containing a β-lactam and transfer the entire gel to bioassay plate. After incubation, a suspension of bacteria with a suitable indicator organism (*E. coli* DH10B or DH5alpha) is plated across the agar, and the plate is incubated overnight. An area of growth is seen over the β-lactamase able to hydrolyze the β-lactam in the nutrient agar. To further aid β-lactamase identification, it is sometimes useful to add a β-lactamase inhibitor to the nitrocefin solution, such as 0.3 mmol/L cloxacillin (inhibits class C enzymes) or 0.3 mmol/L clavulanate (inhibits most class A β-lactamases). In this manner, it is possible for the investigator to distinguish between an SHV-related ESBL and a plasmid-born class C enzyme.

DNA Probes

Restriction fragments from β-lactamase genes make effective probes for identifying a particular gene or closely related ones. PCR amplification of a conserved fragment and nonradioactive labeling have simplified this process. Digoxigenin kits and biotin/streptavidin-containing systems are equally effective. In addition, synthetic oligonucleotides can be used as probes. Methods for calculating the optimal hybridization conditions to account for the effect of mismatches have been described. Oligonucleotide probes using nonradioactive labels are preferred.

PCR Detection of β-Lactamase Genes

The PCR method has gained wide acceptance for the rapid detection of β-lactamase genes. In this method, template DNA is readily prepared by boiling a cell suspension of at least 10^4 CFU/mL in TE buffer (1 colony in 100 μL buffer). A positive reaction is noted by the detection of a band of the same size as a positive control on an agarose gel. This is done in a multiplex fashion using multiple β-lactamase primers (260). The examination and comparison of the PCR product to standards helps the investigator determine the number and type of different β-lactamase genes present. Before final report, PCR amplification products should be confirmed by DNA sequencing.

Assays of β-Lactamase Activity

Extraction of β-Lactamase from Gram-negative Bacteria

To extract β-lactamases from cells, bacteria should be grown to logarithmic phase. Logarithmic phase cells have higher β-lactamase–specific activity than stationary phase cells. For aerobic Gram-negative bacteria, all 5–10 mL starter or seed cultures should be grown at 37°C and at 150–200 rpms or more (our incubator shaker is set at 250 rpms). A rich medium is preferred (Luria Bertaini media, 2 YT, or SOB media). After the starter culture is grown overnight, the aliquot is diluted in a larger volume of liquid medium. In a 1.5-L flask, 500 mL of medium are added. The medium should be prewarmed to the same temperature as the starter culture and not exceed 500 mL to ensure proper aeration. If required, selective antibiotics are added. An inducer is added after 90 minutes of growth. For example, cefoxotin (100 μg/mL) is suitable for induction of AmpC β-lactamases in *Enterobacter* spp. After reaching log phase, the cells are harvested by centrifugation at 5000 × g for 15 minutes, still at 4°C. Cell pellets are washed with phosphate buffer saliv (PBS), 20 mmol/L at pH 7.0. The investigator should be aware of two caveats here: if the bacteria possess class B β-lactamases, a 50 mmol/L HEPES buffer, pH 7.2, is preferred; buffers containing chloride ions should be avoided when washing cells containing class D enzymes.

After cells have been pelleted and washed twice the buffer is chilled to 4°C and the β-lactamases are released. Numerous methods exist to aid the investigator in liberating β-lactamases into solution. These include sonication, a French pressurized cell, freeze-thawing, and EDTA-lysozyme treatment. Of all these methods, sonication and a French pressurized cell release most β-lactamases. Freeze-thawing and EDTA/lysozyme treatment, although they release less β-lactamases, yield extracts with less contaminating proteins. Details to assist the investigator have been summarized in previous editions of this textbook. In brief, the freeze-thaw cycle should be performed repeatedly, freezing to –20°C and thawing to room temperature, until the outer membrane ruptures. If the suspension becomes viscous, signifying DNA release, the cycle has been repeated excessively. Hence, the investigator may be forced to use DNAse. If the EDTA-lysozyme method is used, the suspension may be supplemented with 20% (w/v) sucrose, followed by Na_2EDTA and lysozyme to final concentrations of 50 mmol/L and 100 μg/mL, respectively. Sucrose is added to osmotically stabilize the cells. The suspension is maintained at 37°C, and samples are examined by microscopy until spheroplasts dominate the population. We have used a combination of EDTA-lysozyme and freeze-thaw to liberate sufficient quantities of SHV, OXA, and AmpC β-lactamase for investigative purposes. We harvest cells in the manner described, perform an overnight freeze, and liberate β-lactamases using lysozyme-EDTA the next morning (256).

Once satisfactory release of the enzymes has been obtained, residual material may be further removed by ultracentrifugation at 100,000 × g for 30 minutes at 4°C. The supernatant is then retained at –20°C or at 4°C. In some instances it will require performing experiments to determine optimal storage conditions. Standard protein purification methods such as ion exchange chromatography, preparative isoelectric focusing, gel filtration, and chromato-focusing are often employed to yield pure enzyme for analysis. Phenylboronic acid affinity chromotagraphy columns can be used to purify class A, class C, and class D β-lactamases (56). It should be noted that phenylboronic acid columns will not separate out mixtures of β-lactamases, as the serine β-lactamases will all bind to the boronic acid side chain.

Types of β-Lactamase Assays

Spectrophotometry and pH-stat titration are typically used to assay β-lactamase activity.

Spectrophotometric Assays

In the main, hydrolysis of β-lactams is accompanied by a reduction in UV absorption (170,363). The exceptions to this rule are the chromogenic cephalosporins. Hydrolysis rates are determined by adding a 10- to 100-μL aliquot of β-lactamase solution to a prewarmed β-lactam solution in phosphate buffer in a quartz cuvet (we use a 1-cm path length). The time course of absorbance is monitored with a spectrophotometer and compared with a simultaneous blank run. Although variations of this method exist, it is generally very reliable. Caution should be exercised in using buffers containing chloride ions for the evaluation of Class D enzymes. It is also sometimes necessary to assay class B β-lactamases in HEPES buffer. Table 10.6 lists the wavelengths for different β-lactams and the drug concentrations that should be used. Many investigators have determined specific extinction coefficients ($\Delta\epsilon$) for each β-lactam used.

To calculate the rate of reaction, v, a tangent is drawn to the first part of the reaction trace, and the rate of change in optical density (OD) per unit time per volume of enzyme is calculated. This value is converted to moles of substrate hydrolyzed per minute per volume of enzyme using the following equation:

$$V = \Delta OD/\text{unit time} \times N/\Delta OD_{\text{totol}}$$

Here, OD_{total} is the total change in absorbance if the reaction proceeds to completion, and N is the molar amount of β-lactam present. For any given combination of drug and light path, the ratio of N to OD is constant.

Automated pH-Stat Titration

Because hydrolysis of a β-lactam ring yields an acid, it is usually accompanied by a reduction of the pH, which can be monitored in a pH-stat titrator (157). Twenty milliliters of β-lactam substrate in 50 mmol/L KCl is introduced into a temperature-controlled cuvet under nitrogen gas. Enzyme is next added to hydrolyze 2 to 10 mmol/L of β-lactam per minute. The pH-stat titrator monitors the hydrogen-ion concentration and adds 40 mmol/L per liter of KOH at whatever rate is demanded to keep the pH constant. This rate equals the rate of hydrolysis. This assay is preferred for penicillins in lieu of cephalosporins. Occasionally, certain β-lactams will distort this pH determination because they have buffering capacity.

Calculation of β-Lactamase Kinetics

If a sufficiently high substrate concentration is used, the reaction velocity will approach $V_{\max}$. It is desirable to measure $V_{\max}$, as it can be used to determine the concentration of substrate that is required to achieve half the maximum velocity or the K_m. Accurate $V_{\max}$ and K_m values can be obtained by determining V for at least 10 different substrate concentrations and graphing S/V versus S. This depiction is a Hanes plot. The intercept of the x axis corresponds to $-K_m$ and the gradient is $1/V_{\max}$. It is also possible to derive $V_{\max}$ and K_m values from single-reaction progress curves (240). The treatment of such phenomena is beyond the scope of this chapter.

β-Lactamase Inhibition

Although the chemistry of β-lactamase inhibition is quite complex, the ability of certain compounds to inhibit β-lactamases can be easily measured (52,53). This can be done using an indicator substrate such as cephaloridine, penicillin, or nitrocefin. Incubating the inhibitor with the enzyme for a period of time before the indicator substrate is added will result in a reduction in substrate hydrolysis rate. In the preincubated system, an identical volume of enzyme is added to a mixture of inhibitor solution and buffer. After 5 minutes of incubation, an indicator substrate is added to the test solution. The decline in absorbance is monitored, and the percentage inhibition is calculated through comparison with the decline when the inhibitor solution is replaced with buffer. If the percentage inhibition values for the incubated and nonincubated solutions are equal, the inhibition is reversible. If the inhibition is greater after preincubation, the inhibition is irreversible. If the inhibition is reduced after preincubation, the inhibitor is a substrate.

Quantifying Inhibition

The most convenient measure of β-lactamase inhibitory power is the IC_{50}, defined as the concentration resulting in a 50% reduction in enzyme activity under specified conditions. Usually, IC_{50} values are obtained by performing

TABLE 10.6

Wavelengths of Different β-Lactam Drugs*

Substrate	Wavelength (nm)	MW
Cephaloridine	255	415
Cephalothin	262	396
Cefotaxime	255	455
Ceftriaxone	257	554
Cefoxitin	260	427
Ceftazidime	257	546
Benzylpenicillin	235	334
Ampicillin	240	349
Piperacillin	235	517
Carbenicillin	235	378
Oxacillin	263	401
Imipenem	297	299
Meropenem	297	399
Aztreonam	315	435
Nitrocefin	482	516

*The reader is referred to the 4th edition of this text for a more complete listing of wavelengths and MW of β-lactam compounds.

preincubation-type inhibition assays. Percent inhibition on the linear y-axis is plotted against inhibitor concentration on a logarithmic x-axis. A sigmoidal relationship is observed and the IC_{50} can be derived. IC_{50} values are most useful for comparing different inhibitors against the same enzyme. Another measure of β-lactamase inhibition is the determination of the disassociation constant of noncovalent inhibitor complex (K_i). It is not always appropriate for irreversible inhibitors but is useful as a measure of affinity.

Quantitation of β-Lactamase Activity

The amount of enzyme produced affects the degree of resistance expressed. Hence, it is often desirable to measure the amount of enzyme activity related to the amount of protein. Such measurements are necessary to quantify β-lactamase induction (200). In this measurement, 10 mL of cells are grown. β-Lactam antibiotics are added after 90 minutes and are best used at fractions or multiples of their MICs (e.g., 0.0625 × MIC, 0.25 × MIC, 1 × MIC, and 4 × MIC). At the end of the incubation period, cells are harvested by centrifugation, and β-lactamases are released in the manner described earlier. Activity is assayed using nitrocefin. The hydrolysis rates obtained are standardized against the protein concentration of the extracts. Specific activity is defined as β-lactamase activity per milligram of protein per volume.

Molecular Weight of β-Lactamases

The molecular weight of β-lactamases can be estimated by SDS-PAGE of purified proteins. Mass spectrometry cav offer a more accurate determination.

Other Miscellaneous Tests

Two variations of PCR have been applied to the typing of ceftazidime-resistant, ESBL-producing organisms: randomly amplified polymorphic DNA (RAPD), which is also known as arbitrarily primed PCR (AP-PCR), and PCR based on repetitive chromosomal sequences (rep-PCR) (255). Of these, RAPD (AP-PCR) has been by far the most popular method for evaluating the genetic relatedness of ESBL-producing strains. rep-PCR is extremely valuable and easy to perform (repetitive extragenic polindromic), but it has not been used as extensively as PFGE. The PAGE method is based on the observation that short primers (around 10 bp) whose sequence is not directed to any known genetic locus will regardless hybridize at random chromosomal sites with sufficient affinity to permit the initiation of polymerization. If two such sites are located within a few kilobases of each other on opposite DNA strands and in the proper orientation, then amplification of the intervening fragment will occur. The number and locations of these random sites (and therefore the number and sizes of the fragments) will vary among different strains of the same species (255).

Restriction site insertion PCR (RSI-PCR) is a recently developed technique to detect mutations of the SHV genes and so identify ESBLs. RSI-PCR uses amplification primers designed with one to three base mismatches near the 3′ end of the primer to engineer a desired restriction site. Chanawong et al. (58) demonstrated that the combination of PCR-restriction fragment length polymorphism (PCR-RFLP) and RSI-PCR techniques can be readily applied to the epidemiological study of SHV β-lactamases. Another useful tool for the detection of certain SHV variants is the combination of PCR–single-strand conformational polymorphism (PCR-SSCP) and PCR-RFLP (59). Through the use of PCR-SSCP and PCR-RFLP with DdeI and NheI digestion, the genes encoding SHV-1, SHV-2a, SHV-3, SHV-4, SHV-5, SHV-11, and SHV-12 were distinguishable (58).

Ligase chain reaction (LCR) is a recently developed technique also used to discriminate SHV variants. LCR uses a thermostable ligase and biotinylated LCR primers. It can detect single base pair changes (176).

A very promising method marries the sensitivity of PCR with fluorescent-labeled probes. Randeggar and Haechler developed a technique using real-time PCR monitored with fluorescently labeled hybridization probes, followed by melting curve analysis (272). Their technique was able to differentiate SHV variants and to discriminate between non-ESBLs and ESBLs. This technique, termed the *SHV melting curve mutation detection method*, promises to save investigators hours of time.

APPENDIX VII: BACTERIAL CELL WALL SYNTHESIS*

It is now well established that β-lactam antibiotics inhibit the synthesis of bacteria cell wall peptidoglycan (333,364,365). Peptidoglycan is a complex repeating unit of the amino acids and sugars that maintain the cell wall shape and structure and protect the bacterium against external osmotic changes (88,219). The ability of peptidoglycan to maintain cell wall architecture is dependent on a multipart network of interconnecting sugar chains (N-acetyl glucosamine and N-acetyl muramic acid) cross-linked by amino acids. In Gram-positive bacteria, peptidoglycan typically forms a thick layer external to the cytoplasmic membrane. This layer usually represents 50% of the bacterial cell dry weight. By contrast, in Gram-negative bacteria, peptidoglycan forms a relatively

**The following discussion summarizes material presented in the 4th edition of this text (Chapter 12). It is included here to serve as background for understanding PBP analysis.*

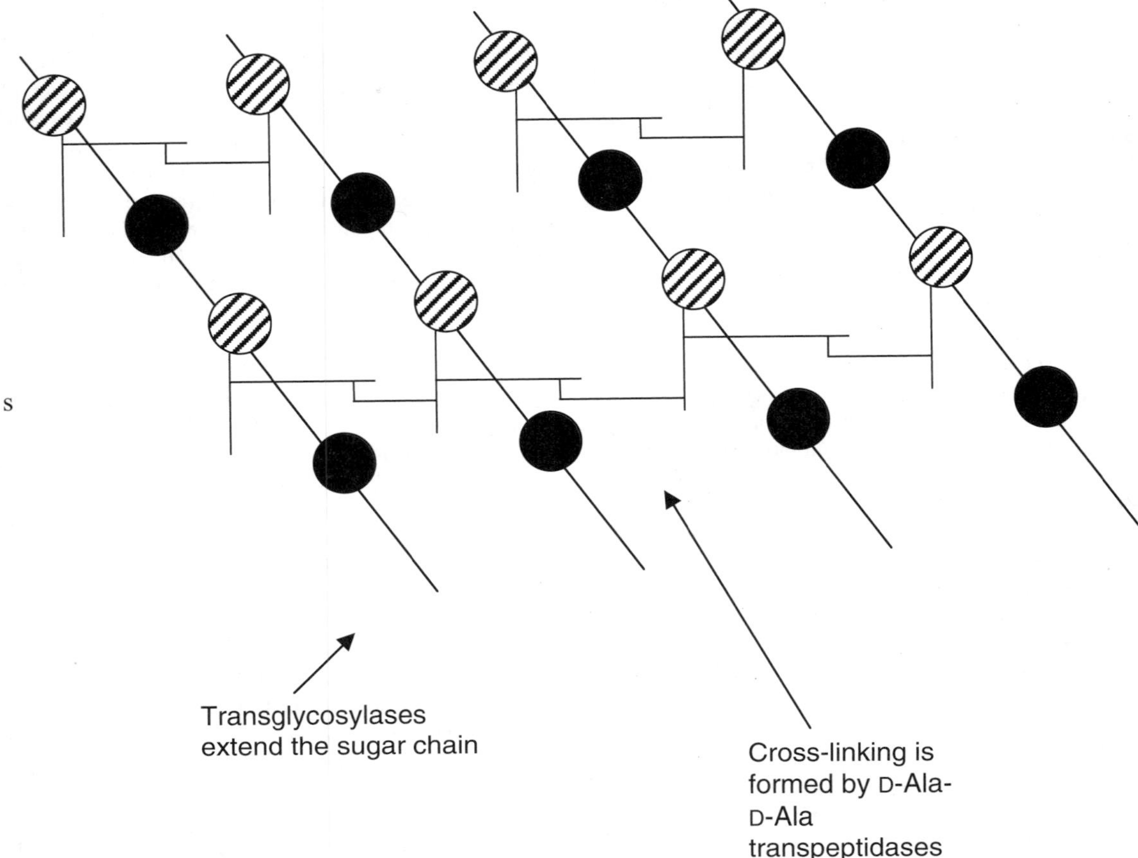

FIGURE 10.11 ● Illustration of interconnecting sugar chains (solid, *N*-acetylglucosamine; striped, *N*-acetylmuramic acid) with pentapeptides attached (vertical lines) and cross-linking of pentapeptide chains (horizontal staggered lines).

thin layer. Gram-negative peptidoglycan is generally positioned between the outer and inner cytoplasmic membranes.

The synthesis of peptidoglycan requires the coordination of a number of bacterial enzymes. The precursor molecule is uridine diphosphate (UDP) which is linked to the *N*-acetylmuramic (NAM) acid pentapeptide. The amino acid sequence of the pentapeptide that stems from *N*-acetylmuramic acid is unique to the particular species being studied. However, it is well recognized that the two terminal residues are D-alanine and the third residue is L-lysine or *m*-diaminopimelic acid. These precursors, which are produced in the cytoplasm of the cell, are transferred from UDP to an isoprenoid carrier located in the cytoplasmic membrane. An *N*-acetylglucosamine sugar (NAG) is next added to yield "disaccharide pentapeptide," which is transported across the membrane and inserted into the existing murein sacculus by transglycosylation (attachment of disaccharides) and transpeptidation (cross-linking of peptides in a plane perpendicular to the glycosidic chain) (Figs. 10.11 and 10.12). Transglycosylation extends sugar chains by attaching the muramyl residue of a new precursor to a free *N*-acetlglucosamine residue on the existing peptidoglycan. These two functions, transglycosylation and transpeptidation, often exist at separate sites of the same cell wall–synthesizing proteins. Most bacteria possess multiple peptidoglycan transglycosylation/transpeptidation proteins. As a rule, these complex enzymes contain a lipophilic anchor that attaches them to the cytoplasmic membrane and allows particular activities to be localized. In the main, these enzymes are referred to as penicillin-binding proteins (PBPs) (333, 364,365).

In addition to PBPs, autolysins or peptidoglycan hydrolases are also present in bacteria, and in much greater amounts (98,220,339,340) (Fig. 10.13). Autolysins degrade and remodel PBPs to provide sites for new peptidoglycan, but they may also assist in daughter cell cleavage, autolysis, and flagellar extrusion. Degraded peptidoglycan fragments are absorbed and recycled. The

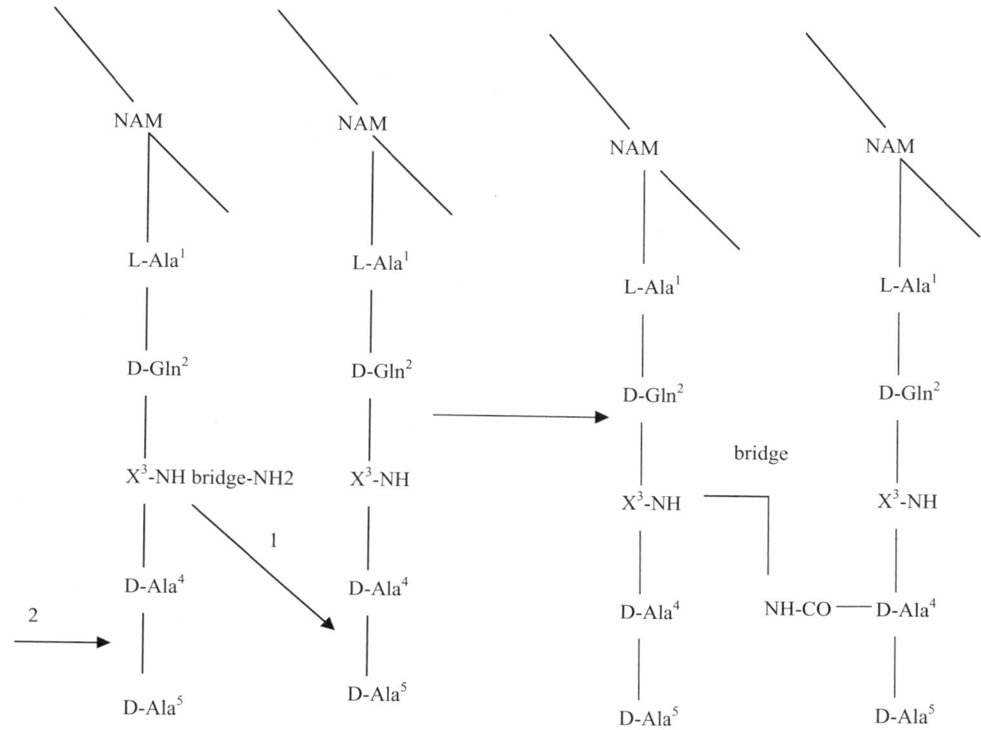

FIGURE 10.12 ● Detail illustration of the cross-linking process in cell wall synthesis. **1.** Action of D-Ala-D-Ala transpeptidases; **2.** action of D-Ala-D-Ala carboxypeptidases. The third amino acid of the peptide, X-NH2, has a bridge of additional amino acids. This free amino group is linked to the carboxy group of the penultimate D-Ala of the second side chain.

enzymes defined as autolysins include D,D-endopeptidases, *N*-acetylmuramyl-L-alanine amidase, lytic glycosylases, β-*N*-acetylglucosaminidases, and β-*N*-acetylmuramidases. Autolysins are strategically located on the bacterial cell inner membrane and hydrolyze the sugar backbone of peptidoglycan.

Mechanism of Action of β-Lactam Antibiotics

β-Lactam antibiotics inhibit D-alanyl-D-alanine transpeptidase activities by acylation, forming stable esters with the opened lactam ring attached to the hydroxyl group of the enzyme's active-site serine (333,339,364,365). These esters have hydrolysis half-lives of less than an hour, so inactivation is effectively permanent for the bacteria cell. In general, β-lactam antibiotics do not interfere with transglycosylation. The ability of β-lactams to inhibit the D-alanyl-D-alanine trans- and carboxypeptidases depends on conformational similarity between the amide bond of the β-lactam ring and the peptide link of D-alanyl-D-alanine. By inhibiting bacteria transpeptidases and cell wall synthesis, autolysins cause bacterial cells walls to degrade. In this fractured state, the cell walls cannot withstand osmotic forces. Evidence of this view comes from the occurrence of "tolerant" mutants, particularly Gram-positive cocci that are inhibited but not killed by β-lactam antibiotics. In this case, both cell wall synthetic enzymes and cell wall–degrading enzyme functions are repressed. β-Lactams may also "trigger" deregulation of autolysins, initiating lysis. It has been suggested that release of lipoteichoic acid is the trigger for lysis in pneumococci. Whether this is relevant to other species remains to be determined. The mutational loss of a cytoplasmic *N*-acetylmuramyl-L-alanine amidase autolysin is the cause of β-lactamase depression in *C. freundii*.

D-Alanyl-D-Alanine Trans- and Carboxypeptidases as PBPs

Virtually all Gram-negative bacteria have seven PBPs, designated, in order of descending molecular weight, 1a, 1b, 2, 3, 4, 5, and 6. Occasionally, two other PBPs, 7 and 8, are described. Exceptions include: *Neisseria* organisms have three PBPs, and *Haemophilus* and *Acinetobacter* have five to eight, numbered differently. The functions, as well as the patterns, of the PBPs of Gram-negative bacilli are better characterized than those of other bacteria, because of the relationship between

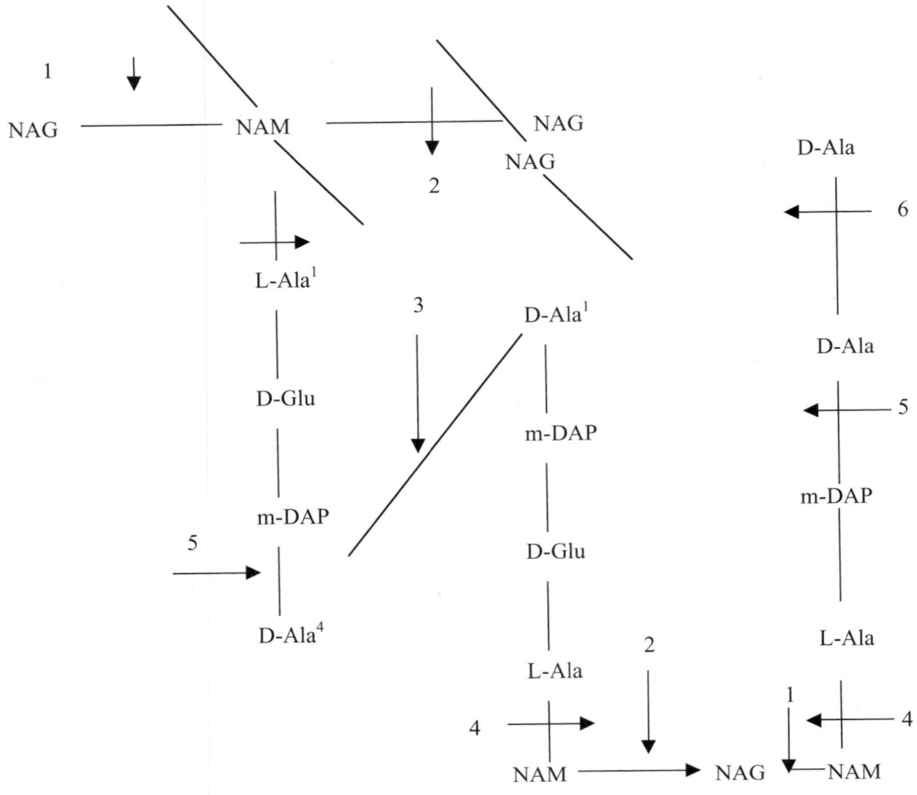

FIGURE 10.13 ● Action of autolysins. **1.** β-*N*-acetylglucosaminidase. **2.** Lytic transglycosylase and β-*N*-acetylmuraminidase (lysozyme). **3.** D, D, endopeptidase; **4.** *N*-acetylmuramyl-*L*-alanine amidase. **5.** L,D-carboxypeptidase. **6.** D,D-carboxypeptidase.

PBP function in β-lactam binding. Of the seven components present in Gram-negative bacilli, PBP1a and -1b are bifunctional D-alanyl-D-alanine transpeptidases/transglycosylases. These serve to insert new disaccharide pentapeptide units between existing peptidoglycan units. PBP2 functions as a bifunctional transglycosylase to extend the glycan chains between PBP1a and -1b. PBP3 is a multienzyme complex with proteins FtsA, FtsW, FtsQ, FtsZ, and FtsL as components. These components lay down monolayers of peptidoglycan as the first step in bacteria cell wall septation. Other PBPs, such as PBP4, -5, and -6, are nonessential.

In contrast, PBP1a, -1b, -2, and -3 of Gram-negative bacteria are absolutely essential for bacterial survival (referred to as *essential PBPs*). Inactivation of PBP-1a and -1b leads to the phenomenon of spheroplasting, which is rapidly followed by cell lysis and cell death. Inactivation of PBP3 results in bacteria growing as long nonseptate filaments, which are lysed only slowly.

It should be stressed that many β-lactam antibiotics bind to multiple PBPs and have different effects depending on their concentrations in the external periplasmic space of the bacteria. It is of interest that agents that preferentially bind to PBP3 (i.e., most penicillins and aminothiazolyl cephalosporins) allow a considerable increase in bacteria biomass before bacteriolysis becomes predominant. As the large number of filaments lyse, there is a massive release of endotoxin. In contrast, carbapenems that bind to PBP1a, -1b, and -2 do not carry this risk because they allow little increase in biomass before cell lysis (246).

Antibacterial Kinetics of β-Lactams

The relationship between PBP inhibition, autolysins, and bactericidal action has been discussed. Unless a particular PBP target is in place, the bactericidal rate of β-lactam–induced cell death is concentration-independent above the MIC (time-dependent killing), whereas that of aminoglycosides and quinolones, for example, increases with the concentration (i.e., is concentration-dependent). A curious phenomenon known as the *Eagle effect* is often observed with certain β-lactam antibiotics. In the Eagle effect, the bactericidal rate declines once the drug concentration is raised above a certain limit. Possible explanations for this effect are that (a) overall the inhibition of PBP activity at high concentrations is less favorable to bacteriolysis than at lower concentrations and (b) autolysins are triggered at low but not high β-lactam concentrations or are inhibited at high β-lactam concentrations.

The activities of β-lactam antibiotics strongly depend on the growth rate. Chemostat studies show that rapidly growing cells are killed more quickly than slowly growing cells (78). Many β-lactams demonstrate postantibiotic effects (PAEs) for Gram-positive bacteria, but PAEs for Gram-negative bacteria are seen only with carbapenem and penem antibiotics. It is often challenging to reproduce PAEs in animal models.

Resistance to β-Lactams

The classical mechanisms of resistance to β-lactams are (a) modification of normal PBP, (b) use of alternative peptidoglycan transpeptidases, (c) impermeability, and (d) production of β-lactamases (see previous section). Most recently, efflux has been suggested as an additional mechanism of resistance.

Among the pneumococci and other α-hemolytic streptococci, modification of bacterial PBPs is the sole cause of resistance to β-lactam antibiotics (97,330) (Fig. 10.14). This "intrinsic" resistance has been demonstrated in *Neisseria* spp and *H. influenzae*. This may be also true in certain *Acinetobacter* isolates, but its general importance is uncertain in this genus. The organisms in which PBP modification is of proven importance (i.e., α-hemolytic streptococci, *H. influenzae,* and *Neisseria* spp) are known to be transformable with naked DNA (see above). These species require fragments of PBP genes from other organisms with inherent or acquired β-lactam resistance to insert into their own PBP genes (330 and 330a). These "mosaic" genes result in PBPs that are β-lactam–resistant. The mosaic gene formation is best understood for *N. meningitides*. In *N. meningitidis,* penicillin nonsusceptible strains have alterations in only PBP2. In the *pbp2* gene, there are regions of normal meningococcal sequence interspersed with inserts of 14% to 23% divergence. These inserts closely resemble the *pbp2* gene of *Neisseria flavescens* and *Neisseria cinerea,* which are throat commensals that are inherently resistant to penicillin. Penicillin-resistant gonococci have mosaic *pbp-2* genes with inserts identical to those in resistant meningococci.

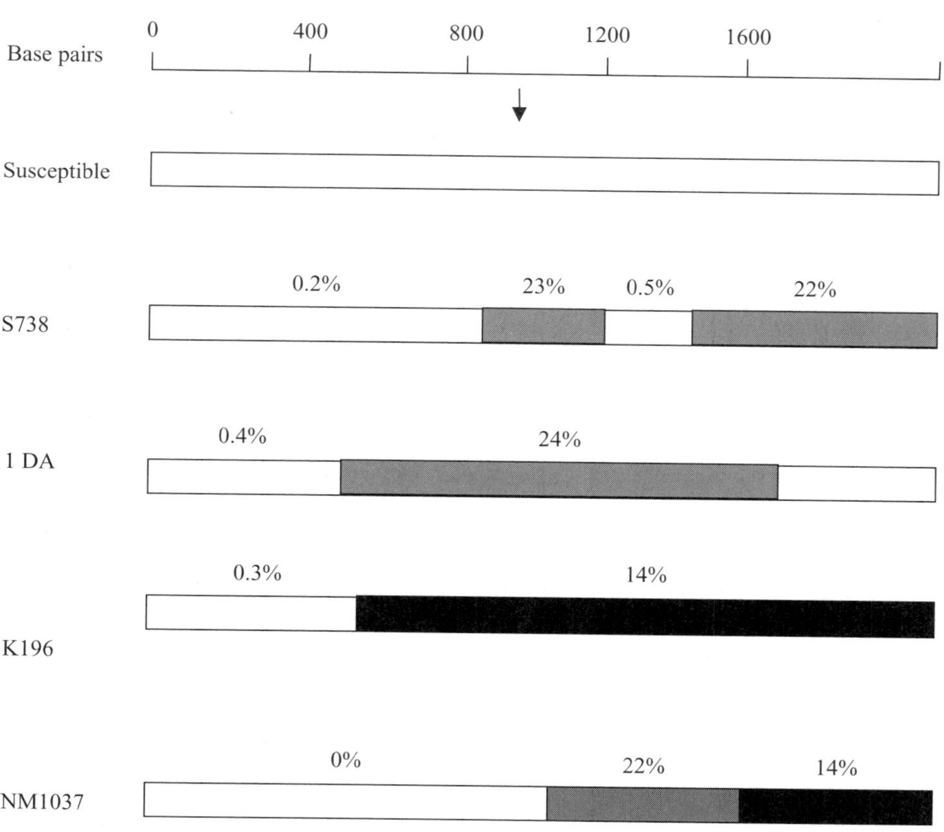

FIGURE 10.14 ● Mosaic genes for PBP2 in a susceptible *N. meningitidis* strain compared to four penicillin-resistant *N. meningitidis* strains. The clear boxes represent areas of normal sequence. The gray boxes are derived from *N. flavescens*. The black boxes are dervied from *N. cinerea*. The percentage designations indicate the degree of divergence from the normal sequence. The arrow shows the position of the active site Adopted from Spratt (330).

Mosaic gene formation has also been extensively studied in pneumococci. The recombination events between penicillin-resistant *Streptococcus pneumoniae* and *Streptococcus mitis* are implicated, but their direction is uncertain. In pneumococci, mosaic gene formation of PBP1a, -2x, -2a, and -2b is established. In contrast, mosaic gene formation has not yet been proven in *H. influenza* isolates.

Pneumococci with low-level penicillin resistance were first recorded in 1967, and pneumococci with high-level resistance were found approximately 10 years later. The number of resistant isolates has since increased, particularly in Spain and Hungary, where they account for to 50% to 60% of all penicillin-resistant pneumococci. The extent of penicillin resistance obviously varies with mosaic gene formation in each of these isolates. In gonococci, the modal benzylpenicillin MIC for β-lactamase nonproducers is now approximately 0.25 μg/mL, compared with 0.004 μg/mL when penicillin entered use.

From a therapeutic standpoint, extended-spectrum cephalosporins and meropenem often remain clinically active against pneumococci, hemophili, and pathogenic *Neisseria* species with altered PBPs; nevertheless, their MICs are higher than those of normal isolates. Unlike penicillin resistance, which requires the alterations of four PBPs, cephalsosporin resistance requires the alteration of only two PBPs.

Alternative Routes of Peptidoglycan Synthesis ("Bypass Resistance")

The most important mechanism of bypass resistance is demonstrated by methicillin-resistant staphylococci. Staphylococci normally have two essential PBPs: PBP2 and PBP3. Methicillin-resistant *S. aureus* (MRSA) organisms manufacture an additional transglycosylase/ transpeptidase, PBP-2′ (PBP-2a), encoded by the *mecA* gene (144). PBP2′ continues to function when PBP1, -2, and -3 have been inactivated. By itself, PBP2′ can yield a stable peptidoglycan, albeit with many fewer cross-links than in normal cells. The *mecA* gene is encoded by a chromosomal insert called the *mec* determinant, which originated outside staphylococci, perhaps via fusion of a β-lactamase gene and a PBP gene. The *mec* determinant is not readily self-transmissible but has spread within *S. aureus* and several coagulase-negative species, indicating that some horizontal transfer is possible.

Expression of *mecA* and, consequently, resistance vary among and within staphylococcal strains. Many strains show "heteroresistance" (303a). This heteroresistance reflects the genetic background of host staphylococci strains, not the gene of the mec determinant itself. Several chromosomal genes have been indicated in the control of *mecA*, including those in the *fem* cluster, particularly *femA*, as well as a recently described determinant, *chr**. Curiously, loss of β-lactamase from MRSA causes *mecA* to be homogeneously expressed. This suggests there is a linkage between the two resistance determinants. Expression of *mecA* and of resistance is induced by β-lactams and is also influenced by environmental conditions such as high osomolalty, low temperature, and neutral to alkaline pH. These conditions play a role in testing for methicillin and are best achieved with methicillin or oxacillin at 30°C on Mueller-Hinton or Iso-Sensitest agar supplemented with 5% to 7% NaCl.

It is known that β-lactams do not bind to PBP2′. Consequently, staphylococci resistant to oxacillin or methicillin are resistant to *all* β-lactam antibiotics. It should be emphasized that when staphylococci are not resistant to methicillin or oxacillin, treatment with β-lactamase–stable β-lactams, such as oxacillin, is to be preferred to vancomycin therapy. Use of these β-lactams minimizes the selection pressure contributing to the spread of glycopeptide resistance and ensures β-lactams achieve higher therapeutic concentrations than glycopeptides and result in greater bactericidal activity.

Special note should be made of PBP-5 of *E. faecium* and the novel occurrence of community-acquired MRSA (CA-MRSA). Bypass resistance is important in *E. faecium* though it is uncommon in *E. faecalis*. *E. faecium* has six PBPs, with PBP-3 serving as the main transpeptidase. This PBP3 is inhibited by penicillins and carbapenems but not by cephalosporins. At low temperature, or following significant mutation, *E. faecium* can switch to using PBP5 as the principal transpeptidase. PBP5 is universal in *E. faecium*, and its permanent expression requires only a regulatory mutation, not acquisition of foreign DNA. CA-MRSA strains differ from hospital-acquired MRSA strains in that they are generally susceptible to most antibiotics except β-lactams. These strains share the presence of staphylococcal cassette chromosome *mec* (*SCCmec*) type IV in their genomes, are frequently virulent, and predominantly cause skin and soft tissue infections. Many CA-MRSA strains are susceptible to clindamycin (305).

PBP Detection

Current methods to detect and analyze PBPs in bacterial cells are here summarized. In the past, radiolabeling penicillin has been the classic method to detect PBPs. But now it appears this approach is being replaced by colorimeteric or fluorometeric methods.

To prepare PBPs from Gram-negative bacteria, a starter culture is grown overnight with appropriate antibiotic selection. After shaking at 37°C for 18 hours, three 1-L volumes of cells are grown in 2-L conical flasks, and incubation is maintained until an optical density of 0.8–0.9 is achieved. At that point, the cells are harvested, centrifuged down to 5,000 × *g* at 4°C, and washed in 100 mL of cold 0.1 mol/L phosphate buffer or phosphate buffer saline, pH 7.0. This phosphate buffer should be supplemented with a minimal amount of β-mercaptoethanol, and resuspended in 20 mL. The cells are then sonicated or passed through a French press. Sonication includes three to five 30-second bursts, and the French press alternative includes subjection to a pressure of 12,000 lb/in^2.

Residual cells and debris are removed by centrifugation at 5,000 × *g* for 10 minutes at 4°C, after which the membranes are harvested by ultracentrifugation at 100,000 × *g* for 30 minutes at 4°C. They are then washed in 10 mmol/L phosphate buffer, pH 7.0, and resuspended in 8 to 10 mL of the same buffer. A sample of protein is withdrawn for Bradford or Lowry analysis (for determination of the protein concentration). It should be kept in mind that the addition of a small amount of β-mercaptoethanol (BME) or dithiothreitol (DTT) protects PBPs from oxidation inactivation. Protein preps containing Gram-negative membranes and PBPs should be stored at –70°C. When thawed for use, these aliquots are diluted with the same buffer to a protein concentration of 10 mg/mL.

To prepare PBPs from staphylococci and enterococci, a slightly different procedure is employed (125). Organisms are grown overnight, with shaking and at 37°C, in 100-mL amounts of a rich broth (BMI agar or a similar medium) and then diluted into 10 L of fresh rich broth. Next, the incubated cells are shaken until the OD reaches 0.8, after which the cells are harvested by centrifugation at 5,000 × *g* and 4°C for 10 minutes. The pellet is suspended and washed in 500 mL of 50 mmol/L phosphate buffer, pH 7.0, containing 0.01 mol/L $MgCl_2$ and 140 mmol/L β-mercaptoethanol, and is then resuspended in 60 mL of the same buffer. This suspension is divided into two 30-mL amounts, mixed with 25 mL of glass beads (0.1- to 0.11-mm diameter), and subjected to violent shaking for 5 minutes in a Mickle disintegrator (H. Mickle Laboratory Engineering Co., Gomshall, UK). Residual cells are removed by centrifugation. Subsequently, the membranes are pelleted at 100,000 × *g* for 30 minutes at 4°C, washed in 15 mL of 0.01 mol/L phosphate buffer, pH 7.0, resuspended in 5 mL of the same buffer, and stored as four 1.25-mL aliquots at –70°C. When thawed for use, these aliquots are diluted with the same buffer to a protein concentration of 10 mg/mL.

Radiolabeling Membranes to Detect PBPs

This method is appropriate for all β-lactamase nonproducers. If a β-lacatamase is present in the staphylococcus or enterococcus, it will destroy the labeled penicillin. Depending on the species and phenotype, this problem can be overcome by adding clavulanate or tazobactam to the membrane preparations before use. If this is done, competition assays with clavulanate or tazobactam as the test β-lactam should be undertaken for β-lacatamase nonproducers of the same species in order to determine the extent to which these inhibitors bind to the PBPs (as controls).

Direct Labeling

The process of direct labeling involves a doubling-dilution sequence of the labeled β-lactam. Generally a solution of β-lactam from 320 to 0.15 μg/mL is prepared in 10 mmol/L phosphate buffer, pH 7.0, and 10-μL amounts are distributed in 1.5-mL Eppendorf tubes, held in a water bath at 30°C. Aliquots of the membrane preparations are added, followed 10 minutes later by 10 μL of 120 mg/mL unlabeled aqueous benzylpenicillin. After an additional 5 minutes, 10 μL of 20% aqueous sodium lauroyl sarkosinate (sarkosyl) is added. So that precise reaction times are maintained, it is convenient to work along the row of tubes, at timed intervals, with each successive addition.

Competitive Labeling

This method overcomes the fact that, aside from benzylpenicillin, radiolabeled β-lactams rarely are available. A doubling-dilution sequence of unlabeled test β-lactam, generally from 320 to 0.15 μg/mL, is prepared in 10 mmol/L phosphate buffer, pH 7.0, and 10-μL amounts are distributed in 1.5-mL Eppendorf tubes, held in a water bath at 30°C. Aliquots (90 μL) of the membrane preparations are added, followed 10 minutes later by 10 μL of 120 mg/mL unlabeled aqueous benzylpenicillin. After an additional 5 minutes, 10 μL of 20% aqueous sarkosyl is added. So that the precise reaction times are maintained, it is convenient to work along the rows of tubes, at timed intervals, with each successive addition. In a competition assay, one takes advantage of the fact that only labeled benzylpenicillin is used. A doubling-dilution sequence of unlabeled test β-lactam, generally from 320 to 0.15 μg/mL, is prepared in 10 mmol/L phosphate buffer, pH 7.0, and 10-μL amounts are distributed in 1.5-mL Eppendorf tubes, held in a water bath at 30°C. Tubes with 10 μL of buffer are included as controls. Aliquots (90 μL) of the membrane preparations are added, followed 10 minutes later by 10 μL of a PBP-saturating concentration of C14 benzylpenicillin with the specified activity units. After an additional 10 minutes, 10 μL of 120 mg/mL unlabeled aqueous benzylpenicillin is added, and, finally, after 5 minutes, 10 μL of 20% aqueous sarkosyl is added.

To determine the saturating concentration of radioactive penicillin, it is first necessary to perform a direct assay, as described above. In general, 32 μg/mL of benzylpenicillin (1.05 mL of phosphate buffer, pH 7.0, added to a 50-μCi vial of benzylpenicillin to give a 350 μg/mL solution, which is further diluted 11–fold when added to the membranes) is sufficient to saturate the PBPs of Gram-negative bacilli, but higher concentration or longer incubation periods are needed for very low-affinity proteins such as PBP-2′ of methicillin-resistant staphylococci or PBP-5 of *E. faecium*.

After preparation as above, the sarkosyl-treated reaction mixtures are held for 20 minutes at room temperature to solubilize the PBPs and then are centrifuged for 30 minutes at 100,000 × *g* and 15°C (sarkosyl precipitates below 10°C). The supernatants are retained, and 75-μL amounts are mixed with 12.5-μL volumes of β-mercaptoethanol and 25 μL of the same buffer, which is prepared by mixing 2 mL of glycerol, 2 mL of 10% aqueous sodium dodecyl sulfate (SDS), 2.5 mL of 0.5 mol/L Tris-HCl, pH 6.8, and 100 μL of 0.5% (w/v) bromphenol blue. These mixtures are then heated to 100°C for 2 minutes.

Gels are prepared by running SDS-polyacrylamide gel standards for fluorography.

Currently rapid PBP assays are more in favor than using radiolabeled penicillin. However, faster PBP methods have been reported and are outlined below. These include the biotinylated and digoxigenin methods, which appear most promising (Weigel, 1994, #23; Lakaye, 1994, #8; Dargis, 1994, #1). Before these methods are used, it is important to perform validation studies by direct labeling to confirm that the agent binds to all PBPs and to determine the concentration needed for saturations. The time-honored biotinylated method of using β-lactams to measure PBPs is similar to the labeling methods. In this method, 4 mL of the *N*-hydroxysuccinimide ester of biotin (NHS-LC-biotin, Pierce Chemical, Rockford, IL) are added, in fivefold molar excess, to 3 mg/mL solution of a β-lactam with a free amino group (ampicillin or 6APA), dissolved in 0.1 mol/L phosphate buffer, pH 7.2 to 7.8, in a microfuge tube. The reaction is stopped by addition of Affi-Gel 102 (Bio-Rad), and an additional 30-minute incubation is allowed. The mixture is then centrifuged, and the supernatant, containing the biotinylated β-lactam, is retained. This method allows the preparation of a higher final concentration of biotinylated ampicillin. When prepared from a freshly acquired NHS-LC-biotin reagent, the biotinylated β-lactams provide high PBP-labeling specificity and can be kept in aliquots at –80°C for more than 6 months.

Digoxigenin-labeled ampicillin detects PBPs also. It can be prepared directly using ampicillin and a variety of buffers such as borate-buffered saline and 1 mg/mL of digoxigenin-*N*-hydroxysuccinimide ester.

Our laboratories favor the use of fluorescent PBP detection methods. Carboxyfluorescein is attached, via its free carboxyl group, to the free amino group of 6APA or to the α-amino group of ampicillin. The fluorescein-tagged penicillin, which is purified by HPLC, is than used as a competition agent in PBP assays, as described. Our laboratories have a preference for using Bocillin as the indicator penicillin (384).

REFERENCES

1. Adams V, Lyras D, Farrow KA, et al. The clostridial mobilisable transposons. *Cell Mol Life Sci* 2002;59:2033–2043.
2. Aendekerk S, Ghysels B, Cornelis P, et al. Characterization of a new efflux pump, MexGHI-OpmD, from *Pseudomonas aeruginosa* that confers resistance to vanadium. *Microbiol* 2002;148:2371–2381.
3. Aires JR, Kohler T, Nikaido H. Involvement of an active efflux system in the natural resistance of *Pseudomonas aeruginosa* to aminoglycosides. *Antimicrob Agents Chemother* 1999;43:2624–2628.

3a. Alvarez M, Tran JH, Chow N, Jacoby GA. Epidemiology of conjugative plasmid-mediated AmpC beta-lactamases in the United States. *Antimicrob Agents Chemother* 2004 Feb;48(2):533–537.

4. Ameyama S, Onodera S, Takahata M, et al. Mosaic-like structure of penicillin-binding protein 2 gene (penA) in clinical isolates of *Neisseria gonorrhoeae* with reduced susceptibility to cefixime. *Antimicrob Agents Chemother* 2002;46:3744–3749.
5. Arathoon EG, Hamilton JR, Hench CE, et al. Efficacy of short courses of oral novobiocin-rifampin in eradicating carrier state of methicillin-resistant *Staphylococcus aureus* and in vitro killing studies of clinical isolates. *Antimicrob Agents Chemother* 1990;34:1655–1659.
6. Archer GL, Niemeyer DM. Origin and evolution of DNA associated with resistance to methicillin in staphylococci. *Trends Microbiol* 1994;2:343–347.
7. Arlet G, Rouveau M, Casin I, et al. Molecular epidemiology of *Klebsiella pneumoniae* strains that produce SHV-4 β-lactamase and which were isolated in 14 French hospitals. *J Clin Microbiol* 1994;32:2553–2558.
8. Aronoff SC, Shlaes DM. Factors that influence the evolution of β-lactam resistance in β-lactamase–inducible strains of *Enterobacter cloacae* and *Pseudomonas aeruginosa*. *J Infect Dis* 1987;155:936–941.
9. Arthur M, Andremont A, Courvalin P. Distribution of erythromycin esterase and rRNA methylase genes in members of the family Enterobacteriaceae highly resistant to erythromycin. *Antimicrob Agents Chemother* 1987;31:404–409.
10. Arthur M, Depardieu F, Molinas C, et al. The *vanZ* gene of Tn*1546* from *Enterococcus faecium* BM4147 confers resistance to teicoplanin. *Gene* 1995;154:87–92.
11. Arthur M, Depardieu F, Snaith HA, et al. Contribution of VanY D,D-carboxypeptidase to glycopeptide resistance in *Enterococcus faecalis* by hydrolysis of peptidoglycan precursors. *Antimicrob Agents Chemother* 1994;38:1899–1903.
12. Arthur M, Molinas C, Depardieu F, et al. Characterization of Tn1546, a Tn3-related transposon conferring glycopeptide resistance by synthesis of depsipeptide peptidoglycan precursors in *Enterococcus faecium* BM4147. *J Bacteriol* 1993;175:117–127.
13. Arthur M, Molinas C, Dutka-Malen S, et al. Structural relationship between the vancomycin resistance protein VanH and 2-hydroxycarboxylic acid dehydrogenases. *Gene* 1991;103:133–134.
14. Arthur M, Quintiliani R Jr. Regulation of VanA- and VanB-type glycopeptide resistance in enterococci. *Antimicrob Agents Chemother* 2001;45:375–381.
15. Arthur M, Reynolds P, Courvalin P. Glycopeptide resistance in enterococci. *Trends Microbiol* 1996;4:401–407.
16. Bakken JS, Sanders CC, Thomson KS. Selective ceftazidime resistance in *Escherichia coli*: association with changes in outer membrane proteins. *J Infect Dis* 1987;155:1220–1225.
17. Balfour JA, Figgitt DP. Telithromycin. *Drugs* 2001;61:815–829.
18. Banerjee A, Dubnau E, Quemard A, et al. *inhA*, a gene encoding a target for isoniazid resistance in *Mycobacterium tuberculosis*. *Science* 1994;263:227–230.
19. Baptista M, Depardieu F, Reynolds P, et al. Mutations leading to increased levels of resistance to glycopeptide antibiotics in VanB-type enterococci. *Mol Microbiol* 1997;25:93–105.
20. Barnes DM, Whittier S, Gilligan PH, et al. Transmission of multidrug-resistant serotype 23F *Streptococcus pneumoniae* in group day care: evidence suggesting capsular transformation of the resistant strain in vivo. *J Infect Dis* 1995;171:890–896.
21. Bartlett JG, Chang TW, Gurwith M, et al. Antibiotic-associated pseudomembranous colitis due to toxin-producing clostridia. *N Engl J Med* 1978;298:531–534.
22. Beaber JW, Burrus V, Hochhut B, et al. Comparison of SXT and R391, two conjugative integrating elements: definition of a genetic backbone for the mobilization of resistance determinants. *Cell Mol Life Sci* 2002;59:2065–2070.

23. Bebrone C, Moali C, Mahy F, et al. CENTA as a chromogenic substrate for studying beta-lactamases. *Antimicrob Agents Chemother* 2001;45:1868–1871.
24. Bennett AD, Shaw WV. Resistance to fusidic acid in *Escherichia coli* mediated by the type I variant of chloramphenicol acetyltransferase. *Biochem J* 1983;215:29–38.
25. Bennett, PM. Integrons and gene cassettes: a genetic construction kit for bacteria. *J Antimicrob Chemother* 1999;43:1–4.
26. Bennett PM, Chopra I. Molecular basis of β-lactamase induction in bacteria. *Antimicrob Agents Chemother* 1993;37:153–158.
27. Berg CM, Berg DE, Groisman EA. Transposable elements and genetic engineering of bacteria. In: Berg DE, Howe MM, eds. *Mobile DNA*. Washington, DC: American Society for Microbiology, 1989;879–925.
28. Berg DE. Transposon Tn5. In: Berg DE, Howe MM, eds. *Mobile DNA*. Washington, DC: American Society for Microbiology, 1989:185–210.
29. Bergstrom S, Olsson O, Normark S. Common evolutionary origin of chromosomal beta-lactamase genes in enterobacteria. *J Bacteriol* 1982;150:528–534.
30. Billot-Klein D, Gutmann L, Sablé S, et al. Modification of peptidoglycan precursors is a common feature of the low-level vancomycin-resistant VANB-type Enterococcus D366 and of the naturally glycopeptide-resistant species *Lactobacillus casei, Pediococcus pentosaceus, Leuconostoc mesenteroides* and *Enterococcus gallinarum*. *J Bacteriol* 1994;176:2398–2405.
31. Birnboim HC. A rapid alkaline extraction method for the isolation of plasmid DNA. *Methods Enzymol* 1983;100:243–255.
32. Bissonnette L, Champetier S, Buisson JP. Characterization of the nonenzymatic chloramphenicol resistance (cmlA) gene of the In4 integron of Tn1696: similarity of the product to transmembrane transport proteins. *J Bacteriol* 1991;173:4493–4502.
33. Blanche F, Cameron B, Bernard FX, et al. Differential behaviors of *Staphylococcus aureus* and *Escherichia coli* type II DNA topoisomerases. *Antimicrob Agents Chemother* 1996;40:2714–2720.
34. Blumberg HM, Rimland D, Carroll DJ, et al. Rapid development of ciprofloxacin resistance in methicillin-susceptible and -resistant *Staphylococcus aureus*. *J Infect Dis* 1991;163:1279–1285.
35. Bolton LF, Kelley LC, Lee MD, et al. Detection of multidrug-resistant *Salmonella enterica* serotype Typhimurium DT104 based on a gene which confers cross-resistance to florfenicol and chloramphenicol. *J Clin Microbiol* 1999;37:1348–1351.
36. Bonfiglio G, Livermore DM. Beta-lactamase types amongst *Staphylococcus aureus* isolates in relation to susceptibility to beta-lactamase inhibitor combinations. *J Antimicrob Chemother* 1994;33:465–481.
37. Bonnet R. Growing group of extended-spectrum beta-lactamases: the CTX-M enzymes. *Antimicrob Agents Chemother* 2004;48:1–14.
38. Boyce JM, Mermel LA, Zervos MJ. Controlling vancomycin-resistant enterococci. *Infect Control Hosp Epidemiol* 1995;16:634–637.
39. Boyce JM, Opal SM, Chow JW, et al. Outbreak of multidrug-resistant *Enterococcus faecium* with transferable *vanB* class vancomycin resistance. *J Clin Microbiol* 1994;32:1148–1153.
40. Bradford PA. Extended-spectrum beta-lactamases in the 21st century: characterization, epidemiology, and detection of this important resistance threat. *Clin Microbiol Rev* 2001;14:933–951.
41. Bradford PA, Sanders CC. Development of a test panel of β-lactamases expressed in a common *Escherichia coli* host background for evaluation of new β-lactam antibiotics. *Antimicrob Agents Chemother* 1995;39:308–313.
42. Brannigan JA, Tirodimos IA, Zhang QY, et al. Insertion of an extra amino acid is the main cause of the low affinity of penicillin-binding protein 2 in penicillin-resistant strains of *Neisseria gonorrhoeae*. *Mol Microbiol* 1990;4:913–919.
43. Brantl S, Behnke D, Alonso JC. Molecular analysis of the replication region of conjugative *Streptococcus agalactiae* plasmid pIP501 in *Bacillus subtilis*: comparison with plasmids pAMβ1 and pSM19035. *Nucleic Acids Res* 1990;18:4783–4790.
44. Breeze AS, Obaseiki-Ebor EE. Nitrofuran reductase activity in nitrofurantoin-resistant strains of *Escherichia coli* K-12: some with chromosomally-determined resistance and others carrying R plasmids. *J Antimicrob Chemother* 1983;21:543–547.
45. Brenwald NP, Appelbaum P, Davies T, et al. Evidence for efflux pumps, other than PmrA, associated with fluoroquinolone resistance in *Streptococcus pneumoniae*. *Clin Microbiol Infect* 2003;9:140–143.
46. Brown GM. The biosynthesis of folic acid. II. Inhibition by sulfonamides. *J Biol Chem* 1962;237:536–540.
47. Bryson V, Szybalski W. Microbial selection. *Science* 1952;11:45–51.
48. Burdett V. Purification and characterization of TET(M), a protein that renders ribosomes resistant to tetracycline. *J Biol Chem* 1991;266:2872–2877.
49. Burns JL, Smith AL. A major outer membrane protein functions as a porin in *Haemophilus influenzae*. *J Gen Microbiol* 1987;133:1273–1277.
50. Burrus V, Pavlovic G, Decaris B, et al. Conjugative transposons: the tip of the iceberg. *Mol Microbiol* 2002;46:601–610.
51. Bush K. New beta-lactamases in Gram-negative bacteria: diversity and impact on the selection of antimicrobial therapy. *Clin Infect Dis* 2001;32:1085–1089.
52. Bush K, Sykes RB. Beta-lactamase inhibitors in perspective. *J Antimicrob Chemother* 1983;11:97–107.
53. Bush K, Sykes RB. Methodology for the study of beta-lactamases. *Antimicrob Agents Chemother* 1986;30:6–10.
54. Carias LL, Rudin SD, Donskey CJ, et al. Genetic linkage and cotransfer of a novel, *vanB*-containing transposon (Tn*5382*) and a low-affinity penicillin-binding protein 5 gene in a clinical vancomycin-resistant *Enterococcus faecium* isolate. *J Bacteriol* 1998;180:4426–4434.
55. Carter PE, Abadi FJR, Yakubu DE, et al. Molecular characterization of rifampin-resistant *Neisseria meningitidis*. *Antimicrob Agents Chemother* 1994;38:1256–1261.
56. Cartwright SJ, Waley SG. Purification of beta-lactamases by affinity chromatography on phenylboronic acid-agarose. *Biochem J* 1984;221:505–512.
57. Catlin BW. Iodometric detection of *Haemophilus influenzae* beta-lactamase: rapid presumptive test for ampicillin resistance. *Antimicrob Agents Chemother* 1975;7:265–270.
58. Chanawong A, M'Zali FH, Heritage J, et al. Characterisation of extended-spectrum beta-lactamases of the SHV family using a combination of PCR–single strand conformational polymorphism (PCR-SSCP) and PCR–restriction fragment length polymorphism (PCR-RFLP). *FEMS Microbiol Lett* 2000;184:85–89.
59. Chang S, Sievert DM, Hageman JC, et al. Infection with vancomycin-resistant *Staphylococcus aureus* containing the vanA resistance gene. *N Engl J Med* 2003;348:1342–1347.
60. Chen HY, Yuan M, Livermore DM. Mechanisms of resistance to beta-lactam antibiotics amongst *Pseudomonas aeruginosa* isolates collected in the UK in 1993. *J Med Microbiol* 1995;43:300–309.

61. Chirurgi VA, Oster SE, Goldberg AA, et al. Nosocomial acquisition of β-lactamase–negative, ampicillin-resistant enterococcus. *Arch Int Med* 1992;152:1457–1461.
62. Chomczynski P, Sacchi N. Single-step method of RNA isolation by acid guanidinium thiocyanate-phenol-chloroform extraction. *Anal Biochem* 1987;162:156–159.
63. Chopra I. Mechanism of resistance to fusidic acid in *Staphylococcus aureus*. *J Gen Microbiol* 1976;96:229–238.
64. Chopra I. Penetration of antibiotics to their target sites. *Antimicrob Agents Chemother* 1990;26:607–611.
65. Chopra I, Hawkey PM, Hinton M. Tetracyclines: molecular and clinical aspects. *J Antimicrob Chemother* 1992;29:245–277.
66. Chopra I, Roberts M. Tetracycline antibiotics: mode of action, applications, molecular biology, and epidemiology of bacterial resistance. *Microbiol Mol Biol Rev* 2001;65:232–260.
67. Chuanchuen R, Narasaki CT, Schweizer HP. The MexJK efflux pump of *Pseudomonas aeruginosa* requires OprM for antibiotic efflux but not for efflux of triclosan. *J Bacteriol* 2002;184:5036–5044.
68. Clark N, Jevitt L, Kellum M, et al. Presented at the 42nd Interscience Conference on Antimicrobial Agents and Chemotherapy; San Diego, CA; 2002.
69. Clewell DB. Plasmids, drug resistance and gene transfer in genus *Streptococcus*. *Microbiol Rev* 1981;45:409–436.
70. Clewell DB, Dunny GM. Conjugation and genetic exchange in enterococci. In: Gilmore MS, ed. *The enterococci: pathogenesis, molecular bioloigy and antibiotic resistance.* Washington, DC: ASM Press, 2002;265–300.
71. Coetzee JN, Datta N, Hedges RW. R factors from *Proteus rettgeri*. *J Gen Microbiol* 1972;72:543–552.
72. Coetzee JN, Datta N, Hedges RW. R factors from *Proteus rettgeri*. *J Gen Microbiol* 1972;72:543–552.
73. Cohen SP, Hachler H, Levy SB. Genetic and functional analysis of the multiple antibiotic resistance (*mar*) locus in *Escherichia coli*. *J Bacteriol* 1993;175:1484–1492.
74. Cole ST. *Mycobacterium tuberculosis*: drug-resistance mechanisms. *Trends Microbiol* 1994;2:411–415.
75. Collis CM, Grammaticopoulos G, Briton J, et al. Site-specific insertion of gene cassettes into integrons. *Mol Microbiol* 1993;9:41–52.
76. Collis CM, Hall RM. Expression of antibiotic resistance genes in the integrated cassettes of integrons. *Antimicrob Agents Chemother* 1995;39:155–162.
76a. Couture F, Lachapelle J, Levesque RC. Phylogeny of LCR-1 and OXA-5 with class A and class D beta-lactamases. *Mol Microbiol* 1992 Jun;6(12):1693–1705.
77. Couturier M, Bex F, Bergquist PL, et al. Identification and classification of bacterial plasmids. *Microbiol Rev* 1988;52:375–395.
78. Cozens RM, Tuomanen E, Tosch W, et al. *Evaluation of the bactericidal activity of beta-lactam antibiotics on slowly growing bacteria cultured in the chemostat. Antimicrob Agents Chemother* 1986;29:797–802.
79. Cui L, Ma X, Sato K, et al. Cell wall thickening is a common feature of vancomycin resistance in *Staphylococcus aureus*. *J Clin Microbiol* 2003;41:5–14.
80. Cui L, Murakami H, Kuwahara-Arai K, et al. Contribution of a thickened cell wall and its glutamine nonamidated component to the vancomycin resistance expressed by *Staphylococcus aureus* Mu50. *Antimicrob Agents Chemother* 2000;44:2276–2285.
81. Dabbs ER, Yazawa K, Mikami Y, et al. Ribosylation by mycobacterial strains as a new mechanism of rifampin resistance. *Antimicrob Agents Chemother* 1995;39:1007–1009.
82. Darini AL, Palepou MF, Woodford N. Effects of the movement of insertion sequences on the structure of VanA glycopeptide resistance elements in *Enterococcus faecium*. *Antimicrob Agents Chemother* 2000;44:1362–1364.
83. Daum RS, Ito T, Hiramatsu K, et al. A novel methicillin-resistance cassette in community-acquired methicillin-resistant *Staphylococcus aureus* isolates of diverse genetic backgrounds. *J Infect Dis* 2002;186:1344–1347.
84. Davies J. Aminoglycoside-aminocyclitol antibiotics and their modifying enzymes. In: Lorian V, ed. *Antibiotics in laboratory medicine,* 3rd ed. Baltimore: Williams & Wilkins, 1991.
85. Davies J. Another look at antibiotic resistance. *J Clin Microbiol* 1992;138:1553–1559.
86. Davies J. Inactivation of antibiotics and the dissemination of resistance genes. *Science* 1994;264:375–382.
87. Davis BD. Gene variation and transfer. In: Davis BD, Dulbecco R, Eisen HN, et al., eds. *Microbiology,* 4th ed. Philadelphia: JB Lippincott, 1990;123–142.
88. de Jonge BL, et al. Peptidoglycan composition in heterogeneous Tn551 mutants of a methicillin-resistant *Staphylococcus aureus* strain. *J Biol Chem* 1992;267:797–802.
89. de la Puente-Redondo VA, del Blanco NG, Gutierrez-Martin CB, et al. Comparison of different PCR approaches for typing of *Francisella tularensis* strains. *J Clin Microbiol* 2000;38:1016–1022.
90. De Lorenzo V, Herrero M, Jakubzik U, et al. Mini-Tn*5* transposon derivatives for insertion mutagenesis, promoter probing, and chromosomal insertion of cloned DNA in Gram-negative eubacteria. *J Bacteriol* 1990;172:6568–6572.
91. Dessen A, Quemard A, Blanchard A, et al. Crystal structure and function of isoniazid target of *Mycobacterium tuberculosis*. *Science* 1993;267:1638–1641.
92. Donskey CJ, Chowdhry TK, Hecker MT, et al. Effect of antibiotic therapy on the density of vancomycin-resistant enterococci in the stool of colonized patients. *N Engl J Med* 2000;343:1925–1932.
93. Donskey CJ, Hanrahan JA, Hutton RA, et al. Effect of parenteral antibiotic administration on persistence of vancomycin-resistant *Enterococcus faecium* in the mouse gastrointestinal tract. *J Infect Dis* 1999;180:384–390.
94. Douthwaite S, Hansen LH, Mauvais P. Macrolide-ketolide inhibition of MLS-resistant ribosomes is improved by alternative drug interaction with domain II of 23S rRNA. *Mol Microbiol* 2000;36:183–193.
95. Dowson CG, Coffey TJ, Spratt BG. Origin and molecular epidemiology of penicillin-binding–protein-mediated resistance to β-lactam antibiotics. *Trends Microbiol* 1994;2:361–366.
96. Dowson CG, Hutchison A, Brannigan JA, et al. Horizontal transfer of penicillin-binding protein genes in penicillin-resistant clinical isolates of *Streptococcus pneumoniae. Proc Natl Acad Sci USA* 1989;86:8842–8846.
97. Dowson CG, Hutchison A, Woodford N, et al. Penicillin-resistant viridans streptococci have obtained altered penicillin-binding protein genes from penicillin-resistant strains of *Streptococcus pneumoniae. Proc Natl Acad Sci USA* 1990;87:5858–5862.
98. Doyle RJ, Chaloupka J, Vinter V. Turnover of cell walls in microorganisms. *Microbiol Rev* 1988;52:554–567.
99. Dubois V, Arpin C, Melon M, et al. Nosocomial outbreak due to a multiresistant strain of *Pseudomonas aeruginosa* P12: efficacy of cefepime-amikacin therapy and analysis of beta-lactam resistance. *J Clin Microbiol* 2001;39:2072–2078.
100. Dulbecco R. Lysogeny and transducing bacteriophages. In: Davis BD, Dulbecco R, Eisen HN, et al., eds. *Microbiology,* 4th ed. Philadelphia: JB Lippincott, 1990;817–832.
101. Duma RJ, Kinz LJ. Simple test for identifying penicillinase-producing staphylococci. *Appl Microbiol* 1968;16:1261–1262.
102. Dunny GM. Electroporation of enterococci, streptococci

and bacilli. In: Dunny GM, Patrick P, Cleary LL, eds. *Genetics and molecular biology of streptococci, lactococci and enterococci.* Washington, DC: American Society for Microbiology, 1991;302.

103. Dunny GM, Leonard BA. Cell-cell communication in Gram-positive bacteria. *Annu Rev Microbiol* 1997;51:527–564.
104. Eady EA, Ross JI, Cove JH. Multiple mechanisms of erythromycin resistance. *J Antimicrob Chemother* 1990;26:461–471.
105. Edwards DI. Nitroimidazole drugs: action and resistance mechanisms. I. Mechanisms of action. *J Antimicrob Chemother* 1993;31:9–20.
106. Edwards DI. Nitroimidazole drugs: action and resistance mechanisms. II. Mechanisms of resistance. *J Antimicrob Chemother* 1993;31:201–210.
107. Ehrenfeld EE, Clewell DB. Transfer functions of the *Streptococcus faecalis* plasmid pAD1: organization of plasmid DNA encoding response to sex pheromone. *J Bacteriol* 1987;169:3473–3481.
108. Eickhoff TC, Finland M. Polymixin B and colistin in vitro activity against *Pseudomonas aeruginosa. Am J Med Sci* 1965;249:172–174.
109. Eliopoulos GM, Farber BF, Murray BE, et al. Ribosomal resistance of clinical enterococcal isolates to streptomycin. *Antimicrob Agents Chemother* 1984;25:398–399.
110. Evers S, Courvalin R. Regulation of VanB-type vancomycin resistance gene expression by the vanSB-VanRB two component regulatory system in *Enterococcus faecalis* V583. *J Bacteriol* 1996;178:1302–1309.
111. Faruki H, Kohmescher RN, McKinney WP, et al. A community-based outbreak of infection with penicillin-resistant *Neisseria gonorrhoeae* not producing penicillinase (chromosomally-mediated resistance). *N Engl J Med* 1985;313:607–611.
112. Fernandez-Rodriguez A, Canton R, Perez-Diaz JC, et al. Aminoglycoside-modifying enzymes in clinical isolates harboring extended-spectrum β-lactamases. *Antimicrob Agents Chemother* 1992;36:2536–2538.
113. Ferretti JJ, Gilmore KS, Courvalin P. Nucleotide sequence of the gene specifying the bifunctional 6′-aminoglycoside acetyltransferase-2″ aminoglycoside phosphotransferase enzyme in *Streptococcus faecalis* and identification and cloning of the gene regions specifying the two activities. *J Bacteriol* 1986;167:631–638.
114. Fey PD, Said-Salim B, Rupp ME, et al. Comparative molecular analysis of community- or hospital-acquired methicillin-resistant *Staphylococcus aureus. Antimicrob Agents Chemother* 2003;47:196–203.
115. Fitzgerald JR, Sturdevant DE, Mackie SM, et al. Evolutionary genomics of *Staphylococcus aureus*: insights into the origin of methicillin-resistant strains and the toxic shock syndrome epidemic. *Proc Natl Acad Sci USA* 2001;98:8821–8826.
116. Flannagan SE, Chow JW, Donabedian SM, et al. Plasmid content of a vancomycin-resistant *Enterococcus faecalis* isolate from a patient also colonized by *Staphylococcus aureus* with a VanA phenotype. *Antimicrob Agents Chemother* 2003;47:3954–3959.
117. Flannagan SE, Zitzow LA, Su YA, et al. Nucleotide sequence of the 18-kb conjugative transposon Tn*916* from *Enterococcus faecalis. Plasmid* 1994;32:350–354.
118. Fraimow HS, Junkind DL, Lander DW. Urinary tract infection with an *Enterococcus faecalis* isolate that requires vancomycin for growth. *Ann Int Med* 1994;121:22–26.
119. Galas DJ, Chandler M. Bacterial insertion sequences. In: Berg DE, Howe MM, eds. *Mobile DNA.* Washington, DC: American Society for Microbiology, 1989;109–162.

119b. Galleni M, Lamotte Brasseur J, Rossolini GM, Spencer J, Dideberg O, Frere JM; Metallo-beta-lactamases Working Group. Standard numbering scheme for class B beta-lactamases. *Antimicrob Agents Chemother* 2001 Mar;45(3):660–663.

119c. Garau G, Garcia-Saez I, Bebrone C, Anne C, Mercuri P, Galleni M, Frere JM, Dideberg O. Update of the standard numbering scheme for class B beta-lactamases. *Antimicrob Agents Chemother* 2004 Jul;48(7):2347–2349.

120. Gill MJ, Simjee S, Al-Hattawi K, et al. Gonococcal resistance to beta-lactams and tetracycline involves mutation in loop 3 of the porin encoded at the penB locus. *Antimicrob Agents Chemother* 1998;42:2799–2803.

120a. Girlich D, Naas T, Nordmann P. OXA-60, a chromosomal, inducible, and imipenem-hydrolyzing class D beta-lactamase from Ralstonia pickettii. *Antimicrob Agents Chemother* 2004 Nov;48(11):4217–4225.

121. Gold HS. Vancomycin-resistant enterococci: mechanisms and clinical observations. *Clin Infect Dis* 2001;33:210–219.
122. Gonzales RD, Schreckenberger PC, Graham MB, et al. Infections due to vancomycin-resistant *Enterococcus faecium* resistant to linezolid. *Lancet* 2001;357:1179.
123. Gordon DM. Rate of plasmid transfer among *Escherichia coli* strains isolated from natural populations. *J Gen Microbiol* 1992;138:17–21.
124. Gouby A, Neuwirth C, Bourg G, et al. Epidemiologic study by pulsed-field gel electrophoresis of an outbreak of extended-spectrum β-lactamase-producing *Klebsiella pneumoniae* in a geriatric hospital. *J Clin Microbiol* 1994;32:301–305.
125. Granier B, et al. Serine-type D-Ala-D-Ala peptidases and penicillin-binding proteins. *Methods Enzymol* 1994;244:249–266.
126. Grebe T, Hakenbeck R. Penicillin-binding proteins 2b and 2x of *Streptococcus pneumoniae* are primary resistance determinants for different classes of β-lactam antibiotics. *Antimicrob Agents Chemother* 1996;40:829–834.
127. Green M, Shlaes JH, Barbadora K, et al. Bacteremia due to vancomycin-dependent *Enterococcus faecium. Clin Infect Dis* 1995;20:712–714.
128. Grohmann E, Muth G, Espinosa M. Conjugative plasmid transfer in Gram-positive bacteria. *Microbiol Mol Biol Rev* 2003;67:277–301.
129. Gutmann L, Chabbert TA. Different mechanisms of resistance to latamoxef (moxalactam) in *Serratia marcescens. J Antimicrob Chemother* 1984;13:15–22.
130. Gutmann L, Williamson R, Moreau N, et al. Cross-resistance to nalidixic acid, trimethoprim, and chloramphenicol associated with alterations in outer membrane proteins of *Klebsiella, Enterobacter* and *Serratia. J Infect Dis* 1985;151:501–507.
131. Haggoud A, M'Hand RA, Reysset G, et al. Prevalence and characteristics of nim genes encoding 5-nitroimidazole resistance among Bacteroides strains isolated in Morocco. *Microb Drug Resist* 2001;7:177–181.
132. Haggoud A, Reysset G, Azeddoug H, et al. Nucleotide sequence analysis of two nitroimidazole resistance determinants from *Bacteroides* strains and of a new insertion sequence upstream of the gene. *Antimicrob Agents Chemother* 1994;38:1047–1051.
133. Hagman KE, Pan W, Spratt BG, et al. Resistance of *Neisseria gonorrhoeae* to antimicrobial hydrophobic agents is modulated by the mtrRCDE efflux system. *Microbiology* 1995;141[Pt 3]:611–622.
134. Hall RM. Mobile gene cassettes and integrons: moving antibiotic resistance genes in Gram-negative bacteria. *Ciba Found Symp* 1995;207:192–202.
135. Hall RM, Brookes DE, Stokes HW. Site-specific insertion of genes into integrons: role of the 59-base element and determination of the recombination crossover point. *Mol Microbiol* 1991;5:1941–1959.

136. Hall RM, Collis CM. Mobile gene cassettes and integrons: capture and spread of genes by site-specific recombination. *Mol Microbiol* 1995;15:593–600.
137. Hamer L, DeZwaan TM, Montenegro-Chamorro MV, et al. Recent advances in large-scale transposon mutagenesis. *Curr Opin Chem Biol* 2001;5:67–73.
138. Hanahan D. Studies on transformation of *Escherichia coli* with plasmids. *J Mol Biol* 1983;166:577–580.
139. Hancock R, Bellido F. Antibiotic uptake: unusual results for unusual molecules. *J Antimicrob Chemother* 1992;29:235–243.
140. Handwerger S. Alterations in peptidoglycan precursors and vancomycin susceptibility in Tn*917* insertion mutants of *Enterococcus faecalis* 221. *Antimicrob Agents Chemother* 1994;38:473–475.
141. Handwerger S, Pucci MJ, Volk KJ, et al. The cytoplasmic peptidoglycan precursor of vancomycin-resistant *Enterococcus faecalis* terminates in lactate. *J Bacteriol* 1991;174:5982–5984.
142. Hanrahan J, Hoyen C, Rice LB. Geographic distribution of a large mobile element that transfers ampicillin and vancomycin resistance between *Enterococcus faecium* strains. *Antimicrob Agents Chemother* 2000;44:1349–1351.
143. Hansen JB, Olsen RH. Isolation of large bacterial plasmids and characterization of the P2 incompatibility group plasmids pMG1 and pMG5. *J Bacteriol* 1978;135:227–238.
144. Hartman BJ, Tomasz A. Low-affinity penicillin-binding protein associated with beta-lactam resistance in *Staphylococcus aureus*. *J Bacteriol* 1984;158:513–516.
145. Hayden MK, Trenholm GM, Schultz JE, et al. In vivo development of teicoplanin resistance in a VanB *Enterococcus faecium* isolate. *J Infect Dis* 1993;167:1224–1227.
146. Heisig P, Schedletzky H, Falkenstein-Paul H. Mutations in the *gyrA* gene of a highly fluoroquinolone resistant clinical isolate of *Escherichia coli*. *Antimicrob Agents Chemother* 1993;37:696–701.
147. Heisig P, Tschorny R. Characterization of fluoroquinolone resistant mutants of *Escherichia coli* selected in vitro. *Antimicrob Agents Chemother* 1994;38:1284–1291.
148. Helfand MS, Bonomo RA. Beta-lactamases: a survey of protein diversity. *Curr Drug Targets Infect Disord* 2003;3:9–23.
149. Herrero IA, Issa NC, Patel R. Nosocomial spread of linezolid-resistant, vancomycin-resistant *Enterococcus faecium*. *N Engl J Med* 2002;346:867–869.
150. Hershberger E, Donabedian S, Konstantinou K, et al. Quinupristin-dalfopristin resistance in Gram-positive bacteria: mechanism of resistance and epidemiology. *Clin Infect Dis* 2004;38:92–98.
151. Hirt H, Erlandsen SL, Dunny GM. Heterologous inducible expression of Enterococcus faecalis pCF10 aggregation substance asc10 in *Lactococcus lactis* and *Streptococcus gordonii* contributes to cell hydrophobicity and adhesion to fibrin. *J Bacteriol* 2000;182:2299–306.
152. Hochhut B, Lotfi Y, Mazel D, et al. Molecular analysis of antibiotic resistance gene clusters in *Vibrio cholerae* 0139 and 01 SXT constins. *Antimicrob Agents Chemother* 2001;45:2991–3000.
153. Hodgson JE, Curnock SP, Dyke KGH, et al. Molecular characterization of the gene encoding high-level mupirocin resistance in *Staphylococcus aureus* J2870. *Antimicrob Agents Chemother* 1994;38:1205–1208.
154. Hoeprich PD. The polymixins. *Med Clin North Am* 1970;54:1251–1265.
155. Honore N, Cole ST. Molecular basis of rifampin resistance in *Mycobacterium leprae*. *Antimicrob Agents Chemother* 1993;37:414–418.
156. Hooper DC. Emerging mechanisms of fluoroquinolone resistance. *Emerg Infect Dis* 2001;7:337–341.
157. Hou JP, Poole JW. Measurement of beta-lactamase activity and rate of inactivation of penicillins by a pH-stat alkalimetric titration method. *J Pharm Sci* 1972;61:1594–1598.
158. Hughes J, Mellows G. On the mode of action of pseudomonic acid: inhibition of protein synthesis in *Staphylococcus aureus*. *Biochem J* 1978;176:305–318.
159. Huovinen P. Resistance to trimethoprim-sulfamethoxazole. *Clin Infect Dis* 2001;32:1608–14.
160. Huovinen P. Trimethoprim resistance. *Antimicrob Agents Chemother* 1987;31:1451–1456.
161. Huovinen P, Sundstrom L, Swedberg G, et al. Trimethoprim and sulfonamide resistance. *Antimicrob Agents Chemother* 1995;39:279–289.
162. Ike Y, Clewell DB. Genetic analysis of the pAD1 pheromone response in *Streptococcus faecalis*, using transposon Tn*917* as an insertional mutagen. *J Bacteriol* 1984;158:777–783.
163. Ike Y, Craig RA, White BA, et al. Modification of *Streptococcus faecalis* sex pheromones after acquisition of plasmid DNA. *Proc Natl Acad Sci USA* 1983;80:5369–5373.
164. Ike Y, Flannagan SE, Clewell DB. Hyperhemolytic phenomena associated with insertions of Tn*916* into the hemolysin determinant of *Enterococcus faecalis* plasmid pAD1. *J Bacteriol* 1992;174:1801–1809.
165. Ince D, Hooper DC. Quinolone resistance due to reduced target enzyme expression. *J Bacteriol* 2003;185:6883–6892.
166. Ito T, Katayama Y, Asada K, et al. Structural comparison of three types of staphylococcal cassette chromosome mec integrated in the chromosome in methicillin-resistant *Staphylococcus aureus*. *Antimicrob Agents Chemother* 2001;45:1323–1336.
167. Jacob AE, Hobbs SJ. Conjugal transfer of plasmid-borne multiple antibiotic resistance in *Streptococcus faecalis* var. *zymogenes*. *J Bacteriol* 1974;117:360–372.
168. Jacobs C, Joris B, Jamin M, et al. AmpD, essential for both β-lactamase regulation and cell wall recycling, is a novel cytosolic *N*-acetylmuramyl-L-alanine amidase. *Mol Microbiol* 1995;15:553–559.
169. Jacoby GA, Medeiros AA. More extended-spectrum β-lactamases. *Antimicrob Agents Chemother* 1991;35:1697–1704.
170. Jansson JA. A direct spectrophotometric assay for penicillin beta-lactamase (penicillinase). *Biochim Biophys Acta* 1965;99:171–172.
171. Jarlier V, Nicolas M-H, Fournier G, et al. Extended broad-spectrum β-lactamases conferring transferable resistance to newer β-lactam agents in Enterobacteriaceae: hospital prevalence and susceptibility patterns. *Rev Infect Dis* 1988;10:867–878.
172. Jin DJ, Gross CA. Mapping and sequencing of mutations in the *Escherichia coli rpoB* gene that leads to rifampicin resistance. *J Mol Biol* 1988;202:45–58.
173. Judson N, Mekalanos JJ. Transposon-based approaches to identify essential bacterial genes. *Trends Microbiol* 2000;8:521–526.
173a. Karabinis A, Paramythiotou E, Mylona Petropoulou D, Kalogeromitros A, Katsarelis N, Kontopidou F, Poularas I, Malamou Lada H. Colistin for Klebsiella pneumoniae-associated sepsis. *Clin Infect Dis* 2004 Jan 1;38(1):e7–9. Epub 2003 Dec 04.
174. Karanfil LV, Murphy M, Josephson A, et al. A cluster of vancomycin-resistant *Enterococcus faecium* in an intensive care unit. *Infect Control Hosp Epidemiol* 1992;13:195–200.
175. Kawalec M, Gniadkowski M, Hryniewicz W. Outbreak of

vancomycin-resistant enterococci in a hospital in Gdansk, Poland, due to horizontal transfer of different Tn1546-like transposon variants and clonal spread of several strains. *J Clin Microbiol* 2000;38:3317–3322.

176. Kim J, Lee HJ. Rapid discriminatory detection of genes coding for SHV beta-lactamases by ligase chain reaction. *Antimicrob Agents Chemother* 2000;44:1860–1864.
177. Klare I, Badstubner D, Konstabel C, et al. Decreased incidence of VanA-type vancomycin-resistant enterococci isolated from poultry meat and from fecal samples of humans in the community after discontinuation of avoparcin usage in animal husbandry. *Microb Drug Res* 1999;5:45–51.
178. Klare I, Heier H, Claus H, et al. *vanA*-mediated high-level glycopeptide resistance in *Enterococcus faecium* from animal husbandry. *FEMS Microbiol Lett* 1995;125:165–172.
179. Kleckner N. Transposon Tn*10*. In: Berg DE, Howe MM, eds. *Mobile DNA*. Washington, DC: American Society for Microbiology, 1989:227–268.
180. Ko WC, Paterson DL, Sagnimeni AJ, et al. Community-acquired *Klebsiella pneumoniae* bacteremia: global differences in clinical patterns. *Emerg Infect Dis* 2002;8:160–166.
181. Kollef MH, Fraser VJ. Antibiotic resistance in the intensive care unit. *Ann Intern Med* 2001;134:298–314.
182. Kreiswirth B, Kornblum J, Arbeit RD, et al. Evidence for a clonal origin of methicillin resistance in *Staphylococcus aureus*. *Science* 1993;259:227–230.
183. Kwon DH, Dore MP, Kim JJ, et al. High-level beta-lactam resistance associated with acquired multidrug resistance in *Helicobacter pylori*. *Antimicrob Agents Chemother* 2003;47:2169–2178.
184. Landman D, Mobarakai NV, Quale JM. Novel antibiotic regimens against *Enterococcus faecium* resistant to ampicillin, vancomycin and gentamicin. *Antimicrob Agents Chemother* 1993;37:1904–1908.
185. Landman D, Quale JM, Mayorga D, et al. Citywide clonal outbreak of multiresistant *Acinetobacter baumannii* and *Pseudomonas aeruginosa* in Brooklyn, NY: the preantibiotic era has returned. *Arch Intern Med* 2002;162:1515–1520.
186. Laurberg M, Kristensen O, Martemyanov K, et al. Structure of a mutant EF-G reveals domain III and possibly the fusidic acid binding site. *J Mol Biol* 2000;303:593–603.
187. Lawley TD, Klimke WA, Gubbins MJ, et al. F factor conjugation is a true type IV secretion system. *FEMS Microbiol Lett* 2003;224:1–15.
188. LeBlanc DL, Lee LN. Rapid screening procedure for the detection of plasmids in streptococci. *J Bacteriol* 1979;140:1112–1115.
189. Leclercq R. Mechanisms of resistance to macrolides and lincosamides: nature of the resistance elements and their clinical implications. *Clin Infect Dis* 2002;34:482–492.
190. Leclerq R, Carlier C, Duval J, et al. Plasmid-mediated resistance to lincomycin by inactivation in *Staphylococcus haemolyticus*. *Antimicrob Agents Chemother* 1985;28:421–424.
191. Leclerq R, Courvalin P. Bacterial resistance to macrolide, lincosamide, and streptogramin antibiotics by target modification. *Antimicrob Agents Chemother* 1991;35:1267–1272.
192. Leclerq R, Courvalin P. Intrinsic and unusual resistance to macrolide, lincosamide and streptogramin antibiotics in bacteria. *Antimicrob Agents Chemother* 1991;35:1273–1276.
193. Leclerq R, Dutka-Malen S, Brisson-Noel A, et al. Resistance of enterococci to aminoglycosides and glycopeptides. *Clin Infect Dis* 1992;15:495–501.
194. Leonard BA, Podbielski A, Hedberg PJ, et al. *Enterococcus faecalis* pheromone binding protein, PrgZ, recruits a chromosomal oligopeptide permease system to import sex pheromone cCF10 for induction of conjugation. *Proc Natl Acad Sci USA* 1996;93:260–264.
195. Lety MA, Nair S, Berche P, et al. A single point mutation in the embB gene is responsible for resistance to ethambutol in *Mycobacterium smegmatis*. *Antimicrob Agents Chemother* 1997;41:2629–2633.
196. Levy S. Active efflux mechanisms for antimicrobial resistance. *Antimicrob Agents Chemother* 1992;36:695–703.
197. Levy SB, McMurry LM, Barbosa TM, et al. Nomenclature for new tetracycline resistance determinants. *Antimicrob Agents Chemother* 1999;43:1523–1524.
198. Li Y, Mima T, Komori Y, et al. A new member of the tripartite multidrug efflux pumps, MexVW-OprM, in *Pseudomonas aeruginosa*. *J Antimicrob Chemother* 2003;52:572–575.
199. Livermore DM. Interplay of impermeability and chromosomal β-lactamase activity in imipenem-resistant *Pseudomonas aeruginosa*. *Antimicrob Agents Chemother* 1992;36:2046–2048.
200. Livermore DM, Yang YJ. Comparative activity of meropenem against *Pseudomonas aeruginosa* strains with well-characterized resistance mechanisms. *J Antimicrob Chemother* 1989;24 [Suppl A]:149–159.
201. Livornese LLJ, Dias S, Samel C. Hospital-acquired infection with vancomycin-resistant *Enterococcus faecium* transmitted by electronic thermometers. *Ann Int Med* 1992;117:112–116.
202. Lobritz M, Hutton-Thomas R, Marshall S, et al. Recombination proficiency influences frequency and locus of mutational resistance to linezolid in *Enterococcus faecalis*. *Antimicrob Agents Chemother* 2003;47:3318–3320.
203. Lyon BR, Skurray R. Antimicrobial resistance in *Staphylococcus aureus:* genetic basis. *Microbiol Rev* 1987;51:88–134.
204. Lyras D, Rood JI. Genetic organization and distribution of tetracycline resistance determinants in *Clostridium perfringens*. *Antimicrob Agents Chemother* 1996;40:2500–2504.
205. Ma XX, Ito T, Tiensasitorn C, et al. Novel type of staphylococcal cassette chromosome mec identified in community-acquired methicillin-resistant *Staphylococcus aureus* strains. *Antimicrob Agents Chemother* 2002;46:1147–1152.
206. MacVanin M, Johanson U, Ehrenberg M, et al. Fusidic acid-resistant EF-G perturbs the accumulation of ppGpp. *Mol Microbiol* 2000;37:98–107.
207. Mahairas GG, Lyon BR, Skurray RA, et al. Genetic analysis of *Staphylococcus aureus* with Tn*4001*. *J Bacteriol* 1989;171:3968–3972.
208. Manavathu EK, Fernandez CL, Cooperman BS, et al. Molecular studies of the mechanism of tetracycline resistance mediated by TET(O). *Antimicrob Agents Chemother* 1990;34:71–77.
209. Maness MJ, Foster GC, Sparling PF. Ribosomal resistance to streptomycin and spectinomycin in *Neisseria gonorrhoeae*. *J Bacteriol* 1974;120:1293–1299.
210. Manges AR, Johnson JR, Foxman B, et al. Widespread distribution of urinary tract infections caused by a multidrug-resistant *Escherichia coli* clonal group. *N Engl J Med* 2001;345:1007–1013.
211. Marshall SH, Donskey CJ, Hutton-Thomas R, et al. Gene dosage and linezolid resistance in *Enterococcus faecium* and *Enterococcus faecalis*. *Antimicrob Agents Chemother* 2002;46:3334–3336.
212. Martin JM, Green M, Barbadora KA, et al. Erythromycin-resistant group A streptococci in schoolchildren in Pittsburgh. *N Engl J Med* 2002;346:1200–1206.
213. Maseda H, Yoneyama H, Nakae T. Assignment of the

substrate-selective subunits of the MexEF-OprN multidrug efflux pump of *Pseudomonas aeruginosa*. *Antimicrob Agents Chemother* 2000;44:658–664.

214. Maslow JN, Mulligan ME, Arbeit RD. Molecular epidemiology: application of contemporary techniques to the typing of microorganisms. *Clin Infect Dis* 1993;17:153–164.

215. Masuda G, Tomioka S, Hasegawa M. Detection of beta-lactamase production by Gram-negative bacteria. *J Antibiot* (Tokyo) 1976;29:662–664.

216. Masuda N, Sakagawa E, Ohya S, et al. Substrate specificities of MexAB-OprM, MexCD-OprJ, and MexXY-oprM efflux pumps in *Pseudomonas aeruginosa*. *Antimicrob Agents Chemother* 2000;44:3322–3327.

217. Matagne A, Dubus A, Galleni M, et al. The beta-lactamase cycle: a tale of selective pressure and bacterial ingenuity. *Nat Prod Rep* 1999;16:1–19.

218. Mates SM, Patel L, Kaback HR, et al. Membrane potential in anaerobically growing *Staphylococcus aureus* and its relationship to gentamicin uptake. *Antimicrob Agents Chemother* 1983;23:526–530.

219. Matsuhashi M. Utilization of lipid-linked precursors and the formation of peptidoglycan in the process of cell growth and division: membrane enzymes involved in the final steps of peptidoglycan synthesis and the mechanism of their regulation. In: Ghuysen JM, Hackenbeck R, eds. *Bacterial cell wall*. New York: Elsevier Science, 1994;55–71.

220. McDowell TD, Reed KE. Mechanism of penicillin killing in the absence of bacterial lysis. *Antimicrob Agents Chemother* 1989;33:1680–1685.

221. McMurry LM, Levy SB. Tetracycline resistance in Gram-positive bacteria. In: Fischetti VA, Novick RP, Ferretti JJ, et al., eds. *Gram-positive pathogens*. Washington, DC: American Society for Microbiology, 2000;660–677.

222. Medeiros AA, O'Brien RF, Rosenberg EY, et al. Loss of OmpC porin in a strain of *Salmonella typhimurium* causes increased resistance to cephalosporins during therapy. *J Infect Dis* 1987;156:751–757.

223. Medical Research Council. Streptomycin treatment of pulmonary tuberculosis. *Br Med J* 1948;2:769–782.

224. Meier A, Kirschner P, Bange F-C, et al. Genetic alterations in streptomycin-resistant *Mycobacterium tuberculosis:* mapping of mutations conferring resistance. *Antimicrob Agents Chemother* 1994;38:228–233.

225. Mercier J, Lachapelle J, Couture F, et al. Structural and functional characterization of *tnpI*, a recombinase locus in Tn*21* and related β-lactamase transposons. *J Bacteriol* 1990;172:3745–3757.

226. Mine T, Morita Y, Kataoka A, et al. Expression in *Escherichia coli* of a new multidrug efflux pump, MexXY, from *Pseudomonas aeruginosa*. *Antimicrob Agents Chemother* 1999;43:415–417.

227. Mongkolrattanothai K, Boyle S, Kahana MD, et al. Severe *Staphylococcus aureus* infections caused by clonally related community-acquired methicillin-susceptible and methicillin-resistant isolates. *Clin Infect Dis* 2003;37:1050–1058.

227a. Montero A, Ariza J, Corbella X, Domenech A, Cabellos C, Ayats J, Tubau F, Borraz C, Gudiol F. Antibiotic combinations for serious infections caused by carbapenem-resistant Acinetobacter baumannii in a mouse pneumonia model. *J Antimicrob Chemother* 2004 Nov 16; [Epub ahead of print]

228. Moreira B, Boyle-Vavra S, deJonge BL, et al. Increased production of penicillin-binding protein 2, increased detection of other penicillin-binding proteins, and decreased coagulase activity associated with glycopeptide resistance in *Staphylococcus aureus*. *Antimicrob Agents Chemother* 1997;41:1788–1793.

229. Morlock GP, Metchock B, Sikes D, et al. ethA, inhA, and katG loci of ethionamide-resistant clinical *Mycobacterium tuberculosis* isolates. *Antimicrob Agents Chemother* 2003;47:3799–3805.

230. Morris AB, Brown RB, Sands M. Use of rifampin in nonstaphylococcal, nonmycobacterial disease. *Antimicrob Agents Chemother* 1993;37:1–7.

231. Morris JG, Shay DK, Hebden JN, et al. Enterococci resistant to multiple antimicrobial agents, including vancomycin: establishment of endemicity in a university medical center. *Ann Int Med* 1995;123:250–259.

232. Mullany P, Roberts AP, Wang H. Mechanism of integration and excision in conjugative transposons. *Cell Mol Life Sci* 2002;59:2017–2022.

233. Murakami S, Nakashima R, Yamashita E, et al. Crystal structure of bacterial multidrug efflux transporter AcrB. *Nature* 2002;419:587–593.

234. Murray BE, Singh KV, Markowitz SM, et al. Evidence for clonal spread of a single strain of β-lactamase–producing *Enterococcus (Streptococcus) faecalis* to six hospitals in five states. *J Infect Dis* 1991;163:780–785.

235. Naimi TS, LeDell KH, Boxrud DJ, et al. Epidemiology and clonality of community-acquired methicillin-resistant *Staphylococcus aureus* in Minnesota, 1996–1998. *Clin Infect Dis* 2001;33:990–996.

236. Naimi TS, LeDell KH, Como-Sabetti K, et al. Comparison of community- and health care–associated methicillin-resistant *Staphylococcus aureus* infection. *JAMA* 2003;290:2976–2984.

237. Nakanishi N, Yoshida S, Wakebe H, et al. Mechanisms of clinical resistance to fluoroquinolones in *Staphylococcus aureus*. *Antimicrob Agents Chemother* 1991;35:2562–2567.

237a. National Committee for Clinical Laboratory Standards. 1999. Performance standards for antimicrobial susceptibility testing. NCCLS approved standard M100-S9. National Committee for Clinical Laboratory Standards, Wayne, PA

238. Navarro F, Courvalin P. Analysis of genes encoding D-alanine-D-alanine ligase-related enzymes in *Enterococcus casseliflavus* and *Enterococcus flavescens*. *Antimicrob Agents Chemother* 1994;38:1788–1793.

239. Neyfakh AA, Borsch CM, Kaatz GW. Fluoroquinolone resistance protein NorA of *Staphylococcus aureus* is a multidrug efflux transporter. *Antimicrob Agents Chemother* 1993;37:128–129.

240. Nichols WW, Hewinson RG. Rapid and automated measurement of Km and specific Vmax values of beta-lactamases in bacterial extracts. *J Antimicrob Chemother* 1987;19:285–295.

241. Nikaido H. Molecular basis of bacterial outer membrane permeability revisited. *Microbiol Mol Biol Rev* 2003;67:593–656.

242. Nikaido H. Multiple antibiotic resistance and efflux. *Curr Opin Microbiol* 1998;1:516–523.

243. Nikaido H. Prevention of drug access to bacterial targets: permeability barriers and active efflux. *Science* 1994;264:382–8.

244. Nikaido H. Role of the outer membrane of Gram-negative bacteria in antimicrobial resistance. In: Bryan LE, ed. *Handbook of experimental pharmacology: microbial resistance to drugs*, vol. 91. Berlin: Springer-Verlag, 1989;1–34.

245. Nilsson AI, Berg OG, Aspevall O, et al. Biological costs and mechanisms of fosfomycin resistance in *Escherichia coli*. *Antimicrob Agents Chemother* 2003;47:2850–2858.

246. Noguchi H, Matsuhashi M, Mitsuhashi S. Comparative studies of penicillin-binding proteins in *Pseudomonas aeruginosa* and *Escherichia coli*. *Eur J Biochem* 1979;100:41–49.

246b. Nordmann P, Poirel L. Emerging carbapenemases in Gram-negative aerobes. *Clin Microbiol Infect* 2002 Jun;8(6):321–331.

247. O'Callaghan CH, Morris A, Kirby SM, et al. Novel method for detection of β-lactamases by using a chromogenic cephalosporin substrate. *Antimicrob Agents Chemother* 1972;1:283–288.
248. Ochs MM, McCusker MP, Bains M, et al. Negative regulation of the *Pseudomonas aeruginosa* outer membrane porin OprD selective for imipenem and basic amino acids. *Antimicrob Agents Chemother* 1999;43:1085–1090.
249. Okuma K, Iwakawa K, Turnidge JD, et al. Dissemination of new methicillin-resistant *Staphylococcus aureus* clones in the community. *J Clin Microbiol* 2002;40:4289–4294.
250. Pai MP, Rodvold KA, Schreckenberger PC, et al. Risk factors associated with the development of infection with linezolid- and vancomycin-resistant *Enterococcus faecium*. *Clin Infect Dis* 2002;35:1269–1272.
251. Pang Y, Brown BA, Steingrube VA, et al. Tetracycline resistance determinants in *Mycobacterium* and *Streptomyces* species. *Antimicrob Agents Chemother* 1994;38:1408–1412.
252. Pangon B, Bizet C, Bure A, et al. In vivo selection of a cephamycin-resistant, porin-deficient mutant of *Klebsiella pneumoniae* producing a TEM-3 -lactamase. *J Infect Dis* 1989;159:1005–1006.
253. Parenti MA, Hatfield SM, Leyden JJ. Mupirocin: a topical antibiotic with a unique structure and mechanism of action. *Clin Pharmacol* 1987;6:761–770.
254. Paterson DL. Extended-spectrum beta-lactamases: the European experience. *Curr Opin Infect Dis* 2001;14:697–701.
255. Paterson DL, Bonomo RA. Extended-spectrum β-lactamases: a review. *J Clin Microbiol* (in press).
256. Paterson DL, Hujer KM, Hujer AM, et al. Extended-spectrum beta-lactamases in *Klebsiella pneumoniae* bloodstream isolates from seven countries: dominance and widespread prevalence of SHV- and CTX-M-type beta-lactamases. *Antimicrob Agents Chemother* 2003;47:3554–3560.
257. Paterson DL, Rice LB, Bonomo RA. Rapid method of extraction and analysis of extended-spectrum beta-lactamases from clinical strains of *Klebsiella pneumoniae*. *Clin Microbiol Infect* 2001;7:709–711.
258. Patterson JE, Hardin TC, Kelly CA. Association of antibiotic utilization measures and control of multiple-drug resistance in *Klebsiella pneumoniae*. *Infect Control Hosp Epidemiol* 2000;12:455–458.
259. Paulsen IT, Banerjei L, Myers GS, et al. Role of mobile DNA in the evolution of vancomycin-resistant *Enterococcus faecalis*. *Science* 2003;299:2071–2074.
260. Perez-Perez FJ, Hanson ND. Detection of plasmid-mediated AmpC beta-lactamase genes in clinical isolates by using multiplex PCR. *J Clin Microbiol* 2002;40:2153–2162.
261. Petinaki E, Spiliopoulou I, Kontos F, et al. Clonal dissemination of mupirocin-resistant staphylococci in Greek hospitals. *J Antimicrob Chemother* 2004;53:105–108.
262. Pillai SK, Sakoulas G, Wennersten C, et al. Linezolid resistance in *Staphylococcus aureus*: characterization and stability of resistant phenotype. *J Infect Dis* 2002;186:1603–1607.
263. Pittet D, Hugonnet S, Harbarth S, et al. Effectiveness of a hospital-wide programme to improve compliance with hand hygiene. Infection Control Programme. *Lancet* 2000;356:1307–1312.
263b.Philippon A, Arlet G, Jacoby GA. Plasmid-determined AmpC-type beta-lactamases. *Antimicrob Agents Chemother* 2002 Jan;46(1):1–11.
264. Podbielski A, Schonling J, Melzer B, et al. Different promoters of SHV-2 and SHV-2a beta-lactamase lead to diverse levels of cefotaxime resistance in their bacterial producers. *J Gen Microbiol* 1991;137[Pt 7]:1667–1675.
265. Podglajen I, Breuil J, Bordon F, et al. A silent carbapenemase gene in strains of *Bacteroides fragilis* can be expressed after a one step mutation. *FEMS Microbiol Lett* 1992;70:21–29.
266. Podglajen I, Breuil J, Collatz E. Insertion of a novel DNA sequence, 1S1186, upstream of the silent carbapenemase gene cfiA, promotes expression of carbapenem resistance in clinical isolates of *Bacteroides fragilis*. *Mol Microbiol* 1994;12:105–114.
267. Podlesek Z, Comino A, Herzog-Velikonja B, et al. The role of the bacitracin ABC transporter in bacitracin resistance and collateral detergent sensitivity. *FEMS Microbiol Lett* 2000;188:103–106.
267a.Poirel L, Heritier C, Tolun V, Nordmann P. Emergence of oxacillinase-mediated resistance to imipenem in Klebsiella pneumoniae. *Antimicrob Agents Chemother* 2004 Jan;48(1):15–22.
268. Prado D, Murray BE, Cleary TG, et al. Limitations of using plasmid pattern as an epidemiologic tool for clinical isolates of *Shigella sonnei*. *J Infect Dis* 1987;155:314–316.
269. Prystowsky J, Siddiqui F, Chosay J, et al. Resistance to linezolid: characterization of mutations in rRNA and comparison of their occurrences in vancomycin-resistant enterococci. *Antimicrob Agents Chemother* 2001;45:2154–2156.
270. Puzniak LA, Mayfield J, Leet T, et al. Acquisition of vancomycin-resistant enterococci during scheduled antimicrobial rotation in an intensive care unit. *Clin Infect Dis* 2001;33:151–157.
271. Rahal JJ, Urban C, Segal-Maurer S. Nosocomial antibiotic resistance in multiple Gram-negative species: experience at one hospital with squeezing the resistance balloon at multiple sites. *Clin Infect Dis* 2002;34:499–503.
272. Randegger CC, Hachler H. Real-time PCR and melting curve analysis for reliable and rapid detection of SHV extended-spectrum beta-lactamases. *Antimicrob Agents Chemother* 2001;45:1730–1736.
273. Rasheed JK, Jay C, Metchock B, et al. Evolution of extended-spectrum β-lactam resistance (SHV-8) in a strain of *Escherichia coli* during multiple episodes of bacteremia. *Antimicrob Agents Chemother* 1997;41:647–653.
274. Rather PN, Orosz E. Characterization of *aarA*, a pleiotropic negative regulator of the 2′-*N*-acetyltransferase in *Providencia stuartii*. *J Bacteriol* 1994;176:5140–5144.
275. Rather PN, Orosz E, Shaw KJ, et al. Characterization and transcriptional regulation of the 2′-*N*-acetyltransferase gene from *Providencia stuartii*. *J Bacteriol* 1993;175:6492–6498.
276. Rauch PJG, DeVos WM. Characterization of a novel nisin-sucrose conjugative transposon Tn*5276* and its insertion in *Lactococcus lactis*. *J Bacteriol* 1992;174:1280–1287.
277. Raynaud C, Laneelle MA, Senaratne RH, et al. Mechanisms of pyrazinamide resistance in mycobacteria: importance of lack of uptake in addition to lack of pyrazinamidase activity. *Microbiology* 1999;145[Pt 6]:1359–1367.
278. Reynolds PE, Depardieu F, Dutka-Malen S, et al. Glycopeptide resistance mediated by enterococcal transposon Tn*1546* requires production of VanX for hydrolysis of D-alanyl-D-alanine. *Mol Microbiol* 1994;13:1065–1070.
279. Rhinehart E, Smith NE, Wennersten C, et al. Rapid dissemination of β-lactamase–producing, aminoglycoside-resistant *Enterococcus faecalis* among patients and staff on an infant-toddler surgical ward. *N Engl J Med* 1990;323:1814–1818.
280. Rice LB. Tn*916*-family conjugative transposons and dissemination of antimicrobial resistance determinants. *Antimicrob Agents Chemother* 1998;42:1871–1877.
281. Rice LB. Emergence of vancomycin-resistant enterococci. *Emerg Infect Dis* 2001;7:183–187.

282. Rice LB. Association of different mobile elements to generate novel integrative elements. *Cell Mol Life Sci* 2002;59:2023–2032.
283. Rice LB. Controlling antibiotic resistance in the ICU: different bacteria, different strategies. *Cleve Clin J Med* 2003;70:793–800.
284. Rice LB, Carias LL. Studies on excision of conjugative transposons in enterococci: evidence for joint sequences composed of strands with unequal numbers of nucleotides. *Plasmid* 1994;31:312–316.
285. Rice LB, Carias LL. Transfer of Tn*5385*, a composite, multiresistance element from *Enterococcus faecalis*. *J Bacteriol* 1998;180:714–721.
286. Rice LB, Carias LL, Etter L, et al. Resistance to cefoperazone-sulbactam in *Klebsiella pneumoniae*: evidence for enhanced resistance resulting from the coexistence of two different resistance mechanisms. *Antimicrob Agents Chemother* 1993;37:1061–1064.
287. Rice LB, Carias LL, Hujer AM, et al. High-level expression of chromosomally encoded SHV-1 β-lactamase and an outer membrane protein change confer resistance to ceftazidime and piperacillin-tazobactam in a clinical isolate of *Klebsiella pneumoniae*. *Antimicrob Agents Chemother* 2000;44:362–367.
288. Rice LB, Carias LL, Hutton-Thomas R, et al. Penicillin-binding protein 5 and expression of ampicillin resistance in *Enterococcus faecium*. *Antimicrob Agents Chemother* 2001;45:1480–1486.
289. Rice LB, Eckstein EC, DeVente J, et al. Ceftazidime-resistant *Klebsiella pneumoniae* isolates recovered at the Cleveland Department of Veterans Affairs Medical Center. *Clin Infect Dis* 1996;23:118–124.
290. Rice LB, Eliopoulos GM, Wennersten C, et al. Chromosomally-mediated β-lactamase production and gentamicin resistance in *Enterococcus faecalis*. *Antimicrob Agents Chemother* 1991;35:272–276.
291. Rice LB, Marshall SH, Carias LL. Tn*5381*, a conjugative transposon identifiable as a circular form in *Enterococcus faecalis*. *J Bacteriol* 1992;174:7308–7315.
292. Rice LB, Marshall SH, Carias LL, et al. Sequences of MGH-1, YOU-1 and YOU-2 extended-spectrum β-lactamase genes. *Antimicrob Agents Chemother* 1993; 37:2760–2761.
293. Rice LB, Willey SH, Papanicolaou GA, et al. Outbreak of ceftazidime resistance caused by extended-spectrum β-lactamases at a Massachusetts chronic care facility. *Antimicrob Agents Chemother* 1990;34:2193–2199.
294. Ridenhour MB, Fletcher HM, Mortensen JE, et al. A novel tetracycline-resistant determinant, tet(U), is encoded on the plasmid pKq10 in *Enterococcus faecium*. *Plasmid* 1996;35:71–80.
295. Roberts AP, Johanesen PA, Lyras D, et al. Comparison of Tn5397 from *Clostridium difficile*, Tn916 from *Enterococcus faecalis* and the CW459tet(M) element from *Clostridium perfringens* shows that they have similar conjugation regions but different insertion and excision modules. *Microbiology* 2001;147:1243–1251.
296. Roberts M. Epidemiology of tetracycline resistance determinants. *Trends Microbiol* 1994;2:353–357.
297. Roberts RB, de Lancastre A, Eisner W, et al. Molecular epidemiology of methicillin-resistant *Staphylococcus aureus* in 12 New York hospitals. *J Infect Dis* 1998;178:164–171.
297a. Rodriguez-Hernandez MJ, Jimenez-Mejias ME, Pichardo C, Cuberos L, Garcia-Curiel A, Pachon J. Colistin efficacy in an experimental model of Acinetobacter baumannii endocarditis. *Clin Microbiol Infect* 2004 Jun;10(6):581–584.
298. Rosdahl VT, Knudsen AM. The decline of methicillin resistance among Danish *Staphylococcus aureus* strains. *Infect Control Hosp Epidemiol* 1991;12:83–88.
299. Rosenau A, Labigne A, Escande F, et al. Plasmid-mediated ROB-1 beta-lactamase in *Pasteurella multocida* from a human specimen. *Antimicrob Agents Chemother* 1991;35:2419–2422.
300. Roux KH, Dhanarajan P. A strategy for single site PCR amplification of dsDNA: priming digested cloned or genomic DNA from an anchor modified restriction site and a short internal sequence. *Biotechniques* 1990;8:48–57.
301. Rowe-Magnus DA, Guerout AM, Ploncard P, et al. The evolutionary history of chromosomal super-integrons provides an ancestry for multiresistant integrons. *Proc Natl Acad Sci USA* 2001;98:652–657.
302. Rowland SJ, Dyke KGH. Tn*552*, a novel transposable element from *Staphylococcus aureus*. *Mol Microbiol* 1990;4:961–975.
303. Rubin LG, Medeiros AA, Yolken RH, et al. Ampicillin treatment failure of apparently beta-lactamase-negative *Haemophilus influenzae* type b meningitis due to novel beta-lactamase. *Lancet* 1981;2:1008–1010.
303a. Ryffel C, Strassle A, Kayser FH, Berger Bachi B. Mechanisms of heteroresistance in methicillin-resistant Staphylococcus aureus. *Antimicrob Agents Chemother* 1994 Apr;38(4):724–728.
304. Sahm DF, Marsilio MK, Piazza G. Antimicrobial resistance in key bloodstream bacterial isolates: electronic surveillance with The Surveillance Network Database–USA. *Clin Infect Dis* 1999;29:259–263.
305. Said-Salim B, Mathema B, Kreiswirth BN. Community-acquired methicillin-resistant *Staphylococcus aureus*: an emerging pathogen. *Infect Control Hosp Epidemiol* 2003;24:451–455.
306. Sakoulas G, Eliopoulos GM, Moellering RC Jr. *Staphylococcus aureus* accessory gene regulator (agr) group II: is there a relationship to the development of intermediate-level glycopeptide resistance? *J Infect Dis* 2003;187:929–938.
307. Sakoulas G, Eliopoulos GM, Moellering RC Jr, et al. Accessory gene regulator (agr) locus in geographically diverse *Staphylococcus aureus* isolates with reduced susceptibility to vancomycin. *Antimicrob Agents Chemother* 2002;46:1492–1502.
308. Sande MA, Mandell GL. The aminoglycosides. In: Gilman AG, Rall TW, Nies AS, et al., eds. *The pharmacologic basis of therapeutics,* 8th ed. New York: Pergamon Press, 1990;1098–1116.
309. Sanders CC, Watanakunakorn C. Emergence of resistance to β-lactams, aminoglycosides and quinolones during combination therapy for infection due to *Serratia marcescens*. *J Infect Dis* 1986;153:617–619.
310. Santagati M, Iannelli F, Cascone C, et al. The novel conjugative transposon Tn1207.3 carries the macrolide efflux gene mef(A) in *Streptococcus pyogenes*. *Microb Drug Resist* 2003;9:243–247.
311. Saurina G, Quale JM, Manikal VM, et al. Antimicrobial resistance in Enterobacteriaceae in Brooklyn, NY: epidemiology and relation to antibiotic usage patterns. *J Antimicrob Chemother* 2000;45:895–898.
312. Schouten MA, Willems RJ, Kraak WA, et al. Molecular analysis of Tn1546-like elements in vancomycin-resistant enterococci isolated from patients in Europe shows geographic transposon type clustering. *Antimicrob Agents Chemother* 2001;45:986–989.
313. Scott JR, Kirchman PA, Caparon MG. An intermediate in the transposition of the conjugative transposon Tn*916*. *Proc Natl Acad Sci USA* 1988;85:4809–4813.
314. Scott KP. The role of conjugative transposons in spreading

antibiotic resistance between bacteria that inhabit the gastrointestinal tract. *Cell Mol Life Sci* 2002;59:2071–2082.

315. Shaw JH, Clewell DB. Complete nucleotide sequence of macrolide-lincosamide-streptogramin B resistance transposon Tn*917* in *Streptococcus faecalis*. *J Bacteriol* 1985; 164:782–796.
316. Shaw KJ, Rather PN, Hare RS, et al. Molecular genetics of aminoglycoside resistance genes and familial relationships of the aminoglycoside-modifying enzymes. *Microbiol Rev* 1993;57:138–163.
317. Shaw WV, Leslie AGW. Chloramphenicol acetyltransferase. In: Bryan LE, ed. *Handbook of experimental pharmacology: microbial resistance to drugs*, vol. 91. Berlin: Springer-Verlag, 1989;313–324.
318. Sherratt D. Tn*3* and related transposable elements: site-specific recombination and transposition. In: Berg DE, Howe MM, ed. *Mobile DNA*. Washington, DC: American Society for Microbiology, 1989;163–184.
319. Shinabarger DL, Marotti KR, Murray RW, et al. Mechanism of action of oxazolidinones: effects of linezolid and eperezolid on translation reactions. *Antimicrob Agents Chemother* 1997;41:2132–2136.
320. Shlaes DM, Binczewski B, Rice LB. Emerging antimicrobial resistance and the immunocompromised host. *Clin Infect Dis* 1993;17[Suppl 2]:S527–536.
321. Sieradzki K, Roberts RB, Haber SW, et al. The development of vancomycin resistance in a patient with methicillin-resistant Staphylococcus aureus infection. *N Engl J Med* 1999;340:517–523.
322. Sloan J, McMurry LM, Lyras D, et al. The *Clostridium perfringens* Tet P determinant comprises two overlapping genes: tetA(P), which mediates active tetracycline efflux, and tetB(P), which is related to the ribosomal protection family of tetracycline-resistance determinants. *Mol Microbiol* 1994;11:403–415.
323. Small PM, Shafer RW, Hopewell PC, et al. Exogenous reinfection with multidrug-resistant *Mycobacterium tuberculosis* in patients with advanced HIV infection. *N Engl J Med* 1993;328:1137–1144.
324. Soares S, Kristinsson KG, Musser J, et al. Evidence for the introduction of a multiresistant clone of serotype 6B *Streptococcus pneumoniae* from Spain to Iceland in the late 1980s. *J Infect Dis* 1993;168:158–163.

324a. Sobieszczyk ME, Furuya EY, Hay CM, Pancholi P, Della-Latta P, Hammer SM, Kubin CJ. Combination therapy with polymyxin B for the treatment of multidrug-resistant Gram-negative respiratory tract infections. *J Antimicrob Chemother* 2004 Aug;54(2):566–569. Epub 2004 Jul 21.

325. Soltani M, Beighton D, Philpott-Howard J, et al. Mechanisms of resistance to quinupristin-dalfopristin among isolates of *Enterococcus faecium* from animals, raw meat, and hospital patients in Western Europe. *Antimicrob Agents Chemother* 2000;44:433–436.
326. Song MD, Wachi M, Doi M, et al. Evolution of an inducible penicillin-target protein in methicillin-resistant *S. aureus* by gene fusion. *FEBS Lett* 1987;221:167–171.
327. Speer BS, Bedzyk L, Salyers AA. Evidence that a novel tetracycline resistance gene found in two *Bacteroides* transposons encodes an NADP-requiring oxidoreductase. *J Bacteriol* 1991;173:176–183.
328. Speer BS, Shoemaker NB, Salyers AA. Bacterial resistance to tetracyclines: mechanisms, transfer, and clinical significance. *Clin Microbiol Rev* 1992;5:387–399.
329. Spencer RC. The emergence of epidemic multi-antibiotic-resistant *Stenotrophomonas maltophilia* and *Burkholderia cepacia*. *J Hosp Infect* 1995;30[Suppl]:453–464.
330. Spratt BG. Resistance to antibiotics mediated by target alterations. *Science* 1994;264:388–393.

330a. Spratt BG. Properties of the penicillin-binding proteins of Escherichia coli K12,. *Eur J Biochem* 1977 Jan;72(2):341–352.

331. Storrs MJ, Poyart-Salmeron C, Trieu-Cuot P, et al. Conjugative transposition of Tn*916* requires the excisive and integrative activities of the transposon encoded integrase. *J Bacteriol* 1991;173:4347–4352.
332. Stover CK, Pham XQ, Erwin AL, et al. Complete genome sequence of *Pseudomonas aeruginosa* PA01, an opportunistic pathogen. *Nature* 2000;406:959–964.
333. Strominger JL, Tipper DJ. Bacterial cell wall synthesis and structure in relation to the mechanism of action of penicillins and other antibacterial agents. *Am J Med* 1965;39:708–721.
334. Stull TL, Lipuma JJ, Edlind TD. A broad-spectrum probe for molecular epidemiology of bacteria: ribosomal RNA. *J Infect Dis* 1988;157:280–285.
335. Swinfield T-J, Oultram JD, Thompson DE, et al. Physical characterization of the replication region of *Streptococcus faecalis* plasmid pAMβ1. *Gene* 1990;87:79–90.
336. Takahashi S, Nagano Y. Rapid procedure for isolation of plasmid DNA. *J Clin Microbiol* 1984;20:608–613.
337. Telenti A, Imboden P, Marchesi F, et al. Detection of rifampicin-resistance mutations in *Mycobacterium tuberculosis*. *Lancet* 1993;341:647–650.
338. Thomson KS, Sanders CC. Detection of extended-spectrum beta-lactamases in members of the family Enterobacteriaceae: comparison of the double-disk and three-dimensional tests. *Antimicrob Agents Chemother* 1992;36:1877–1882.
339. Tomasz A. The mechanism of the irreversible antimicrobial effects of penicillins: how the beta-lactam antibiotics kill and lyse bacteria. *Annu Rev Microbiol* 1979;33:113–137.
340. Tomasz A, Holtje JV. Murein hydrolases and the lytic and killing actions of penicillin. In: Schlesinger D, ed. *Microbiology*. Washington, DC: American Society for Microbiology, 1977;202–215.
341. Tomich PK, An FY, Clewell DB. Properties of erythromycin-inducible transposon Tn*917* in *Streptococcus faecalis*. *J Bacteriol* 1980;141:1366–1374.
342. Toscano WA Jr, Storm DR. Bacitracin. *Pharmacol Ther* 1982;16:199–210.
343. Tran JH, Jacoby GA. Mechanism of plasmid-mediated quinolone resistance. *Proc Natl Acad Sci USA* 2002; 99:5638–5642.
344. Trias J, Nikaido H. Outer membrane protein D2 catalyzes facilitated diffusion of penems and carnbapenems through the outer membrane of *Pseudomonas aeruginosa*. *Antimicrob Agents Chemother* 1990;34:52–57.
345. Trieu-Cuot P, Carlier C, Poyart-Salmeron C, et al. An integrative vector exploiting the transposition properties of Tn*1545* for insertional mutagenesis and cloning of genes from Gram-positive bacteria. *Gene* 1991;106:21–27.
346. Trieu-Cuot P, deCespedes G, Bentorcha F, et al. Study of heterogeneity of chloramphenicol acetyltransferase (CAT) genes in streptococci and enterococci by polymerase chain reaction: characterization of a new CAT determinant. *Antimicrob Agents Chemother* 1993;37:2593–2598.
347. Triglia T, Peterson MG, Kemp DJ. A procedure for in vitro amplification of DNA segments that lie outside the boundaries of known sequences. *Nucleic Acids Res* 1988;16:8186.
348. Tsiodras S, Gold HS, Sakoulas G, et al. Linezolid resistance in a clinical isolate of *Staphylococcus aureus*. *Lancet* 2001;358:207–208.
349. Tu Y, McCalla DR. Effect of activated nitrofurans on DNA. *Biochim Biophys Acta* 1972;402:142–149.

350. Unal S, Hoskins J, Flokowitch JE, et al. Detection of methicillin-resistant staphylococci by using polymerase chain reaction. *J Clin Microbiol* 1992;30:1685–1691.
351. Unal S, Werner K, DeGirolami P, et al. Comparison of tests for detection of methicillin-resistant *Staphylococcus aureus* in a clinical microbiology laboratory. *Antimicrob Agents Chemother* 1994;38:345–347.
352. Urban C, Meyer KS, Mariano N, et al. Identification of TEM-26 β-lactamase responsible for a major outbreak of ceftazidime-resistant *Klebsiella pneumoniae. Antimicrob Agents Chemother* 1994;38:392–395.
352a. Urban C, Segal-Maurer S, Rahal JJ. Considerations in control and treatment of nosocomial infections due to multidrug-resistant Acinetobacter baumannii. *Clin Infect Dis* 2003 May 15;36(10):1268–1274. Epub 2003 May 01.
353. Vakulenko SB, Mobashery S. Versatility of aminoglycosides and prospects for their future. *Clin Microbiol Rev* 2003;16:430–450.
354. Van Bambeke F, Balzi E, Tulkens PM. Antibiotic efflux pumps. *Biochem Pharmacol* 2000;60:457–70.
355. Van Bambeke F, Chauvel M, Reynolds PE, et al. Vancomycin-dependent *Enterococcus faecalis* clinical isolates and revertant mutants. *Antimicrob Agents Chemother* 1999;43:41–47.
356. Van Belkum A. DNA fingerprinting of medically important microorganisms by use of PCR. *Clin Microbiol Rev* 1994;7:174–184.
357. Vancomycin-resistant *Staphylococcus aureus*—Pennsylvania, 2002. *MMWR* 2002;51:902.
358. van der Auwera P, Pensart N, Korten V, et al. Influence of oral glycopeptides on the fecal flora of human volunteers: selection of highly glycopeptide-resistant enterococci. *J Infect Dis* 1996;173:1129–1136.
359. van der Wouden EJ, Thijs JC, Kusters JG, et al. Mechanism and clinical significance of metronidazole resistance in *Helicobacter pylori. Scand J Gastroenterol [Suppl]* 2001;10–14.
360. Varon E, Gutmann L. Mechanisms and spread of fluoroquinolone resistance in *Streptococcus pneumoniae. Res Microbiol* 2000;151:471–3.
361. Veal WL, Nicholas RA, Shafer WM. Overexpression of the MtrC-MtrD-MtrE efflux pump due to an mtrR mutation is required for chromosomally mediated penicillin resistance in *Neisseria gonorrhoeae. J Bacteriol* 2002;184:5619–5624.
362. Vecoli C, Prevost FE, Ververis JJ, et al. Comparison of polyacrylamide and agarose gel thin-layer isoelectric focusing for the characterization of β-lactamases. *Antimicrob Agents Chemother* 1983;24:186–189.
363. Waley SG. A spectrophotometric assay of beta-lactamase action on penicillins. *Biochem J* 1974;139:789–790.
364. Waxman DJ, Strominger JL. Penicillin-binding proteins and the mechanism of action of beta-lactam antibiotics. *Annu Rev Biochem* 1983;52:825–869.
365. Waxman DJ, Yocum RR, Strominger JL. Penicillins and cephalosporins are active site-directed acylating agents: evidence in support of the substrate analogue hypothesis. *Philos Trans R Soc Lond B Biol Sci* 1980;289:257–271.
366. Webber MA, Piddock LJ. The importance of efflux pumps in bacterial antibiotic resistance. *J Antimicrob Chemother* 2003;51:9–11.
367. Weigel LM, Clewell DB, Gill SR, et al. Genetic analysis of a high-level vancomycin-resistant isolate of *Staphylococcus aureus. Science* 2003;302:1569–1571.
368. Weisblum B. Erythromycin resistance by ribosome modification. *Antimicrob Agents Chemother* 1995;39:577–585.
369. Weisblum B. Insights into erythromycin action from studies of its activity as inducer of resistance. *Antimicrob Agents Chemother* 1995;39:797–805.
370. White DG, Hudson C, Maurer JJ, et al. Characterization of chloramphenicol and florfenicol resistance in *Escherichia coli* associated with bovine diarrhea. *J Clin Microbiol* 2000;38:4593–4598.
371. Whittle G, Shoemaker NB, Salyers AA. The role of Bacteroides conjugative transposons in the dissemination of antibiotic resistance genes. *Cell Mol Life Sci* 2002;59:2044–2054.
372. Willetts N, Skurray R. Structure and function of the F factor and mechanisms of conjugation. In: Neidhardt FC, Ingraham JL, Low KB, et al., eds. *Escherichia coli and Salmonella typhimurium: cellular and molecular biology.* Washington, DC: American Society for Microbiology, 1987;1110–1133.
373. Williams DR, Thomas CM. Active partioning of bacterial plasmids. *J Gen Microbiol* 1992;138:1–16.
374. Williams RJ, Livermore DM, Lindridge MA, et al. Mechanisms of beta-lactam resistance in British isolates of *Pseudomonas aeruginosa. J Med Microbiol* 1984;17:283–293.
375. Williamson R, Calderwood SB, Moellering RCJ, et al. Studies on the mechanism of intrinsic resistance to β-lactam antibiotic in Group D streptococci. *J Gen Microbiol* 1983;129:813–822.
376. Wilson K. Large scale CsCl prep of bacterial genomic DNA. In: Ausebel FM, Brent R, Kingston RE, et al., eds. *Current protocols in molecular biology.* Brooklyn, NY: Green Publishing Assoc, 1987;2.4.3–2.4.5.
377. Wong RS, McMurry LM, Levy SB. "Intergenic" blr gene in *Escherichia coli* encodes a 41-residue membrane protein affecting intrinsic susceptibility to certain inhibitors of peptidoglycan synthesis. *Mol Microbiol* 2000;37:364–370.
378. Yang YJ, Livermore DM, Williams RJ. Chromosomal beta-lactamase expression and antibiotic resistance in *Enterobacter cloacae. J Med Microbiol* 1988;25:227–233.
378a. Yoon J, Urban C, Terzian C, Mariano N, Rahal JJ. In vitro double and triple synergistic activities of Polymyxin B, imipenem, and rifampin against multidrug-resistant Acinetobacter baumannii. *Antimicrob Agents Chemother* 2004 Mar;48(3):753–757.
379. Yoneyama H, Nakae T. Mechanism of efficient elimination of protein D2 in outer membrane of imipenem-resistant *Pseudomonas aeruginosa. Antimicrob Agents Chemother* 1993;37:2385–2390.
380. Yu EW, McDermott G, Zgurskaya HI, et al. Structural basis of multiple drug-binding capacity of the AcrB multidrug efflux pump. *Science* 2003;300:976–980.
381. Zalacain M, Cundliffe E. Methylation of 23S rRNA caused by *tlrA (ermSF),* a tylosin resistance determinant from *Streptomyces fradiae. J Bacteriol* 1989;171:4254–4260.
382. Zervos MJ, Kaufman CA, Therasse PM. Nosocomial infection by gentamicin-resistant *Streptococcus faecalis*: an epidemiologic study. *Ann Int Med* 1987;106:687–691.
383. Zhanel GG, Homenuik K, Nichol K, et al. The glycylcyclines: a comparative review with the tetracyclines. *Drugs* 2004;64:63–88.
384. Zhao G, et al. Bocillin FL, a sensitive and commercially available reagent for detection of penicillin-binding proteins. *Antimicrob Agents Chemother* 1999;43:1124–1128.
385. Zhong P, Shortridge VD. The role of efflux in macrolide resistance. *Drug Resist Update* 2000;3:325–329.
386. Zscheck KK, Murray BE. Genes involved in the regulation of β-lactamase production in enterococci and staphylococci. *Antimicrob Agents Chemother* 1993;37:1966–1970.
387. Zygmunt DJ, Stratton CW, Kernodle DS. Characterization of four β-lactamases produced by *Staphylococcus aureus. Antimicrob Agents Chemother* 1992;36:440–445.

CHAPTER 11

Molecular Methods for the Detection of Antibacterial Resistance Genes

Margareta Ieven

GENETIC METHODS AND THEIR IMPORTANCE FOR THE DETECTION OF RESISTANCE

Resistance genes or mutations in the bacterial chromosome are the identifiable antibiotic resistance determinants. Resistance genes are stretches of DNA coding for an altered antibiotic target or antibiotic efflux or antibiotic inactivation, detectable by appropriate probes, most frequently after *in vitro* amplification of part of the resistance gene.

Mutations in the bacterial chromosome equally give rise to an altered antibiotic target but result from a modified sequence in the genome, to be identified, after *in vitro* amplification of part of the bacterial chromosome involved, by DNA sequencing or an alternative method.

There are only a few instances in which a probe hybridization assay is sufficiently sensitive for clinical use, for example, the EVIGENE MRSA test for staphylococci and the fluorescent hybridization test for clarithromycin resistance in *Helicobacter pylori*.

In all other instances, resistance genes or chromosomal mutations are detected after molecular amplification of the target by PCR (146) and more recently by the real-time formats of PCR (177) or by amplification of the probe, as in the cycling probe assay (29).

Resistance genes are identified after PCR by hybridization of the amplicons with appropriate probes in liquid medium or on a solid surface. In real-time PCR formats, probes are labeled with a fluorophore, and the progress of the reaction is followed by monitoring the increase in fluorescence.

Chromosomal mutations are detected, after genetic amplification, by DNA sequencing, single-strand conformational polymorphism (SSCP) (53,118), or hybridization by fluorescent probes in real-time assays.

In clinical microbiology, the application of molecular methods for the detection of resistance is limited to the group of combinations of antibiotics and microorganisms (a) for which a relatively few genetic polymorphisms are known to be associated with a prevalent pattern of antimicrobial resistance and (b) that have a high degree of clinical importance (38).

There are several reasons to detect microbial antibiotic resistance through molecular techniques. Phenotypic tests do not always produce straightforward results. Bacterial populations may be heterogeneous in that not all individual cells carry the resistance determinant or not all individual cells express it. The resistant fraction of the population may be less vigorous (47) and grow more slowly in the presence of low inhibitory concentrations of the drug tested so that colonies only appear on solid media after prolonged incubation. Phenotypic tests based on growth in the presence of an antibiotic of an isolate obtained from a clinical sample in most cases require a subculture and thus additional time. The time factor is particularly relevant for slowly growing organisms such as *Mycobacterium tuberculosis*.

Genetic tests are particularly useful for the detection of antibiotic resistance in bacterial species with a high potential for hospital epidemics such as *Staphylococcus aureus* and enterococci. They are equally useful for slowly growing *M. tuberculosis*, the antibiotic resistant strains spreading between the moment of first patient contact and the moment of diagnosis of antibiotic resistance.

Screening for colonization of resistant organisms in several body sites may be considerably shortened by testing selective enrichment broths by molecular techniques, resulting in considerable savings in relation to patient isolation measures.

Bacterial resistance for the different antibiotic classes may result from a single molecular mechanism, from one of a variety of molecular mechanisms, or, exceptionally, from a combination of two different mechanisms.

When a variety of resistance mechanisms is possible, as in the case of macrolides and aminoglycosides, identification of the particular mechanism is important for surveillance purposes and might lead to general recommendations on empyric antibiotic use.

The molecular characterization of the resistance determinant may also be epidemiologically important if different mutations result phenotypically in an identical resistance pattern.

The extended-spectrum β-lactamases (ESBLs) occupy a special place in this respect. The responsible mechanisms are widely diverse. Therefore, for practical reasons, their detection relies almost exclusively on phenotypic tests, but because the resistance determinants are located in plasmids, they may spread rapidly among bacterial strains and even species. The epidemiological surveillance of ESBLs through phenotypic tests is thus more pressing, and uncovering the underlying molecular mechanisms can offer detailed epidemiological insight.

It should be remembered that not all types of resistance have been elucidated at the genetic level, particularly resistance resulting from permeability barriers.

Each bacterial species for which resistance determinants are sought has its proper clinical and epidemiological conditions requiring strategies adapted to each application. These will be discussed for some resistance determinants individually.

DETECTION OF METHICILLIN RESISTANCE IN STAPHYLOCOCCI

Since the introduction of methicillin into clinical use, the occurrence of methillin-resistant *Staphylococcus aureus* (MRSA) has steadily increased, mainly in hospitals and nursing homes, and nosocomial infections caused by such isolates have become a serious concern (87).

Methicillin resistance in *S. aureus* primarily results from the presence of the *mecA* gene, which codes for the modified penicillin-binding protein 2a (PBP2a), involved in the bacterial cell wall synthesis (17,52). The *mecA* gene is located on the chromosome. Expression of *mecA* either is constitutive or inducible by some β-lactam antibiotics (but not methicillin or oxacillin) or is heterogeneous (11).

MRSA strains are resistant against all β-lactam antibiotics, β-lactam–β-lactamase inhibitor combinations, the cephalosporins, and the carbapenems. Whatever the results of *in vitro* susceptibility tests, every MRSA strain is to be reported as resistant to all β-lactam antibiotics.

Conventional detection of methicillin resistance, however, is complicated by the fact that its phenotypic expression in many strains is heterogenous. This occurs when only a small fraction of the population tested expresses resistance though all cells may possess the *mec*A-gene (17,52,135). Also, other mechanisms may lead to low-level methicillin resistance (26).

Therefore, susceptibility test conditions have been adapted to enhance the expression of resistance, such as incubation at $\leq 35°C$, addition of NaCl to the growth medium, and prolonged incubation (9,18,51,143,166).

Several alternatives for the phenotypic detection of methicillin resistance in *S. aureus* have been developed. These include automated microdilution systems such as the Vitek GPS-SA card (BioMérieux Vitek, Hazelwood, MO) and the rapid ATB Staph system (BioMérieux, 09280 NARCY L'etoile, France). Such systems provide rapid results (77,164).

The MRSA screen test (Mastalex-MRSA, Mast Group, Bootle, England; DenkaSeiken Co., Tokyo) is a latex agglutination test (15) based on the reaction of latex particles sensitized with monoclonal antibodies against PBP2a of *S. aureus* or other staphylococci that react with PBP2a extracted from test colonies. The test is easy to perform, and results can be obtained within half an hour. The test has a sensitivity of 97% to 98.5% (166,184,187). Its specificity is 100% and is superior to that of any single phenotype-based susceptibility testing method (147).

Another commercially available fluorescence test (the BBL Crystal MRSA ID System, Becton, Dickinson, and Co., Franklin Lakes N.J.) can detect methicillin resistance in both *S. aureus* and coagulase-negative staphylococci (CoNS) within 4 hours with a sensitivity of 98.5% (61).

The limitation of all these methods is that they are phenotypic methods and their level of accuracy can be influenced by the prevalence of strains that express heterogenous resistance.

Furthermore, certain *S. aureus* strains lack the *mec*A gene but demonstrate low-level resistance to methicillin and other penicillin-related antibiotics (99,101). These strains are designated borderline methicillin-resistant *S. aureus* (BORSA) and may also be mistaken for MRSA strains using conventional methods (78). Therefore, the gold standard for the identification of MRSA is molecular detection of the *mecA* gene by a DNA hybridization assay (17) or by PCR.

PROBE TESTS

Probe tests have been available since 1989 and have been applied in dot blot assays (5,84). Recently, a more user-friendly probe test has been commercialized.

The EVIGENE MRSA detection kit (Statens Serum Institute, Copenhagen) is a molecular probe test that allows the simultaneous detection of the *mecA* gene, part of the 16Sr RNA gene of *Staphylococcus* spp and the *nuc* gene specific to *S. aureus*. The assay performed on a suspension of a colony requires 3–4 hours to complete. It has been applied to blood cultures positive for Gram-positive cocci after an additional incubation of 3 hours. The sensitivity was found to be 100% and the specificity 99.5% (83,132,162).

PCR-DIRECTED TESTS

Detection by PCR is done using either a gel-based assay already described in 1991 (80,103,134) or a more recently developed real-time assay (34,50,138,167). As other methicillin resistance–associated genes are known to exist in clinical isolates of *S. aureus* (59,104), it may be useful to apply a multiplex reaction in which a gene identifying *S. aureus* is simultaneously detected, such as the *nuc* gene (coding for nuclease) (10,50,138), the *fem* gene (79), the *coa* gene (72) or the Sa422 gene (50,138), because many CoNS may carry the *mec* gene and be methicillin resistant. Cycling probe technology is now commercially available and has also been used to detect the *mecA* gene in *S. aureus*. (10,21,39).

The increase of CoNS as a cause of bacteremia has increased the need to identify methicillin resistance in these organisms. Since many strains of CoNS are more heterogenous than *S. aureus* strains and only a few cells carry the *mecA* gene, phenotypic detection is even more problematic (60). The MRSA screen test is slightly less sensitive for the detection of PBP2a in CoNS. The test should be applied to CoNS after overnight induction with oxacillin, though detection of the *mecA* gene by an amplification reaction remains the reference standard (60).

POSSIBLE STRATEGIES FOR THE MOLECULAR DETECTION OF THE *mecA* GENE

An antibiotic susceptibility test using an oxacillin disk may reveal methicillin resistance, and multiresistance is a warning signal of possible methicillin resistance. When methicillin resistance is suspected, a MRSA screen test is performed and usually gives a definite result. Susceptibility tests based on MIC values may be used for confirmation.

Exceptionally, *S. aureus* isolates for which the MICs are between 2 and 8 μg/mL may produce very low amounts of PBP2 and contain the *mecA* resistance gene, or they may be so-called BORSAs, producing high levels of β-lactamase but not carrying the *mecA* gene. Molecular detection of the *mecA* gene will be necessary in these exceptional cases only. A number of different methods are summarized in Table 11.1. A detailed protocol used in our laboratory is also presented (adapted from Predari, 134).

TABLE 11.1

Amplification Techniques Applied for the Detection of *mecA* Gene in *Staphylococcus aureus*

Substrate	Gene(s) Detected	Extraction Method	Amplification Reaction	Detection Method	Reference
Agar grown cultures	*mecA*	Achromopeptidase	PCR	AG + H	Murakami 1991 (102)
Agar grown cultures	*mecA, femA, femB*	Achromopeptidase	PCR	AG	Kobayashi 1994 (80)
Agar grown cultures	*mecA* coa IC		Multiplex PCR		Kearns 1999 (72)
Agar grown cultures	*mecA*	Achromopeptidase	CPT	PG	Cloney 1999 (21)
Agar grown cultures	*mecA*	Achromopeptidase	CPT	EIA	Bekkaoui 1999 (10)
Agar grown cultures	*mecA*	Achromopeptidase	CPT	Strip	Fong 2000 (39)
Agar grown cultures	*mecA*, Sa422	Heating	RT-PCR	LightCycler	Reischl 2000 (138)
Blood culture	*mecA*	DNA purification capture kit	RT-PCR	LightCycler	Tan 2001 (167)
Agar grown cultures	*mecA*, Sa422	Automatic device			
			RT-PCR	LightCycler	Grisold 2001 (50)
Broth culture	*mecA, nuc*	Heating	RT-PCR	LightCycler	Fang 2003 (34)

AG, agarose gel electrophoresis; PG, polyacrylamide gel electrophoresis; IC, internal control; CPT, cycling probe technique; EIA, enzyme immunoassay; H, hybridization.

Rapid PCR may play an important role in infection control, particularly in the screening of surveillance cultures to determine appropriate isolation measures. Samples are inoculated in an enrichment broth, then plated on an Oxascreen plate. Alternatively, an aliquot of the enrichment broth may be tested by PCR for the presence of the *nuc* and *mec* genes. If the PCR is performed in a real-time format, the result may be available in less than 24 hours. The EVIGENE test is also probably suitable for this purpose and provides even more rapid results. In circumstances of low prevalence of MRSA, this test can identify MRSA-negative patients rapidly and economically (34).

PROTOCOL FOR THE DETECTION OF THE *mecA* GENE

DNA Extraction

The strain to be tested is grown overnight at 37°C on a blood agar plate. With a sterile 10-μL disposable loop, colonies are scraped from the plate. A full loop of bacteria is suspended in 150 μL sterile distilled water in a screw cap tube, vortex-mixed firmly for homogenization, and incubated for 10 minutes in boiling water. After centrifugation for 15 minutes at 13,000 rpm in an Eppendorf centrifuge, the supernatant is used for PCR. For each extraction series, a negative control—sterile distilled water subjected to the whole process of extraction without the addition of bacteria—is included.

Amplification

The sequences of the primers used for amplification of the *mecA* gene are listed in Table 11.2. For each reaction, a premix solution of 20 μL is prepared; it contains 1 μL of each of the two primer solutions at a concentration of 10 pmol/μL, 1 μL 25 mmol/L $MgCl_2$, and 17 μL sterile distilled water. A bulk premix for 100 reactions is prepared and can be stored up to one year at 4°C.

A hot start PCR reaction is set up by mixing 25 μL of HotStarTaq Master Mix containing 2.5 units of HotStarTaq DNA polymerase, 400 μmol/L of dNTP and of 2 × PCR buffer with 3 mmol/L $MgCl_2$ (Qiagen, Westburg, Netherlands), 20 μL of the premix solution (see previous paragraph), and 5 μL of DNA.

The cycling process consists of an initial incubation of 15 minutes at 95°C, 40 cycles of 30 seconds at 92°C, 30 seconds at 55°C, and 30 seconds at 72°C, followed by a final 10-minute incubation at 72°C and cooling.

For each amplication series, a negative control of the extraction (5 μL of sterile distilled water; see "DNA Extraction") and a negative control of the amplification are included. A positive control, consisting of extracted DNA from an MRSA strain, is also included.

TABLE 11.2

Primers Used for Amplification of the mecA Gene

Primer	Sequence	Reference
mecAf	5′ GGGATCATAGCGTCATTATTC 3′	1
mecAr	AACGATTGTGACACGATAGCC 3′	1

Note. For detection of the amplicons, 20 μL of the amplified material is analyzed by agarose gel electrophoresis on a 2% agarose gel in 0.089 M Tris-borate, 0.002 mol/L EDTA, containing 0.5 μg/mL ethidium bromide. The length of the amplicons is determined by comparison with a molecular weight marker (100 bp DNA step ladder, Promega Benelux BV, Netherlands) that is loaded in one of the lanes of the gel. Predari et al. (134).

DETECTION OF GENES CODING FOR GLYCOPEPTIDE RESISTANCE

Glycopeptide-resistant Enterococci

Glycopeptide resistance in enterococci has emerged as a serious clinical problem in hospitals, especially in the United States, where up to or more then 20% of enterococcal isolates are vancomycin-resistant (86,105). In Europe, the incidence remains low: 3.8% in *Enterococcus faecium* and 0.06% in *E. faecalis* (49,157).

Glycopeptide antibiotics interfere with peptidoglycan biosynthesis in Gram-positive bacteria. They are inactive against Gram-negative organisms because they cannot penetrate the outer cell-wall membrane. Glycopeptide resistance in enterococci results from the presence of an alternative pathway for cell wall precursors: the D-Ala-D-Ala termini are replaced by D-Ala-D-Lac or D-Ala-D-Ser ligases, which bind glycopeptides poorly and are coded for by *van* gene clusters. Resistance to glycopeptides is phenotypically and genotypically heterogeneous (16,105).

Eight genotypes of glycopeptide resistance have been described in enterococci; these differ in resistance level, the range of glycopeptides to which the strains are resistant, and their transferability (Table 11.3). Five are acquired (A, B, D, E, G) and three are intrinsic (C1, C2, C3). There is sequence diversity within the *vanB* genotype, with three subtypes that show some nucleotide divergence. These alleles have been designated *vanB1*, *vanB2*, and *vanB3*. They are important for the development of highly sensitive amplification tests (45).

The VanA is the most frequently encountered glycopeptide-resistant phenotype in enterococci. It is associated with inducible high-level resistance to

TABLE 11.3

Types of Glycopeptide Resistance in Entercocci

Characteristic	Phenotype				
	VanA	VanB	VanC	VanD	VanE/G
Vancomycin MIC (μg/mL)	64–>1000	4–>1000	2–32	16–64	16
Teicoplanin MIC (μg/mL)	16–512	0.5 > 32[a]	0.5 –1	2–4	0.5
Ligase gene	*vanA*	*vanB*	*vanD*	*vanE*	*vanC*
Ligase product	D-Ala-D-Lac	D-Ala-D-Lac	D-Ala-D-Lac	D-Ala-D-Ser	D-Ala-D-Ser
Most frequent enterococcoal species	*E. faecium*, *E. faecalis*	*E. faecalis*, *E. faecium*	*E. gallinarum*, *E. casseliflavus*/ *E. flavescens*	*E. faecium* *E. faecium* Acquired	*E. faecalis* *E. faecalis* Acquired
Genetic determinant	Acquired	Acquired	Intrinsic species characteristic		
Transferable	Yes	Yes	No	No	No

[a] Most *vanB*-containing isolates are susceptible to teicoplanin on testing, but the development of resistance *in vivo* and *in vitro* has been documented.

vancomycin (MIC >128μg/mL) and resistance to teicoplanin (MIC >8μg/mL). The VanB strains have variable levels of resistance to vancomycin (MIC = 4–1000 μg/mL), but most strains remain susceptible to teicoplanin (MIC = 0.5 – 1 μg/mL). They are induced by vancomycin but not by teicoplanin.

The VanC type is expressed by the *vanC1* and the *vanC2* genes specific to the species *E. gallinarum* and *E. casseliflavus* (111). *E. flavescens* and its gene *vanC3* are so closely related to *E. casseliflavus* and *vanC2* that different names are probably not warranted. VanC enterococci characterized by a lower level of resistance to only vancomycin (MIC = 2–32 μg/mL) are rarely responsible for human infections. Some strains of *E. gallinarum* and *E. casseliflavus* have been found that carry both *van*C and *van*A genes. VanD-type enterococci are resistant to variable levels of vancomycin (MIC = 16–64 μg/mL) and teicoplanin (MIC = 2–4 μg/mL). Only a few such strains have been found (119,126). The VanE and VanG types are characterised by a low level of inducible resistance to vancomycin (MIC = 16 μg/mL) and susceptibility to teicoplanin (MIC = 0.5 μg/mL). The VanE type has been detected in one strain of *E. faecalis* only and the VanG type in four isolates of *E. faecalis* (37,93).

VanA is the most widespread resistance gene and has been detected in a large variety of enterococcal species (45,106), whereas *vanB* is generally limited to *E. faecalis* and *E. faecium* (45,105). Most outbreaks of infection or colonization of glycopeptide-resistant enterococci in hospitals involve the *vanA* type (41). Most glycopeptide-resistant *Enterococcus* strains are *E. faecium* strains, whereas *E. faecalis* strains most often cause infections (104).

The *vanA* and *vanB* gene clusters are carried on transposons of the 1546 family (45,105), the latter being part of a larger element carrying PBP5 (penicillin-binding protein) and mediating high-level penicillin resistance. This is particularly the case for *E. faecium* (in more than 60% of the strains).

High-level aminoglycoside resistance mediated by aminoglycoside-modifying enzymes has been found in up to 50% of enterococcal isolates (67). Resistance to virtually all other antibiotics may result from chromosomal mutations.

Spread of vancomycin resistance may occur either by clonal dissemination of resistant strains or by dissemination of plasmids or transposons to different clones (16).

VanA and *vanB* gene clusters also are transferable to several other Gram-positive species, such as *Streptococcus bovis*, and experimentally to *S. aureus* (113, 126,133).

Human infections caused by vancomycin-resistant Gram-positive bacteria other than enterococci—for example, coagulase-negative staphylococci, streptococci, and some aerobic and anaerobic Gram-positive rods—have been described in immunosuppressed patients (123).

At present, gastrointestinal colonization by vancomycin-resistant enterococci (VRE) appears to be the major form of infection by these organisms (16).

Possible Strategies for the Molecular Detection of *van* Genes

Early detection of infections by VRE in the hospital is essential.

Culture based-detection methods for VRE take 2–5 days to complete and do not clearly distinguish the different Van phenotypes.

High-level VanA-mediated glycopeptide resistance can be detected easily. However, low-level VanB- and VanC-mediated resistance, often inducible, may be difficult to detect by phenotypic procedures or by the use of automated equipment (66,172).

The agar screening test on brain-heart infusion agar containing 6 μg/mL of vancomycin is a simple, sensitive, and reliable test for the detection of vancomycin resistance. The disk diffusion method allows accurate detection of vancomycin resistance if the plates are read under strong transmitted light. The Etest is an accurate alternative. All tests, including MIC determinations by macro or micro techniques, require incubation for a full 24 hours. Some of the fully automatic methods are unreliable, especially in detecting VRE isolates containing the *van*B resistance determinant (33). Testing isolates for susceptibility to teicoplanin by the disk diffusion method will differentiate between *vanA* (teicoplanin-R) and *vanB* (teicoplanin-S) in most instances, although exceptions have been reported (16).

PCR assays designed to detect the genes responsible for glycopeptide resistance are the most specific and are preferably applied to all clinical isolates expressing low-level resistance.

In hospitals with a high prevalence of glycopeptide-resistant enterococci, screening programs may be implemented: when based on culture detection methods, these are too slow to allow the rapid application of adequate control measures. The advent of real-time PCR technology offers the possibility of an early yes or no answer concerning the presence of VRE. Surveillance cultures may be done by spreading an aliquot of a broth enrichment culture (enterococcosel broth with 6 mg/mL vancomycin) on a vancomycin agar screen plate, followed by amplification of the *vanA*, *vanB*, and *vanC* genes of suspected colonies in a multiplex PCR or in separate amplification reactions (62). Both gel-based and real-time formats are available. A more rapid strategy involves gene amplification, preferably in a real-time format, of the enrichment broth after 15–18 hours of incubation. Amplification of stool samples results in frequent inhibition of the reaction. The combination of incubation in enrichment broth followed by amplification tests is optimal in terms of sensitivity and speed (122).

Several protocols for the detection and identification of *van* genes in entercocci have been developed, and some include the detection of a species-specific gene for the identification of *E. faecalis* or *E. faecium* (*ddl* genes) or a genus-specific gene, (*tuf*). These additional gene targets are particularly useful when surveillance enrichment cultures are tested to ensure that the *van* genes detected are associated with enterococci or at least with some enterococcal species.

A number of different methods are summarized in Table 11.4. A detailed protocol used in our laboratory is also included.

All described protocols have been evaluated on known susceptible and resistant enterococcal strains and/or on clinical specimens in comparison with *in vitro* susceptibility tests.

A cycling probe assay has also been applied to the detection of *vanA* and *vanB* genes in enterococci (98).

The only study in which different amplification protocols were compared with each other involved a comparison of multiplex real-time amplification and gel-based PCR (121).

Glycopeptide-resistant *Staphylococcus aureus*

Some isolates of *S. aureus* show an intermediate resistance to vancomycin (MIC = 8–16 μg/mL). They are sometimes referred to as VISA (vancomycin intermediate *S. aureus*) or GISA (glycopeptide intermediate *S. aureus*) (171). The mechanism of resistance is related to alterations in the cell wall metabolism for which no genetic determinant has yet been identified. Genotypic detection of VISA isolates therefore is not yet practical. However, two vancomycin-resistant isolates carrying the *van*A gene identical to that present in *E. faecium* from the same patient have been cultured. The MIC for vancomycin of this isolate is >2 μg/mL.The *vanA* gene is detected by a PCR identical to that applied to enterococci (48).

PROTOCOL FOR THE DETECTION OF *vanA*, *vanB*, *vanC1*, AND *vanC2* GENES

DNA Extraction

The strain to be tested is grown overnight at 37°C on a blood agar plate. With a sterile 10-μL disposable loop, colonies are scraped from the plate. A full loop of bacteria is suspended in 150 μL of sterile distilled water in a screw cap tube, vortex-mixed firmly for homogenization, and maintained for 10 minutes in boiling water. After centrifugation for 15 minutes at 13,000 rpm in an Eppendorf centrifuge, the supernatant is used for PCR. For each extraction series, a negative control—sterile distilled water subjected to the whole process of extraction without the addition of bacteria—is included.

TABLE 11.4

Amplification Techniques Applied for the Simultaneous Detection of Different Glycopeptide Resistance Genes

Substrate	Genes Detected	Extraction Method	Amplification Reaction	Detection	Reference
Agar grown cultures	*vanA, vanB, vanC*	10′ 95°	PCR	AG/H	Clark 1993 (20)
Agar grown cultures	*vanA, vanB, vanC1, vanC2/C3* ddl *E. faecium* ddl *E. faecalis*	Lysozyme	Single and multiplex PCR	AG	Dutka-Malen 1995 (30)
Rectal swabs Enrichment broth Agar grown cultures	*vanA, vanB, vanC1, vanC2* ddl *E. faecium* ddl *E. faecalis*	Proteinase K	Multiplex PCR Multiplex PCR	AG	Satake 1997 (153)
		Satake 1997 (153)			
Rectal swabs Stool specimens	*vanA, vanB*	XTRAX	Multiplex PCR	EIA	Petrich 1999 (127)
Agar grown cultures	*vanA, vanB, vanC2/C3 ddl E. faecalis ddl E. faecium* 22s 16SrRNA	Chelex	Multiplex PCR	AG	Kariyama 2000 (70)
Agar grown cultures	*vanA, vanB ddl E. faecalis ddl E. faecium vanC1, vanC2/C3*		Multiplex PCR Multiplex PCR	AG 16S rRNA sequencing	Angeletti 2001 (4)
Agar grown cultures	*vanA, vanB, vanC1, vanC2/C3 tuf*	Boiling	Multiplex PCR	AG	Perez-Hernandez 2002 (125)
Agar grown cultures	*vanA, B*	Chelex	Multiplex RT-PCR		Palladino 2003 (121)

Amplification

The sequences of the primers used for *vanA, vanB, vanC1,* and *vanC2* are listed in Table 11.5.

Premix solutions are made for a duplex amplification of *vanA* and *vanB* genes, on the one hand, and a duplex amplification of *vanC1* and *vanC2* genes, on the other hand. These 20-μL premix solutions contain 1 μL of each of the 4 primer solutions at a concentration of 10 pmol/μL, 1 μL of 25 mmol/L $MgCl_2$, and 15 μL sterile distilled water. A bulk premix for 100 reactions is prepared and can be stored up to one year at 4°C.

A hot start PCR reaction is set up by mixing 25 μL of HotStarTaq Master Mix containing 2.5 units of HotStarTaq DNA polymerase, 400 μmol/L of dNTP and of 2 × PCR buffer with 3 mmol/L $MgCl_2$ (Qiagen), 20 μL of premix solution (see Table 11.4), and 5 μL of DNA.

The cycling process consists of an initial incubation of 15 minutes at 95°C, 40 cycles of 30 seconds at 92°C, 30 seconds at 55°C, and 30 seconds at 72°C, followed by a final 10-minute incubation at 72°C and cooling.

For each amplification series, a negative control of the extraction (5 μL of sterile distilled water) and a negative control of the amplification are included.

For *vanA-vanB* duplex PCR, a positive control for *vanA* (extracted DNA of *E. faecium* strain IOWA1) and a positive control for *vanB* (extracted DNA of *E. faecium* strain IOWA2) are included. For *vanC1-vanC2* duplex PCR, a positive control for *vanC1* (extracted DNA *from E. gallinarum*) and a positive control for *vanC2* (extracted DNA from *E. casselliflavus*) are included.

Detection of Macrolide, Lincosamide, and Streptogramin B (MLS_B) Resistance Genes

Macrolides are composed of 14-membered lactones (erythromycin and clarithromycin), 15-membered lactones (azithromycin), and 16-membered lactones (josamycin, spiramycin, and tylosin), to which are attached amino and/or neutral sugars via glycosidic bonds.

Macrolides act by blocking protein synthesis on assembled and functioning 50S rRNA subunits and by inhibiting the assembly of new 50S ribosomal subunits.

TABLE 11.5

Primers Used for Amplification of *vanA*, *vanB*, *vanC1* and *vanC2* Genes

Primer	Sequence	Reference
vanAf	5′ CATGAATAGAATAAAAGTTGCAATA 3′	1
vanAr	5′ CCCCTTTAACGCTAATACGATCAA 3′	1
vanBf	5′GTGACAAACCGGAGGCGAGGA 3′	1
vanBr	5′ CCGCCATCCTCCTGCAAAAAA 3′	1
vanC1f	5′ GAAAGACAACAGGAAGACCGC 3′	1
vanC1r	5′ ATCGCATCACAAGCACCAATC 3′	1
vanC2f	5′ CTCCTACGATTCTCTTG 3′	2
vanC2r	5′ CGAGCAAGACCTTTAAG 3′	2

Note. For detection of the amplicons, 20 μL of the amplified material is analyzed by agarose gel electrophoresis on a 2% agarose gel in 0.089 mol/L Tris-borate, 0.002 mol/L EDTA, containing 0.5 μg/mL ethidium bromide. The length of the amplicons is determined by comparison with a molecular weight marker (100 bp DNA step ladder, Promega Benelux BV, The Netherlands) that is loaded in one of the lanes of the gel.
Adapted from Clark et al. (20) and Dutka-Malen et al. (30).

Macrolide resistance is clinically most important in *S. pneumoniae* and *S. pyogenes* and secondarily in *S. aureus* and *H. pylori*.

Gram-positive and Gram-negative Cocci

Three different mechanisms of macrolide resistance are known: (a) target-site alteration, (b) efflux of the antibiotic, and (c) antibiotic inactivation. Four different phenotypes with resistance to macrolides (M), lincosamides (L), and streptogramins type B (S_B) have been reported: MLS_B, L, MS_B, and M. Phenotype L is due to lincosamide inactivation (*lnu* gene) (82,124).

The most widespread mechanism of macrolide resistance is methylation- or mutation-caused target-site modification preventing the binding of the antibiotics to the ribosomal target (192). Since the binding site in the 50S ribosomal subunit for erythromycin overlaps the binding site of the newer macrolides as well as the structurally unrelated lincosamides (lincomycin, clindamycin) and streptogramin Bs (pristinamycin IA, virginiamycin S) antibiotics, ribosomal modification reduces the binding of all three classes of antibiotics, which results in resistance against macrolide, lincosamide, and streptogramin B antibiotics (MLS_B). Methylation of the ribosomal target is mediated by methylases encoded by a variety of *erm* (*e*rythromycin *r*ibosome *m*ethylase) genes that are borne on transposons and plasmids and tend to be relatively specific, though not strictly confined to a bacterial genus. A nomenclature system for the *erm* genes proposed by Roberts et al. (142) distinguishes 21 types, of which the most frequently found are *ermA, ermB, ermC,* and *ermF. Erm*-mediated resistance resulting in the MLS_B phenotype could either be inducibly or constitutively expressed (Table 11.6). For instance, the *ermA* and *ermC* genes found predominantly in staphylococci (*ermA* in MRSA and in coagulase-negative staphylococci, *ermC* in methicillin-sensitive *S.aureus* [85,165]) confer the MLS_B inducible phenotype, which demonstrates resistance to the "inducers" i.e., the 14- and 15-membered macrolides) and susceptibility to the 16-membered macrolides, lincosamides, and streptogramin Bs. Susceptibility to the latter three groups, however, might be compromised in the presence of the inducers. The *ermB* and *ermTR* genes, which from a subset of *ermA* (158) genes, predominantly mediate macrolide resistance in streptococci (*S. pyogenes* and *S. pneumoniae*) (35) and enterococci. Although both genes can code for the MLS_B inducible phenotype and give rise to a variety of phenotypes—high- or low-level erythromycin resistance with susceptibility or resistance to clindamycin—*ermB* is also associated with the MLS_B constitutive phenotype, which demonstrates high-level resistance to macrolides, lincosamides, and streptogramin Bs. *Listeria monocytogenes* and other *Listeria* species may carry *ermC* genes (139), and the *ermF* gene has been found in *Treponema denticola* (140). Various *erm* genes have been found in *Neisseria gonorrhoeae,* such as *ermB* and *ermF,* and in some strains two or even three different *erm* genes are present simultaneously (141).

Note, however, that erythromycin resistance in *N. gonorrhoeae* strains has also been found to result from mutations in the target site in the V domain of the 23S rRNA (112,141).

Mutations are also found in Gram-positive cocci. These mutations are studied only in research settings.

Antibiotic efflux is the second mechanism of macrolide resistance. In staphylococci, efflux is caused by the presence of *msrA* or *msrB* genes specific to 14- and 15-membered macrolides and type B streptogramins, resulting in an MS_B phenotype. The *msr* genes are not found in streptococci. The *mefA* gene in *S. pyogenes* and in enterococci and the *mefE* gene in *S. pneumoniae* encode the efflux pump affecting only 14- and 15-membered macrolides, resulting in an M phenotype. The genetic determinants for the macrolide efflux system are present on mobile genetic elements (82,151,152). A combination of several resistance-coding genes may sometimes be found.

Unlike target modification and efflux, the mechanism of antibiotic inactivation confers resistance on structurally related antibiotics only. This mechanism is not considered clinically important yet, as among Gram-positive organisms only a few strains of *S. aureus* have been found to produce inactivating enzymes, such as esterases (encoded by an *ere*-like gene ([195]), phosphotransferases (encoded by *mph* genes), nucleotidyltransferases (14), and

TABLE 11.6

Phenotypes and Genotypes of Macrolide Resistance Determinants in Gram-positive Cocci[a]

Species	Gene Class	Mechanism	Phenotype Designation	Phenotype of Resistance		
				14-, 15-M	16-M	Cli
Staphylococcus spp	*erm*	Target methylation	MLS_B inducible	R	s	s
			MLS_B constitutive	R	R	R
	msr(A)	Efflux	MS_B	R	S	S
	lnu(A)	Lincosamide inactivation	L	S	S[b]	S
Streptococcus spp and	*erm*(A)	Target methylation	MLS_B inducible	R/I	R/I/s	R/I/s
			MLS_B constitutive	R	R	R
Enterococcus spp	*mef*(A)	Efflux	M	R/I	S	S
Enterococcus faecium	*lnu*(B)	Lincosamide inactivation	L	S	S[b]	S

Cli, clindamycin; 14-, 15-M, 14- and 15-membered rings; I, intermediate; L, lincosamides; MLS_B, macrolides, lincosamides, and streptogramins B; MS_B, macrolides, streptogramins B; R, resistant; S, susceptible; s, susceptible *in vitro*, but risk of selection of constitutive mutants *in vivo*; 16-M, 16-membered ring.

[a] Adapted from Leclercq (82).

[b] Diminished bactericidal activity.

streptogramin B hydrolases (encoded by the *sbh* or *vga* gene ([3,53]), that elicit resistance to any macrolide, lincosamide, streptogramin B antibiotic.

Thus, from the clinical point of view, the *erm* and *mef* genes are the most important macrolide resistance mechanisms in streptococci, though the prevalence of these genes exhibits considerable variation geographically (71). Erythromycin resistance induced by *erm* genes is higher (MIC > 128 mg/mL) than that induced by the *mef* gene (MIC = 2–16 mg/mL), but because differences in MIC are not always easy to determine, only gene amplification is an accurate method of identifying the genes that are present.

Helicobacter pylori

In *H. pylori,* resistance to clarithromycin is the most important type of macrolide resistance because this antibiotic is the key component of many combination therapies used to eradicate *H. pylori* and because resistance to it is the most significant cause of treatment failure (57). Macrolide resistance results from the lack of binding of macrolides to the 23S rRNA components of the bacterial ribosome due to point mutations in the peptidyltransferase region (2,40,92,129,189). The small number of mutations described (six) allows molecular detection of resistance by PCR (182). Several protocols have been published, but Lascols et al. (81) propose a LightCycler PCR to detect *H. pylori* and clarithromycin resistance mutations simultaneously in gastric biopsy specimens.

The same mutations are also possible in *Mycobacterium avium-intracellulare* (94,109).

Possible Strategies for the Molecular Detection of MLS Resistance

Molecular methods for the detection of MLS_B resistance genes are not routinely used for diagnostic purposes and instead are restricted mainly to epidemiological and research studies. The main exception is the detection of point mutations in the 23S rRNA of *H. pylori* that result in macrolide resistance. A number of different protocols are summarized in Table 11.7.

PCR detection of resistance genes in staphylococci is mostly done by multiplex reactions targeted at *ermA, ermC, msrA,* and *msrB*. In *S. pyogenes*, the targets are the *ermB, ermTR,* and *mefA* genes; in *S. pneumoniae,* the *ermA, ermTR,* and *mefE* genes. Conserved primers for the simultaneous amplification of several classes of the *erm* gene are available (8,165).

Rapid detection of macrolide resistance in *H. pylori* may be clinically important for treatment-resistant or

TABLE 11.7

Amplification Techniques for the Detection of Macrolide and Lincosamide Resistance Genes

Substrate	Genes Detected	Extraction Method	Amplification Technique	Selection Method	Reference
Agar grown cultures	*ermA, ermB, ermC, msr ereA, ereB, mphA, mef*		Multiplex PCR Multiplex PCR followed by single if necessary	AG AG	Sutcliffe 1996 (165)
Agar grown cultures	*ermA, ermAH, ermC, msrA, msrB, ereA, ereB*	Heat	PCR	AG	Shortridge 1996 (161)
Agar grown cultures	*ermA, ermB, ermC erm TR, mefA/E*	Intragene matrix system	single PCR	AG + H	Portillo 1999 (131)
Agar grown cultures	23S rRNA	Q/Amp tissue kit	PCR	AG/RFLP	Matsuoka 1999 (92)
Agar grown cultures	*ermA, ermB, ermC, ermTR, mefA ermB, mefA,* 16S rRNA *ermA, ermC,* 16S rRNA *ermA, ermTR,* 16S sRNA	Lysostaphyin	Multiplex PCR Multiplex PCR I Multiplex PCR II Multiplex PCR III	H/EIA	Farrell 2001 (35)
Agar grown *H. pylori*	23S rRNA	Phenol-chloroform	PCR	AG and RFLP	Occhiliani 1997 (116)
Agar grown *H. pylori*	23S rRNA	Phenol-chloroform	PCR	AG/H	Pina 1998 (129)
Agar grown *H. pylori*	23S rRNA	Cetyltrimethyl, ammonium bromide	RT-PCR	LightCycler	Gibson 1999 (46)
Agar grown *H. pylori*	23S rRNA	Proteinase K	PCR	Line probe H	Van Doorn 1999 (182)
Gastric biopsies	23S rRNA	Proteinase K	RT-PCR	LightCycler	Chisholm 2001 (19)
Gastic biopsy *H. pylori*	23S rRNA	Q/Amp	RT-PCR	LightCycler	Oleastro 2003 (117)

AG, agarose gel electrophoresis; H, hybridization.

relapsing peptic ulcer cases. Detection of clarithromycin resistance in *H. pylori* isolates can be done by amplification of a 23S rRNA gene fragment encompassing the frequently mutated sites, followed by hybridization with corresponding probes (129) or by sequencing of the amplicons (92).

The mutations responsible for clarithromycin resistance have also been detected by PCR followed by a line probe (reverse hybridization) assay (183) or by real-time amplification and thermal analysis of a fragment of the 23S rRNA (46,117,145). To produce results more rapidly, PCR, either conventional (91) or real-time, can be applied to gastric biopsy specimens (19), or *H. pylori* and its resistance mutations can be simultaneously detected by a real-time procedure (117).

The same techniques can be applied to *Mycobacterium avium-intracellulare* (94,109).

PROTOCOL FOR THE DETECTION OF THE MACROLIDE RESISTANCE GENES

DNA extraction

The strain to be tested is grown overnight at 37°C on a blood agar plate, and genomic DNA is extracted by the alkaline lysis method. With a sterile disposable loop, 4 to 5 colonies are suspended in 20 μL lysis buffer (0.25% sodium dodecyl sulfate, 0.05 N NaOH) and heated at 95°C for 5 minutes. After centrifugation for 1 minute at 13,000 rpm in an Eppendorf centrifuge, 180 μL of dd H_2O are added to resuspend the clot, and the suspension is used to perform PCR. For each extraction series, a negative control—lysis buffer subject to the whole process of extraction without the addition of bacteria—is included. The bacterial DNA extraction is confirmed by performing a PCR for housekeeping genes (e.g., the 16S rRNA or *gyrA* gene).

Amplification

The sequences of the primers used for amplification of the *ermA*, *ermB*, and *mefA* genes are listed in Table 11.8.

For the *ermB* and *mefA* genes, amplification is performed in 50 μL of solution containing 50 mmol/L KCl, 10 mmol/L Tris-HCl (pH 9.0), 2.5 mmol/L $MgCl_2$, 0.1% Triton X-100, 0.01% gelatin, 200 μmol/L deoxynucleoside triphosphates, 100 pmol of both primers, 0.45 U SuperTaq polymerase (Enzyme Technologies Ltd, UK), and 2 μL template DNA. The PCR cycling process comprises an initial cycle consisting of 3 minutes of denaturation at 93°C; followed by 35 cycles consisting of 1 minute of denaturation at 93°C, 1 minute of annealing at 52°C, and 1 minute of elongation at 72°C; followed by 1 cycle consisting of 5 minutes of elongation at 72°C (3).

For the *ermA* gene, amplification is performed in 50 μL of solution containing 50 mmol/L KCl, 10 mmol/L Tris-HCl (pH 9.0), 0.1% Triton X-100, 0.01% gelatin, 200 μmol/L dNTPs, 1.5 mmol/L $MgCl_2$, 20 pmol of each primer, 0.45 U SuperTaq polymerase (Enzyme Technologies Ltd, UK), and 2 μL template DNA. The PCR cycling process comprises an initial cycle consisting of 5 minutes of denaturation at 94°C; 35 cycles consisting of 30 seconds of denaturation at 90°C, 60 seconds of annealing at 60°C, and 90 seconds of extension at 72°C; followed by 1 cycle consisting of 5 minutes of extension at 72°C (1). Please see also chapter 5, Antimycobacterial Agents.

TABLE 11.8

Primers Used for Amplification of the *erm*(A), *erm*(B), and *mef*(A/E) Genes

Primer	Sequence	Reference
erm(A)Fw	5′ CCCGAAAAATACGCAAAATTTCAT 3′	1
erm(A)Rev	5′ CCCTGT TTACCCATTTATAAACG 3′	1
erm(B)Fw	5′ GAAAAGGTACTCAACCAAATA 3′	2
erm(B)Rev	5′ AGTAACGGTACTTAAATTGTTTAC 3′	2
mef(A/E)Fw	5′ AGTATCATTAATCACTAGTGC 3′	2
mef(A/E)Rev	5′ TTCTTCTGGTACTAAAAGTGG 3′	2

Note. After amplification, the amplicon is mixed with 20 μL loading buffer (50% glycerol, bromophenol blue 0.8 mg/mL), 30 μL of which is electrophoresed in a 1.5% Pronarose D1 gel (Sphaero Q, Burgos, Spain) for 1 hour at 150 V in 0.5 x TBE (45 mmol/L Tris–HCl, 45 mmol/L boric acid, 1 mmol/L EDTA) containing ethidium bromide 0.05 mg/L. Visualization and image acquisition are carried out using the Gel Doc 1000 documentation system (Bio-Rad Laboratories, Nazareth, Belgium) (3).
Descheemaeker et al. (28), Malhotra-Kumar et al. (90), and Sutcliffe et al. (165).

DETECTION OF RIFAMPIN RESISTANCE IN *MYCOBACTERIUM TUBERCULOSIS*

Rifampin and isoniazid are the key components of tuberculosis treatment regimens. The detection of resistance against these drugs is therefore crucial. All susceptibility tests for *Mycobacterium tuberculosis* are dependent on its long generation time (about 24 hours). This prolongs the time required for its detection by culture as well as for the susceptibility tests. Although the susceptibility tests have been thoroughly validated, they require an incubation time of 10 to 30 days, depending on whether a solid or liquid medium is used. Thus the importance of molecular tests for the detection of drug resistance in *M. tuberculosis*, for they hold the promise of delivering results significantly more rapidly. Rifampin binds to the β subunit of the DNA-dependent RNA polymerase coded for by the *rpoB* gene, resulting in inhibition of transcription and cell death. Specific mutations in the *rpoB* gene apparently diminish rifampin binding on the RNA polymerase. More than 95% of rifampin-resistant *M. tuberculosis* strains are associated with mutations within a 81-bp core region of the *rpoB* gene (69, 170). Exceptionally, mutations are located at other codons (54,55). The resistance mechanism for the small proportion ($\pm$4%) of rifampin-resistant strains remains unknown (69,100,106,170,194). Some mutations do not result in rifampin-resistant (so-called silent mutations) but are responsible for a possible discrepancy between the detection of an undefined mutation by a molecular genetic test and the phenotypic susceptibility of the strain (73).

Molecular detection of isoniazid resistance is not straightforward because neither the bacterial target nor the mode of action is well understood (106,163). Mutations associated with isoniazid resistance are located at widely separated regions of the *M. tuberculosis* genome (128). Mutations in a relatively large number of genes have been associated with isoniazid resistance: *katG, inhA, kasA*, and *ahpC* (137,163). Isoniazid resistance is most frequently associated with mutations in *katG* (50% to 60%), though the mechanism of isoniazid resistance in some strains remains to be determined (137).

M. tuberculosis strains resistant to isoniazid and rifampin are known as multidrug-resistant (MDR) strains. Rifampin resistance can be used as a marker for isoniazid resistance, as most rifampin resistance develops in patients whose bacteria previously developed isoniazid resistance. Monoresistance to isoniazid is observed whereas monoresistance to rifampin is extremely rare. Isoniazid monoresistance has also less therapeutic consequences than rifampin monoresistance.

The great majority of rifampin susceptibility assays are performed on subcultures of isolates from clinical specimens; only a few assays can presently be performed on clinical specimens without a primary culture. This is because commensal bacteria in clinical specimens may harbor a *rpoB* region coding for rifampin (74), particularly nontuberculous mycobacteria (193). Specimens containing a pure culture of *M. tuberculosis,* if sufficiently rich in bacteria, can be genotypically tested for rifampin resistance without prior cultivation; examples include cerebrospinal fluid (154), as well as "rapid" cultures in liquid medium. Identification of the strain under investigation may be obtained by amplification of the *M. tuberculosis*–specific insertion fragment IS6110 in a separate PCR or amplification of *hsp65* (68).

All genotypic assays depend on the amplification of the mutation prone 816bp segment of the *rpoB* gene.The diversity stems from the procedures used to identify the mutant amplicons. There is no evidence in *M. tuberculosis* of extra chromosomal resistance determinants.

The gold standard for rifampin resistance detection is DNA sequencing. Although automatic sequencers are increasingly available, they are not routinely used in diagnostic microbiology laboratories.

The first assays used in practice were based on SSCP (single-strand conformation polymorphism) (69,169,194). This technique does not give any information concerning the type of mutation or silent mutations being detected as well (73). It is inexpensive, relatively quick, and does not require complex devices, but not all nucleotidic changes are well detected, and in certain cases interpretation is difficult (43).

In an effort to apply the SSCP method directly to clinical samples, Whelen et al. (193), Felmlee et al. (36), and Scarpellini et al. (154) developed modifications of the original assay, but their versions have not gained general acceptance. Kim et al. (74), to apply the assay directly to sputum specimens, proposed a nested format in which a *rpoB* sequence specific to *M. tuberculosis* was amplified in the second reaction.

Hybridization-based techniques have found a wide application. The INNO-LiPA test, developed by Innogenetics, Ghent, Belgium (in US, Innogenetics, Alpharetta, GA), employs strips in which a set of ten oligonucleotide probes have been immobilized: five of these are homologous with five subregions that together make up the *rpoB* region, four are homologous with frequent rifampin resistance mutations, and the tenth is an amplification control for *M. tuberculosis* complex. The *rpoB* region of the strain under examination is amplified by PCR with biotin-labeled primers, and the amplicons are hybridized under stringent conditions with the probes on the strip. If any of the five probes homologous with the wild-type sequences fail to hybrdize, a mutation is suspected. If any of the probes homologous with a mutation gives a positive hybridization signal, it is possible to specify the mutation type. The application of INNO-LiPA test to clinical isolates shows excellent correlation with DNA sequencing: only 2% to 4% discrepancies were noted (27,56,144,191).

Several real-time PCR assays for the detection of rifampin resistance have been developed. Some of these have been applied to a moderate number of samples, others are still to be considered experimental. The procedures for detecting the mutations are different in the assays described. Most assays are designed to detect rifampin resistance and isoniazid resistance simultaneously; however, as mentioned earlier, there is less need for the detection of both resistance determinants in the clinical laboratory. The assays could be limited to the detection of rifampin resistance only.

In the assay described by Torres et al. (175), the principle is to use two labeled hybridization probes that recognize adjacent sequences in the amplicon in the reaction mixture. The shorter detection probe covers the predicted mutation site, and the longer probe produces the fluorescent signal. After annealing, the fluorophores are in close proximity and fluoresce, providing the real-time monitoring. After completion of the PCR, the temperature is increased, and fluorescence is used to monitor the melting temperature of the probe-amplicon duplexes, each genotype producing a characteristic melting profile.

Piatek et al. (128) used molecular beacons to achieve simultaneous detection of rifampin and isoniazid resistance. The assay is performed in a multiwell plate using several primer sets for isoniazid determinants and for *rpoB*; added to each well is a primer set for the amplification of part of the 16S rRNA gene of *M. tuberculosis.* Molecular beacons are designed to hybridize to targets not affected by resistance mutations, drug resistance being indicated by the absence of a fluorescence signal (but in the presence of a positive fluorescence for *M. tuberculosis*). Five molecular beacons were used to hybridize to a single *rpoB* amplicon spanning the entire region. The sensitivity of the assay for rifampin resistance was 98% on 149 isolates with a high prevalence of rifampin resistance. The assay can be completed in 3 hours. This assay could also be performed for rifampin resistance only.

El-Hajj et al. (32) performed PCR in a single tube, adding five different molecular beacons, each complementary to a different wild-type sequence of the entire *rpoB* gene and labeled with a differently colored fluorophore. The presence of any mutation in the amplicon prevents binding of one of the molecular beacons, resulting in the absence of one of the five fluorescent colors.The sensitivity of the assay was 96.9% on 148 isolates, of which 65 were rifampin-resistant. The assay could also be performed on smear-positive sputum samples.

Garcia (43) performed isoniazid and rifampin resistance detection in a single tube using fluorescence resonance energy transfer (FRET) probes in the LightCycler instrument. Two adjacent pairs of dual-sensor FRET probes were designed to cover the entire *rpoB* region. The detection of mutations is based on the differential patterns of denaturation of the probes bound to either homologous sequences or to sequences with a mutation. There was 100% agreement with sequencing data on 33 rifampin-resistant strains. No mention is made of the application of the assay to sputum specimens.

Edwards et al. (31) used fluorescent-labeled biprobes that fluoresce when bound to double-stranded DNA. Determination of the melting curves can detect the presence of mutations. There is as yet no large-scale evaluation of this assay.

The latest development is the micoarray technique. Sets of oligonucleotides of different lengths, each one corresponding to a different variant of the *rpoB* mutations, are immobilized on a glass substrate. The *rpoB* region from the analysis strain is amplified, fluorecent-labeled during PCR, and hybridized to the microarray oligonucleotides. Fluoresence is higher for the homologous amplicons, and relative fluorescence intensity between the different positions in the microarray defines the pattern of mutations. The procedure remains to be validated (95,176).

POSSIBLE STRATEGIES FOR THE MOLECULAR DETECTION OF RESISTANCE IN *MYCOBACTERIUM TUBERCULOSIS*

In testing for *M. tuberculosis*, the need to shorten the time between submission of a clinical specimen—typically a sputum specimen– and delivery of the result has been answered by growing cultures in liquid media rather than on solid media and in some cases by the application of nucleic acid amplification tests. The Centers for Disease Control produced a recommendation for the application of nucleic acid amplfication tests for the detection of *M. tuberculosis* (1).

Rifampin susceptibility tests should be performed for patients who had tuberculosis in the past, patients who recently came from or recently traveled to areas with a known high prevalence of drug-resistant tuberculosis, and patients who are failing to respond to therapy or have contact with a known drug-resistant patient.

All molecular susceptibility assays depend on a preliminary PCR, and therefore, if applicable to clinical specimens, they are limited to smear positive specimens because of the lack of sensitivity of nucleic amplifications performed on smear negative clinical samples. A number of possible protocols are summarized in Table 11.9.

The INNO-LiPA test is particularly suited for smaller laboratories because it does not require special apparatus, but it is rather expensive (approximately $20 per test). The SSCP-based test, which is not applicable to sputum specimens, will certainly be replaced by real-time tests except in those laboratories that do not have the necessary equipment. Such tests remain to be validated.

DETECTION AND IDENTIFICATION OF GENES CODING FOR EXTENDED-SPECTRUM β-LACTAMASES

The first plasmid-mediated β-lactamase in Gram-negative organisms, TEM-1, was described in 1965 (24). Within a few years of its first isolation, TEM-1 spread worldwide in *enterobacteria, Haemophilus influenzae, N. gonorrhoeae,* and *Pseudomonas aeruginosa.* TEM-1 is able to hydrolyze penicillins and the early cephalosporins, such as cephalothin and cephaloridine. Another common plasmid-mediated β-lactamase found in *Klebsiella pneumoniae* and *Escherichia coli* is SHV-1, chromosomally encoded in the majority of *K. pneumoniae* isolates but plasmid-mediated in *E. coli.* The widespread occurrence of plasmid-mediated β-lactamases was therapeutically resolved by the introduction of new β-lactam antibiotics and broad-spectrum cephalosporins, such as cefotaxime and the monobactams, designed to be resistant to the action of β-lactamases. However, Gram-negative bacteria quickly acquired resistance to these expanded-spectrum β-lactam antibiotics by acquisition of new plasmid-encoded β-lactamases. The first enzyme capable of hydrolyzing the newer β-lactams, SHV-2, was isolated in 1985 in Germany. Because of its increased spectrum of activity, this enzyme was called extended-spectrum β-lactamase (ESBL). Mutations in TEM-1 gave rise to TEM-2 and TEM-3. TEM-3, originally reported in 1989, was the first TEM-type β-lactamase that displayed the ESBL phenotype (13).

With few exceptions, the majority of ESBLs are derived from either the TEM family or the SHV family of β-lactamases. They are located on plasmids and are usually found in *enterobacteria.* Although TEM-type β-lactamases are most often found in *E. coli* and *K. pneumoniae,* they are also found in other species of Gram-negative bacteria, and with increasing frequency (13).

TABLE 11.9

Amplification Techniques for the Detection of RMP and RMP-INH Resistance Determinants in *Mycobacterium tuberculosis*

Substrate	Target	Extraction	Amplification	Detection	Reference
Sputum	*rpoB*	Bead-beat	PCR	AG and SSCP	Telenti 1993 (169)
Cultures	*rpoB*	Bead-beat	PCR	Sequencing	Kapur 1994 (69)
Cultures	*rpoB*	Freeze-thawing	PCR	SSCP, sequencing	Williams 1994 (194)
Cultures, sputum	*rpoB*	Bead-beat/boiling	Heminested, single-tube PCR	AG/H and SSCP	Whelen 1995 (193)
Cultures, specimens	*rpoB*	Bead-beat/boiling	Heminested, single-tube PCR	SSCP, sequencing	Felmlee 1995 (36)
Cultures	*rpoB, katG, ahpC, inhA*	Boiling	PCR	SSCP	Telenti 1997 (168)
CSF, culture	*rpoB*	Boom	PCR	AG and SSCP, sequencing	Scarpellini 1997 (154)
Cultures	*rpoB*	Heat	PCR	Strip, reverse hybridization	Rossau 1997 (144)
	rpoB, hsp65		PCR	Sequencing	Kapur 1995 (68)
Cultures	*rpoB*, IS6110	Boom	PCR	DG-DGGE denaturing gel gradient electrophoresis	Scarpellini 1999 (155)
Cultures	*rpoB, katG*	Chelex	RT-PCR (multiplex)	LightCycler	Torres 2000 (175)
Cultures	*rpoB, katG, inhA, ahpC-oxyR*	Boiling	RT-PCR (multiplex)	Perkin-Elmer Cycler	Piatek 2000 (128)
Cultures, sputum	*rpoB*, I6SRNA	Boiling	RT-PCR	Molecular beacons	El Hajj 2001 (32)
Cultures	*rpoB*		RT-PCR	LightCycler	Edwards 2001 (31)
Sputum	*rpoB*,[a]	Phenol-chloroform bead-beat	nPCR	SSCP, sequencing	Kim 2001 (74)
Cultures, liquid cultures	*rpoB, katG*	boiling	RT-PCR	LightCycler	Garcia de Viedma 2002 (44)

[a] Nested reaction using a *M. tuberculosis*–specific *rpoB* sequence.

At present, more than 90 TEM derivatives have been described, along with and more than 25 SHV-type enzymes.

New families of ESBLs have also appeared, including the CTX-M and OXA-type enzymes as well as novel, unrelated β-lactamases (13).

ESBLs hydrolyze broad-spectum cephalosporins and monobactams, including oxyimino-cephalosporins (e.g., ceftazidime, cefotaxime, and ceftriaxone) and older β-lactam drugs. Most are susceptible to cefoxitin and cefotetan and are inhibited by clavulanic acid.

That the ESBLs are located on plasmids and transferable to other bacterial species is reason for great medical concern. Bacterial strains expressing ESBLs will present considerable therapeutic challenges in the future.

The increased prevalence of ESBL-producing enterobacteria creates the need for laboratory testing methods that can accurately identify these enzymes in clinical isolates.

A variety of clinical microbiologic tests have been proposed based on antibiotic disk diffusion tests (22,63,65,174).

Disk diffusion and broth microdilution screening breakpoints for aztreonam and cefalosporins were recently introduced by NCCLS in order to improve the detection of ESBL-producing strains (110). The screening breakpoints described work well for identifying ESBL-producing *K. pneumoniae*. They are much less specific for *E. coli*.

The sensitivity and specificity of susceptibility tests to detect ESBLs vary with the cephalosporin tested.

At present, NCCLS recommends an initial screening in which one of five expanded-spectrum β-lactam antibiotics are tested. A positive result is to be reported as indicative of the presence of an ESBL (110). This screen is then followed by a phenotypic confirmatory test that consists of determining the MICs of either ceftazidime or cefotaxime with and without the presence of clavulanic acid (4 μg/mL). A decrease in the MIC equal to or greater than 3 twofold dilutions in the presence of clavulanate is indicative of the presence of an ESBL. If an ESBL is detected, the strain should be reported as nonsusceptible to all expanded-spectrum cephalosporins and aztreonam regardless of the susceptibility testing result (110).

The commercially available Etest ESBL detection method (AB Biodisk, Solna, Sweden) employs a two-sided strip containing a gradient of ceftazidime at one end and ceftazidime plus clavulanate at the other end. A test is positive for an ESBL if there is more than a three-dilution reduction in the MIC of ceftazidime in the presence of clavulanic acid.

The automated microbial susceptibility test system Vitek (Biomerieux, Hazlewood, MO) includes an ESBL test that utilizes either ceftazidime or cefotaxime alone and in combination with clavulanic acid (4 μg/mL). In a study of *Klebsiella* spp and *E. coli* expressing well-characterized β-lactamases, Sanders et al. showed that the Vitek ESBL test was 99% sensitive and specific for the detection of ESBLs (148,149).

Another automatic ESBL detection test, the Phoenic ESBL test (Becton Dickinson Biosciences, Sparks, MD), was positively evaluated by Sanguinetti et al. (150), who found it to have a sensitivity of 100% and a specificity of 98.9%, with 0.6% false positives and no false negatives. It produces results within 6 hours.

None of the methods can accurately detect all ESBL producers, which highlights the need for improved detection of ESBLs in clinical isolates of *enterobacteria*. In our laboratory, we showed that the Etest ESBL test with ceftazidime detected only 81% of ESBLs, compared with 97% and 91% for the double-disk test and the three-dimensional test, respectively (188). The Etest method was convenient and easy to use, but reading of the results is sometimes difficult when the MICs of ceftazidime are low, as the clavulanate may diffuse over to the side of the strip containing ceftazidime alone.

POSSIBLE METHODS FOR THE MOLECULAR DETECTION OF ESBLs

The great diversity of ESBL genes has resulted in a multitude of molecular techniques to detect and to identify TEM, SHV, OXA, and CTX-M genes (Table 11.10). However, these methods belong to the domain of the reference laboratory. Early detection of β-lactamase genes was performed using DNA probes that were specific to TEM and SHV enzymes (7,42,58).

PCR can detect β-lactamases belonging to a family of enzymes using primers specific to a β-lactamase gene and intended to anneal to regions where point mutations are not known to occur (the primers can be chosen from a database such as Genbank). Several methods allow the differentiation of ESBLs.

TEM variants can be identified by using specific probes (88,173), by restriction fragment length polymorphism (RFLP) of the amplicons (7), by PCR-RFLP (115), and by PCR single-strand conformational polymorphism (SSCP) (107,108).

Ligase chain reaction, which allows the discrimination of DNA sequences differing by a single base pair, has been applied to distinguish variants of SHV (75).

PCR-RLFP has also been applied to OXA-type genes (178).

Nucleotide sequencing remains the standard for determining the specific β-lactamase gene present in a strain.

TABLE 11.10

Molecular Detection of ESBLs[a]

Substrate	Amplification Reaction	Target Advantages	Target Disadvantages	Reference
Agar grown cultures	DNA probes	Specific for gene family (e.g., TEM or SHV)	Labor intensive, cannot distinguish between ESBLs and non-ESBLs, cannot distinguish between variants of TEM or SHV	Huovinen 1988 (58), Gallego 1990 (42), Arlet 1991 (7).
Agar grown cultures	PCR	Easy to perform, specific for gene family (e.g., TEM or SHV)	Cannot distinguish between ESBLs and non-ESBLs, cannot distinguish between variants of TEM or SHV	Courvalin 1991 (23), Mabilat 1993 (89), Nüesch-Inderbinen 1996 (115)
Agar grown cultures	Oligotyping	Detects specific TEM variants	Requires specific oligonucleotide probes, labor intensive, cannot detect new variants	Ouellette 1988 (120)
Agar grown cultures	PCR-RFLP	Easy to perform, can detect specific nucleotide changes	Nucleotide changes must result in altered restriction site for detection	Nüesch-Inderbinen 1996 (115)
Agar grown cultures	PCR-SSCP	Can distinguish between a number of SHV variants	Requires special electrophoresis conditions	M'Zali 1996 (107), M'Zali 1998 (108)
Agar grown cultures	LCR	Can distinguish between a number of SHV variants	Requires a large number of oligonucleotide primers	Kim 2000 (76)
Agar grown cultures	Nucleotide sequencing	The gold standard; can detect all variants	Labor intensive, can be technically challenging, can be difficult to interpret manual methods	Bradford 1999 (12)

[a] Adapted from Bradford (2001).

However, it too can give variable results depending on the method used (12).

DETECTION OF GENES CODING FOR AMINOGLYCOSIDE RESISTANCE

Aminoglycosides have ribosome as the primary target, inhibiting one or more of the biochemical steps involved in the translation of ribosome.

Several resistance mechanism have been discovered, including decreased antibiotic uptake and accumulation, modification of the ribosomal target, efflux of the antibiotic, and enzymatic modification of aminoglycosides.

The major mechanism of aminoglycoside resistance in both Gram-positive and Gram-negative organisms is enzymatic modification of the antibiotic (180).

The three routes of inactivation are phosphorylation by phosphotransferases (APH) adenylation by nucleotransferases (ANT), and acetylation by acetyltransferases (AAC). Over 50 different enzymes have been identified as aminoglycoside modifiers, including a fusion of an AAC enzyme and an APH enzyme that is widely distributed in staphylococci and enterococci (96). A nomenclature has been proposed by Shaw (160). A number with or without either a prime or double prime denotes the position of the modification on the substrate.

Recent surveys of aminoglycoside resistance show the emergence of complex phenotypes and a multiplicity of genotypes (97).

With the development of molecular techniques, a large number of resistance-conferring genes have been identified (97) so that each resistant phenotype has been associated with the expression of several distinct proteins with the same aminoglycoside-modifying activity. Single amino acid changes in the protein can alter the substrate profile of an enzyme.

POSSIBLE METHODS FOR THE MOLECULAR DETECTION OF AMINOGLYCOSIDE GENES CODING FOR AMINOGLYCOSIDE RESISTANCE

As the DNA sequences of many genes encoding aminoglycoside modifying enzymes have been determined, primers for PCR detection of these enzymes have been proposed (114,130,136). Some bacterial strains harbor two aminoglycoside resistance genes. The presence of different aminoglycoside resistance genes has also been used for epidemiological typing, particularly in *Acinetobacter* strains (114,159,190).

PCR has been shown to be a reliable tool for the detection of aminoglycoside-modifying enzyme genes in staphylococci (185).

In *S. aureus,* the most prevalent aminoglycoside resistance gene is *aac(6′)-Ie+aph(2″),* found in 76% of MRSA and 50% of MSSA, isolates; the least common is *aph(3′)IIIa,* found in 7% of MRSA and 13% of MSSA isolates (156). Because of the limited number of aminoglycoside resistance–encoding genes, molecular assays can be useful for the detection of these genes.

Molecular assays for the detection of aminoglycoside resistance in enterococci and streptococci are only used in epidemiological studies.

A study by van Asselt et al. (181) showed that with a limited number of PCR assays a clear picture of the distribution of genes responsible for high-level resistance in enterococci and streptococci could be obtained.

PCR and hybridization were used in an epidemiological study in Spain for the detection of the *aac*(6′)-*aph*(2″) gene (25).

A multiplex PCR was used in the study by Kobayashi (79) that showed that the *aac*(6′)-*aph*(2″) was present at a higher frequency in *E. faecalis* than in *E. faecium,* but this study indicates mainly that there is a variety of distribution profiles for aminoglycoside-modifying enzymes in enterococci.

A more recent study (179) also describes a multiplex PCR for accurately detecting several aminoglycoside resistance genes in enterococci.

A number of studies have focused on aminoglycoside resistance among Gram-negatives bacteria. In a study by Vanhoof et al., PCR was used to detect 179 aminoglycoside resistance mechanisms (i.e., 150 genes encoding modifying enzymes and 29 permeability mechanisms) in 148 isolates (186). The *aac*(6′)-*I* genes were found to be the most predominant resistant mechanisms, followed by the *aac*(3) genes and permeability mechanisms.

Several studies focused on the detection of aminoglycoside resistance in *Acinetobacter* spp. In one of the first studies (130), both hybridization and PCR were used and led to the same results.

Seward et al. described the presence of entirely different genes from those found in a study by Ploy (159).

Although a clear explanation cannot be given, geographical differences may play a role. In any case, results from one study cannot automatically be extrapolated to other situations.

An epidemiological study of the genes encoding for aminoglycoside-modifying enzymes was also done by Noppe-Leclerq et al. (114) using three multiplex assays covering a total of seven aminoglycoside resistance genes and the 16S rRNA genes. The authors conclude that the technique was useful as an epidemiological tool.

One of the major challenges of aminoglycoside resistance is the large number and diversity of the modifying enzymes. The multitude of different aminoglycoside resistance genes involved makes full coverage by molecular techniques a difficult exercise. The application of molecular assays for the detection of aminoglycoside resistance has therefore received only limited attention and is restricted to epidemiological studies. A possible solution may be provided by DNA chips, as all genes can be concentrated on one single chip. However, the cost of this technology will be a limiting factor for routine use.

REFERENCES

1. Anonymous. Update: nucleic acid amplification tests for tuberculosis. *MMWR* 2000;49:593–594.
2. Alarcon T, Vega AE, Domingo D, et al. Clarithromycin resistance among *Helicobacter pylori* strains isolated from children: prevalence and study of mechanism of resistance by PCR-restriction fragment length polymorphism analysis. *J Clin Microbiol* 2003;41:486–499.
3. Allignet J, Loncle V, Mazodier P, et al. Nucleotide sequence of a staphylococcal plasmid gene, vgb, encoding a hydrolase inactivating the B components of virginiamycin-like antibiotics. *Plasmid* 1988;20:271–275.
4. Angeletti S, Lorino G, Gherardi G, et al. Routine molecular identification of enterococci by gene-specific PCR and 16S ribosomal DNA sequencing. *J Clin Microbiol* 2001;39:794–797.
5. Archer GL, Pennell E. Detection of methicillin resistance in staphylococci by using a DNA probe. *Antimicrob Agents Chemother* 1990;34:1720–1724.
6. Arlet G, Brami G, Decre D, et al. Molecular characterisation by PCR-restriction fragment length polymorphism of TEM beta-lactamases. *FEMS Microbiol Lett* 1995;134:203–208.
7. Arlet G, Phillipon A. Construction by polymerase chain reaction and intragenic DNA probes for three main types of transferable beta-lactamases (TEM, SVH, CARB). *FEMS Microbiol Lett* 1991;82:19–26.
8. Arthur M, Andremont A, Courvalin P. Distribution of erythromycin esterase and rRNA methylase genes in members of the family Enterobacteriaceae highly resistant to erythromycin. *Antimicrob Agents Chemother* 1987;31:404–409.

9. Baker CN, Huang MB, Tenover FC. Optimizing testing of methicillin-resistant Staphylococcus species. *Diagn Microbiol Infect Dis* 1994;19:167–170.
10. Bekkaoui F, McNevin JP, Leung CH, et al. Rapid detection of the mecA gene in methicillin resistant staphylococci using a colorimetric cycling probe technology. *Diagn Microbiol Infect Dis* 1999;34:83–90.
11. Berger-Bächi B. Update on methicillin resistance mechanisms in staphylococci. *Chemotherapy* 1996;42[Suppl. 2]:19–26.
12. Bradford PA. Automated thermal cycling is superior to traditional methods for nucleotide sequencing of bla(SHV) genes. *Antimicrob Agents Chemother* 1999;43:2960–2963.
13. Bradford PA. Extended-spectrum beta-lactamases in the 21st century: characterization, epidemiology, and detection of this important resistance threat. *Clin Microbiol Rev* 2001;14:933–951, table.
14. Brisson-Noel A, Delrieu P, Samain D, et al. Inactivation of lincosaminide antibiotics in *Staphylococcus*: identification of lincosaminide O-nucleotidyltransferases and comparison of the corresponding resistance genes. *J Biol Chem* 1988;263:15880–15887.
15. Cavassini M, Wenger A, Jaton K, et al. Evaluation of MRSA-Screen, a simple anti-PBP 2a slide latex agglutination kit, for rapid detection of methicillin resistance in Staphylococcus aureus. *J Clin Microbiol* 1999;37:1591–1594.
16. Cetinkaya Y, Falk P, Mayhall CG. Vancomycin-resistant enterococci. *Clin Microbiol Rev* 2000;13:686–707.
17. Chambers HF. Methicillin resistance in staphylococci: molecular and biochemical basis and clinical implications. *Clin Microbiol Rev* 1997;10:781–791.
18. Chambers HF, Hackbarth CJ. Effect of NaCl and nafcillin on penicillin-binding protein 2a and heterogeneous expression of methicillin resistance in *Staphylococcus aureus*. *Antimicrob Agents Chemother* 1987;31:1982–1988.
19. Chisholm SA, Owen RJ, Teare EL, et al. PCR-based diagnosis of *Helicobacter pylori* infection and real-time determination of clarithromycin resistance directly from human gastric biopsy samples. *J Clin Microbiol* 2001;39:1217–1220.
20. Clark NC, Cooksey RC, Hill BC, et al. Characterization of glycopeptide-resistant enterococci from U.S. hospitals. *Antimicrob Agents Chemother* 1993;37:2311–2317.
21. Cloney L, Marlowe C, Wong A, et al. Rapid detection of mecA in methicillin resistant *Staphylococcus aureus* using cycling probe technology. *Mol Cell Probes* 1999;13:191–197.
22. Cormican MG, Marshall SA, Jones RN. Detection of extended-spectrum beta-lactamase (ESBL)–producing strains by the Etest ESBL screen. *J Clin Microbiol* 1996;34:1880–1884.
23. Courvalin P. Genotypic approach to the study of bacterial resistance to antibiotics. *Antimicrob Agents Chemother* 1991;35:1019–1023.
24. Datta N, Kontomichalou P. Penicillinase synthesis controlled by infectious R factors in Enterobacteriaceae. *Nature* 1965;208:239–241.
25. del Campo R, Tenorio C, Rubio C, et al. Aminoglycoside-modifying enzymes in high-level streptomycin and gentamicin resistant Enterococcus spp. in Spain. *Int J Antimicrob Agents* 2000;15:221–226.
26. de Lencastre H, Sa Figueiredo AM, Urban C, et al. Multiple mechanisms of methicillin resistance and improved methods for detection in clinical isolates of *Staphylococcus aureus*. *Antimicrob Agents Chemother* 1991;35:632–639.
27. de Oliveira MM, da Silva RA, Cardoso OM, et al. Rapid detection of resistance against rifampicin in isolates of *Mycobacterium tuberculosis* from Brazilian patients using a reverse-phase hybridization assay. *J Microbiol Methods* 2003;53:335–342.
28. Descheemaeker P, Chapelle S, Lammens C, et al. Macrolide resistance and erythromycin resistance determinants among Belgian *Streptococcus pyogenes* and *Streptococcus pneumoniae* isolates. *J Antimicrob Chemother* 2000;45:167–173.
29. Duck P, Alvarado-Urbina G, Burdick B, et al. Probe amplifier system based on chimeric cycling oligonucleotides. *Biotechniques* 1990;9:142–148.
30. Dutka-Malen S, Evers S, Courvalin P. Detection of glycopeptide resistance genotypes and identification to the species level of clinically relevant enterococci by PCR. *J Clin Microbiol* 1995;33:24–27.
31. Edwards KJ, Metherell LA, Yates M, et al. Detection of rpoB mutations in *Mycobacterium tuberculosis* by biprobe analysis. *J Clin Microbiol* 2001;39:3350–3352.
32. El Hajj HH, Marras SA, Tyagi S, et al. Detection of rifampin resistance in *Mycobacterium tuberculosis* in a single tube with molecular beacons. *J Clin Microbiol* 2001;39:4131–4137.
33. Endtz HP, van den BN, van Belkum A, et al. Comparison of eight methods to detect vancomycin resistance in enterococci. *J Clin Microbiol* 1998;36:592–594.
34. Fang H, Hedin G. Rapid screening and identification of methicillin-resistant *Staphylococcus aureus* from clinical samples by selective-broth and real-time PCR assay. *J Clin Microbiol* 2003;41:2894–2899.
35. Farrell DJ, Morrissey I, Bakker S, et al. Detection of macrolide resistance mechanisms in *Streptococcus pneumoniae* and *Streptococcus pyogenes* using a multiplex rapid cycle PCR with microwell-format probe hybridization. *J Antimicrob Chemother* 2001;48:541–544.
36. Felmlee TA, Liu Q, Whelen AC, et al. Genotypic detection of *Mycobacterium tuberculosis* rifampin resistance: comparison of single-strand conformation polymorphism and dideoxy fingerprinting. *J Clin Microbiol* 1995;33:1617–1623.
37. Fines M, Perichon B, Reynolds P, et al. VanE, a new type of acquired glycopeptide resistance in *Enterococcus faecalis* BM4405. *Antimicrob Agents Chemother* 1999;43:2161–2164.
38. Fluit AC, Visser MR, Schmitz FJ. Molecular detection of antimicrobial resistance. *Clin Microbiol Rev* 2001;14:836–871, table.
39. Fong WK, Modrusan Z, McNevin JP, et al. Rapid solid-phase immunoassay for detection of methicillin-resistant *Staphylococcus aureus* using cycling probe technology. *J Clin Microbiol* 2000;38:2525–2529.
40. Fontana C, Favaro M, Minelli S, et al. New site of modification of 23S rRNA associated with clarithromycin resistance of *Helicobacter pylori* clinical isolates. *Antimicrob Agents Chemother* 2002;46:3765–3769.
41. French GL. Enterococci and vancomycin resistance. *Clin Infect Dis* 1998;27[Suppl 1]:S75–83.
42. Gallego L, Umaran A, Garaizar J, et al. Digoxigenin-labeled DNA probe to detect TEM type beta-lactamases. *J Microb Meth* 1990;11:261–267.
43. Garcia de Viedma D. Rapid detection of resistance in *Mycobacterium tuberculosis:* a review discussing molecular approaches. *Clin Microbiol Infect* 2003;9:349–359.
44. Garcia de Viedma D, del Sol Diaz Infantes M, Lasala F, et al. New real-time PCR able to detect in a single tube multiple rifampin resistance mutations and high-level isoniazid resistance mutations in *Mycobacterium tuberculosis*. *J Clin Microbiol* 2002;40:988–995.

45. Gholizadeh Y, Courvalin P. Acquired and intrinsic glycopeptide resistance in enterococci. *Int J Antimicrob Agents* 2000;16[Suppl 1]:S11–17.
46. Gibson JR, Saunders NA, Burke B, et al. Novel method for rapid determination of clarithromycin sensitivity in *Helicobacter pylori*. *J Clin Microbiol* 1999;37:3746–3748.
47. Gillespie SH. Evolution of drug resistance in *Mycobacterium tuberculosis*: clinical and molecular perspective. *Antimicrob Agents Chemother* 2002;46:267–274.
48. Gonzalez-Zorn B, Courvalin P. VanA-mediated high level glycopeptide resistance in MRSA. *Lancet Infect Dis* 2003;3:67–68.
49. Goossens H. The epidemiology of vancomycin-resistant enterococci. *Curr Opin Inf Dis* 1999;12:537–541.
50. Grisold AJ, Leitner E, Muhlbauer G, et al. Detection of methicillin-resistant *Staphylococcus aureus* and simultaneous confirmation by automated nucleic acid extraction and real-time PCR. *J Clin Microbiol* 2002;40:2392–2397.
51. Hackbarth CJ, Chambers HF. Methicillin-resistant staphylococci: detection methods and treatment of infections. *Antimicrob Agents Chemother* 1989;33:995–999.
52. Hackbarth CJ, Chambers HF. Methicillin-resistant staphylococci: genetics and mechanisms of resistance. *Antimicrob Agents Chemother* 1989;33:991–994.
53. Hayashi K. PCR-SSCP: a simple and sensitive method for detection of mutations in the genomic DNA. *PCR Methods Appl* 1991;1:34–38.
54. Heep M, Brandstatter B, Rieger U, et al. Frequency of rpoB mutations inside and outside the cluster I region in rifampin-resistant clinical *Mycobacterium tuberculosis* isolates. *J Clin Microbiol* 2001;39:107–110.
55. Heep M, Rieger U, Beck D, et al. Mutations in the beginning of the rpoB gene can induce resistance to rifamycins in both *Helicobacter pylori* and *Mycobacterium tuberculosis*. *Antimicrob Agents Chemother* 2000;44:1075–1077.
56. Hirano K, Abe C, Takahashi M. Mutations in the rpoB gene of rifampin-resistant *Mycobacterium tuberculosis* strains isolated mostly in Asian countries and their rapid detection by line probe assay. *J Clin Microbiol* 1999;37:2663–2666.
57. Houben MH, Van der Beek D, Heusen EF, et al. A systematic review of *Helicobacter pylori* eradication therapy, the impact of antimicrobial resistance on eradication rates. *Aliment Pharmacol Ther* 2003;13:1047–1055.
58. Huovinen S, Huovinen P, Jacoby GA. Detection of plasmid-mediated beta-lactamases with DNA probes. *Antimicrob Agents Chemother* 1988;32:175–179.
59. Hurlimann-Dalel RL, Ryffel C, Kayser FH, et al. Survey of the methicillin resistance–associated genes mecA, mecR1-mecI, and femA-femB in clinical isolates of methicillin-resistant *Staphylococcus aureus*. *Antimicrob Agents Chemother* 1992;36:2617–2621.
60. Hussain Z, Stoakes L, Massey V, et al. Correlation of oxacillin MIC with mecA gene carriage in coagulase-negative staphylococci. *J Clin Microbiol* 2000;38:752–754.
61. Ieven M, Jansens H, Ursi D, et al. Rapid detection of methicillin resistance in coagulase-negative staphylococci by commercially available fluorescence test. *J Clin Microbiol* 1995;33:2183–2185.
62. Ieven M, Vercauteren E, Descheemaeker P, et al. Comparison of direct plating and broth enrichment culture for the detection of intestinal colonization by glycopeptide-resistant enterococci among hospitalized patients. *J Clin Microbiol* 1999;37:1436–1440.
63. Jacoby GA, Han P. Detection of extended-spectrum beta-lactamases in clinical isolates of Klebsiella pneumoniae and Escherichia coli. *J Clin Microbiol* 1996;34:908–911.
64. Jacoby GA, Medeiros AA. More extended-spectrum beta-lactamases. *Antimicrob Agents Chemother* 1991;35:1697–1704.
65. Jarlier V, Nicolas MH, Fournier G, et al. Extended broad-spectrum beta-lactamases conferring transferable resistance to newer beta-lactam agents in Enterobacteriaceae: hospital prevalence and susceptibility patterns. *Rev Infect Dis* 1988;10:867–878.
66. Jones ME, Gesu G, Ortisi G, et al. Proficiency of Italian clinical laboratories in detecting reduced glycopeptide susceptibility in Enterococcus and Staphylococcus spp. using routine laboratory methodologies. *Clin Microbiol Infect* 2002;8:101–111.
67. Kanematsu E, Deguchi T, Yasuda M, et al. Alterations in the GyrA subunit of DNA gyrase and the ParC subunit of DNA topoisomerase IV associated with quinolone resistance in *Enterococcus faecalis*. *Antimicrob Agents Chemother* 1998;42:433–435.
68. Kapur V, Li LL, Hamrick MR, et al. Rapid Mycobacterium species assignment and unambiguous identification of mutations associated with antimicrobial resistance in *Mycobacterium tuberculosis* by automated DNA sequencing. *Arch Pathol Lab Med* 1995;119:131–138.
69. Kapur V, Li LL, Iordanescu S, et al. Characterization by automated DNA sequencing of mutations in the gene (rpoB) encoding the RNA polymerase beta subunit in rifampin-resistant *Mycobacterium tuberculosis* strains from New York City and Texas. *J Clin Microbiol* 1994;32:1095–1098.
70. Kariyama R, Mitsuhata R, Chow JW, et al. Simple and reliable multiplex PCR assay for surveillance isolates of vancomycin-resistant enterococci. *J Clin Microbiol* 2000;38:3092–3095.
71. Kataja J, Huovinen P, Seppala H. Erythromycin resistance genes in group A streptococci of different geographical origins. The Macrolide Resistance Study Group. *J Antimicrob Chemother* 2000;46:789–792.
72. Kearns AM, Seiders PR, Wheeler J, et al. Rapid detection of methicillin-resistant staphylococci by multiplex PCR. *J Hosp Infect* 1999;43:33–37.
73. Kim BJ, Kim SY, Park BH, et al. Mutations in the rpoB gene of *Mycobacterium tuberculosis* that interfere with PCR–single-strand conformation polymorphism analysis for rifampin susceptibility testing. *J Clin Microbiol* 1997;35:492–494.
74. Kim BJ, Lee KH, Park BN, et al. Detection of rifampin-resistant *Mycobacterium tuberculosis* in sputa by nested PCR–linked single-strand conformation polymorphism and DNA sequencing. *J Clin Microbiol* 2001;39:2610–2617.
75. Kim J, Kwon Y, Pai H, et al. Survey of *Klebsiella pneumoniae* strains producing extended-spectrum beta-lactamases: prevalence of SHV-12 and SHV-2a in Korea. *J Clin Microbiol* 1998;36:1446–1449.
76. Kim J, Lee HJ. Rapid discriminatory detection of genes coding for SHV beta-lactamases by ligase chain reaction. *Antimicrob Agents Chemother* 2000;44:1860–1864.
77. Knapp CC, Ludwig MD, Washington JA. Evaluation of differential inoculum disk diffusion method and Vitek GPS-SA card for detection of oxacillin-resistant staphylococci. *J Clin Microbiol* 1994;32:433–436.
78. Knapp CC, Ludwig MD, Washington JA, et al. Evaluation of Vitek GPS-SA card for testing of oxacillin against borderline-susceptible staphylococci that lack mec. *J Clin Microbiol* 1996;34:1603–1605.
79. Kobayashi N, Alam M, Nishimoto Y, et al. Distribution of aminoglycoside resistance genes in recent clinical isolates of Enterococcus faecalis, Enterococcus faecium and Enterococcus avium. *Epidemiol Infect* 2001;126:197–204.

80. Kobayashi N, Wu H, Kojima K, et al. Detection of mecA, femA, and femB genes in clinical strains of staphylococci using polymerase chain reaction. *Epidemiol Infect* 1994;113:259–266.
81. Lascols C, Lamarque D, Costa JM, et al. Fast and accurate quantitative detection of *Helicobacter pylori* and identification of clarithromycin resistance mutations in *H. pylori* isolates from gastric biopsy specimens by real-time PCR. *J Clin Microbiol* 2003;41:4573–4577.
82. Leclercq R. Mechanisms of resistance to macrolides and lincosamides: nature of the resistance elements and their clinical implications. *Clin Infect Dis* 2002;34:482–492.
83. Levi K, Towner KJ. Detection of methicillin-resistant Staphylococcus aureus (MRSA) in blood with the EVIGENE MRSA detection kit. *J Clin Microbiol* 2003;41:3890–3892.
84. Ligozzi M, Rossolini GM, Tonin EA, et al. Nonradioactive DNA probe for detection of gene for methicillin resistance in *Staphylococcus aureus*. *Antimicrob Agents Chemother* 1991;35:575–578.
85. Lina G, Quaglia A, Reverdy ME, et al. Distribution of genes encoding resistance to macrolides, lincosamides, and streptogramins among staphylococci. *Antimicrob Agents Chemother* 1999;43:1062–1066.
86. Low DE, Keller N, Barth A, et al. Clinical prevalence, antimicrobial susceptibility, and geographic resistance patterns of enterococci: results from the SENTRY Antimicrobial Surveillance Program, 1997–1999. *Clin Infect Dis* 2001;32[Suppl 2]:S133–145.
87. Lowy FD. *Staphylococcus aureus* infections. *N Engl J Med* 1998;339:520–532.
88. Mabilat C, Courvalin P. Development of "oligotyping" for characterization and molecular epidemiology of TEM beta-lactamases in members of the family Enterobacteriaceae. *Antimicrob Agents Chemother* 1990;34:2210–2216.
89. Mabilat C, Goussard S. PCR detection and identification of genes for extended-spectrum beta-lactamases. In: Persing DH, Smith TF, Tenover TC, eds. *Diagnostic molecular microbiology*. Washington, DC: American Society for Microbiology, 1993;553–559.
90. Malhotra-Kumar S, Wang S, Lammens C, et al. Bacitracin-resistant clone of *Streptococcus pyogenes* isolated from pharyngitis patients in Belgium. *J Clin Microbiol* 2003;41:5282–5284.
91. Marais A, Monteiro L, Occhialini A, et al. Direct detection of *Helicobacter pylori* resistance to macrolides by a polymerase chain reaction/DNA enzyme immunoassay in gastric biopsy specimens. *Gut* 1999;44:463–467.
92. Matsuoka M, Yoshida Y, Hayakawa K, et al. Simultaneous colonisation of *Helicobacter pylori* with and without mutations in the 23S rRNA gene in patients with no history of clarithromycin exposure. *Gut* 1999;45:503–507.
93. McKessar SJ, Berry AM, Bell JM, et al. Genetic characterization of vanG, a novel vancomycin resistance locus of *Enterococcus faecalis*. *Antimicrob Agents Chemother* 2000;44:3224–3228.
94. Meier A, Kirschner P, Springer B, et al. Identification of mutations in 23S rRNA gene of clarithromycin-resistant *Mycobacterium intracellulare*. *Antimicrob Agents Chemother* 1994;38:381–384.
95. Mikhailovich V, Lapa S, Gryadunov D, et al. Identification of rifampin-resistant *Mycobacterium tuberculosis* strains by hybridization, PCR, and ligase detection reaction on oligonucleotide microchips. *J Clin Microbiol* 2001;39:2531–2540.
96. Miller GH, Sabatelli FJ, Hare RS, et al. The most frequent aminoglycoside resistance mechanisms—changes with time and geographic area: a reflection of aminoglycoside usage patterns? Aminoglycoside Resistance Study Groups. *Clin Infect Dis* 1997;24[Suppl 1]:S46–62.
97. Mingeot-Leclercq MP, Glupczynski Y, Tulkens PM. Aminoglycosides: activity and resistance. *Antimicrob Agents Chemother* 1999;43:727–737.
98. Modrusan Z, Marlowe C, Wheeler D, et al. CPT-EIA assays for the detection of vancomycin resistant vanA and vanB genes in enterococci. *Diagn Microbiol Infect Dis* 2000;37:45–50.
99. Montanari MP, Massidda O, Mingoia M, et al. Borderline susceptibility to methicillin in *Staphylococcus aureus*: a new mechanism of resistance? *Microb Drug Resist* 1996;2:257–260.
100. Morris S, Bai GH, Suffys P, et al. Molecular mechanisms of multiple drug resistance in clinical isolates of *Mycobacterium tuberculosis*. *J Infect Dis* 1995;171:954–960.
101. Mulligan ME, Murray-Leisure KA, Ribner BS, et al. Methicillin-resistant *Staphylococcus aureus*: a consensus review of the microbiology, pathogenesis, and epidemiology with implications for prevention and management. *Am J Med* 1993;94:313–328.
102. Murakami K, Minamide W, Wada K, et al. Identification of methicillin-resistant strains of staphylococci by polymerase chain reaction. *J Clin Microbiol* 1991;29:2240–2244.
103. Murakami K, Tomasz A. Involvement of multiple genetic determinants in high-level methicillin resistance in *Staphylococcus aureus*. *J Bacteriol* 1989;171:874–879.
104. Murray BE. The life and times of the Enterococcus. *Clin Microbiol Rev* 1990;3:46–65.
105. Murray BE. Vancomycin-resistant enterococcal infections. *N Engl J Med* 2000;342:710–721.
106. Musser JM. Antimicrobial agent resistance in mycobacteria: molecular genetic insights. *Clin Microbiol Rev* 1995;8:496–514.
107. M'Zali FH, Gascoyne-Binzi DM, Heritage J, et al. Detection of mutations conferring extended-spectrum activity on SHV beta-lactamases using polymerase chain reaction single strand conformational polymorphism (PCR-SSCP). *J Antimicrob Chemother* 1996;37:797–802.
108. M'Zali FH, Heritage J, Gascoyne-Binzi DM, et al. PCR single strand conformational polymorphism can be used to detect the gene encoding SHV-7 extended-spectrum beta-lactamase and to identify different SHV genes within the same strain. *J Antimicrob Chemother* 1998;41:123–125.
109. Nash KA, Inderlied CB. Genetic basis of macrolide resistance in *Mycobacterium avium* isolated from patients with disseminated disease. *Antimicrob Agents Chemother* 1995;39:2625–2630.
110. National Committee for Clinical Laboratory Standards. Methods for dilution antimicrobial susceptibility tests for bacteria that grow aerobically. Approved standard M7-A5 and informational supplement M100-S13. Wayne, PA: National Committee for Clinical Laboratory Standards, 2003.
111. Navarro F, Courvalin P. Analysis of genes encoding D-alanine-D-alanine ligase-related enzymes in *Enterococcus casseliflavus* and *Enterococcus flavescens*. *Antimicrob Agents Chemother* 1994;38:1788–1793.
112. Ng LK, Martin I, Liu G, et al. Mutation in 23S rRNA associated with macrolide resistance in *Neisseria gonorrhoeae*. *Antimicrob Agents Chemother* 2002;46:3020–3025.
113. Noble WC, Virani Z, Cree RG. Co-transfer of vancomycin and other resistance genes from *Enterococcus faecalis* NCTC 12201 to *Staphylococcus aureus*. *FEMS Microbiol Lett* 2003;93:195–190.
114. Noppe-Leclercq I, Wallet F, Haentjens S, et al. PCR detection of aminoglycoside resistance genes: a rapid molecular

typing method for Acinetobacter baumannii. *Res Microbiol* 1999;150:317–322.

115. Nüesch-Inderbinen MT, Hachler H, Kayser FH. Detection of genes coding for extended-spectrum SHV beta-lactamases in clinical isolates by a molecular genetic method, and comparison with the Etest. *Eur J Clin Microbiol Infect Dis* 1996;15:398–402.
116. Occhialini A, Urdaci M, Doucet-Populaire F, et al. Macrolide resistance in *Helicobacter pylori*: rapid detection of point mutations and assays of macrolide binding to ribosomes. *Antimicrob Agents Chemother* 1997;41:2724–2728.
117. Oleastro M, Menard A, Santos A, et al. Real-time PCR assay for rapid and accurate detection of point mutations conferring resistance to clarithromycin in *Helicobacter pylori*. *J Clin Microbiol* 2003;41:397–402.
118. Orita M, Iwahana H, Kanazawa H, et al. Detection of polymorphisms of human DNA by gel electrophoresis as single-strand conformation polymorphisms. *Proc Natl Acad Sci USA* 1989;86:2766–2770.
119. Ostrowsky BE, Clark NC, Thauvin-Eliopoulos C, et al. A cluster of VanD vancomycin-resistant *Enterococcus faecium*: molecular characterization and clinical epidemiology. *J Infect Dis* 1999;180:1177–1185.
120. Ouellette M, Paul GC, Philippon AM, et al. Oligonucleotide probes (TEM-1, OXA-1) versus isoelectric focusing in beta-lactamase characterization of 114 resistant strains. *Antimicrob Agents Chemother* 1988;32:397–399.
121. Palladino S, Kay ID, Costa AM, et al. Real-time PCR for the rapid detection of vanA and vanB genes. *Diagn Microbiol Infect Dis* 2003;45:81–84.
122. Palladino S, Kay ID, Flexman JP, et al. Rapid detection of vanA and vanB genes directly from clinical specimens and enrichment broths by real-time multiplex PCR assay. *J Clin Microbiol* 2003;41:2483–2486.
123. Patel R. Enterococcal-type glycopeptide resistance genes in non-enterococcal organisms. *FEMS Microbiol Lett* 2003;185:1–7.
124. Pechere JC. Macrolide resistance mechanisms in Gram-positive cocci. *Int J Antimicrob Agents* 2001;18[Suppl 1]: S25–28.
125. Perez-Hernandez X, Mendez-Alvarez S, Claverie-Martin F. A PCR assay for rapid detection of vancomycin-resistant enterococci. *Diagn Microbiol Infect Dis* 2002;42:273–277.
126. Perichon B, Reynolds P, Courvalin P. VanD-type glycopeptide-resistant *Enterococcus faecium* BM4339. *Antimicrob Agents Chemother* 1997;41:2016–2018.
127. Petrich AK, Luinstra KE, Groves D, et al. Direct detection of vanA and vanB genes in clinical specimens for rapid identification of vancomycin resistant enterococci (VRE) using multiplex PCR. *Mol Cell Probes* 1999;13:275–281.
128. Piatek AS, Telenti A, Murray MR, et al. Genotypic analysis of *Mycobacterium tuberculosis* in two distinct populations using molecular beacons: implications for rapid susceptibility testing. *Antimicrob Agents Chemother* 2000;44:103–110.
129. Pina M, Occhialini A, Monteiro L, et al. Detection of point mutations associated with resistance of *Helicobacter pylori* to clarithromycin by hybridization in liquid phase. *J Clin Microbiol* 1998;36:3285–3290.
130. Ploy MC, Giamarellou H, Bourlioux P, et al. Detection of aac(6′)-I genes in amikacin-resistant Acinetobacter spp. by PCR. *Antimicrob Agents Chemother* 1994;38:2925–2928.
131. Portillo A, Lantero M, Gastanares MJ, et al. Macrolide resistance phenotypes and mechanisms of resistance in *Streptococcus pyogenes* in La Rioja, Spain. *Int J Antimicrob Agents* 1999;13:137–140.
132. Poulsen AB, Skov R, Pallesen LV. Detection of methicillin resistance in coagulase-negative staphylococci and in staphylococci directly from simulated blood cultures using the EVIGENE MRSA Detection Kit. *J Antimicrob Chemother* 2003;51:419–421.
133. Poyart C, Pierre C, Quesne G, et al. Emergence of vancomycin resistance in the genus Streptococcus: characterization of a vanB transferable determinant in *Streptococcus bovis*. *Antimicrob Agents Chemother* 1997;41:24–29.
134. Predari SC, Ligozzi M, Fontana R. Genotypic identification of methicillin-resistant coagulase-negative staphylococci by polymerase chain reaction. *Antimicrob Agents Chemother* 1991;35:2568–2573.
135. Quintiliani R Jr, Courvalin P. Mechanisms of resistance to antimicrobial agents. In: Murray PR, Barron EJ, Pfaller MA, et al., eds. *Manual of clinical microbiology*. Washington, DC: American Society for Microbiology, 1995;1308–1326.
136. Rainey FA, Lang E, Stackebrandt E. The phylogenetic structure of the genus *Acinetobacter*. *FEMS Microbiol Lett* 1994;124:349–353.
137. Ramaswamy S, Musser JM. Molecular genetic basis of antimicrobial agent resistance in *Mycobacterium tuberculosis*: 1998 update. *Tuber Lung Dis* 1998;79:3–29.
138. Reischl U, Linde HJ, Metz M, et al. Rapid identification of methicillin-resistant *Staphylococcus aureus* and simultaneous species confirmation using real-time fluorescence PCR. *J Clin Microbiol* 2000;38:2429–2433.
139. Roberts MC, Facinelli B, Giovanetti E, et al. Transferable erythromycin resistance in *Listeria* spp. isolated from food. *Appl Environ Microbiol* 1996;62:269–270.
140. Roberts MC, Chung WO, Roe DE. Characterization of tetracycline and erythromycin resistance determinants in *Treponema denticola*. *Antimicrob Agents Chemother* 1996;40:1690–1694.
141. Roberts MC, Chung WO, Roe D, et al. Erythromycin-resistant *Neisseria gonorrhoeae* and oral commensal *Neisseria* spp. carry known rRNA methylase genes. *Antimicrob Agents Chemother* 1999;43:1367–1372.
142. Roberts MC, Sutcliffe J, Courvalin P, et al. Nomenclature for macrolide and macrolide-lincosamide-streptogramin B resistance determinants. *Antimicrob Agents Chemother* 1999;43:2823–2830.
143. Rohrer S, Tschierske M, Zbinden R, et al. Improved methods for detection of methicillin-resistant *Staphylococcus aureus*. *Eur J Clin Microbiol Infect Dis* 2001;20:267–270.
144. Rossau R, Traore H, De Beenhouwer H, et al. Evaluation of the INNO-LiPA Rif. TB assay, a reverse hybridization assay for the simultaneous detection of *Mycobacterium tuberculosis* complex and its resistance to rifampin. *Antimicrob Agents Chemother* 1997;41:2093–2098.
145. Russmann H, Adler K, Haas R, et al. Rapid and accurate determination of genotypic clarithromycin resistance in cultured *Helicobacter pylori* by fluorescent in situ hybridization. *J Clin Microbiol* 2001;39:4142–4144.
146. Saiki RK, Scharf S, Faloona F, et al. Enzymatic amplification of beta-globin genomic sequences and restriction site analysis for diagnosis of sickle cell anemia. *Science* 1985;230:1350–1354.
147. Sakoulas G, Gold HS, Venkataraman L, et al. Methicillin-resistant *Staphylococcus aureus*: comparison of susceptibility testing methods and analysis of mecA-positive susceptible strains. *J Clin Microbiol* 2001;39:3946–3951.
148. Sanders CC, Barry AL, Washington JA, et al. Detection of extended-spectrum-beta-lactamase–producing members of

the family Enterobacteriaceae with Vitek ESBL test. *J Clin Microbiol* 1996;34:2997–3001.

149. Sanders CC, Peyret M, Moland ES, et al. Ability of the VITEK 2 advanced expert system to identify beta-lactam phenotypes in isolates of Enterobacteriaceae and *Pseudomonas aeruginosa*. *J Clin Microbiol* 2000;38:570–574.
150. Sanguinetti M, Posteraro B, Spanu T, et al. Characterization of clinical isolates of Enterobacteriaceae from Italy by the BD Phoenix extended-spectrum beta-lactamase detection method. *J Clin Microbiol* 2003;41:1463–1468.
151. Santagati M, Iannelli F, Cascone C, et al. The novel conjugative transposon tn1207.3 carries the macrolide efflux gene mef(A) in *Streptococcus pyogenes*. *Microb Drug Resist* 2003;9:243–247.
152. Santagati M, Iannelli F, Oggioni MR, et al. Characterization of a genetic element carrying the macrolide efflux gene mef(A) in *Streptococcus pneumoniae*. *Antimicrob Agents Chemother* 2000;44:2585–2587.
153. Satake S, Clark N, Rimland D, et al. Detection of vancomycin-resistant enterococci in fecal samples by PCR. *J Clin Microbiol* 1997;35:2325–2330.
154. Scarpellini P, Braglia S, Brambilla AM, et al. Detection of rifampin resistance by single-strand conformation polymorphism analysis of cerebrospinal fluid of patients with tuberculosis of the central nervous system. *J Clin Microbiol* 1997;35:2802–2806.
155. Scarpellini P, Braglia S, Carrera P, et al. Detection of rifampin resistance in *Mycobacterium tuberculosis* by double gradient-denaturing gradient gel electrophoresis. *Antimicrob Agents Chemother* 1999;43:2550–2554.
156. Schmitz FJ, Verhoef J, Fluit AC. Comparative activity of 27 antimicrobial compounds against 698 *Streptococcus pneumoniae* isolates originating from 20 European university hospitals. SENTRY Participants Group. *Eur J Clin Microbiol Infect Dis* 1999;18:450–453.
157. Schouten MA, Voss A, Hoogkamp-Korstanje JA. Antimicrobial susceptibility patterns of enterococci causing infections in Europe. European VRE Study Group. *Antimicrob Agents Chemother* 1999;43:2542–2546.
158. Seppala H, Skurnik M, Soini H, et al. A novel erythromycin resistance methylase gene (ermTR) in *Streptococcus pyogenes*. *Antimicrob Agents Chemother* 1998;42:257–262.
159. Seward RJ, Lambert T, Towner KJ. Molecular epidemiology of aminoglycoside resistance in Acinetobacter spp. *J Med Microbiol* 1998;47:455–462.
160. Shaw KJ, Rather PN, Hare RS, et al. Molecular genetics of aminoglycoside resistance genes and familial relationships of the aminoglycoside-modifying enzymes. *Microbiol Rev* 1993;57:138–163.
161. Shortridge VD, Flamm RK, Ramer N, et al. Novel mechanism of macrolide resistance in *Streptococcus pneumoniae*. *Diagn Microbiol Infect Dis* 1996;26:73–78.
162. Skov RL, Pallesen LV, Poulsen RL, et al. Evaluation of a new 3-h hybridization method for detecting the mecA gene in *Staphylococcus aureus* and comparison with existing genotypic and phenotypic susceptibility testing methods. *J Antimicrob Chemother* 1999;43:467–475.
163. Slayden RA, Barry CE III. The genetics and biochemistry of isoniazid resistance in mycobacterium tuberculosis. *Microbes Infect* 2000;2:659–669.
164. Struelens MJ, Nonhoff C, van der AP, et al. Evaluation of Rapid ATB Staph for 5-hour antimicrobial susceptibility testing of *Staphylococcus aureus*. Groupement pour le Depistage, L'Etude et la Prevention des Infections Hospitalieres–Groep ter Opsporing, Studie en Preventie van Infecties in de Ziekenhuizen. *J Clin Microbiol* 1995;33:2395–2399.
165. Sutcliffe J, Grebe T, Tait-Kamradt A, et al. Detection of erythromycin-resistant determinants by PCR. *Antimicrob Agents Chemother* 1996;40:2562–2566.
166. Swenson JM, Spargo J, Tenover FC, et al. Optimal inoculation methods and quality control for the NCCLS oxacillin agar screen test for detection of oxacillin resistance in *Staphylococcus aureus*. *J Clin Microbiol* 2001;39:3781–3784.
167. Tan TY, Corden S, Barnes R, et al. Rapid identification of methicillin-resistant *Staphylococcus aureus* from positive blood cultures by real-time fluorescence PCR. *J Clin Microbiol* 2001;39:4529–4531.
168. Telenti A, Honore N, Bernasconi C, et al. Genotypic assessment of isoniazid and rifampin resistance in *Mycobacterium tuberculosis*: a blind study at reference laboratory level. *J Clin Microbiol* 1997;35:719–723.
169. Telenti A, Imboden P, Marchesi F, et al. Direct, automated detection of rifampin-resistant *Mycobacterium tuberculosis* by polymerase chain reaction and single-strand conformation polymorphism analysis. *Antimicrob Agents Chemother* 1993;37:2054–2058.
170. Telenti A, Imboden P, Marchesi F, et al. Detection of rifampicin-resistance mutations in *Mycobacterium tuberculosis*. *Lancet* 1993;341:647–650.
171. Tenover FC, Lancaster MV, Hill BC, et al. Characterization of staphylococci with reduced susceptibilities to vancomycin and other glycopeptides. *J Clin Microbiol* 1998;36:1020–1027.
172. Tenover FC, Swenson JM, O'Hara CM, et al. Ability of commercial and reference antimicrobial susceptibility testing methods to detect vancomycin resistance in enterococci. *J Clin Microbiol* 1995;33:1524–1527.
173. Tham TN, Mabilat C, Courvalin P, et al. Biotinylated oligonucleotide probes for the detection and the characterization of TEM-type extended broad spectrum beta-lactamases in Enterobacteriaceae. *FEMS Microbiol Lett* 1990;57:109–115.
174. Thomson KS, Sanders CC. Detection of extended-spectrum beta-lactamases in members of the family Enterobacteriaceae: comparison of the double-disk and three-dimensional tests. *Antimicrob Agents Chemother* 1992;36:1877–1882.
175. Torres MJ, Criado A, Palomares JC, et al. Use of real-time PCR and fluorimetry for rapid detection of rifampin and isoniazid resistance-associated mutations in *Mycobacterium tuberculosis*. *J Clin Microbiol* 2000;38:3194–3199.
176. Troesch A, Nguyen H, Miyada CG, et al. Mycobacterium species identification and rifampin resistance testing with high-density DNA probe arrays. *J Clin Microbiol* 1999;37:49–55.
177. Tyagi S, Kramer FR. Molecular beacons: probes that fluoresce upon hybridization. *Nat Biotechnol* 1996;14:303–308.
178. Vahaboglu H, Ozturk R, Akbal H, et al. Practical approach for detection and identification of OXA-10–derived ceftazidime-hydrolyzing extended-spectrum beta-lactamases. *J Clin Microbiol* 1998;36:827–829.
179. Vakulenko SB, Donabedian SM, Voskresenskiy AM, et al. Multiplex PCR for detection of aminoglycoside resistance genes in enterococci. *Antimicrob Agents Chemother* 2003;47:1423–1426.
180. Vakulenko SB, Mobashery S. Versatility of aminoglycosides and prospects for their future. *Clin Microbiol Rev* 2003;16:430–450.
181. van Asselt GJ, Vliegenthart JS, Petit PL, et al. High-level aminoglycoside resistance among enterococci and group A streptococci. *J Antimicrob Chemother* 1992;30:651–659.
182. van Doorn LJ, Debets-Ossenkopp YJ, Marais A, et al. Rapid detection, by PCR and reverse hybridization, of mutations

in the *Helicobacter pylori* 23S rRNA gene, associated with macrolide resistance. *Antimicrob Agents Chemother* 1999;43:1779–1782.

183. van Doorn LJ, Glupczynski Y, Kusters JG, et al. Accurate prediction of macrolide resistance in *Helicobacter pylori* by a PCR line probe assay for detection of mutations in the 23S rRNA gene: multicenter validation study. *Antimicrob Agents Chemother* 2001;45:1500–1504.
184. van Griethuysen A, Pouw M, van Leeuwen N, et al. Rapid slide latex agglutination test for detection of methicillin resistance in *Staphylococcus aureus*. *J Clin Microbiol* 1999;37:2789–2792.
185. Vanhoof R, Godard C, Content J, et al. Detection by polymerase chain reaction of genes encoding aminoglycoside-modifying enzymes in methicillin-resistant *Staphylococcus aureus* isolates of epidemic phage types. Belgian Study Group of Hospital Infections (GDEPIH/GOSPIZ). *J Med Microbiol* 1994;41:282–290.
186. Vanhoof R, Nyssen HJ, Van Bossuyt E, et al. Aminoglycoside resistance in Gram-negative blood isolates from various hospitals in Belgium and the Grand Duchy of Luxembourg. Aminoglycoside Resistance Study Group. *J Antimicrob Chemother* 1999;44:483–488.
187. van Leeuwen WB, van Pelt C, Luijendijk A, et al. Rapid detection of methicillin resistance in *Staphylococcus aureus* isolates by the MRSA-screen latex agglutination test. *J Clin Microbiol* 1999;37:3029–3030.
188. Vercauteren E, Descheemaeker P, Ieven M, et al. Comparison of screening methods for detection of extended-spectrum beta-lactamases and their prevalence among blood isolates of *Escherichia coli* and *Klebsiella* spp. in a Belgian teaching hospital. *J Clin Microbiol* 1997;35:2191–2197.
189. Versalovic J, Shortridge D, Kibler K, et al. Mutations in 23S rRNA are associated with clarithromycin resistance in *Helicobacter pylori*. *Antimicrob Agents Chemother* 1996;40:477–480.
190. Vila J, Ruiz J, Navia M, et al. Spread of amikacin resistance in *Acinetobacter baumannii* strains isolated in Spain due to an epidemic strain. *J Clin Microbiol* 1999;37:758–761.
191. Watterson SA, Wilson SM, Yates MD, et al. Comparison of three molecular assays for rapid detection of rifampin resistance in *Mycobacterium tuberculosis*. *J Clin Microbiol* 1998;36:1969–1973.
192. Weisblum B. Erythromycin resistance by ribosome modification. *Antimicrob Agents Chemother* 1995;39:577–585.
193. Whelen AC, Felmlee TA, Hunt JM, et al. Direct genotypic detection of *Mycobacterium tuberculosis* rifampin resistance in clinical specimens by using single-tube heminested PCR. *J Clin Microbiol* 1995;33:556–561.
194. Williams DL, Waguespack C, Eisenach K, et al. Characterization of rifampin-resistance in pathogenic mycobacteria. *Antimicrob Agents Chemother* 1994;38:2380–2386.
195. Wondrack L, Massa M, Yang BV, et al. Clinical strain of *Staphylococcus aureus* inactivates and causes efflux of macrolides. *Antimicrob Agents Chemother* 1996;40:992–998.

CHAPTER 12

Molecular Mechanisms of Action for Antimicrobial Agents: General Principles and Mechanisms for Selected Classes of Antibiotics

Charles W. Stratton

INTRODUCTION

Dawn of the Antimicrobial Era

The close of the 19th and the beginning of the 20th century brought forth a series of events in science that forever changed the interaction between humans and microbes (191,290). These events began during the 1860s, when Joseph Lister was the first scientist to study the inhibitory effect of chemicals on bacteria and to directly apply this knowledge to the practice of medicine. Lister used phenol to sterilize surgical instruments and in doing so greatly reduced the morbidity and mortality rates associated with surgery at that time (12). This early event marks the dawn of the antimicrobial era.

Another early scientist, Paul Ehrlich, recognized the interaction of chemical agents with microorganisms and began to evaluate various chemical agents that he hoped would have selective inhibitory effects on invading microorganisms but not harm the human host. Among the chemicals Ehrlich screened were arsenic compounds, and in 1910 the 606th arsenic compound tested was found to be active against the treponemal cause of syphilis. This compound became the drug of choice for treating syphilis until replaced by penicillins in the 1940s (118).

The discovery of penicillin in 1929 by Fleming (90) led to Chain and colleagues demonstrating in 1940 that crude penicillin cured streptococcal and staphylococcal infections in mice (1). Successful clinical use in humans soon followed.

In 1932 Domagk (73) reported that the azo dye prontosil rubrum also was able to cure streptococcal infections in mice. It was this antimicrobial agent that in 1937 became the first to be used in the United States (41). Thus began the sulfonamide class of antibiotics.

Resistance: A Neglected Tenet of Antimicrobial Usage and the Seed of Destruction

The clinical success associated with the use of antimicrobial agents was truly amazing and resulted in these drugs being hailed as miracle drugs. Until recently, the continued success of these agents blinded scientists and laypersons alike to the possibility that such success might not continue indefinitely. Unfortunately, as medicine enters the 21st century with 50 years of almost complete control over bacterial infections, antimicrobial resistance has emerged as a major threat (142,152,190,270,290).

One reason for this turn of events is that the only effects of antimicrobial agents on microbes that were seriously considered were their inhibitory or lethal effects. However, there is another possible effect of antimicrobial agents on microbes: the emergence of resistance. This is a tenet of antimicrobial use that has been neglected. The topic of resistance is covered elsewhere in this book.

Although it seems paradoxical that excessive use of antibiotics as miracle drugs has the potential to destroy the miracle, the tenet of antimicrobial use would predict this exact result, because within this use lies the seed of destruction, resistance (152,270). As a result, the arrival of the postantibiotic era is anticipated less than a century after the dawn of the antimicrobial era (10).

Importance of Understanding the Molecular Basis of Antimicrobial Action

Antimicrobial action can be defined as the interaction of the drug with the microorganism, the result of which may be inhibition or death of the organism or instead the emergence of resistance that negates the effect of the antibiotic (260,270). Although the emergence of resistance may well be an inevitable result of the use of antimicrobial agents, the understanding and application of the molecular basis of antimicrobial action can minimize the degree of resistance that occurs (82,234). Moreover, appreciation of the molecular basis of antimicrobial action allows better understanding of resistance mechanisms, which, in turn, allows these resistance mechanisms themselves to be targeted by antimicrobial agents (214). The therapy of tuberculosis serves as an example, in that the use of combination therapy with different classes of antimycobacterial agents as well as specific therapeutic approaches (e.g., directly observed therapy) can lead to differing rates of resistance (296). It is therefore the purpose of this chapter to review general principles for understanding the molecular basis of antimicrobial action and then to review mechanisms of action for selected classes of antimicrobial agents.

GENERAL PRINCIPLES OF ANTIMICROBIAL ACTION

Antimicrobial Mechanisms of Action in Relationship to the Cellular Structure and Physiology of Microbes

Importance of Microbial Physiology in Antimicrobial Action

The importance of the microbial growth phase for the *in vitro* effects of antimicrobial action has long been appreciated in clinical microbiology (161). However, this is only a small part of the microbial physiology that must be understood for the optimal use of antimicrobial agents. Microbial physiology is a complex subject with important implications for the effectiveness of antimicrobial agents, implications that are only now becoming appreciated. Fortunately, there has been a great deal of progress made in understanding microbial physiology and its influence on antimicrobial action. It is important to appreciate that microorganisms have mechanisms for replication, including synthesis of the cell wall, an important target of antimicrobial therapy. In addition to synthesis of the cell wall, a microorganism must also be able to focally lyse its cell wall so that replication can occur (249). The enzymes that mediate cell wall lysis must be tightly controlled, as they could cause destruction of the cell. These enzymes are preformed and are diffusely present in the cell wall until focally activated (250). Moreover, these enzymes can be globally activated as part of programmed cell death (i.e., apoptosis) (225). Microorganisms have evolved compensatory mechanisms to deal with times of starvation; these mechanisms ensure that the genome of some microorganisms survive until better times (232). Such mechanisms include quorum sensing, which may activate programmed cell death as the microbial population increases and nutrients become sparse (154). Microorganisms also have repair mechanisms; failing repair, programmed cell death is likely to occur (289). Finally, microorganisms often live in microcolonies in biofilm, and the behavior of a cell is greatly influenced by the location of the cell within the microcolony (58). Into this complex environment, antimicrobial agents are introduced. Attempting to understand the mechanism of action of these agents without understanding microbial physiology is futile. Accordingly, microbial physiology will be discussed in some detail.

The specific physiologic state of the microorganism, particularly its surface properties and rate of cell replication, markedly influences the activity of antimicrobial agents and partially determines whether they are bactericidal or bacteriostatic as well as their rate of killing (33–35). It has become clear that the pure *in vitro* broth culture, albeit the mainstay of antimicrobial susceptibility testing, is an artifact emphasizing free-floating mobile (planktonic) cells, which exist primarily in the laboratory setting and not in nature (i.e., infections) (161). This discriminates against the adherent (sessile) cells present in biofilm, which has now been acknowledged as the predominant growth form in natural ecosystems, including most infections (58,59,75,255). Moreover, microbial growth forms in biofilm have been associated with persistent infections and microbial resistance (33,59,255). Although noted long ago, it is no less true today: a solid support surface for the growth of bacteria provides a better approximation of the *in vivo* state than does broth medium (161).

Cellular Physiology of Microbial Life and Death

The growth of microorganisms in natural environments is characterized by periods of nutrient starvation, which results in growth rates that approximate zero (232). Nonetheless, bacteria are able to survive for prolonged periods of time despite the relative absence of nutrients. The survival of bacteria under these starvation conditions involves induction of a number of genes or proteins that mediate physiologic changes that enable the survival of some of the cells (53,232). These physiologic changes also can be seen as a microorganism transitions from the logarithmic phase of growth to the stationary phase, during which time the expression levels of a number of gene products produce marked phenotypic changes (21,176,254). Finally, these changes are seen after exposure of the microorganism to antimicrobial agents (246,251). The following examples are illustrative. Nutrient limitation in isolates of *Pseudomonas aeruginosa* has been shown to result in increased synthesis of exopolysaccharides (66,226). This phenotypic change, in turn, results in increased biofilm that appears to decrease the antimicrobial activity of a number of agents (81,256), including β-lactam agents such as piperacillin (4). In response to a broad range of environmental stresses, wild-type strains of *Escherichia coli* become short coccobacillary forms that exhibit resistance (116). These changes in *E. coli* are associated with alterations in the expression of penicillin-binding proteins (PBPs), with an increase seen in the amount of PBP6 and a decrease in PBP3 (77). Similar changes in the PBPs of *Streptococcus pyogenes* (254) and *Haemophilus influenzae* (176) during the stationary phase have been reported. This suggests some common effects for PBPs during the stationary phase on microorganisms. Lack of certain nutrients may also play a role (171). For example, limitation of choline in the teichoic acids of *Streptococcus pneumoniae* results in replacement by ethanolamine, which subsequently inhibits the growing cells from splitting into diplococci (292). All of these changes and more appear to be triggered by limitation of nutrients (185) and to be essential for continued cell survival during prolonged periods in the stationary phase (53,69,137,302).

Among other changes that occur under starvation conditions are those associated with the stringent response (97). The stringent response is an adaptation to conditions of amino acid starvation. This response includes induction of specific enzymes such as guanosine tetraphosphate in the initial stage, which then increases the transcription of both inducible and repressible enzyme operons involved in the stringent response (97,171). Examples of the stringent response include phenotypic changes seen in marine bacterial cells (185). These changes are characterized by rapid multiple divisions of starved cells, leading to the formation of ultramicrobacteria (less than 0.3 μm in diameter), which are also called dwarf forms. Rapid formation of multiple copies is presumed to improve the chances of individual genomes surviving. These cells are dormant forms and are quite resistant to many antimicrobial agents as well as to osmotic stress.

Starvation conditions are not the only conditions that may induce the stringent response. Other conditions that appear to induce the stringent response are exposure to certain antibiotics, including β-lactam agents. Lorian (160,162,163) demonstrated that staphylococci, when exposed to subinhibitory concentrations of penicillin, produced abnormally large cells that were actually clusters of smaller dwarf staphylococci crowded together within a single surrounding thickened cell wall and prevented from separating by the presence of many wide cross-walls. Comparison of the ultrastructure of staphylococci following penicillin exposure with that of staphylococci isolated from osteomylitis in animal models revealed morphologies that were virtually indistinguishable (93). When incubated on drug-free media, these clusters of staphylococci separated into smaller clusters and eventually become normal-sized individual cells.

These dwarf forms of staphylococci crowded together within a single thickened surrounding cell wall are likely to be dormant forms produced by the stringent response due to limited cell wall damage caused by subinhibitory concentrations of β-lactam agents. In contrast, higher levels of β-lactam agents cause enough cell wall damage to activate autolytic mechanisms (202). These differences, thus, may simply reflect a difference in the physiological response to cell wall damage: limited cell wall damage triggers a stringent response whereas extensive damage triggers apoptosis.

Similar multicellular forms of staphylococci are seen in mutant staphylococci that have had their *scdA* gene inactivated (36). This aberrant cellular morphology is similar to those of staphylococci carrying *femA* and *femB* mutations (117). This suggests that the transient changes described by Lorian and colleagues may become permanent after mutation of specific genes involved in this cellular morphology. Multiple dwarf copies of a microorganism within one thickened cell wall would presumably be more resistant to antimicrobial agents or other noxious substances and also would increase the chance of the genome surviving.

Similar effects have been described for other microorganisms. *Helicobacter pylori*, for example, has been shown to produce coccoid forms, which have been attributed to environmental stress such as starvation (21,45). These coccoid forms have also been found to emerge after exposure to antibiotics such as amoxicillin (24). They are not culturable *in vitro* but revert to culturable forms in mice (47). In *Bilophila wadsworthia*, subinhibitory concentrations of imipenem have been shown by scanning and transmission electron microscopy to result in large multilobate cells, suggesting that new growth of cells was initiated while cell division or separation was inhibited (266). A similar effect of imipenem has been reported for *P. aeruginosa* isolates, where large spheroplasts with evidence of cross-wall formation are seen just before lysis occurs after exposure to concentrations of imipenem greater that the relevant minimal inhibitory concentrations (MICs) (85). This effect presumably extends to the newer carbapenems such as meropenem. Dwarf forms of *P. aeruginosa* have been observed in microcolonies within the lung tissue of patients with cystic fibrosis (57,136,144). Each of these aberrant forms described most likely represents the entry of the microorganism into the stringent response phase.

It is of interest that, while long-starved cells are resistant to cell wall–active agents as well as agents that inhibit DNA synthesis, they remain somewhat susceptible to certain agents that inhibit protein synthesis (253). *Staphylococcus aureus* exposed to subinhibitory concentrations of antimicrobial agents that interfere with protein synthesis develop a thick cell wall (93) with one or two thick cross-walls, except in the case of tetracycline, where no cross-wall formation has been observed (112). This older observation has greater significance with the more recent demonstration of successful *in vivo* therapy of methicillin-resistant *S. aureus* endocarditis with minocycline in the clinical setting (146) as well as in an experimental model (196). In the experimental endocarditis model, minocycline was as effective as vancomycin. Recognition of the bactericidal effects of minocycline on microorganisms in a dormant phase may ultimately result in an additional antimicrobial agent for the therapy of methicillin-resistant staphylococci (309). This observation may become more important as the incidence of vancomycin-resistant staphylococci increases.

Cellular Physiology of Microbial Apoptosis and Repair

There are a number of physical or chemical agents in the natural environment of microbes that can cause damage to cells (121). The most vulnerable portions of microbial cells are the cell wall/membrane and the cell genome. Therefore, it is not surprising that microbial cells have evolved repair systems for these vulnerable targets. If the damage to the microbial cell is severe and cannot be repaired, an apoptosis (programmed cell death) mechanism is activated (19,120,225). Programmed cell death may, for example, play a role in the elimination of bacterial cells that are damaged by cell wall–active agents such as penicillins (18,154). The balance between repair and programmed cell death may well be an unappreciated target of antimicrobial therapy. Moreover, it is likely that rapid killing of microbes involves activation of apoptotic mechanisms. Such apoptotic mechanisms may also explain species-specific bactericidal activity. For example, chloramphenicol kills certain species such as *S. pneumoniae* and *H. influenzae* but not *E. coli*. This may simply reflect differences in the activation of apoptotic mechanisms.

Prevention of damage to vital portions of the microbial cell is clearly an important prelude to cellular repair. Accordingly, microbial cells have developed an effective protective barrier for their cell wall/membrane called biofilm. Biofilm is discussed in the next two sections. Repair of this biofilm and of the underlying cell wall/membrane structure when damage occurs is an important microbial function. Biofilm repair involves synthesis of the precursors within the cytoplasm, translocation of these precursors to the outer portions of the cell wall/membrane, and final assembly of the biofilm matrix. Studies have shown that biofilm repair is dependent on a carbohydrate source, an energy source, certain enzymes, and functioning efflux pumps. With these components available, repair occurs very quickly (148). There is now intriguing evidence that macrolides interfere with the synthesis and repair of biofilm and with the elaboration of exotoxins by means of codon-anticodon interactions that inhibit the translation of messenger RNA (mRNA) for inducible enzymes (105,133,179,189,224,305). This important topic is discussed in the following sections.

Repair of any damage to the cell wall/membrane of microbes appears to be most easily accomplished by replication, provided the damage is not extensive. This may be an important factor in combination antimicrobial therapy specifically directed at creating a physiological conflict for the infectious microbes. Such an approach might involve the use of cell wall disrupters combined with agents active against replicating microorganisms.

The repair of structural damage to DNA is also of considerable importance to the microbe, because this damage (and the repair) might result in mutations that could be lethal. Accordingly, the response to DNA damage by the microorganism is complex (289). There are three important mechanisms of DNA repair in microorganisms: (a) direct repair, which restores the original structure; (b) indirect repair, in which one DNA strand is bypassed during replication or is excised and then rebuilt by copying the intact strand; and (c) postreplication repair, in which the damage is eliminated by recombination between the sister strands after replication.

A major mechanism for indirect repair of damage that blocks chain elongation during replication is that provided by the SOS system (156). The SOS system is a set of approximately 20 damage-inducible (*din*) genes. The SOS response is controlled by two regulatory proteins, which are the products of the *lexA* and *recA* genes. The first protein product of the gene *lexA* normally represses the SOS response. Upon SOS induction, the *recA* gene produces RecA protein. Damaged DNA, in the presence of the single-strand–binding protein, binds RecA protein in a way that changes its configuration so that it becomes a protease that cleaves *lexA*. This results in derepression of the other genes. The induction of RecA protein can be inhibited by antimicrobial agents such as chloramphenicol, erythromycin, and tetracycline, which have codon-anticodon interactions that inhibit the translation of mRNA needed for the synthesis of inducible enzymes.

Once activated, the SOS response has several effects. One of these is induction of DNA polymerases, which will be needed when cell division resumes (306). Another is cell division inhibition mediated by *sfiA* and *sfiC*, which target the *ftsZ* gene and protein, important factors in cell separation (56). Overproduction of the ftsZ protein has been shown to produce ultramicrobacteria. The SOS response is primarily involved in DNA repair. The major mechanism of repair of the activated SOS system is bypass repair. This particular mechanism of DNA repair tends to be error-prone and often results in mutants (291).

Cell Wall/Biofilm Structures of Gram-Positive and Gram-Negative Microorganisms

The cell walls of both Gram-positive (Fig. 12.1) and Gram-negative (Fig. 12.2) bacteria are similar, in that both possess inner cytoplasmic membranes as well as outer peptidoglycan (murein) layers (228). Gram-negative bacteria also have an additional outer cell membrane, which covers the peptidoglycan layer (25,166). Finally, the cell walls of both Gram-positive and Gram-negative bacteria interface with the external milieu via biofilm, which is a matrix-supported gel (58). Each of these structures plays a critical role in the interaction of antimicrobial agents with the microorganism.

The cytoplasmic membrane in each group of bacteria is a semipermeable membrane that regulates molecular flow, in turn determining pH (30,205), osmotic pressures (31), and availability of essential substances. The peptidoglycan layer in each group is a continuous cross-linked mesh that forms a polyionic and amphoteric network. The peptidoglycan mesh is composed of linear glycan chains that are interlinked by short peptides (282). This shell surrounds the entire microorganism, is known as a sacculus, and is found exclusively in eubacteria. The peptidoglycan sacculus is not a rigid shell but instead is elastic and flexible. This relatively porous peptidoglycan sacculus (exclusion limits of 100,000 Da) serves as a mechanical "exoskeleton" that helps to maintain the microorganism's shape, rigidity, and osmotic stability. The exoskeleton of Gram-positive bacteria is thicker than that of Gram-negatives, thus providing more rigidity. Although this polyanionic sacculus might appear to be an exclusion barrier, the exclusion limits of 100,000 Da make this meshwork very coarse and thus allow molecules of lesser size, such as antimicrobial agents, which have sizes of 300–700 Da, to readily diffuse through the layer. Finally, the peptidoglycan structure is involved in the cell division process (188).

The molecular structures of the cytoplasmic membranes of Gram-positive and Gram-negative bacteria are essentially the same, consisting of lipid bilayers containing phospholipids and membrane proteins (228). There are, however, important differences in the peptidoglycan wall and the biofilm for these two groups of bacteria. Gram-positive bacteria have a relatively simple but thick cell wall constructed of peptidoglycan and teichoic acids, which are long-chain polymers consisting of glycerol or ribitol residues with phosphodiester links and various substituents such as uronic acids (248,292). Teichoic acids are found as either cell-bound or free soluble acids. The cell wall of Gram-positive bacteria contains two forms of the cell-bound teichoic acid. In one form, lipoteichoic acid, one end of the chain is anchored to phospholipids in the

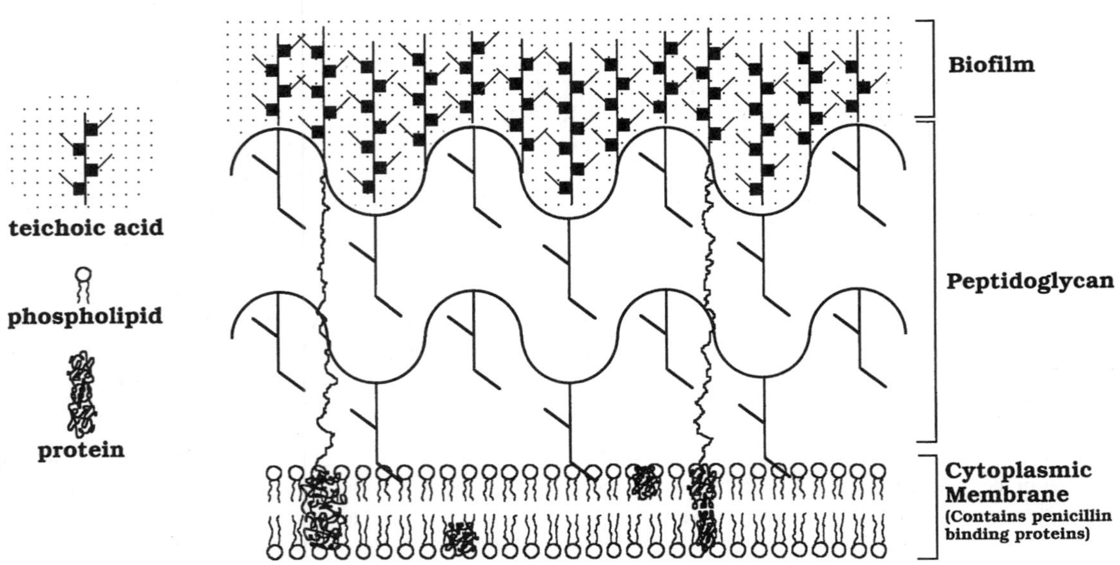

FIGURE 12.1 ● Schematic representation of the cell wall of Gram-positive microorganisms.

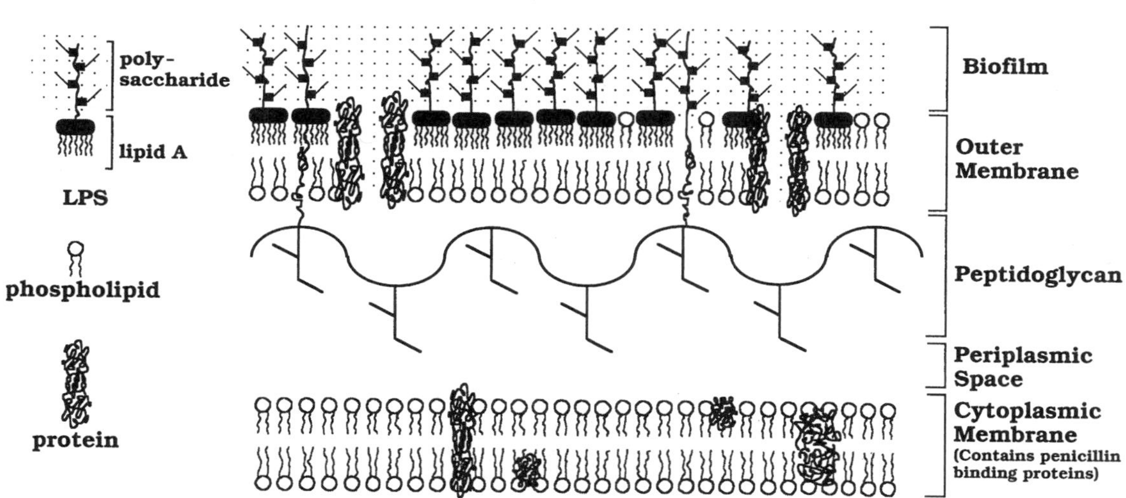

FIGURE 12.2 ● Schematic representation of the cell wall of Gram-negative microorganisms. LPS, lipopolysaccharide.

cytoplasmic membrane while the other end transverses the peptidoglycan layer in such a way that it protrudes at the cell surface. In the second, a cell wall teichoic acid, one end is attached to *N*-acetylmuramyl residues in the peptidoglycan layer and the free end protrudes at the cell surface. Finally, free, soluble teichoic acid is present in large amounts in the outer portion of the cell wall.

At the surface of the Gram-positive cell wall, the protruding teichoic acids can be linked with one another via branching polysaccharides to form a matrix. The cross-linking of the biofilm matrix is accomplished using polysaccharides with repeating units of two or three sugars. The variety of possible hexose stereoisomers and of linkages, as well as the potential incorporation of unusual sugar residues, results in thousands of different trisaccharides in the matrix. Because the polysaccharide chains in the matrix are hydrophilic, water is absorbed into the matrix and transforms this outer layer into a gel. This matrix-supported gel (99% water) is known by a variety of names, including *biofilm, glycocalyx, slime, alginate,* and *capsule*.

One of the key components of the biofilm is phospholipids because of the covalent bonding they provide. In addition, this hydrated matrix depends on calcium and magnesium cations to maintain the negatively charged ends of the polysaccharides in close approximation. The availability of phospholipids and divalent cations in the medium greatly influences the final composition of the cell wall. This can be appreciated by considering the Gram-positive cell wall. Under conditions of magnesium limitation, Gram-positive bacteria increase the amount of teichoic acid produced while decreasing the amount of alanyl ester substitutions, which results in fewer polysaccharides present in the matrix and hence less biofilm. Phosphate limitation results in the replacement of teichoic acids by teichuronic acids, which have less covalent bonding. Starvation conditions, then, would be predicted to result in cell walls with minimal biofilm.

The cell walls of Gram-negative bacteria differ from those of Gram-positive bacteria in a number of ways (166). First, they have a relatively thin peptidoglycan layer, which provides less rigidity. Gram-negative cell walls also have an additional outer cell membrane (25,107) that serves as an effective permeability barrier (149,198). This outer cell membrane is composed of two layers. The inner layer consists largely of glycerophospholipid molecules with two covalently linked fatty acid chains, a molecular structure that is fairly common in membranes in general. The outer layer is somewhat unique among membranes and contains lipopolysaccharides with six or seven covalently linked fatty acid chains. The fatty acids present in the lipopolysaccharides are saturated. This results in the interior of the lipid bilayer being less fluid, because there is no packing of carbons, as seen when the fatty acids are unsaturated (198). This serves to make this barrier more restrictive to hydrophilic agents.

Areas of adhesion between the outer cell membrane and the inner cytoplasmic membrane, called Bayer's junctions, have been described by a number of investigators. These adhesions of the inner cytoplasmic membrane to the cell peptidoglycan/outer membrane are probable sites of synthesis of the outer membrane and biofilm as well as synthesis of other substrates to be pumped from the cell cytoplasm into the periplasmic space or from the cell cytoplasm directly into the biofilm.

Gram-negative bacteria, like Gram-positive bacteria, are surrounded by a polyanionic polysaccharide matrix, which differs mainly by being anchored by the lipo-oligosaccharides rather than by lipoteichoic acids. In some instances, the attachment is to the peptidoglycan layer, whereas in others the lipid A is anchored to the inner cytoplasmic membrane. This lipopolysaccharide matrix of Gram-negative bacteria is also thought to provide some selectivity/hindrance via negative ionic charges and/or steric hindrance (239).

Biofilms of both Gram-positive and Gram-negative bacteria are essentially anionic polymeric diffusion barriers and can be thought of as an ion-exchange resin of almost infinite surface area. In addition, the biofilm protects the microorganism from heavy metal toxicity, from most bacteriophages, from phagocytic white blood cells, from antibodies and/or complement, and from an inhospitable milieu such as osmotic, pH, or enzymatic dangers. The interface of the biofilm with the aqueous phase can be altered by methylation of fatty acids or by sulfonation of polysaccharides, which increases the barrier to water-soluble agents (167). Bacteria are able to excrete into their biofilm and the surrounding medium several different classes of molecules, including exopolysaccharides (the building blocks of biofilm), siderophores, protein enzymes, and toxins (107). Biofilms also appear to serve as a repository for defensive substances such as β-lactamase (98).

In human infections, microbial cells are most often found with biofilm, even though microscopic examination may not readily reveal this. In clinical microbiology laboratories, the optimal growth conditions sought by microbiologists are far from the near-starvation circumstances the bacteria encounter in their natural environments. This is particularly true for broth media (161). However, the growth of Gram-positive and Gram-negative bacteria on agar plates in the laboratory may reflect, in part, the presence or absence of biofilm. Smooth colonies have more biofilm than do rough colonies, while mucoid or slimy colonies have the most. Deep rough colonies, on the other hand, have the smallest amount of biofilm, if any at all. These deep rough mutants have most of the core lipid A eliminated. Such strains are more susceptible to lysozyme and more permeable to hydrophobic antibiotics. Finally, in clinical microbiology laboratories, biofilm may be recognized and described microscopically as capsule.

Consequences of Biofilm Disruption

The disruption of the bacterial cell wall often results in the death of the microorganism (121). This is well appreciated by clinicians. Less well appreciated is that the disruption of biofilm surrounding an individual microbial cell is not without consequences (280). These may be related to osmotic pressure and the shifting of cell peptidoglycan by that pressure. There is a higher hydrostatic pressure within the cytoplasmic space of a microbe than that which is exerted on the cell by the external milieu. The presence of the biofilm matrix seems to assist in keeping this internal pressure in check (281). When a portion of the gel is removed, however, the internal pressure shifts the cell wall/membrane so that it protrudes through this disrupted area, resulting in a fingerlike projection containing cytoplasmic contents (130,240,307). Extrusion of this portion of the cell wall/membrane through the hole in the biofilm is a result of the cell wall/membrane shifting to adjust to the focused pressure directed at the area of disrupted biofilm. This shift in turn activates autolytic enzymes to dissolve the peptidoglycan component of the cell wall as the wall shifts during replication (272). This causes dissolution of cell wall peptidoglycan in this area, which, in conjunction with the high, focused internal pressure, effectively severs this protruding bleb (229), leaving a transient hole. If enough holes are formed, leakage of cytoplasmic contents results in cellular death (71). The results of this process can be demonstrated by electron microscopy, which makes visible a range of ultrastructural changes, including narrow fingerlike projections, blebs, and extracellular cytoplasmic-filled vesicles. Disruption of the entire biofilm matrix, in contrast, tends to equalize the pressure over the entire cell wall/membrane. Consequently, when the autolytic enzymes dissolve the peptidoglycan of the entire cell, the result may be lysis of the entire cell or the creation of a spheroplast if the osmolarity of the external milieu is sufficiently high. When lysis is seen, it occurs rapidly, in contrast to the lysis seen after exposure to penicillin, where cells continue to grow for approximately half a generation before lysis (119,229). Finally, it appears that Gram-negative bacteria are more susceptible to the effects of biofilm disrupters, perhaps because of their less rigid cell walls.

Disruption of biofilm can be accomplished by a number of physicochemical mechanisms (167). This disruption can be best appreciated by electron microscopy. The ultrastructure of normal cells of Gram-negative or Gram-positive bacteria has a slightly undulating smooth surface, which is transformed to a surface with blebs and tubular projections after displacement of Ca^{2+} and Mg^{2+} from the biofilm. Displacement of these cations from the biofilm by chelating agents such as ethylenediaminetetraacetic acid (EDTA) (148,229) or by polycationic agents (281) such as polymyxin B (130,240) and aminoglycosides (126,169) has been shown to be an effective way to disrupt biofilm, although this mechanism can be countered by the presence of excessive amounts of calcium and magnesium cations in the milieu (192,194,278). However, adding these cations after the damage has been done has no effect. The ultrastructural changes seen by electron microscopy are accompanied by a functional change, namely, increased permeability to hydrophobic agents such as antibiotics (106,107,280).

If the changes induced by the disruption of biofilm are not rapidly fatal and the cells are allowed to grow, the permeability barrier is repaired in about two-thirds of a generation (148). The addition of chloramphenicol or tetracycline or the omission of required amino acids does not affect the repair rate. A proton pump inhibitor such as 2,4-dinitrophenol, however, prevents repair. The activity of omiprazole and lansorprazole against *H. pylori* (233) may be related to their inhibitory effect on certain cellular membrane pumps. Omitting glucose also prevents biofilm repair. Interestingly, the addition of macrolides decreases the repair rate, possibly because of its inhibition of mRNA translation (177).

Effects of Antimicrobial Agents on the Production of Biofilm

Antimicrobial agents, not unexpectedly, can either increase or decrease the production of biofilm. This effect, in part, appears species-specific. For example, fluoroquinolones at concentrations of one half the MIC of *Staphylococcus epidermidis* decrease the production of slime (i.e., biofilm) (216). On the other hand, exposure of *Klebsiella pneumoniae* to a fluoroquinolone such as ciprofloxacin (114) has been shown to increase the amount of biofilm by more than 100-fold. Similarly, exposure of many microorganisms to β-lactam agents results in increased production of biofilm (114). Reduction of biofilm can be seen with other agents such as salicylates (74). The reduction of biofilm appears to occur concomitantly with a decrease in porin proteins (40,238,265). If these porins are being utilized to pump the biofilm precursors to the cell wall outer surface for final assembly, the two events are probably cause and effect. The decrease in biofilm and porin protein has been shown to result in resistance (40,231). This phenomenon has been shown to inhibit the activity of cephalosporins (91), aminoglycosides (74), and carbapenems (265). If biofilm is increased by exposure to β-lactam agents, then antimicrobial agents that have an effect on biofilm should be enhanced by preexposure of the bacteria to β-lactam agents. Indeed, this has been reported in both *in vitro* (15) and *in vivo* (103) studies.

Effects of Biofilm on Antimicrobial Action

The establishment of biofilm is an important aspect of cell wall physiology for individual cells and is equally important for microorganisms collectively. Bacteria that live and metabolize in these dense biofilm-encased microcolonies gain a number of the advantages enjoyed by multicellular life forms. One such advantage is a circulatory system (although primitive) with which to receive nutrients and into which to discharge metabolic wastes. This circulatory system consists of permeable channels that pass through less dense areas of biofilm interspersed within the dense microcolonies (58). Along these channels live river populations of microorganisms. These channels have convective flow patterns that permit the penetration and distribution into the biofilm matrix of large (2000-Da) molecules. Dissolved oxygen is another critical commodity that is distributed within the biofilm through these channels. Microelectrodes have determined that the concentrations of dissolved oxygen in dense microcolonies approach zero at the center, owing to diffusion limitations and oxygen utilization (227). Such direct observations explain the need for anaerobic pathways for microorganisms that are considered to be strict aerobes. Similar redox-sensitive chemical probes and autoradiography (257) have been used to detect metabolic activity and have demonstrated that, within a microcolony, the majority of cells are metabolically active. Although metabolically active, bacteria within biofilm colonies grow very slowly and are considered to resemble stationary-phase cultures (33). Moreover, those microorganisms downriver receive fewer substrates and may therefore become nutritionally starved, setting into motion the complex set of events (34,35) described in the preceding section.

Changes in microbial growth rate and nutrient limitation have long been recognized to cause changes in cell envelope components, which, in turn, influence the susceptibility of the microbes to antimicrobial agents (34,35,119,277). Establishment of biofilm is a growth-related factor that influences the susceptibility of the microbes to antimicrobial agents (88). For example, exposure of planktonic cells of *P. aeruginosa* to a biofilm surface produced by cells of the same species triggers the expression of at least two genes, *algC* and *algG* (66). This influences the susceptibility of these cells to antimicrobial agents, because sessile cells encased in biofilm are phenotypically different from planktonic cells of the same species (101).

The presence of biofilm at the individual cellular level contributes to changes in the overall susceptibility patterns of microorganisms involved in chronic infections, because the encasement by biofilm allows aggregates of cells to exist together in microcolonies. In mature biofilms, bacterial cells occupy only 5% to 35% of the biofilm mass. There are currently two leading hypotheses for the persistence of chronic biofilm-associated infections: (a) decreased concentrations of antibiotics caused by impaired transport to some regions of the biofilm (141,255,297) or by a dilutional effect (255) and (b) physiologic differences of sessile cells (101). A biofilm accumulation model has predicted that both mechanisms would result in reduced antimicrobial susceptibilities of 7-day-old biofilms compared with those of 2-day-old films (255). Growth rate–dependent killing was predicted to be decreased in thicker biofilms because of oxygen depletion, leading to reduced growth rates. The model also predicted resistance to the antibiotic due to depletion caused by increased biomass. The explanation was not that the antibiotic would fail to penetrate the biofilm but instead that the drug would be diluted in the bulk fluid. The binding of agents to biofilm is related to two factors: the relative availability of drug and the relative proximity. Relative availability is proportional to the amount of drug, whereas relative proximity is proportional to the concentration of the drug. The total amount of drug may remain the same as the biomass of polysaccharide increases, but the relative proximity decreases. Finally, many of the factors affecting antimicrobial susceptibility may change over time as the biofilm colony matures, because maturation alters the milieu for many microorganisms within the microcolony. For example, colonies deep within thick, mature biofilm may have reached the starvation stage.

Mechanisms of Antimicrobial Uptake

A factor that is clearly of great importance for effective antimicrobial action against bacteria is the penetration of the antimicrobial agent into the microbial cell. In order to understand the mechanics of antimicrobial uptake, it is useful to understand the physiology of transport systems located on microbial cell membranes.

In all microorganisms, the cytoplasmic membrane provides an osmotic barrier that is permeable to very few substances. It is porous to water and to uncharged organic molecules up to the size of glycerol. Gram-negative bacteria have an additional cell membrane, the outer membrane, which also acts as an effective barrier against antibiotics. In particular, hydrophobic antibiotics diffuse relatively poorly through the outer cell membrane in Gram-negative bacteria in comparison with diffusion through the cytoplasmic membrane. This is due to the lack of glycerophospholipid in the outer portion of the cell bilayer, which instead consists largely of lipopolysaccharides.

Antimicrobial agents derived from microorganisms bear little resemblance to natural substrates brought into the bacterial cell but instead are more akin to metabolites excreted by cells (108). Therefore, with few exceptions (e.g., fosfomycin, which uses a stereospecific nutrient transport system (128), antibiotics do not utilize active transport mechanisms for substrate uptake into bacteria.

There are three general mechanisms for substrate uptake into the bacterial cell: simple diffusion, facilitated diffusion, and active transport (9). There is a fourth mechanism known as the self-promoted uptake pathway, which is used by certain bacteria. Each is discussed.

Simple or passive diffusion is defined as movement of molecules across a permeable membrane in which the flux in either direction is proportional to the concentration on the entering side and the rate of net transfer is proportional to the concentration differences between the two sides. An important factor in this type of diffusion is the partitioning coefficient, which essentially indicates the ability of the substrate to dissolve into the membrane interior (i.e., permeability). Simple diffusion kinetics are seen with nonpolar organic molecules such as tetracycline, which penetrates by dissolving in the lipid of the membrane, as well as with antimicrobial agents that move across the membrane through pores. Fluoroquinolones, for example, are taken into bacteria by passive diffusion through porins in a passive diffusion process that exhibits nonsaturable kinetics. Fluoroquinolones are amphoteric molecules and have both zwitterionic and uncharged forms at neutral pH. Generally, only uncharged molecules are involved in the passive diffusion process, with the amount of uncharged forms greatly influencing the penetrating ability of these agents. Charged molecules can also exhibit passive diffusion, provided there is an electrical gradient across the membrane (170).

Facilitated diffusion in theory involves a barrier-insoluble substance reacting with a carrier within the barrier to form a complex that can shuttle across the membrane, where the substance is then released. This type of diffusion exhibits saturable Michaelis kinetics with a K_m and a V_{max}, but the K_m is the same on both sides of the membrane because this mechanism is not linked to an energy source. Another name for this type of uptake pathway is a passive carrier–mediated system. Facilitated diffusion is seen in yeasts but has not yet been identified in bacteria.

Active transport means that the bacterial cell has the ability to concentrate molecules within the cell. This ability can be turned on or off (i.e., is inducible) and is linked to an energy source. Without this energy source, the molecules cannot pass across the membrane. The kinetics of active transport exhibit a K_m and a V_{max}, like the activity of an enzyme, and the carrier system can be saturated.

The self-promoted uptake pathway has been described for Gram-negative bacteria and involves binding of the antibiotic to the lipopolysaccharide in the outer membrane (127,211). This is followed by outer displacement, by the antimicrobial agent, of magnesium and possibly calcium ions in the lipopolysaccharide matrix of the biofilm (109). This causes instability of the biofilm matrix, as described earlier, and leads to increased permeability (123). The presence of additional divalent cations prevents this by stabilizing the complex. The self-promoted pathway was first described as an uptake mechanism in *P. aeruginosa* for polycationic antibiotics such as polymyxin and the aminoglycosides (109). More recently it has been noted for azithromycin in *E. coli* (89).

Cell membranes of microorganisms must be energized in order to concentrate nutrients needed for growth. The electrochemical gradient–induced proton motive force is a key factor in these energized cytoplasmic membranes. Microbial cell membranes are intrinsically impermeable to protons yet must move protons in or out of the cell. For example, any change in the intracellular pH of the microorganism would need to be absorbed by the buffering capacity of the cytoplasm (30) unless there was some method for expelling protons. Such a pH-homeostatic method exists and involves membrane-bound proton pumps (205). Proton-driven translocation of molecules is facilitated by reduced pH (174). These pumps may at times be responsible for the efflux of antibiotics by pumping out protons that are complexed with a negatively charged antibiotic.

The uptake of antimicrobial agents into bacterial cells can be greatly influenced by efflux mechanisms that may concomitantly act to remove the agent (31,198, 199,208,217). In fact, the antimicrobial activity may be determined by the race between uptake and efflux. It is useful to appreciate the mechanisms of efflux, because these should themselves prove to be excellent targets for antimicrobial agents (158,159).

Membrane-bound proton pumps may be readily overcome by compounds with uncoupling activity (208). Classic uncouplers include carbonyl cyanide-*m*-chlorophenylhydrazine and 2,4-dinitrophenol (235). These uncouplers result in the abolition of respiratory control in the bacteria. This, in turn, results in stimulation of respiratory activity.

Inhibitory or Lethal Antimicrobial Activity versus Physiologic Conflict in Microbes

Inhibitory and Lethal Effects

The goal of antimicrobial therapy, as appreciated by Lister and Ehrlich, is to destroy the invading microorganism without harming the host. The effectiveness of an antimicrobial agent has traditionally been measured by its ability to inhibit and kill bacteria. In theory, there are three basic ways to kill a bacterial cell: by causing irreparable damage to its genome, to its envelope, and to certain classes of its proteins (121). Antimicrobial agents have been developed that attempt to kill bacteria in each of these ways. Often several antibiotics that use two of these three different ways are combined to enhance the lethal effect. Yet, as already noted, bacteria are not particularly easy to kill. This fact has not escaped microbiologists. It is well known that most antimicrobial agents exert their lethal effects on bacteria during the growth phase (61,119,277). Therefore, microbiologists have designed routine susceptibility tests to measure antimicrobial activity during the logarithmic growth phase in media that provide all of the ingredients for optimal growth (259). However, this is not the usual state of microorganisms in infected tissues. For example, *S. aureus* isolates from tissue-cage infections in rats have been shown to be in a state of dormancy and thus are relatively resistant to most antimicrobial agents (52). Perhaps the closest that broth susceptibility testing comes to mimicking a clinical infection is in the case of acute bacterial meningitis. Even then, there clearly is room for improvement (261). Susceptibility testing must be repositioned to provide test results that correlate with the clinical infection. This must be done as a part of larger programs aimed at controlling resistance.

Physiologic Conflict

Most clinical infections involve bacteria in a sessile state, as opposed to a planktonic state. However, antimicrobial agents that are able to kill bacteria in their sessile state are few in number (86,276). Of those agents currently available for clinical use, imipenem and the fluoroquinolones have the greatest lethal effect against sessile bacteria—a lethal effect more readily obtained against Gram-negative isolates than against Gram-positive ones. This *in vitro* bactericidal activity, often defined as a = 3 $\log_{10}$ decrease in colony-forming units over a 24-hour period (259), may not be sufficient for total microbial killing against certain microorganisms. Total and rapid microbial killing is important in acute bacterial meningitis as well as in acute sepsis in immunodeficient hosts (61,62). Even the most rigorous *in vitro* susceptibility test methods, including time-kill kinetic methodology, may provide misinformation if the growth phase of the microorganism and the clinically desired endpoint are not correlated with the test method. This is shown by a report by investigators who found that clarithromycin, like other macrolides, demonstrated *in vitro* bactericidal activity against pneumococci by time-kill kinetic methodology (241). However, in a rabbit model for pneumococcal meningitis, clarithromycin was unable to cure pneumococcal meningitis despite susceptible isolates and cerebrospinal fluid levels of clarithromycin comparable to those used to achieve *in vitro* killing (241). In chronic infections such as endocarditis and osteomyelitis, where involvement of biofilm is almost always present, rapid microbial killing is usually not achievable due to factors such as decreased biofilm penetration/dilutional effects and dormant growth phase. Total microbial killing, on the other hand, is a well-recognized goal when treating these particular infections.

The accumulated knowledge of antimicrobial mechanisms of action, or lack thereof, on different growth phases of bacteria has reached a point where it can provide an alternate approach to antimicrobial therapy. This approach involves creating physiological conflict for the infecting microorganism. Physiological conflict directed at the microorganism often can be achieved by using knowledge of the various physiological states that microorganisms turn to for survival combined with knowledge of specific antimicrobial agents that interfere with each of the altered physiological states. When these agents are combined for initial therapy, their use creates a physiological conflict for the microorganism when it seeks an altered physiological state. Although increased killing as defined by synergy may not be detected, enhancement of total killing may be measured.

Physiological conflict as a therapeutic tenet is already in use but is not well appreciated. The therapy of tuberculosis is one of the oldest examples of this tenet, for in such therapy multiple antituberculous agents create a physiological conflict by inhibiting the mycolic acid/lipid layer and minimizing the emergence of resistance. An example of this therapeutic approach is the recognition of the lethal effect of metronidazole on dormant forms of *Mycobacterium tuberculosis* (294). This lethal activity appears to be related to the fact that the dormant state requires anaerobic pathways, which then provide the necessary electrons to activate metronidazole to its electrophilic degradation products. Exposing *M. tuberculosis* in its dormant state to metronidazole either kills the organism or forces it back to aerobic respiration. The return to aerobic pathways does not occur independently but instead occurs with resumption of mycobacterial replication. Thus, combining metronidazole or similar agents with agents that interfere with this replicating stage creates a physiological conflict that prevents the mycobacterium from remaining in either growth phase.

Another example of physiological conflict is the use of an aminoglycoside with a β-lactam agent for the therapy of infections such as bacterial endocarditis caused by *P. aeruginosa*. The increased effectiveness of this combination is due to the disruption of the biofilm by the aminoglycoside (169,193), which enhances the β-lactam agent in two ways. The first is when disruption provides holes in the bacterial cell wall that allow increased penetration of the β-lactam agent. The second is when the dormant form is forced to replicate in an attempt to fix the damaged cell wall, thus providing a target for the β-lactam agent.

Other chronic infections that might benefit from an approach that creates physiological conflict include pulmonary infections caused by *P. aeruginosa* in patients with cystic fibrosis. These infections involve the establishment in lung tissue of biofilm-encased microcolonies in which are found some dwarf forms, which may represent dormant forms that are utilizing anaerobic pathways (57,136,144). Clinical cure of these *Pseudomonas* pulmonary infections is rarely achieved (136). This is consistent with the *in vitro* observation that total microbial killing of sessile strains of *P. aeruginosa* is extremely difficult to achieve after the biofilm has matured for 5 to 7 days (88). Neither older synergistic combinations such as tobramycin and piperacillin (4) nor newer synergistic combinations such as fosfomycin and ofloxacin (140) are able to achieve total killing.

There are, however, some approaches that may create physiological conflict. The use of aerosolized tobramycin (219) is one of these; it provides greater concentrations of this biofilm disrupter, which enhances the use of other antipseudomonal agents. The prolonged use of aminoglycosides in chronic *Pseudomonas* infections is known to be followed by the emergence of aminoglycoside-resistant *Pseudomonas* strains characterized by a deep rough colony morphology on agar plates due to the lack of biofilm (193). The lack of a lipopolysaccharide/biofilm target for the primary action of the aminoglycoside is the mechanism of resistance, because these strains do not exhibit altered ribosomes or produce aminoglycoside-inactivating enzymes. The outer cell walls of these aminoglycoside-resistant strains are characterized by the lack of lipopolysaccharide and a marked increase in the amount of OprH outer membrane protein (193). Overproduction of this outer cell membrane protein decreases the accumulation of polymyxin and gentamicin by the self-promoted pathway (123). However, overproduction of OprH is associated with increased susceptibility to fluoroquinolone antibiotics (308). It appears that the overproduction of OprH is a mechanism that minimizes biofilm in order to counter the effects of biofilm disruption by polycationic agents, but in doing so the altered cell wall seems to offer increased diffusion of lipophilic fluoroquinolones into the cytoplasm. The use of a fluoroquinolone and an antipseudomonal β-lactam agent along with the aerosolized aminoglycoside thus creates a physiological conflict. Moreover, the addition of a macrolide such as erythromycin, azithromycin, or clarithromycin to this regimen may prove useful. These macrolides have been shown to decrease the production of both biofilm (122,305) and exoenzymes (133) by *P. aeruginosa*, which creates yet another biofilm-related conflict while preventing further pulmonary damage by the exoenzymes (76,122,139,179,181,236,237). Finally, if the dwarf forms represent dormant forms that utilize anaerobic pathways, the addition of metronidazole might also prove useful. Although these may seem to be only theoretical approaches for antimicrobial combinations, there currently are sufficient data to initiate *in vitro* investigations that could be followed by animal studies (62) and then by clinical trials if warranted.

There are other examples of physiological conflict in microbes that can be purposely created by the selective use of antibiotics. A number of these are discussed. Temofloxacin has been shown to be effective in the therapy of experimental streptococcal endocarditis, and studies have found it to penetrate vegetations in a homogeneous manner (63). Dextranase is an enzyme capable of hydrolyzing 20% to 90% of streptococcal glycocalyx (biofilm). When used alone, dextranase has no *in vitro* antimicrobial effect on viridans streptococci, nor does it have a beneficial effect on experimental streptococcal endocarditis (65). When dextranase is used in combination with temofloxacin, it significantly potentiates the effect of temofloxacin *in vivo* by reducing the amount of bacterial biofilm in infected vegetations and by altering the metabolic status of the microorganisms (180). The same effect has been seen when dextranase and penicillin have been combined in the treatment of experimental streptococcal endocarditis (65). Finally, an animal model for experimental *P. aeruginosa* endocarditis has shown an identical effect for alginase combined with amikacin (17). Of importance is the lack of beneficial effect demonstrated when the vegetation size is reduced by fibrinolytic therapy (39,70). The results of these studies are consistent with the theory that the bacteria in microcolonies embedded in biofilm have a lower metabolic rate. Reducing the amount of biofilm results in both an increased metabolic rate and increased replication, which each increase the antimicrobial activity of most antibiotics.

Another approach to disrupting the biofilm as a method for creating physiological conflict is to use the proteolytic enzyme serratiopeptidase (178). Serratiopeptidase is a metalloprotease produced by a strain of *Serratia* that is only partially inhibited by *in vivo* protease inhibitors and has been used as an antiinflammatory drug because of its ability to increase the penetration of antibiotics into infected sites (304). This protease has been found to enhance the activity of ofloxacin on sessile cultures of *P. aeruginosa* and *S. aureus* (243).

Another commonly used drug with the potential for creating biofilm-related physiological conflict in microbes is aspirin. Aspirin has been noted to be a cell wall permeabilizer for *P. aeruginosa* (106). This role as a cell wall permeabilizer may be related to its effect on biofilm. Aspirin has been shown to cause a dose-dependent reduction in the weight of aortic vegetations in experimental endocarditis (197). In addition, when combined with vancomycin, aspirin improves the sterilization rate of aortic valve vegetations infected with *S. aureus*. These effects are similar to those of dextranase (180) and the protease of *Serratia* (243) and may be a result of physiological conflict. Aspirin has been found to diminish the amount of microbial biofilm in a number of other studies (74). Salicylates are also known to depress the synthesis of porins in *E. coli*, *K. pneumoniae*, *Serratia marcescens*, *Burkholderia cepatia*, and *P. aeruginosa* (40,91,238,265). If these depressed porins are involved in the efflux of biofilm precursors as a part of biofilm maintenance, these two phenomena may be related.

Another commonly used agent that seems to create a physiological conflict when combined with certain antimicrobial agents for the treatment of chronic *P. aeruginosa* infections in patients with cystic fibrosis is ascorbic acid. Ascorbic acid is a weak acid that has been shown to have a bactericidal effect alone and acts to increase the permeability of the cell membrane at nonbactericidal concentrations (221). These effects are interfered with by magnesium ions. Because ascorbic acid does not chelate magnesium to form a detectable complex, it is thought that the ascorbic acid displaces the magnesium ions in a manner similar to that of polycations. The permeabilization of the *Pseudomonas* cell wall renders the organism susceptible to antimicrobial agents such as sulfamethoxazole/trimethoprim, erythromycin, and chloramphenicol, which are usually not active against this pathogen (222,223). The combination of erythromycin and ascorbic acid has been evaluated in a mouse model and found to be effective, whereas sulfamethoxazole/trimethoprim/ascorbic acid has been found to diminish by 10- to 100-fold the number of viable *P. aeruginosa* organisms in the sputum in patients with cystic fibrosis (222).

There is another combination of antimicrobial agents that recently has been used for chronic infections of prosthetic devices and that may owe its somewhat surprising efficacy in these difficult-to-treat infections to physiological conflict. This is the combination of rifampin with the fluoroquinolones. There are several studies worth reviewing. In the first, therapy with 900 mg/day rifampin plus 600 mg/day ofloxacin for 6 months was used for patients with prosthetic implants infected with *Staphylococcus* spp. The overall success rate was 74% among 47 patients, with 62% of patients being cured without removal of their orthopedic device (80). The success rate was 81% for the hip prosthesis group, 69% for the knee prosthesis group, and 69% for the osteosynthesis device group. A total of eight treatment failures were related to the isolation of a resistant microorganism. In an earlier study (298), 10 patients with *Staphylococcus* spp–infected orthopedic implants were treated with various antibiotic regimens, all of which included rifampin. Of these patients, 8 were cured.

A rat model of chronic staphylococcal foreign-body infection (52) demonstrated that antimicrobial combinations of fleroxacin plus vancomycin and vancomycin plus fleroxacin and rifampin were highly effective and superior to single drugs. Further, the three-drug therapy decreased bacterial counts more rapidly than the two-drug therapy and was curative in most cases (92% for three drugs versus 41% for two and less than 6% for monotherapy). No mutants resistant to these three agents were detected with combination therapy.

The success of this approach to the therapy of infected prosthetic devices may once again be due to a biofilm-related physiological conflict. Fluoroquinolones have been shown to decrease the production of slime (biofilm in more polite company) by *S. epidermidis* (216), and it is likely that rifampin, through inhibition of protein synthesis, may decrease or prevent the availability of critical enzymes needed for ongoing maintenance of biofilm. As the biofilm microcolonies attached to the prosthetic device or glued into the bone begin to be slowly disrupted by the lack of ongoing maintenance, the staphylococci are forced to replicate, which further enhances the antimicrobial action of each antibiotic.

MECHANISMS OF ACTION FOR SELECTED CLASSES OF ANTIMICROBIAL AGENTS

Antimicrobial Classes in Current Clinical Use

β-Lactam Agents

As mentioned previously, the main structural features of the peptidoglycan sacculus are linear glycan chains interlinked by short peptide bridges. A number of enzymatic activities are involved in the biosynthesis of the sacculus: catalyzation by glycosyltransferase enzymes of the formation of the linear glycan chains, cross-linking of the glycan chains by transglycosylase enzymes, and cross-linking via peptide bridges by transpeptidase enzymes (282). The latter peptide cross-links provide mechanical strength against osmotic pressure forces. Peptidoglycan structural modifications of completed cell wall are required in replicating cells as they grow, and each microorganism therefore possesses specific peptidoglycan hydrolases that are responsible for such structural adjustments (249,250). It is these transpeptidases/hydrolases, as well as other factors such as activation of newly recognized apoptotic death pathways, that appear to be the target(s) of β-lactam agents (202,273,274).

The mechanism of action of β-lactam agents is more complex than initially thought and likely involves three interrelated cellular processes. The first of these cellular processes is transpeptidation, which initially was thought to be the sole target of β-lactam agents (273). Penicillins, because of their structural similarity to the C-terminal D-alanyl-D-alanine end of the peptide stem, react chemically with the transpeptidases, also known as PBPs, to form stable acyl-enzymes, inactivating the PBPs and preventing further cross-linking. The inhibition of glycan cross-linking then leads to a weakened cell wall, which eventually ruptures due to osmotic pressure. However, it was noted that penicillins were able to cause inhibition of growth in certain bacteria without bacteriolysis. Therefore, triggering of autolytic cell wall enzymes was considered as a second and separate target of β-lactam agents (134,184,274). However, the mechanism for control of the autolytic system and how it was activated during treatment with β-lactam agents remained unknown until recently, when a number of observations have suggested several possibilities. The electophysiological state of the cellular membrane is thought to be a factor in the regulation of bacterial cell wall autolysis (111,125). There is some evidence that β-lactam agents may depolarize the membrane potential as a signal to induce autolysis (210). Moreover, there are a number of regulatory genes that are involved in bacterial autolysis (36,37,102). These genes may be activated after exposure to a sufficient concentration of β-lactam agent to cause irreparable damage (95,102). For example, a signal transduction pathway involved in regulating apoptotic death in pneumococci has been described (202). One of the death signals appears to be a peptide, which may function in a quorum-sensing manner. This pathway is modulated by the stringent response in a manner yet to be detailed. Modulation of the stringent response under antimicrobial selection appears to create mutants that are virulent and not killed by a broad spectrum of antimicrobial agents. This resistance phenomenon has been described as physiological tolerance (200,275).

Penicillins

Penicillins are characterized by a four-membered β-lactam ring fused to a five-membered thiazolidine ring containing a side chain (303). Manipulations of this side chain have been important in the pharmacokinetics and pharmacodynamics of penicillins. The ability to produce 6-aminopenicillanic acid (6-APA) by fermentation allowed chemists to replace the amino group of 6-APA with a large number of altered side chains, thus producing many different semisynthetic penicillins. The streric hinderance around the amide bond produced by bulky side chains such as carbocyclic or heterocyclic rings with substituents at the ortho- position of the 6-APA site produced the first semisynthetic penicillins with increased stability against staphylococal β-lactamase. A number of such antistaphylococcal penicillins with bulky side chains have been synthesized, including methicillin; nafcillin; and the isoxazolyl penicillins, oxacillin, cloxacillin, dicloxacillin, and flucloxacillin.

Semisynthetic penicillins also include those created by a simple replacement of the α-carbon of the hydrophobic side chain at position 6 of benzylpenicillin by an amino (e.g., ampicillin), a carboxyl (e.g., carbenicillin), a ureido (e.g., mezlocillin), or a piperazino (e.g., piperacillin) group. The result was the development of the extended-spectrum penicillins, which have been grouped as aminopenicillins, carboxypenicillins, and ureidopenicillins. Such substitutions provided improved penetration through the outer cell membrane of Gram-negative microorganisms as well as increased stability against β-lactamases produced by these pathogens. In particular, penetration through the restrictive pores of *P. aeruginosa* resulted in antipseudomonal activity for the carboxypenicillins (e.g., carbenicillin and ticarcillin) and the ureidopenicillins (e.g., mezlocillin, azlocillin, and piperacillin). Because the stability against β-lactamases did not include staphylococcal β-lactamase, a number of these extended-spectrum penicillins were combined with a β-lactamase inhibitor (e.g., clavulanate, sulbactam, or tazobactom) and are known as β-lactam/β-lactamase inhibitor combinations (147). To date, these combinations include amoxicillin/clavulanate, ampicillin/sulbactam, ticarcillin/clavulanate, and piperacillin/tazobactam.

Cephalosporins

Cephalosporins are characterized by a four-membered β-lactam ring fused to a sulfur-containing ring-expanded system (168). One of the first cephalosporins, cephalosporin C, possessed an aminoadipic side chain, which could easily be chemically removed to give rise to 7-aminocephalosporonic acid (7-ACA), which is analogous to 6-APA. From 7-ACA came the first-generation semisynthetic cephalosporins such as cefazolin. Substitutions at the C7 position as well as at the C3 position of the dihydrothiazine ring allow greater variation of semisynthetic cephalosporins than can be achieved with the penicillins. Consequently, more cephalosporins have been developed, and detailed reviews of these agents are available (11,168). Side chain substitution in the cephalosporins is built on the experience with penicillins and includes thiazolyl and phenylglycyl side chains. The substitutions at the C7 position are of particular importance in governing stability against β-lactamases. For example, substitution at the C7-α position of cephalosporins with a methoxy group (e.g., cefoxitin and cefotetan, which are second-generation cephalosporins) resulted in the cephamycins, which have increased stablility against β-lactamases, including those of the *Bacteroides fragilis* group. Substitution at the C7-β position with a methoxyimino group (e.g., cefotaxime, which is a third-generation cephalosporin) also increased the resistance of these agents to β-lactamases. Acyl side chains used with cephalosporins include aminothiazole oximes, which may have charged carboxylates (e.g., ceftazidime, which is a third-generation cephalosporin) that improve penetration through Gram-negative bacterial outer membranes. Cefepime, a fourth-generation cephalosporin, also has a positively charged quaternary ammonium in position C3, which creates a zwitterion that allows increased penetration of the Gram-negative bacterial outer membrane. The 2-aminothiazolylacetamido group found in cefepime provides increased stability against β-lactamases.

Carbapenems

Carbapenems differ from conventional penicillins in having no sulfur atom in their five-membered ring and in having a double bond between carbons 2 and 3 (115). This stearically alters the cis/trans configuration of the molecule in comparison with other β-lactam agents and places the amide bond away from the water-containing groove of the serine-based β-lactamases. However, carbapenems are susceptible to hydrolysis by metallo-β-lactamases. Three carbapenems (imipenem, meropenem, and ertapenem) are approved for clinical use in the United States.

Monobactams

There are two monocyclic β-lactams produced by microorganisms that possess antimicrobial activity, nocardicins and monobactams (29). The monobactam nucleus of these compounds exhibits only weak antimicrobial activity, and they, like the penicillins and cephalosporins, must have substitution around the central nucleus to achieve clinically useful antimicrobial activity. Side chain structure-activity relationships in monobactams parallel those of penicillins and cephalosporins. There is only one monobactam antibiotic, aztreonam, that has an 3-acyl aminothiazole-oxime side chain identical to that of ceftazidime, while the lactam ring has a *N*-sulfonate substituent on the other side (11,29,115). The *N*-sulfonate substituent is essential for β-lactamase stability. Like ceftazidime, aztreonam is useful only against Gram-negative pathogens, with good activity against *P. aeruginosa*.

Aminoglycosides

All aminoglycoside antibiotics contain two or more amino sugar residues linked to a central, six-membered aminocyclitol ring by glycosidic bonds. Spectinomycin is, strictly speaking, also an aminocyclitol but lacks amino sugars and glycosidic bonds. The primary mechanism of action of aminoglycosides is a decrease in protein synthesis after the drug has bound to the bacterial 30S subunit of the ribosome (44,138,285). Aminoglycosides are hydrophilic sugars with multiple amino groups that function as polycations. Their polycationic nature allows binding to the polyanionic 16S rRNA on the 30S ribosome at the A site for aminoacyl-tRNA binding. Analysis by X-ray crystallography suggests that the polycation contacts are to the RNA bases rather than to backbone atoms. Attachment at the A site suggests that aminoglycosides block a required transformational transition during the peptide bond–forming translocation process, bringing the translocation steps of protein synthesis in the ribosome to a halt.

The polycationic nature of aminoglycosides also accounts for their recognized effect on biofilm and cell membranes (281). Aminoglycosides are bactericidal agents and often exhibit a rapid lethal effect on susceptible aerobic Gram-negative bacilli. Such a rapid lethal effect has been noted to be contrary to the expected effect of agents acting on ribosomal targets (169). This lethal effect of aminoglycosides against aerobic Gram-negative bacilli, moreover, is concentration-dependent, with increasing concentrations achieving increased killing. Their effect against Gram-positive cocci is, at best, inhibitory, unless a β-lactam agent is used in combination with the aminoglycoside.

Inhibition of protein synthesis, however, usually does not produce a bactericidal effect, let alone a rapid one. Therefore, binding to the 30S ribosome may not be the only mechanism of antimicrobial action for aminoglycosides; in fact, many susceptible Gram-negative bacilli

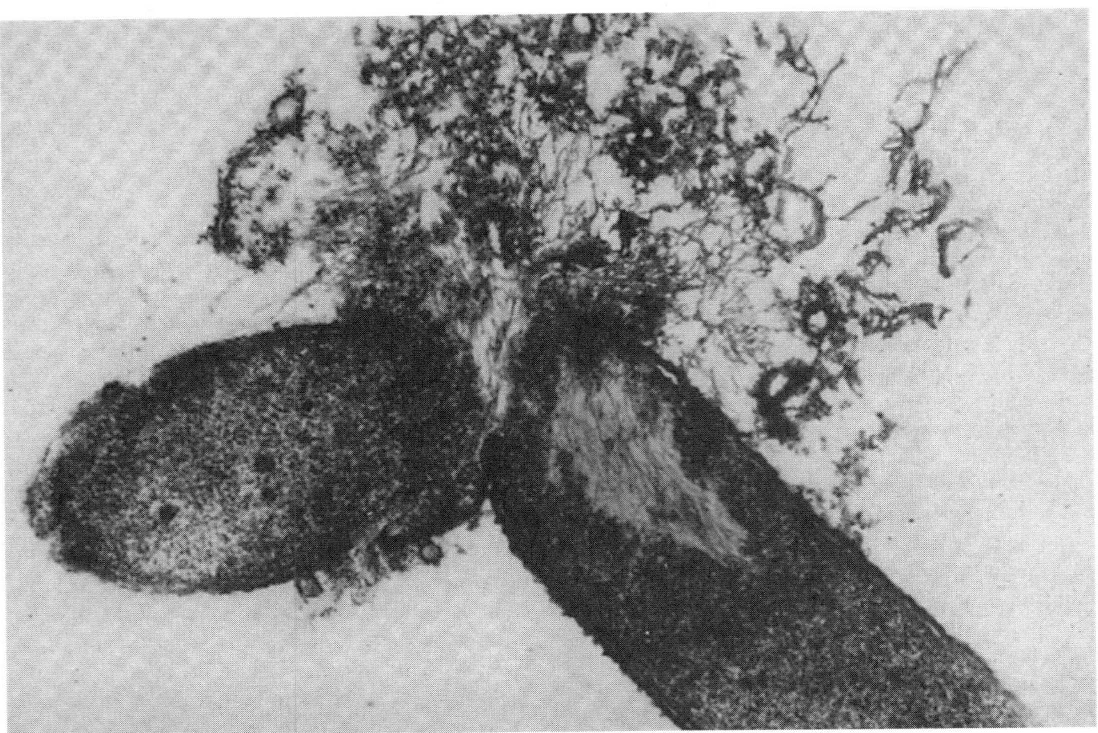

FIGURE 12.3 ● *P. aeruginosa* exposed to amikacin at 5 times the MIC for 5 hours. Note the break in the cell wall, allowing the extrusion of the cell contents. Reproduced with permission from Lorian V, Effects of low concentrations of antibiotics, in Lorian V, ed. Antibiotics in Laboratory Medicine, 4th ed. 1996 p. 416.

may be dead long before the drug arrives at the 30S ribosome (126,127,169). It is now recognized that aminoglycosides competitively displace cell biofilm–associated Mg^{2+} and Ca^{2+} that link the polysaccharides of adjacent lipopolysaccharide molecules (109,126,127,211). The result is shedding of cell membrane blebs, with formation of transient holes in the cell wall and disruption of the normal permeability of the cell wall (126,169,229). This action alone may be sufficient to kill many susceptible Gram-negative bacteria before the aminoglycoside has a chance to reach the 30S ribosome (Fig. 12.3). The surface effect of gentamicin has been investigated using bovine serum albumin–gentamicin complexes (126), which have been shown to be bactericidal against *P. aeruginosa*. These findings are in agreement with similar studies done with other immobilized surface agents (107,113,145,230).

Increased understanding of the mechanisms of action of aminoglycosides brought with it the realization that aminoglycosides have a concentration-dependent bactericidal effect (183) as well as a considerable postantibiotic effect (61). This allowed the dosing schedule to be modified to once per day (96). The modification integrated both pharmacokinetic and pharmacodynamic properties and offered the potential for greater efficacy and less toxicity (83,96). There has now been considerable experience with once-daily aminoglycoside regimens (96,195). Such regimens indeed appear to be clinically effective while reducing the incidence of nephrotoxicity (195). Moreover, they reduce the cost by decreasing ancillary service time and the need for serum aminoglycoside determinations.

Another question about the optimal utilization of aminoglycosides can be addressed. This concerns the timing of the doses when both an aminoglycoside and a β-lactam agent are administered. *In vitro* (15) and *in vivo* (103) studies have clearly demonstrated a remarkable advantage gained from nonsimultaneous administration of aminoglycosides and β-lactam agents when they are used in combination. The main benefit is a marked delay in bacterial regrowth regardless of the order in which the agents are given. However, the initial bactericidal effect is greater when the aminoglycoside is given first. The minimum time interval between doses of the aminoglycoside and the β-lactam agent for maximum delay of regrowth is 2 hours.

The reason for this phenomenon is clear if one accepts the premise that the aminoglycoside has its primary antimicrobial effect on biofilm. This effect would be greatest when there was no prior or concomitant use of cell wall–active agents, which have been shown to markedly affect the bacterial cell surfaces (85) and would thus lessen the opportunity for the aminoglycoside to have the optimal biofilm targets.

The bactericidal effects of aminoglycosides combined with β-lactam agents *in vitro* have been shown to be dependent on the concentrations of β-lactam agents used. If the concentration of the β-lactam agent is not optimized for bactericidal activity (i.e., four- to eightfold higher than the MIC), the effect of the β-lactam on the test microorganism is to stimulate increased production of biofilm (114) and thus enhance the effect of the aminoglycoside by providing a better target. This has been nicely demonstrated by Lorian and Ernst (164). If, on the other hand, the concentration of the β-lactam agent is high enough to disrupt the cell wall morphology (85), then the biofilm target is lessened, which in turn lessens the lethal effect of the aminoglycoside (88,126). These two effects are exactly the opposite of what would be predicted to occur if the target of the aminoglycoside was the ribosome rather than biofilm. Importantly for clinical use of these β-lactam–aminoglycoside combinations, the overall lethal effect *in vivo* is enhanced by administering the aminoglycoside first (103).

Macrolides, Azolides, Lincosamides, Ketolides, and Streptogramins

The macrolides, azolides, lincosamides, ketolides, and streptogramins are grouped together despite structural differences because of similar biologic properties, including their mechanism of action against the 50S subunit of the bacterial ribosomes. The specific target for these agents appears to be domain V of the 23S rRNA, which is the peptidyltransferase center (78). Macrolides block the approach to the exit tunnel for elongating peptides and thus prevent polypeptide translation, causing premature release of peptidyl-tRNA intermediates. Lincosamides, however, inhibit the initiation of peptide chain formation (224), and the effect of the other macrolides is to prevent the extension of the growing peptide chain. Macrolides also block assembly of 50S subunits by their interaction with the 23S rRNA.

Ketolides are the latest members of the macrolide group and are novel semisynthetic 14-membered–ring macrolides in which the main structural innovations are the lack of the neutral sugar cladinose in position C3 as well as a C11/C12 carbamate (38,311). When the C3 cladinose sugar moiety is removed, the resulting 3-hydroxy group is oxidized to a 3-keto group, hence the name *ketolide*. The macrolides, azolides, lincosamides, and ketolides all appear to bind to the same site or contiguous sites on the ribosome and so they may become competitive inhibitors if used together (55,311,312). This mechanism of action, inhibition of protein synthesis, results in bacteriostatic activity against most bacteria by all of these agents except ketolides, which have bactericidal activity (311). Inhibition of critical proteins in certain microbial species does, however, result in bactericidal activity. Such species-specific bactericidal activity is seen *in vitro* with the macrolide clarithromycin against *S. pneumoniae* but is less evident *in vivo* (241).

Macrolide antibiotics such as erythromycin, clarithromycin, and azithromycin appear to have the ability to decrease sputum production in patients with chronic respiratory infections (99,236,237,269). This has been attributed to a direct effect on the production of sputum (99) but may instead be due to inhibition of biofilm production by respiratory pathogens (122,236). Macrolides have been shown to markedly reduce the biofilm structure of microorganisms in their sessile phase (305) and to reduce the amount of virulent exotoxins (133,179). These microorganisms include *S. epidermidis* and *P. aeruginosa*. The mechanism seems to involve the suppression of a step or steps in the synthesis of monosaccharides, probably as a result of the suppression of mRNA (105). The use of macrolides such as erythromycin or azithromycin has been beneficial in chronic respiratory tract infections caused by *P. aeruginosa* (139,236).

Erythromycin

Erythromycin is a metabolic product of *Streptomyces erythreus* and consists of a 14-member lactone ring to which are attached two deoxy-sugars, desosamine and cladinose. The macrocyclic lactone ring is the source of the class name, *macrolide*. Erythromycin, like most macrolides, appears to act by binding in the ribosomal tunnel through which the nascent peptide moves and thus can be considered a peptidyltransferase inhibitor (105). Against some rapidly replicating bacteria, erythromycin exhibits *in vitro* bactericidal activity, but overall it is considered to be bacteriostatic in clinical use.

Clarithromycin

Clarithromycin, like erythromycin, has a 14-member lactone ring structure that has been altered by the addition of a methoxy group at C6 of the lactone ring (189,312). This substitution primarily results in better oral absorption, with little effect on the spectrum of activity. In fact, erythromycin, clarithromycin, and azithromycin appear to bind to the same receptor on the bacterial 50S ribosome subunit. Clarithromycin, like the other macrolides, has species-specific bactericidal activity, as defined by *in vitro* methods of assessment where a $\geq$3-$\log_{10}$ decrease in colony-forming units over a 24-hour period is defined as bactericidal (232). The species usually considered to be killed by macrolides are *S. pneumoniae, S. pyogenes,* and *H. influenzae*. However, the bactericidal activity of clarithromycin against susceptible strains of *S. pneumoniae,* as demonstrated *in vitro* by time-kill kinetic curves, has been found to lack correlation with results from the rabbit model for pneumococcal meningitis (241). The use of an *in vitro* method to measure total microbial killing has been suggested as a way to better assess the bactericidal activity of antimicrobial agents used in bacterial meningitis (261).

Azithromycin

Azithromycin is derived from erythromycin and differs in having a methyl-substituted nitrogen in its 15-membered lactone ring (14,312). This class of drugs receives its name, *azolides,* from the presence of the nitrogen group. Azithromycin has the same mechanism of action as erythromycin, and these two drugs bind so close to each other on the ribosome that they are considered competitive inhibitors. Azithromycin, like erythromycin and other macrolides, is a bacteriostatic agent. Azithromycin, however, has a major advantage, namely, its absorption and prolonged intracellular/interstitial fluid levels. In particular, the intracellular levels should greatly enhance the therapy of infections caused by intracellular pathogens.

Dirithromycin

Dirithromycin is a semisynthetic derivative of erythromycin that is converted during absorption and distribution to an active metabolite 9-(*S*)-erythromyclamine, which is the predominant agent found in plasma and extravascular tissues (132,300). This macrolide demonstrates high and prolonged tissue concentrations, allowing once-daily dosing. The mechanism of action is identical to that of the other macrolides. The result is bacteriostatic activity against logarithmically growing microorganisms and may include bactericidal activity against bacteria in a static growth phase. Dirithromycin, like azithromycin, does not inhibit cytochrome P450 enzymes and thus does not cause clinically important drug-drug interactions, although its gastrointestinal side effects are similar to those of other macrolides (293,312). Macrolides appear to be able to suppress the initiation of mRNA synthesis (177) and thereby inhibit the production of biofilm (305), exoenzymes (179), and other such virulence factors by a diverse group of pathogens, including *P. aeruginosa* (133,181). If this proves to be clinically effective in chronic infections, a once-daily dosing that achieves high and prolonged tissue concentrations and has no significant drug-drug interactions will be extremely useful.

Telithromycin

Telithromycin is a ketolide in which the C11/C12 carbamate residue includes a butyl chain linking an imidazole ring and a pyridine ring (3,38). The most important factors in terms of the structure and activity of telithromycin are the lack of the neutral sugar cladinose in position C3 as well as a C11/C12 carbamate group, which together markedly increase the affinity of telithromycin for its microbial target, the 23S ribosomal drug-binding pocket (78,110). Telithromycin interacts with the 23S rRNA portion of the 50S subunit in the upper portion of the peptide exit channel close to the peptidyl transferase center and prevents the peptide chain from passing through the peptide exit channel (78,110). The increased affinity of telithromycin for the 23S rRNA is seen even in macrolide-resistant strains (79) and also results in concentration-dependent bactericidal activity and a prolonged postantimicrobial effect against important respiratory tract pathogens. The microbiological spectrum of activity for telithromycin includes *S. pneumoniae, S. pyogenes, H. influenzae, Moraxella catarrhalis, Legionella* species, *Mycoplasma pneumoniae,* and *Chlamydia pneumoniae,* which suggest that telithromycin will play an important clinical role in the empirical treatment of community-acquired respiratory tract infections. The pharmacokinetic profile of telithromycin demonstrates that this drug can be administered once daily without regard for meals and requires no dose reduction in elderly patients or those having hepatic impairment. Telithromycin is well absorbed after oral administration, rapidly penetrates into respiratory tissues and fluids, and is highly concentrated within white blood cells. Integration of pharmacokinetic and pharmacodynamic properties reveals that telithromycin has a high AUC:MIC ratio compared with macrolide antimicrobial agents, which results in enhanced efficacy. Resistance, although rare to date, can occur (284). Finally, telithromycin is well tolerated and has a low propensity for drug interactions.

Clindamycin

Clindamycin is a member of the lincosamides, which are chemically unrelated to the macrolides. Lincosamides consist of an amino acid linked to an amino sugar. Clindamycin is a 7-deoxy-7-chloro derivative of lincomycin, the first member of the lincosamide class. These two agents, like the macrolides, act on the peptidyltransferase center of the 50S subunit of bacterial ribosomes (224). Clindamycin may exhibit *in vitro* bactericidal activity against susceptible microorganisms such as *S. aureus* and *B. fragilis,* but its *in vivo* activity is considered bacteriostatic. The reason for this species-specific bactericidal activity is unknown but may reflect differences in the apoptotic mechanisms of these microorganisms.

Streptogramins

The streptogramin group of antibiotics includes the mikamycins, the pristinamycins, the oestreomycins, and the virginiamycins. These compounds are classified into two main groups: polyunsaturated cyclic peptidolides and cyclic hexadepsipeptides. Both groups possess a wide variety of chemical functions. Quinupristin/dalfopristin (Synercid) is a semisynthetic antibiotic consisting of two water-soluble streptogramin components: pristinamycin IA, a peptidic macrolactone, and pristinamycin IIA, a polyunsaturated macrolactone (8,67). These two macrolactones are modified to be water-soluble and together demonstrate synergistic and concentration-independent lethal activity against Gram-positive pathogens, including *S. aureus*, in contrast to the individual components, which are only inhibitory (129). This bactericidal effect is seen clinically as well, as evidenced by the successful treatment of bacterial endocarditis. It is thought that this activity is related to irreversible binding to ribosomes (13). The 70S ribosomal subunit appears to be the target, with binding closing or narrowing the extrusion channel. This combination also demonstrates a postantibiotic

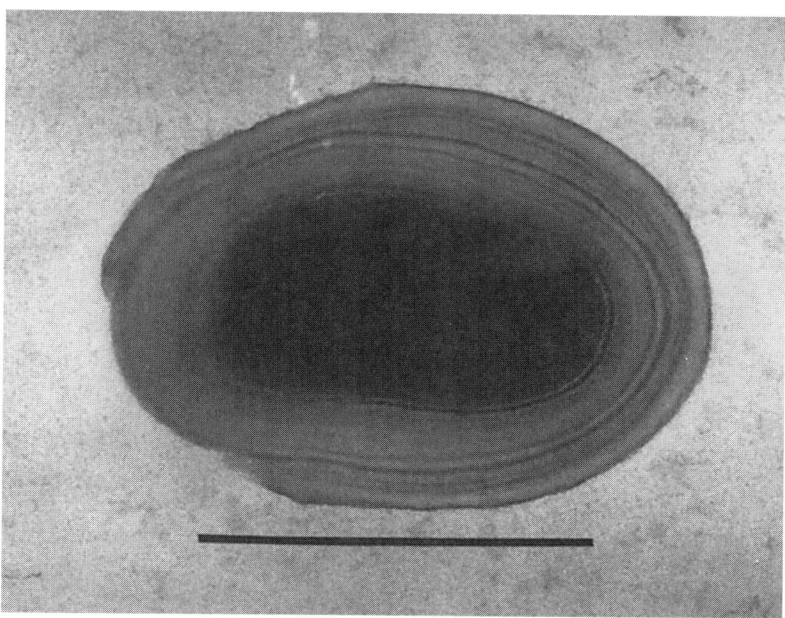

FIGURE 12.4 • *S. aureus* exposed to pristinamycin I and II in combination. Six layers of the cell wall are shown (original magnification ×100,000). Reproduced with permission from Lorian V, Modes of Action of Antibiotics and Bacterial Structure: Bacterial Mass Versus their Numbers in Zack, O *Handbook of Animal Models of Infection* 1999;105–116.

effect (201). Moreover, each component diffuses throughout cardiac vegetations and is more concentrated in these vegetations than in cardiac tissue. The peptide macrolactone is distributed homogeneously throughout each vegetation, while the polyunsaturated macrolactone reaches the core, with a gradient of decreasing concentrations from the periphery.

Exposure of *S. aureus* to quinupristin/dalfopristin results in two major cell alterations: an increase in cell size and an increase in the thickness of the cell wall. Some cells exhibit multilayered cell walls with as many as six layers (162) (Fig. 12.4), which is considerably thicker than the two- or three-layer cell wall that has been seen with exposure of *S. aureus* to chloramphenicol (93). This alteration is likely to be a stringent response.

Quinolones

The fluoroquinolones are synthetic antimicrobial agents that inhibit topoisomerases. Within several decades these agents have proven their usefulness as a major class of broad-spectrum agents and have therapeutic potential yet to be realized. The first member of this group was nalidixic acid. The newer fluoroquinolones are all structurally similar to nalidixic acid and have a common skeleton, the four-quinolone planar heterocycle nucleus. Most also have a fluorine atom at position C6 of the structure (hence the name *fluoroquinolones*). Substitution on this skeleton is greatly aided by the vast knowledge accumulated regarding the structure-activity relationships, and the optimal groups for each position, in terms of size, shape, and electrical properties, have been well defined (51,72,172). Specific structural features that enhance the activity of fluoroquinolones are listed in Table 12.1.

These features can be used to predict the best configuration for a specific microorganism. For example, there are a number of new antibiotics that have demonstrated activity against *Mycobacterium* species (131). Among these are fluoroquinolones. These fluoroquinolones can be evaluated by predicting their active structures (135). In addition, the most beneficial substituent of quinolones today holds not only for Gram-positive and Gram-negative bacteria but also for *M. avium* (135); an N-substitution offers the greatest enhancement (104). This may be related to two factors: the amine groups may allow a greater concentration of the uncharged species to exist at neutral pH, and the N1-cyclopropylamine may also serve as a suicide inhibitor of redox enzymes, such as cytochrome P450 and methylamine dehydrogenase, which are present in bacteria. Alkylation of the N1-substituted moiety increased the activity of these agents against mycobacteria (104).

Fluoroquinolones interact with either or both of two topoisomerases, topoisomerase II and IV (22,60,247). Topoisomerase II, or DNA gyrase, is a vital bacterial enzyme that catalyzes the introduction of negative superhelical twists in circular DNA. Negative superhelical twists in circular DNA are needed for the following reasons. In

TABLE 12.1

Summary of Structure-Activity Relationships for Fluoroquinolone Antimicrobial Agents

Structure	Position	Activity
Halogen (F or Cl)	Position 6	Enhances overall effect
Pyrrolidine ring	Position 7	Enhances effect on Gram-positive organisms
Piperazine ring	Position 7	Enhances effect on Gram-positive organisms
Cyclopropyl ring	Position N1	Enhances overall effect
Amino group	Position 5	Enhances overall effect
Alkylation	Pyrrolidine or piperazine ring	Enhances effect on Gram-positive organisms
Second halogen	Position 8	Enhances effect on anaerobic organisms

order for DNA replication or transcription to take place, the two strands of double-helical DNA must first be separated. Separation, however, results in excessive positive supercoiling of the DNA in front of the point of separation. The bacterial enzyme DNA gyrase prevents this positive supercoiling by introducing negative supercoils into DNA. Gyrase consists of two functional subunits, the A subunit and the B subunit. The first catalyzes the step involving the passage of a segment of DNA through a double-stranded DNA break held open by the enzyme and then reseals the break. The second is responsible for adenosine triphosphate (ATP) hydrolysis, which is required for catalytic supercoiling by gyrase. Topisomerase IV decatenates DNA and removes positive and negative supercoils: as in the case of topoisomerase II, there are two subunits involved.

Fluoroquinolones are bactericidal agents that exhibit concentration-dependent killing with little postantibiotic effect at concentrations ranging from those equal to the MIC (1 times the MIC) up to approximately 10- to 20-fold higher (10 to 20 times the MIC). At these higher concentrations, the SOS response appears to be evoked (153). This results in a secondary bactericidal effect that is accompanied by a longer postantibiotic effect and a decrease in the emergence of resistant clones (43,212). This secondary bactericidal effect may involve a signal to the apoptotic mechanism of the microbial cell, ultimately leading to apoptosis.

DNA gyrase is the target of an increasing number of antibiotic classes. One of these classes consists of the synthetic quinolones, which act by interfering with the DNA-rejoining step involving the A subunit, while another class consists of the natural coumarin-type compounds, which compete with ATP for binding to the B subunit of the enzyme. A related class, consisting of the 2-pyridones, is discussed later, in "Antimicrobial Classes with Potential for Future Use."

Novobiocin

Novobiocin is a glycosylated dihydroxycoumarin derivative of the natural coumarin-type antibiotics produced by streptomycetes. Natural coumarin-type antibiotics to date include only two agents, the novobiocin precursor and coumermycin, which is almost a dimer of novobiocin. These agents act on the B subunit of DNA gyrase and interfere with ATP hydrolysis (54). Like the fluoroquinolones, novobiocin exhibits bactericidal activity *in vitro* and *in vivo*. Perhaps their greatest benefit would come from combining them with other DNA gyrase inhibitors (60) in order to decrease the selection of resistant mutants.

Sulfonamides

The sulfonamides were the first effective chemotherapeutic agents to be used for the systemic therapy of bacterial infections in humans. Domagk (73) recognized this potential with Prontosil, which has sulfanilamide as its active metabolite, and later received the Nobel Prize in Medicine for this discovery. *Sulfonamide* is the generic name for derivatives of *p*-aminobenzenesulfonamide. These agents owe their activity to their being structural analogs and competitive antagonists of *p*-aminobenzoic acid; this antagonism is in part due to the attachment of the sulfa molecule directly to the benzene ring. The result is competitive inhibition of dihydropteroate synthase, the bacterial enzyme that catalyzes the incorporation of *p*-aminobenzoic acid into dihydropteroic acid, the immediate precursor of folic acid (2,301). The *in vitro* and *in vivo* effects of this inhibition are bacteriostatic.

Trimethoprim

Trimethoprim chemically is 2,4-diaminopyrimidine and was specifically synthesized as an inhibitor of dihydrofolate reductase. This antibiotic thus inhibits folic acid synthesis, acting on the enzyme step that immediately follows that blocked by sulfonamides. The folic acid pathway is a small portion of a more complex pathway known as the aromatic biosynthetic pathway. Trimethoprim, like the sulfonamides, is bacteriostatic when used alone. The combination of these two inhibitors of folic acid synthesis, however, produces a bactericidal effect.

Chloramphenicol

Chloramphenicol, also called chloromycetin, is a broad-spectrum antibiotic produced by a variety of *Streptomyces* species, including *S. venezuelae* (16,215). This antimicrobial agent is unique among natural compounds in that it contains a nitrobenzene moiety that is connected to propanol as well as an amino group binding a derivative of dichloroacetic acid (16,286). These latter moieties, propanol and dichloroacetic acid, must be intact for antimicrobial activity to occur, although substitution of the dichloroacetamide side chain is possible. A common mechanism of resistance is the acetylation of one or both hydroxyl groups on the propanediol moiety. These hydroxyl groups, however, cannot be substituted to prevent this type of resistance. The chloramphenicol molecule is one of the simplest antibiotic structures and was quickly and easily synthesized (16), becoming the first antibiotic whose chemical synthesis was feasible for large-scale commercial production.

Chloramphenicol is a small, uncharged, nonpolar molecule and readily diffuses through the cell wall/membrane. Although early work suggested that chloramphenicol is actively taken up by *E. coli*, later studies showed that there is actually an endogenous active efflux that depends on the proton motive force (151).

Chloramphenicol inhibits the peptidyltransferase reaction in bacterial protein synthesis by reversibly binding to the peptidyltransferase center of the 50S subunit of the 70S ribosome (213). This attachment prevents the attachment of the amino acid–containing end of the amino acyl–tRNA complex to the ribosome, thereby inhibiting the formation of a peptide bond. The site of action is near that of the macrolide antibiotics and clindamycin, which it inhibits competitively. This inhibition of protein synthesis in most susceptible microorganisms results in a bacteriostatic effect, although certain microbial pathogens, such as *H. influenzae*, *S. pneumoniae*, and *Neisseria meningitidis*, are readily killed *in vivo* by clinically achievable concentrations (218). This bactericidal activity may be due to the triggering of apoptotic mechanisms in these pathogens.

Chloramphenicol has other inhibitory effects in bacterial cells that are not related to inhibition of protein synthesis. Perhaps the most important effect is that on the bacterial translocase reaction in certain microorganisms. Chloramphenicol strongly inhibits the synthesis of teichoic acid in *Bacillus licheniformis* by inhibiting the function of undecaprenol-P (258).

Chloramphenicol is among the few agents that retain antimicrobial activity against bacteria in the stringent response phase (86). It therefore has potential for being combined with other agents that have similar effects, such as metronidazole and the macrolides. Susceptibility testing methods, however, must reflect the nonreplicating growth phase when evaluating these combinations.

Rifampin

The rifamycins are a group of structurally similar macrocyclic antimicrobial agents produced by *Nocardia mediterranei* (244). The basic structure of rifamycins is a naphthalene ring spanned by a long aliphatic loop. Rifampin is a semisynthetic derivative with modifications at the 4-position on the naphthalene ring of one of these natural agents, rifamycin B. Rifampin acts by inhibiting DNA-dependent RNA polymerase by binding to the β-subunit of the enzyme (42,295). The final result is inhibition of protein synthesis by prevention of chain initiation. Rifampin is a bactericidal agent *in vivo* as well as *in vitro*, but because of the high rate of resistant mutants, this antibiotic is always used in combination with another agent when treating serious infections.

Tetracyclines

The tetracyclines are broad-spectrum antibiotics discovered in the late 1940s following the isolation of chlortetracycline from *Streptomyces aureofaciens* (50). These agents were the first broad-spectrum antibiotics to be widely used in the therapy of bacterial infections in humans.

Tetracycline antibiotics consist of a hydronaphthacene nucleus with four fused rings. Substitutions on this fused ring structure at carbons 4, 5, and 6 have resulted in semisynthetic agents; two of these are doxycycline and minocycline. These semisynthetic compounds are more lipophilic than their precursors and hence are more active.

At physiological pH, many tetracyclines can exist in a mixture of two forms, a nonionized lipophilic form and a zwitterionic hydrophilic form. The lipophilic form assists passage through the cell membrane, while the hydrophilic form assists diffusion through the biofilm and the cytoplasm. Passage of tetracycline itself through Gram-negative outer membranes involves the porins, with a preference for OmpF. OmpF porins are cation-selective, and tetracycline may pass through these channels as a cationic chelate of magnesium. The uptake of tetracycline across the cell membrane has been shown to involve an energy-dependent process that is now thought to be the result of a pH gradient. After tetracyclines enter bacteria via diffusion through the cell wall/membrane, these agents remain as a magnesium chelate or are complexed as such within the cytoplasm. These tetracycline/magnesium-chelated complexes, once inside the cytoplasm, appear to be membrane-impermeable.

Tetracycline derivatives can be classified into two categories based on their mechanism of action. The traditional tetracyclines, including tetracycline, chlortetracycline, minocycline, and doxycycline, inhibit protein synthesis at the ribosomal level due to disruption of codon-anticodon interactions between tRNA and mRNA in which binding of amino acyl tRNA to the ribosomal acceptor site is prevented. This interaction appears to be reversible and is thought to account for the bacteriostatic nature of these agents.

In the atypical tetracyclines, substituents are introduced at carbon 9 without alteration of the basic structure of the classical tetracyclines, with the result that the primary target is not the ribosome but the cytoplasmic membrane. These modifications also allow the molecule to avoid recognition by a tetracycline efflux protein [TetA(B)]. The atypical tetracyclines may exist primarily in the nonionized lipophilic form, which allows them to remain in the cell membranes. The interaction of these tetracycline analogs with the cell membrane is lethal, resulting in cellular lysis (203,220).

Nitroimidazoles and Nitrofurans

Nitroimidazoles and nitrofurans are synthetic antimicrobial agents that are grouped together because both are nitro group (-NO_2)–containing ringed structures having similar antimicrobial effects. These effects require degradation of the agent within the microbial cell so that electrophilic radicals are formed. These reactive electrophilic intermediates then damage nucleophilic sites, including ribosomes, DNA, and RNA. The effect *in vitro* and *in vivo* against susceptible microorganisms is bactericidal.

Nitroimidazoles

The nitroimidazoles are organic nitroaromatic derivatives that are activated within the cytoplasm of microorganisms by electrons in order to exert their antimicrobial effect. The key to the antimicrobial activity of this class of drugs is the nitro group, which acts as a preferential electron acceptor (124). Electrons are needed to reduce the nitro group (-NO_2) to an amine or amino group (-NH_2). The reduction, however, does not proceed along the classical reduction pathway seen with nitrobenzene or its derivatives, such as chloramphenicol. Instead, the reduction leads to nitro radical anions, which undergo rapid decomposition to a nitrite ion and an imidazole radical. These short-lived electrophilic reduction products of the nitroimidazoles are produced within the microbial cell by enzymatic pathways utilized in anaerobic metabolism. Anaerobes depend on the ferredoxin-linked pyruvate oxidoreductase system as a major route of ATP generation. These pyruvate oxidoreductase pathways utilize ferredoxin, or similar electron transfer proteins, as electron acceptors from the oxidation of an enzyme-thiamine-pyrophosphate complex. The reduced ferredoxin normally transfers electrons to hydrogenase, but in the presence of nitroimidazoles those electrons are transferred to the latter. Electrons from hydrogenase can also be transferred to nitroimidazoles. This transfer initiates the decomposition of the nitroimidazoles to radical electrophilic products. These products, most likely nitrite radicals, then react with nucleophilic protein sites and, among other effects, oxidize DNA, causing strand breaks and subsequent cell death.

Nitrofurans

Nitrofuran compounds consist of a primary nitro group (-NO_2) joined to a heterocycle ring. Susceptible microorganisms have been shown to possess reductases that reduce nitrofurans to reactive electrophilic metabolites, and an inverse correlation exists between reductase levels and MICs (175). These electrophilic metabolites produce a qualitatively nonspecific attack on nucleophilic sites, including ribosomal proteins and mRNA.

Metronidazole

Metronidazole is a nitroheterocyclic compound belonging to the nitroimidazole group of antimicrobial agents, and it was the first of this group of drugs to show useful clinical activity (124). This antibiotic has two metabolic derivatives, a hydroxy metabolite with significant antimicrobial activity and an acid metabolite with relatively little activity (209). The activity of metronidazole, like other members of the nitroimidazole group, is related to the production of nitrite radicals. Metronidazole is rapidly bactericidal, and its high anaerobe killing rate is not affected by nutrients or growth rates.

Several studies demonstrated that anaerobic preincubation markedly increased the susceptibility of metronidazole-resistant strains of *H. pylori*, suggesting that sufficient anaerobic metabolism must occur before there are enough electrons on the ferredoxin electron transfer protein to decompose a sufficient amount of metronidazole to kill the microorganism (46). The length of time for anaerobic preincubation is undoubtedly related to the amount of electrons produced and transferred to ferredoxin; it may take a number of generations undergoing anaerobic metabolism before the ferredoxin has acquired enough electrons to cause sufficient degradation of metronidazole to kill the microorganism.

Nitrofurantoin

Members of the nitrofuran class include nitrofurantoin and furazolidone, the latter being available only in Europe. Nitrofurantoin is metabolized by bacterial reductases, resulting in electrophilic radicals that nonspecifically attack nucleophilic sites and inhibit protein synthesis. In addition, nitrofurantoin appears to have another important mechanism of action. Nitrofurantoin has been found to increase the levels of Gp4, an enzyme implicated in the induction of the stringent response (175). At the same time, nitrofurans, including nitrofurantoin, have specific interactions with ribosome sites such as S18 in the platform region of the 30S subunit, which disrupts codon-anticodon interactions and thereby prevents mRNA translation (55,175). Therefore, it is possible that nitrofurantoin acts to induce Gp4 while preventing translation of the Gp4-stimulated mRNAs for inducible enzymes (55,175).

This would effectively prevent bacterial entry into the stringent response and thus impair viability.

Glycopeptides

Glycopeptide antimicrobial agents currently include vancomycin, teicoplanin, daptomycin, and ramoplanin. Vancomycin was originally isolated from the fermentation broths of *Amycolatopsis orientalis* (100), while teicoplanin was obtained from *Actinoplanes teichomyceticus* (299). Both agents possess a heptapeptide backbone but differ in substituents.

Both glycopeptides achieve their antimicrobial activity by binding to the terminal amino acyl-D-alanyl-D-alanine, which prevents the transfer of cell wall components from the lipid carrier to cell wall growth points (187). Therefore, they share similar antimicrobial spectra and potencies, which are essentially confined to Gram-positive bacteria. Their activities are, however, not identical. There are several explanations for this fact. The two agents differentially bind to other peptide components of preformed peptidoglycan, which has no direct effect but reduces the available drug. In addition, structure-activity relationships for these two glycopeptide agents (vancomycin and teicoplanin) suggest dimerization of these antibiotics as a potentially important factor in their activity. Such dimerization has been shown to enhance the binding affinities of most glycopeptides for the peptidyl-D-alanyl-D-alanine sequence present in the growing cell wall, the notable exception being teicoplanin (20). Teicoplanin is unique among the glycopeptides in that it demonstrates no measurable propensity for dimerization (94). A dimerized agent has enhanced activity because the second binding event is essentially intramolecular, whereas the activity of an agent with a lipid anchor requires two steps for the same effect. Although perhaps subtle, this difference may account for some of the difference in the activities of these two agents against certain species of enterococci. The fatty acid chain that teicoplanin carries may diminish this difference by acting as a membrane anchor, thus increasing the affinity of the antimicrobial agent for the growing cell wall.

Vancomycin

Vancomycin is a narrow-spectrum antimicrobial agent that is mainly active against Gram-positive cocci. It is a large, complex, tricyclic antibiotic with a molecular mass of 1449 Da. Within the chlorine face of this large molecule, there is a pocket into which the D-alanyl-D-alanine precursor of the cell wall peptidoglycan is complexed, preventing polymerization of undecaprenyl pyrophosphoryl-*N*-acetylmuramyl-pentapeptide (UDP-MurNAc-pentapeptide) and *N*-acetylglucosamine into peptidoglycan (186). The *in vitro* and *in vivo* results of this inhibition of peptidoglycan synthesis, like that caused by a β-lactam agent, are bactericidal. However, it is important to appreciate that this bactericidal effect of vancomycin (and teicoplanin) is much slower than that of the β-lactam agents (150,262). Vancomycin, therefore, should be substituted for antistaphylococcal penicillins such as nafcillin only when absolutely necessary, as in cases of penicillin allergy or methicillin resistance.

Teicoplanin

Teicoplanin differs chemically from vancomycin in a number of ways. First, teicoplanin has different carbohydrate substituents: D-glycosamine and D-mannose versus D-glucose and vancosamine in vancomycin. Next, teicoplanin has two dihydroxyphenylglycines rather that aspartic acid and *N*-methylleucine. Finally, teicoplanin is unique among the glycopeptides in having an acyl substituent, which is a fatty acid. This fatty acid makes teicoplanin much more lipophilic than vancomycin, accounting for its greater tissue and cellular penetration. This same property accounts for its activity against *M. tuberculosis*. The actual mechanism of action is identical to that of vancomycin, although the activity of these two agents is not always identical. Like vancomycin, teicoplanin is slowly bactericidal, in comparison with antistaphylococcal penicillins.

Phosphonomycins

Fosfomycin is a phosphoenolpyruvate analog that irreversibly inhibits enolpyruvate transferase. This agent is a unique antimicrobial agent unrelated to any other recognized class and is the only member, to date, of the phosphonomycin class. Fosfomycin is a broad-spectrum antibiotic produced by some strains of *Streptomyces* and by *Pseudomonas syringae*. The structure of fosfomycin is characterized by an epoxide ring and a carbon-phosphorus bond. This agent has an extremely low molecular mass of 138 Da and has been found to be nonreactive with negatively charged glycocalyx such as that produced by *P. aeruginosa*. This agent enters bacterial cells by active transport through the L-glycerophosphate and the hexose-6-phosphate uptake systems. Within the cell, fosfomycin blocks peptidoglycan synthesis through inhibition of the bacterial enzyme *N*-acetylglucosamine-3-*O*-enolpyruvyl transferase, which prevents the formation of *N*-acetylmuramic acid, an essential element of the peptidoglycan cell wall (128). The *in vitro* and *in vivo* results of this inhibition of polypeptide chain elongation are bactericidal.

Fusidanes

Fusidanes are a family of naturally occurring tetracyclic triterpenoid antibiotics, of which fusidic acid is the only therapeutic representative. Fusidic acid is derived from the fungus *Fusidium coccineum*. This antibiotic exhibits a steroidlike structure but has no steroidlike activity due to the stereochemistry of the molecule. The mechanism of action for this antimicrobial agent appears to involve binding to elongation factor G, thus inhibiting polypeptide chain elongation (287). The *in vitro* and *in vivo* results of this inhibition of polypeptide chain elongation are bactericidal. Fusidic acid is most active against *S. aureus*, including methicillin-resistant isolates (283). The MICs for methicillin-resistant isolates range from 0.03 to 1.0 g/mL. Although resistance can occur, it is rare. Fusidic acid was introduced into clinical practice in 1962, and despite more than three decades of use, the resistance rate is still below 2% (245). Fusidic acid is not available in the United States for general use.

Polymyxins and Colistin

The polymyxins are a group of polypeptide antibiotics that have molecular masses of approximately 1000 Da and are isolated from different strains of *Bacillus*. These antimicrobial agents are characterized by a heptapeptide ring, a high content of diaminobutyric acid, and a side chain ending in fatty acid residues. Only polymyxin B and colistin are currently used clinically. All of the polymyxins are cationic detergents that disrupt biofilm and result in altered membrane permeability. Colistin also is a polymyxin B nonapeptide derivative, lacking the fatty acid tail. Polymyxin B covalently attached to agarose inhibits the respiration and growth of Gram-negative bacteria but not Gram-positive bacteria. Also, spheroplasts of *E. coli* are seen after exposure to immobilized polymyxin B (145,230,240). This is interpreted as indicating the activity is directed at the outer cell membrane. The effects of immobilized polymyxin B are identical to the effects of EDTA (148). The target, like that of EDTA, is most likely the biofilm via displacement of magnesium and calcium ions. This effect can be reversed by an excess of these divalent cations (130,192).

Daptomycin

Daptomycin is a semisynthetic cyclic lipopeptide antibiotic that appears to dissipate membrane potential (5,267). The evidence for this is the activity of daptomycin on L forms of *S. aureus,* which results in the leakage of intracellular potassium. In addition, scanning electron microscopy has shown gross morphologic alterations in the cytoplasmic membrane (288) that are consistent with disruption of the biofilm or cell wall/membrane (126,130,230,240). Finally, a number of reports have noted that daptomycin is capable of calcium-dependent interactions with bilayer membranes (7,143). Daptomycin thus may exert its rapid bactericidal effect (261) by dissipating the transmembrane electrochemical potential via either biofilm disruption or inhibition of the proton pump. In either case, the rapid killing may be due to activation of apoptotic mechanisms. A similar phenomenon of dissipation of membrane potential has been described for gentamicin and *S. aureus* (170).

Oxazolidinones

Oxazolidinones are a new class of synthetic bacterial protein synthesis inhibitors (157). These agents are multicyclic compounds, some with fused rings, that represent a new series of antimicrobial agents unrelated by chemical structure to any other currently available antibiotics. Like the fluoroquinolones, another class of multicyclic compounds with fused rings, oxazolidinones are synthetic agents that offer many substitution sites for chemical modifications, as dictated by structure-activity relationships. Also like the fluoroquinolones, some oxazolidinones have D- and L-isomers, only the latter of which is active against microorganisms (87). Salient structural features of representative agents in this class include tricyclic fused rings, which exhibit potent activity against methicillin-resistant *S. aureus* and *S. epidermidis*; an appended thiomorpholine moiety, which confers potent *in vitro* activity against *M. tuberculosis*; fluorine substitution on the generic aromatic ring, which enhances activity against Gram-positive cocci; and the addition of a piperazine ring, which also increases potency against Gram-positive cocci (64,87). The spectrum of activity of oxazolidinones includes Gram-positive microorganisms such as *Enterococcus* spp, *M. tuberculosis*, and *Bacteroides* spp (64,157,252).

The mechanism of action is thought to be inhibition of protein synthesis because oxazolidinones inhibit ribosomal protein synthesis in a cell-free system (64,207). Like many antimicrobial agents that inhibit protein synthesis, oxazolidinones are bacteriostatic. However, their inhibition of protein synthesis is somewhat novel in that the oxazolidinones do not inhibit the peptide elongation step (64). Instead, the initial step of protein synthesis is inhibited, which in turn leads to codon-anticodon interactions where translation of mRNA for inducible enzymes is inhibited. In this respect, oxazolidinones are similar in action to lincosamides (224). This effect over time may result in cell death; both oxazolidinones and lincosamides are slowly bactericidal to certain microorganisms.

Resistance to oxazolidinones can occur by a single-step selection process, but this occurs at a frequency of less than 1 in 10^9. Resistance, when seen, is not associated with cross-resistance to other classes of antimicrobial agents.

Finally, oxazolidinones can be administered by both intravenous and oral routes. Peak levels in humans given 1 g orally reach 6 to 7 μg/mL, while the half-lives range from 2.4 to 12 hours (136). Oxazolidinones are metabolized by free radicals as well as excreted in the urine, with 40% to 60% of the drug intact.

Antimicrobial Classes with Potential for Future Use

Glycylcyclines

Glycylcyclines are a new class of semisynthetic tetracyclines (48,49,263,264,268) that contain the

N,N-dimethylglycylamido substituent at the 9-position of minocycline and 6-demethyl-6-deoxytetracycline. The presence of this substituent overcomes the two major mechanisms responsible for tetracycline resistance in a wide variety of bacterial pathogens: active efflux of the drug out of the cell and protection of the ribosomes by the production of cytoplasmic proteins (23,263,264). Glycylcyclines have a higher binding affinity for ribosomes than earlier tetracyclines, which is thought to explain why cytoplasmic ribosomal protection proteins are unable to confer resistance to glycylcyclines (23). This accordingly extends the spectrum of these new agents to include multiresistant strains, including *Neisseria gonorrhoeae*, and in addition significantly improves their activity (at least fourfold), compared with the activity of minocycline and tetracycline (271).

2-Pyridones

The 2-pyridones are a new class of broad-spectrum antimicrobial agents that inhibit bacterial DNA gyrase (84,155). These compounds are similar to fluoroquinolones but differ by placement of the nitrogen atom in the ring juncture. Because the basic ring structure of the molecule is different from that of the quinolones or naphthyridines, 2-pyridones appear to bind differently at the DNA gyrase site. Accordingly, these agents have been found to be active against fluoroquinolone-resistant bacteria (6). The 2-pyridones exhibit *in vitro* bactericidal activity. Like fluoroquinolones, these agents are water soluble and thus have excellent bioavailability when taken orally. Hundreds of 2-pyridones have been synthesized and evaluated *in vitro* and *in vivo*, with selected agents now moving toward human clinical trials (155).

Lantibiotics

Lantibiotics are a diverse group of antimicrobial peptides that contain the thioether amino acids lanthionine and/or 3-methyllanthionine (173,206). Wide ranges of bacteria, including a variety of lactic acid bacteria, produce lantibiotics (26,279). Lantibiotics are primarily active against Gram-positive bacteria (173,182) via a number of diverse mechanisms. Some of these peptides—type A lantibiotics such as Pep5—are positively charged, amphiphilic molecules that exert their primary bactericidal action on the cell membrane by causing pores (173). Type B lantibiotics such as cinnamycin possess globular shapes and no net charge or a negative charge. These globular lantibiotics appear to inhibit phospholipases by binding phosphoethanolamine (206). A third group of lantibiotics includes mersacidin and actagardine; these lantibiotics inhibit peptidoglycan synthesis, probably on the level of transglycosylation by complexing lipid II (32,206). The latter two groups of lantibiotics appear to be bacteriostatic.

Cationic Peptides

Cationic peptides, also called defensins, are polycationic peptides that function as an important mechanism of innate immunity in plants and animals (92). These antimicrobial peptides are produced by phagocytic cells and lymphocytes as well as by the epithelial cell lining of the gastrointestinal and genitourinary tracts, the tracheobronchial tree, and keratinocytes (204). There are more than 800 sequences of antimicrobial peptides from the plant and animal kingdoms (27). Examples of these agents include cecropins (28), melittin (68), magainins (310), and epidermin (242). The main targets of these antimicrobial peptides are the bacterial cell membranes, with cell death resulting from increased permeability. Polycations have long been known to affect the outer membranes of Gram-negative bacteria (281) and have been thought to do so by crossing the outer membrane by the self-promoted uptake pathway (108). Aminoglycosides exemplify this mechanism. It is likely that the primary effect of these cationic peptides, like that of aminoglycosides, is the disruption of the biofilm caused by these agents displacing Mg^{2+} and Ca^{2+}. Evidence for this is found in the fact that a number of these antimicrobial peptides have been noted to be active as insoluble complexes (113). This suggests that surface activity on the targeted microorganism is sufficient for lethal activity. Moreover, the interaction of antimicrobial peptides with biofilm is well served by the fact that these agents possess both amphipathic and hydrophobic portions, which facilitates the passage of the molecule from the aqueous phase to the biofilm phase, where it displaces magnesium and calcium cations. Finally, some antimicrobial peptides are multifunctional and can enhance both cellular (Th1-dependent) and humoral (Th2-dependent) cytokine production and immune responses (204).

REFERENCES

1. Abraham EP. Fleming's discovery. *Rev Infect Dis* 1980;2:140–141.
2. Achari A, Somers DO, Champness JN, et al. Crystal structure of the anti-bacterial sulfonamide drug target dihydropteroate synthase. *Nat Struct Biol* 1997;4:490–497.
3. Ackermann G, Rodloff AC. Drugs of the 21st century: telithromycin (HNR 3647)—the first ketolide. *J Antimicrob Chemother* 2003;51:497–511.
4. Ahnwar H, Strap JL, Costerton JW. Dynamic interactions of biofilms of mucoid *Pseudomonas aeruginosa* with tobramycin and piperacillin. *Antimicrob Agents Chemother* 1992;36:1208–1214.
5. Alborn WE Jr, Allen NE, Preston DA. Daptomycin disrupts membrane potential in growing *Staphylococcus aureus*. *Antimicrob Agents Chemother* 1991;35:2282–2287.
6. Alder J, Clement J, Meulbroek J, et al. Efficacies of ABT-719 and related 2-pyridones, members of a new class of antibacterial agents, against experimental bacterial infections. *Antimicrob Agents Chemother* 1995;39:971–975.
7. Allen NE, Alborn WE Jr, Hobbs JN Jr. Initiation of membrane potential–dependent amino acid transport by

daptomycin. *Antimicrob Agents Chemother* 1991;35:2639–2642.

8. Allington DR, Rivey MP. Quinupristin/dalfopristin: a therapeutic review. *Clin Ther* 2001;23:24–44.
9. Ames GF. Bacterial periplasmic transport systems: structure, mechanism, and evolution. *Annu Rev Biochem* 1986;55:397–425.
10. Amyes SGB. *Magic bullets, lost horizons: the rise and fall of antibiotics*. New York: Taylor & Francis, 2001.
11. Asbel LE, Levison ME. Cephalosporins, carbapenems, and monobactams. *Infect Dis Clin North Am* 2000;14:435–447.
12. Ashhurst AP. The centenary of Lister (1827–1927): a tale of sepsis and antisepsis. *Ann Med Hist* 1927;9:205–211.
13. Aumercier M, Bouhallab S, Capmau ML, et al. RP 59500: a proposed mechanism for its bactericidal activity. *J Antimicrob Chemother* 1992;30[Suppl A]:9–14.
14. Ballow CH, Amsden GW. Azithromycin: the first azalide antibiotic. *Ann Pharmacother* 1992;26:1253–1261.
15. Barclay ML, Begg EJ, Chambers ST, et al. Improved efficacy with nonsimultaneous administration of first doses of gentamicin and ceftazidime in vitro. *Antimicrob Agents Chemother* 1995;39;132–136.
16. Bartz QR. Isolation and characterization of chloromycetin. *J Biol Chem* 1948;172:445–450.
17. Bayer A, Susan P, Ramos MC, et al. Effects of alginase on the natural history and antibiotic therapy of experimental endocarditis caused by mucoid *Pseudomonas aeruginosa*. *Infect Immun* 1992;60:3979–3985.
18. Bayles KW. The bacterial action of penicillin: new clues to an unsolved mystery. *Trends Microbiol* 2000;8:274–278.
19. Bayles KW. Are the molecular strategies that control apoptosis conserved in bacteria? *Trends Microbiol* 2003;11:306–311.
20. Beauregard DA, Williams DH, Gwynn MN, et al. Dimerization and membrane anchors in extracellular targeting of vancomycin group antibiotics. *Antimicrob Agents Chemother* 1995;39:781–785.
21. Benaissa M, Babin P, Quellard N, et al. Changes in *Helicobacter pylori* ultrastructure and antigens during conversion from the bacillary to the coccoid form. *Infect Immun* 1996;64:2331–2335.
22. Berger JM, Gamblin SJ, Haarrison SC, et al. Structure and mechanism of DNA topoisomerase II. *Nature* 1996;379:225–232.
23. Bergeron J, Ammirati M, Danley D, et al. Glycylcyclines bind to the high-affinity tetracycline ribosomal binding site and evade Tet(M) and Tet(O)-mediated ribosomal protection. *Antimicrob Agents Chemother* 1996;40:2226–2228.
24. Berry V, Jennings K, Woodnutt G. Bactericidal and morphological effects of amoxicillin on *Helicobacter pylori*. *Antimicrob Agents Chemother* 1995;39:1859–1861.
25. Beveridge TJ. Structures of Gram-negative cell walls and their derived membrane vesicles. *J Bacteriol* 1999;181:4725–4733.
26. Bierbaum G, Sahl H-G. Lantibiotics: unusually modified bacteriocin-like peptides from Gram-positive bacteria. *Zentralbl Bakteriol Paraitenkd Infektionskr Hyg Abt I Orig* 1993;278:1–22.
27. Boman HG. Antibacterial peptides: basic facts and emerging concepts. *J Intern Med* 2003;254:197–215.
28. Bomam HG, Faye I, Gudmundsson GH, et al. Cell-free immunity in *Cecropia*: a model system for antibacterial proteins. *Eur J Biochem* 1991;201:23–31.
29. Bonner DP, Sykes RB. Structure activity relationship among the monobactams. *J Antimicrob Chemother* 1984;14:313–327.
30. Booth IR. Regulation of cytoplasmic pH in bacteria. *Microb Rev* 1985;49:359–378.
31. Borges-Walmsley MI, Walmsley AR. The structure and function of drug pumps. *Trends Microbiol* 2001;9:71–79.
32. Brotz H, Bierbaum G, Markus A, et al. Mode of action of the lantibiotic mersacidin: inhibition of peptidoglycan biosynthesis via a novel mechanism. *Antimicrob Agents Chemother* 1995;39:714–719.
33. Brown MRW, Allison DG, Gilbert P. Resistance of bacterial biofilms to antibiotic: a growth-rate related effect? *J Antimicrob Chemother* 1988;22:777–783.
34. Brown MRW, Williams P. Influence of substrate limitation and growth phase on sensitivity to antimicrobial agents. *J Antimicrob Chemother* 1985;15[Suppl A]:7–14.
35. Brown RW, Collier PJ, Gilbert P. Influence of growth rate on susceptibility to antimicrobial agents: modification of the cell envelope and batch and continuous culture studies. *Antimicrob Agents Chemother* 1990;34:1623–1628.
36. Brunskill EW, Bayles KW. Identification and molecular characterization of a putative regulatory locus that affects autolysis in *Staphylococcus aureus*. *J Bacteriol* 1996;178:611–618.
37. Brunskill EW, de Jonge BLM, Bayles KW. The *Staphylococcus aureus scdA* gene: a novel locus that affects cell division and morphogenesis. *Microbiol* 1997;143:2877–2882.
38. Bryskier A. Ketolides-telithromycin, an example of a new class of antibacterial agents. *Clin Microbiol Infect* 2000;6:661–669.
39. Buiting AGM, Thompson J, Emeis JJ, et al. Effects of tissue-type plasminogen activator (t-PA) on the treatment of experimental *Streptococcus sanguis* endocarditis. *J Infect Dis* 1989;159:780–784.
40. Burns JL, Clark DK. Salicylate-inducible antibiotic resistance in *Pseudomonas cepacia* associated with absence of a pore-forming outer membrane protein. *Antimicrob Agents Chemother* 1992;36:2280–2285.
41. Carithers HA. The first use of an antibiotic in America. *Am J Dis Child* 1974;128:207–211.
42. Campbell EA, Korazheva N, Mustaev A, et al. Structural mechanism for rifampin inhibition of bacterial RNA polymerase. *Cell* 2001;104:901–912.
43. Carrer G, Flandrois JP, Lobry JR. Biphasic kinetics of bacterial killing by quinolones. *J Antimicrob Chemother* 1991;27:319–327.
44. Carter AP, Clemons WM, Brodersen DE, et al. Functional insights from the structure of the 30S ribosomal subunit and its interactions with antibiotics. *Nature* 2000;407:340–348.
45. Catrenich C, Makin K. Characterization of the morphological conversion of *Helicobacter pylori* from bacillary to coccoid form. *Scand J Gastroenterol* 1991;26[Suppl 181]:58–64.
46. Cederbrant G, Kahlmeter G, Ljungh A. Proposed mechanism for metronidazole resistance in *Helicobacter pylori*. *J Antimicrob Chemother* 1992;29:115–120.
47. Cellini L, Allocati N, Angelucci D, et al. Coccoid *Helicobacter pylori* not culturable in vitro reverts in mice. *Microbiol Immunol* 1994;38:843–850.
48. Chopra I. Glycylcyclines: third generation tetracycline antibiotics. *Curr Opin Microbiol* 2001;1:464–469.
49. Chopra I. New developments in tetracycline antibiotics: glycylcyclines and tetracycline efflux pump inhibitors. *Drug Resist Updat* 2002;5:119–125.
50. Chopra I, Roberts M. Tetracycline antibiotics: mode of action, applications, molecular biology, and epidemiology of bacterial resistance. *Microbiol Mol Biol Rev* 2001;65:232–260.

51. Chu DTW, Fernandes PB. Structure-activity relationships of the fluoroquinolones. *Antimicrob Agents Chemother* 1989;33:131–135.
52. Chuard C, Herrmann M, Vaudaux P, et al. Successful treatment of experimental chronic foreign body infection due to methicillin-resistant *Staphylococcus aureus* by antimicrobial combinations. *Antimicrob Agents Chemother* 1991;35:2611–2616.
53. Colwell RR. Viable but nonculturable bacteria: a survival strategy. *J Infect Chemother* 2000;6:121–125.
54. Contreras A, Maxwell A. *GyrB* mutations which confer resistance also affect DNA supercoiling and ATP hydrolysis by *Escherichia coli* DNA gyrase. *Mol Microbiol* 1992;6:1617–1624.
55. Contreras A, Vasquez D. Cooperative and antagonistic interactions of peptidyl-tRNA and antibiotics with bacterial ribosomes. *Eur J Biochem* 1977;74:539–547.
56. Corton JC, Ward JE Jr, Lutherhaus J. Analysis of cell division gene *ftsZ* (*sulB*) from Gram-negative and Gram-positive bacteria. *J Bacteriol* 1987;169:1–7.
57. Costerton JW, Lam K, Chan R. The role of the microcolony in the pathogenesis of *Pseudomonas aeruginosa*. *Rev Infect Dis* 1983;5[Suppl]:S867–S873.
58. Costerton JW, Lewandowski Z, Caldwell DE, et al. Microbial biofilms. *Annu Rev Microbiol* 1995;49:711–745.
59. Costerton JW, Stewart PS, Greenberg EP. Bacterial biofilms: a common cause of persistent infections. *Science* 1999;284:1318–1322.
60. Couturier M, el Bahassi M, Van Melderen L. Bacterial death by DNA gyrase poisoning. *Trends Microbiol* 1998;6:269–275.
61. Craig WA, Ebert SC. Killing and regrowth of bacteria in vitro: a review. *Scand J Infect Dis Suppl* 1991;74:63–70.
62. Craig WA, Leggett K, Totsuka K, et al. Key pharmacokinetic parameters of antibiotic efficacy in experimental animal infections. *J Drug Dev* 1988;1:7–15.
63. Cremieux AC, Saleh-Mghir A, Vallois JM, et al. Efficacy of temofloxacin in experimental *Streptococcus adjacens* endocarditis and autoradiographic diffusion pattern of [^{14}C]temofloxacin in cardiac vegetations. *Antimicrob Agents Chemother* 1992;36:2216–2221.
64. Daley JS, Eliopoulos GP, Reiszner E, et al. Activity and mechanism of action of DuP 105 and DuP 721, new oxazolidone compounds. *J Antimicrob Chemother* 1988;21:721–730.
65. Dall L, Barnes WG, Lane JW, et al. Enzymatic modification of glycocalyx in the treatment of experimental streptococcal endocarditis due to viridans streptococci. *J Infect Dis* 1987;156:736–740.
66. Davies DG, Chakrabarty AM, Geesey GG. Exopolysaccharide production in biofilms: substratum activation of alginate gene expression by *Pseudomonas aeruginosa*. *Appl Environ Microbiol* 1993;59:1181–1186.
67. Delgado G Jr, Neuhauser MM, Bearden DT, et al. Quinpristin-dalfopristin: an overview. *Pharmacotherapy* 2000;20:1469–1485.
68. Dempsey CE. The actions of melittin on membranes. *Biochim Biophys Acta* 1990;1031:143–161.
69. Denome SA, Elf PK, Henderson TA, et al. *Escherichia coli* mutants lacking all possible combinations of eight penicillin binding proteins: viability, characteristics, and implications for peptidoglycan synthesis. *J Bacteriol* 1999;181:3981–3993.
70. Dewar HA, Jones MR, Barnes WS, et al. Fibrinolytic therapy in bacterial experimental studies in dogs. *Eur Heart J* 1986;7:520–527.
71. Dixon RA, Chopra I. Leakage of periplasmic proteins from *Escherichia coli* mediated by polymyxin B nonapeptide. *Antimicrob Agents Chemother* 1986;29:781–788.
72. Domagala JM. Structure-activity and structure-side-effect relationships for the quinolone antibacterials. *J Antimicrob Chemother* 1994;33:685–706.
73. Domagk G. Ein Beitrag zur Chemotherapie der Bakteriellen Infektionen. *Dtsch Med Wochenschr* 1935;61:250–253.
74. Domenico P, Hopkins T, Schoch PE, et al. Potentiation of aminoglycoside inhibition and reduction of capsular polysaccharide production in *Klebsiella pneumoniae* by sodium salicylate. *J Antimicrob Chemother* 1990;25:205–214.
75. Donlan RM, Costerton JW. Biofilms: survival mechanisms of clinically relevant microorganisms. *Clin Microbiol Rev* 2002;15:167–193.
76. Doring G, Goldstein A, Roll A. Role of *Pseudomonas aeruginosa* exoenzyme in lung infections of patients with cystic fibrosis. *Infect Immun* 1985;49:557–562.
77. Dougherty T, Pucci MJ. Penicillin-binding proteins are regulated by *rpoS* during transitions in growth states of *Escherichia coli*. *Antimicrob Agents Chemother* 1994;38:205–210.
78. Douthwaite S, Champney WS. Structures of ketolides and macrolides determine their mode of interaction with the ribosomal target site. *J Antimicrob Chemother* 2001;48[Topic T1]:T1–8.
79. Douthwaite S, Hansen LH, Mauvais P. Macrolide-ketolide inhibition of MLS-resistant ribosomes is improved by alternative drug interaction with domain II of 23S rRNA. *Mol Microbiol* 2000;36:183–193.
80. Drancourt M, Stein A, Argenson JN, et al. Oral rifampin plus ofloxacin for the treatment of *Staphylococcus*-infected orthopedic implants. *Antimicrob Agents Chemother* 1993;37:1214–1218.
81. Drenkard E, Ausubel FM. *Pseudomonas* biofilm formation and antibiotic resistance are linked to phenotypic variation. *Nature* 2002;416:740–743.
82. Drlica K. Antibiotic resistance: can we beat the bugs? *Drug Discov Today* 2001;6:714–715.
83. Ebert SC, Craig WA. Pharmacodynamic properties of antibiotics: application to drug monitoring and dosage regimen design. *Infect Control Hosp Epidemiol* 1990;11:319–326.
84. Eliopoulos GM, Wennersten CB, Cole G, et al. In vitro activity of A-86719.1, a novel 2-pyridone antimicrobial agent. *Antimicrob Agents Chemother* 1995;35:850–853.
85. Elliot TS, Greenwood D. The morphological response of *Pseudomonas aeruginosa* to aztreonam, cefoperazone, ceftazidime, and formimidoyl thienamycin. *J Med Microbiol* 1984;17:159–169.
86. Eng RHK, Padberg FT, Smith SM, et al. Bactericidal effects of antibiotics on slowly growing and non-growing bacteria. *Antimicrob Agents Chemother* 1991;35:1824–1828.
87. Eustice DC, Brittelli DR, Feldman PA, et al. An automated pulse labelling method for structure-activity relationship studies with antibacterial oxazolidinones. *Drugs Exp Clin Res* 1990;16:149–155.
88. Evans DJ, Brown MRW, Allison DG, et al. Susceptibility of bacterial biofilms to tobramycin: role of specific growth rate and phase in division cycle. *J Antimicrob Chemother* 1990;25:585–591.
89. Farmer S, Li Z, Hancock REW. Influence of outer membrane mutations on susceptibility of *Escherichia coli* to the dibasic macrolide azithromycin. *J Antimicrob Chemother* 1992;29:27–33.
90. Fleming A. On the antibacterial action of cultures of a penicillium, with special reference to their use in the isolation of *B. influenzae*. *Br J Exp Pathol* 1929;10:226–236.

91. Foulds J, Murray DM, Chai T, et al. Decreased penetration of cephalosporins through the outer membrane of *Escherichia coli* grown in salicylate. *Antimicrob Agents Chemother* 1989;33:412–417.
92. Ganz T. Defensins: antimicrobial peptides of innate immunity. *Nat Rev Immunol* 2003;3:710–720.
93. Gemmell CG, Lorian V. Effects of low concentrations of antibiotics on bacterial ultrastructure, virulence, and susceptibility of immunodefenses: clinical significance. In: Lorian V, ed. *Antibiotics in laboratory medicine,* 4th ed. Baltimore: Williams & Wilkens, 1996;397–452.
94. Gerhard U, Mackay JP, Maplestone RA, et al. The role of the sugar and chlorine substituents in the dimerizatiion of vancomycin antibiotics. *J Am Chem Soc* 1993;115:232–237.
94a. Giesbrecht P. Zur Norphogenase der Zellwand von Staphylokoken. *Mikroskopie* 1972;28:323–342.
95. Giesbrecht P, Kersten T, Maidhof H, et al. Staphylococcal cell wall: morphogenesis and fatal variations in the presence of penicillin. *Microbiol Mol Biol Rev* 1998;62:1371–1414.
96. Gilbert DN. Once-daily aminoglycoside therapy. *Antimicrob Agents Chemother* 1991;35:399–405.
97. Gilbert P, Collier PJ, Brown MRW. Influence of growth rate on susceptibility to antimicrobial agents: biofilms, cell cycle, dormancy and stringent response. *Antimicrob Agents Chemother* 1990;34:1865–1868.
98. Giwercman B, Jensen ET, Hiby N, Kharazmi A, Costerton JW. Induction of beta-lactamase production in *Pseudomonas aeruginosa* biofilm. *Antimicrob Agents Chemother* 1991;35:1008–1010.
99. Goswami SK, Kivity S, Marom Z. Erythromycin inhibits respiratory glycoconjugate secretion from human airways in vitro. *Am Rev Respir Dis* 1990;141:72–78.
100. Griffith RS, Peek FB. Vancomycin, a new antibiotic: preliminary clinical and laboratory studies. In: Welch H, Martini-Ibanez, F. eds. *Antibiotics annual 1955–1956.* New York: Medical Encyclopedia, 1956;619–622.
101. Gristina AG, Hobgood CD, Webb LX, et al. Adhesive colonization of biomaterials and antibiotic resistance. *Biomaterials* 1987;8:423–426.
102. Groicher KH, Friek BA, Fujimoto DF, et al. The *Staphylococcus aureus* irgAB operon modulates murein hydrolase activity and penicillin tolerance. *J Bacteriol* 2000;182:1794–1801.
103. Guggenbichler JP, Allerberger F, Dierich MP, et al. Spaced administration of antibiotic combinations to eliminate *Pseudomonas* from sputum in cystic fibrosis. *Lancet* 1988;2:749–750.
104. Haemers A, Leysen DC, Bollaert W, et al. Influence of N substitution on antimycobacterial activity of ciprofloxacin. *Antimicrob Agents Chemother* 1990;34:496–497.
105. Haight TH, Finland M. Observations on mode of action of erythromycin. *Proc Soc Exp Biol Med* 1952;81;188–193.
106. Hancock REW. Alterations in outer membrane permeability. *Annu Rev Microbiol* 1984;38:237–264.
107. Hancock REW. Bacterial outer membranes: evolving concepts. *ASM News* 1991;57:175–182.
108. Hancock REW, Bellido F. Antibiotic uptake: unusual results for unusual molecules. *J Antimicrob Chemother* 1992;29:235–243.
109. Hancock REW, Raffle VJ, Nicas TI. Involvement of the outer membrane in gentamicin and streptomycin uptake and killing in *Pseudomonas aeruginosa*. *Antimicrob Agents Chemother* 1981;19:777–785.
110. Hansen LH, Mauvais P, Douthwaite S. The macrolide-ketolide antibiotic binding site is formed by structures in domains II and V of 23S ribosomal RNA. *Mol Microbiol* 1999;31:623–631.
111. Harold FM. Ion currents and physiological functions in microorganisms. *Ann Rev Microbiol* 1977;31:181–203.
112. Hash JH, Davis MC. Electron microscopy of *Staphylococcus aureus* treated with tetracycline. *Science* 1962;138: 8–28.
113. Haynie SL, Crum GE, Doele BA. Antimicrobial activities of amphiphilic peptides covalently bonded to a water-insoluble resin. *Antimicrob Agents Chemother* 1995;39:301–307.
114. Held TK, Adamczik C, Trautmann M, et al. Effects of MICs and sub-MICs of antibiotics on production of capsular polysaccharide of *Klebsiella pneumonia*. *Antimicrob Agents Chemother* 1995;39:1093–1096.
115. Hellinger WC, Brewer NS. Carbapenems and monobactams: imipenem, meropenem, and aztreonam. *Mayo Clin Proc* 1999;74:420–434.
116. Henge-Aronis R. Survival of hunger and stress: the role of *rpoS* in early stationary phase gene regulation in *E. coli*. *Cell* 1993;72:165–168.
117. Henze U, Sidow T, Wecke J, et al. Influence of *femB* on methicillin resistance and peptidoglycan metabolism in *Staphylococcus aureus*. *J Bacteriol* 1993;175:1612–1620.
118. Himmelweith F, ed. *The collected papers of Paul Ehrlich*. London: Pergamon Press, 1960;505–510.
119. Hobby GL, Dawson MH. Effect of growth rate of bacteria on action of penicillin. *Proc Soc Exp Biol* 1944;56:181–184.
120. Hochman A. Programmed cell death in prokaryotes. *Crit Rev Microbiol* 1997;23:207–214.
121. Hugo WB, ed. *Inhibition and destruction of the bacterial cell*. New York: Academic Press, 1971.
122. Ichimiya T, Takeoka K, Hiramatsu K, et al. The influence of azithromycin on the biofilm formation of *Pseudomonas aeruginosa* in vitro. *Chemotherapy* 1996;42:186–191.
123. Iida K, Koike M. Cell wall alterations in Gram-negative bacteria by aminoglycoside antibiotics. *Antimicrob Agents Chemother* 1974;5:95–97.
124. Ingham HR, Selkon JB, Hale JH. The antibacterial activity of metronidazole. *J Antimicrob Chemother* 1975;1:355–361.
125. Jolliffe LK, Doyle RJ, Steips UN. The energized membrane and cellular autolysis in *Bacillus subtillis*. *Cell* 1981;25:753–763.
126. Kadurugamuwa JL, Clarke AJ, Beveridge TJ. Surface action of gentamicin on *Pseudomonas aeruginosa*. *J Bacteriol* 1993;175:5798–5805.
127. Kadurugamuwa JL, Lam JS, Beveridge TJ. Interaction of gentamicin with the A band and B band lipopolysaccharides of *Pseudomonas aeruginosa* and its possible lethal effect. *Antimicrob Agents Chemother* 1993;37:715–721.
128. Kahan FM, Kahan JS, Cassidy PJ, et al. The mechanism of action of fosfomycin. *Ann NY Acad Sci* 1974;235:364–385.
129. Kang L, Rybak MJ. Pharmacodynamics of RP 595000 alone and in combination with vancomycin against *Staphylococcus aureus* in an in vitro–infected fibrin clot model. *Antimicrob Agents Chemother* 1995;39:1505–1511.
130. Kaye JJ, Chapman GB. Cytological aspects of antimicrobial antibiosis. III. Cytologically distinguishable stages in antibiotic action of colistin sulfate on *Escherichia coli*. *J Bacteriol* 1963;86:536–543.
131. Khardoli N, Nguyen H, Rosenbaum B, et al. In vitro susceptibilities of rapidly growing mycobacteria to newer antimicrobial agents. *Antimicrob Agents Chemother* 1994;38:134–137.

132. Kirst HA, Creemer LC, Paschal JW, et al. Antimicrobial characterization and interrelationships of dirithromycin and epidirithromycin. *Antimicrob Agents Chemother* 1995;39:1436–1441.
133. Kita E, Sawaki M, Nishikawa F, et al. Suppression of virulence factors of *Pseudomonas aeruginosa* by erythromycin. *J Antimicrob Chemother* 1991;27:273–284.
134. Kitano K, Tomasz A. Triggering of autolytic cell wall degradation in *Escherichia coli* by beta-lactam antibiotics. *Antimicrob Agents Chemother* 1979;16:838–848.
135. Klopman G, Li J-Y, Wang S, et al. In vitro anti–*Mycobacterium avium* activities of quinolones: predicted active structures and mechanistic considerations. *Antimicrob Agents Chemother* 1994;38:1794–1802.
136. Koch C, Hiby N. Pathogenesis of cystic fibrosis. *Lancet* 1993;341:1065–1069.
137. Kolter R. Life and death in stationary phase. *ASM News* 1992;58:75–79.
138. Kotra LP, Haddad J, Mobashery S. Aminoglycosides: perspectives on mechanisms of action and resistance and strategies to counter resistance. *Antimicrob Agents Chemother* 2000;44:3249–3256.
139. Kudoh S, Azuma A, Yamamoto M, et al. Improvement of survival in patients with diffuse panbronchiolitis treated with low-dose erythromycin. *Am J Respir Crit Care Med* 1998;157:1829–1832.
140. Kumon H, Ono N, Iida M, et al. Combined effect of fosfomycin and ofloxacin against *Pseudomonas aeruginosa* growing in a biofilm. *Antimicrob Agents Chemother* 1995;39:1038–1044.
141. Kumon H, Tomochika K, Matunaga T, et al. A sandwich cup method for the penetration assay of antimicrobials through *Pseudomonas* exopolysaccharides. *Microbiol Immunol* 1994;38:615–619.
142. Kunin CM. Resistance to antimicrobial drugs a worldwide calamity. *Ann Intern Med* 1993;118:557–561.
143. Lakey JH, Ptak M. Fluorescence indicates a calcium-dependent interaction between the lipopeptide antibiotic LY146032 and phospholipid membranes. *Biochemistry* 1988;27:4639–4645.
144. Lam JS, Chan R, Lam K, et al. The production of mucoid microcolonies by *Pseudomonas aeruginosa* within infected lungs in cystic fibrosis. *Infect Immun* 1980;28:546–556.
145. LaPorte DC, Rosenthal KD, Storm DR. Disruption of *Escherichia coli* growth and respiration by polymyxin B covalently attached to agarose beads. *Biochemistry* 1977;16:1642–1648.
146. Lawlor MT, Sullivan MC, Levitz RE, et al. Treatment of prosthetic valve endocardidtis due to methicillin-resistant *Staphylococcus aureus* with minocycline. *J Infect Dis* 1990;161:812–814.
147. Lee N, Yuen KY, Kumana CR. Clinical role of beta-lactam/beta-lactamase inhibitor combinations. *Drugs* 2003;63:1511–1524.
148. Leive L. Studies on the permeability change produced in coliform bacteria by ethylenediaminetetraacetate. *J Biol Chem* 1968;243:2373–2380.
149. Leive L. The barrier function of the Gram-negative envelope. *Ann NY Acad Sci* 1974;235:109–129.
150. Levine DP, Fromm BS, Reddy BR. Slow response to vancomycin or vancomycin plus rifampin in methicillin-resistant *Staphylococcus aureus* endocarditis. *Ann Intern Med* 1991;115:674–680.
151. Levy SB. Active efflux mechanisms for antimicrobial resistance. *Antimicrob Agents Chemother* 1992;36:695–703.
152. Levy SB. *The antibiotic paradox: how miracle drugs are destroying the miracle.* New York: Plenum, 1992.
153. Lewin CS, Howard BMA, Ratclife NT, et al. 4-Quinolones and the SOS response. *J Med Microbiol* 1989;29:139–144.
154. Lewis K. Programmed cell death in bacteria. *Microbiol Mol Biol Rev* 2000;64:503–514.
155. Li Q, Mitscher LA, Shen LL. The 2-pyridone antibacterial agents: bacterial topoisomerase inhibitors. *Med Res Rev* 2000;20:231–293.
156. Little JW, Mount DW. The SOS regulatory system of *Escherichia coli*. *Cell* 1982;29:11–22.
157. Livermore DM. Linezolid in vitro: mechanism and antibacterial spectrum. *J Antimicrob Chemother* 2003;51[Suppl 2]: S9–S16.
158. Lomovskaya O, Warren MS, Lee A, et al. Identification and characterization of inhibitors of multidrug resistance efflux pumps in *Pseudomonas aeruginosa*: novel agents for combination therapy. *Antimicrob Agents Chemother* 2001;45:105–116.
159. Lomovskaya O, Watkins W. Inhibition of efflux pumps as a novel approach to combat drug resistance in bacteria. *J Mol Microbiol Biotechnol* 2001;3:225–236.
160. Lorian V. Some effects of subinhibitory concentrations of penicillin on the structure and division of staphylococci. *Antimicrob Agents Chemother* 1975;7:864–870.
161. Lorian V. In vitro simulation of in vivo conditions: physical state of the culture medium. *J Clin Microbiol* 1989;27:2403–2406.
162. Lorian V, Atkinson B. Effects of subinhibitory concentrations of antibiotics on cross walls of cocci. *Antimicrob Agents Chemother* 1976;9:1043–1055.
163. Lorian V, Atkinson B, Lim Y. Effect of rifampin and oxacillin on the ultrastructure and growth of staphylococci. *Rev Infect Dis* 1983;5[Suppl]:S419–S427.
164. Lorian V, Ernst J. Activity of amikacin and ampicillin in succession and in combination. *Diagn Microbiol Infect Dis* 1988;11:163–169.
165. Lorian V, Esanu Y, Amaral L. Ultrastructure alterations of *Staphylococcus aureus* exposed to RP 59500. *J Antimicrob Chemother* 1994;33:625–628.
166. Lugtenberg B, Van Alphen L. Molecular architecture and functioning of the outer membrane of *Escherichia coli* and other Gram-negative bacteria. *Biochim Biophys Acta* 1983;737:511–515.
167. Magnusson K-E. Physiochemical properties of bacterial surfaces. *Biochem Soc Trans* 1989;17:454–458.
168. Marshall WF, Blair JE. The cephalosporins. *Mayo Clin Proc* 1999;74:187–195.
169. Martin NL, Beveridge TJ. Gentamicin interaction with *Pseudomonas aeruginosa*. *Antimicrob Agents Chemother* 1986;29:1079–1087.
170. Mates SM, Eisenberg ES, Mandel LJ, et al. Membrane potential and gentamicin uptake in *Staphylococcus aureus*. *Proc Natl Acad Sci USA* 1982;79:6693–6697.
171. Matin A. The molecular basis of carbon-starvation-induced general resistance in *Escherichia coli*. *Mol Microbiol* 1991;5:3–10.
172. Maxwell A. The molecular basis of quinolone action. *J Antimicrob Chemother* 1992;30:409–416.
173. McAuliffe O, Ross RP, Hill C. Lantibiotics: structure, biosynthesis and mode of action. *FEMS Microbiol Rev* 2001;25:285–308.
174. McLaughlin SGA, Dilger JP. Transport of protons across membranes by weak acids. *Physiol Rev* 1980;60:825–863.
175. McOster CC, Fitzpatrick PM. Nitrofurantoin: mechanism of action and implications for resistance development in common uropathogens. *J Antimicrob Chemother* 1994;33:23–33.
176. Mendelman PM, Chaffin DO. Two penicillin binding proteins of *Haemophilus influenzae* are lost after cells

enter stationary phase. *FEMS Microbiol Lett* 1985;30: 399–402.
177. Menninger JR. Functional consequences of binding macrolides to ribosomes. *J Antimicrob Chemother* 1985;16[Suppl A]:23–24.
178. Miyata K, Maejima K, Tomada K, et al. *Serratia* protease. I. Purification and general properties of the enzyme. *Agric Biol Chem* 1970;34:310–318.
179. Mizukane R, Hirakata Y, Kaku M, et al. Comparative in vitro exoenzyme-suppressing activities of azithromycin and other macrolide antibiotics against *Pseudomonas aeruginosa*. *Antimicrob Agents Chemother* 1994;38:528–533.
180. Moghir AS, Crmieux AC, Jambou R, et al. Dextranase enhances antibiotic efficacy in experimental viridans streptococcal endocarditis. *Antimicrob Agents Chemother* 1994;38:953–958.
181. Molinari G, Guzmn A, Pesce A, et al. Inhibition of *Pseudomonas aeruginosa* virulence factors by subinhibitory concentrations of azithromycin and other macrolide antibiotics. *J Antimicrob Chemother* 1992;31:681–688.
182. Moll GN, Roberts GC, Konings WN, et al. Mechanism of lantibiotic-induced pore-formation. *Antonie Van Leeuwenhoek* 1996;69:185–191.
183. Moore RD, Lietman PS, Smith CR. Clinical response to aminoglycoside therapy: importance of the ratio of peak concentration to minimal inhibitory concentration. *J Infect Dis* 1987;155:93–99.
184. Moreillon P, Markiewicz Z, Machman S, et al. Two bactericidal targets for penicillin in pneumococci: autolysis-dependent and autolysis-independent killing mechanisms. *Antimicrob Agents Chemother* 1990;34:33–39.
185. Moyer CL, Morita RY. Effect of growth rate and starvation-survival on the viability and stability of a psychrophilic marine bacterium. *Appl Environ Microbiol* 1989;55:1122–1127.
186. Nagarajan R. Antibacterial activities and modes of action of vancomycin and related glycopeptides. *Antimicrob Agents Chemother* 1991;35:605–609.
187. Nagarajan R. Structure-activity relationships of vancomycin-type glycopeptide antibiotics. *J Antibiot* (Tokyo) 1993; 46:1181–1195.
188. Nanninga N. Morphogenesis of *Escherichia coli*. *Microbiol Mol Biol Rev* 1998;62:110–129.
189. Neu HC. The development of macrolides: clarithromycin in perspective. *J Antimicrob Chemother* 1991;27[Suppl 4]: 19.
190. Neu HC. The crisis in antibiotic resistance. *Science* 1992;257:1064–1073.
191. Neu HC. Antimicrobial chemotherapy, 1934–1994. *Antimicrob Infect Dis Newslett* 1994;13:18.
192. Newton BA. Reversal of the antimicrobial activity of polymyxin by divalent cations. *Nature* 1953;172:160–161.
193. Nicas TI, Hancock REW. Outer membrane protein H1 of *Pseudomonas aeruginosa*: involvement in adaptive and mutational resistance to ethylenediaminetetraacetate, polymyxin B, and gentamicin. *J Bacteriol* 1980;143:872–878.
194. Nicas TI, Hancock REW. Alteration of susceptibility to EDTA, polymyxin B and gentamicin in *Pseudomonas aeruginosa* by divalent cation regulation of outer membrane protein H1. *J Gen Microbiol* 1983;129:509–517.
195. Nicolau DP, Freeman CD, Belliveau PP, et al. Experience with a once-daily aminoglycoside program administered to 2,184 adult patients. *Antimicrob Agents Chemother* 1995;39:650–655.
196. Nicolau DP, Freeman CD, Nightingale CH, et al. Minocycline versus vancomycin for treatment of experimental endocarditis caused by oxacillin-resistant *Staphylococcus aureus*. *Antimicrob Agents Chemother* 1994;38:1515–1518.
197. Nicolau DP, Marangos MN, Nightingale CH, et al. Influence of aspirin on development and treatment of experimental *Staphylococcus aureus* endocarditis. *Antimicrob Agents Chemother* 1995;39:1748–1751.
198. Nikaido H. Prevention of drug access to bacterial targets: role of permeability barriers and active efflux. *Science* 1994;264:382–388.
199. Nikaido H. Antibiotic resistance caused by gram-negative multidrug efflux pumps. *Clin Infect Dis* 1998;27[Suppl 1]: S32–41.
200. Normark BH, Normark S. Antibiotic tolerance in pneumococci. *Clin Microbiol Infect* 2002;8:613–622.
201. Nougayrede A, Berthaud N, Bouanchaud DH. Post-antibiotic effects of RP 59500 with *Staphylococcus aureus*. *J Antimicrob Chemother* 1992;30[Suppl A]:101–106.
202. Novak R, Charpentier E, Braun JS, et al. Signal transduction by a death signal peptide: uncovering the mechanism of bacterial killing by penicillin. *Mol Cell* 2000;5:49–57.
203. Oliva B, Gordon G, McNicholas P, et al. Evidence that tetracycline analogs whose primary target is not the bacterial ribosome cause lysis of *Escherichia coli*. *Antimicrob Agents Chemother* 1992;36:913–919.
204. Oppenheim JJ, Biragyn A, Kwak LW, et al. Roles of antimicrobial peptides such as defensins in innate and adaptive immunity. *Ann Rheum Dis* 2003;62[Suppl 2]:17–21.
205. Padan E, Schuldiner S. Intracellular pH regulation in bacterial cells. *Methods Enzymol* 1986;25:337–352.
206. Pag U, Sahl HG. Multiple activities in lantibiotics: models for the design of novel antibiotics? *Curr Pharm Des* 2002;8:815–833.
207. Patel U, Yan YP, Hobbs FW, et al. Oxazolidinones' mechanism of action: inhibition of the first peptide bond formation. *J Biol Chem* 2001;276:37199–37205.
208. Paulsen IT, Brown MH, Skurray RA. Proton-dependent multidrug efflux systems. *Microbiol Rev* 1996;60:575–608.
209. Pendland SL, Piscitelli SC, Schreckenberger PC, et al. In vitro activities of metronidazole and its hydroxy metabolite against *Bacteroides* spp. *Antimicrob Agents Chemother* 1994;38:2106–2110.
210. Penyige A, Matko J, Deak E, et al. Depolarization of the membrane potential by beta-lactams as a signal to induce autolysis. *Biochem Biophys Res Comm* 2001;290:1169–1175.
211. Peterson AA, Hancock REW, McGroaty EJ. Binding of polycationic antibiotics and polyamines to lipopolysaccharide of *Pseudomonas aeruginosa*. *J Bacteriol* 1985;164:1256–1261.
212. Piddock LJV, Walters RN. Bactericidal activities of five quinolones for *Escherichia coli* strains with mutations in genes encoding the SOS response or cell division. *Antimicrob Agents Chemother* 1992;36:819–825.
213. Pongs O, Bald R, Erdmann VA. Identification of chloramphenicol-binding protein in *Escherichia coli* ribosomes by affinity labeling. *Proc Natl Acad Sci USA* 1973;70:2229–2233.
214. Poole K. Overcoming antimicrobial resistance by targeting resistance mechanisms. *J Pharm Pharmacol* 2001;53:283–294.
215. Powell DA, Nahata MC. Chloramphenicol: new perspectives on an old drug. *Drug Intell Clin Pharm* 1982;16:295–300.

216. Prez-Giraldo C, Rodriguez-Benito A, Noran FJ, et al. In-vitro slime production of *Staphylococcus epidermidis* in the presence of subinhibitory concentrations of ciprofloxacin, ofloxacin, and sparfloxacin. *J Antimicrob Chemother* 1994;33:845–848.
217. Putman MY, van Veen HW, Konings WN. Molecular properties of bacterial multidrug transporters. *Microbiol Mol Biol Rev* 2000;64:672–693.
218. Rahal JJ, Simberkoff MS. Bactericidal and bacteristatic action of chloramphenicol against meningeal pathogens. *Antimicrob Agents Chemother* 1979;16:13–18.
219. Ramsey BW, Dorkin HL, Eisenberg JD, et al. Efficacy of aerosolized tobramycin in patients with cystic fibrosis. *N Engl J Med* 1993;328:1740–1746.
220. Rasmussen B, Noller HF, Doubresse G, et al. Molecular basis of tetracycline action: identification of analogs whose primary target is not the bacterial ribosome. *Antimicrob Agents Chemother* 1991;35:2306–2311.
221. Rawal BD. Bactricidal action of ascorbic acid on *Pseudomonas aeruginosa*: alteration of cell surface as a possible mechanism. *Chemotherapy* 1978;24:166–171.
222. Rawal BD, Charles BG. Inhibition of *Pseudomonas aeruginosa* by ascorbic acid-sulphamethoxazole-trimethoprim combination. *Southeast Asian J Trop Med Public Health* 1972;3:225–228.
223. Rawal BD, McKay G, Blackhall MI. Inhibition of *Pseudomonas aeruginosa* by ascorbic acid acting singly and in combination with antimicrobials: in-vitro and in-vivo studies. *Med J Aust* 1974;1:169–174.
224. Reusser F. Effect of lincomycin and clindamycin on peptide chain initiation. *Antimicrob Agents Chemother* 1975;7: 32–37.
225. Rice KC, Bayles KW. Death's toolbox: examining the molecular components of bacterial programmed cell death. *Mol Microbiol* 2003;50:729–738.
226. Robertson JA, Trulear MG, Characklis WG. Cellular reproduction and extracellular polymer formation by *Pseudomonas aeruginosa* in continuous culture. *Biotechnol Bioeng* 1984;26:1409–1417.
227. Rodriguez GG, Phipps D, Ishiguro K, et al. Use of a fluorescent redox probe for direct visualization of actively respiring bacteria. *Appl Environ Microbiol* 1992;58:1801–1808.
228. Rogers HJ, Perkins HR, Ward JB. *Microbial cell walls and membranes*. London: Chapman & Hall, 1980.
229. Rogers SW, Gilleland HE, Eagon RG. Characterization of a protein-lipopolysaccharide complex released from cell walls of *Pseudomonas aeruginosa* by ethylenediaminetetraacetic acid. *Can J Microbiol* 1964;15:743–748.
230. Rosenthal KS, Storm DR. Disruption of the *Escherichia coli* outer membrane permeability barrier by immobilized polymyxin B. *J Antibiot* (Tokyo) 1977;30:1087–1092.
231. Rosner JL. Nonheritable resistance to chloramphenicol and other antibiotics induced by salicylates and other chemotactic repellents in *Escherichia coli* K-12. *Proc Natl Acad Sci USA* 1985;82:8771–8774.
232. Roszak DB, Colwell RR. Survival strategies of bacteria in the natural environment. *Microb Rev* 1987;51:365–379.
233. Rubinstein G, Dunkin K, Howard AJ. The susceptibility of *Helicobacter pylori* to 12 antimicrobial agents, omeprazole and bismuth salts. *J Antimicrob Chemother* 1994;34:409–413.
234. Russell AD, Chopra I. *Understanding antimicrobial action and resistance*, 2nd ed. New York: Ellis Horwood, 1996.
235. Russell JB. Another explanation for the toxicity of fermentation acids at low pH: anion accumulation versus uncoupling. *J Appl Bacteriol* 1992;73:363–370.
236. Saiman L, Marshall BC, Mayer-Hamblett N, et al. Azithromycin in patients with cystic fibrosis chronically infected with *Pseudomonas aeruginosa*. *JAMA* 2003; 290:1749–1756.
237. Sawaki M, Mikami R, Mikasa K, et al. The long-term chemotherapy with erythromycin in chronic lower respiratory tract infections second report: including cases with *Pseudomonas* infections. *J Jpn Assoc Infect Dis* 1986;60:45–50.
238. Sawal T, Hirano S, Yamaguchi A. Repression of porin synthesis by salicylate in *Escherichia coli*, *Klebsiella pneumoniae* and *Serratia marcesans*. *FEMS Microbiol Lett* 1987;40:233–237.
239. Schearer BG, Legakis NJ. *Pseudomonas aeruginosa*: evidence for the involvement of lipopolysaccharide in determining outer membrane permeability to carbenicillin and gentamicin. *J Infect Dis* 1985;152:351–355.
240. Schindler PRG, Teuber M. Action of polymyxin B on bacterial membranes: morphological changes in the cytoplasm and in the outer membrane of *Salmonella typhimurium* and *Escherichia coli* B. *Antimicrob Agents Chemother* 1975;8:95–104.
241. Schmidt T, Froula J, Tauber MG. Clarithromycin lacks bactericidal activity in cerebrospinal fluid in experimental pneumococcal meningitis. *J Antimicrob Chemother* 1993;32:627–632.
242. Schnell N, Entian K-D, Schneider U, et al. Prepeptide sequence of epidermin, a ribosomally synthesized antibiotic with four sulphide-rings. *Nature* 1988;333:276–278.
243. Selan L, Berlutti F, Passariello C, et al. Proteolytic enzymes: a new treatment strategy for prosthetic infections? *Antimicrob Agents Chemother* 1993;37:2618–2621.
244. Sensi P. History of the development of rifampin. *Rev Infect Dis* 1983;5[Suppl]:S402–S406.
245. Shanson DC. Clinical relevance of resistance to fusidic acid. *J Antimicrob Chemother* 1990;25[Suppl B]:15–21.
246. Shaw KJ, Miller N, Liu X, et al. Comparison of the changes in global gene expression of *Escherichia coli* induced by four bactericidal agents. *J Mol Microbiol Biotechnol* 2003;5:105–122.
247. Shen LL, Mitscher LA, Sharma PN, et al. Mechanism of inhibition of DNA gyrase by quinolone antibacterials: a cooperative drug-DNA binding model. *Biochemistry* 1989;28:3886–3894.
248. Shockmann GD, Barrett JF. Structure, function, and assembly of cell walls of Gram-positive bacteria. *Ann Rev Microbiol* 1983;37:501–527.
249. Shockman GD, Daneo-Moore L, Higgins ML. Problems of cell wall and membrane growth, enlargement, and division. *Ann NY Acad Sci* 1974;235:161–197.
250. Shockman GD, Holtje J-V. Microbial peptidoglycan (murein) hydrolases. In: Ghuysen JM, Hakenbeck R, eds. *Bacterial cell wall*. Amsterdam: Elsevier, 1994;131–166.
251. Singh VK, Jayaswal RK, Wilkinson BJ. Cell wall–active antibiotic-induced proteins of *Staphylococcus aureus* identified using a proteomic approach. *FEMS Microbiol Lett* 2001;199:79–84.
252. Slee AM, Wuonola MA, McRipley RJ, et al. Oxazolidines, a new class of synthetic antibiotic agents: in vitro and in vivo activities of DuP 105 and DuP 721. *Antimicrob Agents Chemother* 1987;31:1791–1797.
253. Sterstrom T-A, Conway P, Kjelleberg S. Inhibition by antibiotics of the bacterial response to long-term starvation of *Salmonella typhimurium* and the colon microbiota of mice. *J Appl Bacteriol* 1989;67:53–59.

254. Stevens DL, Sizhuang Y, Bryant AE. Penicillin-binding protein expression at different growth stages determines penicillin efficacy in vitro and in vivo: an explanation for the inoculum effect. *J Infect Dis* 1993;167:1401–1405.
255. Stewart PS, Costerton JW. Antibiotic resistance of bacteria in biofilms. *Lancet* 2001;358:135–138.
256. Stewart PS. Biofilm accumulation model that predicts antibiotic resistance of *Pseudomonas aeruginosa* biofilms. *Antimicrob Agents Chemother* 1994;38:1052–1058.
257. Stewart PS, Karel SF, Robertson CR. Characterization of immobilized cell growth rates using autoradiography. *Biotechnol Bioeng* 1991;37:824–833.
258. Stow M, Starkey BJ, Hancock IC, et al. Inhibition by chloramphenicol of glucose transfer in teichoic acid biosynthesis. *Nature* 1971;229:56–57.
259. Stratton CW. Bactericidal testing. *Med Clin North Am* 1993;7:445–459.
260. Stratton CW. Dead bugs don't mutate: susceptibility issues in the emergence of bacterial resistance. *Emerging Infect Dis* 2003;9:10–16.
261. Stratton CW, Aldridge KE, Gelfand MS. In vitro killing of penicillin-susceptible, -intermediate, and -resistant strains of *Streptococcus pneumonia* by cefotaxime, ceftriaxone, and ceftizoxime: a comparison of bactericidal and inhibitory activity with CSF levels. *Diagn Microbiol Infect Dis* 1995;22:35–42.
262. Stratton CW, Liu C, Weeks LS. Bactericidal activity of daptomycin compared with methicillin, cefazolin, cefamandole, cefuroxime, ciprofloxacin, and vancomycin against staphylococci as determined by kill-kinetic studies. *Antimicrob Agents Chemother* 1987;31:1210–1215.
263. Sum PE, Lee VJ, Testa RT. Glycyclines. I. A new generation of potent antimicrobial agents through modification of 9-aminotetracyclines. *J Med Chem* 1994;37:184–188.
264. Sum PE, Sum FW, Projan SJ. Recent developments in tetracycline antibiotics. *Curr Pharm Des* 1998;4:119–132.
265. Sumita Y, Fukasawa M. Transient carbapenem resistance induced by salicylate in *Pseudomonas aeruginosa* associated with suppression of outer membrane protein D2 synthesis. *Antimicrob Agents Chemother* 1993;37:2743–2746.
266. Summanen F, Wexler HM, Lee K, et al. Morphological response of *Bilophia wadsworthia* to imipenem: correlation with properties of penicillin-binding proteins. *Antimicrob Agents Chemother* 1993;37:2638–2644.
267. Tally FP, DeBruin MF. Development of daptomycin for gram-positive infections. *J Antimicrob Chemother* 2000;46:523–526.
268. Tally FP, Ellestad GA, Testa RT. Glycylcyclines: a new generation of tetracyclines. *J Antimicrob Chemother* 1995;35:449–452.
269. Tamaoki J, Takeyama K, Tagaya E, et al. Effect of clarithromycin on sputum production and its rheological properties in chronic respiratory tract infections. *Antimicrob Agents Chemother* 1995;39:1688–1690.
270. Tenover FC. Development and spread of bacterial resistance to antimicrobial agents: an overview. *Clin Infect Dis* 2001;33[Suppl 3]:S108–S115.
271. Testa RT, Petersen PJ, Jacobus NV, et al. In vitro and in vivo antibacterial activities of the glycylcyclines, a new class of semisynthetic tetracyclines. *Antimicrob Agents Chemother* 1993;37:2270–2277.
272. Tetsuaki T, Svarachorn A, Soga H, et al. Lysis and aberrant morphology of *Bacillus subtilis* cells caused by surfactants and their relation to autolysin activity. *Antimicrob Agents Chemother* 1990;34:781–785.
273. Tipper DJ, Strominger JL. Mechanism of action of penicillins: a proposal based on their structural similarities to acyl-D-alanyl-D-alanine. *Proc Natl Acad Sci USA* 1965;54:1133–1141.
274. Tomasz A. The mechanism of the irreversible antimicrobial effects of penicillins: how the beta-lactam antibiotics kill and lyse bacteria. *Annu Rev Microbiol* 1979;33:113–137.
275. Tuomanen E. Phenotypic tolerance: the search for beta-lactam antibiotics that kill nongrowing bacteria. *Rev Infect Dis* 1986;8[Suppl 3]:S279–S291.
276. Tuomanen E. Antibiotics which kill non-growing bacteria. *Trends Pharmacol Sci* 1987;8:121–122.
277. Tuomanen E, Cozens R, Tosch W, et al. The rate of killing of *Escherichia coli* by beta-lactam antibiotics is strictly proportional to growth rate. *J Gen Microbiol* 1986;132:1297–1304.
278. Turakhia MH, Characklis WG. Activity of *Pseudomonas aeruginosa* in biofilms: effect of calcium. *Biotechnol Bioeng* 1989;33:406–414.
279. Twomey D, Ross RP, Ryan M, et al. Lantibiotics produced by lactic acid bacteria: structure, function and applications. *Antonie Van Leeuwenhoek* 2002;82:165–185.
280. Vaara M. Polycations sensitize enteric bacteria to antibiotics. *Antimicrob Agents Chemother* 1983;24:107–113.
281. Vaara M, Vaara T. Polycations as outer membrane-disorganizing agents. *Antimicrob Agents Chemother* 1983;24:114–122.
282. van Heijenoort J. Formation of the glycan chains in the synthesis of bacterial peptidoglycan. *Glycobiology* 2001;11:25–36.
283. Verbist L. The antimicrobial activity of fusidic acid. *J Antimicrob Chemother* 1990;25[Suppl B]:1–15.
284. Vester B, Douthwaite S. Macrolide resistance conferred by base substitutions in 23S rRNA. *Antimicrob Agents Chemother* 2001;45:1–12.
285. Vicens Q, Westhof E. RNA as a drug target: the case of aminoglycosides. *Chembiochem* 2003;4:1018–1023.
286. Vining LC, Stuttard C. Chloramphenicol. *Biotechnology* 1995;28:505–530.
287. Von Daehne W, Godtfredsen WO, Rasmussen RR. Structure-activity relationships on fusidic acid–type antibiotics. *Adv Appl Microbiol* 1979;25:95–146.
288. Wale LJ, Shelton AP, Greenwood D. Scanning electron microscopy of *Staphyococcus aureus* and *Enterococcus faecalis* exposed to daptomycin. *J Med Microbiol* 1989;30:45–49.
289. Walker GC. Understanding the complexity of an organism's responses to DNA damage. *Cold Springs Harb Symp Quant Biol* 2000;65:1–10.
290. Walsh C. *Antibiotics: actions, origins, resistance.* Washington, DC: ASM Press, 2003.
291. Walthers RN, Piddock LJV, Wise R. The effect of mutations in the SOS response on the kinetics of quinolone killing. *J Antimicrob Chemother* 1989;24:863–873.
292. Ward JB. Teichoic and teichuronic acids: biosynthesis, assembly, and location. *Microbiol Rev* 1981;45:211–243.
293. Watkins VS, Polk RE, Stotka JL. Drug interactions of macrolides: emphasis on dirithromycin. *Ann Pharmacother* 1997;31:349–356.
294. Wayne LG, Sramek HA. Metronidazole is bactericidal to dormant cells of *Mycobacterium tuberculosis. Antimicrob Agents Chemother* 1994;38:2054–2058.
295. Wehrli W. Rifampin: mechanisms of action and resistance. *Rev Infect Dis* 1983;5[Suppl 3]:S407–S411.
296. Weis SE, Slocum PC, Blais FX, et al. The effects of directly observed therapy of the rates of drug resistance and relapse in tuberculosis. *N Engl J Med* 1994;330:1247–1251.

297. Westrin BA, Axelsson A. Diffusion in gels containing immobilized cells: a critical review. *Biotechnol Bioeng* 1991;38:439–446.
298. Widmer AF, Gaechter A, Ochsner PE, et al. Antimicrobial treatment of orthopedic implant–related infections with rifampin combinations. *Clin Infect Dis* 1992;14:1251–1253.
299. Williams AH, Gruneberg RN. Teicoplanin. *J Antimicrob Chemother* 1984;22:397–401.
300. Wintermeyer SM, Abdel-Rahman SM, Nahata MC. Dirithromycin: a new macrolide. *Ann Pharmacother* 1996;30:1141–1149.
301. Woods DD. Relation of *p*-aminobenzoic acid to mechanism of action of sulphanilamide. *Br J Exp Pathol* 1940;21:74–90.
302. Wrangstadh M, Conway PL, Kjelleberg S. The role of an extracellular polysaccharide produced by the marine *Pseudomonas* sp. S9 in cellular detachment during starvation. *Can J Microbiol* 1989;35:309–312.
303. Wright AJ. The penicillins. *Mayo Clin Proc* 1999;74:290–307.
304. Yamazaki H, Tsjuji H. Anti-inflammatory activity of TSP, a protease produced by a strain of *Serratia*. *Folia Pharmacol Jpn* 1967;63:302–314.
305. Yasuda H, Ajiki Y, Koga T, et al. Interaction between biofilms formed by *Pseudomonas aeruginosa* and clarithromycin. *Antimicrob Agents Chemother* 1993;37:1749–1755.
306. Yeiser B, Pepper ED, Goodman MF, et al. SOS-induced DNA polymerases enhance long-term survival and evolutionary fitness. *Proc Natl Acad Sci USA* 2002;99:8737–8741.
307. Yoshida T, Hiramatsu K. Potent bactericidal activity of polymyxin B against methicillin-resistant *Staphylococcus aureus* (MRSA). *Microbiol Immunol* 1993;31:853–859.
308. Young M, Hancock REW. Fluoroquinolone supersusceptibility mediated by outer membrane protein OprH overexpression in *Pseudomonas aeruginosa*: evidence for involvement of a non-porin pathway. *Antimicrob Agents Chemother* 1992;36:2365–2369.
309. Yuk JH, Dignani MC, Harris RL, et al. Minocycline as an alternate antistaphylococcal agent. *Rev Infect Dis* 1991;13:1023–1024.
310. Zasloff M. Magainins, a class of antimicrobial peptides from *Xenopus* skin: isolation, characterization of two active forms and partial cDNA sequence of a precursor. *Proc Natl Acad Sci USA* 1987;84:5449–5453.
311. Zhanel GG, Walters M, Noreddin A, et al. The ketolides: a critical review. *Drugs* 2002;62:1771–1804.
312. Zuckerman JM, Kaye KM. The newer macrolides, azithromycin and clarithromycin. *Infect Dis Clin North Am* 1995;9:731–745.

CHAPTER 13

The Antivirogram and the Modes of Action of Antiviral Agents, HIV, Hepatitis, Influenza, and Cytomegalovirus

Pierre Dellamonica, Vincent Calvez, Anne-Geneviève Marcelin, Albert Tran, Pierre-Marie Roger, Marie-Christine Mazeron, Bruno Lina

Antiviral agents have been available for approximately the past 10 years. As was the case for antibiotics, the question of their evaluation in clinical practice has arisen; i.e., the correlation between their activity tested *in vitro* on cell cultures and that observed in human disease. While the initial approach for antibiotics was to identify a phenotype, antiviral evaluation was conducted using genotypic testing. This was made possible through sequencing techniques that were applied to portions of viral RNA and DNA related to the targets of available compounds. Phenotypic testing is a more complex, time-consuming, and costly procedure. The first clinical trial that demonstrated the practical utility of human immunodeficiency virus (HIV) genotype identification was conducted by our team (1). We showed that adapting the treatment strategy to the HIV genotype significantly improved results.

Currently, aside from spontaneous mutations, most of the available compounds are able to induce mutations, at least at their active site, resulting in a modified viral replication capacity. This varies according to the mutations, some of which may be beneficial in reducing viral replication (viral fitness). However, reciprocal interaction between mutations can only be measured by phenotypic testing. Resistance testing is currently used in clinical practice for HIV infection. These mutations in proviral DNA are being investigated. For the other viral infections presented in this chapter, i.e., hepatitis B (HBV) and C, cytomegalovirus (CMV) and influenza, sequencing procedures for clinical practice are still at the early stage, and are restricted to treatment failure, but rarely for treatment choice, for lack of a significant number of available compounds. However, their use for epidemiological purposes has been amply demonstrated. This has provided data on viral variability among different countries. These reflections will probably also be applied to the prions PrP. The prions (PrP) show remarkable resistance to treatment that is expected to inactivate nucleic acid (virus). Prions consist principally of an abnormal isoform of a host-encoded protein obtained by a posttranslational mechanism. Genotyping and sequencing will allow not only molecular diagnosis of prion disease, but also its subclassification according to specific mutations. Such techniques aimed at determining resistance will have to be further developed in the context of widening therapeutic options.

SUSCEPTIBILITY TESTING IN HUMAN IMMUNODEFICIENCY VIRUS

Considerable progress has been made in defining the indications for resistance testing and determining the cost-effectiveness of strategies that use testing in the management of HIV-infected individuals. Prospective, randomized trials have shown at least short-term virological benefits for resistance testing (1). Moreover, emerging data indicate that viral drug resistance is a problem whenever treatment is used, and it may be increasing in importance. It has also become clear that knowledge concerning patterns of resistance and cross-resistance is critical to the development of successful sequential antiretroviral regimens.

In developed countries, resistance testing has been adopted as the standard of care in case of failure to antiretroviral treatments of HIV infection (2,3). Drug-resistance testing became an essential tool to assist clinicians in the selection of potent antiretroviral drug regimens that will enhance the likelihood of favorable treatment responses. Two different approaches are used to assess HIV drug resistance: genotyping and phenotyping. Understanding the characteristics, performances, and the interpretation of these assays is needed to use them optimally (4–6). Genotypic assays detect mutations resulting in amino acid changes that have been shown to correlate with *in vitro* and/or *in vivo* resistance to a particular drug or class of drugs. Phenotypic assays provide quantitative measure of drug susceptibility by determining the concentration of drug required to inhibit virus replication in cell culture.

Antiretroviral resistance due to viral gene mutations accounts for a large portion of treatment failures. The emergence of these genetic changes in HIV type 1 (HIV-1) is fostered by ongoing viral replication in the presence of subinhibitory concentrations of antiretrovirals. Poor penetration of drugs into certain body compartments (sanctuary sites), inadequate adherence, and variable pharmacokinetic factors may contribute to subtherapeutic drug levels *in vivo*. This, in turn, may allow for selection of either preexisting (archived) or newly generated drug-resistant mutants. The critical problem in the clinical setting is that a mutant selected by a failing regimen may have some degree of cross-resistance to other drugs in the same class that have not yet been prescribed to that patient. The development of cross-resistance may lead to a reduced virological or immunological response to subsequent regimens. As scientists develop new agents active against resistant virus, clinical medicine is also implementing diagnostic strategies designed to detect antiretroviral resistance and individualize subsequent regimens.

Antiretroviral resistance develops when viral replication continues in the presence of the selective pressure of drug exposure. For some drugs, such as the nucleoside reverse-transcriptase inhibitor (NRTI) lamivudine and all available non-nucleoside reverse transcriptase inhibitors (NNRTIs), a single mutation induces high-grade resistance in a predictable manner. For others such as zidovudine, abacavir, tenofovir, and most of the protease inhibitors (PIs), high-grade resistance requires the serial accumulation of multiple mutations and is thus slower to emerge.

Nucleoside and Nucleotide Reverse-Transcriptase Inhibitors

Although most of the mutations associated with NRTI resistance are not at the active site of the enzyme, they do lead to conformational changes that affect the active site aspartate residues. Different mutations lead to two different mechanisms for resistance: decreased substrate binding and increased phosphorolysis (removal of the chain-terminating substrate that has already been incorporated into the growing proviral DNA chain). Both mechanisms lead to an overall net decrease in termination of the elongating chain of HIV DNA by the NRTI.

Nonnucleoside Reverse-Transcriptase Inhibitors

Two patterns of multi-NNRTI resistance have been described. One is the K103N reverse-transcriptase mutation. This single mutation confers resistance to all currently available NNRTIs, presumably by stabilizing the closed-pocket form of the enzyme, thus inhibiting the binding of the drug to its target. The fact that all available agents in this class bind to the same domain explains the broad pattern of cross-resistance and has prompted the development of new agents that interact with this domain more favorably. Indeed, another pattern of multi-NNRTI resistance is the accumulation of multiple mutations, including L100I, V106A, Y181C, G190S/A, and M230L. Rarely, Y188L causes multi-NNRTI resistance.

Enhanced susceptibility to NNRTIs (i.e., hypersusceptibility) has been described in association with multiple mutations confering broad cross-resistance to NRTIs and a lack of NNRTI resistance mutations. Longer duration of NRTI use, prior use of zidovudine, and abacavir or zidovudine resistance have all been associated with hypersusceptibility. This phenomenon appears to have biological significance, with its presence enhancing the response to efavirenz-based regimens. A significantly greater short-term reduction in plasma HIV-1 RNA level, showing hypersusceptibility to efavirenz, was noted in patients who received that drug for salvage therapy.

Protease Inhibitors

The sequential use of certain PIs may be possible in some situations because several drugs in this class have distinctive major resistance mutations. This is particularly true for nelfinavir and has been suggested for atazanavir. All other PIs retain activity *in vitro* and *in vivo* against D30N isolates selected by nelfinavir. Less commonly, nelfinavir failure is associated with L90M, which is more likely to add to cross-resistance to other PIs. The I50V amprenavir resistance mutation alters the hydrophobic interaction with the target and had been thought to alter the binding of other drugs in this class only minimally. Clinical evidence to support particular PI sequencing, except that for nelfinavir, is lacking.

The presence of two key mutations (e.g., D30N, G48V, I50V, V82A/F/T/S, I84V, and L90M) generally confers broad cross-resistance to most currently available PIs. One strategy to avoid the accumulation of multiple mutations is to use low-dose ritonavir to increase the circulating levels (or "boost") of other PIs (e.g., lopinavir, indinavir, amprenavir, and saquinavir), which may result in higher and more prolonged drug concentrations and greater suppression of viral variants that contain a limited number of mutations. Thus, resistance depends not only on intrinsic properties of the virus but also on the achievable plasma levels of the drug.

Entry Inhibitors

Entry of HIV-1 into target cells is a multistep process involving attachment (mediated by gp120 binding to CD4), chemokine co-receptor binding, and association of two trimeric helical coils (HR-1 and HR-2) located in the ectodomain of gp41 into a six-helix bundle that brings the virus and cell membranes into close approximation, allowing membrane fusion to occur. A number of drugs currently in development block HIV-1 infection by interfering with one of these steps. The recently approved fusion inhibitor enfuvirtide (known as T-20) blocks the association of HR-1 with HR-2 by binding to the trimeric HR-1 complex, thereby inhibiting fusion and blocking virus entry [56]. Mutations in HR-1 that reduce enfuvirtide susceptibility are selected by *in vitro* passage of HIV-1 in the presence of the drug and have been identified in isolates obtained from patients receiving enfuvirtide in clinical trials.

Identification of the presence of drug resistance by means of genotypic or phenotypic resistance assays can help a health-care provider select a combination of antiretrovirals that is likely to suppress HIV-1 replication (i.e., "active drugs" to which that patient's virus population is not cross-resistant). To maximize the therapeutic benefit and minimize toxicity, information collected from the viral genotype or phenotype must be used in conjunction with the patient's antiretroviral treatment history, response to past regimens, immunological status, pharmacological data, and the clinician's own knowledge of antiretroviral drugs. Knowing when and how to use resistance testing in a clinical practice will lead to better clinical management of HIV-1-infected patients.

METHODS

Resistance assays use different technologies that provide complementary information about antiretroviral resistance. The two different types of drug resistance tests available are assays for genotype and assays for phenotype. Genotype assays provide information about viral mutations that may result in changes in viral susceptibility to particular drugs or classes of drugs. Phenotype assays directly quantitate the level of susceptibility of a patient's virus sample to specific drugs *in vitro*. The values measured from the patient sample are compared with values measured from a standard wild-type reference strain. The degree of phenotypic resistance is the difference in susceptibility to a particular drug between the patient sample and the reference strain. In most cases, both genotype and phenotype testing methods require the use of polymerase chain reaction (PCR) technology to amplify the HIV-1 genes of interest (PR and RT) from patients' plasma samples. However, there are numerous differences between these two resistance testing methods.

Phenotypic Testing

Drug susceptibility assays report the concentration of drug required to inhibit 50% or 90% (IC_{50} and/or IC_{90} [inhibitory concentration 50% and/or 90%]) of the *in vitro* virus replication.

In the late 1980s, the first developed phenotypic assays were peripheral blood mononuclear cell (PBMC) assays that required isolation of the virus by cocultivating patient's PBMCs with mitogen-stimulated PBMCs obtained from HIV-seronegative donors, then titration of the virus stock. Subsequently, the inhibition of virus growth, in the presence of several concentrations of the drug, was evaluated by measurement of p24 Ag or RT (reverse transcriptase) activity in comparison with the replication in the absence of drug (7,8). These PBMC assay methods had several limitations as regards the difficulties in standardization, the interassay variability, and the high workload. Overall, the PBMC compartment does not represent the actively replicating virus population present in the plasma compartment.

The development of recombinant virus assay method (RVA), first described in 1994 (9), enabled the measurement of phenotypic resistance on a large scale. Since 1998, two companies have developed RVA assays: Antivirogram (Virco BVBA; Mechelen, Belgium) (Fig. 13.1) and PhenoSense (ViroLogic, Inc., San Francisco, CA) (Fig. 13.2) (10). Antivirogram was the first RVA adapted to commercial development. The overall approach of the three commercial phenotypic assays is similar, but each assay is performed using different protocols (extraction, amplification) and reagents (viral vectors, cell lines, titration of the virus) (Table 13.1). Assays use PCR to amplify the entire protease, much of RT and a part of the 3′ end of *gag* gene, including cleavage sites (p4/p2, p2/p7, p7/p1, p1/p6) from HIV-1 RNA extracted from patient plasma. Phenotypic PI resistance may be modulated by mutations at *gag-pol* cleavage sites, and four of the nine cleavage sites in the recombinant virus come from the patient virus and five from the laboratory virus construct. The amplified material is incorporated into vectors that derive from full-length molecular clones of HIV-1 but lack the protease and RT regions of the *pol* gene to create a recombinant HIV-1 isolate. After amplification two strategies have been used to insert patient PR and RT sequences into vectors: the Antivirogram test uses homologous recombination following co-transfection of cell lines while the PhenoSense assay uses site-specific endonuclease cleavage and direct ligation. Ligation products that are capable of propagating the vectors to high copy number are then

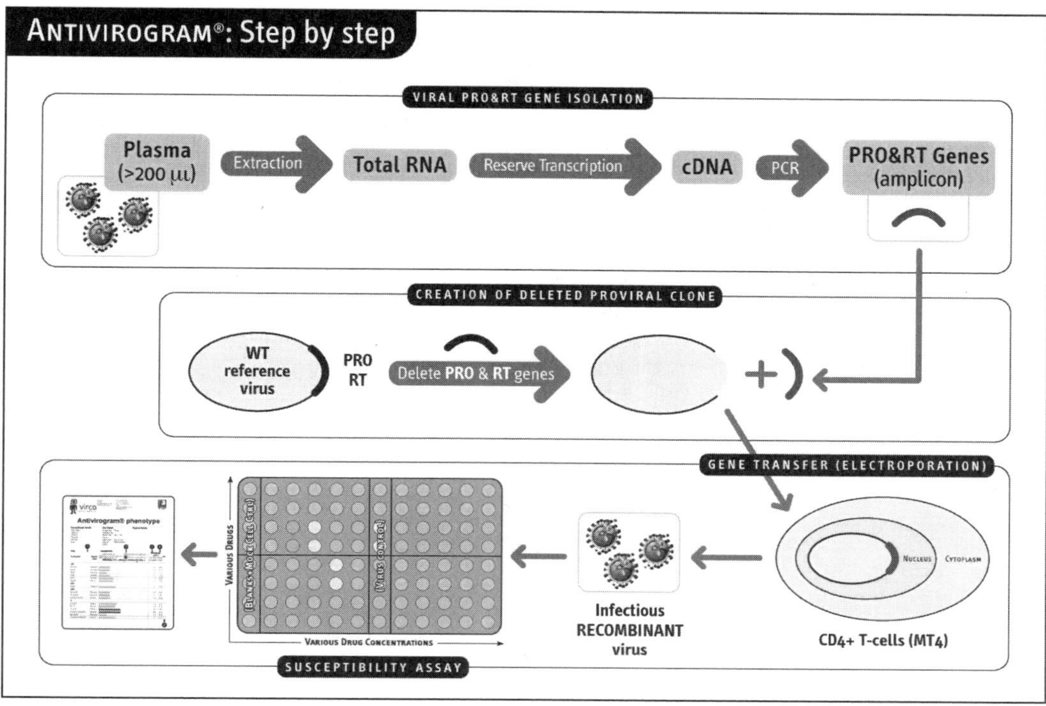

FIGURE 13.1 • Schematic representation of the Antivirogram from Virco, Mechelen, Belgium.

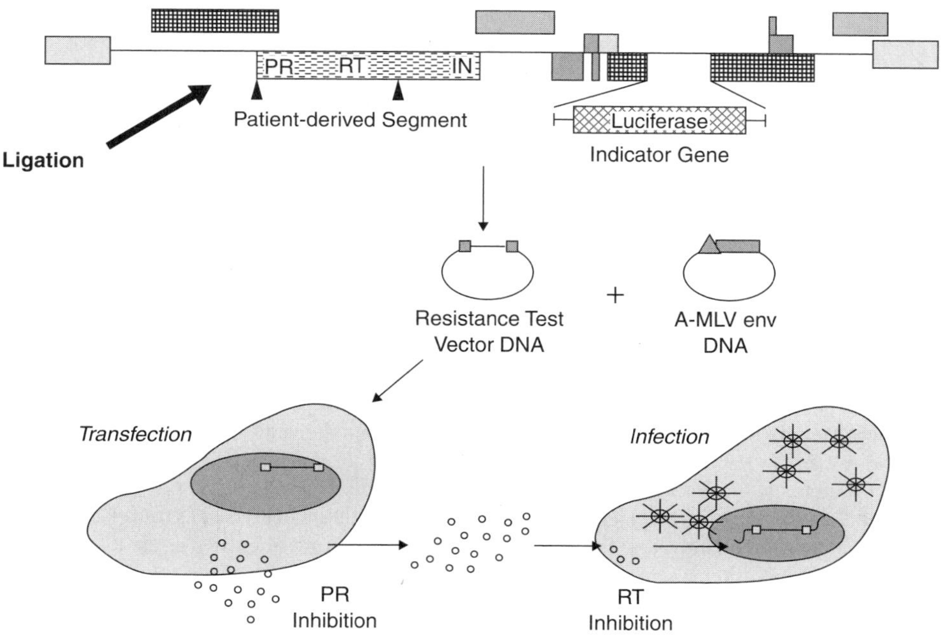

FIGURE 13.2 • Schematic representation of PhenoSense from ViroLogic, Inc., San Francisco. See text for details.

TABLE 13.1

Characteristics of Commercial Phenotypic Resistance Assays[a]

	Antivirogram (Virco)	PhenoSense (ViroLogic)
Requirements:		
Viral load	• 1000 copies/mL	• 500 copies/mL
Volume	• <500 μL (ideal, 3 mL)	• 1 ml
Amplification of PR and RT	• RT-PCR (two rounds, PCR) • PR/RT amplified together PR (10–99), RT (1–500)	• Purification of viral RNA • RT-PCR (one round, PCR) • PR/RT amplified together: 3'gag, PR (1–99), RT (1–305)
Assembly of recombinant virus	Transfected producer cells: MT4 and homologous recombination between: • PR/RT products (2.2kB) • infectious ΔPR/RT HIV vector	DNA ligation between: • PR/RT products (1.5 kB) • ΔPR/RT HIV vector with luciferase gene in envelope. Propagation of retroviral vector as bacterial plasmid
Preparation of virus stock	Multiple rounds of replication competent virus in MT4 after homologous recombination	Single burst of virus after transfection of HEK293 cells by: • recombinant vector • plasmid encoding the envelope of A-MLV
Drug susceptibility	• Titration of recombinant viruses using cells containing a fluorescent reporter gene	• PI added to transfected cells • RT added at the infection step (fresh HEK293)
Assay readout	Fluorescent readout of indicator cells	Luciferase indicator gene in virus vector; bioluminescence readout
Turnaround time	3–4 weeks	2 weeks

[a] PCR, polymerase chain reaction; HEK293, human embryonic kidney 293 cell line; A-MLV, amphotropic murine leukemia virus.

introduced into bacterial cells. High virus stocks are generated by transfecting the recombinant viral vector DNA.

PhenoSense assay is a single-cycle assay using recombinant viruses that are limited to a single round of viral replication by a specific deletion in the HIV *env* gene of the vector. In this assay, evaluation of reverse-transcriptase inhibitors (RTI) involve serial dilutions of drugs added to the target cell line at the time of virus inoculation to block RT activity at the cell entry. PIs are evaluated by adding serial dilutions of drug to the transfected cells producing the virus stocks. In the Antivirogram assay, generation of high virus stocks is obtained by cultivating the recombinant viruses for several replication cycles (1 to 2 weeks). Then the virus stock is titrated before testing for drug susceptibility. Either PIs or RTIs can be evaluated using the same format by adding serial dilutions of drug to the cultures at the time of virus inoculation.

Commercially available RVA systems exploit the use of sensitive reporter genes that have been engineered into the target cells or the retroviral vector. Transcription of the reporter gene is placed under the regulatory control of the HIV-1 promoter/enhancer within the Long Terminal Repeat (LTR). With infection with the recombinant virus, reporter gene expression is transactivated by the HIV-1 tat protein that is produced early in the HIV-1 replication cycle.

Drug susceptibility is assessed by comparing the IC_{50} of the patient virus to the IC_{50} of a drug susceptible reference strain derived from the NL4–3 or HXB2 strain. Assay data are analyzed by plotting the percent inhibition of virus replication versus the $\log_{10}$ drug concentration. The final results are expressed as fold change or resistance indices, which are calculated as the IC_{50} of the patient virus divided by the IC_{50} of the reference virus. The Antivirogram assay results report IC_{50} values with graphically and numerically fold change values.

These phenotypic methods have been adapted to measure drug susceptibility to the entry inhibitors (11). The first results showed a very large variability in the IC_{50} of isolates from drug-naïve patients. Such variability of up to three logs difference in IC_{50} is not yet explained.

Studies evaluating the comparative performances of the different phenotyping assays are limited. Excellent concordance was observed between the Antivirogram and PhenoSense assays (12) but the majority of the viruses tested were of the wild type.

TABLE 13.2

Commercial Phenotypic Assays: Biological or Clinical Cutoffs

Drug	Antivirogram (TVirco)	PhenoSense (ViroLogic)
Zidovudine	4.0	2.2
Lamivudine	4.5	2.5
Didanosine	3.5	1.7[a]
Zalcitabine	3.5	1.7
Stavudine	3.0	1.7[a]
Abacavir	3.0	4.5–6.5[a,b]
Tenofovir	4.0[a]	1.4–4[a,b]
Nevirapine	8.0	2.5
Delavirdine	10.0	2.5
Efavirenz	6.0	2.5
Indinavir	3.0	2.5
Ritonavir	3.5	2.5
Nelfinavir	4.0	2.5
Saquinavir	2.5	2.5
Amprenavir	2.5	2.5
Lopinavir	10.0[a]	10.0[a]

[a] Clinical cutoff.
[b] The lowest cutoff corresponds to a possible virological response and the highest to the absence of response.

Genotypic Testing

The presence of resistance mutations by genotypic assays is identified by DNA sequencing or point mutation assays such as hybridization assays. Most diagnostic laboratories developed their own assays, which are referred to as "home-brew" assays. All genotypic assays require extraction of the virus genome, usually from the plasma specimen, then retrotranscription of the viral RNA in cDNA. Subsequently, the DNA is amplified in a single or nested PCR. Dideoxynucleotide sequencing is the standard approach to HIV genotyping (13).

Mutations in the nucleic acid sequence cause amino acid substitutions when mRNA is translated into protein. Some mutations are "silent mutations"; that is, the nucleic acid changes do not alter the amino acid sequence. Mutations are designated in a shorthand format using single-letter abbreviations for the amino acids encoded by a particular triplet of nucleotides (a codon). The normal, or wild-type, amino acid present at a particular location in a protein is given, followed by the location (amino acid position, or codon number), followed by the new amino acid that has replaced the wild-type amino acid. The designation L90M, for example, indicates that the amino acid methionine (M) has been substituted for the wild-type amino acid leucine (L) at position 90, which is one of the codons in the region that codes for the protease enzyme, and is designated PR. The region that codes for the reverse-transcriptase enzyme is designated RT.

In 2001, a commercial HIV-1 RT and protease genotyping kit (TruGene; Visible Genetics, Inc., Toronto, Canada) was approved by the FDA (US Food and Drug Administration) and EMEA (European Medical Evaluation Agency) for use in clinical settings. A second kit (ViroSeq; Applied Biosystems, Foster City, CA) was FDA- and EMEA-approved in 2002 (Table 13.2). The advantages of using approved kits include standardization and consistency of results across laboratories, making them preferable to home-brew methods in local laboratories with low experience in molecular biology. However, the commercial kits are more expensive and may not provide the flexibility of home-brew methods.

Brief Description of a Home-Brew Sequencing Method: HIV-1 RNA Extraction, cDNA Synthesis, Amplification, and Sequencing

Plasma HIV-1 RNA extractions are performed using HIV Roche extraction kit (Roche Diagnostic Systems, Inc., Branchburg, NJ) on 200 μL following the kit manufacturer's recommendations. HIV-1 RNA is resuspended in 50 μL of distilled Rnase-free water. RT PCR is performed on 5 μL of the HIV-1 RNA solution using Titan One Tube RT-PCR System (Boehringer, Ingelheim, Germany). The primers used for the reactions are MJ3 (5′-AGTAGGACCTACACCTGTCAAC-3′) and MJ4 (5′-CTGTTAGTGCTTTGGTTCCTCT-3′). The cycling conditions on a thermocycler (model 9600; Perkin-Elmer, Paris) are 50°C for 30 minutes, one cycle; 94°C for 2 minutes; 55°C for 30 seconds; 68°C for 3 minutes, 40 cycles. Then 5 μL of the outer PCR product is used in a 50-μL nested PCR with primers A 35 (5′-TTG GTT GCA CTT TAA ATT TTC CCA TTA GTC CTA TT-3′) and NE1 35 (5′-CCT ACT AAC TTC TGT ATG TCA TTG ACA GTC CAG CT-3′). The cycling conditions on a thermocycler (model 9600; ABI, Foster City, CA) are 94°C for 1 minute, 55°C for 1 minute, 72°C for 1 minute, 40 cycles. The inner PCR products are analyzed by agarose electrophoresis with ethidium bromide staining to check for the presence of a sufficient quantity of DNA and the absence of non-specific bands. Then the PCR products are purified before sequencing, using Microcon (Millipore, Billerica, MA) following the kit manufacturer's recommendations, and directly sequenced, using ABI Prism BigDye Terminator Cycle Sequencing Ready Reaction Kit (ABI, Foster City, CA), on an automated DNA sequencer (ABI 3100, ABI, Foster City, CA). Sample files are aligned by use of autoassembler software "Sequence Navigator" (ABI, Foster City, CA) to generate a deduced nucleotide sequence, which is transtranslated to yield the amino acid sequence with respect to the sequence of the wild-type virus HXB2. All sequences are proofread manually.

Hybridization can be used to detect specific resistance mutations. Point mutation assays are more sensitive at detecting minor populations of resistant viruses, but have difficulties in managing the background sequence variability. The INNO-LIPA HIV-1 line probe assays (Innogenetics, Ghent, Belgium) have specific probes for some wild-type and mutant codons attached to a nitrocellulose strip. The hybridization of the labeled RT-PCR product from the patient sample to the strip is revealed using an enzymatic colorimetric system. This assay is limited because it only detects a subset of drug resistance mutations and has a 10% rate of uninterpretable results due to poor hybridization (14).

The gene chip was divided in several thousand segments, each containing millions of similar probes designed to interrogate every nucleotide position in a test DNA or RNA molecule. Prior knowledge of the sequence is required to design probes that can bind to nucleotides adjacent to the position being interrogated. DNA chips seem to be less capable of detecting insertions or deletions in viral sequences and of sequencing viral subtypes other than subtype B (15,16). DNA chips are not currently available for HIV drug resistance testing in clinical practice.

Quality control measures are needed to ensure the accuracy of testing. Sequence quality control should avoid PCR contamination and sample mix-ups to prevent sample contamination with DNA from other sources. The VGI system (Visible Genetics, Inc. Suwance, GA) employs a genetic fingerprinting function for the detection of potential contamination, sample mix-up, or misidentification prior to result reporting. The sequence analyzed is compared with other sequences generated by the laboratory. Controlling PCR contamination with the ABI system (ABI, Foster City, CA) is addressed through the use of uracil *N*-glycosilase (UNG), which destroys PCR products previously amplified by the system and that may contaminate the current specimen. This process controls for in-run PCR contaminants during the test as a result of laboratory error. However, cross-contamination from a source other than previous amplification reactions is not detectable. Laboratories should use standard physical precautions, run negative controls with each PCR step, and examine their final sequence results for the possibility of contamination with other samples sequenced at the same time. These analyses should compare each new sequence with other recently generated sequences to look for unexpectedly similar isolates. If a sequence is incompatible with the patient's treatment history, sequencing should be repeated on a new clinical sample.

Several studies evaluated the reproducibility of DNA sequence analysis using either cultural PBMC pellets or clinical plasma specimens (17,18). The participating laboratories used different methods. The overall rate of discrepant nucleotide assignments was low (0.1% to 0.29%) over several thousands of nucleotide positions analyzed. Discordances appear more related to variations in plasma sampling than to technical errors (17).

It is critical for laboratories performing genotypic sequencing to participate in repeated quality assurance programs. The first international approaches were based on the use of plasmid constructs containing different concentrations of mutant viruses (19,20). Only half of the laboratories were able to detect the mutations when present as 50% mixtures. These studies demonstrated that the presence of resistance mutations is frequently underestimated, while a pure wild-type genotype was correctly identified by the majority of the laboratories. Performances were related to the experience level of the laboratory and independent of the type of genotypic assay. The use of clinical plasma specimens in the quality control assessment enables monitoring of the quality of all the sequencing steps and is more close to real-life genotyping situations (21,22). The major difficulty is to define the reference amino acid sequence. The quality control assessment must include HIV-negative control, specimens with low viral load, specimens in duplicate, samples with a high number of mutations, and the most prevalent HIV-1 subtypes circulating in the country where the laboratories are located.

INTERPRETATION OF DRUG-RESISTANCE ASSAYS

Appropriate interpretation of the results of drug-resistance testing is a challenging problem for both phenotype and genotype assays (2). These interpretation tools show variability, which may modulate the choice of drugs to be used and therefore affect the therapeutic outcome. More attention is being focused on the importance of a standardized approach to interpret resistance results. Interpretation of resistance testing and choice of new therapy must be performed in light of all clinical information, including past therapies, previous viral load and immunological responses, adherence, tolerance, and toxicities. Previous resistance test results must be considered when available.

Phenotypic Assays

Phenotypic drug susceptibility assay results are interpreted by comparing the replication of patient-derived viruses to replication of well-characterized laboratory strains at equivalent drug concentrations. The phenotypic assay cutoffs (change in IC_{50}) defining whether the patient viral strain is susceptible or resistant are evolving. Former assays used "technical" cutoffs that refer to the interassay variability of the controls (one- to twofold for PhenoSense and two- to fourfold for Antivirogram). The "biological" cutoff was obtained by testing a large number of viruses from treatment-naïve individuals and defining the natural distribution of drug susceptibility in HIV-1 strains. The most relevant interpretation of phenotypic assay results is based on "clinical" cutoffs, which are distinct for each antiretroviral drug and different for each assay system. Clinically relevant cutoffs available for a limited number of drugs are based on analysis of the relationship between baseline phenotype and reduction in viral load (Table 13.3).

In the Antivirogram assay, biological cutoff values are the basis for reporting assay results for all drugs tested except tenofovir and lopinavir/ritonavir, which are based on clinical response data. In the PhenoSense assay results for lopinavir/ritonavir (23), abacavir (24), tenofovir (25), stavudine and didanosine (26,27) are reported using clinically derived cutoffs. The PhenoSense assay can also measure increased susceptibility, often referred to as hypersusceptibility. This phenomenon has been mainly described for Non Nucleoside Reverse Transcriptase Inhibitor NNRTI drugs and is associated with resistance to nucleoside analogs (28). In a retrospective analysis of virological outcome in patients who were NNRTInaïve and NRTIexperienced, increased susceptibility to efavirenz (as defined as less than 0.4-fold in susceptibility) was independently predictive of reduction in virological failure (29). Even partial activity may be clinically useful when treatment options are limited (23).

There are ongoing efforts to develop clinical cutoffs for all approved antiretroviral drugs, but some clinical cutoffs are difficult to establish as they are too close to the technical cutoff or the variability of the assay (30). When interpreting the results of phenotypic assay, the clinician should consider how each cutoff was derived (Table 13.2).

Genotypic Assays

The interactions between different mutations complicate the interpretation of genotypic assays. Mutations are designated by the wild-type amino acid present at a particular position of the RT or protease gene, followed by the amino acid position, then by the new amino acid that has replaced the wild-type amino acid. For example, M184V indicates that the methionine (M) wild-type amino acid at position 184 of the RT gene is replaced by the valine (V) amino acid. A large number of genotypic-resistance interpretation tools have been developed in recent years. These include mutation lists, rule-based algorithms, and interpretations based on databases correlating genotypes with corresponding phenotypic susceptibilities. The listing of mutations associated with resistance is available through the expert panel of International AIDS Society (IAS)-USA (http://www.iasusa.org) or Los Alamos National Laboratory (http://hiv-web.lanl.gov).

The interpretation of genotypic assays is based on interpretation systems called algorithms. They have the objective, in treated patients, to predict the response to each antiretroviral according to the combination of mutations present on the RT and protease genes. More than

TABLE 13.3

Characteristics of Commercial HIV-1 Genotypic Assays

	TRUGENE HIV-1 Genotyping Kit (Visible Genetics)	ViroSeq HIV-1 Genotyping System (Celera Diagnostics)
Requirements	1,000 copies/mL	1,000 copies/mL
Sequenced region	RT: codons 39–244 PR: codons 1–99	RT: codons 1–335 PR: codons 1–99
Contents of the kit	• RT-PCR • Clip sequencing • Electrophoresis • Software for interpretation	• RNA extraction • RT-PCR • Sequencing • Software for interpretation
Interpretation and reporting	• List of resistance mutations • Interpretation by rules-based algorithm available in the package	• List of resistance mutations • List of unknown mutations as compared with HXB2 • Interpretation by proprietary algorithm

20 algorithms are available from different sources. Some algorithms are public and available on web sites such as the algorithms from Stanford University (http//hivdb.Stanford.edu), the Rega Institute (http://www.kuleuven.ac.be), and the Agence nationale du Sida (http://www.hivfrenchresistance.org).

The early approach to interpreting genotypes was based on the *in vitro* correlation studies relating genotype with phenotype. However, recent data showed difficulty in determining reliable phenotypic cutoffs for some drugs such as stavudine, didanosine, and amprenavir (30,31). Correlation studies analyzing the virological response in treatment-experienced patients according to the genotypic profile at baseline should provide the most relevant information for establishing algorithms. Such algorithms are still limited and available for some antiretroviral drugs such as abacavir (32), stavudine (33,34), amprenavir (35), lopinavir (23,36,37) and tenofovir (25). The method issues for correlating baseline phenotype with virological response also apply to analyses of baseline genotype and response. To build up such algorithms a strict method is needed that is not standardized. Multivariate analyses must show the predictive value of the algorithm when there are confounding factors such as viral load at baseline, previous drug history, duration of past treatment, and new drugs in the regimen (38). Then the validation step must confirm that the algorithm is also predictive of the virological response in a different data set (33). These correlation studies are based on retrospective analyses of patients enrolled in therapeutic trials that are sometimes several years old. The accuracy of these algorithms depends on the prevalence of specific resistant mutations at baseline; some mutations, relevant to the resistance but underrepresented in the genotype profile will be ignored by the algorithm.

No single study can be expected to provide a full picture of the relationship between genotype and response. The genotypic profile of patients is changing as new drugs as new drugs become available that may select for previously unknown mutations. There is a need for wide-ranging databases containing appropriately quality controlled data from genotypic resistance assays, and international efforts to be developed to pool databases and to establish standardized analyses for constructing algorithms that need to be frequently refined.

Different reporting formats and interpretation systems are provided by the wide diversity of clinical virology laboratories providing HIV genotyping. Laboratories using home-brew assays have different approaches to reporting the results. Some laboratories provide only a list of mutations, and readability is poor. In addition to listing each resistance mutation detected in RT and PR genes, the interpretation must be provided with the precise indication of the algorithm used.

Reports of genotypic resistance usually score virus isolates as "resistant," "possible resistant," or "no evidence of resistance." Some algorithms classify patient isolates in four or five categories. Possible resistance corresponds to different situations according to the algorithm and the drugs: the detected mutations may have been associated with diminished virologic response in some but not all patients. This classification may also refer to a limited knowledge on resistance to this particular drug.

The use of expert advice in interpreting a genotype result has been shown to lead to a better choice in the alternative regimen compared with a regimen chosen in the absence of expert advice (39). Unfortunately, such expert advice is not always available. The role of the expert is to know the bases of the algorithm and to modulate the interpretation according to the clinical and immunological parameters of the patient.

The discordances in interpretations seem to be drug-related, low for NNRTI, and more important for some antiretrovirals such as stavudine, didanosine, abacavir, and amprenavir (40,41). Several studies retrospectively analyzed the relationship between the different interpretations of resistance genotypes by several algorithms and the outcome of salvage treatment in cohorts of drug-experienced patients (41,42). These studies show generally significant discordances between available algorithms that are associated with different predictions of subsequent virological outcomes.

Virtual Phenotype

Another approach to interpreting genotype is employed by Virco (43). This company maintains a large proprietary database of specimens for which both genotype and phenotype are known for each drug. From this database, viruses with the same genotype as that of the patient's virus are identified and the average IC_{50} of these matching viruses is calculated, estimating the likely phenotype of the patient's virus. Several reports support the validity of the virtual phenotype for interpreting genotypes (44). However, the accuracy of the predicted phenotype depends on the number of database matches with the patient's isolate. For the new or investigational agents the system is delayed by the need to accumulate genotype-phenotype data; with the availability of new drugs and the selection of new mutations, the number of matches may decrease.

Discordances between Genotype and Phenotype Results

Several studies comparing phenotype and genotype results on a large number of clinical samples showed that discordances between results are not uncommon (45,46). The clinical usefulness of genotypic testing has been demonstrated in most prospective, randomized studies; in contrast, phenotypic testing has been shown to be clinically useful in a few prospective studies. Genotypic testing is also used more commonly than phenotypic testing because of its lower cost, wider availability, and shorter turnaround time. Unlike genotyping assays, phenotyping assays involving sophisticated laboratory procedures are not available as test-kits for widespread distribution.

Genotypic testing may detect a single drug-resistance mutation within a virus population that will affect the virological response but will not reduce phenotypic drug susceptibility. For example, the Y181C mutation confers *in vitro* susceptibility to efavirenz (47) but is associated with absence of clinical response to this drug (48). Genotypic assays detect mutations present as mixtures even if the mutation is present at a level that is too low to affect drug susceptibility in a phenotypic assay, and identify reversal mutations that do not cause phenotypic drug resistance but indicate the presence of previous drug pressure. Decreased phenotypic susceptibility to some drugs may be suppressed (resensitization) by other mutations in the sequence. In the presence of thymidine mutations that decrease susceptibility to zidovudine, the presence of M184V or L74V or K65R may restore the *in vitro* susceptibility to this drug. Such *in vitro*-increased susceptibility has not been proved to be clinically relevant.

Phenotypic testing in research settings is essential for establishing genotype-phenotype correlations, which provide the first bases for interpreting genotype tests and for designing new antiviral drugs that are effective against existing drug-resistance strains.

Relating Genotype and Phenotype Results to Drug Levels

Virus drug susceptibility is likely to be a continuous phenomenon because of partial remaining activity of the drugs against mutant viruses and variability of drug exposure.

Data correlating drug concentrations with virological response have been generated for most protease inhibitors and NNRTIs. The concept of inhibitory quotients (IQs) characterizes the relationship between drug exposure and drug susceptibility of the virus and is defined as the C_{min} of drug divided by measure of resistance either by phenotype (IQ: C_{min}/IC_{50}), "virtual" phenotype (vIQ:C_{min}/value of IC_{50} according to the virtual phenotype), or genotype (GIQ: C_{min}/number of mutations). This concept has begun to be applied to prediction of response to protease inhibitor (49). The concept is particularly suitable for PIs that exhibit very large interindividual drug-concentration variability. Although IQs have yet to be prospectively evaluated as a tool for managing HIV infection, they have been shown to be better predictors of virological response, in treatment-experienced patients receiving lopinavir boosted by ritonavir, than plasma drug concentrations and/or resistance testing alone (49). The virtual IQ was the best predictor of viral load reduction in response to ritonavir boosting indinavir-based therapy in patients with ongoing viremia (50). The accurate adjustment of the *in vitro*-calculated IC_{50} to the *in vivo* protein binding remains to be determined. In PI-experienced patients receiving boosted amprenavir, the genotype IQ, using the C_{min} measured at week 8 and the number of PI resistance mutations evaluated at baseline, was the best predictor of the virological response at week 12 (51). These approaches need to be validated in prospective clinical trials.

PRACTICAL CONSIDERATIONS

All genotypic and recombinant phenotypic assays use initial amplification through RT-PCR as the first step in the process. Because these assays require amplification of a larger segment of the HIV-1 genome than assays designed only to detect the presence of HIV-1 RNA, they are generally less sensitive than viral load assays and require samples with at least 1,000 copies per milliliter of HIV-1 RNA to obtain amplification from plasma, although amplification is possible in some samples at lower viral load.

Plasma is the main source of virus used for testing HIV-1 drug resistance in the clinical setting. Because the half-life of HIV-1 in plasma is approximately 6 hours, only actively replicating virus can be isolated from this source; thus, the sequence of plasma virus represents the quasispecies most recently selected by antiretroviral drugs (52). Specialized testing for research purposes can use a variety of other tissue compartments such as cerebrospinal fluid, genital secretions, PBMCs, or lymph nodes.

Blood samples may be drawn in either EDTA or acid citrate dextrose vacutainers. Heparin must be avoided as it inhibits PCR reactions. Plasma separation should be performed within a maximum of 6 hours after blood collection. Sample volume consists of 1 to 3 mL of plasma that can be stored at –80°C. Samples taken for viral load should be stored frozen within the laboratory in order that retrospective resistance testing can be undertaken.

These tests are technically demanding, and external quality control is essential. This is addressed by national and international pathology laboratory accreditation programs. Laboratories undertaking resistance testing should provide clinical support to HIV clinics and demonstrate participation in external quality control programs and accreditation by national and international agencies. In addition to quality assurance of the assay, quality assurance of the laboratory performing the assay is also required. Currently, all the laboratories in the United States that perform genotyping or phenotyping assays must have certification according to the Clinical Laboratory Improvement Act (CLIA) 1988 indicating some level of review of the laboratory's performance standard (CLIA Related Federal Register, FDA, 1995. Available at: http//www.fda.gov/cdrh/clia/fr/hsq230n.html). In Europe, some hospital laboratories participate in proficiency testing programs for genotyping.

Drug costs are driving the overall total cost of HIV-1 care in developed countries. A National Institutes of Allergy and Infectious Diseases and Centers for Disease Control and Prevention-funded study analyzed cost-effectiveness in genotypic resistance testing using an HIV-1 stimulation model of one million patients (53). The authors reported that the cost-effectiveness of genotypic resistance is similar or better than that of recommended interventions for HIV-1-infected patients, such as *Mycobacterium avium* complex prophylaxis.

There is large geographical variability in reimbursement of HIV drug resistance assays. Lack of or low levels of reimbursement may still limit access in some areas or countries. However, proper implementation of resistance assays may reduce the overall cost of patient management by prompting more appropriate choices in therapy and avoiding drugs that are likely to induce toxicities.

LIMITATIONS OF RESISTANCE TESTING

Quasispecies

Resistance testing has technical limitations. Both genotypic and phenotypic testing depend on PCR amplification of virus from plasma, and therefore do not address the properties of different virus components (i.e., whole virus vs. viral genome alone). The likelihood of generating sufficient genome product to undertake further analysis depends on the starting concentration of virus. The nature of direct PCR sequencing techniques limits the detection of minority strains of virus within the plasma virus population to 20% (19,54–57). Smaller proportions of mutant virus may contribute to subsequent therapy failure and will not be detected. This limitation is particularly troublesome in patients with complicated treatment histories or in those who have discontinued one or more antiretroviral drugs. To maximize the likelihood of identifying drug-resistance mutations present within the virus population of a patient, it is important to analyze plasma samples for resistance testing before changing or stopping antiretroviral therapy and to consider the patient's treatment history when interpreting the results of resistance testing.

Direct PCR is done in clinical settings because it is quicker and more affordable than testing multiple clones individually. Clonal sequencing of individual strains is performed in research settings to answer questions about the pathways and evolution of HIV-1 drug resistance. Multiple quasispecies with distinct resistance genotypes coexist at any given time and some initially minority populations, with or without additional changes, can subsequently emerge as majority populations (58).

Technologies that reliably detect small genetic changes in a large sea of closely related viral quasispecies need to be available. GENE-CODE technology is a novel, closed-tube, single-vessel RT-PCR method made possible through the use of an expanded genetic alphabet. This technology is capable of detecting one copy of mutant 184V per 10,000 wild-type M184 RNA copies in a reaction containing 1.5×10^7 total target molecules (59). However, detecting minority mutant species has not yet been proved to be clinically relevant.

Cellular Reservoirs

The evolution of HIV-1 drug resistance mutations in proviral DNA in PMBCs lags behind that in plasma HIV-1 RNA. In patients with multiple virological failures, proviral DNA may contain multiple archived mutations that are not present in plasma (60–63). Discrepancies in protease and RT resistance profiles have been described between plasma and other compartments such as cerebrospinal fluid or semen. The variable penetration of antiretroviral drugs into sanctuary sites may contribute to the differential evolution of HIV and the emergence of drug resistance (64–66). However, the utility of sequencing virus from PBMC or from other sanctuary sites has not been evaluated in either prospective or retrospective clinical trials.

Non-B Subtypes

HIV-1 group M has evolved into multiple subtypes that differ from one another by 10% to 30% along their genomes. In North America and Europe, most HIV-1 isolates belong to subtype B. However, subtype B accounts for only a small proportion of HIV-1 isolates worldwide, and non-B isolates are being identified with increasing frequency in Europe. Technically, primers used for RT, PCR, and sequencing may have a lower rate of annealing for non-B compared with subtype B templates. The performances of the different phenotypic and genotypic assays are currently being investigated. The ViroSeq HIV-1 genotyping system was used to determine protease and RT sequences from a panel of 126 non-B subtypes isolates. Four specimens that could not be amplified included three subtype D isolates and one CRF02-AG isolate (67). The TruGene assay using prototype 1.5 RT-PCR primers and the ViroSeq assay were both successful for sequencing 34 non-B isolates, although five isolates (two belonging to subtype C, one to subtype B, one to subtype E, and one to subtype H) lacked double-strand sequence coverage in the ViroSeq assay (68).

Another comparison of the performance of two sequence-based, commercially available kits was assessed against a panel of 35 virus isolates from HIV-1 group M. Full-length consensus sequences were generated for 26 of 31 (84%) and 16 of 30 (53%) by the ViroSeq and the TruGene assays, respectively (69).

While the availability of these genotyping systems should facilitate studies of HIV-1 drug resistance in countries in which these subtypes are prevalent, the performance against non-B subtypes needs to be evaluated on larger studies.

HEPATITIS B: STRUCTURE OF THE VIRUS AND DISCUSSION OF ANTIVIRAL AGENTS

Hepatitis B virus was the first of the hepatitis viruses to be discovered. Whereas infection during adulthood is frequently cleared, vertical transmission from mother to child leads to persistent infection. More than *350* million people worldwide are currently persistently infected with HBV and are at risk of developing liver cirrhosis and hepatocellular carcinoma (70).

The asymmetric replication of the HBV genome, via RT of an RNA intermediate, makes it prone to mutations. Although mutations can occur randomly along the HBV genome, the overlapping open reading frames (ORFs) limit the number and location of viable mutations. Viable variants are selected on the basis of replication competence of the virus, selection pressure from the host's immune system, and in some instances exogenous factors such as antiviral therapy. The divergence of HBV sequences results in HBV quasispecies, variants, and genotypes with epidemiological and clinical significance.

The HBV is a noncytopathic, parenteral DNA virus. The outcome of HBV infection depends on the kinetics of the virus-host interaction and particularly on the strength of the innate and adaptive, humoral and cellular immune response. Whereas patients with acute hepatitis B have a vigorous and polyclonal immune response to HBV antigens, individuals with chronic hepatitis B have a weak and restricted immune response to HBV (71). Studies demonstrated that the latent, immune-mediated clearance mechanisms become activated spontaneously in chronically infected individuals undergoing HBeAg clearance (72). In addition, it has been shown that immune clearance of HBV can occur via cytolytic as well as noncytolytic mechanisms (73).

Success in HIV drug development in the 1990s revolutionized treatment of hepatitis B. Several antiviral agents that were developed for the treatment of HIV infection proved to be effective in inhibiting HBV replication. Three medications are now available (interferon-alpha, lamivudine, and adefovir). All three treatments have limited long-term efficacy. Although there have been few direct comparison trials, the short-term efficacy for both HBeAg-positive and HBeAg-negative hepatitis B appears to be comparable with all three medications. Also, factors predictive of response are similar. Thus, the advantages and disadvantages of each treatment, the durability of response, and the patient's preference must be carefully weighed before a decision is made (74).

Structure of Hepatitis B

Virions

The HBV is an enveloped, double-stranded DNA virus that is the prototype member of the family *Hepadnaviridae* (75), which includes genetically similar viruses that infect primates and monkeys, woodchucks and ground squirrels, and herons and ducks. Electron microscopic examination of the serum of a highly viremic carrier reveals three types of virus-associated particles. The HBV virion, which is 42 nm in diameter, comprises an outer envelope formed by the hepatitis B surface antigen (HBsAg). This envelope surrounds an inner nucleocapsid made up of the hepatitis B core antigen (HBcAg) that packages the viral genome and associated polymerase. Abundant spherical particles 17 to 25 nm in diameter in numbers up to 10^{13} per milliliter and less numerous tubular structures or filaments approximately 20 to 22 nm in diameter and of variable length in numbers up to 10^{11} per milliliter do not contain HBV DNA and thus are not infectious.

Viral Genotypes

There are currently seven recognized genotypes of HBV, designated A to G, that vary by 8% at the nucleotide level over the entire genome (76). The HBV genotype designation is based on the entire genomic sequence and thus is more reliable than the serological subtype nomenclature that was used previously, which was based on the immunoreactivity of particular antibodies to a limited number of amino acids in the envelope protein. The relationship between the four major subtypes (*adw, adr, ayw,* and *ayr*) and genotypes has been determined (Table 13.4) (77).

Important pathogenic and therapeutic differences do exist among HBV genotypes (78). For example, genotype C is associated with more severe disease than genotype B, and genotype D is associated with more severe disease than genotype A (79). Genotypes C and D are associated with a lower response rate to interferon therapy than genotypes B and A (77,79). Recombination betweeen two HBV genotypes has been reported for genotypes B and C (80) and genotypes A and D (81), generating more diversity.

Genome and Common Mutants of Hepatitis B Virus

The genome of HBV is a partially double-stranded, relaxed, circular DNA molecule about 3,200 nt (nucleotides) in length (Fig. 13.3) (75). The two linear DNA strands are held in a circular configuration by a 226-base pair (bp) cohesive overlap between the 5′ ends of the two DNA strands that contain 12-nt direct repeats called DR1 and DR2 (75). All known complete HBV genomes are gapped and circular, comprising between 3,181 and 3,221 bases, depending on the genotype (Table 13.4). Within the virion, the minus strand has a

TABLE 13.4

Major Hepatitis B Virus Genotypes

Genotype	Subtype	Genome Length (nt)	Global Distribution
A	*adw2, ayw1*	3,221	USA, Western Europe, Central Africa, India
B	*adw2, ayw1*	3,215	Asia
C	*adw2, adr, ayr*	3,215	East Asia, Polynesia
D	*ayw*	3,182	Mediterranean area, India
E	*ayw*	3,212	West Africa
F	*adw, ayw*	3,215	Central and South America, Polynesia
G	*adw*	3,248	USA, Europe

fixed length with defined 5′ and 3′ ends and a terminal redundancy of 8 to 9 nt (82). The minus strand is not a closed circle and has a nick near the 5′ end of the plus-strand. The viral polymerase is covalently bound to the 5′ end of the minus strand. The 5′ end of the plus strand contains an 18-base-long oligoribonucleotide, which is capped in the same manner as messenger RNA (mRNA) (82). The 3′ end of the plus strand is not at a fixed position, so most viral genomes contain a single-stranded gap region of variable length ranging from 20% to 80% of genomic length that can be filled in by the endogenous viral DNA polymerase.

The minus strand contains four ORFs and carries all the protein-coding capacity of the virus (75). Importantly, these overlap in a frame-shifted manner with one another so that the minus strand is read one and a half times (75). The longest ORF encodes the viral polymerase (POL). The ORF for the envelope (PreS/S) genes is completely located within the POL ORF, and the ORF for the core (PreC/C) and X genes partially overlap with POL ORF. Thus, the HBV encodes more than one protein from one ORF by using multiple internal AUG codons within an ORF, creating additional start sites for protein biosynthesis. Nested sets of proteins with different N-termini are thus synthesized (76).

The HBV mutation frequency has been estimated to be approximately 1.4 to 3.2 × 10^{-5} nucleotide substitution per site per year, approximately tenfold higher than for other DNA viruses (83). The HBV POL is a reverse transcriptase and lacks proofreading function. The mutation rate of HBV is also influenced by the clinical phase of the patients, such as immune-tolerance versus immune elimination, and clinical settings such as immunosuppression and transplantation (84). The predominant HBV exists in an infected individual as the major population of the HBV quasispecies pool. The stability of the predominant HBV within this pool is maintained by particular selection pressures from the host's immune system and the contraints imposed by the overlap in reading frames, viability, and replication competence of the virus. Furthermore, the magnitude and rate of virus replication are important, with the total viral load in serum frequently approaching 10^{11} virions per milliliter. Most estimates place the mean half-life of the serum HBV pool at about 1 to 2 days, so that the daily rate of the de novo HBV production may be as great as 10^{11} virions.

The high viral loads and turnover rates, coupled with poor replication fidelity, all influence mutation generation and the extent of the HBV quasispecies pool. Furthermore, the availability of "replication space" requires that the eventual takeover by a mutant virus depends on the loss of the original wild-type virus, which is itself governed by factors such as replication fitness and the turnover and proliferation of hepatocytes (85,86). Replication space can be understood in terms of the potential of the liver to accommodate new HBV covalently closed circular DNA molecules (cccDNA; see 'Viral Life Cycle'). Synthesis of new cccDNA molecules can occur only if uninfected cells are generated by growth within the liver, hepatocyte turnover, or loss of cccDNA from existing infected hepatocytes (87,88). Thus, the expansion of a (drug-) resistant mutant in the infected liver can be possible only with the creation of new replication space.

Mutations in the Precore/Core Promoter, Precore, and Core Genes

Two major groups of mutations have been identified that result in reduced or blocked HBeAg expression. The first group includes a translational stop codon mutation at nt 1896 of the precore gene (89). The second group of mutations affect the Precore/core (Pre-C/C) promoter, also called basic core promoter, at nt 1762 and nt 1764, resulting in a transcriptional reduction of the Pre-C/C mRNA (Table 13.5).

The single-base substitution (G-to-A) at nt 1896 gives rise to a translational stop codon (TGG to TAG) in the second last codon (codon 28) of the precore gene

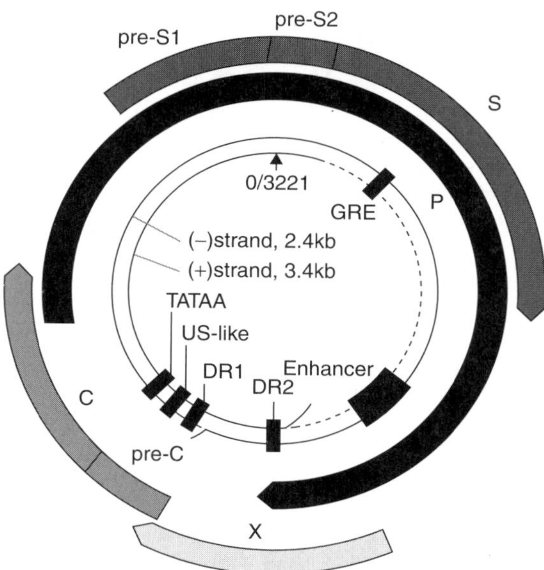

FIGURE 13.3 • The genome of hepatitis B virus (HBV), within virus particles or spherical virion, is composed of relaxed-circular, partially double-stranded DNA. The long, full-length minus-strand is approximately 3,200 nt in length and has a protein (the viral polymerase) covalently bound to its 5′ terminus. The plus-strand, which varies in length depending on species and subtype, has a capped oligoribonucleotide at its 5′ end. The plus-strand maintains genome circularity by a cohesive overlap across the 5′ and 3′ termini of the minus-strand. The HBV genome includes four open reading frames that encode at least seven translation products through the use of varying in-frame initiation codons. These translation products include three surface antigens (HBsAg): the envelope glycoproteins preS1, preS2, and S; core (C) and e antigens (HBcAg and HBeAg); viral polymerase (P); and the X protein (HBx). The genome is also replete with important *cis*-elements required for the regulation of HBV gene expression and replication. These include viral promoters, enhancers, and signal regions. The 5′ terminus of both strands contain regions of short (11-nucleotide) repeats, DR1 and DR2, which are essential for priming the synthesis of their respective DNA strands during replication.

located in the ϵ structure. The ϵ structure is a highly conserved stem loop structure, with the nt G1896 forming a base pair with nt 1858 at the base of the stem loop. In HBV genotypes B, D, E, G, and some strains of genotype C, the nt 1858 is a thymidine (T). Thus, the stop codon mutation created by G1896A (T-A) stabilizes the ϵ structure. In contrast, the precore stop codon mutation is rarely detected in HBV genotype A, F, and some strains of HBV genotype C, as the nt at position 1858 is a cytidine (C), maintaining the preferred Watson-Crick (G-C) base pairing.

Three other mutations (at nt positions 1817, 1874, 1897) that cause truncations in HBeAg have been reported

TABLE 13.5

Main Forms of Hepatitis B Virus Variants/Mutants

Precore gene
G-A at nt 1896, tryptophan-stop at codon 28 (G1896A)
G-A at nt 1899, glycine-aspartate at codon 29 (G1889A)
Precore/Core promoter gene
A-T at nt 1762 and G-A at nt 1764 (A1762T, G1764A)
Envelope gene
Glycine-arginine at codon 145 (sG145R)
Aspartate-alanine at codon 144 (sD144A)
Polymerase gene
Lamivudine-resistant mutants
Methionine-valine or isoleucine at codon 204 (rtM204V/I)
Leucine-methionine at codon 180 (rtL180M)
Adefovir dipivoxil-resistant mutants
Asparagine-threonine at codon 236 (rtN236T)

(84). In addition, changes that affect the initiation codon at nt 1814, 1815, and 1816 have been described. The mutation at G1899A is frequently detected in association with the precore stop mutation of G1896A. Early studies implicated the HBV precore stop codon mutant, leading to HBeAg negativity, as a possible virulence factor for severe liver disease and fulminant hepatitis B (90,91). However, this strain has also been found in asymptomatic carriers (92).

The Pre-C/C promoter mutations, such as A1762T plus G1764A, may be found in isolation or conjunction with precore mutations, depending on the genotype (Table 13.5). The double mutation of A1762T plus G1764A results in a decrease in HBeAg production of up to 70% (93). This mutant strain display reduced binding of liver-specific transcription factors, resulting in less Pre-C/C mRNA transcripts and thus less precore protein. However, this mutation does not affect the transcription of pregenomic RNA or the translation of the core or polymerase protein. Thus, by removing the inhibitory effect of the precore protein on HBV replication, the Pre-C/C promoter mutations appear to enhance viral replication by suppressing Pre-C/C mRNA relative to pregenomic RNA (93). As with the precore mutations, the Pre-C/C promoter mutations have not been conclusively identified as a potential virulence marker.

The core gene possesses both B cell and cytotoxic T lymphocyte epitopes, and for the virus to persist in the infected host, during the elimination phase of hepatitis B, escape mutations within those epitopes are readily selected (84,93). Akarca et al. (94) have demonstrated that the frequency of core gene mutations is associated with the presence of precore stop codon mutations, HBeAg negativity, and active liver disease.

Mutations in the X Gene

Mutations in the X region can involve the regulatory elements that control replication such as the Pre-C/C promoter and the enhancer 1. Because the Pre-C/C promoter encompasses nt 1742 to 1802 and overlaps with the X gene in the concomitant reading frame, the A1762T plus G1764A Pre-C/C promoter mutations also change in the X gene at xK130M and xV131I. A novel class of HBx mutants has been found in patients with hepatocarcinoma exhibiting increased clonal outgrowth and decreased apoptosis, implying a possible role in hepatocarcinogenesis (95).

Mutations in the Envelope Gene

Most hepatitis B vaccines contain the major HBsAg, and an immune response to the major hydrophilic region induces protective immunity. Mutations in this epitope have appeared under pressure generated by vaccine-induced antibodies (96). In addition, mutations have been detected after treatment of liver-transplant patients with hepatitis B immunoglobulin (97). Most isolates have a mutation from glycine to arginine at residue 145 of HBsAg (sG145R) or aspartate to alanine at residue 144 (sD144A) (Table 13.5). The former mutation has been shown to evade the known protective anti-HBs response.

Viral Life Cycle

An understanding of the HBV life cycle is crucial for the identification of potential antiviral targets (98,99). HBV replication begins when the virion attaches to an as yet unidentified receptor on the hepatocyte surface (Fig. 13.4). Following viral entry, the virus uncoats and is transported to the nucleus where the relaxed circular genome is converted by the host cellular machinery to the covalently closed circular DNA (cccDNA); the cccDNA is, in turn, organized into viral minichromosomes. This key replicative intermediate is the transcriptional template for production of the various HBV RNAs, including the pregenomic RNA (pgRNA), that are necessary for viral

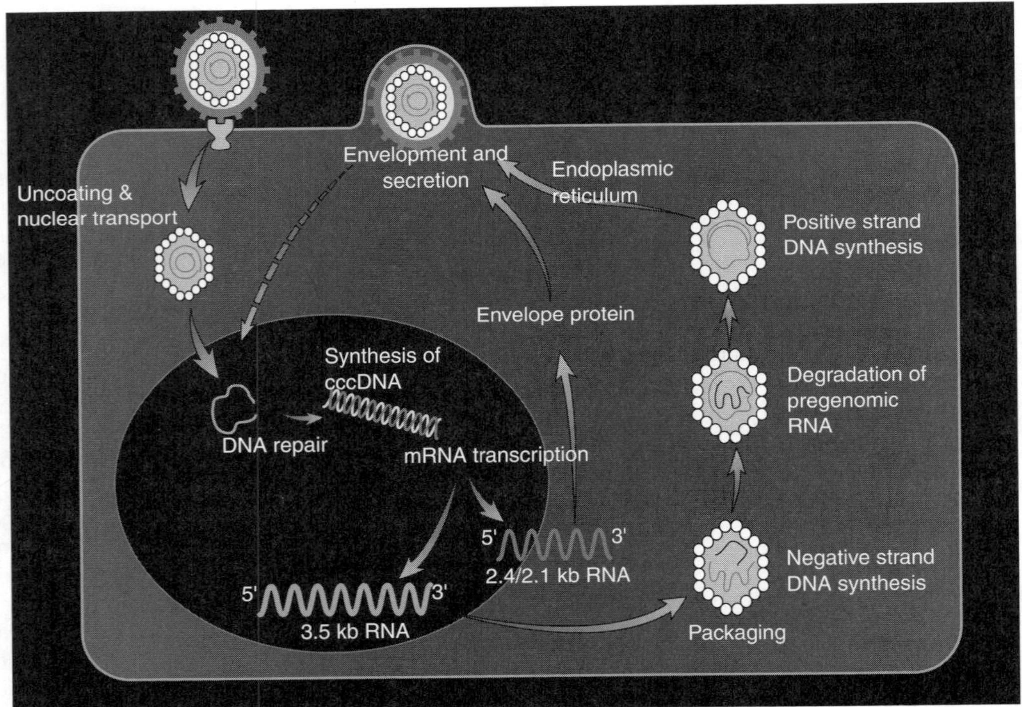

FIGURE 13.4 ● A schematic illustration of the hepatitis B viral infection and replicative cycle within the hepatocyte. Infectious virions attach to a cellular receptor(s) and uncoat, releasing nucleocapsids that migrate to the cell nucleus. The partially double-stranded DNA genome is converted to cccDNA, which is the template for the transcription of four viral transcripts. Translation occurs following transcript export to the cytoplasm. The pregenomic RNA (pgRNA) interacts with two gene products, P and C, to form immature, RNA-packaged, nucleocapsids. The pgRNA is reverse-transcribed into DNA by P. The DNA genome can be either redelivered to the nucleus, or nucleocapsids can be coated by surface glycoproteins (in the Golgi and endoplasmic reticulum) before being exported as enveloped virions.

replication and represents one of the major obstacles in the development of effective treatments for the control of HBV infection. Transcription of the 3.5-kb pgRNA serves three important roles. First, its translation leads to production of the core and POL proteins. Second, it participates in the nucleocapsid packaging reaction, the specificity of which is provided by a unique stem-bulge-stem structure known as epsilon (ϵ) on the 5′ and 3′ ends of the pgRNA (100). Following translation of the pgRNA, the POL protein binds to the 5′-end ϵ. Host proteins such as heat shock protein 90 stabilize this POL-ϵ interaction (100). The *cis*-translated core proteins dimerize around the pgRNA-pol complex and self-assemble to form viral nucleocapsids (101).

Once packaged into a nucleocapsid, the pgRNA serves its third and most important role as the template for reverse transcription and DNA synthesis. The POL protein is bound to the 5′ ϵ-structure and acts as its known primer for initiation and synthesis of the first three nucleotides of the negative-strand DNA (98,99). This nascent DNA is then translocated to the 3′ end of the pgRNA where its binds to the complementary sequence within a 12-nt region known as direct repeat 1 (DR1). From here, negative-strand DNA synthesis proceeds and the RNase H activity of the POL protein degrades all but the last few nucleotides of the template pgRNA. This RNA oligomer is translocated to the 3′ copy of the 12-nt repeat known as DR2, from which point positive-strand DNA synthesis begins. Elongation of the positive-strand DNA proceeds to the 5′ end of the negative strand where a third strand transfer occurs. This is facilated by a short redundancy (r) in the negative-strand DNA template, which anneals to the r region on the 5′ end positive-strand DNA, thereby circularizing the genome (98,99). Premature termination of the positive-strand DNA synthesis by the POL protein results in the characteristic partially double-stranded genome. The HBV nucleocapsid containing the partial double-strand DNA is either recycled back to the nucleus to increase the supply of cccDNA, or undergoes further processing in the endoplasmic reticulum and Golgi for virion assembly. Mature virions are subsequently exported from the cell via the constitutive secretory pathway.

Antiviral Drugs

The review of the HBV life cycle reveals that apart from reverse transcription, most viral processes depend on host-cell machinery. The most important of these is the generation and persistence of cccDNA. Conventional antiviral inhibitors of viral DNA synthesis such as nucleoside/nucleotide analogs (Table 13.6) can prevent or reduce the development of new molecules of cccDNA. However, successful elimination of the existing pool of hepadnaviral cccDNA has only been achieved by either a noncytolytic T helper type 1 (Th1) immune response (102,103) or immune-mediated cell killing followed by hepatocyte division (104,105). In this context, it is important to note that treatment of hepatitis B with nucleoside analogs can result in the partial restoration of specific immunoresponsiveness, which appears necessary for durable host-mediated control of infection (106). Thus, the concept of successful therapy for hepatitis B is converging on the use of both antiviral and immunomodulating approaches. For this chapter, we only focus on antiviral drugs.

Lamivudine and adefovir are now licensed for therapy of hepatitis B in various parts of the world.

TABLE 13.6

Antiviral Drugs for Treatment of Chronic Hepatitis B

Antiviral drugs
Lamivudine
Adefovir dipivoxil
Entecavir
Clevudine
Emtricitabine
β-L-nucleosides (L-dT, L-dC, L-dA)
Tenofovir
Future approaches
Phenylpropenamide derivates
Gene therapy
RNA interference

Evaluation of Drug Efficacy

The major role of serum HBV DNA assays in patients with hepatitis B is to assess HBV replication and candidacy for antiviral therapy. Tests for HBV DNA in serum are also important in assessing the response to antiviral treatment. Serum HBV DNA levels can be quantified by molecular hybridization or signal amplification assays, which have sensitivity limits of 10^5 to 10^6 viral copies per milliliter. PCR assays are more sensitive and capable of detecting fewer than 10^2 copies per milliliter. The appropriate HBV DNA assay to use for the initial evaluation of patients with hepatitis B has not been determined. An arbitrary value of more than 10^5 viral copies per milliliter has been chosen as a diagnostic criterion for hepatitis B (74). However, this definition is not perfect. The assays for HBV DNA quantification are not well standardized (Table 13.7). In some patients with chronic hepatitis, the HBV DNA levels may fluctuate and at times fall below 10^5 viral copies per milliliter.

At a recent National Institutes of Health workshop on the management of hepatitis B, it was proposed that the

TABLE 13.7

Comparison of Hepatitis B Virus DNA Quantification Assays

Assay (Manufacturer)	Sensitivity pg/mL	Sensitivity copies/mL	Linearity (copies/mL)
Branched DNA (Bayer Diagnostics, Tarrytown, NY)	2.1	7×10^5	7×10^5–5×10^9
Liquid hybridization (Abbott Laboratories, Abbott Park, IL)	0.02	5×10^3	5×10^3–3×10^6
Hybrid capture (Digene Corporation, Gaithersburg, MD)	0.5	1.4×10^5	2×10^5–1×10^9
Amplicor PCR (Roche Diagnostics, Basel, Switzerland)	0.001	4×10^2	4×10^2–1×10^7 Cobas: 10^2–10^5 Taqman: 10^2–10^{10}
Molecular beacons		< 50	50–1×10^9

definitions and criteria of the response to antiviral therapy of hepatitis B be standardized. The proposal categorized responses as biochemical, virological or histological, and as on-therapy or sustained off-therapy (74) (Table 13.8).

Lamivudine and Virogram

Hepadnaviruses replicate through an RNA template that requires RT activity. HBV DNA polymerase was shown to share homologies with the RT from retroviruses. Inhibitors for RT of oncogenic RNA viruses may suppress HBV DNA replication. Lamivudine (Epivir) is the minus enantiomer of 2′,3′-dideoxy-3′-thiacytidine (3TC). It was developed as an RTI for use in HIV infection. Lamivudine has been shown to be a potent inhibitor of HBV replication in 2.2.15 cells (107). The 2.2.15 cells were clonal cells derived from Hep G2 cells that were transfected with a plasmid containing HBV DNA. These cells secreted hepatitis B virions. The 2.2.15 cells were maintained in minimal essential medium supplemented with 10% (vol/vol) fetal bovine serum. Cells were incubated at 37°C in a moist atmosphere containing 5% CO_2/95% air. The 2.2.15 cells were inoculated at a density of 3×10^5 cells per 5 mL in a 25-cm^2 flask.

The drugs studied were added to the medium 3 days after the inoculation. Cells were grown in the presence of drugs for 12 days with changes of medium every 3 days. After incubation, the medium was centrifuged (10 minutes at 2,000 × g) and polyethylene glycol (M_r, 8,000) was added to the supernatant to a final concentration of 10% (wt/vol). The virus was pelleted (10 minutes at 10,000 × g). The pellet was resuspended at 1% the original volume in TNE (10 mM Tris HCl, pH 7.5/100 mM NaCl/ 1 mM EDTA). The suspension was adjusted to 1% sodium dodecyl sulfate (SDS) and proteinase K at 0.5 mg/mL and incubated for 2 hours at 55°C. The digest was extracted with phenol/chloroform, 1:1 (vol/vol), and the DNA was precipitated with ethanol. The DNA pellet was dissolved in TE_{80} (10 mM Tris-HCl, pH 8.0/1 mM EDTA) and then electrophoresed in a 0.8% agarose gel followed by blotting onto Hybond-N membrane (Amersham, Buckinghemshire, UK). The blot was hybridized with a ^{32}P-labeled HBV DNA (*Bam*HI insert from plasmid pam6 [American Type Culture Collection]) probe, washed twice with standard saline citrate (SSC)/0.2% SDS at room temperature for 1 hour and 0.1 × SSC/0.2% SDS at 55°C for 30 minutes, and then autoradiographed. The intensity of the autoradiographic bands was quantified by a scanning densitometer. $HBID_{50}$ was defined as the drug concentration that inhibited HBV viral DNA yield in the medium by 50%. The values were obtained by plotting percentage inhibition compared with control versus the drug concentration.

TABLE 13.8

Definition of Response to Antiviral Therapy of Chronic Hepatitis B

Category of Response	Criteria
Biochemical	Decrease in serum ALT to within the normal range
Virologic	Decrease in serum HBV DNA to undetectable levels (<105 copies/mL in unamplified assays) and loss of HBeAg in patients who were initially HbeAg
Histologic	Decrease in histology activity index by at least two points in comparison with pretreatment liver biopsy
Complete	Loss of HBsAg and fulfillment of criteria of biochemical and virologic response

No cell growth retardation or effects on mtDNA was observed after the administration of lamivudine at concentrations at least 100 times higher than concentrations that completely block HBV replication. Lamivudine did not affect the integrated HBV DNAs. Since the RNA replicative intermediates are transcribed from the integrated DNA, it is not surprising that HBV-specific transcripts were not affected by drug treatment. Thus, interruption of drug treatment resulted in a return of HBV virus to intra- and extracellular populations (107). Lamivudine is phosphorylated *in vivo* to the active triphosphate (3TC-TP) that competes with deoxycytidine triphosphate for DNA synthesis. It inhibits DNA synthesis by terminating the nascent proviral DNA chain.

Emergence of the YMDD mutation was associated with duration of therapy. Sixty-seven percent of patients who received lamivudine for 4 years showed evidence of the YMDD mutation, 40% of patients showing evidence after 104 weeks, 31% of patients showing evidence between weeks 52 and 104, and 14% showing evidence after 52 weeks (108,109). Drug resistance can be detected as early as 49 days after taking lamivudine (110), but clinical evidence (phenotypic expression) of drug resistance, which is indicated by a rise in serum alanine transferase (ALT), does not occur before 6 months. Mutations in the catalytic polymerase/RT domain of the gene for HBV polymerase have been associated with lamivudine resistance in patients receiving treatment for HBV infection (111). This is one of the four functional domains of HBV polymerase, which also possesses a priming region, a spacer domain, and a region with ribonuclease H activity (87). The identification of several regions of conserved sequences within the polymerase/RT domain has led to its further subdivision into subdomains A to F. A sequence of four amino acids within the C subdomain consisting of tyrosine (Y) followed by methionine (M) and two aspartic acid (D) residues is highly conserved among viral polymerase/RTs. Termed the "YMDD motif," it is essential for polymerase activity because of its involvement in binding nucleotide substrates in the catalytic site (111). Lamivudine resistance has been associated with substitution of isoleucine (I) or valine (V) for methionine in the YMDD motif at position 552 (rtM204I/V) of HBV polymerase/RT (Table 13.5) (112). *In vitro* assays have confirmed that the YMDD motif mutations conferred reduced susceptibility of HBV to lamivudine (111,113). However, *in vitro* experiments also suggested that YMDD mutant HBV had reduced replicative efficiency in the absence of lamivudine, compared with wild-type HBV (111).

In most cases, YMDD mutations occur in combination with an additional mutation in the B subdomain rtL180M (L528M) that is located in the catalytic site near the YMDD motif in the three-dimensional model of HBV polymerase. The combined L528M/M552I or L528M/M552V mutations have been shown to restore the *in vitro* viral replication capacity of HBV containing YMDD motif mutations (111). These data reaffirm the growing body of clinical data indicating that patients who develop lamivudine-resistant HBV undergo rebound in serum HBV DNA that returns to level similar to those seen prior to therapy with lamivudine (114). Modeling suggests that mutation of the YMDD motif methionine at position 552 to valine or isoleucine causes steric hindrance between the methyl group on the β-branched side chain of valine/isoleucine and the sulfur atom in the unnatural L-oxathiolane ring of lamivudine (87,112). Besides reducing the strength of binding of lamivudine to the polymerase, steric hindrance results in a different orientation of the inhibitor when bound to the mutant enzyme that reduces the efficiency of incorporation of lamivudine triphosphate into replicating viral DNA. Resistance because of steric hindrance may be a problem common to all L-nucleosides (87). These mutations do not affect binding of the natural substrate deoxycytidine triphosphate (dCTP) to the same degree because the deoxyribose ring is in the natural D-configuration. Thus, the effect on natural substrates is small compared with the effect on lamivudine, and the polymerase enzyme can preserve a significant, but decreased, level of activity (112).

Adefovir Dipivoxil

Adefovir dipivoxil is an oral prodrug of adefovir (9-[2-phosphonylmethoxyethyl] adenine, PMEA), a phosphonate nucleotide analog of adenosine monophosphate. It is an acyclic nucleoside phosphonate (ANP) compound (115). The antiviral effect of the ANP analogs is the result of a selective interaction of their diphosphate metabolite with the viral DNA polymerase. Based on the structural resemblance to natural deoxynucleoside triphosphates (i.e., dATP in this case), this diphosphate metabolite acts both as a competitive inhibitor and an alternative substrate during the DNA polymerase reaction. PMEA inhibited HBV release from human hepatoma cell lines Hep G2 2.2.15 and HB611 cells (transfected with human HBV) (116). The cells were seeded in 25 cm^2 tissue culture flasks (Costar) at a density of 4×10^4 cells/cm^2 in Dulbecco's modified Eagle minimum essential medium (EMEM) supplemented with 2 mmol/L L-glutamine (Flow Laboratories, Rockville, MD:), garamycine (40 μg/mL), amphotericin B (2.5 μg/mL), the neomycin analog G418 (360 μg/mL for HepG2 cells; 200 μg/mL for HB611 cells) and 10% fetal bovine serum (FBS; Hyclone Laboratories, Inc., Logas, UT). Medium was changed every 3 days. When cells reached confluency at day 6, FBS concentration was reduced to 2%. Cell cultures were maintained in 5% CO_2 atmosphere at 37°C. At day 3, the culture medium was supplemented with various concentrations of PMEA. Cell culture supernatants and cells were harvested at day 12 and sujected to HBV DNA and HBsAg analysis.

The 50% cytotoxic concentration of PMEA was determined in 24-well tissue plates (cell density: 4×10^4 cells/cm^2) by inhibition of [^{3}H]methyl-dThd incorporation during 24 hours starting at 3 days after seeding.

HBsAg secretion was inhibited by PMEA in a concentration-dependent manner in HB611 cells. Moreover, in congenital duck HBV (DHBV)-infected ducklings, PMEA at a dose of 30 mg/kg^{-1}/day^{-1} was found to effect a marked decrease in DHBV DNA (116). PMEA has been found to have immunostimulating effects in mice, reflected by the induction of interferon (mainly α/β) and a significant enhancement of natural killer cell activity (117,118). The interferon levels induced by PMEA, given for 5 consecutive days at a dose of 25 mg/kg^{-1}, were comparable with those achieved with the known interferon-inducer poly I:C. The natural killer enhancement by PMEA appeared to be coupled, at least in part, to interferon production. However, cytokines other than interferon may be involved, since prolonged administration of PMEA (5 mg/kg^{-1}/day^{-1} for 20 days) resulted in sustained natural killer enhancement in the absence of interferon production.

In two phase III clinical studies, although mutations in the polymerase sites of HBV had been described (rtS119A, rtH133L, rtV214A, rtH234Q) in four of 271 patients treated with adefovir dipivoxil for 48 weeks, no adefovir resistance mutations were identified in this large group of hepatitis B patients (119). However, in one patient during the second year of treatment with adefovir dipivoxil, the rise of HBV DNA and the exacerbation of liver disease led to the identification of a novel asparagine-to-threonine mutation at residue rt236 in domain D of the HBV polymerase (Table 13.5). *In vitro* testing of a laboratory strain encoding the rtN236T mutation and testing of patient-derived virus confirmed that the rtN236T substitution caused a marked reduction in susceptibility to adefovir dipivoxil (120).

Resistance to adefovir dipivoxil is significantly less common than for lamivudine. The emergence of resistance to adefovir dipivoxil appears to be delayed and infrequent. Adefovir is an acyclic nucleotide analog and is smaller than the bulkier oxathiolanes (112). Molecular modeling studies suggest that adefovir can be accommodated more effectively in the more constrained and "crowded" deoxynucleoside triphosphate-binding pocket that carries the rtM204V/I mutations (120). Finally, the adefovir-resistant HBV was sensitive to lamivudine (121).

Other Antiviral Agents

Entecavir

Entecavir, a cyclopentyl guanosine analog, is a potent inhibitor of HBV DNA polymerase, inhibiting both the priming and elongation steps of viral DNA replication (74,122,123). Entecavir is phosphorylated to its triphosphate, the active compound, by cellular kinases. It is a selective inhibitor of HBV DNA. It has little or no inhibitory effect on the replication of other DNA viruses such as herpes simplex, CMV, and RNA viruses such as HIV. Entecavir is also effective against lamivudine-resistant mutants, but less effective than against wild-type HBV (122,124,125). In an *in vitro* assay using Hep G2 2.2.15 human liver cells, the EC_{50} for entecavir was 0.00375 μM compared with 0.116 μM for lamivudine. Therefore, entecavir is 30 times more potent than lamivudine in suppressing viral replication. In woodchucks with chronic woodchuck infection, doses of 0.1 mg/kg of entecavir reduced woodchuck hepatic virus (WHV) titers by seven logs (126). In addition, after 14 months of entecavir therapy, viral core antigen, WHV and cccDNA were undetectable in liver biopsy samples of nine woodchucks (WHV) tested (127). There is also a decrease of the incidence of hepatocellular carcinoma and an increase of survival in treated WHc as compared with untreated WHc.

Entecavir has been evaluated in phase I/II clinical studies. The viral dynamics during and after entecavir therapy were studied in a small number of patients with hepatitis B receiving different doses of entecavir ranging from 0.05 to 1.0 mg/day of entecavir. The median effectiveness in blocking viral production was 96%. The median half-life of viral turnover was 16 hours and the median half-life of infected hepatocytes was 257 hours (10.7 days). Rebound of viral replication also followed a biphasic return to baseline levels (128). During short-term therapy, entecavir seems to show stronger antiviral activity than lamivudine, but this assumption should be validated by head-to-head studies. In addition, entecavir shows continuous activity in patients with detectable lamivudine-induced mutant virus (129).

Until now, no entecavir-resistant viral mutants have been described (123). Prolonged therapy as well as prophylactic therapy, for example in liver-transplant recipients is feasible and not limited by breakthrough infections. Different ongoing multicenter phase III studies are currently evaluating the efficacy and safety of entecavir in HBeAg-positive and -negative patients and in patients resistant to lamivudine. These studies are comparing entecavir with lamivudine for 48 weeks with extended treatment (96 weeks).

Clevudine

Clevudine (L-FMAU; 1-(2-fluoro-5methyl-μ-L-arabinosyl) uracil) is a pyrimidine analog with marked *in vitro* activity against HBV but not HIV (74,130). The active triphosphate inhibits HBV DNA polymerase but is not an obligate chain terminator. Clevudine has *in vitro* an EC_{50} value ranging from 0.02 to 0.15 μM with a mean of 0.08 μM. Clevudine may also be effective against lamivudine-resistant HBV mutants in the *in vitro* studies. In an infected woodchuck model, a once-daily dose of 10 mg/kg of clevudine led to a 9 $\log_{10}$ decrease in viral load. Clevudine also delayed the time to viral recrudescence in a dose-dependent manner (131). Treatment was associated with a decrease in intrahepatic WHV replicative intermediates and woodchuck hepatitis surface and core antigens. No significant side effects were observed in treated animals.

Preliminary results show that clevudine has potent antiviral activity (132) and maintains a sustained posttreatment antiviral effect for at least 6 months after the 28-day treatment period.

Emtricitabine

Emtricitabine (FTC) is a cytosine nucleoside analog with antiviral activity against both HBV and HIV. It differs from lamivudine in having a fluorine at the 5-position of the nucleic acid. In a pilot study, five different doses of emtricitabine were evaluated (25, 50, 100, 200, and 300 mg daily for 8 weeks) in 49 patients with HBeAg-positive hepatitis B (74,130). At the end of treatment, serum HBV DNA decreased by two to three logs in patients receiving the higher doses.

Phase III clinical trials are underway to determine the long-term safety and efficacy of FTC. However, the role of FTC in the treatment of hepatitis B may be limited by its structural similarity to lamivudine and, hence, the potential for cross-resistance and the development of HBV drug-resistant mutants.

Tenofovir

Tenofovir is a nucleotide analog approved for the treatment of HIV infection. It has *in vitro* activity against both wild-type and lamivudine-resistant HBV (133). A report of five patients with HBV and HIV coinfection demonstrated a 4 $\log_{10}$ drop in HBV DNA levels during 24 weeks of treatment (134).

β-L-Nucleosides

The natural nucleosides in the β-L-configuration (β-L-thymidine (L-dT), β-L-2-deoxycytidine (L-dC), and β-L-2-deoxyadenosine [L-dA]) represent a newly discovered class of compounds with potent, selective, and specific activity against hepadnavirus. *In vitro* studies have shown that these compounds are not active against other viruses such as herpes viruses or HIV, but these compounds have marked effects on HBV replication. It is not yet clear if these compounds are active against lamivudine-resistant HBV mutants (74,135–138).

L-dT is at the most developed stage of clinical investigation and has a remarkably clean preclinical toxicology profile. So far, it does not have mitochondria toxicity and it appears not to be mutagenic. After 1 year of therapy, antiviral activity was significantly greater for L-dT compared with lamivudine, and ALT normalization was greatest for L-dT monotherapy (139). Combination treatment (L-dT and lamivudine) was not better than L-dT (140). Phase III trials of L-dT are underway internationally.

Another promising β-L-nucleoside compound is Val-L-dC. Preliminary results in phase I/II testing indicate substantial antiviral activity with a good safety profile (74).

Combinations of β-L-nucleoside appear to have additive or synergistic effect against HBV. *In vitro* studies and animal testing showed that there is no evidence of cellular or mitochondrial toxicity.The combination of L-dT and Val-L-dC was analyzed in a woodchuck study. Over a 12-week treatment period, the combination of L-dT and Val-L-dC cleared WHV DNA in all of the five animals tested with no significant side effects noted.

Future Antiviral Drugs

Several compounds have recently been developed that have a mechanism of HBV inhibition that is unrelated to the viral polymerase. The first of these are the phenylpropenamide derivates, AT-61 and AT-130. King et al. (141) showed that AT-61 did not affect total HBV RNA production or HBV DNA polymerase activity but did significantly reduce the production of encapsidated RNA. Importantly, both AT-61 and AT-130 have identical antiviral activity against wild-type strains as well as a number of different lamivudine-resistant strains of HBV (142). *In vitro* studies using AT-130 showed significant inhibition of the production of encapsidated HBV RNA, but had no effect on total HBV RNA and did not affect core protein or nucleocapsid production, indicating an interference with the encapsidation process itself (143). Steric inhibition or interaction with the host cell chaperone proteins such as Hsp90 may be a possible mechanism. Phenylpropenamides are not water-soluble and have very low bioavailability. Their future successful development as antiviral agents will depend on overcoming potential toxicity and medicinal chemistry issues.

A second class of compounds, the heteroaryldihydropyrimidines, are also potent nonnucleoside inhibitors of HBV replication both *in vitro* and *in vivo* (144). The heteroaryldihydropyrimidine compounds include the candidate molecule Bay 41–4109, and congeners, Bay 38–7690 and Bay 39–5493. Exposure of HBV-infected cells to Bay 41–4109 resulted in increased degradation of core protein through improper formation of viral nucleocapsids. These heteroaryldihydropyrimidine compounds were shown to have efficacy against HBV in the HBV-transgenic mouse model and to possess suitable preclinical pharmacokinetic and toxicology profile (144). Their novel mechanism of action and highly specific antiviral activity indicates that future clinical studies are warranted.

A third compound, LY582563, is a 2-amino-6-arylthio-9-phosphonomethoxyethylpurine bis (2,2,2,-trifluoro-ethyl) ester, a novel nucleotide analog derivative of phosphonomethoxyethyl purine. It belongs to a structural class that is similar to adefovir. This compound has excellent antiviral activity against HBV with a good preclinical toxicity profile (145). It is also effective against lamivudine-resistant HBV (146). Its mechanism of action and early clinical development are under investigation.

Gene therapy is defined as the introduction of new genetic material into a target cell with a therapeutic benefit to the individual (147). Several genetic antiviral strategies including ribozymes, antisense oligonucleotides, interfering peptides or proteins, and therapeutic DNA vaccine have been explored for the molecular therapy of hepatitis B (147,148). A novel molecular strategy that holds promise is the use of small interfering RNAs (siRNA). RNA interference is a cellular process of sequence-specific gene silencing in which small duplexes of RNA target a homologous sequence for cleavage by cellular ribonucleases (149). The introduction of approximately 22-nt siRNAs into mammalian cells can lead to specific silencing of cellular mRNAs without induction of the nonspecific interferon responses that are activated by longer RNA duplexes. Posttranscriptional gene silencing mediates resistance to both endogenous, parasitic, and exogenous pathogenic nucleic acids and can regulate the expression of protein-coding gene (149). This approach has been successfully applied to HBV (150). The siRNA molecules dramatically reduced virus-specific protein expression and RNA synthesis, and these antiviral effects were independent of interferon. Although this approach holds great promise, issues such as gene delivery, stability, toxicity, resistance, and safety need to be resolved.

Conclusions Regarding Hepatitis B

The long-term success of therapy for hepatitis B depends on safe, effective suppression of HBV replication for a long period of time without giving rise to resistant viral strains. As the long-term efficacy of current therapy for hepatitis B is limited, the patient's age, severity of liver disease, and likely response must be weighed against the potential for adverse events and complications before treatment is initiated. Current recommendations for the management of patients with hepatitis B have been recently published by an international panel (151).

In the past 5 years, the treatment of hepatitis B has been improved. It is now possible to contemplate combination therapy for hepatitis B. The future question is which agents to combine: two or more nucleoside/nucleotide analogs or antiviral agents plus immunomodulatory drugs.

HEPATITIS C VIRUS INFECTION: VIROLOGY AND CULTURE SYSTEMS FOR ANTIVIRAL DRUG STUDIES

Hepatitis C virus (HCV) is a major pathogen, harbored by over 250 million people worldwide, with a 70% risk of chronic infection for contaminated individuals (152). Chronic hepatitis may lead to limited histologic lesions in 20% of patients, but also to severe fibrosis and cirrhosis. Among the latter, at least 30% will develop hepatocellular carcinoma in the following 20 years (152,153). Accordingly, HCV chronic infection is the leading cause of liver transplantation throughout the world. Although recent progress has been made in the knowledge of the HCV life cycle, thanks to new experimental tools such as selectable subgenomic replicons, we are still limited in our understanding by the lack of an efficient cell culture system and of an easy-to-use animal model (154). Consequently, the identification of new therapeutic targets is particularly difficult. Currently, interferon alpha (IFN-α) and ribavirin are the only two available therapies for chronic HCV infection. Therapeutic results may appear disappointing as, at best, 50% of the treated patients will have undetectable HCV viremia when these drugs are used in combination therapy (155).

Biology of Hepatitis C Virus

HCV is an enveloped virus containing a single-strand, positive-sense RNA (156). It belongs to the Flaviridae family, also containing two other genera: pestivirus and flavivirus. The most closely related virus is GBC-B, a hepatotropic virus infecting tamarins (157). The HCV genome contains approximately 9,600 nucleotides with one ORF, encoding for a single polyprotein.

Genetic Variability of Hepatitis C Virus

Despite this apparently basic genetic structure, the polyprotein may vary, depending on the genotype. In fact, HCV RNA shows wide genetic variability as the estimated rate of nucleotide change is around 10^3 substitutions per site per year (158), although this rate of nucleotide change depends on the considered genomic region. For example, the polyprotein is flanked by two nontranslated regions that are highly conserved, and in contrast, some hot spots of mutations have been recognized, particularly in the E2 envelope protein, which contains two hypervariable sequences (159). It is noteworthy that this genetic variability complicates study designs of HCV pathogenesis since a single viral protein may lead to different *in vitro* reactivity with host proteins, depending on the amino acid sequence. Thus, over 90 genotypes have been screened around the world, and six main HCV types are now distinguished, according to the proposed classification (160). Prevalence of genotypes may vary around the world; for example, genotype 1b represents more than 45% of the isolates in Europe and only 17% in the United States (161). This genetic variability is obvious within the host, representing quasispecies (162). These facts are, at least in part, related to the high viral turn-over, since the estimated viral production is 10^{12} per day (160,163).

Since infectious virions are permanently selected through their interactions with the host, this may partly explain immune failure to eradicate HCV and resistance to antiviral drugs (154,164). However, the identification of some highly conserved amino acid sequences among both structural and nonstructural proteins suggest essential functions for viral life cycle, and could constitute the target of new antiviral drugs.

Viral Life Cycle

The polyprotein is processed by viral and cellular proteases in ten structural and nonstructural proteins. Structural proteins include the core (i.e., the viral nucleocapsid) and the envelope proteins El and E2. The nonstructural proteins are NS2 to NS5B, required for viral replication. These two groups of proteins are separated by the short membrane peptide p7 (154,165). Very recently, the p7 function appeared to act as an ion channel (166). This assemblage results in a complete virion exhibiting a diameter of 30 to 50 nm (167). However, particles isolated from plasma may vary as a result of complex formation with very low-density lipoproteins or immunoglobulins (168).

The main cellular target for HCV is the hepatocyte (163). But extrahepatic sites allowing viral replication have been identified, such as peripheral blood mononuclear cells (essentially B cells and monocytes), lymph nodes, and possibly biliary cells (163,169,170). More than one cellular receptor should exist for HCV: CD81 was the first one to be discovered (171), but experimental animal models showed that it did not allow viral replication by itself (172). Accordingly, very low-density lipoprotein receptors and glycosaminoglycans are potential co-receptors for HCV (173).

The life cycle of HCV is more hypothetical beyond the stage of target-cell infection because our progress in this field is hampered by the absence of a relevant model for HCV entry, replication, and release. Clearly, El and E2 are involved in membrane fusion operating between the virus and the endoplasmic reticulum (174). For this purpose, these two viral products interact through heterodimerization, allowing endoplasmic reticulum retention (175). Thus, viral RNA translation may proceed, beginning by the internal ribosome entry site binding to ribosome (176,177). The positive-stranded viral RNA serves as a template for the production of RNA negative strands, which allow the synthesis of viral genome, and thus virions, by interactions with copies of the core protein (176). As an example, the core protein produced in bacteria allows the formation of nucleocapsides when incubated with RNA molecules (178). However, nonstructural proteins such as NS3 helicase and NS5B RNA-dependent RNA-polymerase obviously play a major role in this viral life cycle, but our understanding of their molecular interactions needs to be improved (154).

Culture Systems for Anti-viral Drug Study

All this information is required to fully understand the current procedure to study the antiviral effects of licensed drugs. However, the mechanisms accounting for the antiviral activity of both IFN-α and ribavirin are essentially unidentified (152,155,179,180). Interferon alpha is thought to induce an antiviral cellular state and may up-regulate the destruction of infected cells. Ribavirin is a synthetic guanosine analog mostly used for the treatment of respiratory syncytial virus infection. The inhibition of HCV is hypothetical, and it seems that most of its antiviral effect is indirect, through synergic interaction with IFN-α, up-regulating antiviral immune responses (181).

As discussed later, the paucity of information concerning antiviral effects of current drugs labeled for HCV treatment is due to the lack of an appropriate experimental system. HCV protein functions are largely described, and even the crystal structure of the RNA-dependent RNA polymerase has been determined (182). This information should lead to the definition of new therapeutic targets. However, until early in this century, the absence of reliable cellular and/or animal model for stable HCV replication hampered the evaluation of assumed antiviral interventions. Yet, several studies have reported experimental conditions allowing HCV replication, using fetal liver cells, hepatoma cell lines, immortalized T or B cell lines, but in most cases with limited viral replication and low reproducibility (165).

The simian model is the most relevant to study any step of the natural history of HCV infection. However, for obvious reasons, this approach is not available for most of the laboratories involved in HCV research. Animal models have revealed the narrow host range of HCV because only primary hepatocytes from chimpanzees, and not baboons, allow complete HCV replication. Recently, stable HCV replication has been obtained using transgenic mice with chimeric human liver. Mice were infected by intraperitoneal injection of fresh serum from patients, resulting in the production of infectious viral particles (183).

Cultures of primary human hepatocytes infected with HCV-positive serum results in HCV replication as demonstrated by the detection of negative-sense RNA strands (184,185). Nevertheless, HCV replication was of variable levels, depending on hepatocyte donors and viral strains, resulting in heterogeneous results and interlaboratory variability. Accumulation of nucleotide mutations may be observed in these models as well as the concentration-dependent inhibition of HCV replication by IFN-α (the latter leading to a reduction in genome mutations) (184).

Primary cell cultures and immortalized cell lines infected with HCV-containing serum do not allow production of viral infectious particles; thus, taking into account the absence of cellular cytotoxicity of HCV, these experiments require molecular biological methods, such as RT-PCR, to determine the level of replication, implying other technical problems.

Accordingly, Lohmann et al. have developed a cell culture system allowing the replication of subgenomic HCV RNA (186). The structural region was deleted and the gene encoding the neomycin phosphotransferase and the internal ribosome entry site of the encephalomyocarditis virus were inserted. This bicistronic replicon was initially transfected in human hepatocarcinoma cell line Huh-7, in which autonomous replication was observed, resulting in detection of both positive and negative RNA strands. As suggested by previous studies, replicon levels depended on cell metabolism, being minimal at the confluence state. Subsequent analysis showed adaptive mutations in replicons, leading to optimized replication in the Huh-7 cell line exclusively (187). No cytopathogenicity of these HCV replicons has been observed (188). This easy-to-use cellular system that gives access to stable HCV replication may therefore be used for the evaluation of drug efficacy. Accordingly, recent data indicate that IFN-α inhibits the replication of HCV subgenomic replicons (189). However, because structural proteins may influence drug sensitivity, the activity of new compounds will still require validation in animal models allowing full viral production. As an example, very recently an inhibitor of the HCV-encoded NS3 protease has been described, resulting in a significant decrease of viral load (190).

Conclusions Regarding Hepatitis C

Despite many unresolved aspects of HCV infection, considerable efforts have been made since the definitive identification of the virus. A better understanding of HCV epidemiology will allow improved prevention; meanwhile, detection of infected patients is easy to achieve early in the natural history of their disease. Therefore, treatment combinations may be prescribed in cases of mild liver disease, increasing chances of cure for patients. Moreover, current tools for the study of the HCV life cycle should provide the opportunity to develop new antiviral drugs.

RESISTANCE OF HUMAN CYTOMEGALOVIRUS TO ANTIVIRAL DRUGS AND DISCUSSION OF SUSCEPTIBILITY TESTING

Human cytomegalovirus (HCMV), a member of the herpesvirus family, is a ubiquitous agent that commonly infects human beings. As with other herpesviruses, primary infection is followed by latent infection. Recurrent infections are most often caused by reactivation of latent virus but reinfection also occurs. HCMV infections are generally mild or asymptomatic in immunocompetent adults, but HCMV is a major cause of defects in neonates and is a major pathogen in immunosuppressed individuals, including recipients of bone marrow and solid-organ transplants and patients with acquired immunodeficiency syndrome (AIDS). In particular, HCMV was the most common cause of sight- and life-threatening opportunistic infection in patients with AIDS prior to the availability of highly active antiretroviral therapy.

Three compounds are currently approved for the treatment of severe HCMV infections. The compounds include the deoxyguanosine analog ganciclovir and its prodrug valganciclovir, the acyclic nucleoside phosphonate cidofovir, and the pyrophosphate analog foscarnet. All of these compounds are inhibitors of the viral DNA polymerase encoded by gene *UL54*. Ganciclovir must be phosphorylated to ganciclovir triphosphate to exert its antiviral activity. Initial phosphorylation is achieved by the viral protein kinase *UL97* and further phosphorylations are performed by host cellular kinases. Ganciclovir triphosphate is a competitive inhibitor of the natural substrate (deoxyguanosine triphosphate) for the HCMV DNA polymerase. In addition, incorporation of ganciclovir triphosphate onto growing viral DNA causes a slowing, and subsequent cessation, of DNA chain elongation. As cidofovir already contains a phosphate-mimetic group, it needs only two phosphorylation steps to reach the active stage. These phosphorylations are performed by host cellular enzymes. Thus, cidofovir does not depend on the virus-induced kinase to exert its antiviral action. Cidofovir diphosphate interacts as competitive inhibitor with the normal substrate (deoxycytosine triphosphate) for the viral polymerase. Two consecutive incorporations at the 3′ end of the DNA chain are required to efficiently shut off DNA elongation. Incorporation of one cidofovir diphosphate molecule causes a marked decrease in the rate of DNA elongation. Foscarnet does not require intracellular activation to exert its antiviral activity. It is not incorporated into the growing DNA and it reversibly blocks the pyrophosphate binding site of the viral DNA polymerase and inhibits the cleavage of pyrophosphate from deoxynucleoside triphosphates.

Patients receiving long-term suppressive anti-HCMV therapy may develop antiviral resistance. In AIDS patients before the era of highly active antiretroviral therapy, epidemiological studies have shown that the frequency of resistance increased with the duration of therapy and reached 27% of patients after 9 months of ganciclovir (191), 13% of patients after 1 year of valganciclovir (192), and 37% of patients after 1 year of foscarnet (193). In solid-organ recipients, 7% of the HCMV infection were resistant to ganciclovir after a median delay of 10 months (194).

Methods used in the laboratory to determine the susceptibility of HCMV strains to antiviral drugs are classified as phenotypic or genotypic. Phenotypic methods aim to determine the concentration of an antiviral agent that inhibits the virus in culture. Genotypic assays are designed to detect mutations known to confer antiviral resistance in the genome of the viruses being studied.

Phenotypic Antiviral Assays

A variety of phenotypic assays have been used in different studies to determine the antiviral susceptibilities of HCMV strains. Each of these methods measures the inhibition of HCMV growth in tissue cultures in the presence of serial dilutions of antiviral drugs. The 50% inhibitory concentration (IC_{50}) is defined as the concentration of antiviral agent resulting in a 50% reduction in viral growth. The methods usually performed include the plaque-reduction assays that measure the inhibition of replication of infectious virus, the assays based on DNA hybridization that measure the inhibition of viral DNA synthesis, and enzyme-linked immunosorbent- and flow cytometry-based assays that measure production of one or more viral proteins. The IC_{50} values determined with these different phenotypic assays depend on the nature of the replication marker chosen.

Clinical Specimens to Study

HCMV can be recovered from various clinical specimens such as peripheral blood leukocytes, bronchoalveolar liquid, cerebrospinal fluid, organ biopsy, urine samples, and vitreous fluid. Strains recovered from blood are usually chosen to be tested because viremia reflects blood dissemination and active infection. However, resistance profiles of a blood strain may differ from those of strains recovered from other body compartments and directly responsible for the disease because antiviral drug selection pressure may differ from one compartment to another. In addition, patients may shed multiple strains of HCMV either concurrently or sequentially (195).

Constitution of Viral Stocks

All the assay methods require the constitution of viral stocks obtained after sequential passaging of the viral isolate. Viral stocks are constituted by either extracellular virus recovered from culture supernatants or intracellular virus present in infected cells. Constitution of extracellular virus stocks requires at least eight to ten passages and is therefore time-consuming. Moreover, some isolates remain cell-associated and no extracellular virions are produced. On the contrary, constitution of a stock of infected cells may be achieved after only one to three passages; however, it may require more passages (196).

Tissue culture supernatants containing extracellular virus are clarified by centrifugation at 1,000 rpm for 10 minutes and divided into aliquots and kept frozen at −80°C until use. Titers of extracellular virus stocks are determined from a thawed aliquot using a plaque assay or a rapid immunocytochemistry assay. Infected fibroblast monolayers are trypsinized; cells are then counted and used for the phenotypic assay.

Plaque-Reduction Assay

Plaque-reduction assay has been considered as the "gold standard" for antiviral phenotypic testing. A standardized assay has been proposed by Landry et al. (197).

Human fibroblasts grown as just confluent monolayers in 24-well plates are inoculated with a standardized inoculum of a stock virus (50 to 100 plaque-forming units per well). After adsorption for 90 minutes, the medium is aspirated and the wells are overlaid with a 0.4% agarose medium containing serial dilutions of the drug to be tested. Concentrations usually tested are between 1 and 50 μM for ganciclovir, 50 and 800 μM for foscarnet, and 0.1 and 20 μM for cidofovir. Each drug concentration is tested at least in triplicate, as well as controls without drug. The cultures are incubated for 7 days at 37°C. Monolayers are fixed in 10% formalin in phosphate-buffered saline (PBS) and stained with 0.8% crystal violet in 50% ethanol. The IC_{50} of the antiviral agent for the isolate is defined as the concentration causing a 50% reduction in the number of plaques produced as compared with controls. Alternatively, a medium without agarose can be used. The plates are then incubated for 4 days and the foci are revealed by immunoperoxidase staining using monoclonal antibody E-13 (195).

DNA Hybridization Assay

Cell cultures are inoculated with a standardized amount of virus and incubated in the presence of different concentrations of antiviral agent until control wells show 60% to 80% cytopathic effect. Then the cells are lysed and whole DNA is extracted and hybridized to a radiolabelled HCMV probe. Radioactivity is counted. The IC_{50}s of the antiviral agents are the concentrations that reduce by 50% the DNA hybridization values compared with the hybridization values of controls (198).

Detection of Human Cytomegalovirus Antigens

Viral production is measured by using immunofluorescence-, immunoperoxidase-, or flow cytometry-based methods for detection and quantification of cells expressing HCMV antigens or by using enzyme-linked immunosorbent assay-based methods for quantification of HCMV antigens produced in cells (199,200).

Drawbacks of the Phenotypic Assays

Phenotypic assays are limited by the excessive time required to complete the assay (1 to 2 months). To reduce the turnaround time involved in plaque-reduction assays, a modified assay has been performed directly in primary cultures of clinical specimens such as urine, amniotic fluid, and bronchoalveolar lavage samples (201). Blood leukocytes from patients with documented HCMV viremia were also used as inoculum in a plaque-reduction assay (202). These methods provided results within 4 to 6 days. Their major limitation is that the virus titers of the clinical specimens are often too low to allow them to be used.

Resistant strains in a mixture may not be detected because of strain selection that occurs during passaging. Therefore, the virus stock studied may be not representative of the original population of virus. If antiviral drug is added to the cell-culture medium in order to favor growth of mutant virus, *de novo* resistant strains may be selected in cell culture [203].

Interpretation

Dose-inhibition curves are constructed to determine the IC_{50} values of the antiviral agents of the studied strains. The type of cell culture used, the size of the viral inoculum, the method used, and the laboratory performing the test are factors that affect the results. Therefore, there is a significant variability among methods and laboratories. When feasible, a baseline isolate from the same patient should be tested in parallel with the isolate of interest. However, baseline isolates are often missing. Reference susceptible and resistant strains must be included in each susceptibility assay. Antiviral drug IC_{50} values for the isolate to test are compared with the results obtained for the reference strains. A comparison with the results obtained for a panel of susceptible strains tested in the laboratory can assist in the interpretation.

The IC_{50} cutoff values proposed to define resistance to antiviral compounds are as follows: more than 12 μM for ganciclovir, more than 400 μM for foscarnet, and more than 2 or 4 μM for cidofovir. HCMV strains for which ganciclovir IC_{50} is more than 6 μM and less than 12 μM are considered to have decreased susceptibility to ganciclovir (196,197,204). However, cutoff values are to be determined in each laboratory.

Genotypic Antiviral Assays

Ganciclovir resistance results mostly from changes in the *UL97* phosphotransferase responsible for the primophosphorylation of ganciclovir (Table 13.9) (205,206). Mutations in the *UL54* DNA polymerase gene appear after prolonged ganciclovir therapy (207). They contribute to a high level of resistance to ganciclovir and induce cross-resistance to cidofovir. All foscarnet and cidofovir resistance mutations that are currently known map to the *UL54* gene (Table 13.10) (204,208–212).

Viral DNA Extraction

Viral DNA is extracted from cultures in 25-cm^2 flasks using the procedure described by Hirt (213). Briefly, infected cell monolayers exhibiting at least 50% cytopathic effect are washed twice in PBS and then 0.4 mL of Hirt solution (100 mM Tris-HCl, pH 7.5, 10 mM EDTA, 0.5% sodium dodecyl sulfate) is added. After incubation at room temperature for 20 minutes, the lysate is transferred to a microtube, and 0.1 mL of 5 M NaCl solution is added. The mixture is incubated for 12 hours at 4°C and centrifuged at 15,000 rpm for 5 minutes. The resulting supernatant is digested with proteinase K (1 mg/mL) at 56°C for 1 hour and then extracted with phenol chloroform and precipitated with ethanol. By this procedure, a purified DNA preparation enriched in viral DNA is obtained. Alternatively, infected monolayers are trypsinized, washed twice in PBS, and centrifuged. The cell pellet is submitted to lysis in a buffer containing 10 mM Tris-HCl, pH 8.0, 50 mM KCl, 2 mM $MgCl_2$, 0.9% Nonidet P-40, and 100 μg/mL of proteinase K for 1 hour at 56°C (196). The mixture is centrifuged for 5 minutes at 15,000 rpm and the supernatant containing DNA is collected. DNA is extracted from clinical samples using commercially available purification columns (Qiagen, Valencia, CA, or Macherey-Nagel, Düren, Germany) according to the manufacturer's instructions.

Rapid Genotypic Methods

Detection of Ganciclovir Resistance-related Mutations in Gene *UL97*

Rapid screening methods have been designed to detect the mutations at codons 460, 594, 591, 592, 594, 595 (the most frequently observed in clinical isolates) and at codon 520 (214–217). They are based on restriction enzyme analysis of three selected PCR products amplified from HCMV-infected cultures or from clinical samples (Tables 13.11 and 13.12). The PCR reaction mixtures include 5% dimethyl sulfoxide, deoxynucleosides triphosphate at 200 μM each, primers at 1μM each, 2.5 units of Taq polymerase (Roche Diagnostics), and 500 ng of DNA. The reactions are cycled 40 times as follows: 95°C for 1 minute, 55°C for 45 seconds, and 72°C for 45 seconds.

The restriction enzymes, *Nla*III, *Alu*I, *Hha*I, *Mse*I, *Taq*I and *Hae*III are used to digest the PCR products (Table 13.13) (214,216,217). The digests are analyzed on a 15% polyacrylamide gel and stained with ethidium bromide (Table 13.11).

The diagnostic screening assays based on restriction enzyme analysis of selected PCR products allow the detection of the most frequent *UL97* mutations involved in resistance to ganciclovir and can identify minority mutants if they reach 10% of the viral population. The disadvantage of these rapid and simple tests is that they miss specific mutations that do not result in a change in

TABLE 13.9

UL97 Changes in Cytomegalovirus Strains Resistant to Ganciclovir

Role in Conferring Resistance to Ganciclovir	Residue	Amino Acid Change
Proven by marker transfer experiments	460	Methionine to isoleucine/valine
	520	Histidine to glutamine
	590–593	Deletion of alanine-alanine-cysteine-arginine
	591–594	Deletion of alanine-cysteine-arginine-alanine
	594	Alanine to valine/glycine
	595	Deletion of leucine, leucine to serine/phenylalanine
	603	Cysteine to tryptophane
	607	Cysteine to tyrosine
Suspected	590	Alanine to threonine
	591	Alanine to valine/aspartic acid
	592	Cysteine to glycine
	595	Leucine to tryptophane/threonine
	596	Glutamic acid to glycine/aspartic acid
	597	Asparagine to isoleucine
	598	Glycine to valine
	599	Lysine to methionine
	600	Deletion of leucine
	601	Deletion of threonine
	603	Cysteine to tyrosine
	606	Alanine to aspartic acid
	665	Valine to isoleucine

the restriction enzyme pattern and previously unmapped mutations.

Detection of Resistance-related Mutations in Gene *UL54*

Restriction enzyme analysis of PCR fragments have been used to detect the ganciclovir and cidofovir resistance change L501F and the ganciclovir and foscarnet resistance change A809V in the DNA polymerase (209,218).

Sequence Analysis Methods

Sequencing is the nucleotide sequence analysis that is proved to be the most accurate method for genotypic resistance determination of HCMV strains. However, no standardized assay is available to routinely achieve the analysis of the *UL97* and *UL54* genes. The complete genes or the gene regions involved in resistance are amplified by PCR, and then PCR products are directly sequenced (Tables 13.14 through 13.16) (196,219,220). Amplification of *UL97*, either with the primer set CPL97-F and CPL97-R or the primer set HLF97-F and HLF97-R, is performed using the GeneAmp XL PCR kit (Applied Biosystems). The reactions are cycled 30 times as follows: 94°C for 1 minute and 60°C for 10 minutes. The entire gene *UL54* is amplified using the GeneAmp XL PCR kit. The *UL54* region of interest is amplified using high-fidelity polymerase (LA PCR kit, Takara, Shiga, Japan). PCR products are purified using QIAquick PCR purification kits (Qlagen) and are then submitted to sequence reaction. When analysis of sequences are to be performed on an ABI automated DNA sequencer, the purified templates (10 or 20 ng) are sequenced using ABI Prism Big Dye Terminator version 3.0 ready reaction cycle sequencing kit (Applied Biosystems) according to the manufacturer's instructions. Depending on the sequencing method chosen, minority mutants in a mixture can be detected if they reach 20% to 40% of the viral population. Sequences of *UL97* and *UL54* are aligned with the AD169

TABLE 13.10

UL54 Changes in HCMV Strains Resistant to Antiviral Compounds[a]

Region	Modification	Viral Phenotype		
		Ganciclovir	Cidofovir	Foscarnet
ExoI	D301N	R	R	S
IV	N408D	R	R	S
	F412C	R	R	S
	F412V	R	R	S
	D413E	R	R	S
δC	L501I	R	R	S
	K513E	R	R	S
	P522S	R	R	S
	L545S	R	R	S
	D588E	S	S	R
II	T700A	S	S	R
	V715M	S	S	R
	I722V	R	R	S
VI	V781I	S	S	R
III	L802M	R	S	R
	K805Q	S	R	S
	T821I	R	S	R
V	A987G	R	R	S
	Del 981–982	R	R	R
Other	E756D	S	S	R
	E756K	I	I	R

[a] Data derived from Chou et al. (204), Cihlar et al. (210), and Erice (211).
R, resistant; S, sensitive; I, intermediate; del, deletion.

TABLE 13.11

Restriction Enzyme Digestion Screening for *UL97* Mutations Related to Ganciclovir Resistance

PCR Product			Enzyme	*UL97*	Fragment Size (Base Pair)	
Forward Primer	Reverse Primer	Size (Base Pair)		Codon	Wild-type Sequence	Mutant Sequence
CPT1088 M	CPT1619	532	*Nla*III	460	198, 168, 126, 9	324, 168, 9
CPT1088 M	CPT1587 M	501	*Alu*I	520	314, 187	297, 187, 17
CPT1713	CPT1830	118	*Hha*I	594	50, 38, 18, 12	62, 38, 18
			*Mse*I	595 =>F	76, 42	46, 42, 30
			*Taq*I	595 =>S	99, 19	71, 48, 19
			*Hae*III	591 + 592	59, 59	63, 55
			*Hae*III	591		118

TABLE 13.12

Sequence of the Primers Used for Rapid Screening for *UL97* Mutations[a]

Primer	5′-3′ Sequence
CPT 1088	ACGGTGCTCACGGTCTGGAT
CPT 1619	AAACGCGCGTGCGGGTCGCAGA
CPT 1587 M	CTGCAGCGGCATGGGTCGGAAAGCAAG
CPT 1713	CGGTCTGGACGAGGTGCGCAT
CPT 1830 M	AATGAGCAGACAGGCGTCGAAGCA GTGCGTGAGCTTGCCGTTCTT

[a] Isolated base changes have been introduced in primer CPT 1830 to create recognition sites for *Taq* I (TCGA) in S595 mutants and a recognition site for *Mse* I (TTTA) in F595 mutants. Primer CPT 1587 creates an additional *Alu* I site in presence of Q520.

strain reference sequence (EMBL accession no. X17403) using Align Plus, version 4.0 (Scientific and Educational Software, Durham, NC).

The interpretation of genetic assays requires the distinction of resistance-associated mutations to natural interstrain variation. Some of the mutations observed in resistant strains have been validated as resistance markers by a process of marker transfer, but others have not. To date, resistance mutations in *UL97* have been found at one of three sites. At two of those, there are point mutations in a single codon (460 and 520) and at the third site there are point mutations or deletions within the codon range 590 to 607. On the contrary, resistance-associated mutations in *UL54* are widely dispersed across the coding sequence. The interstrain sequence homology is above 98% and 99% for *UL54* and *UL97*, respectively (196,219, 220). *UL54* sequences determined in HCMV isolates sensitive to antiviral drugs have been deposited in GenBank under accession numbers AF133589 through AF133628 and under accession numbers AY422355 through AY422377 (219,220). *UL97* sequences of ganciclovir-sensitive strains have been deposited under accession numbers AF34548 through AF345573 (196).

Conclusions Regarding Human Cytomegalovirus Assays

Phenotypic assays are still important to corroborate genotypic results. However, the time required to perform the assays is too long to provide useful therapeutic information. Results obtained by both types of susceptibility testing are usually concordant. However, it should be noted that viruses harboring mutations responsible for resistance can be classified as susceptible in phenotypic assays. Because some *UL97* or *UL54* mutations are associated with a slow growth of HCMV in culture, it has been proposed that the presence of these mutations could introduce a bias in the phenotypic assays. Moreover, as patients can be infected by multiple HCMV strains, it is possible that tissue-culture based assays will select a different virus population from that selected by PCR-based assays.

ANTIVIRAL AGENTS FOR INFLUENZA VIRUSES: MODE OF ACTION AND ANTIVIRAL RESISTANCE

Influenza is a viral disease of major importance. It is responsible for annual epidemics with significant mortality and morbidity (221). In some rare cases, a pandemic

TABLE 13.13

Rapid Screening for *UL97* Mutations: Conditions of Polymerase Chain Reaction Product Digestion with Restriction Enzymes[a]

Enzyme	Enzyme Unity Number Per Reaction	Incubation	
		Length Time (Hours)	Temperature (°C)
NlaIII	3	2	37
AluI	5	2	37
HhaI	3	2	37
HaeIII	3	2	37
TaqI	3	2	65
MseI	3	2	37

[a] A 10-μL sample of polymerase chain reaction product is digested in a final volume of 20 μL.

TABLE 13.14

Primer Sequences for Polymerase Chain Reaction Amplification of the *UL97* Gene

Fragment Amplified[a]	Sequence	Reference
Entire gene (2,254 bp)	CPL97-F 5′-GGAAGACTGTCGCCACTATGTCC-3′ CPL97-R 5′-CTCCTCATCGTCGTCGTAGTCC-3′	Lurain et al. (196)
Codons 400 to 707 (1,038 bp)	HLF97-F 5′-CTGCTGCACAACGTCACGGTACATC-3′ HLF97-R 5′-CTCCTCATCGTCGTCGTAGTCC-3′	Lurain et al. (196)

[a] bp, base pair.

strain can emerge from the animal reservoir, leading to a devastating influenza with high attack rates (222). This disease is highly contagious, with person-to-person disease spread via aerosol droplets that infect epithelial cells of the respiratory tract (223).

The human and animal influenza viruses belong to the family Orthomyxoviridae. There are three genera, corresponding to influenza virus types A, B, and C (224). The latter is rarely encountered and will not be discussed in this chapter. Influenza A viruses are divided into subtypes based on major antigenic specificities of their surface glycoproteins hemagglutinin (HA) and neuraminidase (NA). To date, 15 different HA have been described and nine different NA. There are no influenza B subtypes (224).

Among influenza viruses, influenza A is the most important, causing (with influenza B) annual outbreaks and epidemics during the winter seasons in temperate climates, but also being responsible for the rare pandemics (225). These pandemics were observed three times during the 20th century (225,226). These influenza A pandemics resulted in a rapid worldwide spread of the emerging influenza A, associated with very high mortality and morbidity (227).

Influenza is associated with nonspecific signs and symptoms (224). The definition for influenza-like illness is the triad associating fever plus one respiratory and one general sign. Briefly, following a short incubation period of 24 to 48 hours, the disease is usually characterized by the sudden onset of high fever with chills,

TABLE 13.15

Primer Sequences for Polymerase Chain Reaction Amplification of the *UL54* Gene

Fragment Amplified[a]	Primer Sequence	Reference
Entire gene (3.7 kbp)	Forward: 5′-GTCAGCCTCTCACGGTCCGCTAT-3′ Reverse: 5′-CTCAGTCTCAGCAGCATCATCAC-3′	Chou et al. (219)
Codons 363 to 1,005 (1,926 bp)	Forward : 5′-ATC TCT TTA CGA TCG GCA CC-3′ Reverse : 5′-ATC CTC AAA GAG CAG GGA GAG-3′	Fillet et al. (220)

[a] bp, base pair.

TABLE 13.16

Primer Sequences for Sequencing of *UL97* and *UL54* Coding Strands[a]

Gene	Sequence	Nucleotide Position	Reference (s)
UL97	5′-ATCGACAGCTACCGACGTGCC-3′	1285–1305	Lurain et al. (196)
	5′-GTCGGAGCTGTCGGCGCTGGG-3′	1651–1671	
UL54	5′-CGCCTCTCACTCGATGAAGT-3′	3708–3727	Sullivan et al. (212), Ducancelle et al. (195), Fillet et al. (220)
	5′-TCAGGAAGACTATGTAGTGG-3′	3260–3279	
	5′-GCCCACAACCTCTGCTACTC-3′	2840–2859	
	5′-CAGCAGATCCGTATCT-3′	2391–2406	
	5′-CGGCCGCCACCAAGGTGTAT-3′	2071–2090	
	5′-AGATCTCGTGCGTGTGCTACG-3′	1627–1647	

[a] *UL97* nucleotides are numbered from codon 1. Nucleotide positions in *UL54* gene are identified according to Kouzarides et al. (*J Virol* 1987;61:125–133).

headache, dry cough, myalgia, nasal congestion with mild or no rhinorrhea, asthenia, and diarrhea (224,228). This disease is observed in all age groups. In some cases, bacterial superinfection can be observed leading to severe pulmonary infection (229). In classic influenza disease, spontaneous recovery is observed after 5 to 7 days of infection, depending on the patient's age, and the immune status (the disease lasts 7 to 8 days in young children and can last several months in immunocompromised patients).

Influenza Virus Structure

Influenza A and B viruses share common features (224). The are pleomorphic, 80- to 120-nm virus particles. The virus contains eight gene segments, each of these coding for one or two proteins whose name and function are listed in Table 13.17. These viruses are enveloped viruses. On the envelope surface are located the two glycoproteins HA and NA. This envelope also contains tetramers of the M2 protein, whose function is described here. Inside the

TABLE 13.17

List of the Different Virus Proteins of Influenza A

Segment	Gene Size in Nucleotides	Protein(s)	Protein Size in Amino Acids	Protein Function
1	2,341	PB2	759	Polymerase (subunit Basic 2)
2	2,341	PB1	757	Polymerase (subunit Basic 1)
		PB1-F1	87	Proapoptotic mitochondrial protein
3	2,233	PA	716	Polymerase (subunit Acidic)
4	1,778	HA	566	Receptor binding site and fusion, main target of neutralizing antibodies
5	1,565	NP	498	Nucleoprotein
6	1,413	NA	454	Sialidase enzymatic activity (virion release)
7	1,027	M1	252	Matrix protein
		M2	97	Proton channel activity
8	890	NS1	230	Interferon inhibitor, gene regulation
		NS2/NEP	121	Nuclear export of viral proteins

virus particle, just within the envelope, lies the M1 matrix protein. This protein is responsible for the stability of the particle and interacts with the virus RNA segments. These single-strand, negative-RNAs are associated with the nucleoprotein and with the three proteins of the polymerase complex (PB1, PB2 and PA). NS1 and NEP cannot be detected in the viral particle.

Protein Function

Hemagglutinin

Hemagglutinin (HA) is encoded from genome RNA segment 4 in influenza A and B viruses (224). HA is a complex protein with key functions in the infectious process (230,231). It is synthetized as a precursor protein HA0 that has to undergo a proteolytic cleavage to become active. This cleavage generates two proteins (HA1 and HA2) bonded by two disufide bonds (Fig. 13.5). HA1 is of globular form and contains the major antigenic sites as well as the receptor binding site, which is highly conserved between types and subtypes (232,233). HA2 is a long, fibrous stem that forms triple-stranded, coiled-coil protein that contains the transmembrane domain and the fusion peptide; this fusion peptide is available after the HAO cleavage (234). At the virus surface, the hemagglutinin glycoproteins are trimeric and very abundant. When submitted to low pH, HA undergoes conformational changes that allow HA-mediated membrane fusion (230). These mechanisms have been intensively analyzed by several investigators.

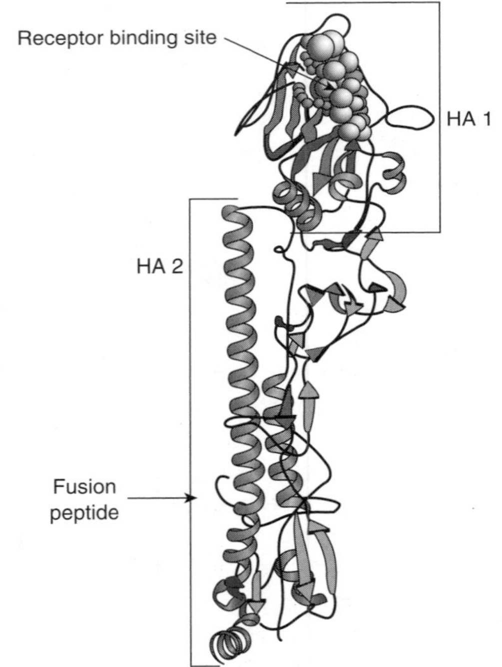

FIGURE 13.5 ● Structure of the hemagglutinin (monomeric).

Neuraminidase

NA is the second surface glycoprotein (224,235). It is encoded from genome RNA segment 6 in influenza A and B viruses. This protein is a sialidase. It is organized into two domains, the stalk and the head. The head of the NA contains the active site of the enzyme (Fig. 13.6). These proteins are organized as homotetramers at the virus surface (224). Among influenza viruses, the structure of the catalytic site of NA is highly conserved. The role of the neuraminidase is to remove sialic acids from glycoproteins. This ensures the proper release of the virions from the host cell surface after budding by preventing virus aggregation and facilitating release of newly produced viruses. After release, NA helps the virus to find the target cell despite the large amount of protein covered with sialic acids in the nasal mucus (235). Compared with influenza A, there is a very low quantity of NA at the surface of the influenza B viruses (approximately 60 proteins).

Matrix 2 Protein

Matrix 2 (M2) is a protein of influenza A viruses only (224,236). This protein has a ion channel activity. To be active, M2 molecules are organized as disulfide-linked tetramers, located as integral membrane proteins, with their N terminus expressed at the virus surface. They are encoded by a spliced mRNA from genome RNA segment 7, the virus (224). During acidification of the endosome, these tetramers form an ion channel between the interior of the virus and its environment, providing a low pH within the virus leading to uncoating. The active part of M2 in the ion channel is located in the 19 residue transmembrane domain.

BM2 Protein

The BM2 protein is an influenza B protein only (224). According to recent data, this protein also acts as an ion channel protein, with an organization different from M2.

Viral Infection and Pathogenic Mechanisms

The first step in cellular infection by influenza viruses is the attachment of the virus to its cellular receptor (224,226,230). These receptors are identical for influenza A and B viruses. This attachment is performed by interaction between the receptor binding site located at the end of the HA and the sialic acids of the target cell. Virus attachment depends on the recognition of the specific sialic acid by the receptor binding site (RBS) (230). There are sialic acids with different structures; the one recognized by human influenza viruses is linked to galactose by an α (2–3) linkage. This attachment mediates endocytosis. After

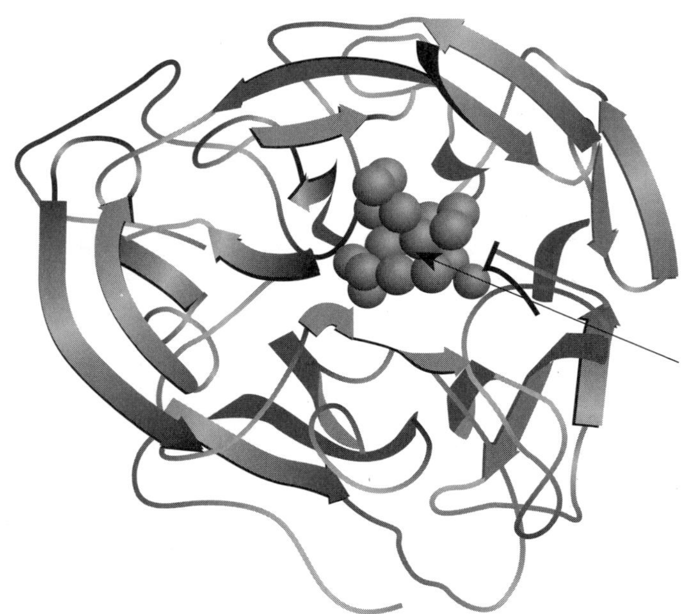

FIGURE 13.6 ● Structure of the neuraminidase (monomeric). Arrow shows sialic acid in the catalytic site of the neuraminidase.

endocytosis, the pH in the endosome is lowered, leading to HA conformational change and subsequent membrane fusion. The fusion peptide of several HA trimers intercalate into lipid bilayers to be efficient (230). Concomitantly, the M2 ion channel conducts H^+ ions inside the viral particle to allow uncoating and subsequent release of viral ribonucleo proteins (RNPs) in the cytoplasm of the infected cell and its transport to the nucleus. The eight vRNAs are then both transcribed into messenger RNAs and replicated.

Viral mRNA synthesis in the nucleus requires initiation by host cell primers. Replication of virion RNA occurs in two steps: the synthesis of the RNA template (full-length copies) and the copy of these templates into vRNAs. The switch from mRNA to vRNA synthesis has been intensively analyzed and is not yet fully understood (224,226). Viral mRNA is translated into viral proteins. HA, NA, and M2 are integral membrane proteins and hence are synthesized in the Golgi apparatus, while M1, NP, PA, PB1, PB2, NS1, and NEP are not. During synthesis in the Golgi apparatus, the M2 protein acts as an ion channel to prevent HA molecules from undergoing early, irreversible, pH-induced conformational changes of the HA. The synthesis of HA in the endoplasmic reticulum (ER) is a step-wise conformational maturation of the protein with independent folding of specific domains in the HA monomer. This is followed by trimerization of the uncleaved HA0 and the completion of the folding to a pH-neutral form of HA. Once properly assembled and folded, it is transported to the Golgi apparatus where oligosaccharide chains are added and HAO cleavage is performed. NA and M2 follow the same pathway and eventually are transported to the cell surface. These integral proteins are expressed at the cell surface, preferentially in the lipid raft microdomains, and can initiate viral budding.

The budding process starts by protein-protein interaction between intracellular domains of the NA, M2, and HA and M1 (237). Subsequently, viral RNPs assemble themselves as a structure of eight RNPs with one of each viral segment; this complex interacts with the M1 monolayer located at the budding area. This initiates the budding process with a proper packaging of eight RNA segments (238). NA is needed to release fully formed virions from the cell surface because these virions are covered with sialic acids and, hence, aggregate, and/or adhere to the cell surface. NA removes these HA-sialic acid links, releasing the viral particle (239). The release of the newly formed viral particles yields between 5 log and 6 log viral particles per milliliter of nasal mucus.

Antiviral Agents for Influenza in Clinical Use

Mechanism of Action of Anti–M2 Products: Amantadine and Rimantadine

The first description of an antiinfluenza activity of amantadine was reported in 1962. Since, the mechanism of action of amantadine and its derivative rimantadine has been analyzed (226). These products are very small molecules (Fig. 13.7) and are active against influenza A viruses only. Both drugs inhibit *in vitro* replication of influenza A viruses at concentrations achievable *in vivo*. The target site is the M2 ion channel protein

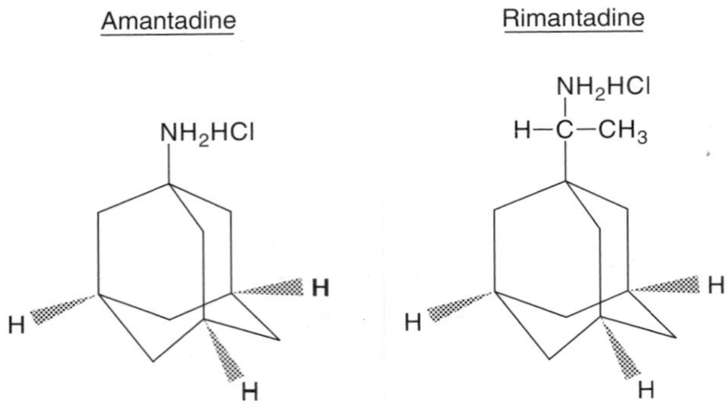

FIGURE 13.7 ● Chemical structure of amantadine (*left*) and rimantadine (*right*).

transmembrane domain (236). The ion channel activity is blocked by amantadine. As a result, M1 protein does not dissociate from the vRNPs (224,226). The drug has a second, late effect on some subtypes of influenza A virus whose HA undergoes fusion-conformational changes at relatively high pH. Amantadine can block the H+ transport from the trans Golgi. This can lead to premature conformational changes of the HA from lack of control of the pH in this intracellular compartment.

As demonstrated by analysis of resistant mutants, altered M2 proteins containing a change in the transmembrane domain display resistant phenotype to amantadine and rimantadine. Sequencing of RNA segment 7 from resistant isolates has demonstrated that nucleotide changes in the transmembrane domain, such as single nucleotide changes at residues 26, 27, 30, 31, and 34, can result in a resistant phenotype (226). Among clinical cases, the most frequent resistant mutation observed is in codon 31. All amino acid residues involved in resistance are located in the drug binding site.

The use of amantadine or rimantadine results in the frequent *emergence of resistant strains* (226,240). This resistance can be observed by day 2, and in up to 45% of treated patients by day 7. These resistant isolates are as contagious and infectious as the suseptible strains.

Both amantadine and rimantadine are available in oral formulation (226). The therapeutic regimen for both drugs is shown in Table 13.18.

These products have similar structures, but different pharmacokinetic patterns. Amantadine taken orally shows a plasmatic peak at 2 to 4 hours and more than 90% of the product is excreted unchanged in the urine. Plasma concentration after a 100-mg dose peaks at 0.2 to 0.3 mg/L, and at 0.5 to 0.7 mg/L with a 200-mg dose. Adequate antiviral levels are obtained in nasal mucus, lung, saliva, and cerebrospinal fluid with these regimens. In the elderly, the peak is twice as high, and excretion is reduced by 50%. Dosage adjustment is required in elderly patients and in patients with impaired renal function.

Rimantadine is also administered orally. The plasma peaks are lower and rimantadine is metabolized and excreted by the kidney; only 10% is excreted unchanged. The half-life is half that of amantadine. However, rimantadine concentration is higher in respiratory secretions.

Both products have frequent side effects; the adverse effects are mainly reported with amantadine. The side effects are frequently minor and include irritability, insomnia, and difficulty in concentrating. These side effects resolve on discontinuation of treatment. Severe adverse events are sometimes observed, including neurological disorders such as seizures and delirium. This type of side effect is less frequently observed with rimantadine.

In Vitro Testing of Anti-M2 Products

In vitro testing is done in cell culture. The first assay described was a plaque-inhibition assay (241). Depending on incubation periods, the plaque-reduction assay showed great variability in the results. Hence, alternative methods that can be easily standardized have been developed (242,243). These techniques are rapid, as compared with plaque-reduction assays, and use an automated colorimetric assay with antibodies that detect virus growth in the inoculated cells (243). Briefly, virus stocks of the tested strains are prepared in cells to obtain a virus titer of approximately 10^4 per milliliter. Each virus stock is subsequently prepared in serial dilutions ranging from 10^{-1} to 10^{-5}; these dilutions are tested against six antiviral concentrations ranging from 40 to 0.0026 μg/mL in fivefold dilutions. The assay is performed in a 96-well microtiter plate and uses a chess-board titration technique that allows simultaneous titration of the virus both in the absence and the presence of increasing antiviral doses (amantadine or rimantadine). Vero or MDCK (Madin-Darby canine kidney) cells can be used, the results obtained with both cells are similar. Table 13.19 provides a summary of the assays.

Briefly, the titrated virus (i.e., 10^4 per milliliter) is used for cell inoculation in 96-well microtiter plates. The microtiter plate is prepared by inoculating 15,000 cells per well. The plates are incubated for 2 days at 35°C with

TABLE 13.18

Amantadine and Rimantadine Treatment Regimens

Drug	Age (Years)			
	1–9	10–13	14–64	>65
Amantadine[a]				
Treatment	5 mg/kg/day, max 150 mg, 75 mg twice daily	100 mg, split in 50 mg twice daily[b]	100 mg, split in 50 mg twice daily[b]	100 mg, split in 50 mg twice daily[b]
Prophylaxis	5 mg/kg/day, max 150 mg, 75 mg twice daily	100 mg, split in 50 mg twice daily[b]	100 mg, split in 50 mg twice daily[b]	100 mg, split in 50 mg twice daily[b]
Rimantadine[c]				
Treatment	NA[d]	NA[d]	100 mg, split in 50 mg twice daily[b]	100 to 200 mg/day[e]
Prophylaxis	5 mg/kg/day, max 150 mg, 75 mg twice daily	100 mg, split in 50 mg twice daily[b]	100 mg, split in 50 mg twice daily[b]	100 to 200 mg/day[e]

[a] Reduce dosage if creatinine clearance is <50 mL/min.
[b] For children 10 to 40 kg, the appropriate dose is 5 mg/kg/day.
[c] Reduce dose to 100 mg/day in case of severe hepatic failure or if creatinine clearance is <10 mL/min.
[d] Not applicable.
[e] Reduce to 100 mg/day in the elderly when side effects are observed with 200 mg/d.

5% CO_2. The assay is performed; the culture medium is removed and 25 μL of the antiviral dilution, 25 μL of the calibrated virus suspension, and 200 μL of Eagle's minimum essential medium (EMEM) plus trypsine (final concentration, 2 μg/mL) are added to each well. Each test is performed in duplicate. After inoculation, the plates are centrifuged at 225 × g for 30 minutes. at room temperature. The plates are subsequently incubated at 35°C in a 5% CO_2 atmosphere for 20 hours for MDCK cells and 44 hours for Vero cells. Subsequently, the medium is removed from each well and the cells are fixed with 200 μL of 0.1% glutaraldehyde prepared in PBS. The fixation is performed for 15 minutes at 20°C. The wells are then washed with 500 μL of PBS. Virus protein detection is performed with a rabbit polyclonal antiserum to the A or B strain and is used to detect a wide range of influenza proteins. Briefly, 50 μL of rabbit antisera prepared in PBS plus 0.5% Bovine serum albumin (BSA) is added in each well and incubated for 90 minutes at 35°C. The wells are then washed with 500 μL of PBS. Next, 50 μL of protein A horseradish peroxidase conjugate is added and the mixture is incubated for 60 minutes at 35°C. The wells are subsequently washed with PBS and 100 μL of the substrate solution is added to reveal the reaction. The substrate is a 2,2-azino-di-(3-ethylbenzthiazoline) sulfonic acid prepared in ABTS buffer. The incubation is performed at 20°C for 60 minutes. The optical densities are read at 405 nm by using a multichannel spectrophotometer; the data provided are analyzed with a microcomputer. For each antiviral concentration, a curve is drawn with the optical density values obtained with the different virus concentrations. This curve is compared with the control without antiviral agents. The antiviral concentration providing a 50% reduction in the production of antigenic material as determined at the optimal virus suspension is the IC_{50} value. This value is calculated from the data provided with the tested antiviral concentrations (Fig. 13.8).

For strains sensitive to rimantadine, the IC_{50} range is from 0.02 to 1 μg/mL. The resistant strains have an IC_{50} ranging from 4 to 28 μg/mL.

Mechanism of Action of Neuraminidase Inhibitors: Zanamivir and Oseltamivir

As explained in the "Protein Function" section earlier, the influenza NA is a sialidase that has a role in the release of the newly assembled virions from infected cells (226,235). This enzyme cleaves the linkage between a terminal sialic acid and the adjacent D-galactose or D-galactosamine. It is responsible for 1) the removal of sialic acids and 2) the release of budding virions. It also enables the transport of the virus through the mucin layer of the respiratory tract to bind to the target epithelial cell.

TABLE 13.19

Summary of the Influenza Virus Amantadine and Rimantadine Assays[a]

	Assay in MDCK Cells	Assay in Vero Cells
Virus titration		
Titration of virus	10^4 per mL	10^4 per mL
Number of cells per well	15,000	15,000
Volume of virus and buffer	25 μL of the calibrated suspension in MEM	25 μL of the calibrated suspension in MEM
Colometric assay		
Volume of virus	25 μL of the calibrated suspension in MEM	25 μL of the calibrated suspension in MEM
Volume of inhibitor	25 μL diluted antiviral (prepared in MEM)	25 μL diluted antiviral (prepared in MEM)
Inhibitor concentration	0.0026–40 μg/mL	0.0026–40 μg/mL
Inhibitor preincubation	30 min at room temperature[b]	30 min at room temperature[b]
Atmospheric condition of the assay	35°C with 5% CO_2	35°C with 5% CO_2
Incubation	20 h at 37°C with 5% CO_2	44 h at 37°C with 5% CO_2
Fixation solution	200 μL of 0.1% glutaraldehyde in PBS 15 min at room temperature	200 μL of 0.1% glutaraldehyde in PBS 15 min at room temperature
Polyclonal antibody used	Rabbit PAb in PBS 0.5% BSA for 90 min at 35°C	Rabbit PAb in PBS 0.5% BSA for 90 min at 35°C
Conjugate	Protein A - horseradish peroxidase for 60 min at 35°C	Protein A - horseradish peroxidase for 60 min at 35°C
Substrate	ATBS[c] in ATBS buffer for 60 min at room temperature	ATBS[c] in ATBS buffer for 60 min at room temperature
Reading	405 nm wavelength	405 nm wavelength
Assay duration	26 h	50 h

[a] MEM, minimal essential medium; PBS, phosphate-buffered saline; BSA, Bovine Serum Albumin.
[b] This incubation is performed during a centrifugation step of 30 min at room temperature at 225 g.
[c] ATBS (Zymed, South San Francisco, CA).

The NA is a homotetramer, and each monomer harbors one catalytic site. This catalytic site is highly conserved among the different A subtypes and the B viruses.

It has long been postulated that a substrate analog inhibitor to sialidases may have antiviral activity (226,235,244,245). This competitive inhibition of NA may result in the inhibition of virus replication and spreading. Since 1999, two NA inhibitors have been licensed for use in several parts of the world and a third one is undergoing phase III clinical trial (235,246). These products have a chemical structure that mimicks a sialic acid (Figs. 13.9 and 13.10).

Both licensed compounds display very effective inhibition of the NA enzymatic activity. The antiviral NA interacts with amino acid residues of the catalytic pocket, especially glutamine 119, aspartate 151, arginine 152, glutamine 227, alanine 246, glutamine 276, and arginine 292. Mutations observed in these residues can confer resistance (245). To date, relatively few viruses with altered susceptibility to NA inhibitors have been identified. These viruses showed mutations in position 119, 152, 274, and 292. In some viruses, these mutations were associated with changes in the HA protein (246). They are beated in or near the receptor binding site and lead to a reduced affinity to sialic acids, to ease virion release when the sialidase activity of the NA is impaired because of mutations. However, reduced binding of HA may occur only for a specific subset of receptors. Receptors

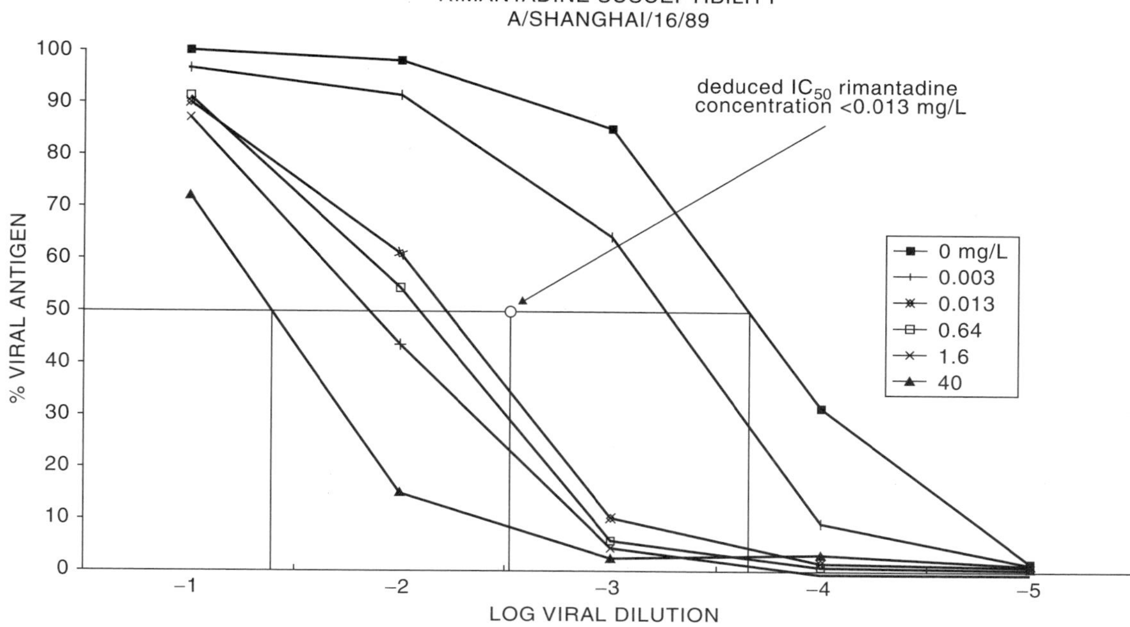

FIGURE 13.8 ● Rimantadine susceptibility.

on MDCK cells, which are most often used for influenza virus growth-inhibiton assays, have both α-2,3- and α-2,6-linked terminal sialic acid residues, whereas human cells have only α-2,6-linked sialic acids (224). Hence, this system may not detect a virus with decreased binding capacities to α-2,6-linked sialic acids.

Resistance has been observed in immunocompromised patients after 14 days of treatment (247). These viruses had reduced fitness and, when used for animal infection, they showed reduced infectivity and pathogenicity. The therapeutic regimen is shown in Table 13.20.

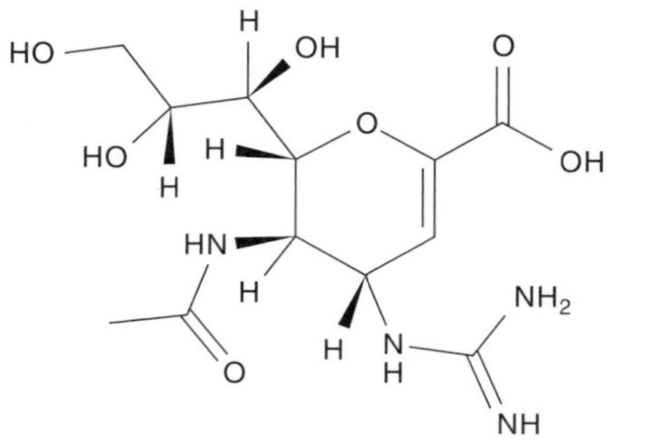

FIGURE 13.9 ● Chemical structure of zanamivir.

Zanamivir is administrated by oral or nasal aerosol. It is poorly absorbed (4% to 17%). It has a half-life of 3.4 hours and it has a bioavailability of 10% to 20% (248). After administration of a single 10-mg dose by using an inhaling device to administer the micronized formulation, the peak is observed at 2.5 hours with a concentration of 34 μg/L, and 78% of the active product is deposited in the oropharynx. As measured in different studies, the pharmacokinetic parameters after a single inhaled dose of 10 mg were area under curve (AUC), 247 μg/L · hour; t_{max}, 0.75 hours; $t_{1/2}$, 3.56 hours; C_{max}, 39 μg/L; and Cl_{ren}, 6.45 liters/hour. Zanamivir is not metabolized, and 90% is eliminated unmetabolized in the urine.

Oseltamivir is given by month. Oseltamivir phosphate (GS 4104) is an ethyl ester prodrug that is hydrolyzed by hepatic esterases to its active form, oseltamivir (GS 4071), specifically, oseltamivir carboxylate (Fig. 13.10). Absolute bioavailability is approximately 80%, with an elimination half-life of oseltamivir carboxylate of 6.7 to 8.2 hours. The prodrug is absorbed at 75%, with this form bound to serum proteins at 43%. Studies in healthy volunteers who received oral oseltamivir, 150 mg, and an intravenous infusion of oseltamivir, 150 mg, showed that the absolute bioavailability of oseltamivir (prodrug) was 79%, with a t_{max} of 5.0 hours and a maximum concentration of 456 μg/L. The metabolite (active drug) had an AUC of 6,834 μg/L · hour, t_{max} of 2.88 hours, V_d of 25.6 liters, $t_{1/2}$ of 1.79 hours, C_{max} of 2,091 μg/L,

TABLE 13.20

Zanamivir and Oseltamivir Treatment Regimens

Drug	Age (Years) 0–1	1–13	>14
Zanamivir[a]			
Treatment	NA[b]	NA	10 mg per day, 5 mg inhaled twice daily for 5 days
Prophylaxis	NA	NA	5 mg inhaled for 7 days
Oseltamivir[c]			
Treatment	NA	<15 kg 30 mg × 2/d 16–23 kg 45 mg × 2/d 23–40 kg 60 mg × 2/d >40 kg 75 mg × 2/d for 5 days	150 mg, split in 75 mg twice daily for 5 days
Prophylaxis	NA	<15 kg 30 mg 16–23 kg 45 mg 23–40 kg 60 mg >40 kg 75 mg for 7 days[d]	75 mg daily for 7 days

[a] Reduce dosage if creatinine clearance is <30 mL/min.
[b] Not applicable.
[c] Reduce dose to 75 mg/d in case creatinine clearance is <30 mL/min; NA if creatinine clearance is <10 mL/min.
[d] Possible seasonal prevention in unvaccinated at-risk patient groups.

Cl of 6.67 liters/hour, and a Cl_{ren} of 18.8 liters/hour, with approximately 93% excreted in the urine. Pharmacokinetics of the active metabolite appeared to be linear up to dose of 500 mg oseltamivir orally twice daily (248).

Both zanamivir and oseltamivir are well tolerated, with only minor side effects (249). However, because of the rare report of exacerbation of asthma in some young asthmatic patients, oseltamivir is not indicated in children with chronic asthma.

In Vitro Testing of Neuraminidase Inhibitors

Several assays are available and have been evaluated for testing NA inhibitors. Today, a cell-based assay is not convenient because of the presence of alternative virus receptors to the α-2,6-linked sugar that is exclusively observed in human cells (250). Enzyme inhibition assays that are not subject to receptor specificity have been developed. These assays can be performed in 96-well microtiter plates. They are biochemical assays developed to determine enzyme inhibition with a substrate that mimicks sialic acids. The most widely used substrate is the fluorogenic reagent 2′MUNANA (methyl umbelliferone *N*-acetyl aquaminic acid), initially described by Potier et al.

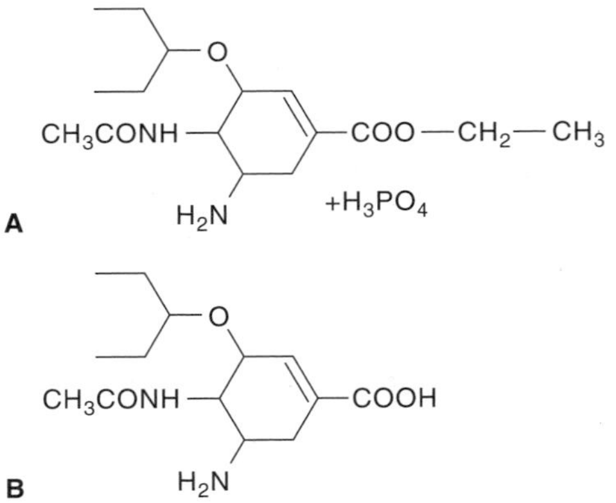

FIGURE 13.10 ● Chemical structures of the prodrug (oseltamivir [phosphate]) **(A)** and the active product (oseltamivir [carboxylate]) of oseltamivir **(B)**.

TABLE 13.21

Summary of the Influenza Virus Neuraminidase Inhibitor Assays

	Chemiluminescent Assay	Fluorometric Assay
Virus titration		
Volume of virus and buffer	50	20
Substrate	5 μL of NA-Star (100 μM)	50 μL of MUNANA (100 μL)
Titration conditions	15 min at 37°C, shaking	1 h at 37°C
Inhibition assay		
Signal-to-noise ratio	40:1	2:1
Volume of virus	40	25
Volume of inhibitor	40	25
Inhibitor concentration	0.028–550	0.0038–1000
Inhibitor preincubation	30 min at room temperature	15 min at 37°C
Substrate	5 μL of NA-Star (100 μM)	50 μL of MUNANA (100 μL)
Incubation	15 min at 37°C, shaking	1 h at 37°C
Stop solution	55 μL of Sapphire II enhancer	150 μL of 50 mM glycin adjusted to pH 10.4 with NaOH
Substrate half-life	5 min	hours
Assay duration	1 h	2 h, 15 min

The drawback of using fluorescent enzymatic assays is that evaluation of strains with poor enzymatic activity can be difficult. Therefore, an alternative chemiluminescent assay has been developed to overcome this problem (252), with a 1,2-dioxetane derivative of sialic acid [NA-Star (Tropix, Bedford, MA)]. Both assays must be performed with the active antivirals zanamivir and oseltamivir carboxylate. These assays are performed in 96-well microtiter plates at room temperature. Both procedures are summarized in Table 13.21.

Fluorometric Neuraminidase Assay Method

The fluorometric assay was first described by Potier et al. (250). The input virus used for the assay must be titrated by making serial twofold dilutions and then graphically determining the virus and enzyme concentrations, which fall into the linear part of the curve for the inhibition assay. A signal-to-noise ratio of 2 or more is considered optimal for use in the inhibition assay. Equal volumes of drug and the appropriate virus dilution are mixed and incubated for 15 minutes at room temperature on 96-well microtiter plates. The final drug concentration uses ranges from 0.0033 to 30,000 nM in serial 1:10 dilutions. The reaction is initiated by the addition of 100 μM MUNANA substrate solution prepared in 2-(*N*-morpholins) ethanesulfonic acid) (MES) buffer $CaCl_2$ (32.5 mM MES, pH 6.5, 4 mM $CaC1_2$). After 1 hour of incubation (37°C, with shaking), the reaction is stopped by the addition of 150 μL of a freshly prepared 50 mM glycin solution whose pH has been equilibrated to 10.4 with NaOH. This buffer is preferred to an alternative 0.14 M NaOH buffer prepared in 83% ethanol, which can result in precipitates in the reacting well.

In our laboratory, the influenza virus NA activity is assayed in the fluorometric test by using a modification of the technique described by Potier et al. (250). The MUN, 2′-(4-methylumbelliferyl)-α-D-*N*-acetylneuraminic acid, sodium salt (MW, 489.4; Sigma-Aldrich Chime), was used as substrate, and 32.5 mM MES [2-(*N*-morpholino) ethanesulfonic acid, sodium salt (MW, 217.2; Sigma-Aldrich Chime), pH 5.8, 4 mM $CaC1_2$] was chosen for the buffer. The 100-μM working solution of MUN was prepared in MES.

Detailed Neuraminidase Activity Assay

Reaction mixtures containing 25 μL of calibrated virus obtained by twofold dilutions, 25 μL of MES $CaC1_2$ and 50 μL of 100 μM MUN working solution are incubated in flat-bottom plates for 1 hour at 37°C. The reaction is terminated by the addition of 150 μL of 50 mM glycine buffer, pH 10.4.

Fluorescence was quantified in an MRX fluorometer (Dynex Technologies Ltd., Worthing, West Sussex, UK) with an excitation wavelength of 355 nm and an emission wavelength of 460 nm. Relative fluorescent units of sample were measured and corrected using the mean value of blank controls obtained when carrying out the reaction in the absence of virus.

The quantitation of NA activity was deduced from comparison of sample values with a standard curve established by using 4-methylumbelliferone (4-Mu) sodium salt. The equation establishing the correlation between free 4-Mu concentration and the amount of fluorescence is written as follows:

$$\text{A (nmol 4} - \text{Mu/hour/mL)} = 22.7\,10^{-3} \times \Delta\ \text{fluorescence} \times \text{dilution}^{-1}$$

(The constant value derived from the slope of the line.)

Detailed Neuraminidase Activity Inhibition Assay

A standard dose of virus (10 nmol/hour/mL) in 25 μL of MES buffer is preincubated with 25 μL of inhibitor dilution for 15 minutes at 37°C with shaking. After addition of 50 μL of 100 μM MUN working solution, the reaction mixture was incubated for 60 minutes at 37°C, with shaking. Finally, the reaction was terminated by adding 150 μL of 50 mM glycine buffer, pH 10.4. The IC_{50} values of inhibitors were further calculated as the inhibitor concentration required for reducing NA activity by 50%.

When used to determine NA activity inhibition assay, the values obtained with sensitive and resistant isolates were easy to interpret (Fig. 13.11). Values of IC_{50} are between 0.05 and 2 nM, with the resistant isolates displaying IC_{50} values beyond 50 nM.

Chemiluminescent Assay

The chemiluminescent assay was developed as an alternative to the fluorometric assay. It is decribed by Buxton et al. (252). It requires the growth of cells and virus in phenol red-free media, since residual phenol red can interfere with the assay. The virus is initially titrated in twofold dilutions in 32.5 MES (pH 6.0)-4 mM $CaCl_2$, and the signal-to-noise ratio of 40 is used for the dilution. Final drug concentrations ranged from 0.028 to 550 nM in serial 1:3 dilutions. The appropriate viral NA dilution (40 μL) was preincubated with 10 μL of drug for 30 minutes at room temperature on white Optiplates (Packard, Meridan, CT). The reaction was started by the addition of 5 μL of a 1:9 dilution of NA-Star prepared in 32.5 mM MES (pH 6.0)-4 mM $CaC1_2$. The final concentration of substrate used in the assay was 100 μM. The reaction mixture was incubated at 37°C for 15 minutes, with shaking. Chemiluminescent light emission was triggered by the addition of 55 μL of Light Emmission Accelerator II (Applied Biosystems) to each well. The half-life of the mixture is 5 minutes, which means that rapid automation is required to optimize sensitivity. All assay results were immediately read with an Applied Biosystems' NORTHSTAR Luminometer.

Fifty percent inhibitory concentration (IC_{50}) values were calculated by using the Robosage Microsoft Excel software add-in for curve fitting and calculation of IC_{50} values. The equation used for the calculation of IC_{50} values was $y = V_{max} \times (1\text{–}[x/K + x])$. This equation describes a simple hyperbolic inhibition curve with a zero baseline. In this equation, x is the inhibitor concentration, y is the response being inhibited (i.e., the velocity of an enzymatic reaction), and V_{max} is the limiting response as x approaches zero. As x increases without bound, y tends toward its lower limit, zero. K is the IC_{50} for the inhibition curve; that is, y is 50% V_{max} when $x = K$. Graphic presentations of the raw data are used to identify possible sources of variability and to characterize any patterns in the data (Fig. 13.11).

The results obtained with both chemiluminescent and fluorometric assays are consistent regarding the values for resistance thresholds in influenza A and B viruses. The IC_{50} values of the resistant isolates are beyond 20 nM for influenza A stains and beyond 40 nM for influenza B. Some differences are observed between IC_{50} values obtained with oseltamivir carboxylate and zanamivir.

Other Antiviral Agents

There are several other anti-M2 and NA inhibitors that attack other targets of influenza virus replication. Binding to cell membrane and penetration of influenza viruses are important stages in the process of virus replication, and several compounds that inhibit these functions have been reported. For example, a polyoxometalate (PM523) was shown to be a potent inhibitor of influenza A viruses by inhibition of membrane fusion between the virus envelope and the cellular membrane. During *in vitro* evaluation, strains had acquired resistance to PM523 by the introduction of mutations in the amino acid substrates in the HA1 head, and amino acid changes occurred in the interface peptide of the trimers of HA. Cap formation of influenza-encoded mRNA is unique; it uses 5′-mGpppXm of host mRNA. Several substances that inhibit this cap formation (namely, inhibitors of the PB2 enzyme activity) were also evaluated. This study is still in its very early stage and these products have yet to be examined for clinical use. Among the putative antiinfluenza agent, ribavirin has been evaluated and has shown some antiinfluenza activity. However, this product has been seldom used because of its toxicity. A metabolic product of ribavirin, 1,2,4-triazole carboxamide (T-CONH2), has been developed and seems to inhibit influenza A growth *in vitro*. Oral administration of TCONH2 also has shown therapeutic effect in an experimental mouse infection model of influenza A virus, as has ribavirin. TCONH2 seems to be less toxic than ribavirin for mice and may be useful as an alternative chemotherapy to ribavirin. No procedure for *in vitro* testing is yet available.

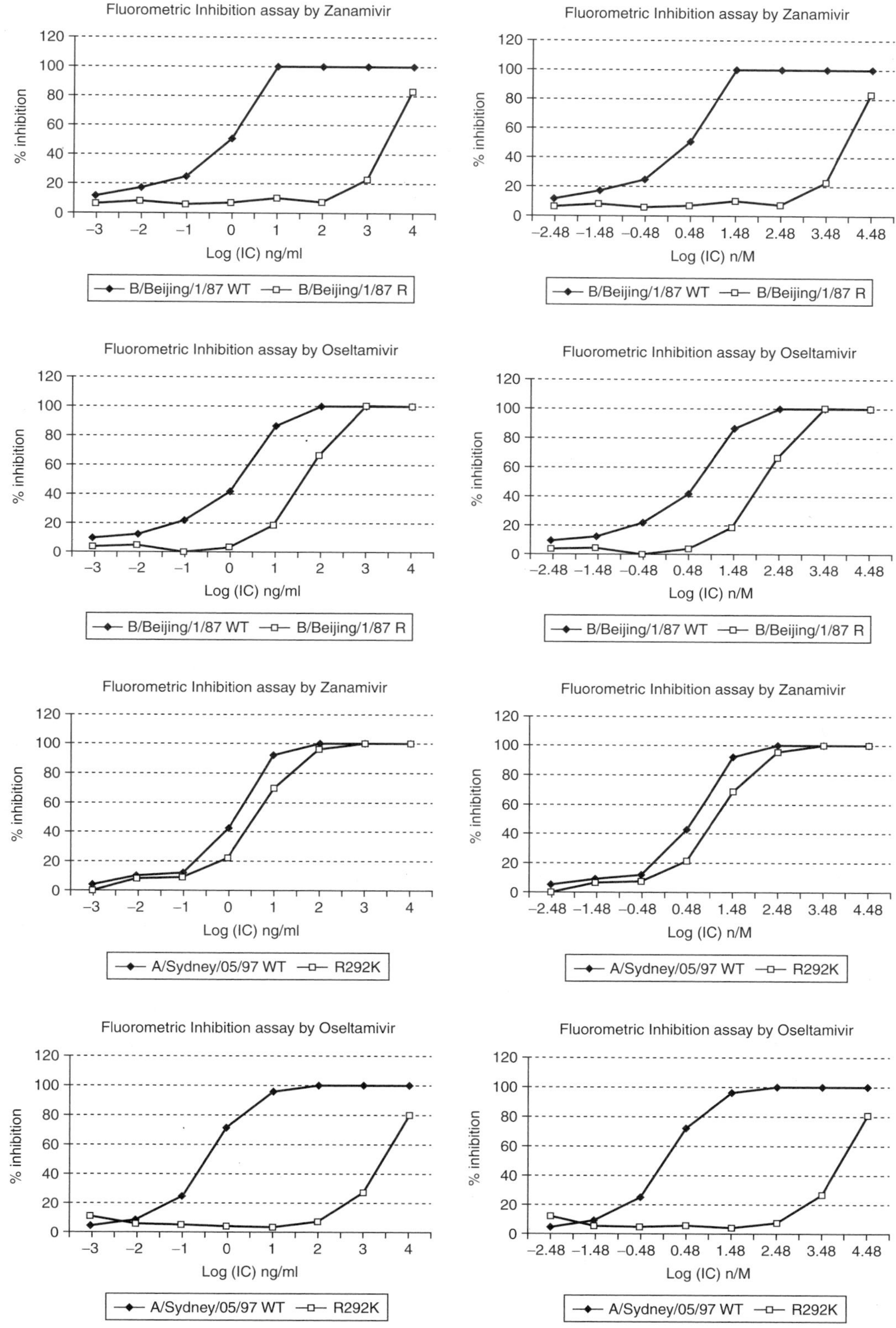

FIGURE 13.11 ● Neuraminidase activity inhibition assay.

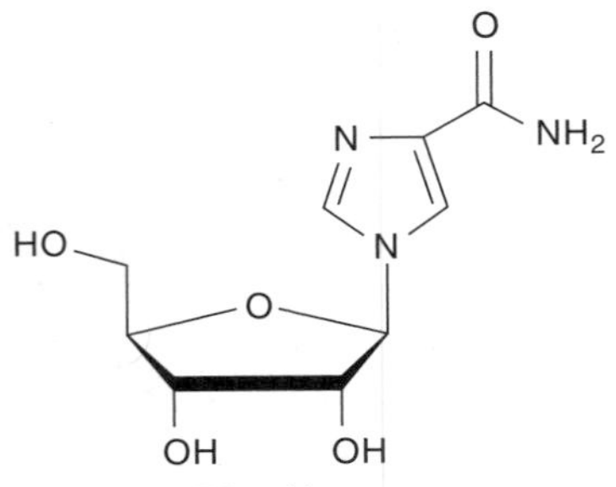

FIGURE 13.12 ● Chemical structure of ribavirin.

Ribavirin

Ribavirin is a synthetic nucleoside analog that has an antiviral activity against influenza A and B viruses (Fig. 13.12) (226,253,254). It inhibits cellular inosine-5′-monophosphate dehydrogenase activity, thereby depleting intracellular pools of guanosine 5′-triphosphate; the addition of guanosine can inhibit the antiviral effect of ribavirin. The phosphorylated ribavirin has a direct inhibitory effect on viral RNA-dependent RNA polymerase activity (254). This product has currently no defined role in the treatment or the prevention of influenza infections in humans. Its activity determined *in vitro* shows that virus growth is inhibited with the antiviral agent with inhibitory levels (3 to 6 μg/mL) that cannot be obtained *in vivo* with a single dose of 400 mg. Hence, this product has inconsistent effects when administered orally. However, when administered through an aerosol, it has a modest but detectable therapeutic effect. The aerosols have been associated with some toxicity, including reticulocytosis, rash, and conjunctivitis. In animals, this product is described as teratogenic, mutagenic, embryotoxic, and possibly carcinogenic (226,255). Its low *in vitro* activity combined with its high toxicity, plus the emergence of new therapeutic agents, make this product unsuitable for the treatment of influenza-related diseases.

In Vitro Testing

In vitro assays have been designed to test the susceptibility of influenza viruses to ribavirin. These assays are performed on cell cultures the procedure is similar to that described for amantadine and rimantadine *in vitro* testing. The cells have to be confluent and are grown in 96-well microtiter plates. The virus must be cultivated in the presence of 2 μg/mL of trypsin. MDCK cells are used for the assay. Cells are cultivated in EMEM supplemented with antibiotics and 10% fetal calf serum. The diluted viral suspensions are inoculated without fetal calf serum. After inoculation, the trays are centrifugated at 700×g for 5 to 30 minutes. The medium is subsequently substituted with a maintenance medium containing the appropriate concentration of the diluted compound (ribavirin). Usually, four to ten wells are used for each concentration. Tenfold serial dilutions of the virus to be tested, prepared in the maintenance medium, are inoculated onto the cell line. The culture plates are then incubated at 37°C in 5% CO_2 for 7 days, until development of cytopathic effect. The maintenance medium is changed at day 3. The evaluation of antiviral activity is based on the use of serial twofold dilutions of ribavirin starting at 200 μM. These antiviral dilutions are prepared in a maintenance medium. Three wells are used per ribavirin dilution. The average value of the EC_{50} for a sensitive strain is 34 μM.

Procedure for *In Vitro* Testing of the Susceptibility of Influenza A Viruses to Neuraminidase Inhibition Fluorometric Neuraminidase Assay Method

Influenza viruses are susceptible to NA inhibition. The fluorometric assay, described here, begins with the collection of nasal swab specimens. This procedure may be adapted to begin with nasal washes or throat swab specimens. Virus isolation must be performed on MDCK cells.

A. Isolation and Culture of Influenza Virus from Clinical Specimens

Clinical isolates are obtained by the culture of virus from clinical specimens on MDCK cells. Alternative culture systems for virus detection that have been proposed are less efficient than the MDCK cell system.

1. MDCK Cell Culture

MDCK cells can be purchased from Cambrex BioScience (Baltimore, MD) (ATCC, CCL34). Cells can be routinely passaged twice weekly in serum-free Ultra-MDCK medium (Cambrex BioScience, Walkersville, MD) supplemented with 2 mM L-glutamine (Sigma), penicillin (225 U/mL), and streptomycin (225 μg/mL) (Cambrex BioScience). Alternatively, the passage medium can be EMEM (Cambrex BioScience) with the same supplementation, and with 2 μ/mL trypsin (Boehringer, ref. 108819).

2. Virus Isolates

Swab samples are removed from the transport tube and expressed in 2.5 mL of EMEM, which has been supplemented with the antibiotic mix (penicillin plus streptomycin). The transport medium is then added. This suspension is inoculated onto MDCK subconfluent monolayers in 24-well microtiter plates. To promote growth of the influenza viruses, the microtiter plates are subsequently centrifuged at 300×g for 30 minutes (255a). The cells are then incubated at 33°C in 5% CO_2 atmosphere. At day 4, the monolayers are checked for cytopathic effect. The supernatant is collected and may be tested for HA activity or blindly passaged. The HA activity of the supernatant must reach a minimum titer of 16 to detect NA activity. At least two passages are necessary to obtain this titer on MDCK cell culture supernatants.

3. Virus Controls

In each assay, a reference-sensitive and reference-resistant isolate are included. (These controls are kindly provided by GlaxoSmithKline, Brentford, UK.) The resistant isolate has a specific resistant mutation in the NA gene (i.e., position R152). The susceptible isolates used were the ongoing vaccine prototype strains. When testing an isolate, the resistant and susceptible controls are from the same subtype. These reference strains are tested in the same conditions as the isolates.

B. Neuraminidase Activity Assay

Influenza virus NA activity is assayed in the fluorometric test by using a modification of the technique previously described by Potier et al. (250). The assay measures 4-methylumbelliferone released from the fluorogenic substrate 2′-MUN (MW, 489.4, Sigma Aldrich Chime) by the influenza virus NA.

1. Reagents

The *buffer* is 32.5 mL of 100 mM MES sodium salt (MW, 217.2; Sigma Aldrich Chime), pH 5.8, and 4 mL of 100 mM $CaCl_2$ made up to a 100-mL final volume with sterile water. Store at 4°C.

The *substrate mix* is 100-μM working solution of MUN prepared in 32.5 mM MES, pH 5.8, 4-mM $CaCl_2$ buffer. Store 500-μL aliquots of 5 mM MUN at −20°C and dilute 1:50 in 32.5 mM MES, pH 5.8, 4 mM $CaCl_2$ buffer immediately prior to assay. This substrate mix must be stored in the dark (wrapped in aluminum foil).

The *stop solution* is 50 mM glycine, pH 10.4 (Sigma Aldrich Chime). Store at 4°C.

2. Titration of Neuraminidase Activity

The assay is performed in 96-well flat-bottom plates to allow optical reading from the bottom. Prior to performing the titration, creation of a standard curve is necessary to control the linearity of the assay within the concentration range used. This is also performed in a 96-well flat-bottom plates.

Standard Curve

Free 4-methylumbelliferone can be used to generate a standard curve and to verify the linearity of the assay. The reagents are 4-methylumbelliferone, sodium salt (Sigma; M-1508, MW 198.2), and a stop solution of 50 mM glycine, pH 10.4 (Sigma Aldrich Chime). Store at 4°C.

For the reagent preparation of 5 mM of 4-methylumbelliferone stock solution, dissolve 9.91 mg in 10 mL of water. Store at 4°C in the dark for up to 2 months. For the preparation of 10 μM of 4-methylumbelliferone standard solution, dissolve 20 μL of stock solution into 10 mL of 50 mM glycine buffer, pH 10.4. Store at 4°C in the dark for up to 2 months. With the standard stock solution, prepare the dilution from 0.2 to 5 μM. Fluorescence is quantified in a Dynex MRX fluorometer with an excitation wavelength of 355 nm and an emission wavelength of 460 nm.

Testing of Isolates

The isolate testing is done in 96-well flat-bottom plates. The reagents are added as follows: 25 μL of serial twofold dilutions (from 1/2 to 1/2,048) of culture supernatant of the controls and the tested isolates (HA titer above 16) prepared in 32.5 mM MES, pH 5.8; 4 mM $CaCl_2$ buffer are added in columns 2 to 12. Then 25 μL of 32.5 mM MES, pH 5.8, and 4 mM $CaCl_2$ buffer are added to each well, except for the well of column 1 where the volume is 50 μL (reaction control). Fifty microliters of substrate are then added in every well to start the reaction. (A freshly made 100-μM working solution of MUN must be prepared in 32.5 mM MES, pH 5.8, and 4 mM $CaCl_2$ buffer.)

The contents of the plates are mixed gently on a mechanical vibrator. The plates are incubated for 1 hour at 37°C. The reaction is then stopped by adding 150 μL of 50 mM glycine buffer, pH 10.4, in each well. Fluorescence can be measured in a Dynex MRX fluorometer with an excitation wavelength of 355 nm and an emission wavelength of 460 nm. If the measure is delayed, the plate must be stored in the dark.

Relative fluorescent units of a sample are measured and corrected using the mean value of blank controls obtained when performing the reaction in the absence of the virus (column 1). The quantification of NA activity is deduced from comparison of sample values with a standard curve established by using 4-Mu sodium salt. The equation establishing the correlation between free 4-Mu concentration and the amount of fluorescence is as follows:

$$\text{A (nmol 4} - \text{Mu/hour/mL)} = 22.7\ 10^{-3} \times \Delta \text{ fluorescence} \times \text{dilution}^{-1}$$

(The constant value is derived from the slope of the line.) The A value obtained by this calculation is used to determine the input of the virus in the NA activity inhibition assay. This input must be 10 nmoL/hour/mL.

3. Neuraminidase Activity Inhibition Assay

The assay is done in 96-well flat-bottom plates to allow optical reading from the bottom. Reagents are added as described:

25 μL of tenfold dilutions of NA inhibitors prepared in 32.5 mM MES, pH 5.8, 4 mM $CaCl_2$ buffer (from 30,000 to 0.003 nM) are added in the wells from columns 1 to 8. Column 9 is used to determine the blank value and contains 50 μL of 32.5 mM MES, pH 5.8, and 4 mM $CaCl_2$ buffer. Twenty-five microliters of a standard dose of virus or control (10 nmoL/hour/mL, as determined in the titration of NA activity) prepared in 32.5 mM MES, pH 5.8, 4 mM $CaCl_2$ buffer is added to each well except well 9. Wells 10 to 12 are used as a control of the standard dose.

The contents of the plates are gently mixed on a mechanical vibrator. The plates are incubated for 15 minutes at 37°C. Then 50 μL of substrate is added in each well to start the reaction. (A freshly made 100-μM working solution of MUN is prepared in 32.5 mM MES, pH 5.8, and 4 mM $CaCl_2$ buffer.) The contents of the plates are gently mixed on a mechanical vibrator and the plates are incubated for 1 hour at 37°C. The reaction is then stopped by adding 150 μL of 50 mM glycine buffer, pH 10.4, in all wells. Fluorescence is immediately quantified by using a Dynex MRX fluorometer with an excitation wavelength of 355 nm and an emission wavelength of 460 nm.

If this measurement is delayed, the plates must be stored in the dark. The IC_{50} values of antiviral agents are calculated according to the concentration required for reducing NA activity by 50%.

CORONAVIRUS RESPONSIBLE FOR SARS

Description of the Virus and Mechanism of Pathogenicity

The severe acute respiratory syndrome (SARS)-related virus was identified as the result of collaborative work among several laboratories. The discovery that a novel coronavirus was the cause of the newly recognized SARS was simultaneously reported by Ksiazek et al. (255) and Drosten et al. This virus was isolated on a specific Vero cell line, the Vero E6 line (256). This virus is one of the most lethal respiratory viruses ever isolated (approximately 10% of the infected persons died of this infection).

Since the global outbreak, the virus has been intensely analyzed, showing that it very likely emerged from a still-unknown animal reservoir (257). Its genetic features revealed a new coronavirus. Despite numerous efforts, no specific treatment has yet been identified for SARS. However, attempts are being made to identify antiviral agents that could be effective in treating the SARS-coronavirus (CoV) infection, and empirical therapeutic regimens have been tried (256,258). The most widely used therapy has been ribavirin. As described previously, this drug has the putative ability to block RNA polymerases and, hence, it may have some benefit for patients infected with SARS-CoV. What can we learn from the literature that has been published internationally that mentions antiviral treatment of SARS? Some studies have reported the clinical outcomes of patients receiving either ribavirin therapy or a combined ribavirin and steroid therapy. Despite reports in which ribavirin was considered to have had some benefit, its effectiveness in the treatment of SARS remains controversial. Randomized clinical studies showed that the drug, given at a low dose (400 to 600 mg/day), was basically ineffective (258,259). Moreover, *in vitro* data showed no effect of ribavirin on the replication of SARS-CoV. However, the nonrandomized studies suggest that the combined treatments, including ribavirin plus steroids and/or interferon, given at quite different doses, might have been effective to some extent. The limited data available suggest that (a) doses lower than 1 g/day are likely to be ineffective and (b) doses of about 2 g/day might not cause severe adverse reactions and might be effective. Therefore, these doses should be considered for further studies if this virus reemerges (257).

Antiviral Agents Presently in Clinical Use

Measurement of *in vitro* susceptibility of SARS-coronavirus to antiviral agents has been done. All assays were performed on cell culture. These assays must be performed in a BioSafely Level (BSL3) facility. The cells used for SARS-CoV culture are Vero E6 cells (260). The antiviral potential of recombinant interferons α, β, and γ has been evaluated against two clinical isolates of SARS-CoV (FFM-1 and Hong Kong) (261). Scored cytopathogenic effects induced by the virus 72 hours after infection in 96-well microplates on confluent layers of Vero E6 cells treated with interferons 24 hours prior to and immediately after virus infection have been measured (mutiplicity of infection 0:01). The selectivity index was defined by the authors as the ratio of the concentration of the interferon that reduced cell viability to 50% (CC_{50}) to the concentration of the compound needed to inhibit the cytopathic effect to 50% of control value (EC_{50}). Interferon β was the most potent inhibitor of SARS-CoV. In Vero cells, the selectivity index of interferon β activity for SARS-CoV strain FFM-1 was 50-fold and 25-fold higher than that of interferon α and interferon γ, respectively. The susceptibility of the Hong Kong isolate was similar to that of the FFM-1 strain. Interferon β (EC_{50}, 105 IU/mL) was more potent than interferons α or γ (EC_{50} 6,500 and 1,700 IU/mL, respectively).

Other products have also been evaluated as antiviral therapy; one such product is glycyrrhizin (262). The mechanism of glycyrrhizin's activity against SARS-CoV is unclear. Glycyrrhizin is known to affect cellular signaling pathways such as protein kinase C, casein kinase II, and transcription factors (activator protein 1 and nuclear factor κB). Furthermore, glycyrrhizin and its main metabolite are known to up-regulate expression of inducible nitric oxide synthase and production of nitric oxide in macrophages (263). This induction of nitric oxide synthase by glycyrrhizin is observed in Vero cells, and virus replication is inhibited when the nitric oxide donor (DETA NONOate) is added to the culture medium (263).

In addition to inhibition of virus replication, glycyrrhizin also inhibits adsorption and penetration of the virus, both early steps of the replicative cycle. The assay was performed as follows: confluent Vero cells were infected with a calibrated suspension of SARS-CoV (262). After 72 to 96 hours of infection, the cells were fixed with 60 parts methanol to 40 parts acetone. Virus growth was detected by specific peroxidase staining using a patient serum. Infected cells were treated with 1,000 or

4,000 mg/L of glycyrrhizin. Expression of viral antigens was much lower in cultures treated with 1,000 mg/L of glycyrrhizin than in any other culture; high concentrations of glycyrrhizin (4,000 mg/L) completely blocked replication of the virus. Glycyrrhizin was less effective when added during the adsorption period than when added after virus adsorption (EC_{50}, 600 vs. 2,400 mg/L, respectively). Glycyrrhizin was most effective when given both during and after the adsorption period (EC_{50}, 300 mg/L).

The antiviral activities of mycophenolic acid have been evaluated against two clinical isolates of coronavirus (FFM-1 and FFM-2) from patients with SARS in Germany. The findings showed that mycophenolic acid had no effect on SARS-CoV replication *in vitro* (261).

REFERENCES

1. Durant J, Clevenbergh P, Halfon P, et al. Drug-resistance genotyping in HIV-1 therapy: the VIRADAPT randomised controlled trial. *Lancet* 1999:353(9171):2195–2199.
2. Hirsch MS, Brun-Vezinet F, Clotet B, et al. Antiretroviral drug resistance testing in adults infected with human immunodeficiency virus type 1: 2003 Recommendations of an International AIDS Society–USA Panel. *Clin Infect Dis* 2003;37:113–128.
3. The Euroguidelines Group for HIV resistance. Clinical and laboratory guidelines for the use of HIV-1 drug resistance testing as part of treatment management: recommendations for the European setting. *AIDS* 2001;15: 309–320.
4. Demeter L, Haubrich R J. Phenotypic and genotypic resistance assays: methodology, reliability, and interpretations. *J Acquir Immune Defic Syndr* 2001;26(Suppl 1):S3–S9.
5. Shafer RW. Genotypic testing for human immunodeficiency virus type 1 drug resistance. *Clin Microbiol Rev* 2002;2:247–277.
6. Vandamme AM, Houyez F, Banhegyi D, et al. Laboratory guidelines for the practical use of HIV drug resistance tests in patient follow-up. *Antivir Ther* 2001;6:21–39.
7. Japour AJ, Fiscus SA, Arduino JM, et al. Standardized microtiter assay for determination of syncytium-inducing phenotypes of clinical human immunodeficiency virus type 1 isolates. *J Clin Microbiol* 1994;32:2291–2294.
8. Brun-Vézinet F, Ingrand D, Deforges L, et al. HIV-1–1 sensitivity to zidovudine: a consensus culture technique validated by genotypic analysis of the reverse transcriptase. *J Virol Methods* 1992;37:177–188.
9. Kellam P, Larder BA. Recombinant virus assay: a rapid, phenotypic assay for assessment of drug susceptibility of human immunodeficiency virus type 1 isolates. *Antimicrob Agents Chemother* 1994;38:23–30.
10. Petropoulos CJ, Parkin NT, Limoli KL, et al. A novel phenotypic drug susceptibility assay for human immunodeficiency virus type–1. *Antimicrob Agents Chemother* 2000;44:920–928.
11. Whitcomb JM, Huang W, Fransen S, et al. Analysis of baseline Enfuvirtide (T20) susceptibility and co-receptor tropism in two-phase III study populations. *Proceedings of 10th conference on retrovirus and opportunistic infections*, Boston, MA, Feb 10–14, 2003. Abstract 557.
12. Qari SH, Respess R, Weinstock H, et al. Comparative analysis of two commercial phenotypic assays for drug susceptibility testing of human immunodeficiency virus type 1. *J Clin Microbiol* 2002;40:31–35.
13. Sanger F, Nicklen S, Coulson AR. DNA sequencing with chain terminating inhibitors. *Proc Natl Acad Sci USA* 1977;74:5463–5467.
14. Servais J, Lambert C, Fontaine E, et al. Comparison of DNA sequencing and a line probe assay for detection of human immunodeficiency virus type 1 drug resistance mutations in patients failing highly active antiretroviral therapy. *J Clin Microbiol* 2001;39:454–459.
15. Vahey M, Nau ME, Barrick S, et al. Performance of the Affymetrix GeneChip HIV PRT 440 platform for antiretroviral drug resistance genotyping of human immunodeficiency virus type 1 clades and viral isolates with length polymorphisms. *J Clin Microbiol* 1999;37:2533–2537.
16. Hanna GJ, Johnson VA, Kuritzkes DR, et al. Comparison of sequencing by hybridization and cycle sequencing for genotyping of human immunodeficiency virus type 1 reverse transcriptase. *J Clin Microbiol* 2000;38:2715–2721.
17. Shafer RW, Hertogs K, Zolopa AR, et al. High degree of interlaboratory reproducibility of human immunodeficiency virus type 1 protease and reverse transcriptase sequencing of plasma samples from heavily treated patients. *J Clin Microbiol* 2001;39:1522–1529.
18. Demeter LM, D'Aquila R, Weislow O, et al. Interlaboratory concordance of DNA sequence analysis to detect reverse transcriptase mutations in HIV-1 proviral DNA. ACTG Sequencing Working Group. AIDS Clinical Trials Group. *J Virol Methods* 1998;75:93–104.
19. Schuurman R, Demeter L, Reichelderfer P, et al. Worldwide evaluation of DNA sequencing approaches for identification of drug resistance mutations in the human immunodeficiency virus type 1 reverse transcriptase. *Clin Microbiol* 1999;37:2291–2296.
20. Schuurman R, Brambilla D, de Groot T, et al. Underestimation of HIV type 1 drug resistance mutations: results from the ENVA-2 genotyping proficiency program. *AIDS Res Hum Retroviruses* 2002;18:243–248.
21. Sayer DC, Land S, Gizzarelli L, et al. Quality assessment program for genotypic antiretroviral testing improves detection of drug resistance mutations. *J Clin Microbiol* 2003;41:227–236.
22. Brun-Vézinet F, Masquelier B, Izopet J, et al. Quality control assessment for HIV-1 genotypic antiretroviral testing (2002). *Antivir Ther* 2003;8:S99.
23. Kempf DJ, Isaacson JD, King MS, et al. Analysis of the virological response with respect to baseline viral phenotype and genotype in protease inhibitor-experienced HIV-1-infected patients receiving lopinavir/ritonavir therapy. *Antivir Ther* 2002;7:165–174.
24. Lanier ER, Hellmann N, Scott J, et al. Determination of a clinically relevant phenotypic resistance cut-off for abacavir using the PhenoSense assay. *Proceedings of the 8th conference on retrovirus and opportunistic infections*, Chicago, IL, Feb 4–8, 2001. Abstract 254.
25. Margot NA, Isaacson E, McGowan I, et al. Genotypic and phenotypic analyses of HIV-1 in antiretroviral-experienced patients treated with tenofovir DF. *AIDS* 2002;16:1227–1235.
26. Katzenstein DA, Bosch RJ, Wang N, et al. Baseline phenotypic suceptibility and virological failure over 144 weeks among NRTI experienced subjects in ACTG 364. *Proceedings of the 9th conference on retrovirus and opportunistic infections*, Seattle, WA, Feb 24–28, 2002. Abstract 591.
27. Shulman NS, Hughes MD, Winters MA, et al. Subtle decreases in stavudine phenotypic susceptibility predict poor virologic response to stavudine monotherapy in

zidovudine-experienced patients. *J Acquir Immune Defic Syndr* 2002;31:121–127.
28. Whitcomb JM, Huang W, Limoli K, et al. Hypersusceptibility to nonnucleoside reverse transcriptase inhibitors in HIV-1: clinical, phenotypic and genotypic correlates. *AIDS* 2002;16:F41–F47.
29. Katzenstein DA, Bosch RJ, Hellmann N, et al. Phenotypic susceptibility and virological outcome in nucleoside-experienced patients receiving three or four antiretroviral drugs. *AIDS* 2003;17:821–830.
30. Haubrich R, Keiser P, Kemper C, et al. CCTG 575: a randomised, prospective study of phenotype versus standard of care for patients failing antiretroviral therapy. *Antivir Ther* 2001;6(Suppl 1):63.
31. Meynard JL, Vray M, Morand-Joubert L, et al. Phenotypic or genotypic resistance testing for choosing antiretroviral therapy after treatment failure: a randomized trial. *AIDS* 2002;16:727–736.
32. Brun-Vézinet F, Descamps D, Ruffault A, et al. Clinically relevant interpretation of genotype for resistance to abacavir. *AIDS* 2003;17:1795–1802.
33. Calvez V, Costagliola D, Descamps D, et al. Impact of stavudine phenotype and thymidine analogue mutations on viral response to stavudine plus lamivudine in ALTIS 2 ANRS trial. *Antivir Ther* 2002;7:211–218.
34. Shulman NS, Machekano RA, Shafer RW, et al. Genotypic correlates of a virologic response to stavudine after zidovudine monotherapy. *J Acquir Immune Defic Syndr* 2001;27:377–380.
35. Descamps D, Masquelier B, Mamet JP, et al. A genotypic sensitivity score for amprenavir based on genotype at baseline and virological response. *Antivir Ther* 2001; 6:S59.
36. Masquelier B, Breilh D, Neau D, et al. Human immunodeficiency virus type 1 genotypic and pharmacokinetic determinants of the virological response to lopinavir-ritonavir-containing therapy in protease inhibitor-experienced patients. *Antimicrob Agents Chemother* 2002;46:2926–2932.
37. Calvez V, Cohen-Codar I, Marcelin AG, et al. Identification of individual mutations in HIV protease associated with virological response to lopinavir/ritonavir therapy. *Antivir Ther* 2001;6 (Suppl 1):64.
38. Van Laethem K, De Luca A, Antinori A, et al. A genotypic drug resistance interpretation algorithm that significantly predicts therapy response in HIV-1-infected patients. *Antivir Ther* 2002;7:123–129.
39. Tural C, Ruiz L, Holtzer C, et al. Clinical utility of HIV-1 genotyping and expert advice: the Havana trial. *AIDS* 2002;216:209–218.
40. Ravela J, Betts BJ, Brun-Vezinet F, et al. HIV-1 protease and reverse transcriptase mutation patterns responsible for discordances between genotypic drug resistance interpretation algorithms. *J Acquir Immune Defic Syndr* 2003;33:8–14.
41. De Luca A, Cingolani A, Di Giambenedetto S, et al. Variable prediction of antiretroviral treatment outcome by different systems for interpreting genotypic human immunodeficiency virus type 1 drug resistance. *J Infect Dis* 2003;187:1934–1943.
42. Schmidt B, Walter H, Schwingel E, et al. Comparison of different interpretation systems for genotypic HIV-1 drug resistance data. *Antivir Ther* 2001;6(Suppl 1):102.
43. Larder BA, Kemp SD, Hertogs K. Quantitative prediction of HIV-1 phenotypic drug resistance from genotypes: the virtual phenotype (*Virtual*Phenotype). *Antivir Ther* 2000;5(Suppl 3):49–50.
44. Perez-Elias MJ, Garcia I, Munoz V. A randomized prospective study of phenotype (P) versus virtual phenotype (virtualP) testing for patients failing antiretroviral therapy. *Proceedings of the 42nd Interscience Conference on Antimicrobial Agents*, San Diego, CA, Sep 27–30, 2002. Abstract H-1079.
45. Parkin N, Chappey C, Maroldo L, et al. Phenotypic and genotypic HIV-1 drug resistance assays provide complementary information. *J Acquir Immune Defic Syndr* 2002;31:128–136.
46. Brun-Vézinet F, Race E, Descamps D, et al. Difference between genotype and phenotype in the Narval trial, ANRS 088. *Antivir Ther* 2000;5 (Suppl 3):78.
47. Bacheler L, Jeffrey S, Hanna G, et al. Genotypic correlates of phenotypic resistance to efavirenz in virus isolates from patients failing nonnucleoside reverse transcriptase inhibitor therapy. *J Virol* 2001;75:4999–5008.
48. Falloon J, Ait-Khaled M, Thomas DA, et al. HIV-1 genotype and phenotype correlate with virological response to abacavir, amprenavir and efavirenz in treatment-experienced patients. *AIDS* 2002;16:387–396.
49. Hsu A, Isaacson J, Brun S, et al. Pharmacokinetic-pharmacodynamic analysis of lopinavir-ritonavir in combination with efavirenz and two nucleoside reverse transcriptase inhibitors in extensively pretreated human immunodeficiency virus-infected patients. *Antimicrob Agents Chemother* 2003;47:350–359.
50. Shulman N, Zolopa A, Havlir D, et al. Virtual inhibitory quotient predicts response to ritonavir boosting of indinavir-based therapy in human immunodeficiency virus-infected patients with ongoing viremia. *Antimicrob Agents Chemother* 2002;46:3907–3916.
51. Marcelin AG, Lamotte C, Delaugerre C, et al. Genotypic inhibitory quotient as predictor of virological response to ritonavir-amprenavir in human immunodeficiency virus type 1 protease inhibitor-experienced patients. *Antimicrob Agents Chemother* 2003;47:594–600.
52. Perelson AS, Neumann AU, Markovitz M, et al. HIV-1 dynamics in vivo: virion clearance rate, infected cell life-span, and viral generation time. *Science* 1996;271:1582–1586.
53. Weinstein MC, Goldie SJ, Losina E, et al. Use of genotypic resistance testing to guide HIV therapy: clinical impact and cost effectiveness. *Ann Intern Med* 2001;134:440–450.
54. Larder BA, Kohli A, Kellam P, et al. Quantitative detection of HIV-1 drug resistance mutations by automated DNA sequencing. *Nature* 1993;365:671–673.
55. Gunthard HF, Wong JK, Ignacio CC, et al. Comparative performance of high density oligonucleotide sequencing and dideoxynucleotide sequencing of HIV type 1 pol from clinical samples. *AIDS Res Hum Retroviruses* 1998;14:869–876.
56. Shafer RW, Warford A, Winters MA, et al. Reproducibility of human immunodeficiency virus type 1 (HIV-1) protease and reverse transcriptase sequencing of plasma samples from heavily treated HIV-1 infected individuals. *J Virol Methods* 2000;86:143–153.
57. D'Aquila RT. Limits of resistance testing. *Antivir Ther* 2000;5:71–76.
58. Charpentier C, Dwyer DE, Lecossier D, et al. Co-evolution and competition of viral populations with distinct resistance genotypes in patients failing treatment with protease inhibitors. *Antivir Ther* 2002;7:S42.
59. Moser MJ, Sharma PL, Nurpeisov V, et al. Using GENE-CODE technology to detect early emerging populations of drug-resistant human immunodeficiency virus Type 1. *Proceedings of the XII International HIV Drug Resistance*

workshop: Basic Principles and Clinical Implications. Los Cabos, Mexico, Jun 10–14, 2003. Abstract 89.

60. Simmonds P, Zhang LQ, McOmish F, et al. Discontinuous sequence change of human immunodeficiency virus (HIV) type 1 env sequences in plasma viral and lymphocyte-associated proviral populations in vivo: implications for models of HIV pathogenesis. *J Virol* 1991;65:6266–6276.
61. Smith MS, Koerber KL, Pagano JS. Zidovudine-resistant human immunodeficiency virus type 1 genomes detected in plasma distinct from viral genomes in peripheral blood mononuclear cells. *J Infect Dis* 1993;167:445–448.
62. Wei X, Ghosh SK, Taylor ME, et al. Viral dynamics in human immunodeficiency virus type 1 infection. *Nature* 1995;373:117–122.
63. Koch N, Yahi N, Ariasi F, et al. Comparison of human immunodeficiency virus type 1 (HIV-1) protease mutations in HIV-1 genomes detected in plasma and in peripheral blood mononuclear cells from patients receiving combination drug therapy. *J Clin Microbiol* 1999;37:1595–1597.
64. Tashima KT, Flanigan TP, Kurpewski J, et al. Discordant human immunodeficiency virus type 1 drug resistance, including K103N, observed in cerebrospinal fluid and plasma. *Clin Infect Dis* 2002;35:82–83.
65. Ghosn J, Viard JP, De Almeida M, et al. HIV-1 resistance pattern may be frequently different than in blood in the male genital compartment of patients with therapeutic failure. *Antivir Ther* 2002;7:S46.
66. Solas C, Lafeuillade A, Halfon P, et al. Discrepancies between protease inhibitor concentrations and viral load in reservoirs and sanctuary sites in human immunodeficiency virus-infected patients. *Antimicrob Agents Chemother* 2003;47:238–243.
67. Marlowe N, Swanson P, Drews B, et al. Performance of Celera Diagnostics ViroSeq HIV-1 genotyping system on genetically diverse HIV-1 strains. *Proceedings of the 10th conference on retroviruses and opportunistic infections.* Boston, MA, Feb 10–14, 2003. Abstract 582.
68. Jagodzinski LL, Cooley JD, Weber M, et al. Performance characteristics of human immunodeficiency virus type 1 (HIV-1) genotyping systems in sequence-based analysis of subtypes other than HIV-1 subtype B. *J Clin Microbiol* 2003;41:998–1003.
69. Beddows S, Galpin S, Kazmi SH, et al. Performance of two commercially available sequence-based HIV-1 genotyping systems for the detection of drug resistance against HIV type 1 group M subtypes. *J Med Virol* 2003;70:337–342.
70. Beasley RP, Lin C-C, Hwang LY, et al. Hepatocellular carcinoma and hepatitis B virus: a prospective study of 22,707 men in Taiwan. *Lancet* 1981;2:1129–1133.
71. Rehermann B, Fowler P, Sidney J, et al. The cytotoxic T lymphocyte response to multiple hepatitis B virus polymerase epitopes during and after acute viral hepatitis. *J Exp Med* 1995;181:1047–1058.
72. Rehermann B, Lau D, Hoofnagle JH, et al. Cytotoxic T lymphocyte responsiveness after resolution of chronic hepatitis B virus infection. *J Clin Invest* 1996;97:1655–1665.
73. Guidotti LG, Chisari FV. To kill or to cure: options in host defense against viral infection. *Curr Opin Immunol* 1996;8:478–483.
74. Lok AS, Heathcote EJ, Hoofnagle JH. Management of hepatitis B: summary of a workshop. *Gastroenterology* 2001;120:1828–1853.
75. Ganem D, Schneider R. Hepadnaviridae: the viruses and their replication. In: Knipe DM, Howley PM, eds. *Fields virology.* Philadelphia: Lippincott-Williams & Wilkins, 2001;2923–2970.
76. Kann M, Gerlich W. Hepadnaviridae: structure and molecular virology. In: Zuckerman A, Thomas H, eds. *Viral hepatitis.* London: Churchill Livingstone, 1998;77–105.
77. Kao JH. Clinical relevance of hepatitis B viral genotypes: a case of déjà vu? *J Gastroenterol Hepatol* 2002;17:113–115.
78. Kao JH. Hepatitis B viral genotypes: clinical relevance and molecular characteristics. *J Gastroenterol Hepatol* 2002;17:643–650.
79. Kao JH, Liu CJ, Chen DS. Hepatitis B viral genotypes and lamivudine resistance. *J Hepatol* 2002;36:303–304.
80. Sugauchi F, Orito E, Ichida T, et al. Hepatitis B virus of genotype B with or without recombination with genotype C over the precore region plus the core gene. *J Virol* 2002;76:5985–5992.
81. Owiredu WK, Kramvis A, Kew MC. Hepatitis B virus DNA in serum of healthy black African adults positive for hepatitis B surface alone: possible association with recombination between genotypes A and D. *J Med Virol* 2001;64:441–454.
82. Will H, Reiser W, Weimer T, et al. Replication strategy of human hepatitis B virus. *J Virol* 1987;61:904–911.
83. Okamoto H, Imai M, Kametani M, et al. Genomic heterogeneity of hepatitis B virus in a 54-year-old woman who contracted the infection through maternal fetal transmission. *Jpn J Exp Med* 1987;57:231–236.
84. Gunther S, Fischer L, Pult I, et al. Naturally occurring variants of hepatitis B virus. *Adv Virus Res* 1999;52:25–137.
85. Zhang YY, Summers J. Enrichment of a precore-minus mutant of duck hepatitis B virus in experimental mixed infections. *J Virol* 1999;73:3616–3622.
86. Zhang YY, Summers J. Low dynamic state of viral competition in a chronic avian hepadnavirus infection. *J Virol* 2000;74:5257–5265.
87. Doo E, Liang TJ. Molecular anatomy and pathophysiologic implications of drug resistance in hepatitis B virus infection. *Gastroenterology* 2001;120:1000–1008.
88. Seeger C, Mason WS. Hepatitis B virus biology. *Microbiol Mol Biol Rev* 2000;64:51–68.
89. Lok AS, Akarca U, Greene S. Mutations in the pre-core region of hepatitis B virus serve to enhance the stability of the secondary structure of the pre-genome encapsidation signal. *Proc Natl Acad Sci USA* 1994;91:4077–4081.
90. Liang TJ, Hasegawa K, Rimon N, et al. A hepatitis B virus mutant associated with an epidemic of fulminant hepatitis. *N Engl J Med* 1991;324:1705–1709.
91. Omata M, Ehata T, Yokosuka O, et al. Mutations in the precore region of hepatitis B virus DNA in patients with fulminant and severe hepatitis. *N Engl J Med* 1991;324:1699–1704.
92. Okamoto H, Yotsumoto S, Akahane Y, et al. Hepatitis B viruses with precore region defects prevail in persistently infected hosts along with seroconversion to the antibody against e antigen. *J Virol* 1990;64:1298–1303.
93. Hunt CM, McGill JM, Allen MI, et al. Clinical relevance of hepatitis B viral mutations. *Hepatology* 2000;31:1037–1044.
94. Akarca U, Lok AS. Naturally occurring hepatitis B virus core gene mutations. *Hepatology* 1995;31:1037–1044.
95. Sirma H, Giannini C, Poussin K, et al. Hepatitis B virus X mutants, present in hepatocellular carcinoma tissue abrogate both the antiproliferative and transactivation effects of HBx. *Oncogene* 1999;18:4848–4859.

96. Carman WF, Zanetti AR, Karayiannis P, et al. Vaccine-induced escape mutant of hepatitis B virus. *Lancet* 1990; 336:325–329.
97. Carman WF, Trautwein C, Van Deursen FJ, et al. Hepatitis B virus envelope variation after transplantation with and without hepatitis B immune globulin prophylaxis. *Hepatology* 1996;24:489–493.
98. Tavis J. The replication strategy of the hepadnaviruses. *Viral Hepatitis Rev* 1996;2:205–218.
99. Nassal M, Schaller H. Hepatitis B virus replication. *J Viral Hepatitis* 1996;3:217–226.
100. Hu J, Toft D, Seeger C. Hepadnavirus assembly and reverse transcription require a multi-component chaperone complex which is incorporated into nucleocapsids. *EMBO* 1997;16:59–68.
101. Von Weizacker F, Kock J, Weiland S, et al. Cis-preferential recruitment of duck hepatitis B virus core protein to the RNA/polymerase preassembly complex. *Hepatology* 2002;35:209–216.
102. Guidotti LG, Rochford R, Chung J, et al. Viral clearance without destruction of infected cells during acute HBV infection. *Science* 1999;284:825–829.
103. Thimme R, Wieland S, Steiger C, et al. CD8+ T cells mediate viral clerance and disease pathogenesis during acute hepatitis B virus infection. *J Virol* 2003;77:68–76.
104. Guo JT, Zhou H, Liu C, et al. Apoptosis and regeneration of hepatocytes during recovery from transient hepadnavirus infections. *J Virol* 2000;74:1495–505.
105. Kajino K, Jilbert AR, Saputelli J, et al. Woodchuck hepatitis virus infections: very rapid recovery after a prolonged viremia and infection of virtually every hepatocyte. *J Virol* 1994;68:5792–5803.
106. Boni C, Bertoletti A, Penna A, et al. Lamivudine treatment can restore T cell responsiveness in chronic hepatitis B. *J Clin Invest* 1998;102:968–975.
107. Doong SL, Tsai CH, Schinazi RF, et al. Inhibition of the replication of hepatitis B virus in vitro by 2,′ 3′-dideoxy-3′-thiacytidine and related analogues. *Proc Natl Acad Sci USA* 1991;88:8495–8499.
108. Liaw YF, Leung NW, Chang TT, et al. Effects of extended lamivudine therapy in asian patients with chronic hepatitis B. Asia hepatitis lamivudine study group. *Gastroenterology* 2000;119:172–180.
109. Leung NW, Lai CL, Chang TT, et al. Extended lamivudine treatment in patients with chronic hepatitis B enhances hepatitis e antigen seroconversion rates: results after 3 years of therapy. *Hepatology* 2001;33:1527–1532.
110. Lewin SR, Ribeiro RM, Walters T, et al. Analysis of hepatitis B viral load decline under potent therapy: complex decay profiles observed. *Hepatology* 2001;34:1012–1020.
111. Ono SK, Kato N, Shiratori Y, et al. The polymerase L528M mutation cooperates with nucleotide binding-site mutations, increasing hepatitis B virus replication and drug resistance. *J Clin Invest* 2001;107:449–455.
112. Das K, Xiong X, Yang H, et al. Molecular modeling and biochemical characterization reveal the mechanism of hepatitis B virus polymerase resistance to lamivudine (3TC) and emtricitabine. *J Virol* 2001;75:4771–4779.
113. Allen MI, Gauthier J, DesLauriers M, et al. Two sensitive PCR-based methods for detection of hepatitis B virus variants associated with reduced susceptibility to lamivudine. *J Clin Microbiol* 1999;37:3338–3347.
114. Lau DTY, Khokhar F, Doo E, et al. Long-term therapy of chronic hepatitis B with lamivudine. *Hepatology* 2000;32:828–834.
115. Naesens L, Snoeck R, Andrei G, et al. HPMPC (cidofovir), PMEA (adefovir) and related acyclic nucleoside phosphonate analogues: a review of their pharmacology and clinical potential in the treatment of viral infections. *Antiviral Chem Chemother* 1997;8:1–23.
116. Heijtink RA, De Wilde GA, Kruining J, Berk L, et al. Inhibitory effect of 9-(2-phosphonylmethoxyethyl) adenine (PMEA) on human and duck hepatitis B virus infection. *Antiviral Res* 1993;21:141–153.
117. Del Gobbo V, Foli A, Balzarini J, et al. Immunomodulatory activity of 9-(2-phosphonylmethoxyethyl) adenine (PMEA), a potent anti-HIV nucleoside analogue, on in vivo murine models. *Antiviral Res* 1991;16:65–75.
118. Calio R, Villani N, Balestra E, et al. Enhancement of natural killer activity and interferon induction by different acyclic nucleoside phosphonates. *Antiviral Res* 1994;23:77–89.
119. Westland CE, Yang H, Delaney IV WE, et al. Week 48 resistance surveillance in two phase 3 clinical studies of adefovir dipivoxil for chronic hepatitis B. *Hepatology* 2003;38:96–103.
120. Angus P, Vaughan R, Xiong S, et al. Resistance to adefovir dipivoxil therapy associated with the selection of a novel mutation in the HBV polymerase. *Gastroenterology* 2003;125:292–297.
121. Westland CE, Villeneuve JP, Terrault N, et al. Resistance surveillance of liver transplantation patients with lamivudine-resistant hepatitis B virus after 96 weeks of adefovir dipivoxil treatment. *Hepatology* 2003;38: 160A.
122. Balfour HHJ. Antiviral drugs. *N Engl J Med* 1999;340: 1255–1268.
123. Honkoop P, De Man RA. Entecavir: a potent new antiviral drug for hepatitis B. *Expert Opin Investig Drugs* 2003; 12:683–688.
124. Yamanaka G, Wilson T, Innaimo S, et al. Metabolic studies on BMS-200475, a new antiviral compound active against hepatitis B virus. *Antimicrob Agents Chemother* 1999;43:190–193.
125. Levine S, Hernandez D, Yamanaka G, et al. Efficacies of entecavir against lamivudine-resistant hepatitis B virus replication and recombinant polymerases in vitro. *Antimicrob Agents Chemther* 2002;46:2525–2532.
126. Marion PL, Salazar FH, Winters MA, et al. Potent efficacy of entecavir (BMS-200475) in a duck model of hepatitis B virus replication. *Antimicrob Agents Chemother* 2002;46:82–88.
127. Colonno RJ, Genovesi EV, Medina I. Long term entecavir treatment results in sustained antiviral efficacy and prolonged life span in the woodchuck model of chronic hepatitis infection. *J Infect Dis* 2001;184:1236–1245.
128. Wolters LMM, Hansen BE, Niesters HGM. Viral dynamics during and after entecavir therapy in patients with chronic hepatitis B. *J Hepatol* 2002;37:137–144.
129. Tassopoulos NC, Hadziyannis SJ, Cianciara J, et al. Entecavir is effective in treating patients with chronic hepatitis B who failed lamivudine therapy. *Hepatology* 2001;34:340A.
130. Hayden FG. Antimicrobial agents (continued) antiviral agents (Nonretroviral). In: Hardman JG, Limbird LE, eds., and Gilman, AG, (consulting ed.). Goodman & Gilman's: The pharmacological basis of therapeutics, 10th ed. New York: McGraw-Hill; 2001;1313–1347.
131. Peek SF, Cote PJ, Jacob JR, et al. Antiviral activity of clevudine against woodchuck hepatitis virus replication and gene expression in chronically infected woodchucks. *Hepatology* 2001;33:254–266.
132. Marcellin P, Sereni D, Scaks S, et al. Anti-HBV activity and tolerability of clevudine, a novel nucleoside analogue.

Initial results of a phase I/II 28 day study. *Hepatology* 2001;34:320A.
133. James JS. Tenofovir approved: broad indication. *AIDS Treat News* 2001;Oct 26(373):2–3.
134. Van Bommel F, Wunsche T, Schurmann D, et al. Tenofovir treatment in patients with lamivudine-resistant hepatitis B mutants strongly affects viral replication. *Hepatology* 2002;36:507–508.
135. Le Guerhier F, Pichoud C, Guerret S, et al. Characterization of the antiviral effect of 2′3′-dideoxy-2′-3′ didehydro-beta-L-5-fluorocytidine in the duck hepatitis B virus infection model. *Antimicrob Agents Chemother* 2000;44:111–122.
136. Balakrishna PSS, Liu H, Zhu YL. Inhibition of hepatitis B virus by a novel L-nucleoside, 2′ fluoro-5-methyl-beta-L-arabinofuranosyl uracil. *Antimicrob Agents Chemother* 1998;40:380–386.
137. Aguesse-Germon S, Liu H, Chevalier M, et al. Inhibitory effect of 2′ fluoro-5-methyl-beta-L-arabinofuranosyl uracil on duck hepatitis B virus replication. *Antimicrob Agents Chemother* 1998;42:369–376.
138. Pierra C, Imbach JL, De Clercq E, et al. Synthesis and antiviral evaluation of some beta-L-2′-3′ dideoxy-5-chloropyrimidine nucleosides and pronucleotides. *Antiviral Res* 2000;45:169–183.
139. Zhou XJ, Lim SG, Lai CL, et al. Phase 1 dose escalation pharmacokinetics of L-deoxithymidine in patients with chronic hepatitis B virus infection. *Hepatology* 2001;34:629A.
140. Lai CL, Leung NW, Teo EK, et al. Results of one year-international phase IIB comparative trial of telbivudine, lamivudine, and the combination, in patients with chronic hepatitis B. *Hepatology* 2003;38 (Suppl 1):262A.
141. King RW, Ladner SK, Miller TJ, et al. Inhibition of human hepatitis B virus replication by AT-61, a phenyl-propenamide derivative, alone and in combination with (−)beta-L-2,′ 3′-dideoxy-3′thiacytidine. *Antimicrob Agents Chemother* 1998;42:3179–3186.
142. Delaney WE IV, Edwards R, Colledge D, et al. The phenylpropenamide derivatives AT-61 and AT-130 inhibit replication of both wild-type and lamivudine resistant strains of hepatitis B virus *in vitro*. *Antimicrob Agents Chemother* 2002;46:3057–3060.
143. Feld J, Colledge D, Sozzi T, et al. The phenylpropenamide derivative AT-130 inhibits HBV replication at viral encapsidation and packaging. *Hepatology* 2002;36:300A.
144. Deres K, Schroder CH, Paessens A, et al. Inhibition of hepatitis B virus replication by drug-induced depletion of nucleocapsids. *Science* 2003;299:893–896.
145. Kamiya N, Kubota A, Iwase Y, et al. Antiviral activities of MCC-478, a novel and specific inhibitor of hepatitis B virus. *Antimicrob Agents Chemother* 2002;46:2872–2877.
146. Ono-Nita SK, Kato N, Shiratori Y, et al. Novel nucleoside analogue MCC-478 (LY582563) is effective against wild-type or lamivudine-resistant hepatitis B virus. *Antimicrob Agents Chemother* 2002;46:2302–2605.
147. Blum HE. Gene therapy of viral hepatitis. In: Tsuji T, Higashi T, Zeniya M, et al., eds. *Molecular biology and immunology in hepatology.* Freiburg, Germany: Elsevier Science, 2002;97–109.
148. Branch A. A hitchhiker's guide to antisense and nonantisense biochemical pathways. *Hepatology* 1996; 24:1517–1529.
149. Hannon GJ. RNA interference. *Nature* 2002;41:244–251.
150. Shlomai A, Shaul Y. Inhibition of hepatitis B virus expression and replication by RNA interference. *Hepatology* 2003;37:764–770.
151. The EASL Jury. EASL international consensus conference on hepatitis B, 13–14 September, 2002, consensus statement. *J Hepatol* 2003;38:533–540.
152. Lauer GM, Walker BD, MD. Hepatitis C virus infection. *N Engl J Med* 2001;345:41–52.
153. Colombo M. Natural history and pathogenesis of hepatitis C virus related hepatocellular carcinoma. *J Hepatol* 1999;31:25–30.
154. Penin F. Structural biology of hepatitis C virus. *Clin Liver Dis* 2003;7:1–21.
155. Glue P, Rouzier-Panis R, Raffanel C, et al. A dose-ranging study of pegylated interferon alfa-2b and ribavirin in chronic hepatitis C. The Hepatitis C Intervention Therapy Group. *Hepatology* 2000;32:647–653.
156. Choo QL, Kuo G, Weiner AJ, et al. Isolation of a cDNA clone derived from a blood-borne non-A, non-B viral hepatitis genome. *Science* 1989;244:359–362.
157. Robertson B, Myers G, Howard C, et al. Classification, nomenclature, and database development for hepatitis C virus (HCV) and related viruses: proposals for standardization. International Committee on Virus Taxonomy. *Arch Virol* 1998;143:2493–2503.
158. Bantef H, Schulze-Ostoff K. Apoptosis in hepatitis C virus infection. *Cell Death Differ* 2003 Jan; 10(Suppl 1): S48–58.
159. Pawlotsky JM, Germanidis G, Frainais PO, et al. Evolution of the hepatitis C virus second envelope protein hypervariable region in chronically infected patients receiving alpha interferon therapy. *J Virol* 1999;73:6490–6499.
160. Simmonds P, Alberti A, Alter HJ, et al. A proposed system for the nomenclature of hepatitis C viral genotypes. *Hepatology* 1994;19:1321–1324.
161. Wasley A, Alter MJ. Epidemiology of hepatitis C: geographic differences and temporal trends. *Semin Liver Dis* 2000;20:1–16.
162. Martell M, Esteban JI, Quer J, et al. Hepatitis C virus (HCV) circulates as a population of different but closely related genomes: quasispecies nature of HCV genome distribution. *J Virol* 1992;66:3225–9.
163. Giannini C, Bréchot C. Hepatitis C virus biology. *Cell Death Differ* 2003;10:27–38.
164. Pawlotsky JM. Hepatitis C virus resistance to antiviral therapy. *Hepatology* 2000;32:889–896.
165. Bartenschlager R, Lohmarm V. Novel cell culture systems for the hepatitis C virus. *Antiviral Res* 2001;52:1–17.
166. Griffin SD, Beales LP, Clarke DS, et al. The p7 protein of hepatitis C virus forms an ion channel that is blocked by the antiviral drug, amantadine. *FEBS Lett* 2003;535:34–38.
167. Kaito M, Watanabe S, Tsukiyama-Kohara K, et al. Hepatitis C virus particle detected by immunoelectron microscopic study. *J Gen Virol* 1994;75:1755–1760.
168. Thomssen R, Bonk S, Thiele A. Density heterogeneities of hepatitis C virus in human sera due to the binding of beta-lipoproteins and immunoglobulins. *Med Microbiol Immunol* 1993;182:329–334.
169. Loriot MA, Bronowicki JP, Lagorce D, et al. Permissiveness of human biliary epithelial cells to infection by hepatitis C virus. *Hepatology* 1999;29:1587–1595.
170. Moldvay J, Deny P, Pot S, et al. Detection of hepatitis C virus RNA in peripheral blood mononuclear cells of infected patients by in situ hybridization. *Blood* 1994;83:269–273.
171. Pileri P, Uematsu Y, Campagnoli S, et al. Binding of hepatitis C virus to CD81. *Science* 1998;282:938–941.
172. Meola A, Sbardellati A, Bruni Ercole B, et al. Binding of hepatitis C virus E2 glycoprotein to CD81 does not correlate with species permissiveness to infection. *J Virol* 2000;74:5933–5938.

173. Flint M, Quinn ER, Levy S. In search of hepatitis C virus receptor(s). *Clin Liver Dis* 2001;5:873–893.
174. Cocquerel L, Wychowski C, Minner F, et al. Charged residues in the transmembrane domains of hepatitis C virus glycoproteins play a major role in the processing, subcellular localization, and assembly of these envelope proteins. *J Virol* 2000;74:3623–3633.
175. Cocquerel L, Op de Beeck A, Lambot M, et al. Topological changes in the transmembrane domains of hepatitis C virus envelope glycoproteins. *EMBO J* 2002;21:2893–2902.
176. Beales LP, Rowlands DJ, Holzenburg A. The internal ribosome entry site (IRES) of hepatitis C virus visualized by electron microscopy. *RNA* 2001;7:661–670.
177. Reed KE, Rice CM. Overview of hepatitis C virus genome structure, polyprotein processing, and protein properties. *Curr Top Microbiol Immunol* 2000;242:55–84.
178. Kunkel M, Lorinczi M, Rijnbrand R, et al. Self-assembly of nucleocapsid-like particles from recombinant hepatitis C virus core protein. *J Virol* 2001;75(5):2119–2129.
179. Fried MW, Shiffman ML, Reddy KR, et al. Peg interferon alfa-2a plus ribavirin for chronic hepatitis C virus infection. *N Engl J Med* 2002;347:975–982.
180. Hay AJ, Wolstenholme AJ, Skehel JJ, et al. The molecular basis of the specific anti-influenza action of amantadine. *EMBO J* 1985;4:3021–3024.
181. Lau JY, Tam RC, Liang TJ, et al. Mechanism of action of ribavirin in the combination treatment of chronic HCV infection. *Hepatology* 2002;35:1002–1009.
182. Bressanelli S, Tomei L, Roussel A, et al. Crystal structure of the RNA-dependent RNA polymerase of hepatitis C virus. *Proc Natl Acad Sci USA* 1999;96:13034–13039.
183. Mercer DF, Schiller DE, Elliott JF, et al. Hepatitis C virus replication in mice with chimeric human livers. *Nat Med* 2001;7:927–933.
184. Castet V, Fournier C, Soulier A, et al. Alpha interferon inhibits hepatitis C virus replication in primary human hepatocytes infected in vitro. *J Virol* 2002;76:189–199.
185. Rumin S, Berthillon P, Tanaka E, et al. Dynamic analysis of hepatitis C virus replication and quasispecies selection in long-term cultures of adult human hepatocytes infected in vitro. *J Gen Virol* 1999;80:3007–3018.
186. Lohmann V, Komer F, Koch J, et al. Replication of subgenomic hepatitis C virus RNAs in a hepatoma cell line. *Science* 1999;285:110–113.
187. Blight KJ, Kolykhalov AA, Rice CM. Efficient initiation of HCV RNA replication in cell culture. *Science* 2000 Dec 8;290:1972–1974.
188. Piertschmann T, Lohmann V, Rutter G, et al. Characterization of cell lines carrying self-replicating hepatitis C virus RNAs. *J Virol* 2001;75:1252–1264.
189. Pawlotsky JM. Mechanisms of antiviral treatment efficacy and failure in chronic hepatitis C. *Antiviral Res* 2003;59: 1–11.
190. Lamarre D, Anderson PC, Bailey M, et al. An NS3 protease inhibitor with antiviral effects in humans infected with hepatitis C virus. *Nature* 2003;426:186–189.
191. Bowen EF, Emery VC, Wilson P, et al. Cytomegalovirus polymerase chain reaction viraemia in patients receiving ganciclovir maintenance therapy for retinitis. *AIDS* 1998;12:605–611.
192. Boivin G, Gilbert C, Gaudreau A, et al. Rate of emergence of cytomegalovirus (CMV) mutations in leukocytes of patients with acquired immunodeficiency syndrome who are receiving valganciclovir as induction and maintenance therapy for CMV retinitis. *J Infect Dis* 2001;184:1598–1602.
193. Weinberg A, Jabs DA, Chou S, et al. for the cytomegalovirus retinitis and viral resistance study group and the adult AIDS clinical trials group cytomegalovirus laboratories. Mutations conferring foscarnet resistance in a cohort of patients with acquired immunodeficiency syndrome and cytomegalovirus retinitis. *J Infect Dis* 2003;187:777–784.
194. Limaye AP, Corey L, Koelle DM, et al. Emergence of ganciclovir-resistant cytomegalovirus disease among recipients of solid-organ transplants. *Lancet* 2000;356:645–649.
195. Ducancelle A, Belloc S, Alain S, et al. Comparison of sequential cytomegalovirus isolates in a patient with lymphoma and failing antiviral therapy. *J Clin Virol* 2004;29:241–247.
196. Lurain NS, Weinberg A, Crumpacker CS, et al. Sequencing of cytomegalovirus UL97 gene for genotypic antiviral resistance testing. *Antimicrob Agents Chemother* 2001;45:2775–2780.
197. Landry ML, Stanat S, Biron K, et al. A standardized plaque reduction assay for determination of drug susceptibilities of cytomegalovirus clinical isolates. *Antimicrob Agents Chemother* 2000;44:688–692.
198. Dankner WM, Scholl D, Stanat SC, et al. Rapid antiviral DNA-DNA hybridization assay for human cytomegalovirus. *J Virol Methods* 1990;28:293–298.
199. McSharry JM, Lurain NS, Drusano GL, et al. Flow cytometric determination of ganciclovir susceptibilities of human cytomegalovirus clinical isolates. *J Clin Microbiol* 1998;36:958–964.
200. Tatarowicz WA, Lurain NS, Thompson KD. In situ ELISA for the evaluation of antiviral compounds effective against human cytomegalovirus. *J Virol Methods* 1991;35:207–215.
201. Pépin JM, Simon F, Dussault A, et al. Rapid determination of human cytomegalovirus susceptibility to ganciclovir directly from clinical specimens primocultures. *J Clin Microbiol* 1992;30:2917–2920.
202. Gerna G, Sarasini A, Percivalle E, et al. Rapid screening for resistance to ganciclovir and foscarnet of primary isolates of human cytomegalovirus from culture-positive blood samples. *J Clin Microbiol* 1995;33:738–741.
203. Eckle T, Prix L, Jahn G, et al. Drug-resistant human cytomegalovirus infection in children after allogeneic stem cell transplantation may have different clinical outcomes. *Blood* 2000;96:3286–3289.
204. Chou E, Lurain NS, Thompson KD, et al. Viral DNA polymerase mutations associated with drug resistance in human cytomegalovirus. *J Infect Dis* 2003;188:32–39.
205. Baldanti F, Michel D, Simoncini L, et al. Mutations in the UL97 ORF of ganciclovir-resistant clinical cytomegalovirus isolates differentially affect GCV phosphorylation as determined in a recombinant vaccinia virus system. *Antiviral Res* 2002;54:59–67.
206. Sullivan V, Talarico CL, Stanat SC, et al. A protein kinase homologue controls phosphorylation of ganciclovir in human cytomegalovirus-infected cells. *Nature* 1992;358:162–164.
207. Smith IL, Cherrington JM, Jiles RE, et al. High-level resistance of cytomegalovirus to ganciclovir is associated with alterations in both the UL97 and DNA polymerase genes. *J Infect Dis* 1997;176:69–77.
208. Chou E, Marousek G, Guentzel S, et al. Evolution of mutations conferring multidrug resistance during prophylaxis and therapy for cytomegalovirus disease. *J Infect Dis* 1997;176:786–789.
209. Chou E, Marousek G, Parenti DM, et al. Mutation in region III of the DNA polymerase gene conferring foscarnet resistance in cytomegalovirus isolates from three

subjects receiving prolonged antiviral therapy. *J Infect Dis* 1998;178:526–530.
210. Cihlar T, Fuller MD, Cherrington J. Characterization of drug resistance-associated mutations in the human cytomegalovirus DNA polymerase gene by using recombinant mutant viruses generated from overlapping DNA fragments. *J Virol* 1998;72:5927–5936.
211. Erice A. Resistance of human cytomegalovirus to antiviral drugs. *Clin Microbiol Rev* 1999;12(Suppl 2):S286–S297.
212. Sullivan V, Biron KK, Talarico CL, et al. A point mutation in the human cytomegalovirus DNA polymerase gene confers resistance to ganciclovir and phosphonylmethoxyalkyl derivatives. *Antimicrob Agents Chemother* 1993;37:19–25.
213. Hirt B. Selective extraction of polyoma DNA from infected mouse cell cultures. *J Mol Biol* 1967;26:365–369.
214. Alain S, Mazeron MC, Pepin JM, et al. Rapid detection of cytomegalovirus strains resistant to ganciclovir through mutations within the gene UL 97. *Mol Cell Probes* 1993;7:487–495.
215. Chou S, Guentzel S, Michels KR, et al. Frequency of UL97 phosphotransferase mutations related to ganciclovir resistance in clinical cytomegalovirus isolates. *J Infect Dis* 1995;172:239–242.
216. Chou S, Erice A, Jordan MC, et al. Analysis of the UL97 phosphotransferase coding sequence in clinical cytomegalovirus isolates and identification of mutations conferring ganciclovir resistance. *J Infect Dis* 1995;171:576–583.
217. Hanson MH, Preheim LC, Chou S, et al. Novel mutation in the UL97 gene of a clinical cytomegalovirus strain conferring resistance to ganciclovir. *Antimicrob Agents Chemother* 1995;39:1204–1205.
218. Harada K, Eizuru Y, Isashiki Y, et al. Genetic analysis of a clinical isolate of human cytomegalovirus exhibiting resistance against both ganciclovir and cidofovir. *Arch Virol* 1997;142:215–225.
219. Chou S, Lurain NS, Weinberg A, et al. Interstrain variation in the human cytomegalovirus DNA polymerase sequence and its effect on genotypic diagnosis of antiviral drug resistance. *Antimicrob Agents Chemother* 1999;43:1500–1502.
220. Fillet AM, Auray L, Alain S, et al. Natural polymorphism of cytomegalovirus DNA polymerase lies in two non-conserved regions spanning between domains delta-C and II and between domains III and I. *Antimicrob Agents Chemother* 2004;48:1865–1868.
221. Zambon MC. Epidemiology and pathogenesis of influenza. *J Antimicrobial Chemother* 1999;44:3–9.
222. Scholtissek C. Source for influenza pandemics. *Eur J Epidemiol* 1994;10:455–458.
223. Aymard M, Valette M, Lina B, et al. Surveillance and impact of influenza in Europe. *Vaccine* 1999;17:S30–S41.
224. Murphy BR, Webster RG. Orthomyxoviruses. In: Fields BN, Knipe DM, Howley PM, eds. *Virology*, 3rd ed. Lippincott-Raven: Philadelphia, 1996;1397–1446.
225. Reid AH, Fanning TG, Hultin JV, et al. Origin and evolution of the 1918 "Spanish" influenza gene. *Proc Natl Acad Sci USA* 1999;96:1651–1656.
226. Stuart-Harris CH, Schild GC, Oxford JS, eds. *Influenza. The virus and the disease*. London: Edward Arnold, 1985;103–117.
227. Oxford J, Sefton A, Jackson R, et al. Who is that lady? *Nature Med* 1999;12:1351–1352.
228. Zambon MC. The pathogenesis of influenza in humans. *Rev Med Virol* 2001;11:227–241.
229. Tong HH, Long JP, Shannon A, et al. Expression of cytokine and chemokine genes by human middle ear epithelial cells induced by influenza A virus and *Streptococcus pneumoniae* opacity variants. *Infect Immun* 2003;71:4289–4296.
230. Whiley DC, Skehel JJ. The structure and function of the hemagglutinin membrane glycoprotein of influenza virus. *Annu Rev Biochem* 1987;56:365–394.
231. Skehel, JJ, Wiley DC. Receptor binding and membrane fusion in virus entry: the influenza hemagglutinin. *Annu Rev Biochem* 2000;69:531–569.
232. Voeten JTM, Bestebroer TM, Nieuwkoop NJ, et al. Antigenic drift in the influenza A virus (H3N2) nucleoprotein and escape from recognition by cytotoxic T lymphocytes. *J Virol* 2000;74:6800–6807.
233. Wiley DC, Wilson IA, Skehel JJ. Structural identification of the antibody-binding sites of Hong Kong influenza haemagglutinin and their involvement in antigenic variation. *Nature* 1981;289:373–378.
234. Zhirnov OP, Ikizler MR, Wright PF. Cleavage of influenza A virus hemagglutinin in human respiratory epithelium is cell associated and sensitive to exogenous antiproteases. *J Virol* 2002;76:8682–8689.
235. Coleman PM. Influenza virus neuraminidase: structure, antibodies, and inhibitors. *Protein Sci* 1994;3:1687–1696.
236. Holsinger LJ, Nichari D, Pinto LH, et al. Influenza A virus M2 ion channel protein: a structure-function analysis. *J Virol* 1994;68:1551–63.
237. Barman S, Ali A, Hui EK, Adhikary L, et al. Transport of viral proteins to the apical membranes and interaction of matrix protein with glycoproteins in the assembly of influenza viruses. *Virus Res* 2001;77:61–69.
238. Kawoka J. Enigmas of influenza. S4–2. Fifth Annual Options for the control of Influenza Conference. Okinawa, Japan. Oct 7–11, 2003.
239. Blick Tj, Sahasrabudhe A, Mcdonald M, et al. The interaction of neuraminidase and haemagglutinin mutations in the influenza virus in resistance to 4-guanadino-Neu5Ac2en. *Virology* 1998;246:95–103.
240. Dolin R, Reichmein RC, Madore HP, et al. A controlled trial of amantadine and rimantadine in the prophylaxis of influenza A infection. *N Engl J Med* 1982;307:580–584.
241. Hayden FG, Cote KM, Douglas GJR. Plaque inhibition assay for drug susceptibility testing of influenza virus. *Antimicrob Agents Chemother* 1980;17:865–870.
242. Belshe RB, Smith MH, Hall CB, et al. Genetic basis of resistance to rimantadine emerging during treatment of influenza virus infection. *J Virol* 1988;62:1508–1512.
243. Valette M, Allard JP, Aymard M, et al. Susceptibilities to rimantadine of influenza A/H1N1 and A/H3N2 viruses isolated during the epidemics of 1988 to 1989 and 1989 to 1990. *Antimicrob Agents Chemother* 1993;37:2239–2240.
244. Palese, P, Compans RW. Inhibition of influenza virus replication in tissue culture by 2-deoxy-2,3-dehydro-N-trifluoro-acetylneuraminic acid (FANA): mechanism of action. *J Gen Virol* 1976;33:159–163.
245. McKimm-Breschin JL. Resistance of influenza viruses to neuraminidase inhibitors: a review. *Antiviral Res* 2000;47:1–17.
246. Wetherall NT, Trivedi T, Zeller J, et al. Evaluation of neuraminidase enzyme assays using different substrates to measure susceptibility of influenza virus clinical isolates to neuraminidase inhibitors: report of the neuraminidase inhibitor susceptibility network. *J Clin Microbiol* 2003;41:742–750.
247. McKimm-Breschkin J, Trivedi T, Hampson A, et al. Neuraminidase sequence analysis and susceptibilities of

influenza virus clinical isolates to zanamivir and oseltamivir. *Antimicrob Agents Chemother* 2003;47:2264–2272.

248. McNicholl IR, McNicholl JJ. Neuraminidase inhibitors: zanamivir and oseltamivir. *Ann Pharmacother* 2001; 35:57–70.
249. Gubareva LV, Kaiser L, Hayden FG. Influenza virus neuraminidase inhibitors. *Lancet* 2000;355:827–35.
250. Potier M, Mameli L, Bélisle M, et al. Fluorometric assay of neuraminidase with a sodium (4-methylumbelliferyl-D-N-acetylneuraminate) substrate. *Anal Biochem* 1979;94:287–296.
251. Barnett JM, Cadman A, Gor D, et al. Zanamivir susceptibility monitoring and characterization of influenza virus clinical isolates obtained during phase II clinical efficacy studies. *Antimicrob Agents Chemother* 2000;44:78–87.
252. Buxton RC, Edwards B, Juo RR, et al. Development of a sensitive chemiluminescent neuraminidase assay for the detection of influenza virus susceptibility to zanamivir. *Anal Biochem* 2000;280:291–300.
253. Stiver G. The treatment of influenza with antiviral drugs. *CMAJ* 2003;168:49–56.
254. Shigeta S. Targets of anti-influenza chemotherapy other than neuraminidase and proton pump. *Antivir Chem Chemother* 2001;12(Supp 1):179–88.
255. Ksiazek TG, Erdman D, Goldsmith CS, et al. SARS Working Group. A novel coronavirus associated with severe acute respiratory syndrome. *N Engl J Med* 2003;348:1953–1966.

255a. Chonel JJ, Pardon D, Thouvenot D, et al. Comparison between three rapid methods for direct diagnosis of influenza and the conventional isolation procedure. *Biologicals* 1991;19:287–292.

256. Drosten C, Gunther S, Preiser W, et al. Identification of a novel coronavirus in patients with severe acute respiratory syndrome. *N Engl J Med* 2003;348:1967–1976.
257. Guan Y, Zheng BJ, He YQ, et al. Isolation and characterization of viruses related to the SARS coronavirus from animals in southern China. *Science* 2003;302:276–278.
258. Booth CM, Matukas LM, Tomlinson GA, et al. Clinical features and short-term outcomes of 144 patients with SARS in the greater Toronto area. *JAMA* 2003;289:2801–2809.
259. Tsui PT, Kwok ML, Yuen H, et al. Severe acute respiratory syndrome: clinical outcome and prognostic correlates. *Emerg Infect Dis* 2003;9:1064–1069.
260. Ng ML, Tan SH, See EE, et al. Proliferative growth of SARS coronavirus in Vero E6 cells. *J Gen Virol* 2003;84:3291–3303.
261. Cinatl J, Morgenstern B, Bauer G, et al. Treatment of SARS with human interferons. *Lancet* 2003;362 (9380):293–294.
262. Cinatl J, Morgenstern B, Bauer G, et al. Glycyrrhizin, an active component of liquorice roots, and replication of SARS-associated coronavirus. *Lancet* 2003;361:2045–2046.
263. Crance JM, Scaramozzino N, Jouan A, et al. Interferon, ribavirin, 6-azauridine and glycyrrhizin: antiviral compounds active against pathogenic flaviviruses. *Antiviral Res* 2003;58:73–79.

CHAPTER 14

Disinfectants and Antiseptics, Modes of Action, Mechanisms of Resistance, and Testing

Joseph M. Ascenzi, Martin S. Favero

The purpose of this chapter is to describe chemical germicides formulated as sterilants, disinfectants, and antiseptics, with a focus on their use in health care facilities. It describes the most widely used active ingredients, their mechanism of action and spectrum of activity, and lastly the development of resistance to these chemicals.

DEFINITIONS

Typically, disinfectants are used in the hospital in several different areas: housekeeping, to clean floors, walls, and other environmental surfaces; in laboratories, to decontaminate reusable instruments; and in departments where reusable instruments do not require sterilization prior to reuse. These chemical germicides are referred to as instrument or environmental surface disinfectants. Disinfection of skin or mucosal membranes is accomplished by antiseptics.

Instrument processing involves a number of steps, including cleaning, decontamination, low-level or high-level disinfection, and sterilization. Cleaning refers to the removal of organic material from an instrument or environmental surface. Decontamination is a process by which a reduction in the number of organisms that remain on an instrument after processing is achieved. Cleaning and decontamination are usually achieved by use of detergents, both enzymatic and nonenzymatic. Low- or intermediate-level disinfection is a process using chemical agents that will kill most vegetative pathogenic bacteria and fungi and nonenveloped viruses. There are many products on the market that fall into this category. High-level disinfection is distinguished by activity to kill or inactivate, in addition to the aforementioned organisms, *Mycobacterium tuberculosis,* enveloped viruses, and bacterial spores. There are several products on the market that will provide this level of activity. The primary active ingredients belong to the chemical classes of aldehydes or oxidizing agents; however, some quaternary ammonium compounds and phenolics have made claims to be high-level disinfectants. Lastly there are the sterilization processes that are used to render material or devices free from all living organisms.

Sterilization is an absolute process whereas the other processes, while effective for their particular uses, may produce instruments that still have some organisms remaining on them. Cleaning and decontamination are processes primarily used to prepare devices for one of the secondary processes of disinfection or sterilization. This chapter focuses on the active ingredients used in high- and intermediate-level disinfectants and antiseptics used in the hospital or medical setting to disinfect medical instruments and skin.

The term *antiseptic* is used to describe a substance that has antimicrobial activity and is formulated for use on or in living tissue to remove, inhibit the growth of, or inactivate microorganisms. Quite often the distinction between an antiseptic and a disinfectant is not made. However, the differences between a disinfectant and an antiseptic are very great, and their applications are significantly different. A disinfectant is a chemical germicide formulated for use solely on inanimate objects or surfaces such as medical instruments or environmental surfaces; an antiseptic is formulated for use solely on or in living tissues. Some chemical agents such as iodophors can be used as active ingredients in chemical germicides formulated as either disinfectants or antiseptics. However, the precise formulations are significantly different, their use patterns are different, and the germicidal efficacy the formulations differs substantially. Consequently, disinfectants should never be used as antiseptics and vice versa. There are a number of active ingredients used in antiseptics, including the iodine/iodophor group, biguanides (chlorhexidine), alcohols (usually ethanol or isopropanol), and phenolics (PCMX and triclosan). Each of these chemical groups has its own features and its own benefits and drawbacks.

DISINFECTANTS AND ANTISEPTICS USED IN HEALTH CARE

The nature of the disinfection or sterilization of medical instruments, devices, or equipment can be understood more readily if these items are divided into general categories based on the risk of infection involved in their use, as first suggested by Dr. E. H. Spaulding (1). Although one runs the risk of oversimplification in dividing medical devices into such categories, we have chosen to retain Dr. Spaulding's general classification system because it is fairly straightforward and logical and has been used by epidemiologists and microbiologists for years when discussing or planning strategies for disinfection and sterilization. The CDC was first to endorse and use this system and basically promulgated its use nationally (2).

Spaulding believed that strategies for sterilization and disinfection could be better understood and implemented if instruments, equipment, and other medically related surfaces for patient treatment and care were categorized by the degree of risk of infection involved in their use. He defined three categories of such items: critical, semicritical, and noncritical.

Critical instruments or devices, the first category, are so called because of the substantial risk of acquiring infection if the item is contaminated with microorganisms at the time of use. These are instruments or objects that are introduced directly into the human body, either into or in contact with the blood stream or normally sterile areas of the body. Examples include needles, scalpels, transfer forceps, cardiac catheters, implants, and also the inner surface components of extracorporeal blood flow devices such as of the heart-lung oxygenator and the bloodside of artificial kidneys (hemodialyzers). These items must be sterilized by heat (steam autoclave or dry heat), ethylene oxide, hydrogen peroxide gas plasma, other low-temperature sterilization methods, or liquid sterilants in between patients.

Instruments or devices in the second category are classified as "semicritical" in terms of the degree of risk of infection. Examples include flexible fiber-optic endoscopes, endotracheal and aspirator tubes, bronchoscopes, laryngoscopes, respiratory therapy equipment, cystoscopes, vaginal specula, and urinary catheters. Although these items come in contact with mucous membranes, they do not ordinarily penetrate body surfaces. Sterilization of many of these items, although desirable and often cost-effective if steam autoclaves can be used, is not absolutely essential. Semicritical instruments or devices should, at a minimum, be subjected to a process of high-level disinfection. As explained later, a high-level disinfectant is usually a liquid chemical germicide formulated as a sterilant but used as a disinfectant, which means the exposure time is relatively short. A high-level disinfectant is a potent formulation that has broad-spectrum activity and can be expected to destroy some bacterial spores; most fungal spores; all ordinary vegetative bacteria, tubercle bacilli, and small or nonlipid viruses; and medium-sized or lipid viruses. In practice, good cleaning followed by a high-level disinfection procedure gives the user a reasonable degree of assurance that the items are free of pathogenic microorganisms.

The third category consists of "noncritical" instruments or devices. These items usually come into direct contact with the patient but in most instances only with unbroken skin. They include facemasks, blood pressure cuffs, most neurologic or cardiac diagnostic electrodes, and certain surfaces of X-ray machines. Depending on the particular item and the nature and degree of contamination during use, simple washing or scrubbing with a detergent and warm water may be sufficient for an adequate level of safety. Because skin is effective barrier for most microorganisms, the risk of infection due to nonsterile items contacting the individual were considered to be minimal; however, more recent studies have indicated that these surfaces harbor such organisms as *Clostridium difficile* (3–6), methicillin-resistant *Staphylococcus aureus* (7–9), and antibiotic-resistant *Enterococcus* strains (US CDC). It should be noted that, in the case of environmental surfaces, transmission of infectious agents to patients typically involves a vector, commonly a health care worker or other personnel (7–9). The reader is referred to Weber and Rutala (10) for a discussion of the role of the reservoir and the source of infection in the transmission of infectious agents from environmental surfaces. Controlling transmission of these pathogens may be accomplished by disinfection of environmental surfaces and use of proper handwashing with products employing an effective active ingredient.

As mentioned previously, we have chosen to expand Dr. Spaulding's original classification of medically related surfaces to define more clearly the relative risks of disease transmission by these surfaces. The added category consists of environmental surfaces, which carry the least risk of disease transmission. This general category encompasses a wide variety of surfaces that do not ordinarily come into direct contact with the patient, but if they occasionally do, it is only with intact skin. Although not directly implicated in transmission of disease within the hospital, these environmental surfaces may potentially contribute to secondary cross-contamination by the hands of health care workers or by contact with medical instruments that will subsequently come into contact with patients. In terms of relative potential for cross-contamination, the category of environmental surfaces may be further divided into at least two major subdivisions: (a) medical equipment surfaces such as frequently touched adjustment knobs or handles on hemodialysis machines, X-ray machines, instrument carts, or dental units, and (b) housekeeping surfaces such as floors, walls, tabletops, window sills, and so forth. As with noncritical medical instruments, adequate levels of safety for surfaces of medical equipment may be achieved by simple cleaning with a detergent and warm water or, depending on the equipment surface and the nature and degree of contamination, cleaning with a detergent germicide or cleaning with soap and water followed by application of an intermediate- to low-level chemical germicide. Controlling contaminants on environmental surfaces is usually accomplished with agents belonging to the quaternary ammonium and phenolic chemical classes.

Housekeeping surfaces have the least potential for cross-contamination among health care personnel, patients, or medical equipment and instruments. Adequate safety levels can be achieved by maintaining these surfaces in a state of visible cleanliness by using water and a detergent or a hospital-grade disinfectant or detergent designed for general housekeeping purposes (as indicated on the product label). Only in those instances in which there has been a significant spill of blood, another potentially infectious body fluid, or a laboratory culture should the added use of an intermediate-level chemical disinfectant be considered to ensure that such a surface is "safe."

The use of effective handwashing, coupled with the use of effective antiseptics in the hospital environment, is probably one of the most important facets of the overall infection control strategy (11). It has been demonstrated numerous times since the 1840s, beginning with the work of Semmelweis, that effective handwashing alone reduces the transmission of infectious agents. When handwashing is accomplished with an effective antimicrobial agent, the reduction of transmission can be amplified (12).

PRODUCT CLAIMS

In the United States, disinfectants are regulated by two government agencies at the national level, with some states having additional regulations. The US Environmental Protection Agency (EPA) regulates low- and intermediate-level disinfectants, and the Food and Drug Administration (FDA) regulates high-level disinfectants. This division of regulatory responsibility mimics the use of the products, that is, for environmental surfaces and for medical devices, respectively. Antiseptics are regulated solely by the FDA as drugs.

Testing Regimens

Testing regimens used for product claims are defined by government agencies with regulatory responsibility (in the United States, the EPA and FDA). In the European Union (EU), requirements are defined in the various EU directives for biocides, disinfectants, and antiseptics. In the United States, test procedures used for meeting data requirements for disinfectants generally are those formulated by the Association of Official Analytical Chemists (AOAC), the American Society for Testing and Materials (ASTM), and the International Organization for Standardization (ISO). Internationally, regulatory agencies in some countries (e.g., Canada, Australia, and Brazil) use these same test methods, either as written or with slight variations. In France, Germany, and Japan, there are specific test methods used as prescribed by each country's regulatory agency (e.g., AFNOR, DGHM, and CEN). Additionally, some regulatory agencies have adapted different endpoints that one must meet to make a claim. For instance, in the United States, the quantitative tuberculocidal test requires a 6 log reduction to make a claim for tuberculocidal activity, while in the EU, using the same procedure, a 5 log reduction is required. Hence, the same product marketed in the United States and the EU may have different claims. This is a result of the requirements of those regulatory agencies for making specific claims. The remainder of this section deals with test methods used for the determination of claims in the United States.

Historically, hospital disinfectants, whether used for noncritical, semicritical, or critical devices, were regulated by the EPA under the authority of the Federal Insecticide, Fungicide and Rodenticide Act (FIFRA), as amended. Test procedures were established for testing disinfectants under the auspices of AOAC. These test methods were primarily potency tests to determine the effectiveness of disinfectants against bacterial spores, fungi, vegetative bacteria, and mycobacteria. In these test procedures, surrogate organisms representing the class of organisms being tested are inoculated onto hard surface carriers, exposed to the disinfectant for a specified period of time, and then cultured for surviving microorganisms. Much has been written about the deficiencies of these tests (13–15). Some of the issues surrounding use of these methods are lack of standardization of inocula; little control of the organisms' resistance; variations due to the porcelain carriers used in the sporicidal tests, including variations associated with the number of times the carriers are reused and how they are processed; and lack of a relationship between the carrier surfaces used in the test methods and those that are disinfected in real-world situations. In response to criticisms of these methods, alternative procedures have been proposed and adopted. The EPA adopted the use of a quantitative suspension test for measuring tuberculocidal activity of disinfectants (16). Methods that improve upon the current procedures have been proposed by Sattar and Springthorpe (17) and adopted by ASTM. The quantitative carrier test has the following advantages:

- It is fully quantitative.
- It minimizes the potential for false positives.
- It measures kill under ideal and stringent conditions.
- It increases the reliability of the results.
- It can be applied to a wide variety of microorganisms, both vegetative and spore forming.

- It eliminates the potential loss of organisms from wash-off during the exposure period.

This test has two separate parts, QCT-1 and QCT-2, which differ in the hard surface used (glass versus stainless steel) and the type of organic soil challenge that is incorporated into the test. QCT-1 tests the disinfectant under more ideal conditions (e.g., it may not include organic soil), while QCT-2 tests the disinfectant under less ideal conditions by incorporating a surface that can have more variability, reduced disinfectant, and an organic challenge added to the suspension. QCT-1 has been validated for use with vegetative bacteria, including mycobacteria, bacterial spores, and fungi, while QCT-2 has been validated for use with viruses and protozoans in addition to the above categories of microorganism. The data obtained from these procedures allows one to calculate a log reduction value for the potency of the germicide. From a regulatory perspective, various regulatory agencies may choose to set their own end point for determining efficacy.

EPA developed a method for evaluating chemical germicides for virucidal activity. This method was later adopted as an ASTM (E-1052–96) method. It is also accepted by the FDA for those products under its regulatory authority. Claims are made based on testing against specific viruses, although recently claims regarding activity against hepatitis B and hepatitis C virus have been allowed based on testing using the surrogate viruses duck hepatitis virus and bovine diaharrea virus, respectively.

Although chemical germicides maybe labeled as sterilants, guidelines from the CDC, FDA, APIC, and other professional organizations do not recommend the use of these germicides for sterilization unless there is no other available technology. Unlike terminal sterilization processes (steam, ethylene oxide, and peroxide gas plasma), where the items can be maintained in a sterile state after sterilization (by packaging), items sterilized using liquid processes cannot be maintained in a sterile state when they are removed from the solution. Sterilization claims can be obtained for these products using the AOAC sporicidal test (18). This test requires the use of hard surface carriers—silk suture and porcelain penicylinders—surfaces that have little relevance to current materials used in medical devices. A recent modification of the method has allowed the substitution of Dacron suture material for silk for the testing of oxidizing germicides. Miner et al. (15) recently reported on the technical problems associated with this method and how these issues affect the results.

In Vivo Methods Used to Evaluate Antiseptics

Boyce (11) makes the point that comparing *in vivo* studies of alcohol-based waterless antiseptics is complicated by the fact that the methods used vary greatly. Special note should be made of (a) whether or not hands are purposely contaminated, (b) the volume of test substance used, (c) the time period the solution is in contact with the skin, (d) the methods used to recover organisms, and (e) the method of expressing efficiency. Because there are many protocols used for determining the effectiveness of antiseptics based on their use, there is no way to summarize this concisely. The reader is referred to an excellent review of method designs by Hobson and Bolsen (19).

ACTIVE INGREDIENTS

Chlorhexidine

Chlorhexidine, a substituted diguanide, has a high degree of antimicrobial activity, low mammalian toxicity, and the ability to bind to the stratum corneum layer of the skin and to mucous membranes (20). The bactericidal activity of chlorhexidine is much greater than that of monomeric biguanides (21). These unique characteristics make it particularly attractive as an active ingredient in antimicrobial skin preparations. Chlorhexidine's general chemical structure is shown Fig. 14.1.

Practically insoluble in water, it will react with acids to form salts with varying degrees of solubility, depending on the salt. Recognized as an effective antimicrobial, chlorhexidine is found as the active ingredient in a number of products used as preoperative skin preparations, surgical hand scrubs, health care personnel handwash products, skin cleansers, acne creams, oral products such as mouthwashes, burn ointments, and wound protectants and is also incorporated into products as a preservative.

Spectrum of Activity

Antimicrobial activity of the active ingredients is measured by determining the minimal inhibitory concentration (MIC) and minimal bactericidal concentration (MBC). For measuring *in vivo* or *in situ* activity, there

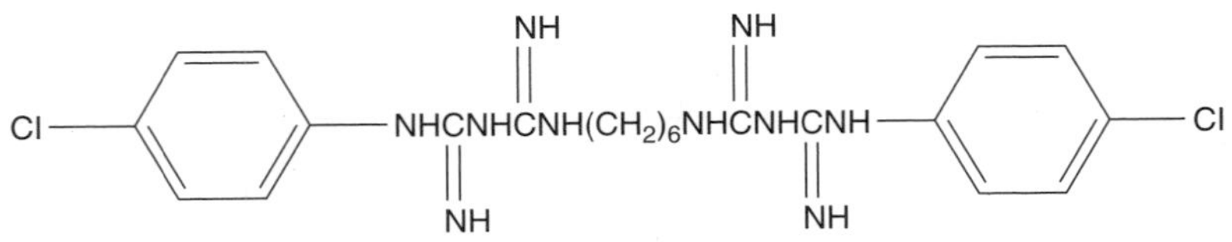

Cl–C₆H₄–NHC(=NH)NHC(=NH)NH$(CH_2)_6$NHC(=NH)NHC(=NH)NH–C₆H₄–Cl

FIGURE 14.1 ● Chemical structure of chlorhexidine.

are several protocols used to test formulations and preparations, as stated in the "Product Claims" section.

A comprehensive study of activity was completed by Denton (20) and published recently, describing both *in vitro* and *in vivo* results. *In vitro* MIC data for bacteria and fungi are presented in Tables 14.1 and 14.2, respectively. These data indicate the broad spectrum of activity of this active ingredient, which is effective against Gram-positive and -negative bacteria, yeasts, and molds.

Studies by Denton (20) determining the bactericidal and fungicidal activity of a 0.05% chlorhexidine solution using the test method described in British Standard 3286 (1960) further confirmed the rapid inactivation of Gram-positive and -negative bacteria, yeasts, and molds. With a 10-minute exposure to this solution at 18°C to 21°C, only *Pseudomonas stuartii, Streptococcus faecalis, Bacillus subtilis,* and *Clostridium difficile* did not show substantial reduction. The MIC values for *B. subtilis* and *Clostridium sporogenes* (Table 14.1) are relatively low, indicating the bacteriostatic effect on these organisms. All of the other 46 bacterial species tested showed >2 $\log_{10}$ reduction in 10 minutes. With the exception of the organisms listed above, Gram-negative bacteria were generally more susceptible (4.0–6.7 $\log_{10}$ reduction) than Gram-positive bacteria (2.1–5.8 $\log_{10}$ reduction) under the conditions tested. Again with the exception of the more resistant organisms listed above, among the Gram-positive bacteria the cocci (2.1–5.8 $\log_{10}$ reduction) were generally more resistant than the bacilli (3.6–4.8 $\log_{10}$ reduction). Holloway et al. (22) demonstrated that treatment of *Escherichia coli* and *Klebsiella pneumoniae* with sublethal concentrations of chlorhexidine resulted in reduction in pathogenicity of these organisms when injected into mice.

As shown in Table 14.1, the MIC for spores is quite low; however, the sporicidal activity is quite low. Data indicate that both *B. subtilis* and *C. difficile* spores show less than 1 $\log_{10}$ reduction when exposed to a 0.05% solution of chlorhexidine. The data indicate that chlorhexidine may be capable of inhibiting spore outgrowth and germination but that it does not kill the spores. Sporicidal activity can be achieved with chlorhexidine at higher temperatures (23).

Chlorhexidine is a moderate surface active agent and as such will interact with lipids. Viruses can be grouped into those that have an outer lipid membrane composed of lipoproteins and glycoproteins around the protein coat (enveloped viruses) and those that are "naked" (i.e., lack a lipid membrane). Chlorhexidine, because of its lipid solubility, is more active against the viruses with a lipid membrane (Table 14.3). Human immunodeficiency virus (HIV), responsible for AIDS, is an enveloped virus.

Studies confirm the supposition that chlorhexidine should be effective against HIV. Several preparations containing chlorhexidine (a 4% and a 0.5% solution in 70% alcohol) were found to be completely effective against HIV-1 after 15 seconds of contact. An aqueous solution of 0.05% was equally effective in 1 minute (24). Aqueous chlorhexidine gluconate at 0.2% was effective but at 0.02% was not effective (25).

In vivo studies using chlorhexidine formulations provide further evidence of the activity of this germicide. The formulation components and the solubility of various chlorhexidine salts can make a difference in the activity of the formulation. Chlorhexidine is incompatible with organic ions such as soaps, sodium lauryl sulfate, sodium carboxymethyl cellulose, alginates, and some dyes. Many of these compounds are commonly used in formulations for antiseptic preparations. There may be no visual evidence of incompatibility, but the antimicrobial activity may be significantly affected, as chlorhexidine may be incorporated into micelles and not be readily available to interact with microorganisms (20).

Many studies have demonstrated the *in vivo* activity of chlorhexidine. Although *in vitro* studies may indicate that various preparations are similar in activity, *in vivo* studies may indicate that the performance of the preparations are not be similar (26). For this reason, one should not rely strictly on data from *in vitro* studies (MIC and MBC data). Chlorhexidine has been incorporated into detergent and alcohol preparations, powders, mouthwashes, and polymeric preparations for a variety of uses. Because of its ability to bind to the stratum corneum layer of the epidermis, chlorhexidine exhibits the phenomenon of persistence and substantivity; that is, it exerts its effect long after it has been used, and the more it is used, the greater the reduction in the resident flora of the skin. This is especially relevant for its use as a surgical scrub and in surgical site preparation formulations.

As a surgical scrub, chlorhexidine has been formulated into 4% and 2% aqueous solutions as well as alcohol-based formulations of different concentrations. Peterson et al. (27) first described the effectiveness of chlorhexidine in removing transient microflora from artificially contaminated hands. They also demonstrated its immediate and long-term (persistent or residual) effects on resident microflora (28). A recent study examining the difference between aqueous formulations and alcohol formulations found that a formulation containing 1% chlorhexidine in 61% ethanol resulted in significantly greater microbial reduction than a 4% aqueous solution or the 61% ethanol vehicle (29). When used as a health care personnel handwash (generally for handwashing done by health care workers between patients), chlorhexidine has typically been employed as the active ingrediant in aqueous or alcohol-based solutions. Larson and Laughon (30) evaluated four chlorhexidine formulations (two 4% aqueous formulations, a 2% aqueous chlorhexidine formulation, and an alcoholic 0.5% chlorhexidine formulation) and compared them to a non-antiseptic soap. After the initial wash with each, there was no difference in microbial reductions; however, as more washes were performed, there was a significant difference between the

TABLE 14.1

Bacteriostatic Activity of Chlorhexidine Gluconate

Test Organism		MIC (mg/L)	
	No. of Strains	Mean	Range
Gram-positive cocci			
Micrococcus flavus	1	0.5	
Micrococcus luteus	1	0.5	
Staphylococcus aureus	16	1.6	1–4
Staphylococcus epidermidis	41	1.8	0.25–8.0
Streptococcus faecalis	5	38.0	32–64
Streptococcus mutans	2	2.5	
Streptococcus pneumoniae	5	11.0	8–16
Streptococcus pyogenes	9	3.0	1–8
Streptococcus sanguis	3	9.0	4–16
Streptococcus viridans	5	25.0	2–32
Gram-positive bacilli			
Bacillus cereus	1	8.0	
Bacillus subtilis	2	1.0	
Clostridium difficile	7	16.0	8–32
Clostridium welchii	5	14.0	4–32
Corynebacterium spp	8	1.6	0.5–8.0
Lactobacillus casei	1	128.0	
Listeria monocytogenes	1	4.0	
Propionibacterium acnes	2	8.0	
Gram-negative bacilli			
Acinetobacter anitratus	3	32.0	16–64
Alkaligenes faecalis	1	64.0	
Bacteroides disastonis	4	16.0	
Bacteroides fragilis	11	34.0	
Campylobacter pyloridis	5	17.0	8–64
Citrobacter freundii	10	18.0	8–32
Enterobacter cloacae	12	45.0	4–32
Escherichia coli	14	4.0	16–64
Gardnerella vaginalis	1	8.0	2–32
Haemophilus influenza	10	5.0	
Klebsiella aerogenes	5	25.0	2–8
Klebsiella pneumoniae	5	64.0	
Proteus mirabilis	5	115.0	82–128
Proteus vulgaris	5	57.0	16–128
Providencia stuartii	5	102.0	32–128
Pseudomonas aeruginosa	15	20.0	64–128
Pseudomonas cepacia	1	16.0	16–32
Pseudomonas fluorescens	1	4.0	

(continued)

TABLE 14.1 (Continued)

Bacteriostatic Activity of Chlorhexidine Gluconate

Test Organism	MIC (mg/L)		
	No. of Strains	Mean	Range
Salmonella bredeney	1	16.0	
Salmonella dublin	1	4.0	
Salmonella galinarum	1	8.0	
Salmonella montivideo	1	8.0	
Salmonella typhimurium	4	13.0	8–16
Salmonella vichow	1	8.0	
Serratia marcescens	10	30.0	16–64

Reprinted from Denton (20).

four chlorhexidine-containing formulations and the soap, though there was no difference between the chlorhexidine formulations.

Incorporation of chlorhexidine into a surgical skin prep (2% chlorhexidine in 70% isopropyl alcohol) proved to be effective. The chlorhexidine solution significantly reduced abdominal and inguinal microbial counts from baseline for up tot 24 hours. It was more persistent in the abdominal region than were two other preparations containing isopropyl alcohol or chlorhexidine alone (31).

Incorporation of chlorhexidine into powders used in routine umbilical decontamination in a neonatal unit indicated continued control of methicillin-resistance *Staphylococcus aureus* (MRSA) (32). Several studies have been done comparing infection rates when chlorhexidine gluconate and povidone-iodine were used as skin preparations in patients with central venous catheters. A comparison of catheter-related bloodstream infections in the studies indicates that chlorhexidine gluconate was superior; however, all the studies were limited by the small numbers of subjects (33–35). A metaanalysis of the data indicates that chlorhexidine reduced the risk of catheter-related bloodstream infections by 50% (36). Catheters impregnated with chlorhexidine and silver sulfadiazine (CHX-SS) were evaluated to determine whether they reduced catheter-related bloodstream infections. Several studies compared the CHX-SS catheters with standard catheters. Again because of the small number of patients involved in each study, the analysis lacked statistical power. When the patients were broken into two groups, those with short-term indwelling catheters (medium duration of 6 days) and those with long-term indwelling catheters (medium duration of 12 days), a metaanalysis of the data from several studies indicated that patients in the former group who used CHX-SS catheters had a significant reduction in the incidence of catheter-related bloodstream infections, while in the later group there was no difference between the CHX-SS catheters and standard catheters (37). *In vitro* studies with CHX-SS supported the data from the *in vivo* studies. Catheters removed from patients showed significant antimicrobial activity against Gram-positive bacteria for as long as 10–14 days, but antimicrobial activity is significantly reduced after the first week (38).

The use of chlorhexidine in dental applications has been explored, including incorporation into mouthwash, varnish, and slow-release materials. The incorporation of chlorhexidine into varnish used on orthodontic patients may help prevent caries lesions. Data indicate that there is a significant reduction in the level of *Streptococcus mutans* 1 week after the application of a sustained-release varnish. The decrease in *S. mutans* was measured for up to 3 weeks after the application. The same results were not obtained with *Actinomyces viscosus* (39). The incorporation of chlorhexidine into mouthwash solutions goes back over 30 years (40). And the incorporation of chlorhexidine into slow-release implantable materials provides for long-term effectiveness. The matrix can influence the overall effectiveness of the chlorhexidine.

Mechanism of Action

The activity of chlorhexidine is related to the interaction of the germicide with the cell membrane. Hugo and Longworth (41–43) designed a series of experiments to elucidate the mode of action of chlorhexidine. The results indicate that chlorhexidine interacts with the cell surface, causing changes in the lipids in the cell membrane. Changes in the integrity of the membrane result in loss of membrane function. The bacterial cell is generally negatively charged, and it has been shown that the charge is rapidly neutralized in the presence of chlorhexidine (20), indicating the reaction of chlorhexidine with

TABLE 14.2

Fungistatic Activity of Chlorhexidine

Organism	No. of Strains	Mean MIC (mg/L)
Mold fungi		
Aspergillus flavus	1	64
Aspergillus fumigatus	1	32
Aspergillus niger	1	16
Penicillium notatum	1	16
Rhizopus sp	1	8
Scopulariopsis spp	1	8
Yeasts		
Candida albicans	2	9
Candida guillermondii	1	4
Candida parapsilosis	2	4
Candida pseudotorpicalis	1	3
Cryptococcus neoformans	1	1
Prototheca zopfii	1	6
Saccharomyces cerevisiae	1	1
Torulopsis glabrata	1	6
Dermatophytes		
Epidermophyton floccosum	1	4
Microsporum canis	2	4
Microsporum fulvum	1	6
Microsporum gypseum	1	6
Trichophyton equinum	1	4
Trichophyton interdigitale	2	3
Trichophyton mentagrophytes	1	3
Trichophyton quinkeanum	1	3
Trichophyton rubrum	2	3
Trichophyton tonsurans	1	3

Reprinted from Denton (20).

the cell membrane. Outer membrane structure in Gram-negative bacteria is stabilized by the interaction of divalent cations and the negative charges associated with lipid A of the lipopolysaccharide (LPS). It is hypothesized that polycationic molecules, such as chlorhexidine, can promote their own uptake by displacement of divalent cations associated with the LPS. Alterations in the LPS can lead to changes in sensitivity to antimicrobials (44). Disruption of the cell membrane results in leakage of cellular material from the cell. The leakage in *E. coli* and *S. aureus* was described by Hugo and Longworth (43) as biphasic with respect to chlorhexidine concentration, and later work with *P. stutzeri* (45) added further evidence of this phenomenon. Experiments using ^{14}C-chlorhexidine indicate that chlorhexidine rapidly enters the cells of both bacteria and yeasts (46,47).

At low concentrations (up to 200 μg/mL), chlorhexidine inhibits membrane enzymes and promotes leakage of cellular constituents. Cells treated with bacteriostatic concentrations lost up to 50% of their K^+ but can recover upon neutralization of excess chlorhexidine (20). At higher concentrations, cytoplasmic contents are coagulated (48), and cells begin to leak higher molecular weight molecules such as nucleotides (20). Uptake of bis-(1,3-dibutylbarturic acid) trimethane oxonal and propidium iodide, which monitor membrane potential and membrane integrity, respectively, was directly related to chlorhexidine concentrations (0.003–0.3 mmol^{-1}), indicating changes in membrane structure with increasing concentrations of chlorhexidine (49).

The effect of chlorhexidine on mycobacterial cells is bacteriostatic, not bactericidal. The treatment of mycobacterial cells with ethambutol (an antituberculosis drug known to inhibit the synthesis of specific components of the mycobacterial cell wall) potentiates the activity of chlorhexidine on *Mycobacterium* spp, indicating that chlorhexidine needs access to the cell membrane to exert its activity (50).

Chlorhexidine has also been shown to damage cytoplasmic membranes in yeast. Treatment of *Saccharomyces cerevisiae* cells with chlorhexidine resulted in the release of pentose (51). In *Candida albicans*, sublethal concentrations of chlorhexidine resulted in loss of cytoplasmic components and coagulation of nucleoproteins (52) and prevented the outgrowth but not the germination of spores (23).

Iodine and Iodophors

Iodine in the form of a tincture has been used in surgery since the early 1900s as a preoperative skin preparation. The problem of local toxicity limited the use of iodine, whether in an aqueous or tincture preparation. The use of iodophors, which are complexes of iodine with a carrier such as polyvinylpyrrolidone (PVP) or poloxamer, allows for the slow release of free iodine, the active species, thereby reducing the preparation's toxicity and staining without limiting the antimicrobial activity of the iodine. Iodophors have been used as both antiseptics and disinfectants in the form of solutions, ointments, and aerosols. As disinfectants, they are usually classified as low- or intermediate-level disinfectants (53) because of they lack activity against spores. An outbreak of bacteremia associated with *Pseudomonas aeruginosa* was traced back to a contaminated 10% PVP-I solution in use at the time (54). Their primary use today is in skin antisepsis, where they have been used as surgical scrubs and skin preparations.

The labeling of iodophor preparations can be misleading in that the concentration of iodophors should not be

TABLE 14.3

Virucidal Activity of Chlorhexidine Gluconate

Virus	Viral Family	Activity[a]	Conc. (%)
Respiratory syncytial virus	Paramyxovirus	+	0.25
Herpes hominis/simplex	Herpesvirus	+	0.02
Poliovirus type 2	Enterovirus	–	0.02
Adenovirus type 2	Adenovirus	–	0.02
Equine infectious anemia virus	Retrovirus	+	2.0
Variola virus (smallpox)	Poxvirus	+	2.0
Herpes simplex types 1 and 2	Herpesvirus	+	0.02
Equine influenza virus	Orthomyxovirus	+	0.001
Hog cholera virus	Togavirus	+	0.001
Bovine viral diarrhea	Togavirus	+	0.001
Parainfluenza virus	Paramyxovirus	+	0.001
Transmissible gastroenteritis virus	Coronavirus	+	0.001
Rabies virus	Rhabdovirus	–	0.001
Canine distemper virus	Paramyxovirus	+	0.01
Infectious bronchitis virus	Coronavirus	+	0.01
Newcastle virus	Paramyxovirus	+	0.01
Pseudorabies virus	Herpesvirus	–	0.01
Cytomegalovirus	Herpesvirus	+	0.1
Coxsackievirus	Picornavirus	–	0.4
Echovirus	Picornavirus	–	0.4
Human rotavirus	Reovirus	–	1.5
HIV type 1	Retrovirus	–	0.2

[a] + indicates activity at concentration stated; – indicates activity not established at concentration stated.
Reprinted from Denton (20).

misconstrued as the concentration of the active ingredient. The amount of free iodine present in iodophors is difficult to determine. Concentrated solutions contain less free iodine than those that are diluted (55), and free iodine is the active species, while the PVP or other molecules with which the iodine is complexed act as carriers. A comparison of several commercial formulations of 10% PVP-I had a two orders of magnitude range of free iodine, hence a wide range of antimicrobial activity (56).

Spectrum of Activity

The antimicrobial activity of iodine and iodine-containing formulations is similar to that of chlorine-releasing compounds: these formulations have broad-spectrum activity against Gram-positive and -negative bacteria, mycobacteria, fungi, and viruses (57). As with most chemical germicides, the activity of iodine is dependent on the concentration of the active ingredient, the formulation, the temperature, the growth conditions of the microorganism, and the presence of organic and inorganic material.

The sporicidal activity of iodine compounds is less than that of the chlorine-releasing compounds. A concentration of 2000–5000 ppm potassium iodine is necessary to produce a 5 $\log_{10}$ reduction in *B. subtilis* spores within 5 minutes. Reports in the literature indicate that iodine solutions are effective in destroying spores of *Bacillus anthracis*, *B. subtilis*, *Bacillus megaterium*, *Bacillus mesentericus*, *Clostridium tetani*, and *Clostridium welchii* (58–60). Generally, disinfectant formulations of iodophors are sporicidal, whereas antiseptic-containing iodophors are not formulated to be sporicidal (61).

The activity of iodine against isolates from a water system (predominantly *Pseudomonas* spp) and *Legionalla pneumophila* was dramatically different if the organisms were grown in water or rich medium, with water-grown organisms showing greater resistance to the iodine

(62,63). Investigations have shown that iodine-containing formulations are more effective against vegetative organisms than are chlorine-based formulations, requiring a less active ingrediant to achieve the same result (57).

Reports on mycobactericidal activity of iodine and iodophors are equivocal. Studies on *Mycobacterium tuberculosis* found that a very low concentration of free iodine (<0.1%) was tuberculocidal with a 5-minute exposure at room temperature (64). Other studies, by Nelson et al. (65), showed that several commercially available iodophor formulations were not effective in killing two strains of *M. tuberculosis* after a 30-minute exposure, and Wright and Mundy (66) showed that thermometers contaminated with *M. tuberculosis* were not effectively disinfected with iodophor solutions. In a comparison of two different iodine formulations, povidone-iodine (1% titratable iodine) and an iodophor (0.008% titratable iodine), it was shown that the later was ineffective in killing >3 $\log_{10}$ cfu *M. tuberculosis* after 1-minute contact in suspension or dried on a carrier, while the former was effective in producing a >3 $\log_{10}$ reduction in a suspension test but not when the organism was dried on carriers in the presence of sputum (67). The iodophor product was also ineffective against *Mycobacterium smegmatis* (68). These data show the lack of consistency regarding the tuberculodcidal activity of iodine and iodophors, which resulted in the removal of these compounds from the category of high-level disinfectants.

Iodine and iodine-containing products have good fungicidal and fungistatic properties. They have been reported to be effective against species of *Trichophyton, Monilia, Epidermophyton, Torula,* and other genera (57).

The information regarding the virucidal activity of iodine and iodophores indicates the effectiveness of these products against a wide range of viruses, including enteroviruses and polio, herpes, vaccinia, rabies, and tobacco mosaic viruses (69–71). Present data show inactivation concentrations of 75–150 ppm for polio type 1, coxsackie B_1, adeno 2, vaccinia, herpes, influenza A, and HIV-1 viruses and 5000 ppm for feline parvovirus. Complete inactivation of cell-free HIV was accomplished using 0.5% PVP-I with a 30- to 60-second exposure. Some preparations of PVP-I have been shown to be active against hepatitis B virus as measured by the morphological alteration test, while other preparations had no activity at all. This variability was also observed with enteroviruses (72). Again, this may be attributable to the amount of free iodine in the preparation.

Iodine-containing solutions have been primarily used as skin prepping/degerming solutions and surgical hand scrubs. In general, most iodine-containing skin prepping and surgical scrubs show rapid reduction in the resident flora of the skin; however, they do not show residual activity. Studies have shown them to be inferior to chlorhexidine gluconate (73). Utilizing the Vienna test method a 3 $\log_{10}$ reduction was achieved after a 2-minute wash with PVP-I while the same effect was achieved with CHG after a 1-minute wash (74). Ayliffe et al (75) confirmed these results testing 14 different iodine preparations. And, in general, PVP-I solutions are more affected by the presence of organic material than are CHG formulations (76,77).

Mechanism of Action

The killing effect of iodine and iodophors is related to the concentration of the free molecular iodine, which is the only species whose concentration correlates with antimicrobial activity (55,78). The exact mechanism of action of iodine is not known. Its ability to penetrate the cell wall rapidly may be the primary mode by which it exerts its antimicrobial activity. The major reactions in which iodine can cause disruption of cells or cellular components are as follows:

- Reactions with N–H groups of amino acids in which N-iodo compounds are formed, resulting in lethal changes to proteins;
- Oxidation of -SH groups of cysteine, which leads to loss of ability to connect protein chains by disulfide (–S–S–) bonds;
- Iodination of phenolic and imidazolic groups of the amino acids tyrosine and histidine and iodination of the pyrimidine derivatives of cytosine and uracil, which lead to steric hindrances in hydrogen bonds and denaturation of DNA; and
- The addition of iodine to unsaturated fatty acids, which leads to changes in the physical properties of lipids and hence membranes.

The first mechanism may be the most important because of the importance of the –SH groups in the cell and the rapid and irreversible nature of the reaction (56,57). The exact mechanism of action is still unknown, partially because of the complex chemistry associated with iodine and iodophors, in which no less than seven spieces are reported to have some antimicrobial activity (79). For a good description of the chemistry, the reader is referred to Gottardi (56).

Alcohols

Alcohols have the general chemical formula R–OH, where R can be any organic structure, such as an alkyl or benzyl molecule. The –OH group is the reactive species, and its reactivity is influenced by the R group attached.

Alcohols have been used for disinfection of both skin and surface. They have been employed as skin disinfectants since antiquity (80). Beck (81) reviewed the use of alcohols as antiseptics. In Europe, the use of ethanol as a skin antiseptic has been the standard, while in the United States, ethanol was used extensively but has been replaced by antiseptic chemicals such as chlorhexidine, povidone-iodine, and triclosan. As skin disinfectants, alcohol preparations have been used as hygienic hand disinfectants, surgical hand disinfectants, and skin disinfectants, each type of disinfectant having its own set of requirements.

Alcohols have also been used as hard surface disinfectants for many years, and appropriately so because of their general antimicrobial properties. However, volatility and flammability can be an issue when using alcohols in this manner. The flash points of ethanol and propanols are below 15°C, requiring caution in their use. On the other hand, these short-chain alcohols can be suitable as disinfectants because they have unlimited solubility in water, have low toxicity, and are fast acting and microbicidal. Because of their polar structure, low-weight alcohols possess less surface tension than water and thus better wetting characteristics, important for antiseptics used on skin or for surface disinfectants used on nonuniform surfaces (80).

Regardless of the application, among isomers the following is the order of antibacterial effect: *n*-primary > *iso*-primary > secondary > tertiary.

Mechanism of Action

It is generally believed that alcohols, like most chemical germicides, act at multiple sites of the cell. The primary mode of action is related to coagulation/denaturation of proteins and their solubility in lipids (82,83). In the absence of water, coagulation will not occur, so higher concentrations of some alcohols are less effective as germicides than lower concentrations (e.g., 70% ethanol is more effective than 95% ethanol). The explanation is that higher concentrations of alcohol may deprive the bacterial cell of water, thereby inducing formation of impermeable protein layers, which then prevent the penetration of alcohol into the cell (80). Hence, with dry cells water in seeded for antimicrobial activity, though this is not true for moist cells.

Coagulation of proteins occurs at the cell wall and the cytoplasmic membrane and within the cell, but does not appear to involve nucleoproteins (84). Obviously, coagulation of enzymatic proteins leads to loss of cellular function; however, there does not appear to be specificity with regard to which enzymes are affected. The work of Sykes (85) with dehydrogenase enzymes from *E. coli* indicates that as the chain length of the alcohol increases, there is a corresponding loss of enzyme function. Bacterial enzymes located in the cell wall were more easily inactivated than intracellular enzymes (86).

Lysis of bacterial cells, including human strains of *Mycoplasma*, has been reported (87,88). Lysis is likely due to disruption of the cell membrane (80).

Spectrum of Activity

Because of the widespread use of alcohols as disinfectants and antiseptics over the last century, there is an abundance of information. This review is confined to the use of alcohols as antiseptics (i.e., their use on skin), as that is the primary use today.

A review of the *in vitro* activity against bacterial spores indicates that alcohols are considered to have little or no activity. As a matter of routine procedures, spore preparations are often kept in 95% ethanol as a means of preventing them from being contaminated by other vegetative organisms. Other published data indicate that the sporicidal activity is related the alcohol itself, the concentration, and the species of organism (80).

There are a number of studies that document the activity of alcohols against Gram-positive and -negative organisms (89–91) and against multidrug-resistant pathogens (92–94). Table 14.4 summarizes the antimicrobial activity of a variety of alcohols against *S. aureus* and *E. coli*.

The data indicate that activity increases with alcohol chain length and that primary and secondary alcohols are more active than tertiary alcohols. This is also true for organisms that are dried on hard surface carriers (Table 14.5).

Ethanol is bacteriostatic and inhibits spore gemination at concentrations around 10% (v/v), is bactericidal at ≥30% (v/v), but loses its activity at ≥90% (v/v), indicating the need for water for biocidal activity. A simple yet elegant experiment by Harrington and Walker (89) demonstrated this phenomenon: *S. aureus* was placed on dry and moist threads and then exposed to various concentrations of ethanol (15% to 99%). On the moist threads, the test organism was killed by the highest concentration within 5 minutes of exposure, whereas on the dry threads, the activity of ethanol was dependent on the amount of water available, with a narrow range of alcohol concentrations being effective. Morton (95) later verified this using other bacterial species.

Alcohol has excellent *in vitro* activity against *M. tuberculosis* and a variety of fungi (80,90,96), but again the role of water in this process is seen in the data presented in Table 14.6. Clinical isolates of *Mycobacterium* have been shown to be resistant to 75% alcohol (the type of alcohol was not identified by the investigators). *M. chelonae* and *M. nonchromogenicum* showed prolonged survival in 75% alcohol as compared with other skin flora (97).

The fungicidal activity of short-chain alcohols, mainly ethanol, against fungi is well established. Table 14.7 summarizes the data from the literature regarding the activity of ethanol against fungal species (80). Most are killed within short exposure periods (5–60 minutes) at concentrations ranging from 35% to 96%. The *Candida* spp and *Aspergillus niger* appear to be very susceptible, with an minimum effective concentration of 35% and an exposure time of 1 minute.

As with other chemical agents, the virucidal activity of alcohols is generally related to the presence or absence of a lipophilic envelope. Among the enveloped viruses,

TABLE 14.4

Comparison of Minimum Microbicidal Concentrations of Various Alcohols in Suspension Tests

		Minimum Effective Concentrations (% v/v)						
		S. aureus				*E. coli*		
Alcohol	**Exposure (Min)**	1	2	2	10	1	2	12
Methanol		65		67[a]		60–65		
Ethanol		50		58[a]		40–50		
Propan-1-ol		20		23[a]		17		
Propan-2-ol		45		46[a]		26		
Butan-1-ol		9		11[a]		5		
Isobutanol		16				6.5		
sec-Butanol		15				11		
tert-Butanol			26	46[b]			14	
Pentan-1-ol					3	2		
Isopentanol			4			2.75		
sec-Pentanol		7.5			4			
tert-Pentanol		15				9		
Hexan-1-ol		0.6[b]	5[b]		0.7			
Heptan-1-ol		0.12[c]						0.12
Octan-1-ol		0.06[c]				0.06		

[a] Converted from % w/w.
[b] In 30 minutes.
[c] In >30 minutes.
Adapted from Rotter (1996).

methanol, at concentrations of 20% to 80%, inactivates viruses in 15 minutes to 24 hours (98,99). Ethanol, on the other hand, inactivates the same viruses in 1 hour at concentrations ranging from 50% to 60% (80). The propanols seem more active, since they require lower concentrations to have the same effect within the same or shorter exposure times (80,100,101).

The naked viruses, however, are much more difficult to kill with the longer chain alcohols than with ethanol. The picornaviruses are of particular note. Against poliovirus type 1, 70% ethanol was effective in 2 minutes (102), though at 25% a 240-minute exposure was necessary for it to be effective. Ninety-five percent 2-propanol, on the other hand, was not effective in 10 minutes against poliovirus type 1 and coxsackievirus type B (101). Echovirus type 6 was inactivated with 50% ethanol in 10 minutes, whereas 90% 2-propanol was not effective. Against hepatitis A, 70% ethanol and 45% 2-propanol were not effective within 1 minute of exposure (103). Hepatitis B, which is normally considered resistant to many chemical germicides, was relatively sensitive to both 70% 2-propanol and 80% ethanol, which were effective in 10 and 2 minutes, respectively (104,105).

There are many studies that document the *in vivo* activity of alcohols. For an excellent review of the subject, the reader is referred to Rotter (80). The microflora of the skin can be divided into two groups: the resident flora (more difficult to remove) and the transient flora (easily removed). The resident microflora not only "reside" there but also replicate on the skin. Health care personnel handwash preparations are designed primarily to remove the transient organisms, whereas surgical scrubs and skin prepping formulations are directed more at reducing the resident flora.

Early studies demonstrated that alcohol rubbed on the skin easily reduced the microbial flora as effectively as a 6-minute scrub with water. Unlike some of the other antiseptics (e.g., chlorhexidine and triclosan), alcohols do not have any residual or substantive properties (see the section on chlorhexidine for a description of substantive effect). However, alcohols appear to have a sublethal effect on the skin microflora that causes it to regrow very slowly

TABLE 14.5

Comparison of Minimum Bactericidal Concentrations (% v/v) of Various Alcohols in Carrier Tests

	S. aureus			*E. coli*		*M. tuberculosis*			
Alcohol	2 min[a]	30 min	30 min	0.25–15 sec	10[b] min	10[b] min	15 min	30 min	120 min
Methanol		57[c]	70	95					90
Ethanol	80	43[c]	60	80	96	80		80	
Propan-2-ol	50		50	50	60			20	
Propan-1-ol		23[c]	30	20	50	50		20	
Butan-1-ol								5	
Isobutanol									10
Propen(1)-ol(3)								20	
Benzyl alcohol							~4		

[a] Length of exposure.
[b] Dried in sputum on glass.
[c] Converted from % w/w.
Adapted from Rotter (80).

TABLE 14.6

Tuberculocidal Effect of Ethanol under Various Conditions

	Tuberculocidal Exposure	
Condition	Conc. (%)	Time
In sputum (wet)	100	30 sec
	95	15 sec
	70	30 sec
	50	60 sec
In water	100	30 sec
	95	15 sec
	70	60 sec
In sputum (dried)		
Thin layer	70	60 sec
	50	60 sec
Thick layer	100	>60 min
	95	30 min
	70	>5 min

Reprinted from Rotter (80).

(79,80). Table 14.8 is a summary of the data demonstrating the efficiency of short-chain alcohols for reducing various bacteria from artificially contaminated hands at various concentrations and exposure times in a hygienic handwash study. The data indicate that the alcohols are fast acting, reducing viable counts released from hands by 2.6–5.8 $\log_{10}$, depending on the type of alcohol and the concentration. In Table 14.9, the effect of alcohol, both immediate and residual, on the resident flora of the skin can be seen. Concentration and exposure time are critical for both immediate and residual activity. 1-Propanol provides good immediate and residual activity. The greatest residual activity is noted when 2-propanol is combined with chlorhexidine.

Health care workers who contacted heavily contaminated patients were less likely to transfer Gram-negative bacilli to urinary catheters when they used 2-propanol as a hand rub rather than washing with soap (106). Data on the reduction of virus release from artificially contaminated hands and fingertips indicates that, compared with a handwash with soap and/or water, ethanol, 1-propanol, and 2-propanol significantly reduce the release of poliovirus type 1 from artificially contaminated hands (80). The data for rhinoviruses is less striking. Seventy percent ethanol in liquid and impregnated into towels was only slightly better than 10% ethanol, and ethanol-2-propanol and ethanol 3% benzyl alcohol were only slightly better than 70% ethanol alone (107).

It has been demonstrated that as many as 10^3–10^4 CFU of skin bacteria escape through pinholes in experimentally punctured gloves during a period of 5 minutes when the

TABLE 14.7

Fungicidal Effect of Ethanol against Various Fungal Species (Minimum Effective Concentration, %)

Fungus	Exposure Times (Min) 1	5	30	60	Not Stated
Yeasts		75			
Candida albicans	35				
Candida krusei	35				
Cryptococcus neoformans	35				
Histoplasma capsulatum					70
Blastomyces dermatitidis					70
Coccidioides immitis					70
Dermatophytes		50			
Microsporum gypseum			80		
(spores)			85		
M. audouini				70	
(on naturally infected hair)					70
Aspergillus niger	35				
Penicillium tardum					90
(conidia)					70–96

Adapted from Rotter (80).

hands had not been scrubbed earlier with a disinfectant. However, when the hands were prepared with a disinfectant scrub prior to donning the gloves, the counts were reduced to no more that 100 cfu, even up to 3–4 hours after the scrub (108). As skin bacteria can be the cause of infection, it is important to limit their access to surgical sites. Thus, surgical personnel should reduce the risk of infection to the patient by reducing the skin bacteria on their hands.

Mixtures of alcohols and agents with a real sustained action, such as chlorhexidine, combine the rapid effect of the alcohol with the substantive activity of the other component (80).

Aldehydes

Formaldehyde and glutaraldehyde have been used in the processes of sterilization and disinfection of medical devices. Although formaldehyde is an excellent biocide, the issues surrounding its toxicity have severally limited its use. Glutaraldehyde was and still is used for the routine disinfection of medical devices, especially flexible fiber-optic endoscopes and other heat-sensitive medical devices. It has excellent biocidal activity and materials compatibility. *ortho*-Phthalaldehyde (OPA) has recently been introduced as a high-level disinfectant. It has the same materials compatibility characteristics of glutaraldehyde and increased antimicrobial properties. Many other aldehydes have antimicrobial activity, but for one reason or another they have not been developed into commercial products.

Mechanism of Action

It has been demonstrated that several different aldehydes have antimicrobial properties, the most widely used being glutaraldehyde and formaldehyde. Other aldehydes showing antimicrobial activity are benzaldehyde, succinaldehyde, malonaldehyde, glyoxal, and several of the β-unsaturated aldehydes (e.g., cinnamaldehyde). OPA has recently been introduced commercially as a high-level disinfectant. Formaldehyde was the first aldehyde to be widely used as an antimicrobial, but because of its toxicity, its use has been somewhat restricted. Glutaraldehyde was first proposed as an antimicrobial by Pepper and Lieberman (109) in their endeavor to find an alternative to formaldehyde sterilization of sutures. The sporicidal properties of alkaline glutaraldehyde were demonstrated by Stonehill et al. (110), making this form preferable as

TABLE 14.8

Efficiency of Short-chain Alcohols to Reduce the Release of Various Test Bacteria from Artificially Contaminated Hands at Various Concentrations and Exposure Times in Hygienic Handrubs[a] (Mean Log Reduction)

Alcohol	Conc. (% w/v)	Test Organism	Exposure Time (Min)			
			0.5	1.0	2.0	4.0
Ethanol	60	*Escherichia coli*		3.8		
	70	*E. coli*	2.6–3.6	3.8–4.3	4.5–5.1	5.4
		Staphylococcus saprophyticus	3.5	4.0		
		Staphylococcus aureus	2.6–3.7			
	80	*E. coli*		4.5		
2-Propanol	50	*E. coli*	3.4	3.9	4.4	
	60	*E. coli*		4.0–4.7		
		Serratia marcescens		4.1		
	70	*E. coli*	3.4–3.5	4.8–4.9		
1-Propanol	40	*E. coli*		4.3		
	50	*E. coli*	3.7	4.7–5.0	4.9	
	60	*E. coli*		5.5		
	100	*E. coli*		5.8		

[a] Tested with comparable methods.
Adapted from Rotter (80).

a chemical sterilant. Until recently, no other aldehydes have been available for routine use as high-level disinfectants or sterilants. The use of OPA is relatively recent, and consequently there is little information on its action. The antimicrobial properties of OPA have recently been described (111), along with its activity and mechanism of action (112–114).

The antimicrobial activity of aldehydes in general is based on the reactivity of the aldehyde group. For a theoretical explanation of the reactivity of the aldehyde group, the reader is referred to Rehn and Nolte (115). The mechanism of action is based on the ability of aldehydes to undergo alkylation reactions. The reactivity of the aldehyde group can be changed by other functional groups on the molecule. Aldehydes tend to become hydrated in aqueous solutions and in equilibrium with the free aldehyde form, which is believed to be the active species. Figure 14.2 depicts the species available when glutaraldehyde is in an aqueous system.

In the case of glutaraldehyde, the monomeric free aldehyde molecule is in equilibrium with the cyclic hemiacetal and acetal polymers, together coexisting with smaller quantities of mono- and dihydrates. This equilibrium appears to be somewhat temperature sensitive, since at higher temperatures there is a shift to the more active monomeric form.

The primary chemical species that aldehydes react with are amines and sulfhydryl groups. The cellular constituents they are most likely to react with are proteins, both enzymes and structural proteins, and nucleic acids. Formaldehyde is known to react with amino groups to bring about intermolecular cross-linking (116) and although it reacts with both RNA and DNA, its reaction with RNA is stronger (117). Glutaraldehyde, like formaldehyde, can cause intramolecular and intermolecular cross-linking of molecules. Understanding the chemistry of aldehydes allows one to speculate as to the cellular sites at which aldehyde germicides work.

Spectrum of Activity

Aldehydes, including formaldehyde, demonstrate activity against both Gram-positive and -negative bacteria. Since the only aldehydes commercially available for hospital use in the United States are glutaraldehyde and OPA, the spectrum of activity of other aldehydes, although of interest, is not dealt with here.

Several publications describe the effectiveness of glutaraldehyde against the Gram-positive and -negative

TABLE 14.9

Efficacy of Alcohol Surgical Handrub on Resident Skin Flora from the Hands

Preparation	Conc. (% v/v)	Time (Min)	Mean Log Reduction after Surgical Handrub	
			Immediate	3 Hours Posttreatment
1-Propanol	60	5	2.5–2.9	1.6–2.4
2-Propanol	70	5	2.4	2.1
		3	1.8	1.2
		2	1.2	0.8
		<1	0.8	
	60	5	1.7	1.0
	50	2	0.7	
Ethanol	95	2	2.1	
	80	5	2.5	
		2	1.5	
	70	5	2.0	
		2	0.6–1.0	0.6
2-Propanol + chlorhexidine gluconate	70.5	5	2.5	2.7
		4	1.7	1.1
		2	1.5	1.0
		<1	0.8	1.2

Adapted from Rotter (80).

bacteria. The rapid bactericidal activity of a 2% glutaraldehyde solution has been documented. Rubo et al. (118) demonstrated the rapid bactericidal activity of 0.02% glutaraldehyde against *S. aureus, E. coli,* and *P. aeruginosa*. In a 20-minute exposure to this low concentration, inactivation of 10^4 cells or more was observed. *P. aeruginosa* appeared to be the most resistant of the three organisms tested. This is supported by additional work by Borick (119), who demonstrated rapid kill (less than 1 minute) of *E. coli, P. aeruginosa, Serratia marcescens, Proteus vulgaris,* and *K. pneumoniae* by 2% glutaraldehyde. *Helicobacter pylori* was rapidly killed by 0.5% glutaraldehyde with exposure as short as 15 seconds (120). OPA was shown to be effective against both vancomycin-resistant enterococci (VRE) and MRSA (121).

The mycobacteria are a heterogeneous group of organisms ranging from the slow-growing *M. tuberculosis* to the more rapidly growing *M. chelonae (*also spelled *chelonei),* from the relatively susceptible *M. fortuitum* to the resistant *M. chelonae*. The one thing they have in common is a cell wall with a high lipid content, which makes them less susceptible to hydrophilic molecules, hence less susceptible to many disinfectants. The surrogate organism used to determine tuberculocidal activity is *M. bovis* var BCG. Collins and Montalbine (122) examined the activity of glutaraldehyde against a variety of mycobacteria, including the virulent strain *M. tuberculosis* H37Rv. The data in Table 14.10 indicate that there is a wide range of susceptibility.

Using a modified Kelsey Maurer procedure, several strains of atypical mycobacteria were tested for susceptibility to glutaraldehyde. It was shown that exposure of strains of *Mycobacterium avium-intracellulare, Mycobacterium gordonae, M. fortuitum,* and *M. chelonae* to 1% glutaraldehyde for 15 minutes resulted in a 4 $\log_{10}$ reduction, and exposure to a 2% solution for 1 minute resulted in 100% kill. In another study, 2% glutaraldehyde tested against several of the same species in a quantitative suspension and carrier test was shown to reduce their populations 5 $\log_{10}$ within 30 minutes in the presence of organic soil and hardwater (123). Further work by the same group showed that endoscopes artificially contaminated with *M. tuberculosis* and *M. avium-intracellulare* in sputum and endoscopes precleaned using a neutral soap could be disinfected with

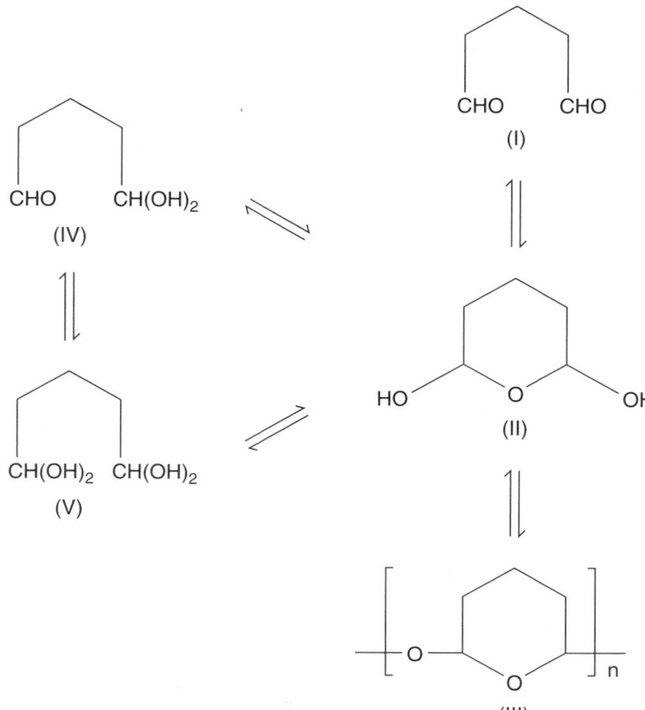

FIGURE 14.2 • Glutaraldehyde species available in aqueous solutions: (I) monomer, (II) cyclic hemiacetal, (III) acetal-like polymer, (IV) monohydrate, and (V) dihydrate.

2% glutaraldehyde in 10 and 20 minutes, respectively (124). The data indicate that there is a range of times for the inactivation of the various species. Collins (125) studied the response of atypical mycobacteria to glutaraldehyde. The most resistant species were *M. gordonae* and members of the *M. avium-intracellulare* group (Table 14.11).

TABLE 14.10

Log Reduction of Mycobacteria Exposed to 1% Alkaline Glutaraldehyde at 18°C

Mycobacterium spp.	Log_{10} Reduction in 5 Min
M. tuberculosis H37Rv	3.7
M. bovis	3.6
M. bovis BCG Montreal	3.9
M. intracellulare	3.2
M. scrofulaceum	>5.0
M. kansasii	>5.0
M. avium	>5.0
M. marinum	>5.0
M. smegmatis	>5.0

Adapted from Collins and Montalbine (1978).

There have been several reports of glutaraldehyde-resistant strains of *M. chelonae* isolated from automated endoscope reprocessors and processed scopes (126–128). Their resistance may be due to the formation of biofilms on the surfaces of the tubing in the machines. Isolation of two *M. chelonae* strains from a scope disinfector and a type strain (NCTC 946) were tested for susceptibility to a wide range of disinfectants, including glutaraldehyde, succinaldehyde, industrial methylated spirits, peracetic acid, chlorine-releasing compounds, and a peroxygen. The type strain, which had never been exposed to disinfectants, was very sensitive to all the disinfectants tested, with the exception of the peroxygen. The isolates from the scope disinfector, however, were less susceptible to the peroxygen and chlorine-releasing compounds and were described as very resistant to 2% glutaraldehyde, with some strains showing a <1 $\log_{10}$ reduction with a 60-minute exposure to 2% glutaraldehyde (129). It was suggested that glutaraldehyde may have selected for the growth of resistant strains of *M. chelonae* (128). Studies have evaluated a variety of disinfectants against several strains of atypical mycobacteria, including glutaraldehyde-resistant strains isolated from washer disinfectors. The data indicate that, as expected, the washer disinfector isolates were extremely resistant to glutaraldehyde, but both acidic OPA and alkaline OPA, under dirty and clean conditions,

TABLE 14.11

Mycobactericidal Activity of 2% Alkaline Glutaraldehyde Solution Tested at 20°C against a Number of Mycobacterial Species

Organism	Inoculum Size (Log)	Rate of Kill (Logs per 10 Min)	ETS[a] (Min)
M. tuberculosis TMC 102[b]	6.10	2.41	25
M. tuberculosis BCG Pasteur TMC 1011	5.92	1.74	30
M. kansasii TMC 1201	4.80	2.50	15
M. kansasii TMC 1203	5.25	2.38	15
M. kansasii TMC 1204	5.35	2.44	15
M. simiae TMC 1226	6.25	2.22	20
M. marinum TMC 1218	5.05	4.33	10
M. avium TMC 706	6.15	1.54	35
M. avium TMC 724	6.21	1.28	40
M. intracellulare TMC 673	6.38	0.44	>60
M. intracellulare TMC 1406	5.75	0.80	60
M. scrofulaceum TMC 1306	6.38	4.05	12
M. gordonae TMC 1327	5.97	0.59	60
M. szulgae TMC 1328	6.24	2.12	20
M. smegmatis TMC 1546	4.86	4.55	10
M. fortuitum TMC 1529	5.70	5.00	10

[a] Estimated time to sterility (<50 CFU/mL).
[b] TMC, Trudeau Mycobacterium Culture Collection number.
Adapted from Collins (125).

were effective (113). It has been shown previously that bacteria isolated from water systems or bacteria that are grown in water are much more resistant to the action of disinfectants than bacteria grown in laboratory media (130,131).

OPA has several advantages over glutaraldehyde, including its superior activity against mycobacteria. Based on the claims for high-level disinfection, a 0.55% solution of OPA is effective in 5 minutes whereas a 2.5% glutaraldehyde solution requires 45 minutes to achieve the same 6 $\log_{10}$ reduction in *M. bovis*.

In general, aldehydes are less effective against bacterial spores than vegetative forms of the same organism and other vegetative organisms. Of all the aldehydes, glutaraldehyde is the only one that has substantial activity against spores. A 2% alkaline glutaraldehyde solution has the same activity as an 8% formaldehyde solution (110,132) and 10 times the activity of glyoxal (ethanedial) (109). The sporicidal activity is also affected by the pH of the solution, and in fact the activity is directly related to the pH. Alkaline solutions have been shown to be more sporicidal. The addition of bicarbonate to glutaraldehyde caused a substantial increase in the sporicidal activity (109). The bicarbonate appears to affect the spore and not the glutaraldehyde molecule, as pretreatment of spores with bicarbonate renders them sensitive to acidic glutaraldehyde. The same effect could not be reproduced with sodium hydroxide (133). In experiments, very high concentrations of glutaraldehyde ($\geq$50%) and glutaraldehyde alkalinized with sodium bicarbonate showed the same pH effect, but formaldehyde did not (132).

C. difficile is a clinically important spore-forming bacterium, especially in aged patients and in conjunction with certain antibiotic therapies (134–137). Data in Table 14.12 indicate the *in vitro* susceptibility of *C. difficile* spores to glutaraldehyde with short exposure periods of 5 to 30 minutes for 0.1% to 2.0% glutaraldehyde. This is in contrast with the longer exposure times required to kill *B. subtilis* and *Bacillus stearothermophilus* spores (138).

A study evaluating the performance of 2% glutaraldehyde against *C. difficile in situ* corroborates the *in vitro* data. Endoscopes contaminated with *C. difficile* were effectively disinfected in 5 minutes (139). A comparison of the sporicidal activity of glutaraldehyde and of OPA indicates that glutaraldehyde is considerably more sporicidal. Two-percent and 3% glutaraldehyde solutions

TABLE 14.12

Sporicidal Activity of Glutaraldehyde against *Clostridium difficile*

Glutaraldehyde Concentration (%)	Spore Challenge	Number of Surviving Organisms (Exposure Time in Min)						
		2	5	10	15	20	25	30
2.0	2×10^3	400	0	0	0	0	0	0
1.0	1×10^4	500	900	0	0	0	0	0
0.2	2×10^3	400	400	400	100	0	0	0
0.1	1×10^4	4000	1400	2900	1000	2100	700	400

Reprinted from Dyas and Das (1986).

achieved a 6 $\log_{10}$ reduction in spores of *B. subtilis* in 6 and 3 hours, respectively, while 0.3% and 0.55% OPA required 72 and 48 hours, respectively. With spores of *C. tetani*, 2% and 3% glutaraldehyde achieved a 2 $\log_{10}$ reduction in 2 minutes, and 0.3% and 0.55% OPA achieved the same results in 20 minutes and 5 minutes, respectively. Finally, with spores of *C. difficile*, 2% and 3% glutaraldehyde achieved a 3 $\log_{10}$ reduction in 15 seconds, whereas 0.3% and 0.55% OPA achieved the same level of sporicidal activity at 2 minutes and 1 minute, respectively (140).

Fungi, both yeasts and molds, are generally susceptible to glutaraldehyde at concentrations sold as high-level disinfectants. The effect of pH again has been demonstrated. A 0.5% solution of alkaline glutaraldehyde was shown to be more effective than an acidic solution at the same concentration at inhibiting spore production and mycelial growth of *A. niger* (141). A 2% acidic glutaraldehyde solution, however, was found to be effective in 15 minutes at 25°C against a wide variety of fungi except *A. niger*, which required 30 minutes for complete kill. The MIC for acidic glutaraldehyde was five times higher than for alkaline glutaraldehyde in inhibiting the growth of *Saccharomyces cerevisiae* (142). Other studies have shown glutaraldehyde to be potent against a wide variety of fungi, including *Trichophyton interdigitale*, *Microsporum gypseum*, *C. albicans*, *Mucor hiemalis*, *Rhizopus stolonifer*, *Penicillium chrysogenum*, and *Byssochlamys fulva* (143). A 10% alkaline glutaraldehyde solution was shown *in vitro* to eradicate *Trichophyton mentagrophytes* and *Cephalosporium* and *Fusarium* spp. (144). *In vivo* activity of glutaraldehyde was demonstrated in the treatment of onychomycoses (145). Isenberg et al. (146) demonstrated the effectiveness of 2% alkaline glutaraldehyde against *C. albicans* and other fast-growing vegetative bacteria after reuse in normal hospital practice. The data in Table 14.13 indicate that, under normal hospital use of a commercially available glutaraldehyde product, the activity of the solution was maintained after reuse of the product for 14 or 28 days.

The virucidal activity of glutaraldehyde has been substantiated in the literature. The work of Klein and Deforest (101) demonstrated the differential activity of glutaraldehyde against enveloped and nonenveloped viruses, the former being more susceptible. Poliovirus type 1, coxsackievirus type B1, and echovirus type 6 were more difficult to inactivate, requiring >1% glutaraldehyde, than were herpes simplex virus, vaccinia virus, Asian influenza virus, and adenovirus. (Although adenovirus is classified as a nonenveloped virus, it does contain lipids absorbed to its protein surface, and they are considered an integral part of the virus structure, as they are with enveloped viruses.) The enveloped viruses and adenovirus required ≥0.2% glutaraldehyde with a 1-minute exposure at room temperature for inactivation. Isolates of echovirus showed differences in susceptibility to glutaraldehyde (147). Table 14.14 lists the viruses susceptible to glutaraldehyde.

OPA is effective against bovine viral diarrhea virus, a surrogate test organism for hepatitis C virus (165), and against duck hepatitis B virus, a surrogate test virus for human hepatitis B virus (166), with an exposure of 5 minutes at 20°C.

Organic soil, which affects the activity of many chemical germicides, has little effect on the virucidal activity of glutaraldehyde (149,150,157,158,163). Saitanu and Lund (149) present data that indicate the activity of glutaraldehyde is faster in the presence of organic soil (10% horse serum and 20% mouse droppings) than in its absence. Glutaraldehyde was also shown to retain its activity against cell-associated HIV in the presence of blood (155).

Mechanism of Action

As stated, protein molecules provide a natural target for the aldehyde-based germicides. Consequently, the cell surface, rich in protein molecules (enzymes, lipoprotein,

TABLE 14.13

Dilution of Commercially Available Glutaraldehyde Solution Required to Inactivate 90% and 99.9% Fast-growing Non-spore-forming Microorganisms

			10 Min		60 Min	
Microorganism	Disinfectant	Condition	90% (24 h)	99.9% (72 h)	90% (24 h)	99.9% (72 h)
Staphylococcus aureus ATCC 653	2% glutaraldehyde	S	32	32	64	64
		U	64	64	128	128
	3.4% glutaraldehyde	S	64	32	128	64
		U	128	64	256	256
Pseudomonas aeruginosa ATCC 15442	2% glutaraldehyde	S	128	64	128	128
		U	256	128	1024	256
	3.4% glutaraldehyde	S	128	64	512	256
		U	256	128	1024	512
Mycobacterium sp MCLO TH7	2% glutaraldehyde	S	8	4	8	4
		U	16	16	16	16
	3.4% glutaraldehyde	S	4	4	8	8
		U	32	32	32	32
Candida albicans ATCC 11651	2% glutaraldehyde	S	512	8	512	8
		U	>1024	8	>1024	16
	3.4% glutaraldehyde	S	16	8	16	8
		U	32	16	64	32

S, stressed; U, fresh disinfectant.
Reprinted from Isenberg (146).

glycoproteins, etc.), is an obvious site for aldehyde germicides to exert their activity, and indeed several experiments show that the cell surface is a potential reactive site for aldehydes (167,168). But although many studies show preferential reaction of glutaraldehyde with the cell surface and indicate this is part of its mechanism of action, there is evidence that there may be other sites involved as well. McGucken and Woodside (169) demonstrated that inhibition of protein, RNA, and DNA synthesis in glutaraldehyde-treated *E. coli* was almost complete within 10 minutes following addition of the aldehyde. This is due to the inhibition of uptake of precursors for synthesis. A direct effect of glutaraldehyde on nucleic acid has not been demonstrated. Transport of low-molecular weight amino acids in glutaraldehyde-treated and untreated *E. coli* shows a reduction of about 50% in the treated cells. One would expect a higher reduction if this was the only mechanism of action (170). Treatment of *Micrococcus lysodeikticus* cells with glutaraldehyde prevented the release of selective enzymes from the periplasmic space of *M. lysodeikticus*, indicating interaction of glutaraldehyde with the outer cell surface (171). Similar phenomena have been observed with formaldehyde-treated *E. coli* (172). Effects on other periplasmic space enzymes have been reported (173,174), including ATPase (175). Cheng et al. (176) showed that glutaraldehyde fixation shifted ATPase from the periplasmic space to the cell surface and that dehydrogenase enzyme activity was inhibited at glutaraldehyde concentrations that did not affect cell viability (177).

In a comparative study of mechanism of action of glutaraldehyde and of OPA on mycobacterial cells, the data suggest that the cross-linking effect of glutaraldehyde on the cell membrane is the mechanism by which glutaraldehyde exerts its antimicrobial action and that the more lipophilic OPA molecule is more efficient at crossing the lipid rich cell surface of the mycobacterial cell and exerting its action internally (178).

The mechanism of action for aldehydes has been extensively studied in bacteria, but little work has been done on viruses and fungi and virtually no data exist relating to protozoans. In some fungal species, glutaraldehyde has been shown to inhibit germination, spore swelling,

TABLE 14.14

Viruses Shown to Be Susceptible to the Activity of Glutaraldehyde

Virus	Reference
Coxsackievirus B1	148
Coxsackievirus B3	149, 150
Human immunodeficiency virus type 1	151, 152, 153, 154, 155
Herpes simplex virus type 2	156, 157
Yellow fever virus	158
Influenza virus PR-8	158
Aphthovirus	150
Pestivirus	150
Iridovirus	150
Hepatitis B virus	104, 105, 159, 160
Hepatitis A virus	103, 161
Duck hepatitis virus	162
Poliovirus type 1	148
Echovirus	148
Rotavirus	163
Feline calcivirus	164

mycelial growth, and sporulation (141). It is proposed that the active site maybe the fungal cell wall, which contains chitin, a compound resembling peptidoglycan, which makes up the bacterial cell wall.

In viruses, the obvious site for glutaraldehyde to react with is the protein capsid or one of the enzymes necessary for the virus to infect cells and replicate. In poliovirus type 1 and echovirus type 25, it was shown that glutaraldehyde reacted with lysine residues in the protein capsid (147). The RNA in poliovirus was resistant to glutaraldehyde concentrations up to 1% (179). With hepatitis A virus (HAV), glutaraldehyde was shown to interact with the surface (163), whereas with hepatitis B virus (HBV), electron micrographs indicate that the virus has a "fixed" appearance (160) and that the DNA polymerase was affected when the virus was exposed to a glutaraldehyde disinfectant (180). Work with *Pseudomonas aeruginosa* phage F116 adds evidence for the theory that the mode of action is at the site of the viral capsid (181–183).

The effect of pH on the activity of aldehydes has been extensively studied. The reaction of glutaraldehyde with protein increases significantly as the pH is increased from 4 to 9 (184). The activity of glutaraldehyde is known to be greater at pH 9–10 than at 6–8, either because of the effect of pH on the bacterial cell or because condensation reactions of aldehydes are catalyzed at alkaline pH. Sodium bicarbonate appears to act on the cell rather than on modification of the glutaraldehyde molecule itself (133). Munton and Russell (185) showed that acidic glutaraldehyde and alkaline glutaraldehyde react with the cell wall to different extents, with alkaline glutaraldehyde showing more immediate reactivity. Uptake isotherms for alkaline glutaraldehyde show initial and secondary increases, suggesting penetration of the glutaraldehyde, presumably aided by the bicarbonate, into reactive sites. The potentiation of glutaraldehyde by cations (Mg, Ca) has also been demonstrated (186).

Glutaraldehyde at low concentrations inhibits germination of *B. subtilis* and *Bacillus pumilus* spores, whereas at higher concentrations it is sporicidal (187). Treatment of spores with glutaraldehyde reduces the release of dipicolinic acid and peroxide-induced lysis of spores, suggesting that glutaraldehyde interacts at the spore surface. Other investigations into the sporicidal activity of glutaraldehyde indicate the protective effect of the spore coat and the role in alkalination of the glutaraldehyde in penetrating this protective barrier (188,189). Differences in uptake of glutaraldehyde suggest that, in contrast to alkaline glutaraldehyde acid, glutaraldehyde may not penetrate beyond the spore coat (190). The spore coat has also been shown to be the structure responsible for resistance to OPA. Resistance to OPA appears at the same time as spore maturation (114).

Peracids

The two peracids that are the most commonly used for the purposes of disinfection and/or sterilization are hydrogen peroxide and peracetic acid. Both of these compounds belong to the group of compounds known as peracids or peroxygen compounds.

Hydrogen peroxide has been used for its antiseptic properties since the 1800s. Early in its evolution, hydrogen peroxide was used for the preservation of milk and water and for the sterilization of certain beverages. As an antiseptic, it has been used in the treatment of periodontal disease and endodontic therapy as well as in topical applications. As a disinfectant, it is used at various concentrations to disinfect materials such as drinking water, medical equipment, and septage, and it was the first nonthermal disinfectant cleared by the FDA for use on contact lenses (191). Its activity is less affected by pH than that of many other disinfectants, such as phenols, organic acids, and glutaraldehyde (192). Hydrogen peroxide is produced naturally in phagocytes, where it acts on bacteria.

Peracetic acid, thought to be a more potent antimicrobial than hydrogen peroxide, has the added advantage of being more lipid soluble and free from the decomposition of catalase and peroxidase (193), which effectively neutralizes the action of hydrogen peroxide. Like hydrogen peroxide, it has been used for the disinfection and sterilization of medical devices (e.g., hemodialyzers) and environmental surfaces. However, it is more resistant than hydrogen peroxide to the neutralizing effect of organic material (79).

Both hydrogen peroxide and peracetic acid have been commercialized in liquid and vapor forms. It is generally accepted that the vapor phase of each compound is more antimicrobial. In the liquid phase, each compound is unstable and requires careful handling and storage to ensure it maintains its level of antimicrobial activity.

Mechanism of Action

The hydroxyl radical is an extremely potent oxidant and is responsible for the killing action of peroxide (194). The hydroxyl radical has the ability to react with various essential components of the cell, such as lipids, proteins, and nucleic acids. Gould and Hitchins (195) suggested that the antimicrobial properties of hydrogen peroxide are due to the oxidation of double bonds in proteins, lipids, and surface membranes. However, it has other known effects, such as dissociation of 70S ribosomal subunits, bringing about cell surface changes and cleavage of the DNA backbone, and damage to spore DNA has been described (196).

The mechanism of action of peracetic acid has not been studied. It is hypothesized that peracetic acid acts by denaturing proteins and enzymes and increasing cell permeability by disrupting sulfhydryl and disulfide bonds (79). Decomposition of peracetic acid produces the highly reactive molecule singlet oxygen, and it has been proposed that this species is responsible for peracetic acid's activity (197). Malachesky (198) reviewed the chemical reactions that peracetic acid can undergo, and it is obvious that many of the functional groups that peracetic acid reacts with are present in living organism; therefore, the mechanism of action is probably not specific to any one cell structure.

Spectrum of Activity

A number of investigators have looked at the activity and disinfecting properties of 3% hydrogen peroxide, expressed as D-values. Table 14.15 lists these values. The data for the bacterial species show rapid disinfection; however, the two fugal species tested show more resistance to the action of 3% peroxide. And there is a large discrepancy between the two studies with regard to the resistance.

C. albicans was very resistant in both studies, indicating that longer disinfection times would be required for this particular organism. D-values for organisms on the surfaces of contact lenses were lower (192). Tables 14.16 and 14.17 indicate the lethality of peroxide toward a number of bacteria, fungi, viruses, and spores at concentrations less than 3%.

Several observations can be made. First, peroxide has a wide spectrum of activity. Its activity is generally better against Gram-negative than Gram-positive organisms. Second, viruses are extremely susceptible, being inactivated at concentrations of 30 ppm or less, although some of the viruses required extended periods of contact. Higher concentrations or temperature would presumably speed the action. Third, most bacteria are easily killed with relatively low concentrations of peroxide and in a relatively short period of time. It is thought the anaerobes are even more susceptible because they lack the enzymes catalase, peroxidase, and superoxide dismutase. Fourth, against spore-forming bacteria the data indicate that high concentrations (i.e., greater than those commercially available) do provide rapid sporicidal activity. However, at lower concentrations (500 ppm or less), the time for lethality is increased significantly to hours. Rutala et al. (199) showed that a 6% solution is an effective sterilant in 6 hours and that it exhibits rapid activity against spores.

Table 14.18 shows the spectrum of activity of peracetic acid (approximately 0.2%) at 50°C in the presence of 5% serum and hard water. The D-values indicate rapid activity against vegetative bacteria, fungi, and spores.

At 50°C, peracetic acid is effective against *M. tuberculosis*, *M. smegmatis* (198), and a variety of clinical isolates of *Mycobacterium* and *Cryptosporidium* spp (200). Table 14.19 presents a comparison between peracetic acid and two other disinfectants commonly used on environmental surfaces. The data for peracetic acid demonstrate the effect of temperature against *Listeria* and *Enterococcus* organisms. The presence of catalase in *S. aureus* may explain the lack of temperature effect. The two other disinfectants tested, chlorine and benzalkonium chloride, show an order of magnitude difference in the time required to achieve the same result as peracetic acid.

TABLE 14.15

D-values for 3% Hydrogen Peroxide against a Variety of Microorganisms

Organism	H_2O_2 Conc. (%)	D-value (Min)
Staphylococcus epidermidis	3	1.7
Pseudomonas aeruginosa	3	1.7
Serratia marcescens	3	3.1
	3	2.8
Aspergillus fumigatus	3	25.1
		11
Candida albicans	3	27.9
		48

Adapted from Lever and Sutton (191).

TABLE 14.16

Antimicrobial Activity of Hydrogen Peroxide toward Bacteria, Yeasts, and Viruses

Organism	Conc. (ppm)	Lethality (Min)	Temp. (°C)
Bacteria			
Staphylococcus aureus	1000	60	NS[a]
Staphylococcus aureus	25.8×10^4	0.2	24
Escherichia coli	1000	60	NS
Escherichia coli	500	10–30	37
Eberthella typhi	1000	60	NS
Aerobacter aerogenes	500	10–30	37
Sarcina spp	500	150	37
Streptococcus lactis	500	150	37
Streptococcus liquifaciens	500	240	37
Micrococcus spp	30	10	NS
Staphylococcus epidermidis	30	10	NS
Yeasts			
Torula spp	500	180–210	37
Oidium spp	500	180–210	37
Viruses			
Orthinosis virus	30	180	NS
Rhinovirus types 1A, 1B, 7	7.5	50–60	37
Rhinovirus types 1A, 1B, 7	15	18–20	37
Rhinovirus types 1A, 1B, 7	30	6–8	37
Poliovirus type 1	15	75	20
Poliovirus type 1	30	75	20

[a] NS, not stated.
Modified from Block (192).

Phenolics

The use of phenol as an antimicrobial dates back to the use of coal tars as antiseptics and disinfectants. However, it was the use of carbolic acid by Lister as an antiseptic in surgery that demonstrated this compound's antimicrobial potential. Phenolic antiseptics and disinfectants make up a large group of compounds whose only commonality is that each is based on the structure of phenol. Phenol itself is the simplest of the group, and more complex compounds include *p-tert*-amylphenol and phenylphenols such as hexachlorophene and triclosan (Fig. 14.3). In general, phenolic compounds are used in the hospital setting as low- to intermediate-level disinfectants (primarily used on environmental surfaces), and in addition 2,4,4′-trichloro-2′-hydroxy-diphenylether (triclosan) and *para*-chloro-*meta*-xylenol (PCMX) have been used in many skin antiseptic formulations. Because of the relatively recent widespread use of triclosan, it is covered in a separate section of this chapter. Phenolic disinfectants are not appropriate for use in disinfecting critical instruments because they are not sporicides and exhibit slow tuberculocidal activity, and their use with semicritical devices is limited because of the difficulty of rinsing them from many materials and because of the tissue irritation caused by residuals (53).

Mechanism of Action

Information on the mode of action of phenolic compounds (with the exception of triclosan) is scarce. The free hydroxyl group is the reactive site of the molecule. Substitution, alkyl or halogen, affects the reactivity of the hydroxyl group. It is the hydrophobic nature of the polar groups that contributes to the membrane active properties of phenolic compounds. Goddard and McCue (201) provide a good

TABLE 14.17

Sporicidal Activity of Hydrogen Peroxide toward Spore-forming Bacteria and Bacterial Spores

Organism	Conc. (ppm)	Lethality (Min)	Temp. (°C)	Comment
Bacillus subtilis	500	420–1080	37	bc
Bacillus cereus	500	420–1080	37	bc
Bacillus megaterium	500	420–1080	37	bc
Bacillus subtilis ATCC 15411[a]	30	1440	37	spores
Bacillus subtilis SA22	25.8×10^4	7.3	24	ss
Bacillus coagulaus	25.8×10^4	1.8	24	ss
Bacillus stearothermophilus	25.8×10^4	1.5	24	ss
Clostridium sporogenes	25.8×10^4	0.8	24	ss
Bacillus subtilis var *globigii*	25.8×10^4	2.0	24	ss
	35×10^4	1.5	24	ss
	41×10^4	0.75	24	ss
Bacillus subtilis SA 22	17.7×10^4	9.4	20	ss
	17.7×10^4	0.53	45	ss
	29.5×10^4	3.6	20	ss
	29.5×10^4	0.35	45	ss
	35.4×10^4	2.3	20	ss
	35.4×10^4	0.19	45	ss

bc, bacterial culture; ss, spore suspension.
[a] Carrier Test.
Adapted from Block (192).

review of the structure-activity relationship of phenolic compounds. Their analysis indicates the following:

- Halogen substitution intensifies the microbicidal activity of the phenol derivative.
- Introduction of aliphatic or aromatic groups into the nucleus of halogen phenols increases bactericidal activity.
- Aliphatic chains on the phenol derivative intensify the bactericidal activity to a greater degree than branched chains or 2-alkyl groups of the same total number of carbon atoms.
- 2-Alkyl derivatives of 4-chlorophenol are more germicidal that 4-alkyl derivatives of 2-chlorophenol.

In general, phenolics exert their biocidal activity by binding to the cell surface, with the primary target being the cell membrane. Subsequent to binding to the membrane surface, interference with membrane-associated functions takes place. Denyer (202) hypothesized that binding to the membrane results in inhibition of respiratory activity, generation of energy, inhibition of substrate oxidation, and inhibition of transport processes. Hexachlorophene was shown to inhibit the membrane-bound part of electron transport near the terminal acceptor (203), and triclosan inhibited uptake of certain amino acids (204). Low concentrations (50% of the MIC) of several compounds increased oxygen uptake, suggesting uncoupling of oxidative phosphorylation (205). This hypothesis was supported by the work of Hugo and Bowen (206), who examined the effects of 4-ethylphenol on *E. coli*, and by studies of the effect of fentichlor on *E. coli* and *S. aureus* (207,208).

The effects of phenolic compounds on cell membrane permeability have been studied. A strong correlation exists between the loss of K^+ and cell viability in *S. marcescens* exposed to phenol (209). Treatment of *Streptococcus faecalis* with 1% phenol produced leakage of amino acids consistent with cell lysis (210). Judis (211,212) substantiated this with experiments that showed leakage of ^{14}C-labeled glutamate, ^{14}C-adenosine, and ^{32}P-phosphate from cells exposed to phenol, along with several other phenolic compounds, including PCMX. The extent of release was directly correlated with the concentration of the biocide. Early events were shown to be reversible, but at some point leakage led to cell death. Commager and Judis (205) proposed that the primary mechanism of action of phenolic compounds is damage to the cytoplasmic membrane. Additional work with

TABLE 14.18

Relative Resistance of Organisms to STERIS 20 Use Dilution in Hard Water (>800 ppm as $CaCO_3$) with 5% Serum at 50°C

Organism	D Value (Sec)
Bacillus stearothermophilus ATCC 7953	14.5
Bacillus circulans ATCC 4513	11.9
Bacillus coagulans ATCC 7050	8.5
Bacillus subtilis ATCC 9372	7.7
Bacillus subtilis ATCC 19659	6.9
Bacillus pumilus ATCC 27142	6.4
Bacillus subtilis var *niger* ATCC 9372	4.9
Bacillus cereus ATCC 11778	4.2
Clostridium sporogenes ATCC 3584	<2.0
Aspergllus fumigatus ATCC 10894	<2.0
Trichophyton mentagrophytes ATCC 9533	<2.0
Aspergillus niger ATCC 16404	<2.0
Candida albicans ATCC 10231	<2.0
Salmonella choleraesuis ATCC 10708	<2.0
Pseudomonas aeruginosa ATCC 15442	<2.0
Staphylococcus aureus ATCC 6538	<2.0

Reprinted from Malchesky (198).

S. aureus indicated that treatment of cells with fentichlor caused leakage of 260 nm of absorbing material from the cells (207,213,214). Similar results were found when *E. coli* was treated with triclosan and *B. megaterium* with hexachlorophene and other bisphenols (204,215). The high lipid content of the mycobacterial cell wall is thought to be the target of phenols against this group of organisms. Rubin (216) has reviewed the effect of phenols on mycobacteria. Phenols are not particularly sporicidal but have been shown to be sporostatic, inhibiting germination and outgrowth. Russell and Chopra (217) suggest that phenol binds loosely to sites on the spore surface, exerting its inhibitory effects. These effects are reversible.

Inhibition of cellular systems by phenolic compounds has also been reported, suggesting that if these compounds do penetrate the cell membrane and enter the cytoplasm, a secondary site of action may be the cytoplasmic enzymes. Treatment of *S. aureus* with a 1:1000 dilution of phenol inhibited the cells' ability to activate several internal metabolites, whereas other systems were only partially inhibited (218,219). Succinate dehydrogenase, a cytoplasmic enzyme, was inactivated by 4-butyl phenol and hexylresorcinol at concentrations higher than those required for microbicidal activity (85). Coagulation of cell protein in phenol-treated cells was observed by Bancroft and Richter (220) and was confirmed by Hugo (221).

Very little information appears in the literature concerning the specific mechanism of action of phenols against fungi and viruses.

Spectrum of Activity

It is difficult to discuss the antimicrobial activity of phenolic compounds as a group because of the variety of

TABLE 14.19

Comparison of Peracetic Acid with Other Disinfectants: Effect of Temperature and Concentration in PPM to Obtain Lethality in 5 Minutes

Organism	Peracetic Acid	Active Chlorine	Benzalkonium Chloride
At 20°C			
Listeria monocytogenes	45	100	200
Staphylococcus aureus ATCC 6538	90	860	500
Enterococcus faecium DSM 2918	45	300	250
At 5°C			
Listeria monocytogenes	90	860	500
Staphylococcus aureus ATCC 6538	90	1100	750
Enterococcus faecium DSM 2918	90	450	500

Reprinted from Block (2001).

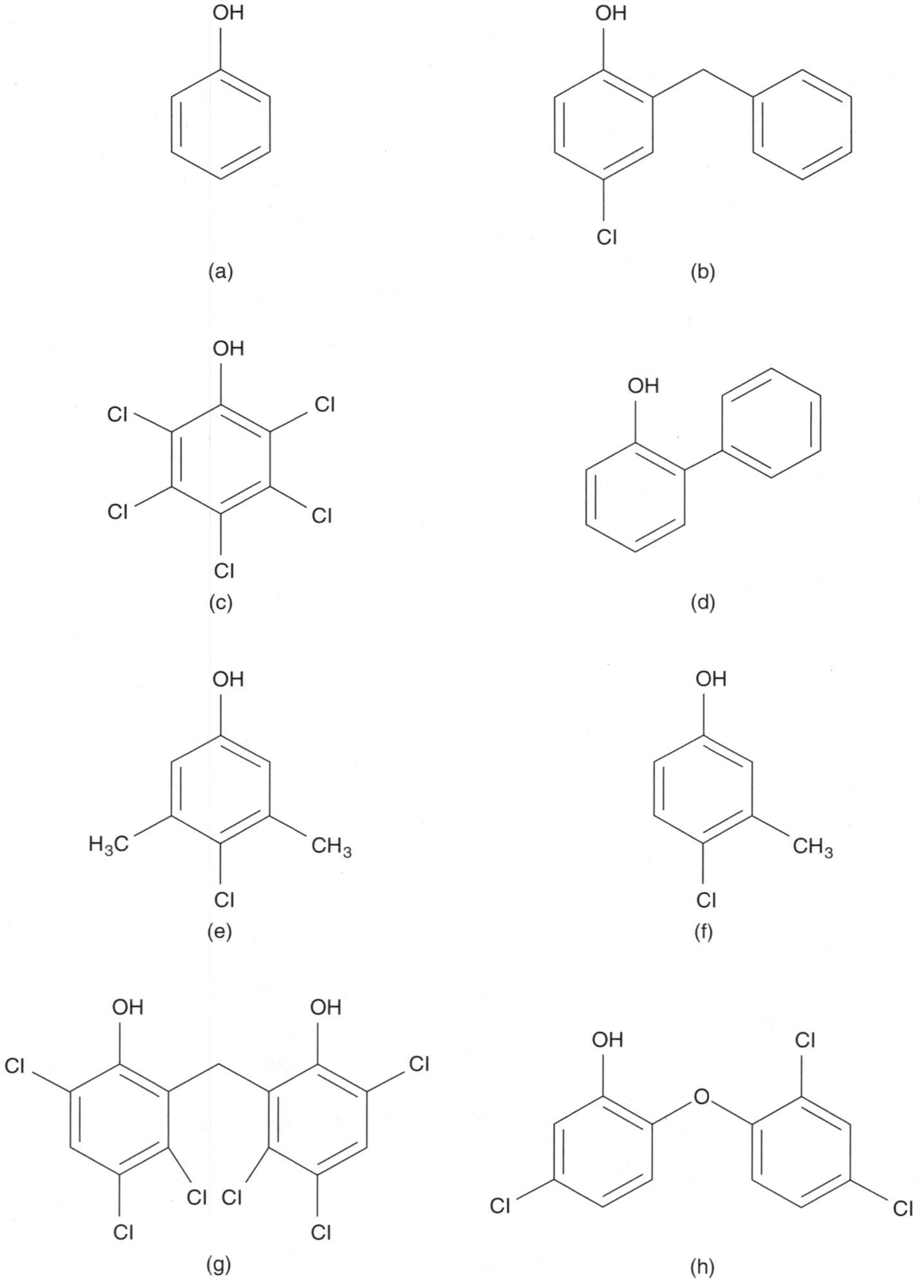

(a)

(b)

(c)

(d)

(e)

(f)

(g)

(h)

FIGURE 14.3 ● Structure of various phenolic compounds typically used in disinfectant and antiseptic preparations: **(a)** phenol, **(b)** 2-benzyl-4-chlorophenol (*o*-benzyl-*p*-chlorophenol), **(c)** pentachlorophenol, **(d)** 2-phenylphenol (*o*-phenylphenol), **(e)** 4-chloro-3,5-dimethylphenol (*p*-chloro-*m*-xylenol, PCMX), **(f)** 4-chloro-3-methylphenol (*p*-chloro-*m*-cresol), **(g)** hexachlorophene, and **(h)** triclosan.

phenolics that exist. Substitution of the ring structure of phenol changes the reactivity and activity of that base compound. Table 14.20 shows the activity of commonly used phenolic compounds. As stated previously, most commercially available phenolic compounds are a mixture of two or more phenolic chemicals. Based on the information in this table, it appears that *Pseudomonas* is more resistant than the other organisms, whereas the other Gram-negative and -positive bacteria and fungi are inhibited at relatively low concentrations.

TABLE 14.20

Minimum Inhibitory Concentration (MIC) of Phenol Derivatives in Nutrient Agar

Organism	OPP	BP	OBPCP	PCMC	PCMX	DC	PCP
Aeromonas punctata	200	100	10	200	100	50	10
Bacillus subtilis	100	100	10	150	75	100	10
Escherichia coli	200	500	3500	250	200	100	500
Leuconostoc mesenteroides	100	100	10	200	100	5	35
Proteus vulgaris	200	200	100	200	200	50	100
Pseudomonas aeruginosa	1500	5000	5000	800	1000	>5000	500
Pseudomonas fluorescens	1500	5000	>5000	800	500	3500	500
Staphylococcus aureus	100	100	20	200	100	5	10
Desulfovibrio desulfuricans	50	100	50	35	50	20	35
Candida albicans	100	100	50	200	75	50	35
Torula rubra	100	100	50	50	100	50	100
Alternaria tenuis	100	75	20	200	75	50	1
Aspergillus flavus	85	200	75	100	100	50	100
Aspergillus niger	75	100	100	100	100	100	50
Aureobasidium pullulans	35	100	20	30	50	35	20
Chaetomium globosum	60	50	20	80	50	20	20
Cladosporium herbarum	60	200	100	200	100	200	50
Coniophora puteana	50	35	5	100	35	2	35
Lentinus tigrinus	100	75	20	3500	75	5	10
Paecilomyces variotii	100	100	50	200	100	50	50
Penicillium citrinum	35	100	75	100	50	50	50
Penicillium glaucum	80	100	50	100	35	50	50
Polyporus versicolor	65	100	50	5000	75	50	20
Rhizopus nigricans	50	100	50	100	100	35	15
Sclerophoma pityophila	100	100	20	100	75	20	10
Stachybotrys atracorda	50	35	20	100	35	15	15
Tricoderma viride	75	200	100	140	100	50	200
Trichophyton pedis	20	20	10	100	50	10	10

OPP, 2-phenylphenol; BP, benzylphenol; OBPCP, 2-benzyl-4-chlorophenol; PCMC, 4-chloro-3-methylphenol; PCMX, 4-chloro-3,5-dimethylphenol; DC, 5,5′-dichloro-2,2′-dihydroxy-diphenyl methane; PCP, pentachlorophenol.
From Goddard and McCue (201).

Studies with PCMX formulated for use in topical preparations confirm this (222). However, higher resistance, as demonstrated by MIC and MBC data, may not be important, as most commercially available products are formulated at concentrations much higher than these values.

Improved antimicrobial activity has been achieved with the combination of *ortho*-phenylphenol and *ortho*-benzyl-*para*-chlorophenol, which is commonly used in hospital disinfectants. Yet there is still little evidence to suggest that these compounds have substantial activity against mycobacteria, including *M. tuberculosis* and *M. smegmatis* (67,68,223), and for this reason they are generally not classified as high-level disinfectants.

Commercially available phenolic disinfectants completely inactivated cell-free HIV and cell-associated HIV in culture medium, but HIV suspended in blood was not completely inactivated when exposed to the same formulations (224,225). Phenolic compounds generally require long exposure times and high concentrations to be effective against hepatitis B virus (72).

Triclosan

Although triclosan is a phenolic, because of its recent pervasive use in home products (toys, kitchen utensils, etc.) and its use in cosmetics and oral hygiene and dermatological preparations as well as health care personnel handwashes, it is dealt with separately. Triclosan, chemically, is 2,4,4′-trichloro-2′-hydroxy-diphenyether.

Mechanism of Action

Activity of triclosan is related to its ability to affect fatty acid synthesis. Bacteria utilize what is known as dissociative fatty acid synthesis (FAS) or type II FAS (FAS-II), as opposed to the single multifunctional enzyme system in associative FAS or type I FAS (FAS-I) present in animal cells as well as fungi. Recently, the FAS-II system has also been identified in *Plasmodium fulciparum* (226).

McMurray et al. (227,228) showed that a mutation in the gene responsible for the enzyme enol-reductase resulted in an increase in the tolerance of *M. smegmatis* and *E. coli* to triclosan. The *fabI* gene encodes the NADH-dependent *trans*-2-enoyl-acyl carrier protein reductase of bacterial FAS. This enzyme catalyzes the last step in the elongation step of fatty acid biosynthesis. The *inhA* gene in mycobacteria is the homologue of the *fabI* gene in *E. coli*. Triclosan is known to be very effective against *S. aureus*, including MRSA, by inhibiting *de novo* fatty acid biosynthesis (229). Heath et al. (230,231) demonstrated that the *fabI* gene product is also the target for triclosan in this organism. Triclosan and two analogs of triclosan were shown to bind to the 50-kDa protein endcoded for by the enoyl acyl carrier protein reductase gene from *P. falciparum*. Inhibition is thought to occur by mimicking the natural substrate of the reductase enzyme This is further substantiated by the fact that the three-dimensional structure of the enoyl reductase enzyme binds to triclosan (232). The conventional wisdom previously was that phenolic compounds exerted their activity through disruption of cellular membranes. These studies suggest there are other mechanisms involved. At higher concentrations, as available in commercial products, cell membrane disruption may be the primary mechanism of action.

Spectrum of Activity

Triclosan has been shown to have antimicrobial activity against a wide variety of microorganisms, including anaerobic and anaerobic bacteria and fungi (233), including the multidrug-resistant *S. aureus*. Determination of MIC with clinical strains of *S. aureus* indicated that these strains were highly susceptible ($MIC_{90} = 0.12\ \mu g/mL$) compared with *S. epidermidis* ($MIC_{90} = 8\ \mu g/mL$) (234). Triclosan was recommended for use in the control of MRSA after several reports of its successful use in controlling MRSA outbreaks in a neonatal nursery and cardiothoracic surgical unit (235). The daily use of triclosan in patient baths resulted in isolation of MRSA with significantly higher MIC to the germicide than sensitive strains of MRSA, and the transfer of resistance was associated with plasmid-mediated mupirocin resistance (236). When 1% triclosan was introduced into a hospital ward, there was a reduction in MRSA infections over a 7-week period, from 3.4 to 0.14 cases per week, but there was no change in the control ward (237). It is generally accepted that triclosan is not effective against *Pseudomonas* spp (238).

Like chlorhexidine, triclosan binds to the skin and has a moderate degree of substantivity, hence its use in surgical preparation formulations and health care personnel handwash preparations (239). Triclosan, along with PCMX, was shown to be less effective as a skin degerming agent than formulations containing chlorhexidine. Larson (240) classified the rapidity of triclosan's antimicrobial action as intermediate.

Recently, triclosan was shown to be a systemic bacterial agent in a mouse model. Mice were injected intraperitoneally with 10^7 CFU/mL *E. coli* 055:B5 and were treated with 40 mg/kg triclosan subcutaneously 2 hours prior to infection and every 12 hours thereafter. The mean survival of these mice was 48 hours (±5 hours). Infected mice treated with ampicillin and tetracycline survived 28 hours (±3 hours) and 24 hours (±2 hours), respectively. The IC_{50} and MIC_{50} for triclosan for this particular organism were 150 nM and 600 nM, respectively (241). Studies on oral preparations containing triclosan indicate that in an *in vitro* system simulating a periodontal disease–like state, exposure of organisms to triclosan or triclosan monophosphate (a more soluble form) caused Gram-negative anaerobic organisms to be affected to a greater extent than Gram-positive organisms (242). In studies utilizing pure cultures of oral microorganisms, the results indicate the same trend, with streptococci and lactobacilli being the least susceptible and the organisms *Neisseria subflava, Prevotella nigrescens*, and *Porphyromonas gingivalis* being highly susceptible to 0.6 mg/mL triclosan (243).

Quaternary Ammonium Compounds

Quaternary ammonium compounds (QAC) are widely used as disinfectants but should not be used as antiseptics. The elimination of such solutions as antiseptics on skin and tissue was recommended by the Centers for Disease Control (244) because of several outbreaks of infection associated with in-use contamination. There have also been a few reports of nosocomial infections associated with contaminated QAC when used to disinfect patient care supplies or equipment such as cystoscopes or cardiac catheters (245,246). The quaternaries are good cleaning agents, but water hardness and materials such as cotton and gauze pads may make them less microbicidal, for these materials absorb the active ingredients. As with several other disinfectants (e.g., phenolics and iodophors), Gram-negative bacteria have been found to survive or grow in QAC (247).

Chemically, the quaternaries are organically substituted ammonium compounds in which the nitrogen atom has a valence of 5, four of the substituted radicals (R1–R4) are alkyl or heterocyclic radicals of a given size or chain length, and the fifth (X^-) is a halide, sulfate, or similar radical. Each compound exhibits its own antimicrobial characteristics, hence the search for one compound with outstanding antimicrobial properties. The chemical names of quaternary ammonium compounds used in hospitals include *alkyl dimethyl benzyl ammonium chloride, alkyl didecyl dimethyl ammonium chloride,* and *dialkyl dimethyl ammonium chloride*. The newer (fourth-generation) quaternary ammonium compounds, referred to as twin-chain or dialkyl quaternaries (e.g., didecyl dimethyl ammonium bromide and dioctyl dimethyl ammonium bromide), purportedly remain active in hard water and are tolerant of anionic residues (248).

Mode of Action

The bactericidal action of the quaternaries has been attributed to the inactivation of energy-producing enzymes, denaturation of essential cell proteins, and disruption of the cell membrane. Evidence offered in support of these and other possibilities is provided by Sykes (83) and Merianos (248).

Microbicidal Activity

Manufacturers' data sheets and results from published studies indicate that the quaternaries sold as hospital disinfectants are generally fungicidal, bactericidal, and virucidal against lipophilic viruses; they are not sporicidal and generally not tuberculocidal or virucidal against hydrophilic viruses. Best et al. (67) demonstrated the low level of effectiveness of quaternary ammonium compounds against mycobacteria.

Attempts to reproduce the bactericidal and tuberculocidal results claimed by manufacturers using the AOAC tests with a limited number of QAC have failed on occasion (249,250).

The quaternaries are commonly used in ordinary environmental sanitation of noncritical surfaces such as floors, furniture, and walls.

RESISTANCE

Resistance to antibiotics is well understood. The mechanisms generally fall into one of three categories: (a) altered targets, (b) production of enzyme(s) that degrade the active molecule, and (c) decreased ability to take up the compound. The resistance to many antibiotics is genetically controlled, that is, linked to the cell's chromosome or a plasmid (251,252). Unlike in the case of antibiotics, the mechanisms of action of chemical germicides, whether antiseptics or disinfectants, are in most instances, at the use concentration, not specific for a target molecule. In fact, they may act at several sites in the cell. The response of cells to exposure to disinfectants is not likely to be as specific as the response to antibiotics. There is evidence that organisms develop resistance to various chemicals due to their heavy use and then revert to a normal state after the removal of the active ingredient. There is some evidence that there is an association between plasmid-linked antibiotic resistance and resistance to disinfectants (253–255). Concern has been expressed over use of disinfectants and antiseptics and the possible implications for antibiotic resistance (256). Increased resistance to germicides used in the sanitization of environmental surfaces has also been implicated in the outbreak of *Listeria monocytogenes* in food-processing plants, which has led to recalls (257).

McDonnell and Russell (79) emphasized that increased resistance to disinfectants and germicides does not necessarily result in their failure to act as intended. Unlike in the case of antibiotics, where an increase in an MIC can have a significant therapeutic impact, increased MIC values for antiseptics and disinfectants may not have a noticeable effect. This is due to the fact the antibiotics work on specific targets within the cell, and therefore changes in the MIC of an antibiotic indicate that the target has changed. With antiseptics and disinfectants, which generally work on the principles of chemical reactions (e.g., oxidation, alkylation, and detergency), many cell components may be susceptible to the action of these germicides.

Resistance of microorganisms to chemical germicides can be the result of several mechanisms; that is, it can be intrinsic resistance or acquired. Acquired resistance is generally thought of as resistance obtained by a change to the genetic makeup of the cell either by mutation or by acquisition of genes by way of plasmids. Intrinsic resistance is resistance consistently demonstrated by naturally occurring isolates. Intrinsic resistance is genetically controlled and may be constitutive (i.e., the normal state of the cell) or inducible or adaptive (i.e., in response to exposure to an agent). Intrinsic resistance may be by way of adaptive changes in the cell wall and/or outer membrane structure in response to exposure to germicides or it may be the natural state of the organism, such as the resistance of members of the genus *Mycobacterium* to antibiotics and germicides attributable to the impenetrable high lipid content in the cell wall (258). Another form of intrinsic resistance worth mentioning is biofilm production because it has been associated with increased resistance of organisms to germicides. Biofilm production is usually associated with adherence of microorganisms to a surface and production of extensive layers of exopolysaccharide exopolymer (259,260). Biofilms have been found on inplantable devices and are a major component of dental plaque. However, there is no evidence that cells form biofilms in response to exposure to germicides. The resistance of biofilms is primarily a physical phenomenon

TABLE 14.21

Mechanisms of Intrinsic Resistance

Phenotype	Example	Mechanism
Impermeability		
Gram-positive bacteria	QUATs, triclosan	Barrier by outer membrane may prevent uptake of antiseptic or disinfectant; glycocalyx may also be involved
	Chlorhexidine	Glycocalyx/mucopolysaccharide may be associated with reduced diffusion of antiseptic
Mycobacteria	Chlorhexidine, QUATs	Waxy cell wall of mycobacteria prevent entry into cell
	Glutaraldehyde	*Mycobacterium chelonae*
Bacterial spores	Chlorhexidine, QUATs, phenolics	Spore coat and cortex present barrier
Inactivation	Chlorhexidine	Breakdown of chlorhexidine molecule may be responsible
Efflux pumps	QUATs	*mdrL* gene encodes for efflux pump, conferring resistance in *Listeria monocytogenes*

Modified from McDonnell and Russell (70).

in which cells are protected from the activity of chemical germicides by the production of extracellular components, which either inhibit access of the biocide to the cells or interact with the biocide to effectively neutralize it. Although the biofilm formed by a consortium of microorganisms maybe resistant to a given germicide, once the biofilm is disrupted and the cells are subcultured, they do not show the same level of resistance, further indicating the mechanism of resistance of the biofilm to be primarily a physical one (261).

Intrinsic resistance to chemical germicides may occur as a result of several different mechanisms (Table 14.21), the two most prominent of which are reduced permeability to the agent due to changes in the exterior layers of the cell (cell wall and/or outer membrane) and efflux mechanisms (262,263) that prohibit or reduce internal concentration of the germicide. A third mechanism, degradation of the germicide by enzymatic activity and rendering of the active ingrediant ineffective, has been reported as a mechanism of resistance (264) but not extensively.

Intrinsic Resistance

Bacterial spores, known to be resistant to many chemical and physical agents, exemplify resistance by impermeability. *Bacillus* and *Clostridium* spores are known to be the most resistant to antiseptics and disinfectants (79), and, as stated earlier, *C. difficile* is a major cause of infections in hospitals and other health care facilities. Some chemical germicides are known to be sporicidal (glutaraldehyde, peracetic acid, and peroxide), but they require high concentrations and/or long periods of contact and/or high temperatures to be effective. The resistance of spores to chemical and physical agents is well understood and documented. Many treatises have been devoted to this subject. Russell and collaborators have elucidated the development of resistance to a number of germicides during sporulation (23,265,266). As sporulation proceeds (stages 0 through VI), spores become increasingly resistant to germicides in the following order: formaldehyde, sodium lauryl sulfate, phenol, *m*-cresol, chlorocresol, chlorhexidine gluconate, cetylpyridinium chloride, sodium dichloroisocyanurate, and glutaraldehyde. The development of resistance to germicides occurs primarily during stages IV through VII, correlating with the start of cortex development, coat synthesis, maturation, and release of mature spores. Spore coat formation plays a significant role in the resistance of spores to chlorine-containing compounds (267,268) and formaldehyde, while the criticality of cortex formation in conferring resistance to quatenary ammonium compounds (QACs), chlorhexidine and glutaraldehyde has been demonstrated (266). There is evidence of other factors (small acid-soluble proteins) being involved in the resistance of spores to chemical agents (269,270).

In the scheme of resistance to antiseptics and disinfectants, the mycobacteria as a group are more resistant than other vegetative bacteria and less resistant than bacterial spores. *Mycobacterium* spp represent a unique class of bacteria in that they possess high lipid content in the cell walls. It has been proposed that these lipids interfere with the uptake or penetration of hydrophilic molecules into the cell. Support for this hypothesis can be found in the relative sensitivity of mycobacteria to various disinfectants. Two dialdehydes, glutaraldehyde and *ortho*-phthalaldehyde, have vastly different activities against mycobacteria. Glutaraldehyde is a highly water-soluble compound, with solubility approaching 50% in water, whereas *ortho*-phthalaldehyde is hydrophobic in nature, with water solubility reaching a maximum at 5%, though it is highly soluble in alcohol and other organic solvents. *ortho*-Phthalaldehyde is at least 5–8 times more active against mycobacteria than is glutaraldehyde when tested under the same conditions (112). This increased activity may be attributable to the hydrophobicity of the molecule and its ability to penetrate the cell wall layer. The same case could be made for phenol and phenolic compounds, which also exhibit better activity against the mycobacteria than the more hydrophilic compounds. Several studies evaluating the role of the mycobacterial cell wall support the cell wall barrier hypothesis. The treatment of *M. avium* and *M. tuberculosis* with ethambutol (which acts by inhibiting a component of the mycobacterial cell wall) renders these organisms more susceptible to the activity of chlorhexidine and the QAC cetylpyridinium chloride (50).

Gram-negative organisms in general are less susceptible to germicides than are Gram positive-bacteria, most likely due to the outer membrane in Gram-negative organisms and its protective effect, limiting penetration of chemicals into the cell (see reference 79 for a general discussion of this). The role of extracellular material in the protection of cells is further supported by the existence of mucoid and nonmucoid strains of *S. aureus:* the nonmucoid cells are more susceptible to several commonly used germicidal agents (271). The cell wall of Gram-positive bacteria may act as an important mechanism in the resistance of these bacteria to chemical agents, although this mechanism is not uniform across all species (272).

This mechanism is generally thought to be related to the existence of the outer membrane in Gram-negative bacteria, based on data between Gram-negative and Gram-positive organisms and using mutants of Gram-negative organisms defective in outer membrane structure (see McDonnell and Russell [79] for discussion of this). It has been demonstrated that changes in the composition of the cell surface, especially the lipopolysaccharides and lipids, can reduce or prevent the penetration of QACs into Gram-negative cells (273).

Recent studies on the adaptive resistance of *Salmonella enterica* and *E. coli* 0157 and cross-resistance to antimicrobial agents reported that *E. coli* 0157 exhibited a high level of resistance to triclosan after exposure to just two sublethal doses. This was accompanied by decreased susceptibility to a number of antibiotics, including chloramphenicol, erythromycin, tetracycline, trimethoprim, and imipenem. Cross-resistance in *S. enterica* was also demonstrated (274).

In *Pseudomonas aeruginosa,* which is intrinsically resistant to many antimicrobial agents, both germicides and antibiotics, a chromosomal DNA fragment conferring triclosan resistance has been isolated. The *mexJK* operon is responsible for the efflux mechanism for triclosan and, in conjunction with the outer membrane channel protein OprM, for erythromycin. Triclosan can select for mutants that are cross-resistant to antibiotics (275). Growth of *Pseudomonas fluoresences* in gradually higher concentrations of didecyl dimethylammonium chloride resulted in higher resistance and cross-resistance to several antibacterial agents. Microscopic observation of cells indicated loss of flagella and slime formation. Removal of the slime layer resulted in loss of resistance (276).

Acquired Resistance

Acquired resistance to germicidal agents may occur through mutation or by acquisition of extrachromosomal DNA (plasmids or transposons). Although the role of plasmids in antibiotic resistance has been known for some time, conventional wisdom until recently was that resistance to chemical germicides was not mediated through plasmids. A number of studies have recently indicated that plasmids do play a role in resistance to chemical germicides.

Staphylococcal resistance to quaternary ammonium compounds has been reported extensively (277–280). Several genes involved in resistance to quaternary ammonium compounds have been isolated from human clinical strains of *S. aureus* and coagulase-negative staphylococcus [*qac A*, *qacB*, and *qacC (smr)*] (281–283). Additionally, two genes, *qacG* and *qacH,* have been isolated from coagulase-negative staphylococcus isolated in the food industry (277,278). A fifth gene encoding for resistance to quaternary ammonium compounds, *qacJ,* has been identified in several species of *Staphylococcus* isolated from horses (284).

Concern has been expressed over emerging cross-resistance or coresistance to widely used disinfectants and antibiotics. The *qac* genes have been located with antibiotic resistance genes for several antibiotics (gentamicin, kanamycin, tobramycin, trimethoprim, and penicillin) on several plasmids (pST6, pSK4, pSK410) and transposons (Tn*552* and Tn*4002*) (279,281,285,286). Sidhu et al. (280) showed that, of 238 clinical isolates of staphylococci, 118 (50%) were resistant to a quaternary ammonium compound, benzalkonium chloride, and in those resistant strains, there was a high frequency of organisms resistant to a range of antibiotics. The plasmid DNA of 78 of the isolates hybridized with one or more of the *qac* genes as well as *blaZ* (which codes for β-lactamase) and *tetK* (which codes for the tetracycline efflux pump). Approximately 34% of the plasmids had both the *qac A/B* and *blaZ* gene. One isolate had a multiresistant plasmid (pMS62) that contained the *qacA/B, blaZ,* and *tetK* genes. Twenty-eight of the benzalkonium chloride–resistant strains also showed low-level resistance to the antiseptic chlorhexidine. In a recent survey of 522 clinical strains of *S. aureus* in Japanese hospitals, 32.6% of the MRSA strains and 7.5% of the methicillin-sensitive *S. aureus* strains contained the *qacA* and *qacB* genes. The *smr* gene was noted at a much lower frequency (287).

Plasmid-mediated resistance to benzalkonium chloride has been demonstrated in *L. monocytogenes* and is transferable with resistance to ethylene bromide (288). A correlation between resistance to QACs and resistance to antibiotics in *L. monocytogenes* has also been reported (257). The genes responsible for this resistance can be plasmid-acquired or chromosomal. The mechanism of resistance to QACs may be similar to that found in *S. aureus*. The *mdrL* gene in *L. monocytogenes* forms a protein that is similar to proteins responsible for efflux mechanisms in *B. subtilis* (289). Originally *mdrL* was reported to be a chromosomal gene (290), making it a case of intrinsic resistance. However, as stated earlier, further work has demonstrated that it may be chromosomal or plasmid-acquired. Chlorhexidine resistance in *Klebsiella pneumoniae* has been linked to the *cepA* gene (associated with the production of cephalosporinase). Transformation of the *cepA* to the *E. coli* XLOLR resulted in chlorhexidine-sensitivity, and retransformation resulted in chlorhexidine-sensitive *K. pneumoniae*. It is hypothesized that the gene product CepA may act as a cation efflux pump. All of these data support the speculation by Russell (291) some time ago that disinfectant resistance may select for antibiotic resistance. The incorporation of triclosan in many household products may contribute to the problem of increased antibiotic resistance (256), yet evidence collected in environmental samples (292,293) and human skin flora (294) does not support this supposition.

REFERENCES

1. Spaulding EH. Chemical disinfection of medical and surgical disinfection of medical and surgical materials. In: Lawerence CA, Block SS, eds. *Disinfection, sterilization and preservation*. Philadelphia: Lea & Febiger, 1968:517–531.
2. Garner JS, Favero MS. Guidelines for handwashing and hospital environmental control, 1985. *Am J Infect Control* 1986;14:110–126.
3. Kim KH, Fekety R, Batts DH, et al. Isolation of *Clostridium difficile* from the environment and contacts of patients with antibiotic-associated colitis. *J Infect Dis* 1981;143:42–50.
4. Larson HE, Barclay FE, Honour P, et al. Epidemiology of *Clostridium difficile* in infants. *J Infect Dis* 1982;146:727–733.
5. Malamou-Ladas H, O'Farrle S, Nash JQ, et al. Isolation of *Clostridium difficile* in hospitalized children: a prospective study. *Acta Paediatr Scand* 1990;79:292–299.
6. Kaatz GW, Gitlin SD, Schaberg DR, et al. Acquisition of *Clostridium difficile* from the hospital environment. *Am J Epidemiol* 1988;127:1289–1294.
7. Boyce JM. Methicillin-resistant *Staphylococcus aureus* in hospitals and long-term care facilities: microbiology, epidemiology, and preventive measures. *Infect Control Hosp Epidemiol* 1992;13:725–737.
8. Boyce JM, Jackson MM, Pugliese G, et al. Methicillin-resistant *Staphylococcus aureus* (MRSA): a briefing for acute care hospitals and nursing facilities. *Infect Control Hosp Epidemiol* 1994;15:105–115.
9. Mulligan ME, Murray-Leisure KA, Ribner BS, et al. Methicillin-resistant *Staphylococcus aureus*: a consensus review of the microbiology, pathogenesis, and epidemiology with implications for prevention and management. *Am J Med* 1993;94:311–328.
10. Weber DJ, Rutala WA. Environmental issues and nosocomial infections. In: Wenzel RP, ed. *Prevention and control of nosocomial infections*, 3rd ed. Baltimore: William & Wilkins, 1997:491–514.
11. Boyce JM. Scientific basis for handwashing with alcohol and other waterless antiseptic agents. In: Rutala WA, ed. *Disinfection, sterilization and antisepsis: principles and practices in healthcare facilities*. Washington, DC: Association for Professionals in Infection Control and Epidemiology, 2001:140–150.
12. Rotter ML. Hand washing, hand disinfection and skin disinfection. Wenzel RP, ed. *Prevention and control of nosocomial infections*, 3rd ed. Baltimore: William & Wilkins, 1997:691–709.
13. Sattar SA, Springthorpe VS. Methods under development for evaluating the antimicrobial activity of chemical germicides. In: Rutala WA, ed. *Chemical germicides in healthcare*, 3rd ed. Morin Heights, Canada: Polyscience and Association for Professionals in Infection Control and Epidemiology, 1994:237–254.
14. Sattar SA. Microbicidal: testing of germicides: an update. In: Rutala WA, ed. *Disinfection, sterilization, and antisepsis in healthcare*. Washington, DC: Association for Professionals in Infection Control and Epidemiology, 1998:227–240.
15. Miner NA, Mulberry GK, Starks AN, et al. Identification of possible artifacts in the Association of Official Analytical Chemists sporicidal test. *Appl Environ Microbiol* 1995;61:1658–1660.
16. Ascenzi JM, Ezzell JM, Wendt TM. A more specific method for measurement of tuberculocidal activity of disinfectants. *Appl Environ Microbiol* 1987;53:2189–2192.
17. Sattar SA, Springthorpe VS. New methods for efficacy testing of disinfectants and antiseptics. In: Rutala WA, ed. *Disinfection, sterilization and antisepsis: principles and practices in healthcare facilities*. Washington, DC: Association for Professionals in Infection Control and Epidemiology, 2001:173–186.
18. Association of Official Analytical Chemists International. *Disinfectants: sporicidal activity of disinfectants*. Washington, DC: Association of Official Analytical Chemists, Official Methods of Analysis, 1998.
19. Hobson DW, Bolsen K. Methods of testing oral and topical antiseptics and antimicrobials. In: Block SS, ed. *Disinfection, sterilization and preservation*, 5th ed. Philadelphia: Lippincott, Williams & Wilkins, 2001:1329–1359.
20. Denton GW. Chlorhexidine. In: Block SS, ed. *Disinfection, sterilization and preservation*, 5th ed. Philadelphia: Lippincott, Williams & Wilkins, 2001:321–336.
21. Davies GE, Field BS. Action of biguanides, phenols, and detergents on *E. coli* and its spheroplasts. *J Appl Bacteriol* 1969;32:233–243.
22. Holloway PM, Bucknall RA, Denton GW. The effect of sub lethal concentrations of chlorhexidine on bacterial pathogenicity. *J Hosp Inf* 1986;8:39–46.
23. Shaker LA, Russell AD, Furr JR. Aspects of the action of chlorhexidine on bacterial spores. *Int J Pharm* 1986;34:51–56.

24. Montefiori DC, Robinson WE, Modliszewski A, et al. Effective inactivation of human immunodeficiency virus with chlorhexidine antiseptics containing detergents and alcohol. *J Hosp Infect* 1990;15:279–282.
25. Harbison MA, Hammer SM. Inactivation of human immunodeficiency virus by Betadine and chlorhexidine. *J AIDS* 1989;2:16–20.
26. Marchetti MG, Kampf G, Finzi G, et al. Evaluation of the bactericidal effect of five products for surgical hand disinfection according to prEN 12054 and prEN 12791. *J Hosp Infect* 2003;54:63–67.
27. Peterson AF, Rosenberg A, Alatary SD. Comparative evaluation of surgical scrub preparations. *Surg Gynecol Obstet* 1978;146:63–65.
28. Wade JJ, Casewell MW. The evaluation of residual antimicrobial activity on hands and its clinical relevance. *J Hosp Infect* 1991;18[Suppl B]:23–28.
29. Mulberry G, Snyder AT, Heilman J, et al. Evaluation of a waterless, scrubless chlorhexidine gluconate/ethanol surgical scrub for antimicrobial efficacy. *Am J Infect Control* 2001;29:377–382.
30. Larson EL, Laughon BE. Comparison of four antiseptic products containing chlorhexidine gluconate. *Antimicrob Agents Chemother* 1987;31:1572–1574.
31. Hibbard JS, Mulberry GK, Brady AR. A clinical study comparing the skin antisepsis and safety of ChloaPrep, 70% isopropyl alcohol, and 2% aqueous chlorhexidine. *J Infus Nursing* 2002;25:244–249.
32. Wilcox MH, Hall J, Gill AB, et al. Effectiveness of topical chlorhexidine powder as an alternative to hexachlorophene for the control of *Staphylococcus aureus* in neonates. *J Hosp Infect* 2004;56:156–159.
33. Maki DG, Ringer M, Alvarado CJ. Prospective randomized trial of povidone-iodine, alcohol, and chlorhexidine for prevention of infection associated with central venous and arterial catheters. *Lancet* 1991;228:339–343.
34. Clemence MA, Walke D, Farr BM. Central venous catheter practices: results of a survey. *Am J Infect Control* 1995;23:5–12.
35. Mimoz O, Pieroni L, Lawerence C, et al. Prospective randomized trial of two antiseptic solutions for prevention of central venous or arterial catheter colonization and infection in intensive care unit patients. *Crit Care Med* 1996;24:1818–1823.
36. Rubinson L, Diette GB. Best practices for insertion of central venous catheters in intensive-care units to prevent catheter-related bloodstream infections. *J Lab Clin Med* 2004;143:5–13.
37. Walder B, Pittet D, Tramer MR. Prevention of bloodstream infections with central venous catheters treated with anti-infective agents depends on catheter type and insertion time: evidence from a meta-analysis. *Infect Control Hosp Epidemiol* 2002;23:748–756.
38. Heard O, Wagle M, Vijayakumar E, et al. Influence of triple lumen catheter venous catheters coated with chlorhexidine and silver sulfadiazine on the incidence of catheter-related bacteremia. *Arch Intern Med* 1998;158:81–87.
39. Beyth N, Redlich M, Harari D, et al. Effect of sustained-release chlorhexidine varnish of *Streptococcus mutans* and *Actinomyces viscosus* in orthodontic patients. *Am J Orthod Dentofacial Orthop* 2003;123:345–348.
40. Magnusson I. Local delivery of antimicrobial agents for the treatment of periodontitis. *Compend Contin Educ Dent* 1998;19:953–956.
41. Hugo WB, Longworth AR. Some aspects of mode of action of chlorhexidine. *J Pharm Pharmacol* 1964;16:655–662.
42. Hugo WB, Longworth AR. Cytological aspects of the mode of action of chlorhexidine. *J Pharm Pharmacol* 1965;17:28–32.
43. Hugo WB, Longworth AR. The effect of chlorhexidine on the electrophoretic mobility, cytoplasmic constituents, dehydrogenase activity and cell walls of *E. coli* and *S. aureus*. *J Pharm Pharmacol* 1966;18:569–578.
44. Tattawasart U, Maillard J-Y, Furr JR, et al. Outer membrane changes in *Pseudomonas stutzeri* resistant to chlorhexidine diacetate and cetylpyridinium chloride. *Int J Antimicrob Agents* 2000;16:233–238.
45. Tattawasart U, Hann AC, Maillard JY, et al. Cytological changes in chlorhexidine-resistant isolates of *Pseudomonas stutzeri*. *J Antimicrob Chemother* 2000;45:145–152.
46. Fitzgerald KA, Davies A, Russell AD. Uptake of ^{14}C-chlorhexidine diacetate to *Escherichia coli* and *Pseudomonas aeruginosa* and its release by azolectin. *FEMS Microbiol Lett* 1989;60:327–332.
47. Hiom SJ, Furr JR, Russell AD. Effects of chlorhexidine diacetate on *Candida albicans, C. glabrata*, and *Saccharomyces cerevisiae*. *J Appl Bacteriol* 1992;72:335–340.
48. Ranganathan NS. Chlorhexidine. In: Ascenzi JM, ed. *Handbook of disinfectants and antiseptics*. New York, Marcel Dekker, 1996:235–264.
49. Sheppard FC, Mason DJ, Bloomfield SF, et al. Flow cytometric analysis of chlorhexidine action. *FEMS Mircobiol Lett* 1997;2:283–288.
50. Broadley SJ, Jenkins PA, Furr JR, et al. Potentiation of the effects of chlorhexidine diacetate and cetylpyridinium chloride on mycobacteria by ethambutol. *J Med Microbiol* 1995;43:458–460.
51. Walters TH, Furr JR, Russell AD. Antifungal action of chlorhexidine. *Microbios* 1983;38:195–204.
52. Bobichon H, Bouchet P. Action of chlorhexidine on budding of *Candida albicans:* scanning and transmission electron microscopic study. *Mycopathologia* 1987;100:27–35.
53. Favero MS, Bond WW. Chemical disinfection of medical and surgical materials. In: Block SS, ed. *Disinfection, sterilization and preservation,* 5th ed. Philadelphia: Lippincott, Williams & Wilkins, 2001:881–918.
54. Craven DE, Moody B, Connolly BS, et al. Pseudobactermia caused by povidone-iodine solution contaminated with *Pseudomonas aeruginosa*. *N Eng J Med* 1981;305:621–623.
55. Berkelmann RI, Holland BW, Anderson RI. Increased bactericidal activity of dilute preparations of povidone-iodine solution. *J Clin Microbiol* 1982;15:635–639.
56. Gottardi W. Iodine and iodine compounds. In: Block SS, ed. *Disinfection, sterilization and preservation,* 5th ed. Philadelphia: Lippincott, Williams & Wilkins, 2001:159–183.
57. Bloomfield SA. Chlorine and iodine formulations. In: Ascenzi JM, ed. *Handbook of disinfectants and antiseptics*. New York: Marcel Dekker, 1996:133–158.
58. Gershenfeld L, Witlin B. Iodine solution as a sporicidal agent. *J Am Pharm Assoc* 1952;41:451–452.
59. Barteltt PG, Schmidt W. Disinfectant iodine complexes as germicides. *J Appl Microbiol* 1957;5:355–359.
60. Sykes G. The sporicidal properties of chemical disinfectants. *J Appl Bacteriol* 1970;33:147–156.
61. Russell AD. Chemical sporicidal and sporostatic agents. In: Block SS, ed. *Disinfection, sterilization and preservation,* 5th ed. Philadelphia: Lippincott, Williams & Wilkins, 2001:529–541.
62. Pyle BH, McFeters GA. Iodine sensitivity of bacteria isolated from iodinated water systems. *Can J Microbiol* 1989;35:520–523.
63. Cargill KL, Pyle BH, Sauer RL, et al. Effects of culture conditions and biofilm formation on iodine susceptibility

of *Legionella pneumophila*. *Can J Microbiol* 1992;38;423–429.
64. Gershenfeld L, Flagg W, Witlin B. Iodine as a tuberculocidal agent. *Mil Surg* 1954;114:172–183.
65. Nelson KE, Larson PA, Schraufnagel DE, et al. Transmission of tuberculosis by flexible fiberbronchoscopes. *Am J Respiratory Dis* 1983;127:97–100.
66. Wright ES, Mundy RA. Studies on disinfection of clinical thermometers. XI. Oral thermometers from tuberculosis sanatorium. *Appl Microbiol Biotechnol* 1961;9:508.
67. Best M, Sattar SA, Springthorpe VS, et al. Efficacies of selected disinfectants against *Mycobacterium tuberculosis*. *J Clin Microbiol* 1990;28:2234–2239.
68. Best M, Sattar SA, Springthorpe VS, et al. Comparative mycobactericidal efficacy of chemical disinfectants in suspension and carrier tests. *Appl Environ Microbiol* 1988;54:2856–2858.
69. Berg G, Chang SL, Harris EK. Devitalization of microorganisms by iodine. *Virology* 1964;22:469–481.
70. Gershenfeld L. Iodine as a virucidal. agent. *J Am Pharm Assoc* 1955;44:177–182.
71. Prince HN, Prince DL. Principles of viral control and transmission. In: Block SS, ed. *Disinfection, sterilization and preservation,* 5th ed. Philadelphia: Lippincott, Williams & Wilkins, 2001:543–571.
72. Thraenhart O, Jursch C. Measures for disinfection and control of viral hepatitis. In: Block SS, ed. *Disinfection, sterilization and preservation,* 5th ed. Philadelphia: Lippincott, Williams & Wilkins, 2001:585–615.
73. Crabtree TD, Pelletier SJ, Pruett TL. Surgical antisepsis. In: Block SS, ed. *Disinfection, sterilization and preservation,* 5th ed. Philadelphia: Lippincott, Williams & Wilkins, 2001:919–934.
74. Rotter ML, Koller W, Wewalka G. Povidone-iodine and chlorhexidine gluconate–containing detergents for disinfection of hands. *J Hosp Infect* 1980;1:149–158.
75. Ayliffe GA, Babb JR, Davies JG, et al. Hand disinfection: a comparison of various agents in laboratory and ward studies. *J Hosp Infect* 1988;11:226–243.
76. Lowbury EJ, Lilly HA. The effect of blood on disinfection of surgeons' hands. *Br Surg J* 1974;61:19–21.
77. Ally R, Maibach H. Comparative evaluation of chlorhexidine gluconate (Hibiclens) and povidone-iodine (E-Z Scrub) sponge/brushes for presurgical hand scrubbing. *Curr Ther Res* 1983;34:740–745.
78. Gottardi W, Puritscher M. Degerming experiments with aqueous povidone-iodine containing disinfecting solutions: influence of the concentration of free iodine on the bactericidal reaction against *Staphylococcus aureus*. *Zentralbl Bakteriol [B]* 1986;182:372–380.
79. McDonnell G, Russell AD. Antiseptics and disinfectants: activity, action, and resistance. *Clin Micriobiol Rev* 1999;12:147–179.
80. Rotter ML. Alcohols for antisepsis of hands and skin. In Ascenzi JM, ed. *Handbook of disinfectants and antiseptics*. New York: Marcel Dekker, 1996:177–233.
81. Beck WC. Disinfection from antiquity to the present. *Guthrie J* 1990;59:191–195.
82. Kamm O. The relation between structure and physiological action of the alcohols. *J Am Pharm Assoc* 1921;10:87–92.
83. Sykes G. *Disinfection and sterilization,* 2nd ed. London: E & FN Spon Ltd, 1965:362–376.
84. Soberheim G. Alkohol als Disinfektionsmittel. *Schweiz Med Wochenschr* 1943;73:1280–1333.
85. Sykes G. Influence of germicides on dehydrogenase of *Bacterium coli:* succinic acid dehydrogenase of *Bacterium coli*. *J Hyg* 1939;59:463–469.
86. Kirschhoff H. Wirkungmechanismem chemischer Desinfektionsmittel. I. Allgemeiner Reaktionsablauf. *Gesundheitwes Desinfekt* 1974;66:125–130.
87. Pulvertaft RJV, Lumb GD. Bacterial lysis and antiseptics. *J Hyg* (London) 1948;46:62–64.
88. Razin S, Argaman M. Lysis of Mycoplasma, bacterial protoplasts, spheroplasts and L-forms by various agents. *J Gen Microbiol* 1963;30:155–172.
89. Harrington C, Walker H. The germicidal activity of alcohol. *Boston Med Surg J* 1903;148:548–552.
90. Coulthard CE, Sykes G. The germicidal effect of alcohol with special reference to its action on bacterial spores. *Pharm J* 1936;137:79–81.
91. Pohle WD, Stuart LS. The germicidal action of cleaning agents: a study of a modification of Price's procedure. *J Infect Dis* 1940;67:275–281.
92. Sakuragi T, Yanagisawa K, Dan K. Bactericidal activity of skin disinfectants on methicillin-resistant *Staphylococcus aureus*. *Anesth Analg* 1995;81:555–558.
93. Kampf G, Jarosch R, Ruden H. Limited effectiveness of chlorhexidine based hand disinfectants against methicillin resistant *Staphylococcus aureus* (MRSA). *J Hosp Infect* 1998;38:297–303.
94. Kampf G, Hofer M, Wendt C. Efficacy of hand disinfectants against vancomycin resistant enterococci. *J Hosp Infect* 1999;42:143–150.
95. Morton HW. Relationship of concentration and germicidal efficacy of ethyl alcohol. *Ann NY Acad Sci* 1950;532:191–196.
96. Ali Y, Dolan MJ, Fendler EJ, et al. Alcohols. In: Block SS, ed. *Disinfection, sterilization and preservation,* 5th ed. Philadelphia: Lippincott, Williams & Wilkins, 2001:229–254.
97. Woo PCY, Leung K-W, Wong SSY, et al. Relatively alcohol-resistant Mycobacteria are emerging pathogens in patients receiving acupuncture treatment. *J Clin Microbiol* 2002;40;1219–1224.
98. Gordon MH. *Studies on viruses of vaccinia and variola*. Privy Council Medical Research Council, Special Reports Series 98.
99. Kuwert EK, Thraendhardt O. Theoretische, Methodische und praktische Probleme der Virusdesinfektion in der Humanmedizin. *Immun Infekt* 1977;4:125–130.
100. Groupe V, Engle CG, Gaffney PE, et al. Virucidal activity of representative antinfective agents against influenza A and vaccinia viruses. *Appl Microbiol* 1955;3:333–339.
101. Klein M, Deforest A. The inactivation of virus by germicides. *Proc Chem Spec Manuf* 1963:116–118.
102. Kewitsch A, Weuffen W. Wirkung chemischer Desinfektionsmittel gegenuber Influenza- Vaccinia- und Poliomyelitisvirus. *Med Welt* 1966;17:76–81.
103. Mbithi JN, Springthorpe VS, Sattar SA. Chemical disinfection of hepatitis A virus on environmental surfaces. *Appl Env Microbiol* 1990;56:3601–3604.
104. Bond WW, Favero MS, Petersen NJ, et al. Inactivation of hepatitis B virus by intermediate-to-high level disinfectant chemicals. *J Clin Microbiol* 1983;18:535–538.
105. Kobayashi H, Tsuzuki M, Koshimizu K, et al. Susceptibility of hepatitis B virus to disinfectants or heat. *J Clin Microbiol* 1984;20:214–216.
106. Ehrenkranz HN, Alfonso BC. Failure of handwashing to prevent hand transfer of patient bacteria to urethral catheters. *Infect Control Hosp Epidemiol* 1991;12:654–658.
107. Handley JO, Mika LA, Gwaltney JM. Evaluation of virucidal compounds for inactivation of rhinovirus on hands. *Antimicrob Agents Chemother* 1978;14:690–694.
108. Furuhashi M, Miyamae T. Effect of pre-operative hand scrubbing and influence of pinholes appearing in surgical

rubber gloves during operations. *Bull Tokyo Med Dent Univ* 1979;26:73–78.

109. Pepper RE, Lieberman ER. Dialdehyde alcoholic sporicidal composition. US Patent 3016328. 1962.
110. Stonehill AA, Krop S, Borick PM. Buffered glutaraldehyde, a new chemical sterilizing solution. *Am J Hosp Pharm* 1963;20:458–465.
111. Gordon MD, Howell R, Bruckner N. Patent No. 4,851,449, July 25, 1989.
112. Walsh SE, Maillard JY, Russell AD. *Ortho*-phthalaldehyde: a possible alternative to glutaraldehyde for high level disinfection. *J Appl Microbiol* 1999;86:1039–1046.
113. Fraud S, Hann AC, Maillard J-Y, et al. Comparison of the mycobactericidal activity of *ortho*-phthalaldehyde, glutaraldehyde and other dialdehydes by a quantitative suspension test. *J Hosp Infect* 2001;48:214–221.
114. Cabrera-Martinez R-M, Setlow B, Setlow P. Studies on the mechanism of the sporicidal action of *ortho*-phthalaldehyde. *J Appl Microbiol* 2002;92:675–680.
115. Rehn D, Nolte H. 1979. Zur antimikrobiellen wirksamkeit substituierter aromatischer aldehyde und alkohole. *Zentrabl Bakteriol Hyg Abt I Orig B* 1979;168:506–516.
116. Fraenkel-Conat H, Cooper M, Olcott HS. The reaction of formaldehyde with proteins. *J Am Chem Soc* 1945;67:950–954.
117. Staehlin M. Reaction of tobacco mosaic virus nucleic acid with formaldehyde. *Biochim Biophys Acta* 1958;29:410–417.
118. Rubo SD, Gardner JF, Webb RL. Biological activities of glutaraldehyde and related compounds. *J Appl Bacteriol* 1967;30:78–87.
119. Borick PM. Chemical sterilizers. *Adv Appl Microbiol* 1968;10:291–312.
120. Akamatsu T, Tabata K, Hironga M, et al. Transmission of *Helicobacter pylori* infection via flexible fiberoptic endoscopy. *Am J Infect Control* 1996;24:396–401.
121. Chan-Myers H, Roberts C, Ascenzi J. Virucidal activity of *o*-phthalaldehyde solutions against drug resistant bacteria. Abstracts of American Society for Microbiology Meeting 2001;Q-64:595.
122. Collins FM, Montalbine V. Mycobactericidal activity of glutaraldehyde solutions. *J Clin Microbiol* 1976;4:408–412.
123. Hernandez A, Martró E, Matas L, et al. In-vitro evaluation of Persafe compared with 2% alkaline glutaraldehyde against *Mycobacterium* spp. *J Hosp Infect* 2003:54:52–56.
124. Hernandez A, Martró E, Puzo C, et al. In-use evaluation of Persafe compared with Cidex in fiberoptic bronchoscope disinfection. *J Hosp Infect* 2003;54:46–51.
125. Collins FM. Bactericidal activity of alkaline glutaraldehyde solution against a number of atypical mycobacterial species. *J Appl Bacteriol* 1986;61:247–251.
126. Nye K, Chadha DK, Hodgkin P, et al. *Mycobacterium chelonei* isolation from bronchoalveolar lavage fluid and its practical implications. *J Hosp Infect* 1990;16:257–261.
127. Fraser VJ, Jones M, Murray PR, et al. Contamination of flexible fiberoptic bronchoscopes with *Mycobacterium chelonae* linked to an automated bronchoscope disinfection machine. *Am Rev Resp Dis* 1992:145:853–855.
128. Griffiths PA, Babb JR, Bradley CR, et al. Glutaraldehyde-resistant *Mycobacterium chelonae* from endoscope washer disinfectors. *J Appl Microbiol* 1997;82:519–526.
129. Lynam P, Babb JR, Fraise AP. Comparison of the mycobactericidal activity of 2% alkaline glutaraldehyde and "Nu-Cidex" (0.35% peracetic acid). *J Hosp Infect* 1995;30:237–240.
130. Carson LA, Favero MS, Bond WW, et al. Factors affecting comparative resistance of naturally occurring and subcultured *Pseudomonas aeruginosa* to disinfectants. *Appl Microbiol Biotechnol* 1972;23:863–869.
131. Carson LA, Petersen NJ, Favero MS, et al. Growth characteristics of atypical mycobacteria in water and their comparative resistance to disinfectants. *Appl Env Microbiol* 1978;36:839–846.
132. Sagripanti J-L, Bonafacino A. Comparative sporicidal effects of liquid chemical agents. *Appl Environ Microbiol* 1996;62:545–551.
133. Gorman SP, Scott EM. Effect of alkalination of the bacterial cell and glutaraldehyde molecule. *Microbios Lett* 1977;6:39–44.
134. Bartlett JG, Onderdonk AB, Cisneros RL, et al. Clindamycin-associated colitis due to toxin-producing species of Clostridium in hamsters. *J Infect Dis* 1977;136:701–705.
135. Bartlett JG, Chang TW, Gurwith M, et al. Antibiotic-associated pseudo-membraneous colitis due to toxin producing clostridia. *N Engl J Med* 1978;298:531.
136. Larson HE, Price AB, Honour P, et al. *Clostridium difficile* and the aetiology of pseudomembranous colitis. *Lancet* 1978;1:1063–1066.
137. Teasley DG, Gerding DN, Olson MM. Prospective randomized trial of metronidazole versus vancomycin for *Clostridium difficile*–associated diarrhea and colitis. *Lancet* 1983;2:1043–1046.
138. Dyas A, Das BC. The activity of glutaraldehyde against *Clostridium difficile*. *J Hosp Infect* 1985;6:41–45.
139. Hughes CE, Gebhard RL, Petersen LR, et al. Efficacy of routine fibreoptic endoscope cleaning and disinfection for killing *Clostridium difficile*. *Gastrointest Endosc* 1986;32:7–9.
140. Oie S, Kamiya A. Sporicidal activity of aldehyde disinfectants. *Env Infect* 2003;18:1–9.
141. Gorman, SP, Scott EM. A quantitative evaluation of the antifungal activity of glutaraldehyde. *J Pharm Pharmacol* 1977;43:83–89.
142. Terleckyj B, Axler DA. Quantitative neutralization assay of fungicidal properties of disinfectants. *Antimicrob Agents Chemother* 1987;31:794–798.
143. Scott EM, Gorman SP. Glutaraldehyde. In: Block SS, ed. *Disinfection, sterilization and preservation,* 5th ed. Philadelphia: Lippincott, Williams & Wilkins, 2001:361–381.
144. Dabrowa N, Landau JW, Newcomer VD. Antifungal activity of glutaraldehyde in vitro. *Arch Dermatol* 1972;105:555–557.
145. Suringa DWR. Treatment of superficial onychomycoses with topically applied glutaraldehyde. *Arch Dermatol* 1970;102:163–167.
146. Isenberg HD, Giugliano ER, France K, et al. Evaluation of three disinfectants after in-use stress. *J Hosp Infect* 1988;11:278–285.
147. Chambon M, Jallat-Archimbaud C, Bailly JL, et al. Comparative sensitivities of Sabin and Mahoney poliovirus type 1 prototype strains and two recent isolates to low concentrations of glutaraldehyde. *Appl Environ Microbiol* 1997;63:3199–3204.
148. Narang HK, Codd AA. Action of commonly used disinfectants against enteroviruses. *J Hosp Infect* 1983;4:209–212.
149. Saitanu K, Lund E. Inactivation of enterovirus by glutaraldehyde. *Appl Microbiol* 1975;29:571–574.
150. Cunliffe HR, Blackwell JH, Walker JS. Glutaraldehyde inactivation of exotic animal viruses in swine heart tissue. *Appl Env Microbiol* 1979;37:1044–1046.
151. Spire B, Montagnier L, Barre-Sinoussi F, et al. Inactivation of lymphadenopathy associated virus by chemical disinfectants. *Lancet* 1984;2:899–901.

152. Hanson PJV, Gor D, Jefferies DJ, et al. Chemical inactivation of HIV on surfaces. *Br Med J* 1989;298:862–864.
153. Hanson PJV, Gor D, Clarke JR, et al. Contamination of endoscopes used in patients with AIDS. *Lancet* 1989;2:86–88.
154. Hanson PJV, Gor D, Jefferies DJ, et al. Elimination if high titre HIV from fibreoptic endoscopes. *Gut* 1990;31:657–660.
155. Druce JD, Jardine D, Locarnini SA, et al. Susceptibility of HIV to inactivation by disinfectants and ultraviolet light. *J Hosp Infect* 1995;30:167–180.
156. Blackwell JH, Chen JHS. Effects of various germicidal chemicals on HEp 2 cell culture and herpes simplex virus. *J Assoc Off Anal Chem* 1970;53:1229–1236.
157. Prince DL, Prince RN, Prince HN. Inactivation of human immunodeficiency virus type 1 and herpes simplex virus type 2 by commercial hospital disinfection. *Chem Times Trends* 1990:13–16.
158. Sable FL, Hellman A, McDade J. Glutaraldehyde inactivation of virus in tissue. *Appl Microbiol* 1969;17:645–646.
159. Seefeld U, Bansky G, Jaeger M, et al. Prevention of hepatitis B virus transmission by gastrointestinal fiberscope: successful disinfection with an aldehyde liquid. *Endoscopy* 1981;13:238–239.
160. Adler-Storthz K, Schulster LM, Dreesman GR, et al. Effect of alkaline glutaraldehyde on hepatitis B virus antigen. *Eur J Clin Microbiol* 1983;2:316–320.
161. Passagot J, Crance JM, Biziagos E, et al. Effect of glutaraldehyde on the antigenicity and infectivity of hepatitis A virus. *J Virol Methods* 1987;16:21–28.
162. Deva AK, Vickery K, Zou J, et al. Evaluation of an in-use testing method for evaluating disinfection of surgical instruments using the duck hepatitis B model. *J Hosp Infect* 1996;33:119–130.
163. Sattar AS, Raphael RA, Lochman H, et al. Rotavirus inactivation by chemical disinfectants and antiseptics used in hospitals. *Can J Microbiol* 1983;29:1464–1469.
164. Doultree JC, Druce JD, Birch CJ. Inactivation of feline calcivirus, a Norwalk surrogate virus. *J Hosp Infect* 1999;41:51–57.
165. Chan Myers H, Roberts C. Virucidal activity of *o*-phthalaldehyde solution against bovine viral diarrhea virus (BVDV). Paper presented at the Association for Professionals in Infection Control Conference; May 2002, Nashville, TN.
166. Roberts C, Chan Myers H. Virucidal activity of *o*-phthalaldehyde solution against duck hepatitis B virus. Paper presented at the Association for Professionals in Infection Control Conference; June 2001, Seaettle, WA.
167. Hughes RC, Thompson PF. Cross linking of bacterial cell walls with glutaraldehyde. *Biochem J* 1970;119:925–926.
168. Munton TJ, Russell AD. Effect of glutaraldehyde on protoplasts of *Bacillus megaterium*. *J Gen Microbiol* 1970;63:367–370.
169. McGucken PV, Woodside W. Studies on the mode of action of glutaraldehyde on *Escherichia coli*. *J Appl Bacteriol* 1973;36:419–426.
170. Gorman SP, Scott EM. Transport capacity, alkaline phosphatase activity and protein content of glutaraldehyde-treated cell forms of *Escherichia coli*. *Microbios* 1977;19:205–212.
171. Ellar DJ, Munoz E, Salton MRJ. The effect of low concentrations of glutaraldehyde on *Micrococcus lysodeikticus* membranes. *Biochim Biophys Acta* 1971;225:140–150.
172. Kubitschek HE. Constancy of uptake during the cell cycle in *Escherichia coli*. *Biophys J* 1968;8:1401–1408.
173. Done J, Shorey CD, Locke JP, et al. The cytochemical localization of alkaline phosphatase in *Escherichia coli* at the electron microscope level. *Biochem J* 1965;96:27c–28c.
174. Wang HJ, Tu J. Modification of glycogen phosphorylase by glutaraldehyde preparation and isolation of enzyme derivatives with enhanced stability. *Biochemistry* 1969;8:4403–4410.
175. Wetzel BK, Spicer SS, Dvorak HF, et al. Cytochemical localization of certain phosphatases *in Escherichia coli*. *J Bacteriol* 1970;104:529–542.
176. Cheng KJ, Ingram JM, Costerton JW. Alkaline phosphates localization and spheroplasts formation of *Pseudomonas aeruginosa*. *Can J Microbiol* 1970;16:1319–1324.
177. Munton TJ, Russell AD. Effect of glutaraldehyde on cell viability, triphenyltrazolium reduction, oxygen uptake and galactosidase activity in *Escherichia coli*. *Appl Microbiol* 1973;36:211–217.
178. Fraud S, Hann AC, Maillard J-Y, et al. Effects of *ortho*-phthalaldehyde, glutaraldehyde and chlorhexidine diacetate on *Mycobacterium chelonae* and *Mycobacterium abscessus* strains with modified permeability. *J Antimicrob Chemother* 2003;51:575–584.
179. Bailey J-L, Chambon H, Peigue-Lafeville H, et al. Activity of glutaraldehyde at low concentrations (<2%) against poliovirus and its relevance to gastrointestinal endoscope disinfection procedures. *Appl Environ Microbiol* 1991;57:1156–1160.
180. Howard CR, Dixon JL, Young P, et al. Chemical inactivation of hepatitis B virus: the effect of disinfectants on virus associated DNA polymerase activity, morphology and infectivity. *J Virol Methods* 1983;7:135–148.
181. Maillard J-Y, Beggs TS, Day MJ, et al. The effects of biocides on transduction of *Pseudomonas aeruginosa* PAO by F116 bacteriophage. *Lett Appl Microbiol* 1995;21:285–292.
182. Maillard J-Y, Beggs TS, Day MJ, et al. The effect of biocides on proteins of *Pseudomonas aeruginosa* PAO by F116 bacteriophage. *J Appl Bacteriol* 1996;80:291–295.
183. Maillard J-Y, Beggs TS, Day MJ, et al. Damage to *Pseudomonas aeruginosa* PAO by F116 bacteriophage DNA by biocides. *J Appl Bacteriol* 1996;80:540–544.
184. Hopewood D, Allen CR, McCabe C. The reactions between glutaraldehyde and various proteins: an investigation of their kinetics. *Histochem J* 1970;2:137–150.
185. Munton TJ, Russell AD. Interaction of glutaraldehyde with spheroplasts of *Escherichia coli*. *J Appl Bacteriol* 1973;36:211–217.
186. Gorman SP, Scott EM. Potentiation and stabilization of glutaraldehyde biocidal activity utilizing surfactant-divalent cation combinations. *Int J Pharm* 1979;4:57–65.
187. Thomas S, Russell AD. Studies on the mechanism of sporicidal action of glutaraldehyde. *J Appl Bacteriol* 1974;37:83–92.
188. McErlean EP, Gorman SP, Scott EM. Physical and chemical resistance of ion-exchange and coat defective spores of *Bacillus subtilis*. *J Pharm Pharmacol* 1980;32:32P.
189. Gorman SP, Scott EM, Hutchinson EP. Interaction of *Bacillus subtilis* spore protoplast, cortex, ion-exchange and coatless forms with glutaraldehyde. *J Appl Bacteriol* 1984;56:95–102.
190. Gorman SP, Hutchison EP, Scott EM, et al. Death, injury and revival of chemically treated *Bacillus subtilis* spores. *J Appl Bacteriol* 1983;54:91–99.
191. Lever AM, Sutton SVW. Antimicrobial effects of hydrogen peroxide as an antiseptic and disinfectant. In: Ascenzi JM, ed. *Handbook of disinfectants and antiseptics*. New York: Marcel Dekker, 1996:159–176.
192. Block SS. Peroxygen compounds. In: Block SS, ed. *Disinfection, sterilization and preservation,* 5th ed.

Philadelphia: Lippincott, Williams & Wilkins, 2001:185–204.

193. Klopotek BB. Peracetic acid methods for preparation and properties. *Chimica Oggi* 1998;16:33–37.
194. Fridovich I. The biology of oxygen radicals. *Science* 1978;201:875–879.
195. Gould GW, Hitchins AD. Sensitization of bacterial spores to lysozyme and hydrogen peroxide with reagents which rupture disulfide bonds. *Nature* 1963;197:622.
196. Russell AD. Similarities and differences in the response of microorganism to biocides. *J Antimicrob Chemother* 2003;52:750–763.
197. Hofmann J, Jusdt G, Pritzkow W, et al. Bleaching activators and mechanism of bleaching activation. *J Prakt Chem* 1992;334:293–297.
198. Malchesky PS. Medical applications of peracetic acid. In: Block SS, ed. *Disinfection, sterilization and preservation,* 5th ed. Philadelphia: Lippincott, Williams & Wilkins, 2001:979–996.
199. Rutala WA, Gergen MF, Weber DJ. Sporicidal activity of chemical sterilants used in hospitals. *Infect Control Hosp Epidemiol* 1993;14:713–718.
200. Holton J, McDonald V. Efficacy of selected disinfectants against *Mycobacteria* and *Cryptosporidium. J Hosp Infect* 1994;27:105–115.
201. Goddard PA, McCue KA. Phenolic compounds. In: Block SS, ed. *Disinfection, sterilization and preservation,* 5th ed. Philadelphia: Lippincott, Williams & Wilkins, 2001:255–281.
202. Denyer SP. Mechanism of action of biocides. *Int Biodeterior Biodegradation* 1990;26:89–100.
203. Fredrick JJ, Corner TR, Gerhardt P. Antimicrobial actions of hexachlorophene: inhibition of respiration in *Bacillus megaterium. Antimicrob Agents Chemother* 1974;6:712–721.
204. Regos J, Hitz HR. Investigations on the mode of action of triclosan, a broad spectrum antimicrobial agent. *Zentralbl Bakteriol* 1974;226:390–401.
205. Commager H, Judis J. Mechanism of action of phenolic disinfectants. VI. Effects on glucose and succinate metabolism of *Escherichia coli. J Pharm Sci* 1965;54:1436–1439.
206. Hugo WB, Bowen JG. Studies on the mode of action of 4-ethylphenol on *Escherichia coli. Microbios* 1973;8:189–197.
207. Hugo WB, Bloomfield SF. Studies on the mode of action of the phenolic antibacterial agent fentichlor against *Staphylococcus aureus* and *Escherichia coli.* III. The effect of fentichlor on the metabolic activities of *Staphylococcus aureus* and *Escherichia coli. J Appl Bacteriol* 1971;34:579–591.
208. Bloomfield SF. The effect of the phenolic antibacterial agent fentichlor on energy coupling in *Staphylococcus aureus. J Appl Bacteriol* 1974;37:117–131.
209. Kroll RG, Anagnostopoulos GD. Potassium leakage as a lethality index of phenol and the effect of solute and water activity. *J Appl Bacteriol* 1981:50:139–147.
210. Gale EF, Taylor ES. Action of tyrocidin and some detergent substances in releasing amino acids from the internal environment of *Streptococcus faecalis. J Gen Microbiol* 1947;1:77–84.
211. Judis J. Studies on the mechanism of action of phenolic disinfectants. I. Release of radioactivity from ^{14}C-labelled *Escherichia coli. J Pharm Sci* 1962;51:261–265.
212. Judis J. Studies on the mechanism of action of phenolic disinfectants. II. Patterns of release of radioactivity from *Escherichia coli* labeled by growth on various compounds. *J Pharm Sci* 1963;52:126–131.
213. Hugo WB, Blolomfield SF. Studies on the mode of action of the phenolic antibacterial agent fentichlor against *Staphylococcus aureus* and *Escherichia coli.* I. The adsorption of fentichlor by the bacterial cell and its antimicrobial activity. *J Appl Bacteriol* 1971;34:557–567.
214. Hugo WB, Blolomfield SF. Studies on the mode of action of the phenolic antibacterial agent fentichlor against *Staphylococcus aureus* and *Escherichia coli.* II. The effect of fentichlor on the bacterial membrane and the cytoplasmic constituents of the cell. *J Appl Bacteriol* 1971;34:569–578.
215. Joswick HL, Corner TR, Silvernale JN, et al. Antimicrobial action of hexachlorophene: release of cytoplasmic materials. *J Bacteriol* 1971;108:492–500.
216. Rubin J. Mycobactericidal disinfection and control. In: Block SS, ed. *Disinfection, sterilization, and preservation,* 4th ed. Philadephia: Lea & Febiger, 1991:331–384.
217. Russell AD, Chopra I. Sporostatic and sporicidal agents: their properties and mechanism of action. In: *Understanding antibacterial action and resistance,* 2nd ed. London: Ellis Horwood, 1996:150–171.
218. Bach D, Lambert J. Action de quelques antiseptiques sur les dehydrogenase du staphylocoque dore. *Compt Rend Soc Biol (Paris)* 1937;126:298–300.
219. Bach D, Lambert J. Action de quelques antiseptiques sur les dehydrogenase du staphylocoque dore; systemes activants le glucose, l'acide formique et un certain nombre d'autres substrates. *Compt Rend Soc Biol (Paris)* 1937;126:300–302.
220. Bancroft WD, Richter GH. The chemistry of disinfection. *J Phys Chem* 1931;35:511–530.
221. Hugo WB. Disinfection mechanisms. In: Russell AD, Hugo WB, Ayliffe GA, eds. *Principles and practices of disinfection, preservation and sterilization,* 3rd ed. Oxford: Blackwell Scientific Publications, 1999:258–283.
222. Bruch M. Chlorxylenol: an old-new chemical. In: Ascenzi JM, ed. *Handbook of disinfectants and antiseptics.* New York: Marcel Dekker, 1996:265–294.
223. Rutala WA, Clontz EP, Weber DI, et al. Disinfection practices for endoscopes and other semicritical items. *Infect Control Hosp Epidemiol* 1991;12:282–288.
224. Martin LS, et al. Disinfection and inactivation of human T-lymphotropic virus type III/lymphadenopathy-associated virus. *J Infect Dis* 1985;2:400–403.
225. Druce JD, Jardine D, Locarnini SA, et al. Syringe cleaning techniques and transmission of HIV. *AIDS* 1995;9:1105–1107.
226. Waller RF, Keeling PJ, Donald RG, et al. Nuclear-encoded proteins target the plastid in *Toxoplasma gondii* and *Plasmodium falciparum. Proc Natl Acad Sci USA* 1998;95:12352–12357.
227. McMurray LA, Oethginger M, Levy SB. Triclosan targets lipid synthesis. *Nature* 1998;394:531–532.
228. McMurray LA, McDermott PT, Levy SB. Genetic evidence that *inhA* of *Mycobacterium smegmatis* is a target for triclosan. *Antimicrob Agents Chemother* 1999;43:711–713.
229. Slater-Radosti C, Van Aller G, Greenwood R. Biochemical and genetic characterization of the action of triclosan on *Staphylococcus aureus. J Biol Chem* 2001:48:1–6.
230. Heath RJ, Yu Y-T, Shapiro MA, et al. Broad spectrum antimicrobial biocides target the FABI component of fatty acid synthesis. *J Biol Chem* 1998;46:30316–30320.
231. Heath RJ, Ronald JR, Holland DR, et al. Mechanism of triclosan inhibition of bacterial fatty acid synthesis. *J Biol Chem* 1999;274:11110–11114.
232. Perozzo R, Kuo M, Sidhu A. Structural elucidation of the specificity of the antibacterial agent triclosan for malarial enoyl acyl carrier protein reductase. *J Biol Chem* 2002;277:13106–13114.

233. Regos J, Zak O, Solf R, et al. Antimicrobial spectrum of triclosan, a broad-spectrum antimicrobial agent for topical applications. II. Comparison with some other antimicrobial agents. *Dermatologica* 1979;158:72–79.
234. Schmid MB, Kaplan M. Reduced triclosan susceptibility in methicillin resistant *Staphylococcus epidermidis*. *Antimicrob Agents Chemother* 2004;48:1397–1399.
235. Suller MTE, Russell AD. Triclosan and antibiotic resistance in *Staphylococcus aureus*. *J Antimicrob Chemother* 2000;46:11–18.
236. Cookson BD, Farrelly H, Stapleton P, et al. Transferable resistance to triclosan in MRSA. *Lancet* 1991;337:1548–1549.
237. Webster J. Handwashing in a neonatal intensive care nursery: product acceptability and effectiveness of chlorhexidine gluconate and triclosan 1%. *J Hosp Infect* 1992;21: 137–141.
238. Furia TE, Schenkel AG. A new, broad-spectrum bacteriostat. *Soap Chem Specialties* 1968;44:47–50, 116–122.
239. Bhargava HN, Leonard PA. Triclosan: applications and safety. *Am J Infect Control* 1996;24:209–218.
240. Larson EL. Guidelines for the use of topical antimicrobial agents. *Am J Infect Control* 1988;8:253–266.
241. Sharma S, Ramya TNC, Surolia A, et al. Triclosan as a systemic antibacterial agent in a mouse model of acute bacterial challenge. *Antimicrob Agents Chemother* 2003:47:3859–3866.
242. Saunders KA, Greenman J, McKenzie C. Ecological effects of triclosan and triclosan monophosphate on defined mixed cultures of oral species grown in continuous culture. *J Antimicrob Chemother* 2000;48:447–452.
243. McBain AJ, Bartolo RG, Catrenich CF, et al. Effects of triclosan-containing rinse on the dynamics and antimicrobial susceptibility of in vitro plaque ecosystems. *Antimicrob Agents Chemother* 2003;11:3531–3538.
244. Simmons BP. Guideline for hospital environmental control. *Am J Infect Control* 1983;11:97–115.
245. Shickman MD, Guze LB, Pearce ML. Bacteremia following cardiac catheterization. *N Engl J Med* 1959;260:1164–1166.
246. Ehrenkranz NJ, Bolyard EA, Wiener M, et al. Antibiotic-sensitive *Serratia marcescens* infections complicating cardiopulmonary operations: contaminated disinfectant as a reservoir. *Lancet* 1980;2:1289–1292.
247. Rutala WA, Cole EC. Antiseptics and disinfectants—safe and effective? *Infect Control* 1984;5:215–218.
248. Merianos JJ. Surface-active agents. In: Block SS, ed. *Disinfection, sterilization and preservation*, 5th ed. Philadelphia: Lippincott, Williams & Wilkins, 2001:283–320.
249. Rutala WA, Cole EC. Ineffectiveness of hospital disinfectants against bacteria: a collaborative study. *Infect Control* 1987;8:501–506.
250. Cole EC, Rutala WA, Samsa GP. Disinfectant testing using a modified use-dilution method: collaborative study. *J Assoc Off Anal Chem* 1988;71:1187–1194.
251. Sasatsu M, Shibata Y, Noguchi N, et al. High-level resistance to ethidium bromide and antiseptics in *Staphylococcus aureus*. *FEMS Microbiol Lett* 1992;93:109–114.
252. Russell AD. Plasmid and bacterial resistance to biocides. *J Appl Microbiol* 1997;82:155–165.
253. Russell AD. The role of plasmids in bacterial resistance to antiseptics, disinfectants and preservatives. *J Hosp Infect* 1985;6:9–19.
254. Moken MC, McMurray LM, Levy SB. Selection of multiple-antibiotic-resistant (mar) mutants of *Escherichia coli* by using the disinfectant pine oil: roles of the *mar* and *acr*AB loci. *Antimicrob Agents Chemother* 1997;41:2770–2772.
255. Price CTD, Singh VK, Jayaswal RK, et al. Pine oil cleaner resistant *Staphylococcus aureus:* reduced susceptibility for vancomycin and oxicillin and involvement of SigB. *Appl Env Microbiol* 2002;68:5417–5421.
256. Levy, SB. Antimicrobial household products: cause for concern. *Emer Infect Dis* 2001;7:512–515.
257. Romanova N, Favrin S, Griffiths MW. Sensitivity of *Listeria monocytogenes* to sanitizers used in the meat processing industry. *Appl Environ Microbiol* 2002;68:6405–6409.
258. Jalier V, Nikaido H. Mycobacterial cell wall: structure and role in natural resistance to antibiotics. *FEMS Microbiol Lett* 1994;123:11–18.
259. Costerton JW, Cheng KJ, Geesey GG, et al. Bacterial biofilms in nature and disease. *Ann Rev Microbiol* 1987;41:435–464.
260. Costerton JD, Lewandowski Z, DeBeer D, et al. Biofilms, the customized niche. *J Bacteriol* 1994;176:2137–2142.
261. Brown, MRW, Gilbert, P. Sensitivity of biofilms to antimicrobial agents. *J Appl Bacteriol Symp Suppl* 1993;74:87S–97S.
262. Russell AD. Mechanism of bacterial resistance to biocides. *Int Biodeterior Biodegradation* 1995;36:247–265.
263. To MS, Favrin S, Romanova N, et al. Postadaptational resistance to benzalkonium chloride and subsequent physiochemical modifications of *Listeria monocytogenes*. *Appl Env Microbiol* 2002;68:5258–5264.
264. Ogase HI, Nigai I, Kameda K, et al. Identification and quantitative analysis of degradation products of chlorhexidine and chlorhexidine-resistant bacteria with three-dimensional high performance liquid chromatography. *J Appl Bacteriol* 1992;73:71–78.
265. Powers EGM, Dancer BN, Russell AD. Emergence of resistance to glutaraldehyde in spores of *Bacillus subtilis*. *FEMS Microbiol Lett* 1988;50:223–226.
266. Knott AG, Russell AD, Dancer BN. Development of resistance to biocides during sporulation of *Bacillus subtilis*. *J Appl Bacteriol* 1995;79:492–498.
267. Bloomfield SF, Arthur M. Interaction of *Bacillus subtilis* spores with sodium hypochlorite, sodium dichloroisocynaurate and chloramine-T. *J Appl Bacteriol* 1992;72:166–172.
268. Bloomfield SF, Arthur M. Mechanism of inactivation and resistance of spores to chemical biocides. *J Appl Bacteriol Symp Suppl* 1994;76:91S–104S.
269. Setlow B, Setlow P. Binding of small, acid-soluble spore proteins to DNA plays a significant role in the resistance of *Bacillus subtilis* spores to hydrogen peroxide. *Appl Environ Microbiol* 1993;59:3418–3423.
270. Sabli MZH, Setlow P, Waites WM. The effect of hypochlorite on spores of *Bacillus subtilis* lacking small acid-soluble proteins. *Lett Appl Microbiol* 1996;22:405–507.
271. Kolawole DO. Resistance mechanism of mucoid-grown *Staphylococcus aureus* to the antibacterial action of some disinfectants and antiseptics. *FEMS Microbiol Lett* 1984;25:205–209.
272. Gilbert P, Brown MRW. Some perspectives on preservation and disinfection in the present day. *Int Biodeterior Biodegradation* 1995;36:219–226.
273. Guerin-Mechin L, Dubois-Brissonnet F, Heyd B, et al. Quaternary ammonium compound stress induces specific variation in fatty acid composition of *Pseudomonas aeruginosa*. *Int J Food Microbiol* 2000;55:157–159.
274. Braoudaki M, Hilton AC. Adaptive resistance to biocides in *Salmonella enterica* and *Escherichia coli* 0157 and cross-resistance to antimicrobial agents. *J Clin Microbiol* 2004;42:73–78.
275. Chuanchuen R, Narasaki CT, Schweizer HP. The MexJK efflux pump of *Pseudomonas aeruginosa* requires OprM for

antibiotic efflux but not for efflux of triclosan. *J Bacteriol* 2002;184:5036–5044.

276. Langsrud S, Sundheim G, Borgman-Strahsen R. Intrinsic and acquired resistance to quaternary ammonium compounds in food related *Pseudomonas* spp. *J Appl Microbiol* 2003;95:874–882.
277. Heir E, Sundheim G, Holck AL. The *Staphylococcus qacH* gene product: a new member of the SMR family encoding multidrug resistance. *FEMS Microbiol Lett* 1998;163:49–56.
278. Heir E, Sundheim G, Holck AL. The *qacG* gene on plasmid pST94 confers resistance to quaternary ammonium compounds in staphylococci isolated from the food industry. *J Appl Microbiol* 1999;86:378–388.
279. Sidhu MS, Heir WE, Sørum H, et al. Genetic linkage between resistance to quaternary ammonium compounds and β-lactam antibiotics in food-related *Staphylococcus* spp. *Microb Drug Resist* 2001;7:363–371.
280. Sidhu MS, Heir E, Leegaard T, et al. Frequency of disinfectant resistance genes and genetic linkage with β-lactamase transposon Tn552 among clinical Staphylococci. *Antimicrob Agents Chemother* 2002;46:2797–2803.
281. Leelaporn A, Firth N, Paulsen IT, et al. Multidrug resistance plasmid pSK108 from coagulase-negative staphylococci; relationship to *Staphylococcus aureus qacC* plasmids. *Plasmid* 1995;34:62–67.
282. Littlejohn TG, DiBerardino, D, Messerotti, LJ, et al. Structure and evolution of a family of genes encoding antiseptic and disinfectant resistance in *Staphylococcus aureus*. *Gene* 1991;101:59–66.
283. Paulsen IT, Brown MH, Littlejohn TG, et al. Multidrug resistance proteins QacA and QacB from *Staphylococcus aureus*: membrane topology and identification of residues involved in substance specificity. *Proc Natl Acad Sci USA* 1996;93:3630–3635.
284. Bjorland J, Steinum T, Sunde M, et al. Novel plasmid-borne *qacJ* mediates resistance to quaternary ammonium compounds in equine *Staphylococcus aureus*, *Staphylococcus simulans*, and *Staphylococcus intermdius*. *Antimicrob Agents Chemother* 2003;47:3046–3052.
285. Lyon BR, Skurray RA. Antimicrobial resistance of *Staphylococcus aureus:* genetic basis. *Microbiol Rev* 1987;51:88–134.
286. Berg, T, Firth, N, Apisirdiej, et al. Complete nucleotide sequence of pSK41: evolution of Staphylococcal conjugative multiresistance plasmids. *J Bacteriol* 1998;180:4350–4359.
287. Alam MM, Kobayashi N, Uehara N, et al. Analysis of distribution and genomic diversity of high-level antiseptic resistance genes *qacA* and *qacB* in human clinical isolates of *Staphylococcus aureus*. *Microb Drug Res* 2003;9:109–121.
288. Lemaitre JP, Echchannaoui H, Michaut G, et al. Plasmid-mediated resistance to antimicrobial agents among listerae. *J Food Prot* 1998;61:1459–1464.
289. Huillet E, Larin S, Pardon P, et al. Identification of a new locus in *Listeria monocytogenes* involved in cellobiose-dependent repression of *hly* expression. *FEMS Microbiol Lett* 1999;174:265–272.
290. Mereghetti L, Quentin R, Marquet-Van Der Mee N, et al. Low sensitivity of *Listeria monocytogenes* to quarternary ammonium compounds. *Appl Env Microbiol* 2000;66:5083–5086.
291. Russell AD. Do biocides select for antibiotic resistance? *J Pharm Pharmacol* 2000;52:227–233.
292. Rutala WA, Stergel MM, Sarubbi FA, et al. Susceptibility of antibiotic-susceptible and antibiotic-resistant hospital bacteria to disinfectants. *Infect Control Hosp Epidemiol* 1997;18:417–421
293. Cole EC, Addison RM, Rubino JR, et al. Investigation of antibiotic and antibacterial agent cross-resistance in target bacteria from homes of antibacterial users and nonusers. *J Appl Microbiol* 2003;95:664–676.
294. Jones RD. Bacterial resistance and topical antimicrobial wash products. *Am J Infect Control* 1999;27:351–363.

CHAPTER 15

Evaluation of Antimicrobials in Experimental Animal Infections

T. O'Reilly, D. A. Andes, Ch. Østergaard, N. Frimodt-Møller

INTRODUCTION

In vitro studies provide important information on the potency and spectrum of activity of new antimicrobials, but animal models form the link between *in vitro* testing and anticipated clinical results. The results of animal studies suggest appropriate indications and clinical trials, uncover potential toxicity problems, and provide insight into the pharmacokinetics (PKs) of new agents in relation to those of known agents. Thus, it is essential that new agents shown to be of interest following *in vitro* evaluation exhibit sufficient activity *in vivo* to justify their continued clinical development. Clinical evaluation guidelines for antiinfective drugs place experimental evaluation of new compounds (or novel combinations or therapeutic modalities) in animals as a prerequisite for clinical trials (43). Specifically, indications of the PKs of new molecules, including their metabolism and pharmacodynamics (PDs) (e.g., the effects of the interaction of drug, host, and infecting microbe, including postantibiotic effects [PAEs] and the efficacy of the drug in animal models mimicking human disease), are required and indeed may assist in the planning of clinical trials of new antibiotics (43).

The present chapter updates the previous chapter (454), and readers are encouraged to consult the earlier work. Additional key reviews include a historical amount of the use of animal models of infection (118); general overviews based on personal experience of animal models of infection and antimicrobial testing (326,506); reviews of animal models of virus infections (601), parasite infections (244), and fungal infections (308a); a review of models of chronic intracellular pathogens (627); a review of the use of animal models for the development of vaccines (397); and a presentation of alternatives to animal testing of antiinfective agents (69). Following a previous edition of the book by Zak and Sande (632), a subsequent "how-to" book was commissioned (633) that covers the technical aspects of almost every major animal model used in infection research.

ETHICAL ASPECTS OF THE USE OF ANIMALS IN ANTIMICROBIAL DRUG DISCOVERY AND DEVELOPMENT

When considering *in vitro* tests, the challenge is to consider whether they are really sufficient indicators of the efficacy and safety of a compound. When considering *in vivo* tests, the challenges include not only assessing whether such tests are reliable indicators of efficacy and safety but also considering the morality of exploitation of animals in research (630). A "practical-minded" discussion of ethics of animal use is available (420). In any discussion of the ethics of animal experimentation, it is critical to expand the discussion to consider the rights of the afflicted, whose suffering may be alleviated based on information gained through animal experimentation (108,441); there is a certain "cost" involved in not using animals, just as there is a cost in their use. Although open and direct discussion between proponents of each view is apparently scarce, it is the key to resolution of this conflict (61,597a). However, because the goal of the animal rights or animal liberation activists is the complete discontinuation of animal experimentation (492,493,538,539), the opposing positions appear fundamentally irreconcilable. What remains clear is that individual researchers remain responsible for their own conduct. In light of this, readers are urged to carefully consider both points of view in order to resolve, as far as possible, this issue for themselves, as well as to provide for themselves a basis for intelligent discussion with fellow biomedical researchers, the general public, and those opposed to vivisection.

Acceptance of the position that it is ethically justified to perform animal experiments does not solve all of the ethical problems associated with such research (441). In answering these questions, it is clear that the bulk of the responsibility again lies with the individual researchers, but the questions should not be decided in isolation. Ethics committees need to be consulted prior to embarking on any experimentation. In brief, the other questions include the following:

- Is this experiment necessary and can it answer the proposed questions? (36)
- Is the welfare of the animals being used in this experiment given due consideration?
- Are the data gained by such experiments being utilized to best advantage?

Perhaps the most difficult issue is the degree of pain and suffering that animals experience during the course of infection. An excellent review of the recognition of pain and distress in animals and the physiologic basis and consequences of pain has been published (202).

Most governments have passed legislation concerning the use of animals in experiments and require that certain basic requirements be met before such experiments can be carried out. Readable synopses of legislation and general approaches to dealing with ethics committees are available (European [147], American [7]).

PRINCIPLES OF ANIMAL CARE

Standards for animal care differ in their details, and various governments have issued guidelines that are periodically updated. Controlling the factors that contribute to animal health will lead to more uniform experimental results (588). The impact of animal health on the outcomes of experiments using infection models has been reviewed (262a,567). Key factors to monitor and control are the environmental conditions the animals are housed under, the adequacy and consistency of the animals' nutritution, and restriction of access to animal rooms in order to protect the animals and minimize risk to the investigator, particularly when animals are experimentally infected.

PRINCIPLES OF PLANNING EXPERIMENTS INVOLVING ANIMAL TESTING

Selecting an Animal Model of Infection

The objectives of a particular study form the basis for model selection, but as complete an understanding of the model as possible is needed to ascertain that the model is appropriate to meet these objectives. Furthermore, at least in testing antimicrobial agents, the choice of model may be dependent on the nature of the compound, the quantities available (in the case of medicinal chemistry programs, the compound supply is limiting at the early stages), and the extent of information available (e.g., the spectrum of action, the PKs). For example, medicinal chemistry programs aimed at discovering a new chemical entity effective against a novel target would normally use a mouse screening model (e.g., thigh infection or peritoneally initiated sepsis with parenteral and oral compound administration–to answer the question: Which of the many newly synthesized compounds that are active *in vitro* are orally active *in vivo*?) early in the program to select compounds for later profiling using the more complex discriminative models needed to provide a basis for clinical trial design (e.g., to determine the PK/PD relationships and demonstrate efficacy in a model closely mimicking a clinical indication so as to discover the best treatment regimen using the selected compound to treat, say, endocarditis alone and in combination with other antibiotics). Therefore, the "ideal" model varies depending on the questions asked. However, the preferred models will be similar to humans in terms of tolerability, drug absorption, distribution, metabolism, and excretion and if possible will demonstrate a pathophysiology of infection similar to that observed in humans. Lastly, using the model should be technically feasible.

Categories of Animal Models of Infection

Animal models of infection have been classified according to the complexity of the model (265). Basic screening models, *ex vivo* models (where implants such as fibrin clots are infected and subsequently removed for further analysis), monoparametric/polyparametric models (which are similar to screening models but where a single parameter or, preferably, many parameters are examined during the experiment), and discriminative models, which are models designed to simulate human infection as closely as possible. A discriminative model is ideal if there is a simple technique of infection; the causative organism, the route of entry, and the spread in the body are identical or at least similar to the human equivalents; the tissue involvement and the severity, course, and duration of the disease should be predictable, reproducible, and amenable to analysis; and the response of the model to chemotherapy should be measurable and reproducible.

Reproducibility of Animal Models

The response (e.g., the rate and extent of bacterial growth or the onset of clinical signs) observed in the control group has to be in the same range every time the experiment is performed. Furthermore, the response to reference compounds should be reliable and dose-dependent. It is difficult and potentially misleading to uncategorically rely on response ranges found in the literature for the interpretation of data collected in a new experiment. For this reason, investigators should establish in-house reference ranges, and these should be periodically reconfirmed. There are many other sources of variation that can affect the results of individual animal experiments and thereby complicate data interpretation. Mainly these are strain and gender differences, age-related changes, animal well-being, and the mode and nature of infection initiation and compound administration.

Limitations of Animal Models

Differences in adsorption, distribution, metabolism, and excretion can be profoundly different, and care has to be taken to study drug doses that are "reasonable" so that the effective dose found in the model is similar to one envisioned for patients; despite the general trend of longer drug half-lives in larger animals, the requirement of large doses in mice is normally a sign that the compound is too weakly active. Ideally, drug exposure should utilize regimens that produce humanlike PK profiles. However, what such a regimen would be is obviously not known for experimental drugs at the preclinical stage. The resulting limitations can be profound and must be taken seriously when performing an animal experiment and interpreting the data obtained. Animal models should be used cautiously, their limitations should be recognized, and only those questions that the models can answer should be asked.

Model Validation

Once the most appropriate model is selected, the next step is to validate model, that is, to establish its the suitability mostly in terms of responsiveness to chemotherapeutic intervention (therapy or prophylaxis). The results of the validation tests must delineate the similarities and differences between the disease as it occurs in the model and in humans. As will be discussed later, redefining or modifying the animal model to better reflect the clinical situation, particularly in terms of response to treatment, apparently seldom occurs but can produce dramatic improvements in the predictive value of the model (see Eichaker et al. [171]). Standard drugs are usually marketed drugs with proven efficacy in patients. Due consideration should be given to devising an appropriate therapeutic regimen so that the outcome in the model is similar to outcome clinically (e.g., creating a severity of infection and devising a treatment regimen that results in a "cure" rate that is similar to the clinical cure rate [see reference 171]).

Validation should be seen as a continuous process. This implies that a positive control (reference compound) should be included as an internal standard every time the model is used. A negative control (vehicle treatment) is almost always needed to account for time-related changes or other "hard-to-control" variables during the experiment.

The nature and extent of variability depends on the homogeneity of the experimental animals used and to a lesser extent on the variability of the analytical methods used. Therefore, experimental animals, especially small rodents, are often derived from inbred populations in order to reduce this variability. Moreover, individual variability due to the physical status of the animals or the procedure itself can occur. Adaptation or acclimatization times may vary depending on the animals used and the time of day of the experiment (many indicators of a disease process are subject to individual circadian rhythms). Differences may be in part controlled by stratifying the treatment groups. In the process of stratification, animals are placed into groups (blocks) based on criteria defined before the experiment, and then the groups are randomized with respect to treatments. However, stratification, though it is likely to reduce variability between groups, may increase variability within groups.

Finally, the use of the most appropriate statistical test to analyze the data is critical to successfully conclude an *in vivo* study. The sizes of the groups of experimental subjects and the exact statistical tests should be chosen based on the expected or desired minimal responses to therapy and the inherent variability of the groups. The downside of these fully justified efforts to minimize variability is that such experiments give no hints of the variability to be expected under clinical conditions, where many factors (e.g., pharmacogenomics, the time of the disease presentation, and the presence of underlying diseases) render extrapolation of preclinical data to the clinical situation more difficult.

Statistics and Experimental Design

The following is extensively based on previous publications (58,59,261,272,322,583,598).

Experimental Design

Any experiment comprises experimental units or subjects, questions posed, experimental design, facilities for performing the experiment, and the logistics of material supply and labor, all of which need to be considered carefully. For several reasons, both ethical and cost-related, *in vivo* pharmacologists have an obligation to consistently use the best possible experimental design. A good experimental design should make efficient use of resources and extract the maximum amount of information from the available material, and the number of animals per group should be neither so small that treatment effects remain undetected and incorrect conclusions are reached, nor so large that animals and other resources are wasted.

Experimental design involves the following:

- The question(s) to be answered must be clearly formulated (but the researchers must be prepared to analyze unexpected observations). The researchers must also recognize the constraints that the model possesses in terms of "relevance" (i.e., they must limit the questions to those that the model can really address).

- Sources of bias must be minimized, normally by including randomization steps.
- The natural subdivisions of experimental subjects (or the treatments) must be accounted for. This is normally accomplished by using specialized experimental designs.
- Whenever possible, the numbers of experimental subjects should be the same in each group to facilitate statistical analysis. Plans for dealing with "dropouts" that reduce the number in a group or cause the loss of data (i.e., censored data) should be in place.
- The researchers must take into account the chronobiological aspects (e.g., orally administered treatments at night will likely be administered to mice with full stomachs).
- They must weigh feasibility versus perfection and the logistics of carrying out the experiment.
- They must plan statistical analyses prior to initiation of the experiment and include questions indicating how large a difference between groups is expected (or desired) and the likely variability of data, both of which are used in estimating the experimental group sizes.
- The researchers must consider the final display of the data. Complex experiments are not easily amenable to graphic display (normally more than 4–5 lines on a single graph are difficult to follow, especially during oral presentations), and therefore it may be necessary to break a single experiment into several parts for effective display of the data.

In a typical experiment only one set of treatments are administered in order to isolate a single variable. However, whenever possible, the design should allow several independent variables (or factors) to be considered simultaneously. Further, the design should be such that each combination of variables is represented in the form of treatments, preferably with replicates in a single experiment. Experimental designs of this type can be used to look at the effect of individual variables but also at possible interactions between the variables. Such "multifactorial" designs clearly require built-in statistical analysis plans (e.g., two-way or three-way ANOVAs). Essential to good experimental design is the inclusion of appropriate controls. Vehicle controls and, if needed, separate controls for each treatment formulation (e.g., saline groups as well as an ethanol group if the test compounds are formulated in saline or ethanol) or each route of administration (e.g., intravenous administration and oral administration) should be included. Controls for the aging of the experimental animals during long-term experiments are often overlooked.

Prevention of bias and appropriate randomization are also important factors to consider. Bias occurs when interfering factors have dissimilar effects on different groups, with the end result that the data are unreliable. The main ways of reducing this are through randomization and elimination of investigator bias through use of blinded treatment and observations. Animals or stratified groups can be assigned to treatments randomly (using random number tables or a computer program). Although somewhat laborious, blinding investigators to treatments by the coding of compounds is recommended, particularly when clinical observation or (histo)pathology is used for the evaluation of effects.

Statistical Analyses

The main purpose of statistical evaluation of animal experiments is to ensure that any findings are not due to chance variation within or between the experimental groups. However, statistical evaluation should also be used to illuminate the data, helping to uncover effects that might otherwise be overlooked. It is critical to understand that statistical analyses do not prove biological "cause and effect" hypotheses, nor do they necessarily prove the biological relevance of an effect of the compound in question. Although statistical significance may be shown, the effect may be so small as to be of little interest biologically (or clinically). A second purpose of statistical analyses is to show that the experiment was carried out so as to be free from the kind of experimental errors that may compromise the data (e.g., placement of all animals having the highest body weight in one group). Statistical analyses should demonstrate that before beginning of the treatment the groups were balanced and that during the course of the experiment no detectable unwanted bias occurred (e.g., high mortality in a treatment group in which the survivors were cured of the disease).

IN VITRO CHARACTERIZATION BEFORE EVALUATING A SUBSTANCE USING ANIMAL MODELS

Owing to both the ethical aspects of animal experimentation and the costs involved in performing an *in vivo* experiment, it behooves researchers to obtain results characterizing the substance(s) *in vitro*. Tests to consider include the following.

Determination of *In Vitro* Antimicrobial Properties

The minimal inhibitory concentration (MIC) and minimal bactericidal concentration (MBC) of a substanced used against a particular microorganism indicate the inherent susceptibility of the microorganism to that substance. When combinations are proposed, potential interactions (interference or antagonism, indifference, additivity, or synergy) should be evaluated by the use of checkerboard titrations. Determination of the MIC and MBC should be considered the minimum prerequisite before proceeding to *in vivo* evaluations. Also, the goal should be to test the *in vitro* activity of antibiotics under conditions likely to exist *in vivo* because environmental factors (e.g., pH, pO_2, and pCO_2) can dramatically affect antibiotic activity (300).

Although requiring specialized equipment that is not always available, the following supplemental experiments may be considered. The activity of antimicrobials against intracellular microorganisms should be determined in specialized models of intracellular growth (e.g., *Mycobacterium avium* growing in J774A cells). Because biofilms have been proposed to be an essential part of the *in vivo* situation (121,122,205), and the activity of antibiotics against adherent bacteria can differ from their activity against planktonic bacteria (526), determination of antimicrobial activity against adherent bacteria using the "Robbins device" (161) or other procedures (15,79,139,166,178,590) may yield insight into the effectiveness of a particular agent. However, at least ciprofloxacin appears to demonstrate growth rate–independent killing of biofilm *S. epidermidis* (166). Furthermore, microorganisms may grow at slower rates *in vivo* than *in vitro* (79,205), and this may affect their susceptibility to antimicrobial agents (79,125,142,205); this can be appropriately determined by evaluation of antimicrobial activity in chemostats, where the growth rate of bacteria can be controlled. Lastly, *in vitro* PK models (63,165) may assist in planning dosing schedules, for such models can be used to predict critical parameters of antimicrobial drug concentration and effectiveness (e.g., time above MIC or peak area) and whether a postantibiotic effect may be a feature of the drug-microbe interaction.

Preparation of Suitable Formulations for Administration of Antimicrobial Agents to Animals

The formulation of compounds may have a profound effect on the activity of antimicrobials. Practical reviews of formulations are available (124; see also 454). Although generally not a problem with well-characterized antiinfective agents, the solubility of novel agents may dictate the routes of administration and the *in vivo* pharmacologic activity of an agent. Generally, the substance should be prepared so that it is in the most soluble form possible. However, specialized delivery systems such as liposomes, depot formulations, or formulations for topical administration may not require highly soluble substances. The choice of formulation ultimately affects the bioavailability and PK attributes of any particular substance, and this should be carefully considered when making comparisons of different chemical classes. In particular, formulations can dramatically affect the oral absorption of compounds and also tissue distribution. Note, however, that formulation effects can differ between species (389), and subtle differences can occur between animal strains (474). Some formulations can also reduce the toxicity of compounds (e.g., cyclodextrin [60]).

When considering oral administration of substances, it is important to recognize that the degree of uptake of antibiotics from the gastrointestinal tract varies between species. For example, *in vitro* tests using intestinal brush-border vesicles to study the kinetics and inhibition of cephalosporin uptake have indicated that the characteristics of transport of β-lactams by brush-border membranes are similar for rat and human tissues but that rabbit tissues possess distinct properties (556). The plasma PKs of amoxicillin are nonlinear in both humans and rats, but rats have lower oral bioavailability (566,567). These studies showed that mathematical modeling could result in predictions of human PKs of amoxicillin in humans from rat plasma profiles (566,567) and also showed that precipitation of a portion of the total orally administered dose in rats may occur in proximal gastrointestinal areas, complicating prediction of human oral bioavailability from data obtained from rats. Furthermore, the lower amoxicillin bioavailability in rats is in part owing to degradation within the intestine (98).

In general, however, use of formulations acceptable for use in humans is recommended whenever possible. When used parenterally, some formulations may provide more of a depot of active substance rather than resulting in immediate high blood levels of the antimicrobial. When comparing a few antimicrobials, the best strategy is to use the best formulation for each compound in order to ensure maximal bioavailability. However, this approach may not be useful for large-scale screening. In this case, a standard formulation optimized for the class of substances to be compared should be used; however, one must accept that some substances may fail due to poor formulation and will be considered poorly active *in vivo*. Adequate formulation of novel antimicrobials is often neglected during *in vivo* evaluations, and following are suggestions that should be considered prior to performing animal experiments. Aqueous solvents are preferred, and poorly soluble substances can be formed into fine suspensions by sonication. At least in initial evaluations, a fine precipitate, if kept in even suspension, can be well tolerated, particularly with oral application. Note, however, that particulate material, especially when administered parenterally, has altered PKs and bioavailability compared with soluble compounds, and this may complicate the interpretation of the findings. Suspensions intended for intravenous application need to consist of nanoparticles (less than 100 nm in diameter), and because this requires specialized technology, suspensions made by sonication should generally not be administered intravenously. Poorly soluble compounds can be prepared using a variety of mixed solvent systems. In these cases, the substance is first dissolved in an organic solvent and then carefully diluted in an aqueous solvent system. For example, a widely suitable method for preparing compounds is to dissolve the substance in *N*-methylpyrrolidine (NMP) and add PEG300 to a final 90% v/v. This procedure can use ethanol (10% v/v) or benzyl alcohol (6% v/v). Mixed solvents may additionally contain tetraglycol (polyethylene glycol monotetrahydrofurfuryl ether), polyethylene glycol 400, or propylene glycol (50% w/v, maximum final concentration). Substances can be dissolved in these solutions (sometimes adding Tween 80 initially) and then diluted in aqueous solutions (e.g., dissolution in PEG300 and then dilution with 0.9% saline to a final 30% PEG30). In all cases, the aqueous solvent should not contain high concentrations of salts, and often physiologic saline is the best cosolvent. Specialized formulations in cyclodextrins, chemically modified celluloses, Gelucire, liposomes, and so on, have been described previously (454).

Stability of Dissolved or Formulated Compounds

Although generally not a problem if compounds are prepared immediately before use, the stability of the compound in solution may become a problem when continuous dosing or prolonged fractional dosing is proposed as an administration technique. Although variations in the biologic activity (MIC/MBC) of the substance when it is stored for varying lengths of time may indicate severe stability problems, chemical assay of the substance (normally by high-performance liquid chromatography) is perhaps best, given the crude activity estimates achievable by *in vitro* activity assessments. Determination of biologic activity may not be appropriate for some formulations (e.g., Gelucire), because this would require rescue of the compound from fine suspensions, which may be incomplete.

ADMINISTRATION OF SUBSTANCES TO ANIMALS

Administration of infectious agents, antimicrobial compounds, or other substances to animals is the central technique in experimental chemotherapy. Excellent introductions to these procedures are available (39,585). Substances are routinely administered subcutaneously (s.c.), intraperitoneally (i.p.), intramuscularly (i.m.), intravenously (i.v.), orally (p.o.), or topically (e.g., on the skin or in a wound). More specialized methods include intranasal, intratracheal, and intragastric, administration and injection directly into the cerebrospinal fluid (CSF) or into the vitreous humor of the eye.

ANESTHESIA AND ANALGESIA

This subject has been thoroughly covered previously (57,202). Anesthetics and analgesics can be of variable duration of action, and care should be taken to provide a suitable period of anesthesia (neither too long nor too short). Postoperative pain relief should be administered, with compensation made in planning the experiment to allow a degree of "washout" of the substance prior to initiation of the experiment, because analgesics may alter normal host responses to infection or provide a source of unwanted drug interaction. However, in certain cases (e.g., models of infection associated with surgery), the use of analgesics may serve to make the models better reflect the clinical situation.

Certain anesthetics may not be applicable to all types of surgical interventions involved in experimental infections, and this should be considered and experimentally tested prior to widespread application. For example, agents that strongly depress respiratory rates (e.g., pentobarbital) are not suitable for pulmonary infection models involving tracheal exposure, and another anesthetic should be used. Furthermore, due consideration should be given to the stress placed on an animal due to anesthesia (long-term depression of normal body function and disorientation of the animal during recovery) versus the stress placed on the animal by not using anesthetics. For example, most routes of compound administration do not require anesthetics, and their use may place additional stress on the animal.

PHARMACOKINETIC PARAMETERS OF ANTIBIOTICS IN ANIMAL MODELS OF INFECTIOUS DISEASE

The MIC (or MBC) provides a good measure of the *in vitro* potency of an antimicrobial. However, PK (as it relates to PD) has long been recognized as the key factor determining the *in vivo* efficacy of antibiotics (10,126,128,129,140,165,211,212,520). *In vivo* models can detail the relationship between antimicrobial concentrations at the site of infection and the drug activity over time (551, but see 437 and 631). A variety of animal models have been used to determine the impact of drug concentration on the rate and extent of antibiotic killing. In addition, these models have been utilized to measure organism growth following drug exposure or postantibiotic effects. The PKs (elimination of antimicrobials from the body) and PDs (antimicrobial action of drugs) of antimicrobial agents have been shown to dramatically affect predictions of *in vivo* efficacy. Modeling of the relationship between drug concentration and efficacy can allow one to determine which PK/PD parameter best correlates with outcome. General background information on PK/PD can be found in several sources (e.g., 10,70,126,128,129,164,211,212,433, 520), and particular issues concerning antimicrobials have been reviewed (41,52,126,128,129,140,327,327a, 509).

Pharmacokinetic Experiments

General Considerations

Analytical Method

The analytical method must be reliably established, balancing sensitivity of detection and robustness of the method. HPLC and mass spectrometric methods have generally surpassed bioassays, but the detection methods that measure the chemical do not indicate biological activity. Control experiments should ideally be performed to ensure that the sample matrices (blood, plasma, or serum or solid tissues) do not interfere with the analyses and that an appropriate extraction method is available and proven. If needed, experiments can be done to ensure stability of the molecule in biological tissues (e.g., loss of esters due to the high-level of serum esterases in mice). Hydrolysis of esters can be prevented by adding eserine to the sample immediately after sample removal from the body (e.g., buffer consisting of 137 mmol/L NaCl, 2.7 mmol/L KCl, and 10 mmol/L phosphate buffer, pH 7.4, containing 2 mmol/L eserine [physostigmine hemisulfate, Sigma product no. P4417]).

Experimental Design

The experimental design should balance the potential use of large numbers of animals with the logistics of completing the experiment. The frequency and number of samples influence the accuracy of the determination of the PK parameters. Given the limitations of the number of samples that can be taken from one animal, it may be necessary to design an experiment in which not all animals are sampled at all time points. Pilot studies are useful to identify optimal sampling approaches, especially if no previous information on the PKs of the compound of interest are available. This should ensure that the number of data points are sufficient for the critical phases of the plasma concentration curve such as the maximal concentration (C_{max}) and the terminal ($t_{1/2}$).

Food can influence the PKs of orally administered compounds, and it must be decided whether the animals should be fasted or not. Clearly, if the intention is to use the PKs to aid in the planning and interpretation of efficacy experiments, then the PK experiments will be done in animals held under the same conditions as those employed in the efficacy experiments. Generally, in nonfasted rodents the PK results vary more than in fasted animals if the oral bioavailability of the test compound is markedly affected by food intake. Some compounds possess intrinsic variability in the extent of absorption, necessitating larger group sizes.

Organ Tissue Sampling

In addition to bloodstream drug levels, tissue concentrations in target organs (and possibly those thought to be target organs for toxicity) should be measured. Correlation of plasma and tissue concentrations with efficacy (e.g., in terms of reduction of tissue bacterial counts) represents the main component of PK/PD relationships. Compounds that are quickly and extensively distributed may still be effective but have relatively low concentrations in the circulation and therefore would limit the usefulness of plasma levels for obtaining PK/PD relationships, the prime example of this being azithromycin (488). Arguably, apart from cases of bacteremia or infections due to intracellular pathogens, the tissue fluid levels of antibiotics are what determine antibiotic efficacy (33,48,89). However, there is still much debate about the relative merits of measuring concentrations in organs or tissue fluid as opposed to the concentration in the circulation (33,89). Whether the concentration in the tissue fluid can be predicted by that in the plasma or serum probably needs to be determined for each compound, although it is probable that at equilibrium the concentrations of unbound drug in plasma and tissue fluids are approximately equal (89). Blood contamination of the organ is inevitable and will lead to an overestimate (especially soon after compound administration, where blood levels may be extremely high) unless a correction is made for the blood content of the organ (e.g., spectrophotometric determination of heme or hemoglobin content [55,494,531]). However, in those circumstances in which the drug concentration in the organ equals or is higher than that in the circulation, the content of the organ *per se* must be higher than the concentration in the circulation, indicating uptake into the organ from the circulation.

It is important to note that the coadministration of any compound along with the test compound (e.g., immunosuppressive agents, analgesics, or even other antibiotics) can affect the PKs of the study compound (e.g., induction of high levels of specific cytochrome p450 family members). This possibility should be evaluated in control experiments.

PK Parameters

Several specialized references on PKs exist (e.g., 105 and 507). There are five key parameters: elimination half-life ($t_{1/2}$), apparent volume of distribution (V), total plasma clearance (C_L), absolute bioavailability (BAV) (relative bioavailability can also be useful), and free fraction of drug. With the exception of free fraction of drug, these parameters can be calculated from data on plasma drug concentrations. Separate parameter estimation for tissues should also be performed, and it can be dramatically different from the estimate for plasma. Such data can be used as "factors" to estimate drug tissue levels in humans based on bloodstream sampling. Commercially available computer programs facilitate such calculations from raw data.

Free Fraction of Drug

Protein constituents of the bloodstream and tissues can have a high capacity to bind drugs. Generally drugs are able to display pharmacological activity, or to be metabolized or excreted, only when free in the plasma (i.e., unbound to blood constituents such as serum albumin). It is therefore important to know the size of the free fraction of drug. Usually determination of plasma concentrations is designed to measure the total drug in the circulation, bound and unbound. The relative amounts of proteins in the circulation and therefore the degree of protein binding can change under certain disease states (640); for example, α-acidic glycoprotein, an acute phase protein, can show high selectivity, avidity, and affinity for binding drugs. Simultaneous administration of drugs with similar protein-binding characteristics can cause changes in the unbound fraction (drug-drug interaction).

Factors Affecting the Pharmacokinetics of Antibiotics in Animals

Effect of Animal Species on Antibiotic Pharmacokinetics

As mentioned previously, the PK parameters for a given compound differ between animal species. For example, rifampicin displays a $t_{1/2}$ of 5.18 hours in mice and 4.72 hours in rats following i.v. administration, but the $t_{1/2}$ in rats is increased to 9.31 hours when the same dose is administered orally, though mice display a more constant $t_{1/2}$ (5.26 hours) (82). Moxifloxacin PK profiles differ between mice and rats (T_{max} values 0.25 and 0.08 hours, C_{max} values of 0.137 and 0.312 mg/L, $t_{1/2}$ values of 1.3 and 1.3 hours, and AUC values of 0.184 and 0.305 mg × h/L, respectively) following administration of 9.2 mg/kg p.o. (535). Following a 200-mg/kg p.o. administration, rats show similar C_{max} values for azithromycin and erythromycin (1.93 and 1.87 mg/L, respectively) but different $t_{1/2}$ values (1.2 and 0.65 hours) and AUC values (41.6 and 29.1 mg × h/L). Administration of 80 mg/kg, p.o. to rabbits produced, for azithromycin and erythromycin, respectively, C_{max} values of 0.69 and 0.12 mg/L, $t_{1/2}$ values of 0.26 and 0.71 hours, and AUC values of 20 and 4 mg × h/L (143). The strain of animal can also affect the PKs of a particular compound. In contrast to BALB/c mice, during multiple administrations of itraconozole, DBA/2 mice display serum levels that are higher and more consistent over time. BALB/c mice initially have lower azole levels than DBA/2 mice but later appear to accumulate azole (365).

Rats display dose-dependent PKs when administered mezlocillin (201,299) i.v. at 20 or 200 mg/kg ($t_{1/2}$ values of 9 and 15 min, AUC values of 431 and 800 mg × m/L, and CL values of 50 and 26 mL/min per kg, respectively [299]). However, they also display concentration-dependent protein binding (20% to 40% bound) that is saturable.

Effect of Infection on Antibiotic Pharmacokinetics

The infection process can have a dramatic effect on the PKs of antibiotics. Perhaps the best example is meningitis, where bacterial-induced blood-brain barrier damage produces a dramatic change in the CSF levels of antibiotics. In rabbits with *Haemophilus influenzae* meningitis, delay in the administration of ceftriaxone results in altered CSF penetration: when determining AUC_{0-12h}, initiating treatment at 6 hours postinfection (mild inflammation) produces a $AUC_{csf}AUC_{plasma}$ of 0.14 ± 0.04 mg×h/L, whereas antibiotic administration at 12 hours postinfection produced higher CSF penetration (AUC_{csf}: AUC_{plasma} = 5.1 ± 1.2) (A. L. Phinney and T. O'Reilly, unpublished).

In a rat model of multiorgan dysfunction, both cefepime and, to a greater extent, amikacin show altered PKs; clearance is slightly reduced for cefepime (7.2 mL/min × kg, normal; 6.7 mL/min × kg, multiorgan dysfunctional) and more pronounced for amikacin (8.7 mL/min × kg, normal; 5.3 mL/min × kg, multiorgan dysfunctional), producing increased $t_{1/2}$ and AUC values (cefepime, $t_{1/2}$ = 0.7 and 0.9 hours, AUC = 116 and 123 mg × h/L, for normal and multiorgan dysfunctional, respectively; amikacin, $t_{1/2}$ = 0.9 and 1.2 hours, AUC = 35 and 57 mg × h/L, for normal and multiorgan dysfunctional, respectively) (400). Rabbits septicemic with *S. pneumoniae* demonstrate altered moxalactam and cefotaxime PKs. Administration of 30 mg/kg i.v. to normal and septicemic rabbits produced the following PK parameters: moxalactam, C_{max} 19 and 13 mg/kg, $t_{1/2}$ = 1.73 and 2.1 hours, AUC_{0-8} = 78 and 65 mg × h/L, for uninfected and septicemic rabbits, respectively; cefotaxime, C_{max} = 19 and 13 mg/kg, $t_{1/2}$ = 1.73 and 2.1 hours, AUC_{0-8} = 78 and 65 mg × h/L, for uninfected and septicemic rabbits, respectively (228).

Rats with endotoxemia show altered clearance of vancomycin and higher kidney levels of vancomycin (in the cortex and medulla but apparently not in the papilla) (432). Endotoxemia reduces gentamicin clearance, and in certain regimens hydrocortisone increases renal levels of gentamicin while increasing clearance (49,50; but see reference 44 for a contrasting view). Endotoxin also exacerbates age-related differences in gentamicin PKs in rats (558). Additionally, it is expected that pyelonephritis would affect drug PKs. In rats with enterococcal pyelonephritis, a single administration of gentamicin (10 mg/kg i.p. 4 days postinfection) produced a serum C_{max} of 11.6 μg/mL (uninfected, 9.7 μg/mL) and urine gentamicin excretion of 91% (infected) and 88% (uninfected). Repeated treatments (0 or 10 mg/kg i.p. twice per day for 7 days) produced a serum C_{max} of 20.6 μg/mL (uninfected, 13 μg/mL) and urine gentamicin excretion of 35% (infected) and 70% (uninfected). Despite kidney infection, renal function remained normal, as indicted by serum creatinine and blood urea nitrogen. Taken together, these data indicate *E. faecalis* pyelonephritis disturbs the renal handling of gentamicin (24).

Effect of Fever on Antibiotic Pharmacokinetics

Fever impacts the PK of antibiotics, though very few systems have been studied in detail (368). Fever can alter drug uptake from the gastrointestinal tract, and protein binding is generally reduced at higher temperatures, thus enhancing distribution of the compound into the peripheral tissues and possibly hastening metabolism (514). Clinically, fever alters cefazolin PKs to increase C_{max}, AUC, and C_{ss} values and tissue distribution and to reduce

C_L (47). Fever associated with acute infection increases V_{ss} and renal clearance of ceftazidime (358,359). Fever reduced serum drug levels in dogs and humans following i.v. administration of gentamicin (473). But the influence of fever on antibiotic PK has not been well studied in experimental models. Amoxicillin demonstrated a lower C_L and higher AUC in febrile dogs than in endotoxin-untreated animals (385). Presumably, in cases where infection and/or endotoxemia altered PKs, fever would be a component in the alteration of antibiotic PKs but was not dissociated from the other physiological effects of endotoxin.

Effect of Animal Age on Antibiotic Pharmacokinetics

Age can have a profound effect on the PK profiles of antibiotics in animals (and humans). Care needs to be taken in extrapolating from the dosages used and results obtained in animals of one age to those of animals of different ages. For example, the plasma PKs of five β-lactams are markedly different in neonatal (1-week-old) and adult (8- to 10-week-old) rats (417). In addition to differences in plasma elimination rates and AUCs following intravenous administration and differences in maximal concentrations, times to maximal concentrations, and AUCs following oral administration, differences in volume of distribution, total body clearance, and bioavailability occur among rats of different ages. Generally, but not uniformly, neonatal rats tend to absorb β-lactams better than adults following oral administration, and the clearance of these drugs is reduced. These differences in oral bioavailability of β-lactam antibiotics are apparently related to more generalized age-dependent gastrointestinal changes (230).

Clear changes in the PKs of antibiotics often occur in the elderly (29,230,334,358,359,521). General physiologic changes associated with aging affect antibiotic absorption, distribution, metabolism, and excretion. As a normal consequence of aging, mice can manifest structural changes in the gastric structure (decreases in the relative volumes of parietal and chief cell components, increases in other components in the lamina propria, but with no change in the relative volume of the mucous cell compartment) beginning about 18 months of age (319). Perhaps the major single factor is the decline in renal function that affects excretion of antibiotics by this route. Despite this, there is apparently little recent research on antibiotic PKs in aged experimental animals. Tanira et al. (558) showed that, compared with adult male Wistar rats (2–3 months), old rats (22–24 months) demonstrate increased bloodstream AUC, prolonged $t_{1/2}$, and increased clearance of gentamicin. Furthermore, endotoxin treatment of adult and old rats also increased bloodstream AUC, prolonged $t_{1/2}$, and increased clearance, with the endotoxin effect being particularly prominent with old rats (319). Young (2- to 3-month) and old (19- to 22-month) Swiss Webster mice bearing experimental *Bacteriodes* abscesses show similar serum but different tissue PKs when treated with trovafloxacin (560). Old mice had a higher C_{max} in the liver, lungs, spleen, and intestine and a higher AUC in the liver, lungs, and spleen than did young mice following a 40-mg/kg i.p. administration of trovafloxacin; the values in serum and abscesses were similar in both ages (560).

Effects of Various Factors on Antibiotic Pharmacokinetics

Gender can also affect PK profiles. For example, following i.v. administration of a unilamellar liposomal preparation of amphotericin B (AmBisome, 20 mg/kg daily for 30 days), the mean plasma amphotericin B levels were 380 μg/mL for female rats and 500 μg/mL for males, the $t_{1/2}$ was 8.7 and 11.2 hours, and clearance was 10.2 and 9.4 mL/h/kg for females and males, respectively (67). Similarly, in contrast to free drug, liposomal ampicillin demonstrated gender differences in PK profiles (466). Female rats demonstrated smaller V_{ss} and higher C_L than male rats; the $t_{1/2}$ values were similar between genders. Furthermore, female rats demonstrated greater tissue distribution of liposomal ampicillin, especially in the spleen and lung (466). G-CSF has been reported to change the PK properties of gentamicin, but not vancomycin, in nude mice (452). Caution should be taken when administering multiple compounds to mice, particularly with oral administration, to avoid drug-drug interactions. For example, rifampicin uptake following oral administration to mice is impaired by ethambutol, pyrazinamide, and in particular the combination of ethambutol, pyrazinamide, and isoniazid (155).

The timing of drug administration can also affect antibiotic PKs. In a study treating rats adjusted to a 12-hours-on, 12-hours-off light cycle (0700 to 1900 on) with a single i.p. administration of 100 mg/kg ceftriaxone at 0400, 1000, 1600, or 2200, the serum PK was determined and analyzed for the presence of a circadian rhythm (490). The C_L rate was strongly affected, being faster during the dark (activity) phase. This suggests that, depending on bacterial sensitivity, the key PK/PD parameter T > MIC (the time serum levels remain above the MIC) may not be reached during the dark part of the cycle. Rebuelto et al. (490) present a set of references concerning circadian rhythms possessed by other antibiotics.

PHARMACOKINETICS OF ANTIBIOTICS: RELATIONSHIP OF EXPERIMENTAL ANIMALS AND HUMANS

The MIC (or MBC) provides a good measure of the *in vitro* potency of an antimicrobial, but it is a static determination that does not reflect the time-influenced processes occurring *in vivo*. However, *in vivo* models can detail the relationship between antimicrobial concentrations at the site of infection and the drug activity over time. A variety of animal models have been used to determine the impact of drug concentration on the rate and extent of antibiotic killing. In addition, these models have been utilized to measure organism growth following drug exposure or postantibiotic effects. Consideration of the PKs (elimination of antimicrobials from the body) and PDs (antimicrobial action of drugs *in vivo*) of antimicrobial agents has been shown to dramatically affect predictions of *in vivo* efficacy. Modeling of the relationship between drug concentration and efficacy can allow one to determine which PK/PD parameter best correlates with outcome. An excellent general discussion of the PKs/PDs of antiinfective therapy can be found in the review by Drusano (164). As guides to performing PK/PD studies, these papers are recommended: 517 (pneumonia in mice) and 10,197,434, and 618 (the thigh infection model in mice). Other key works include a study comparing penicillin PKs/PDs in four different models (182) and of comparison of the PKs/PDs of five fluoroquinolones in neutropenic mice (183).

Perhaps the greatest limitation in the use of animal models for studying chemotherapy—and until recently perhaps the single most ignored parameter—involves differences in the PK parameters of antibiotics between humans and animals. The predominant differences lie in the faster elimination of drugs by small animals, compared with humans (72,146,179,413,414; but see reference 355 for limitations of this approach). Although the dosage of an antimicrobial agent can often be adjusted to mimic the peak serum levels found in humans (e.g., Lister and Sanders [357] administered 40 and 80 mg/kg ampicillin to mice to simulate the peak serum levels obtained with 1.5- and 3-g dosages, respectively, administered to humans), compensating for the faster elimination of most drugs by animals is indeed more difficult. Consideration of these PK differences has led some researchers to adapt antimicrobial dosing to override faster elimination of compounds by animals in order to obtain PKs more similar to the PK expressed by humans. Repeated fractional dosing, renal impairment, and continuous infusion have all been used to mimic in small animals the PK of antimicrobial agents in humans. However, the use of such protocols is limited in experimental evaluations of antibiotics, as they presuppose knowledge of the PK profiles of antibiotics in humans, knowledge that necessarily is obtained late in the development of a new substance. They may retain value in the evaluation of new compounds with unknown human PK profiles when the agents are administered in regimens similar to regimens of standard compounds with established human PK profiles.

Pharmacodynamics examines the relationship between an antimicrobial and the target pathogen over time, determining the effects of variations in drug concentrations on organism killing and growth dynamics. From such determinations, PK/PD indices, such as the area under the serum concentration time curve (AUC) over the minimum inhibitory concentration (MIC) ratio (AUC/MIC), the peak serum level/MIC ratio (peak/MIC), or the time that serum levels remain above the MIC (T > MIC), have been shown to be the primary determinants of *in vivo* efficacy. Such determinations yield some apparently class-specific characteristics: for β-lactams, macrolides, and oxazolidinones, agents for which time-dependent killing and minimally or moderately prolonged postantibiotic effects are inherent properties, T > MIC is the most useful predictor of efficacy; for aminoglycosides, fluoroquinolones, and ketolides, agents with concentration-dependent killing and prolonged postantibiotic effects, the AUC/MIC and C_{max}/MIC parameters appear to be the best predictors. The AUC/MIC ratio can also be used to predict the efficacy of antibiotics with time-dependent killing and prolonged effects, such as azithromycin, the tetracyclines, and the streptogramins (10,11,126,128,164,211,212,433,520).

However, appropriate PD analyses most often account for these differences and allow comparison of data among various *in vivo* models. By correcting for interspecies PK differences, these studies can determine the magnitude of the PK/PD parameter necessary for efficacy across animal species, including humans. This concept should not be surprising, as the target for these drugs is in the pathogen and not in the animal species. Despite the variety of techniques and animal models, there is marked consistency in the PK/PD data in animals. For example, mouse- and rat-dosing studies have demonstrated that amoxicillin treatment regimens achieve serum levels above the MIC for approximately 50% of the dosing interval. Clinical trials using amoxicillin in children with acute otitis media find a similar relationship between efficacy and a 50% time above MIC PK/PD target.

There are several dosing study designs that allow researchers to address many of these PD issues. Dose fractionation studies can be used to determine which PK/PD parameter is most predictive of therapeutic outcome. Dosing regimens that vary the PK/PD parameter magnitude and study against organisms with widely varying *in vitro* susceptibilities can help in identifying a PK/PD target for effect therapy.

Dose Fractionation

Simulation of human serum PKs can be obtained by frequent administration of subsequently smaller doses of drug, thus overriding the faster kinetics of antimicrobial elimination. Gerber et al. (230,231,233) used fractionated dosing protocols to compare simulated human PKs with murine PKs on the clearance of *P. aeruginosa* from infected thighs of normal and granulocytopenic mice. Fractionated dosing prolonged the presence of gentamicin, netilmicin, ticarcillin, and ceftriaxone and was compared to bolus injections that resulted in quantitatively similar AUCs, but of different shapes and with different peak serum levels. Fractionated dosing of β-lactams was considered superior to bolus dosing, suggesting that T > MIC is a critical determinant for this class of compounds. Generally, bolus dosing of aminoglycosides was superior to fractionated dosing, suggesting that peak drug level was the critical determinant for *in vivo* activity (231). Similar experiments were performed using the murine peritonitis model (*P. aeruginosa* suspended in hog gastric mucin with ticarcillin, ceftazidime, and netilmicin) in nonneutropenic hosts (232), confirming the superiority of human-adapted PKs, but in this case the fractional dosing of netilmicin was superior to bolus dosing. Similar experiments were performed using *P. aeruginosa* in a thigh infection in neutropenic mice, with fractional dosing of imipenem designed to mimic serum PKs in humans following intravenous or intramuscular bolus dosing (204). Fractionated dosing provided serum levels over a 6-hour period that inhibited breakthrough bacterial growth and was superior to bolus dosing (murine PKs), despite the fact that bolus doses resulted in peak serum concentrations in excess of 50 times the MIC. The AUCs of imipenem resulting from either administration protocol were similar for the same total dose. Simulation of imipenem levels found after a single intramuscular dose in humans (a fractionated 70 mg/kg dose in mice) was also superior to two 70 mg/kg doses administered to mice simulating imipenem levels following intravenous administration to humans.

Therefore, despite similarities of the AUC between bolus dosing (murine PKs) and fractionated dosing (human PKs), the shape of the curve appeared to have a profound effect on the *in vivo* efficacy of antimicrobial agents, in particular β-lactams. This effect, termed the effect of the shape of the AUC (ESAUC), indicates that careful attention needs to be paid to the PK profile of antimicrobials in animals before extrapolation of results can be made to humans (231).

Additional fractionated dosing studies include those by Hishikawa et al. (274) and Hatano et al. (267).

Renal Impairment

Impairment of kidney function can result in slower elimination of antimicrobials if this is the major clearance organ (e.g., cephalexin [375]). At least in mice, this can be accomplished by the subcutaneous injection of 10 mg/kg uranyl nitrate (234). This technique was utilized by Craig et al. (130) during a study of the effect of total daily dose and dosing frequency on the efficacy of amikacin in mouse models of thigh and lung infections in neutropenic hosts. Uranyl nitrate administration 3 days prior to the injection of the antimicrobial substance increased the half-life, peak level/dose, and AUC/dose of amikacin in neutropenic female ICR mice, compared with normal mice (130). The potency of amikacin (as estimated by PD_{50} value, the total daily dose required to reduce log CFU/g tissue) was 10-fold greater in renally impaired mice, although the maximal amikacin-induced reduction in bacterial load (for any total dose or frequency) was not different. Furthermore, once-daily dosing in mice mimicking human amikacin PKs was more effective than dosing at shorter intervals, which was not the case in renally sufficient mice. The clearance of cephalexin in renally impaired rats has been studied (375). In this model, experimental renal failure in rats was induced by cisplatin (one dose of 5 mg/kg, intraperitoneally, to induce proximal tubular necrosis), 2-bromoethylamine hydrobromide (one dose of 75 mg/kg intravenously to induce papillary necrosis), sodium aurothiomalate (six weekly injections of 0.05 mg/kg intravenously to induce glomerulonephritis), or antirabbit antibodies to rat glomerular basement membrane (single intravenous dose to induce glomerulonephritis).

Continuous Dosing to Achieve Steady-State Antimicrobial Levels

Continuous dosing of antibiotics has been used in several investigations to bypass the effects of rapid antimicrobial clearance by small animals. In such cases, the goal is not to mimic the PK patterns displayed by compounds in humans but rather to maintain a steady-state level of antibiotic in the bloodstream by constant infusion.

Roosendaal et al. (504,505) used this approach to compare the efficacy of intermittently or continuously administered ceftazidime, gentamicin, or ciprofloxacin in leukopenic rats infected endobronchially with an antibiotic-susceptible *Klebsiella pneumoniae* strain. Rather than constant intravenous infusion, those authors exploited a subcutaneous infusion system previously described (563). Continuous infusion resulted in constant serum antibiotic levels as early as 5 hours after the beginning of the infusion, and peak serum levels occurred about 15 minutes after intramuscular injection (505). With the continuous dosing, the serum levels for all compounds were below the MIC at the PD_{50} dose, whereas the intermittent administration mode provided supra-MIC levels, at least initially. Despite the subinhibitory serum concentrations, continuous dosing of ceftazidime was judged more effective than intermittent dosing, whereas the converse was true for gentamicin. Ciprofloxacin was slightly more efficacious when administered intermittently. *In vitro* experiments demonstrated that the bactericidal effect of ceftazidime was slow and independent of concentration but the effect of gentamicin or ciprofloxacin was dose-dependent and rapid. Single-dose (intravenous) studies resulting in clearly supra-MIC serum antibiotic levels confirmed this to be the case also in the killing of *K. pneumoniae* within the lung (505). An earlier study compared continuous versus intermittent (every 6 hours) ceftazidime dosing in treating *K. pneumoniae* pulmonary infection in normal and leukopenic rats (504). There was little difference in the two administration modes in normal rats (PD_{50} of 0.35 and 0.36 mg/kg/day, respectively). However, the PD_{50} value (24.4 mg/kg/day) for intermittent dosing administered to leukopenic rats was about 70 times the PD_{50} in normal rats, but the PD_{50} (1.5 mg/kg/day) for continuous dosing was only about 4 times that in normal rats.

Constant infusion of ampicillin was compared to intermittent dosing in the outcome of endocarditis due to a susceptible strain of *E. faecalis* (562). Continuous administration of ampicillin was at 450 or 4500 mg/kg/day, and intermittent dosing utilized intramuscular injections every 8 hours to deliver 450 mg/kg/day. Treatment began 24 hours after infection and continued for 5 days. Despite high peak serum and cardiac vegetation ampicillin levels, continuous dosing of ampicillin was considered to be superior in terms of promotion of survival of the animals, sterility of blood in survivors, reduction of bacterial load in cardiac vegetations, and number of rats with sterile vegetations. Interestingly, *in vitro* kill-curve tests determined that the *E. faecalis* strain used was more rapidly killed by higher ampicillin concentrations. Coadministration of probenecid (50 mg/kg/day), which increased the serum ampicillin half-life to 1 hour, failed to improve the outcome of intermittent administration (562).

Continuous Dosing to Achieve Steady-State Antimicrobial Levels Using Osmotic Pumps

Osmotic pumps are devices that are designed to provide a constant release of drug over a period of several days. However, osmotic pumps have apparently not been extensively used in experimental treatment of infection. Their advantage lies in their ability to maintain a constant level of antibiotic, thus at least in part overriding differences in elimination between species, and when used in a dose-response curve, they allow determination of the tissue level needed for antibacterial effects. Their disadvantages include the need of the compound to be prepared in a fully soluble, highly concentrated solution; the limited dosing time; and the need for a surgical implant. Before using such devices *in vivo*, it is essential to confirm that the solvent system is compatible with the pump, that the compound is stable at 37°C for the entire administration period (normally 7 to 14 days), that the exit of the compound is constant over time, and that no precipitation of the compound occurs on the outside of the pump once in contact with biological fluids. By immersing a filled pump in a suitable isotonic buffer containing 5% to 50% fetal bovine serum and incubating this at 37°C, followed by periodic sampling, it is usually possible to detect compounds that are incompatible with such a drug delivery device.

Intermittent dosing (mouse PK) was compared to steady-state dosing for the treatment of infections resulting from the implantation of a contaminated suture into mice (429). Thirty minutes prior to infection, all mice received 60 mg/kg cefazolin intraperitoneally, and then *K. pneumoniae*–infected sutures (1 cm of 3–0 cotton) were implanted in the thighs of the animals; the *K. pneumoniae* strain used had a MIC of 8 μg/mL cefazolin. The mice were subsequently treated with 180 mg/kg/day cefazolin either by injection (intraperitoneally, every 8 hours) or by continuous infusion from a peritoneally implanted osmotic pump. Mice receiving intraperitoneal injections of antibiotic demonstrated peak serum cefazolin levels of 74.2 ± 11.9 μg/mL 1 minute after injection, which rapidly declined to nearly undetectable levels (3.9 ± 0.9 μg/mL at 4 hours; limit of detectability, 3 μg/mL). Thigh-muscle cefazolin levels were 7.4 ± 2.2 μg/mL at 1 minute and undetectable at 4 hours. Continuous infusion led to a sustained serum cefazolin level of 17.5 ± 5.1 μg/mL over 3 days without detectable cefazolin within the tissues. These different administration modes were associated with dramatically different outcomes. Ten-day survival rates were 81%, 20%, and 18% for continuous administration, intermittent administration, and saline-treated controls, respectively. Animals treated with intermittent cefazolin had more than log 2 CFU/mL blood on days 2 and 4 after infection, whereas bacteremia was not detected with continuous treatment. Significant reduction in the thigh *K. pneumoniae* occurred only with continuous treatment (4 days after infection: intermittent treatment, $6.9 \pm 2 \times 10^6$ CFU/g muscle; continuous treatment, $1.9 \pm 1.5 \times 10^3$ CFU/g muscle); *K. pneumoniae* regrew to high levels (log 6 CFU/g muscle) in the surviving animals of both groups. Therefore, despite not producing supra-MIC levels, continuous dosing of cefazolin by use of osmotic pumps resulted in a better outcome than achieved with cefazolin administered intermittently.

Other studies that have used osmotic pumps to continuously deliver antibiotics have evaluated the concentration of gentamicin in plasma, endolymph, and perilymph (2-day infusion [571] and 6-day infusion [570]) and in several tissues (569). Furthermore, by using osmotic pumps to establish steady-state serum drug levels, the serum concentrations of clindamycin and the pulmonary clearance of bacteria could be correlated (23).

Continuous Dosing to Mimic Human Pharmacokinetic Profiles

This subject has been thoroughly reviewed by Mizen (405). Continuous- or variable-rate infusion of antibiotics into animals has been used to obtain plasma antibiotic clearance similar to that found in humans administered bolus or drip infusions. Based on careful determination of temocillin PKs in both humans and rabbits, a continuous-rate infusion system was developed to deliver temocillin to rabbits with meningitis due to *K. pneumoniae* in such a manner that human plasma elimination rates following a 2-g dose were obtained (610). The femoral artery was cannulated to allow continuous infusion of antibiotic. Rabbits received first a bolus dose (82 mg/kg) to mimic the temocillin distribution phase and then an infusion of continuously diluted temocillin to mimic the β-elimination phase observed in humans. Phosphate-buffered saline was administered at a constant rate (equivalent to the human temocillin elimination rate corrected for the rate of temocillin elimination by rabbits) into a fixed-volume, stirred reservoir containing temocillin such that the concentration of temocillin infused into the animal was constantly declining. Rabbits receiving infusions were treated with a total of 758 mg/kg temocillin over 12 hours at 2.0 mL/hour. Compared to bolus dosing (82 mg/kg), infusion dosing resulted in a dramatically prolonged temocillin half-life and larger AUC values without altering the percent penetration into the CSF. Note that, after a 2-g dose to humans, the plasma half-life was 5.0 $\pm$ 0.2 hours and the AUC was 784.5 $\pm$ 47.1 μg $\times$ h/mL. However, considering the serum binding of temocillin (60% to 85% in human serum, depending on the temocillin concentration; 35% in rabbit serum, concentration independent), this mode of temocillin administration to rabbits would result in free temocillin concentrations similar to that observed after a 4-g dose to humans. Humanlike PKs resulted in a dramatically improved therapeutic outcome, in that *K. pneumoniae* was rapidly removed from the CSF (to less than log 2 CFU/mL within 6 hours) during infusion but remained essentially unaltered during bolus dosing. The authors did not evaluate the effect of the same total temocillin dose in bolus infusion (610).

This infusion method was adapted to rats in order to mimic the human plasma PKs of cefazolin, piperacillin, and the β-lactamase inhibitor BRL 42715 (609). Rats were infected intraperitoneally with either *E. coli* or *S. marcesens,* and treatment began 1 hour after infection; both microorganisms demonstrated susceptibility to cefazolin or piperacillin only in the presence of BRL 42715 (concentrations more than ~0.1 μg/mL). Simulation of human plasma PKs was obtained. The half-lives for BRL 42715, cefazolin, and piperacillin in humans were 0.6, 1.6, and 1.1 hours, respectively, considerably different from those in rats (0.1, 0.51, and 0.33 hours, respectively). Despite the plasma concentration of the β-lactamase inhibitor falling below the level predicted to be effective within 3 hours, coadministration of BRL 42715 with piperacillin (*E. coli* infection) or cefazolin (*S. marcesens* infection) dramatically improved efficacy in terms of survival and bacterial counts in blood and peritoneal fluid (609); these results indicate that β-lactamase inhibitors need not have plasma PKs identical to those of their partner antibiotics in order to have synergistic effects. Comparison of the effectiveness of human-simulated PKs and the efficacy of these combinations in bolus administration (rat PK) was not reported (609).

A similar approach was used to mimic the PK of 3- and 0.1-g doses of ticarcillin/clavulanic acid and a 2-g dose of ceftazidime administered to humans (405) in rabbits with meningitis due to *K. pneumoniae.* The infusion system was modified to include two pumps, one infusing a constant dose of agent for a short time (to produce a peak serum concentration similar to that seen in humans) and the other constantly infusing a continuously diluted solution of drug (to mimic the serum elimination PKs manifest in humans). This system was successful in overriding the more rapid elimination of ticarcillin, clavulanic acid, and ceftazidime by rabbits. Single doses of ticarcillin/clavulanic acid were able to reduce (by 99% at 4 hours) but not eliminate the drug combination–susceptible *K. pneumoniae* present in the CSF due to regrowth of the organisms after clavulanic acid levels fell below the MBC. Multiple dosing of ticarcillin/clavulanic acid (three doses every 4 hours) according to simulated human PKs resulted in higher AUCs in both plasma and CSF (without altering the CSF penetration) and correspondingly greater antibacterial efficacy (99.99% reduction of CFU/mL in the CSF). Two ceftazidime doses (every 8 hours) reduced the counts of the drug-susceptible microbe below the limit of detectability and sterilized the CSF in two of three rabbits at 12 hours. The efficacy of bolus doses of these drugs (rabbit PKs) was not reported (406).

A computer-controlled, variable-speed pump was used to mimic human serum concentrations of amoxicillin in a study to determine the effectiveness of amoxicillin prophylaxis in preventing streptococcal endocarditis (203). Sterile aortic vegetations were produced by placement of a polyethylene catheter through the right carotid artery across the aortic valve. Amoxicillin was administered by infusion through a Silastic catheter placed into the jugular vein and brought through the skin of the intercapsular region. Intravenous infection with *Streptococcus intermedius* or *Streptococcus sanguis* (1, 10, or 100 $\times$ the 90% inhibitory dose) occurred 1 hour after administration of 40 mg/kg amoxicillin (rat PKs) or amoxicillin dosage to mimic human PKs following a 3-g oral dose. At the time of bacterial challenge, the serum antibiotic levels were similar (bolus dose, 18 $\pm$ 0.3 μg/mL; infusion, 16 $\pm$ 5 μg/mL), but the durations of detectable amoxicillin levels were different (bolus, 4.5 hours; infusion, 9 hours). Simulation of human serum PKs was decidedly more effective than bolus dosing in the protection of rats from developing endocarditis (203). A similar procedure was used to deliver ceftriaxone to obtain humanlike PKs in rats with *S. sanguis* or *Streptococcus mitis* (180) or methicillin-resistant *Staphylococcus epidermidis* (181) endocarditis.

EVALUATION OF ANTIBIOTICS IN ANIMAL MODELS OF INFECTION

Use of animal models in the evaluation of antimicrobial compounds is considered when a clinical study involving humans is not possible because (a) the toxicity of the compound is unknown, (b) its antibacterial ability *in vivo* is unknown, (c) the type of infection under consideration is rarely encountered or impossible to encounter in humans, or (d) the effect parameters needed (e.g., bacterial counts in tissues or fluids) cannot easily be obtained in patients. Otherwise, a clinical study will be the optimal method for studying any drug for clinical use, since it automatically answers the question (which is always asked after an experimental animal study), can the results be extrapolated to the clinic? Animals are always used when new compounds have shown relevant antimicrobial activity *in vitro* and their *in vivo* effects are questioned. Furthermore, experimental animal infections are considered when other important issues need to be solved prior to clinical studies, such as the advantages or disadvantages of the compound in activity, its PK profile (i.e., its dosing advantage), the best mode of administration (i.e., oral or parenteral), and potential toxicity problems (diarrhea, nephrotoxicity, etc.). Given the ethical considerations and government legislation involved, the testing of novel compounds, or novel combinations of known compounds, requires comparative testing in animal experiments in order to indicate efficacy *in vivo*. As in the evaluation of antimicrobials from known classes (e.g., new cephalosporins), the questions include not just whether the agent will be active *in vivo* but how it will compare in spectrum and potency to other antibiotics. β-Lactamase inactivation seen *in vitro* might not occur *in vivo*. In many instances, very low MIC values *in vitro* are not reflected by the *in vivo* results. Thus, for new compounds or derivatives of known antibiotics, the *in vivo* test is also a tool for selecting the potentially best candidate from a number of active agents. The following discussion mostly concerns the evaluation of antibacterial substances in animal models, although examples of antifungal agents, cytokines, and antibiotics are presented; the evaluation of antiviral compounds is not covered. Furthermore, for purpose of simplicity and because they can be obtained elsewhere (632,633), details on the establishment of models have been reduced to a minimum.

General considerations for working safely with infectious agents have been summarized in Richmond and Quimby (497), and readers are encouraged to read this review prior to embarking on establishing animal models of infection in their laboratory.

Factors Influencing Antimicrobial Activity in the *In Vivo* Tests

A number of the factors can influence the activity of antimicrobial agents *in vivo* (e.g., see 214):

- Inoculum size and vehicle. If the inoculum is too small, an infection will not be established; if it is too large, overwhelming endotoxemia can occur.
- Virulence or pathogenicity of the infecting strain. Highly virulent strains may produce rapidly fatal disease, necessitating early treatment initiation.
- Generation time in vivo. Slow-growing bacteria *in vivo* are phenotypically very different from fast-growing bacteria *in vitro*. Similarly, biofilm growth *in vivo* is different from planktonic growth *in vitro*.
- Timing of treatment. A delay in treatment initiation often results in greater difficulty curing the infection.
- Method of antibiotic administration. The lack of oral uptake of a drug highly active *in vitro* may render it inactive *in vivo*.
- The PKs/PDs of the antibiotic. Generally, more rapidly eliminated drugs need to be administered more frequently.
- The development of resistance *in vivo*. Unique resistance patterns *in vivo* may render a drug highly active *in vitro* inactive *in vivo*.
- *In vivo* growth of an intracellular compartment that the drug cannot penetrate.
- Inactivation of the compound *in vivo*. The host metabolism may render a drug highly active *in vitro* inactive *in vivo*.

Inoculum size has a major influence on the *in vivo* activity of antibacterials. An increase of 1 log unit or even less in the challenge dose can render an antibacterial ineffective. In addition, virulence or pathogenicity is closely connected to the inoculum size, since high virulence to a particular animal species often leads to lower inocula being used in order not to induce an overwhelming infection. On the other hand, higher doses are still needed to achieve an effect against a highly virulent strain, compared with strains with lower virulence. For example, the heavily capsulated *Streptococcus pneumoniae* serotype 3 (penicillin MIC, 0.01 mg/L) has an LD_{50} of 10^2 CFU for intraperitoneal infection in CF1 mice, in comparison with 10^7 CFU for *S. pneumoniae* serotype 6B (penicillin MIC, 0.01 mg/L). Still, the ED_{50} for single-dose benzylpenicillin against serotype 3 is 180 mg/kg, in comparison with 0.8–2 mg/kg against serotype 6B strains (215,327a).

For *S. pyogenes*, increasing the *in vitro* starting inoculum (from log 3 to 7 CFU/mL) had no effect on the MIC of cefoxitin (0.5 μg/mL) and mezlocillin (0.05 μg/mL). In contrast, increasing the inoculum of *K. pneumoniae* from log 5 to log 8 CFU/mL had no effect on the MIC of cefoxitin (4 μg/mL) but dramatically altered the MIC of mezlocillin (4 μg/mL at log 5 or 6 CFU/mL, 32 μg/mL at log 7 CFU/mL, and >128 μg/mL at log 9 CFU/mL). Similarly with *in vivo* sensitivity: the ED_{50} of cefoxitin increases with the inoculum (10 × LD_{50}, 2 mg/kg ED_{50}; 1000 × LD_{50}, 190 mg/kg ED_{50}; 1,000,000 × LD_{50}, >1000 mg/kg ED_{50}). Similar results were found for mezlocillin

($10 \times LD_{50}$, 0.4 mg/kg ED_{50}; $1000 \times LD_{50}$, 130 mg/kg ED_{50}; $1{,}000{,}000 \times LD_{50}$, >1000 mg/kg ED_{50}). This effect was more intense with *K. pneumoniae* (cefoxitin: $10 \times LD_{50}$, 140 mg/kg ED_{50}; $100 \times LD_{50}$, 240 mg/kg ED_{50}; $1000 \times LD_{50}$, 400 mg/kg ED_{50}; mezlocillin: $10 \times LD_{50}$, 46 mg/kg ED_{50}; $100 \times LD_{50}$, 420 mg/kg ED_{50}; $1000 \times LD_{50}$, >3000 mg/kg ED_{50}) (631).

Preparation of the microorganism for inoculation in animal experiments can dramatically affect the results obtained, and this fact is often overlooked. Fundamentally, the microbe should be at maximal viability, and care should be taken to obtain suitable cultures for inoculum preparation. Whether the microbe should be taken from the *in vitro* culture in lag phase, log phase, or stationary phase has to our knowledge never been validated. The use of overnight broth cultures may be problematic for bacteria such as *S. pneumoniae* or *H. influenzae*, which undergo autolysis shortly after reaching the stationary phase (456). Agar plate cultures have the advantage that they can be directly studied to determine if any contamination has occurred and whether loss of potential capsule has occurred. Many investigators prefer to bring the microbe into the exponential growth phase in a broth culture prior to its use or inoculation. None has proven, however, that the bacteria will stay in this exponential phase after the procedures used (e.g., washing) to achieve the exact inoculum needed.

An increase in the virulence of certain microorganisms can be achieved in various ways. *In vitro* growth in specialized media can alter virulence. For example, growth of *Neisseria meningitidis* under conditions of low pH and low growth medium iron content increases the virulence of this organism 1200-fold, relative to bacteria grown in neutral-pH, iron-replete medium (74). Growth of uropathogenic *E. coli* in human urine increased siderophore production and renal pathogenicity in ascending pyelonephritis in mice (528). Furthermore, virulence-associated gene expression by *Enterococcus faecalis* is modulated during the growth phase and affected by the growth medium (529). Using the guinea-pig subcutaneous chamber model as a test system, iron-limited gonococci were found to be extremely virulent, whereas cystine-limited (iron-replete) gonococci did not survive in the chambers despite retention of pili. Loss of piliation also occurred during the shift from iron-limited to glucose-limited growth, but the bacteria remained virulent. No change in susceptibility to normal human serum killing occurred, and the lipo-oligosaccharide composition remained similar despite varied culture conditions. Some membrane proteins traditionally associated with iron limitation were produced by cystine- or glucose-limited bacteria (316a). Note, however, that iron restriction apparently does not affect all bacteria. The rate and extent of *in vitro* growth of *S. typimurium* are unaffected by the addition of deferoxamine, and treatment of mice with deferoxime prior to infectious challenge exacerbates *S. typhimurium* infection (110). Virulence can also be enhanced by serial passage in animals; for example, intraperitoneal inoculation with subsequent subculture from peritoneal wash, blood, or organs such as the liver or spleen and use of this growth either directly or after subculture will enhance the virulence of *S. pneumoniae, S. pyogenes,* or *H. influenzae*. In spite of great care taken to standardize the inoculum, one of the major problems encountered in animal experiments is the variation in the virulence and growth of organisms. This problem highlights the need for control groups for every new infection experiment considered rather than relying on historical controls.

Generation time (rate of bacterial cell division) is also a factor of major importance that differs between *in vivo* and *in vitro* test conditions. *In vivo*, the generation time seems to increase progressively during the course of infection and, depending on the site of infection, may last up to 20 hours. Little is known about nutrient limitations on bacterial growth in infected tissues, with the exception of iron, which has been found to limit bacterial growth in serum. It has been demonstrated that prolonged lag phase as well as prolonged generation time may adversely affect the clinical activity of antimicrobials (especially β-lactams) that are most effective against bacterial cells that are rapidly dividing (79,125,205,182). The nature of bacterial growth *in vivo* in tissues is not well studied. Good evidence is available indicating that bacteria grow as biofilms in many urinary tract infections (26,354), cases of otitis media (171a), catheter-related infections (302,303,511), and pulmonary infections (26,100,104,411). For a review, see Costerton et al. (121,122). Further, bacteria growing as biofilm have a dramatically different physiology and antibiotic sensitivity (205). A set of genes are specifically activated during the establishment of a biofilm, both *in vitro* and *in vivo* (583). However, not all bacterial growth *in vivo* occurs as biofilms (208). Multicolor fluorescence microscopy has been used to delineate the nature of *Salmonella enterica* in the livers of infected mice (530). The growth of *Salmonella* occurred by the formation of new foci of infection from initial ones as well as by the expansion of each focus. Each focus consisted of phagocytes containing low numbers of bacteria and of independently segregating bacterial populations. The net increase in bacteria paralleled the increase in the number of infected phagocytes in the tissues (530).

BASIC SCREENING TESTS

Mouse Protection Test

The animal models most frequently used in the evaluation of antibacterials may be categorized as basic screening, *ex vivo*, monoparametric, or discriminative (475,629). For the preliminary evaluation of new agents, the basic screening system is usually employed. The *ex vivo* and monoparametric models are used to measure specific variables (e.g., dosage schedule, serum binding, or penetration into extravascular spaces). The discriminative systems are employed to differentiate the new agents from related or unrelated active agents. Screening models involve simple one-step infections, simple techniques and schedules of treatment, short-duration experiments, reproducible courses of infection, simple evaluation (all-or-nothing models), economy of test drugs, and low costs. These requirements are best met by the mouse protection test, which is the most widely used *in vivo* screening model in antibacterial research. The mouse protection test is suitable for determining the efficacy and toxicity of new antibacterials, and it can indicate whether a drug is likely to be active orally or parenterally. The features and use of the mouse protection test have been previously reviewed (209,210,213).

Various mouse strains are the primary hosts used, for the following reasons: (a) good correlation between the clinical response to an antimicrobial agent and the agent's activity in mice; (b) the ease of obtaining large numbers; (c) the economy of the compound to be tested; (d) the relatively small cost per unit test; and (e) normal use of an outbred strain of mice, which provides a heterogenous population and allows for immunologic and other host factor variations (however, in special situations [e.g., *Mycobacterium* infection models], inbred, genetically defined strains may be required in order to provide a suitably susceptible host). It should be clearly recognized, though, that the mouse protection model represents an unnatural infection in which the host is usually subjected to an overwhelming challenge (134).

Correlation of *In Vitro* and *In Vivo* Results

This subject—the correlation of *in vitro* and *in vivo* activity—has a long history (190) and is critical for a medicinal chemistry program, given the costs of *in vivo* screening.

Many substances that are active *in vivo* are also active *in vitro*; however, the converse is not always true. Many antibacterials that are active *in vitro* either are inactive when tested against systemic infections *in vivo* or are only active in the more sensitive topical infections. Zak and Sande (631) reported a correlation of *in vitro* and *in vivo* activity in only 14.8% of 2000 compounds randomly screened for antimicrobial activity. Of the 2000 compounds, 45.3% were inactive *in vitro* and *in vivo*. Of those inactive *in vitro*, 0.3% showed *in vivo* activity. Of those active *in vitro*, 36.6% were inactive *in vivo*. Of the total, 14.8% displayed activity both *in vitro* and *in vivo*. Given that currently only compounds with *in vitro* activity are tested *in vivo*, recalculation based only on those having *in vitro* activity would change the figures to 73% for *in vitro* activity only and 27% for activity in both tests. The latter percentage is typical of those noted by investigators. Furthermore, a major problem in correlating *in vitro* and *in vivo* results occurs when the agent being tested is very active *in vitro* but inactive or moderately active *in vivo*. Because *in vitro* and *in vivo* tests differ in their general characteristics and specific variables, discrepancies are likely to occur. However, they may be understood and interpreted if the limitations of the tests are taken into account. Causes of missing activity in animal experiments in spite of good activity *in vitro* can include PK factors, such as minimal distribution in the host due to poor uptake and rapid metabolism or other inactivation (e.g., high protein binding) of the drug, resulting in insufficient dosing. Differences in the pharmacology of compounds between humans and animals commonly used for experimentation can lead to effective drugs being wasted because their potential clinical effect is never tested. Beneficial effects of drugs other than their antimicrobial activity (e.g., immunostimulative behavior) have a risk of being overlooked if they do not reach *in vivo* testing (e.g., the potential immunity-stimulating activity of the macrolides has only recently been detected using experimental animal testing).

Commonly used *in vitro* tests do appear to fail to predict outcome in certain types of infections, especially device-related infections (638). Characteristically, bacteria involved in device-related infections are adherent, slow-growing bacteria that are phenotypically distinct from the rapidly multiplying bacteria that grow during *in vitro* susceptibility testing (see 205). Consequently, specialized *in vitro* techniques are needed to obtain a better correlation between *in vitro* and *in vivo* (experimental or clinical) activity. Using a model of *S. aureus* device-related infections (subcutaneous chamber implant) in guinea pigs, Zimmerli et al. (638) found that, as a single agent, only rifampicin was active, in contrast to vancomycin, teicoplanin, ciprofloxacin, and fleroxacin, despite the fact that the *S. aureus* strain was sensitive to all compounds *in vitro* using standard tests. Determination of peak and trough drug levels in tissue cage fluid showed that, at the doses given, the drug levels of rifampicin, vancomycin, and teicoplanin exceeded the MIC constantly throughout the four-day experiment. Further experimentation demonstrated a dramatic loss of drug activity against stationary phase bacteria (the minimal loss occurring with rifampicin) and that testing the killing effect of antibiotics and their combinations against bacteria adherent to glass beads at drug levels achieved *in vivo* did provide an accurate prediction of treatment effect *in vivo*.

Anaissie et al. (8) and Rex et al. (496) have studied the correlation between *in vitro* susceptibility and *in vivo* activity in a candida sepsis model in mice. Lack of *in vitro* susceptibility in a microbroth dilution test correlated well with fungal kidney colonization 4 days postinfection and with prolongation of survival (8). Follow-up studies indicated that MICs determined at 24 hours (as opposed to 48 hours) correlated better with *in vivo* outcomes (496).

Acute Toxicity Assays to Determine Tolerated Doses

Important technical issues that must be considered include the amount of drug administered during a primary screening program and the most suitable route of administration. If possible, some measure of toxicity should be obtained *in vitro*. Although more often done only if anomalous results are obtained, before use in the treatment of infected animals, the maximum tolerated dose of a substance should be determined by administering single injections of the substance to groups of mice ($N = 3$ to 6) by oral, subcutaneous, intraperitoneal routes. The animals are then observed for survival for periods from 24 hours to 7 days. Such acute toxicity studies establish for each route the 100% toxic dose (LD_{100}), the 50% lethal dose (LD_{50}), and the maximum tolerated dose (LD_0)—the dose at which all animals survive. Various methods of determining the LD_{50} (or infectious dose) have been previously reviewed (603). Approximately one-fifth of the maximum tolerated dose of a substance can be well tolerated when treatments are given once daily for 5 days or longer. For 1 to 3 days of treatment, one-half of the maximum dose can usually be given. When using these crude guidelines, it would be reasonable to assume that animals dying after multiple treatments succumb to the effects of the particular infection rather than to drug toxicity.

In addition to initial information on toxicity, some information on oral bioavailability may also be obtained. For example, if a substance is tolerated at 1000 mg/kg when given orally but is toxic when given at a dose of 50 mg/kg intraperitoneally or intravenously, the lack of toxicity by the oral route probably reflects poor oral absorption.

Choice of Organism

In developing an experimental mouse model for *in vivo* testing, it is desirable to use human pathogens whenever possible. It is also desirable to infect with strains of microorganisms that are sufficiently virulent so that conditioning procedures to lower the host's resistance are unnecessary. Natural infections typically result from inoculation with *S. pneumoniae, S. pyogenes,* certain strains of *K. pneumoniae, Salmonella typhi, S. typhimurium, M. tuberculosis,* and *Cryptococcus neoformans.* When reproducible infections cannot be achieved by inoculation of the organisms alone, it is necessary to reduce the resistance of the animal. A common procedure is to suspend the organism in 3% to 10% hog gastric mucin and to administer 0.5 mL amounts by the intraperitoneal route. In the case of infections with *C. albicans* and *Histoplasma capsulatum,* the animals are infected intravenously with virulent strains; for less virulent strains, the animals are conditioned by injection of 0.1 mL of a 1% suspension of cortisone in saline twice daily by the intramuscular route before the introduction of the organisms. Alternatively, immunosuppression can be achieved by rendering the mice leukopenic by administering cyclophosphamide.

Preparation of Inoculum for Infection: Virulence Titration

In order to obtain reproducible infections, it is necessary to determine the degree of virulence of each strain to be studied. To carry out virulence tests, suitable broth cultures (where high viability of the culture is maintained) are serially diluted in broth to obtain 10-fold decreases in the number of organisms. If mucin is to be used, one part of each broth dilution is combined with nine parts of mucin. Groups of four to six mice weighing 18 to 22 g are injected intraperitoneally with 0.5 mL of each dilution. The animals are observed for 3 to 7 days, and the number of survivors at each dilution is noted. The lowest dilution of the organisms at which all of the animals die is defined as the minimal lethal dose (MLD). For chemotherapeutic studies, many investigators use a dilution that is 100 to 1000 times the MLD to ensure that variations in bacterial virulence and animal susceptibility do not result in failure of all control animals to succumb and to ensure that the test antibacterial is not merely marginally effective. Alternatively, in place of MLD, one can use multiples of the challenge dose of organisms that kills 50% of the animals (LD_{50}). The LD_{50} value, as calculated by the Reed and Muench method (491), is based on the same survival rates used for calculating the MLD. Various methods of determining the LD_{50} have been reviewed (603).

The virulence of many organisms is so low for an unnatural animal host that some type of stressing agent or adjuvant is usually required to achieve a reproducible infection. As previously stated, mucin is usually required to provide reproducible bacterial infections in mice. Without mucin, infections would require the large numbers of organisms provided by cultures that are undiluted or only marginally diluted. Such an inoculum may be overwhelming, either because of toxic effects (e.g., endotoxic shock or the introduction of toxic components of spent culture broth) or because the antibacterial would not be able to inhibit the large numbers of organisms (see reference 293). We have found in the past that mucin, at a concentration of 5%, gives consistent results with few deaths directly attributable to the effect of mucin, although with certain batches of mucin an 8% to 10% concentration may be required to give consistent results. The quality of the mucin available is variable, and thus the mucin used should be evaluated in separate experiments. One problem often encountered is contamination of the commercial hog gastric mucin powder. The mucin can be autoclaved without loosing its macrophage-inhibiting abilities. Furthermore, in all experiments, or at least periodically, a group of uninfected animals should receive mucin alone to ensure that deaths are not due to the stressing effects of this adjuvant.

Previous studies (112) clearly show the enhancing effect of mucin on the proliferation of bacteria in the murine host. Mice were infected intraperitoneally with 0.5 mL of an overnight broth culture of *E. coli* 8 either as a saline suspension or in 3% gastric mucin. Groups of five mice were killed, samples of blood were collected from the axillary region at 10 minutes and at hourly intervals after infection, peritoneal lavage was performed, and CFU/mL determinations were made of both fluids. A count of 10^5 CFU/mL was obtained from intraperitoneal washings immediately after infection with bacteria suspended in saline. The count dropped to approximately 10^3 CFU/mL within 10 minutes and remained in this range for the next 7 hours. The viable count in the blood rose to approximately 50 CFU/mL within 10 minutes and then showed little increase over the next 7 hours (approximately 100 CFU/mL). In contrast, when 3% mucin was used as an adjuvant, the initial count in the peritoneal washings of 10^5 CFU/mL increased stepwise with time to a count in excess of 10^9 CFU/mL by the end of 8 hours. The viable count in the blood closely paralleled that seen in the peritoneal washings (increasing from 5×10^3 CFU/mL after 1 hour to 7×10^8 CFU/mL at 8 hours).

For certain slowly growing, fastidious organisms (e.g., *S. pyogenes* and *S. pneumoniae*), mucin is not required in order to obtain a reproducibly virulent infection. The virulence of these organisms is maintained by passage of the cultures in mice. One or two mice are infected intraperitoneally with 1 mL of an overnight broth culture. After 6 to 8 hours, when the animals show signs of illness, they are anesthetized, the hearts are removed aseptically, and several drops of heart blood are added to a tube of appropriate broth medium. For *S. pyogenes* and *S. pneumoniae,* trypticase soy broth containing 10% goat serum is suitable. The serum of other animal species is equally suitable. At the same time, the blood is also streaked on blood agar plates. After overnight incubation, serial 10-fold dilutions of the broth cultures are prepared for use as the infecting inoculum. The blood agar plates are used for confirmation of the purity and identity of the infecting inoculum. The quelling reaction can be used to type the pneumococci, and standard procedures are used to confirm the identity of group A streptococci. *In vivo* passage can dramatically affect the virulence of many other pathogens (e.g., some strains of *H. influenzae*), and this method should be considered for all strains proposed to be used for many experiments. Following *in vivo* passage, stocks of the organisms should be made from exponential-phase cultures of low passage and then stored frozen. If available, liquid nitrogen is preferred; otherwise, a –80°C freezer provides sufficient stability, while storage at –40°C can lead to loss of virulence in *S. pneumoniae* strains often used for animal experiments.

If there is doubt whether animals died from drug toxicity rather than infection, samples of blood from the hearts of dead animals as well as from some of the survivors should be inoculated onto agar plates. The cultures from the dead animals should show the infecting organism, whereas the cultures from surviving animals should be sterile.

The three methods most frequently used for calculating the 50% dose parameter are the method of Reed and Muench (491), the probit method (199), and method of the sigmoidal dose-response (variable slope), also known as the Hill equation (277).

Treatment Routes and Times

By altering the treatment route or schedule, differences in activity can be demonstrated. In addition, the relative efficacy of oral and subcutaneous administration of a substance can be compared (as discussed earlier).

Studies in which mice infected with *S. pneumoniae* serotypes 1 and 2 were treated once, orally or subcutaneously, with doses of ampicillin or amoxicillin demonstrate the influence of the treatment route (282). Treatment by the subcutaneous route was more effective than treatment by the oral route. When administered orally, amoxicillin was more active against the type 1 *S. pneumoniae* than was ampicillin. Otherwise the two agents were equivalent in activity (282).

Tests with ampicillin and amdinocillin (mecillinam) in which the antibacterials were administered to mice subcutaneously immediately (0 hour) or at 1, 2, or 4 hours after infection indicate the potential problems with delay in treatment initiation (282). With treatment 4 hours after inoculation, the regimens were considerably less effective than when administered immediately or at 1 hour (282). Similarly, multiple-dose regimens were more effective than single-dose regimens, which are typical for all β-lactam antibiotics. This can be explained by the importance of T > MIC (i.e., the duration the antibiotic concentration remains above the MIC). Interestingly, the greater effectiveness of multiple dosing was also apparent for ampicillin against enterobacteria resistant toward the drug (282).

For drugs such as the aminoglycosides or the fluoroquinolones, single-dose regimens would result in lower PD_{50}s than those of multiple-dose regimens due to the importance of the AUC/MIC ratio for these types of compounds (e.g., 190). In this manner, PK/PD relationships can be demonstrated by relatively simple dosing experiments using the mouse protection test.

Differences in the PK patterns of various agents may also be determined by prophylactic-type experiments (i.e., treatment before infection). The activities of ceftriaxone and cefotaxime were similar when treatment was administered immediately (0 hour) after treatment (56). However, when treatment was administered at 24 or 8 hours before infection, the activity of ceftriaxone was clearly superior against the Gram-negative bacteria. No such differences were seen against *S. aureus* in this model.

Duration of treatment can affect the outcome (for reviews, see references 439 and 454). For example, extending ciprofloxacin treatment (p.o., 20 mg/kg b.i.d.) of systemic *S. typhimurium*–infected mice from 17 to 28 days improved the outcome (81).

Synergy or Antagonism *In Vivo* in Screening Models

In order to study interaction between two antibiotics *in vivo*, graded doses of the combined agents and the single agents are administered to groups of four to six mice after infection. The PD_{50} can be calculated for the combination and compared to the 50% doses for the single agents. A fractional index (FIC) can be calculated for the combination doses by dividing the PD_{50} value for each of the components in the combination by the PD_{50} value obtained for each component alone and adding the two quotients. Synergy can then be defined using the FIC (e.g., a value of less than or equal to 0.5–0.6), similar to the method of studying synergy *in vitro* (251). Delay of treatment causes loss of synergistic activity.

Setting the PD_{50} value of the combination at one-fourth that of the most active single agent is perhaps an easier way of evaluating the results of the experiments. Combining different dosing regimens over a 24-hour dosing period after inoculation will further allow estimation of the importance of different PK parameters for synergy *in vivo*. This approach has been studied in the neutropenic mouse thigh model (282,422,423) but could also be used in the mouse peritonitis model.

Antagonism between antibiotics *in vivo* has been studied in the mouse peritonitis model (289a). The combination of erythromycin and penicillin against *S. pneumoniae in vivo* resulted in the same mortality as erythromycin alone and significantly higher mortality than penicillin alone. The inhibiting effect of erythromycin on the activity of penicillin could also be demonstrated by *in vivo* time-kill curves of bacterial counts in peritoneal wash. This apparent antagonism between erythromycin and penicillin has been contested by others, at least *in vitro* (153). The use of animal models and PK/PD relationships in determining *in vivo* antibiotic synergy has been reviewed (188,250,251,282,423,522).

Den Hollander et al. (152) used *in vitro*–derived FIC determinations to attain PD parameters of the combination of tobramycin and ceftazidime. They first determined the MICcombi, which is the MIC of tobramycin in the presence of ceftazidime. Using humanlike PK profiles, they then divided the tobramycin and ceftazidime concentrations at each time point along the dosing interval to construct FIC over time curves, which were used to derive PD parameters. $T_{>FICI}$ (time above a specified FIC value during the dosing interval) appears to be the key PD parameter for this combination. Although difficult, to date little application of this methodology has occurred with *in vivo* data.

Systemic Infections in Neutropenic Mice

One desired attribute of any antibacterial agent is its ability to control infections in a host that has a compromised or inoperative phagocytic system. This is especially the case in patients receiving radiation or cancer chemotherapy, whose total white counts are ~1000/mL or less. Mice can be made neutropenic by employing a number of different cytostatic agents such as 5-fluorouracil, methotrexate, and cyclophosphamide. In general, the infections induced in the neutropenic state are more severe than in nonneutropenic animals. Animal survival is shorter and the burden of organisms is greater in neutropenic models. The impact of neutropenia on the growth of organisms *in vivo* varies for different microbial species. For example, the presence of neutrophils in a mouse thigh model enhanced the activity of fluoroquinolone antibiotics against pneumococci nearly sevenfold, though in similar studies with *K. pneumoniae,* the activity was enhanced only twofold. Some microbial species are only able to produce infection in such immunocompromised mice. For example, many strains of *S. pneumoniae* do not grow well in the lungs of nonneutropenic Swiss ICR mice. Therapeutic responses to infection can vary not only among bacterial species but also depending on the class of drug employed. Murine studies in a pneumococcal infection model found that neutropenia reduced the activity of tetracyclines, quinolones, and ketolides four- to eightfold but reduced the activity of the lincomycin clindamycin only twofold.

Neutropenic and nonneutropenic mice were infected with two strains of *K. pneumoniae* and one strain of *S. pneumoniae* and treated with mecillinam and/or amoxicillin. For these experiments, 20-g mice were made neutropenic by intraperitoneal injection of cyclophosphamide (62.5 mg/kg once daily for 5 days). The total number of leukocytes was counted and the mean determined the day after the last cyclophosphamide treatment. White cell counts for nontreated mice were also determined at this time. The mice were then infected with 100 to 1000 times the MLD of the three strains. Treatment was administered once subcutaneously, immediately after infection. The level of antibiotic needed to protect the neutropenic mice was 3 to more than 25 times that needed to protect mice with intact phagocytic systems. For example, *K. pneumoniae*–infected immunocompetent mice (2779 leukocytes/μL) demonstrated PD_{50} values of amdinocillin 10 mg/kg and amoxicillin 10 mg/kg, and neutropenic mice (773 leukocytes/μL) demonstrated values of amdinocillin >250 mg/kg and amoxicillin 54 mg/kg.

Thigh Lesion (Selbie) Model

The thigh lesion model provides a sensitive experimental infection that can be used to evaluate the effectiveness of an antimicrobial and allows the measurement of drug-pathogen interactions and drug PK in the infected host (253). Furthermore, if the animals are made neutropenic, then the thigh model becomes an excellent system for measuring the drug-pathogen interaction with most of the host defense system eliminated (593). This model has been extensively used to determine principles of PK/dosing of antibiotics (253) and to determine the *in vivo* relevance of PAEs (127,252,254).

The method described by Vogelman et al. (593) and reviewed by Gudmundsson and Erlendsdottir (252) illustrates a typical thigh model infection. More recently, investigators have utilized pathogens that have been genetically engineered to produce bioluminescent proteins, allowing live bacteria to be imaged *in vivo*. Bioluminescence decreases with the death of bacteria (206,207). Preliminary treatment studies have demonstrated that this noninvasive monitoring technique correlates well with bacterial numbers grown in homogenate cultures.

FUNGAL INFECTIONS

Animal infection models have been developed for many systemic, mucosal, and cutaneous fungal pathogens. Although many of the described animal infection models involving bacteria can be modified to accommodate fungal infections, a few specific comments are given here (practical descriptions of many models are presented in Zak and Sande [631,633]). Rodents and the rabbit have been most commonly utilized in the analysis of antifungal drug therapies. For systemic fungal pathogens, including yeasts and molds, both disseminated models using intravenous inoculation and site-specific infections of the lung and central nervous system have been developed. Although many fungal species will infect noncompromised animals, the infecting inocula required to produce disease is often quite high (7 to 9 log), and during the study period the organism end-organ pathogen growth in untreated animals is usually small (1 log or less) (141). A variety of methods of immunosuppression have been utilized both to produce a more severe infection in the animals and to mimic the compromised human host. The most common type of immunosuppression in these models is neutropenia induced chemically (by cyclophosphamide or cytarabine). For mold infections, the addition of corticosteroids is often employed as well. Few investigators have utilized specific rodent species devoid of specific immune components (107). For example, SCID mice devoid of B- or T-cell immunity have been used for a mucosal candidosis model to mimic infection in patients with HIV (297). Despite immunosuppression, certain fungi that commonly infect humans, such as *Candida glabrata*, do not produce a severe infection in most animals (75).

For disseminated models, intravenous injection of organisms is used. The level of immunosuppression, the inoculum size, and the specific fungal species will determine the most appropriate duration of study. Large inocula (6–7 log) of *C. albicans* in neutropenic mice will produce a rapidly progressive disseminated infection resulting in animal mortality in 24–72 hours (13). Smaller inocula (4–5 log) can be used in this model to prolong study periods to more than a week (12). Disseminated mold infections in compromised animals require longer periods of time to develop and rarely result in animal mortality before day 7 (87). Smaller inocula of these filamentous pathogens can produce an infection allowing study for more than 30 days (266).

Investigators often also measure antifungal outcomes in several tissues because of concern that antifungal drug PK may vary in different animal tissues. For example, it has been theorized that kidney concentrations may be higher for drugs eliminated primarily by this organ than for drugs that are extensively metabolized or excreted in the bile or intestines. The other commonly utilized internal organs include the liver, spleen, lungs, and brain (597). The burden of organisms in these other tissues is often several logs lower than in the kidneys.

Other than *Candida* species, the major route of systemic infection for fungi is via the lungs. A persistent or progressive infection of the lungs with filamentous pathogens requires neutropenic immunosuppression (597). The addition of corticosteroid therapy preceding infection enhances the severity of infection. Direct instillation of inocula into the trachea or placement of inocula into the nares of anesthetized animals is utilized to produce a fungal pneumonitis. Although the liquid inoculum does not mimic the spore inhalation responsible for infection in humans, histopathologically the disease states are quite similar. Both animal survival and growth of organisms in the lung have been common end points. While therapeutic outcomes using both end points have been similar in the majority of studies, there is concern that during tissue homogenization hyphae are fractured, with each subsequent hyphal piece being capable of producing a fungal colony after plate culture, leading to an overestimation of the fungal burden. Several other therapeutic end points have thus been developed. Both histopathologic and radiographic lung lesion scoring systems have been developed but are obviously labor intensive. More recently, investigators have quantified organism-specific antigen levels or used quantitative determinations of nucleic acid as outcome measures.

Models mimicking fungal meningitis have been developed for a number of fungal pathogens (71,99,106). The rabbit is the most commonly used animal for CNS fungal infection. The fungal inoculum is most often introduced intracisternally. Both animal survival and organism burden in the cerebrospinal fluid and the brain parenchyma are commonly measured therapeutic outcomes.

Both oral and vaginal Candida infection models have been used in the evaluation of antifungal efficacy. A similar range of animal species have been used, but mice are the most common test animals. For oral disease, preceding corticosteroid therapy is typically used to predispose mice to infection. For vaginal disease, a state of pseudoestrus is especially effective in allowing colonization and invasive growth of the organism in vaginal tissues. The state of estrus is induced by removing ovaries and administering estradiol before and throughout the study. The Candida inoculum is introduced by either pipetting it into the cavity, by introducing cotton swabs soaked in the inoculum, or, in the case of oral disease, by placing the organism in the drinking water. Therapy is most often delayed several days to more than 2 weeks to allow the infection to become established. Once antifungal therapy is initiated, it is continued for days to weeks. Organism burden after antifungal therapy is most often quantified in oral or vaginal washes. Histopathologic scoring of tissue sections has also been used.

The efficacy of agents targeted at dermatophytes has been evaluated in cutaneous models of infection in rodents (283). Guinea pigs are commonly utilized. Nail, foot pad, and skin infections can be induced. Most often the tissue bed is mechanically abraded prior to topical inoculation to predispose the tissue to infection. The infecting dermatophytes require several days to weeks to become established prior to the initiation of either topical or systemic antifungal therapy. Therapies are most commonly continued for several weeks, after which tissues are cultured and examined with histopathology.

DISCRIMINATIVE ANIMAL MODELS OF INFECTION

Animal Models of Urinary Tract Infections

The models for experimental acute urinary tract infections (UTIs) that are commonly used to evaluate antibacterials produce either hematogenous or ascending infections, depending on whether the inoculum is administered intravenously or intravesically, with or without the addition of a foreign body (510). Mice and rats are the most common species used in experimental UTIs, and they have been used to determine the pathogenesis of this infection as well as test experimental chemotherapy. Note, however, that naturally occurring vesicoureteral reflux (backflow of the urine from the bladder to the kidneys) normally occurs in rodents but only infrequently in humans (499). Although some bacteria have a trophism for the urinary tract, even when inoculated intraperitoneally (e.g., *Borrelia burgdorferi* [242]), and some models of UTIs utilize bloodstream inoculation with bacteria to generate pyelonephritis (304), normally manipulation of the urinary tract of rodents is a prerequisite for establishing infection. Some of the bacterial virulence factors necessary to establish UTI in humans (e.g., type 1 and type P fimbriae of *E. coli*) are also required to establish ascending UTI in mice and rats with the same binding mechanisms to the epithelium of the urinary tract. With focus on these virulence factors in strains used for inoculation, little manipulation of the urinary tract is actually needed for creating ascending infection in these rodents. In addition to testing antimicrobials, these models have been used to evaluate adjunct antiinflammatory agents (e.g., pentoxifylline [619]). Previous reviews (239,304,486,629) describe additional models for establishing UTI, in particular pyelonephritis.

Ascending Obstructive Pyelonephritis

The original model for pyelonephritis (78) was further developed (239). Rats are operated on and bacteria are inoculated directly into the bladder, whereafter one of the ureters is obstructed by ligation, which is removed 18–24 hours later. This model has been used to demonstrate that, following acute infection, inflammation leading to chronic pyelonephritis is the major contributor to renal damage. Early antibiotic therapy suppresses renal damage (238) by rapid eradication of bacterial infection, but antiinflammatory treatment with dexamethasone failed to suppress renal damage (398). This model has also been used to compare the efficacy of various antibiotics (237).

Chronic Cystitis and Subacute Pyelonephritis

A model of persistent bladder infection has been described that requires placement of a foreign body into the bladder (344). A small cylinder of polyurethane foam (4 $\times$ 2 mm) was introduced into the bladder via a needle pushed bluntly into the bladder via the urethra. Two weeks later, the surgically exposed bladder was inoculated directly with *E. coli*. Chronic bacteriuria ensued for as long as 8 weeks after infection, leading to focal and diffuse inflammation of the bladder wall. Furthermore, bilateral pyelonephritis developed in the majority of the animals. The model is amenable to antimicrobial therapy (344). Several drugs have been tested for 7 days duration, and the effect was measured as reduction of CFU in the bladder wall and kidney homogenates (344).

Acute and Subclinical Pyelonephritis by Intrarenal Infection

This procedure is commonly used to establish kidney infections for the evaluation of antimicrobial agents, usually in rats. The kidney is surgically exposed, and the inoculum (50 to 100 CFU/μL) is injected directly into one (51,343) or both poles (399) of the kidney. Usually only one of the kidneys is used, but infection of the contralateral kidney can ensue (399). The passive infection of the contralateral kidney has been used to study subclinical pyelonephritis in comparison with the acute infection in the directly inoculated kidney (399).

The model has been used to study the effect as well as toxicity of gentamicin (51,343) and the importance of duration of therapy in pyelonephritis (51). Several different antibiotics have been compared in this model (51,344). The most effective drugs have been gentamicin, ceftriaxone, and various fluoroquinolones, while ampicillin and co-trimoxazole have shown lower efficacy (51,344).

Ascending Pyelonephritis Following Direct Bladder Inoculation

Direct inoculation of surgically exposed bladders has long been used to induce experimental UTI. Rodents generally do not need to be water deprived. The urethra is clamped and the bladder exposed by surgical intervention. Bacteria (50–200 CFU/μL) are slowly injected into the bladder, and the urethra remains clamped for 2 to 4 hours in order to avoid discharge of the inoculum. Ascending infection with development of bilateral pyelonephritis will follow. Renal scarring for up to 6 weeks later has been used as a parameter to study interventional therapy (264). Early quinolone treatment eliminated the incidence of renal scarring, while delayed treatment resulted in renal damage in approximately 50% of the animals (264).

Ascending Urinary Tract Infection by Bladder Inoculation via Urethral Catheter

During the last 10–15 years, this model in mice has been the most widely used to study virulence factors and host resistance in UTI. With this model, detailed knowledge of the binding mechanisms between bacteria harboring various virulence traits and epithelial cells in the urinary tract has been discovered, and it has further been utilized to reveal the various facets of the host mechanisms of resistance to infection, both in the bladder and in the kidney. A detailed review of this literature is beyond the scope of this chapter, and the reader is referred to recent reviews (9,425,426,524).

The model is probably by far the easiest to use for the study of UTI when the technique of bladder cauterization has been learned, since no other surgical manipulation is needed. With the correct bacterial strain harboring the virulence factors needed (i.e., type 1 or type P fimbriae of *E. coli* or other enterobacteria), UTI with moderate to high bacterial counts in the urine, bladder wall, and kidneys (40% to 70% of the infected mice) will ensue (259,280,294). The presence of type 1 fimbriae in *E. coli* can easily be tested for by agglutination with *C. albicans* cells or with sheep erythrocytes (318). CFUs appear to decrease after 2–3 weeks, which is why antibiotic treatment studies should preferably be performed 1–8 days after inoculation. Higher colony counts can be obtained by pretreating the mice with 5% glucose in the drinking water starting 3 days prior to infection (294,318).

Antibiotic concentrations can be measured simultaneously in serum, urine and, renal tissue, and these can be related to the effect of the antibiotics according to the MICs of the infecting strains (280,318). PD relationships for dosing of antibiotics in UTI can be studied with this model (212), which has also been used to study antibiotic effect against UTI caused by *E. faecalis* and *P. aeruginosa* (573).

Models of UTIs Associated with Indwelling Catheters

Models of short-term and long-term indwelling catheter infections have been described (291,292). Both long (25-mm) and short (4-mm) segments of tubing have been used in mice, the short not secured and therefore expelled, with 3–7 days serving as a short-term model. When the longer segment has been secured to the bladder, it has been left for up 12 months, thus mimicking a long-term indwelling urinary catheter (292). Spontaneous bacteriuria ($>10^2$ CFU/mL urine) was not reported in the mice with unsecured tubing but occurred intermittently in 44% of the animals with secured bladder catheters and was predominantly due to *Proteus mirabilis*. Apparently no colonization of the kidneys occurred unless the infection was persistent and of high density (10^5 CFU/mL). Postsurgery ampicillin treatment for 7 days and housing on wire platforms reduced the incidence of bacteriuria to 7% over 12 months.

Models of UTI Resulting from Bloodstream Inoculation

Hematogenous infection has been long used to establish UTI (304,628). Normally, no manipulations of the animals are required, but strain selection is essential in order to have selective colonization of the kidneys. Examples of this model have used *E. faecalis* (246,412,512) or *S. aureus* or *K. pneumoniae* (217). Trovafloxacin and rifampin alone or in combination were compared in a rat model against *E. faecalis* pyelonephritis (412). Although antagonism is usually considered the result of combining these two types of antibiotics, no such effect was evident from the reduction in renal colony counts found, which was similar to those achieved with the two drugs given alone. A new cephalosporin with Gram-positive activity was compared with ampicillin and vancomycin against *E. faecalis* in the hematogenous model in mice (246). With the higher doses used, the cephalosporin was as effective as the two other antibiotics.

Animal Models of Foreign Body Infections

Advances in the development of prostheses and a variety of vascular grafts and permanently residing catheters have been limited by problems of bacterial infections, which are exceedingly difficult to cure and often necessitate removal of the device. Reviews of animal models of foreign body infections have appeared (23a,185,636,637), prompting review of strategies for dealing with such infections clinically (148,472).

Prostheses Infections

One of the most common foreign body infection models utilizes the subcutaneous implantation of a perforated plastic cylinder (639). Although commonly used in guinea pigs and rats, this model can also be used in mice. This model is suitable for evaluation of antibiotic treatment, although the infections are difficult to treat. For example, one study demonstrated that only triple therapy with 50 mg/kg vancomycin, 50 mg/kg fleroxacin, and 25 mg/kg rifampin (i.p. every 12 hours for 21 days) provided an adequate response (103).

Infected Sutures

Intramuscular implantation of infected sutures into the thighs of mice has been described (477). Lengths of cotton 2–0 suture are sterilized in broth, which is subsequently inoculated (in this example, with *K. pneumoniae*). The contaminated suture is then attached to a sterile needle and drawn through the thigh muscle of a mouse, the exposed ends are trimmed flush with the skin, and the ends are buried under the skin. Culture of homogenized suture material facilitates determination of the infecting CFU. The infection spreads from the suture to the surrounding muscle, and subsequently a sepsis develops. This model is amenable to antibiotic intervention (429); continuous infusion of 180 mg/kg/day cefazolin by use of intraperitoneally implanted osmotic pumps was superior to an equal amount of antibiotic given by intramuscular bolus dosing (every 8 hours).

Animal Models of Skin, Burn, and Surgical Wound Infections

Several models of infection associated with surgical intervention (in the absence of foreign bodies) have been described and utilized for experimental evaluation of antimicrobial chemotherapy. These models rely on direct inoculation of the wound site and generally achieve simulated prophylaxis of postsurgical infection by administering antibiotics at the time of infection, or just before, and ascertain efficacy of treatment by determining infection remaining at the inoculation site as well as dissemination to internal organs. These models can be used to evaluate oral, parenteral, or topical antibiotic administration. A review of postsurgical infectious complications is available (148). A model of clean wound infections has been described (305).

Models of Infected Burn Wounds

Infections following burns are difficult to treat and have been modeled in several systems. Typically, partial-thickness or full-thickness burn wounds are made on the shaved skin of anesthetized animals by using a metal stamp or by partially immersing the animals in heated water; a minimum of about 30% of the total skin area of the animal needs to be damaged. Normally, the burn wound is then directly inoculated, but translocation of normal intestinal bacteria often follows; interestingly, animal models have demonstrated that infection of a skin burn apparently promotes translocation of intestinal bacteria, compared with that occurring when wounds are kept sterile (159,382). Recent research in this area has evaluated promotion of host resistance to infection by use of cytokines, whose expression in some cases also occurs as part of the normal healing process. In experimental full-thickness murine wounds, the expression of inducible nitric oxide synthase (iNOS) by infiltrating inflammatory cells is not a part of normal repair processes but is a response to bacterial colonization due to *S. aureus* (374).

Animal Models of Pneumonia

Rat Models of Acute Pneumonia

A useful model for production of pneumococcal pneumonia in rats has been described by Ansfield et al. (14). Lung bacterial counts progressively increased, reaching 10^7 CFU per lung within 48 hours. This increase was associated with localized atelectasis and consolidation. Bacterial multiplication could be inhibited with 50 mg/kg tetracycline given once intraperitoneally prior to infection or at 4 or 12 hours after infection. Viable pneumococci were rapidly killed by lung defenses if bacterial multiplication was inhibited within 12 hours of the onset of infection. No change occurred in the bacterial population if tetracycline treatment was delayed until 24 hours after infection.

A similar rat model of pneumococcal pneumonia was used to determine the role of the host defense system in antimicrobial therapy by impairing the phagocytic system by complement depletion using cobra venom factor (28). There was a consistent decrease in body weight with time (approximately 15% to 20% loss by 108 hours postinfection). The temperature was initially elevated (approximately 1–2°C, up from normal levels of 37–37.4°C), but by 108 hours it was depressed (by as much as 4°C). The weight of the left lung increased (from about 0.6 ± 0.15 g to 3–4 g) with the involvement of the lung tissue in the infectious process. Pulmonary lesions were very extensive in the left lung by 108 hours, and the number of pneumococci increased from 6×10^7 CFU to approximately 10^9 CFU per lung. By the end of 108 hours, the infectious process had spread, so that both the blood (approximately 10^3 to 10^6 CFU/mL) and the pleural fluid were positive for pneumococci. Treatment of infected rats with 2 mg/kg penicillin G every 12 hours starting from 36 hours postinfection was very effective in preventing weight loss (only a transient 6% to 8% loss by 36 hours, 0% to 5% by 132 hours), normalizing the temperature (approximately 38–39°C at 36 hours and within normal range from 84 hours onward), and maintaining the weight of the left lung near normal (a transient rise up to 2 g at 36 hours, within the normal ramge from 84 hours, onward). By 84 hours there was a significant but highly variable fall in the number of viable pneumococci, and by 132 hours, all lung, blood, and pleural fluid cultures were sterile. After treatment with cobra venom factor, the whole complement hemolytic activity was decreased to less than 2% of normal values. When cobra venom factor–treated rats were also administered penicillin, the results very closely paralleled the course of infection seen in normal untreated infected rats, indicating the importance of an intact innate immune system for the outcome of antimicrobial therapy (28).

Rat models have also been used to demonstrate that chronic alcohol ingestion increases susceptibility to infection (144), as does liver cirrhosis (396) and neutropenia (596). Intratracheal injection of soft agar (0.7%) encased penicillin-resistant *S. pneumoniae* to create an acute pneumonia model in immunocompetent rats (229a). Lung CFU and mortalities were dependent on the size of the infectious challenge (inocula of 2.9×10^8 or 4.2×10^9 were uniformly fatal, but only the higher inocula produced stable lung CFU of approximately 10^9 CFU/g over 3 days). Despite an *in vitro* MIC of 2 μg/mL for penicillin, 100,000 IU penicillin G/kg every 2 hours for 8 administrations reduced lung CFU (the change was approximately log 2/g versus controls) and promoted survival (13% mortality versus 33% for controls), whereas 250,000 IU/kg reduced the mortality to 7% and the change in CFU/g was approximately log 3. Similar activity was seen with cefpirome (200 mg/kg) and cefotaxime (100 mg/kg). With the latter, the lung CFU/g was similar to that resulting from the penicillin G treatment, but the mortality was apparently higher (19%). Two administrations of 50 mg/kg vancomycin every 8 hours produced a change in CFU/g of log 4 and 7% mortality.

Mouse Models of Acute Pneumonia

A representative method for inducing acute bacterial pneumonia in mice has been previously described (56). Pneumonia was induced by intranasal instillation of *S. pneumoniae* 6301. Infected mice were treated once subcutaneously 24 hours after infection and were sacrificed 48 hours after infection. The lungs were removed aseptically and cultured for the presence of the organism by touching a cut surface of the lung to blood agar (alternatively, the lungs can be homogenized and the CFU/g determined by serially diluting and plating the homogenate). At 48 hours after infection, untreated controls evidenced consolidation of the lungs. Cultures from these animals were strongly positive. Most but not all of the untreated controls died within 96 hours after infection. The PD_{50} values (mg/kg) were as follows: ceftriaxone, 0.88; ampicillin, 11; cefotaxime, 16; piperacillin, 79; cefamandole, 79; and carbenicillin, 84.

Reproducible invasive lung infections are more difficult to induce with some common respiratory pathogens. For example, *H. influenzae* will colonize the respiratory tract of rodents but does not grow in the lungs in untreated control animals over the common 24- to 48-hour study periods. To allow colonization of the organism, infection is often induced after instillation of a chemical irritant such as 1% formalin (404). Similarly, many drug-resistant pneumococci suffer a fitness cost that reduces the growth of organisms in nonneutropenic pneumonia models. For example, in a nonneutropenic mouse pneumonia model, a penicillin-susceptible strain of *S. pneumoniae* grew from 6 log CFU/lung after infection to more than 9 log CFU/lung after 72 hours in the absence of antibiotic therapy. In the same study, bacterial counts of the penicillin-resistant pneumococcus declined from 6 log CFU/lung to less than 4 log CFU/lung over the same study period (220). However, the use of a unique strain of mice, CBA/J, precludes use of neutropenia for the induction of pneumococcal pneumonia, including from drug-resistant strains. There are no defined immune defects in this mouse species.

The majority of pneumonia models initiate infection via direct instillation into the nares or trachea. Lung infection with a number of respiratory pathogens can also be produced in large numbers of mice after aerosolization of a large inocula via a nebulizer into a closed chamber. For example, nebulization of 10^8 CFU/mL of *K. pneumoniae* via a Collison nebulizer for 45 minutes produces a similar degree of pneumonia in up to 100 mice at a time. At the start of antibacterial therapy, 14 hours after inhalation, between 6 and 7 log CFU/lung can be recovered from mice (348).

One mouse bronchopneumonia model used nontypeable (unencapsulated) *H. influenzae* (NTHI) bound to mouse fetal lung (MFL) cells as an infectious inoculum (404). The infection required lung damage to be present by pretreatment of the mice with 40 μL of 1% formalin 3 days before infection. The lung plus tracheal bacterial load increased more than 100 times by day 7 after instillation but declined to the original inoculum size by day 14. Bronchoalveolar infiltration by neutrophils occurred. Serum anti-NTHI IgM levels were maximal on day 7 after infection, then declined, being replaced by IgG.

An acute pneumonia model was used to evaluate the correlation between *in vitro* MIC or MBC level and *in vivo* activity of amoxicillin against several *S. pneumoniae* strains with varied amoxicillin-resistance (408). Mice were rendered neutropenic by cyclophosphamide and infected via intratracheal inoculation. A single administration of amoxicillin was given subcutaneously 1 hour postinfection. Using an E_{max} model, the researchers determined the P_{50} dose (dose required to achieve 50% of the E_{max}) and the P1 dose (dose required to attain a 1 log reduction in CFU/lung), as well as monitoring survival.

The results demonstrated an excellent correlation between *in vitro* and *in vivo* activity against penicillin-sensitive and -resistant strains of *S. pneumoniae.*

A novel formulation, perflubron, appears to be a promising vehicle for local antibiotic administration (termed liquid dose installation), and it allowed high levels of tobramycin to be achieved without systemic toxicity (156,157).

Chronic Pneumonia Models

Chronic lung infection models are usually established as models of infectious exacerbations of chronic obstructive pulmonary diseases (COPD; cystic fibrosis). A major limitation of the models is the absence of underlying disease. Furthermore, infectious exacerbations in patients apparently arise from normal flora (e.g., COPD infections due to unencapsulated *H. influenzae* and initial infections of Cystic Fibrosis (CF) patients involving *S. aureus* and *H. influenzae* prior to *P. aeruginosa*). However, the normal flora of laboratory rodents does not include such microorganisms.

Establishing chronic pneumonia models in animals is very difficult, owing to the rapid clearance of bacteria instilled into the respiratory tract (263,453,565). One method of overcoming this is by encasing the bacterial inoculum in agar or alginate beads to restrict phagocytosis (92), and the use of this animal model has been reviewed (289,424,453). Persistent *P. aeruginosa* pulmonary infection in rats for up to 35 days after inoculation has been achieved. A preparation of the bacteria encased in agar beads is created, and this suspension is then administered intratracheally to anesthetized animals. A modification of this technique was used to establish chronic experimental *H. influenzae* pulmonary infections (453,541).

Although this model has been extensively used to study the pathogenesis of chronic pulmonary infection (453), it has not often been used to evaluate antibiotic chemotherapy. Two studies have evaluated therapeutic antibiotic dosing of chronic *P. aeruginosa* pulmonary infection in guinea pigs (243,523). Monotherapy of infection was initiated 3 days after infection with agar bead–encased bacteria, and compounds were administered subcutaneously once per day for 5 days. Ticarcillin (120 mg/kg) was ineffective, and ciprofloxacin (10 mg/kg) was judged to be superior to tobramycin (1.7 mg/kg) in reducing lung CFU, but these treatments did not completely eradicate the pulmonary infection (523). However, whereas enoxacin (40 mg/kg) was later shown to be as effective as ciprofloxacin (20 mg/kg), only olfloxacin (20 mg/kg) was able to sterilize the lungs after 5 days of treatment (243). A single dose of amoxicillin dramatically reduced the lung burden of *H. influenzae* in chronically infected rats, but regrowth of the bacteria occurred owing to insufficient antibiotic administration (366); such treatment protocols may be used to develop a model of recurrent pulmonary infection occurring as exacerbations of chronic obstructive pulmonary diseases. A specialized liposomal formulation of tobramycin (Fluidosomes, a low-phase transition temperature liposome preparation) was used to treat chronic pulmonary infection due to mucoid *P. aeruginosa.* Intratracheal administration of this preparation was greatly superior to free tobramycin in reducing lung CFU (45).

P. aeruginosa rapidly acquires β-lactamase–mediated ceftazidime resistance *in vitro* and *in vivo* (26). Immunization of rats against *P. aeruginosa* β-lactamase, followed by the establishment of a chronic lung infection with β-lactamase–producing *P. aeruginosa,* allowed the successful use of ceftazidime. The improvement in outcome was related to the intensity of the immune response, with high responders having significantly smaller pathological areas in the lungs and lower CFU/mL lung homogenate than the low responders or uninfected controls (104).

This model has been used to study the effect of subtherapeutic dosages of antibiotics on *in vivo* production of *P. aeruginosa* exoenzymes (248,249,351). The dosages of antibiotics were carefully titrated to achieve subinhibitory levels in tissue that were shown to inhibit the production of exoenzymes (exoenzyme S, phospholipase C, protease, elastase, and exotoxin A), and no reduction of CFU/lung was observed. Subtherapeutic antibiotic treatment reduced lung pathology, with the greatest effects occurring with ciprofloxacin or tobramycin, which correlated with superior inhibition of exoenzymes *in vitro* (248,249). Subtherapeutic tetracycline treatment has been shown to reduce lung pathology, which correlated with the *in vitro* reduction of protease and ferripyochelin-binding protein (351).

This model has also been used to demonstrate the potential of antiinflammatory therapy to reduce lung pathology. Alternate-day subcutaneous administration of methylprednisolone (1 mg/kg) reduced lung pathology, circulating immune complexes and, interestingly, lung *P. aeruginosa* in chronically infected rats (612). Ibuprofen (35 mg/kg administered orally twice per day) was without antibacterial effect but reduced lung pathology in chronically *P. aeruginosa*–infected rats (330).

Animal Models of Otitis Media

Otitis media, an infection of the middle ear, is largely a childhood infection that apparently very people few avoid contracting. Caused chiefly by *H. influenzae* and *S. pneumonia,* the infection, despite being painful, is often self-resolving, and although antibiotic therapy hastens its resolution, recurrence is common. Spread of the infection from the ear to produce sepsis and/or meningitis can occur, as can damage to the ear, suggesting that antibiotics still have a role in its treatment. Antibiotic treatment often results in the transformation of acute otitis media (AOM) into sterile otitis media with effusion (OME). However, culture-negative OME fluid may contain viable bacteria (479–481), likely due to the growth of bacteria as biofilm

(171a,479–481), which conveys different physiological character to the bacteria, including antibiotic-sensitivity.

Excellent technical descriptions of the models are available for the chinchilla (260), guinea pig (186), and gerbil (30). Briefly, anesthetized animals have their ear canals thoroughly cleaned and are infected by direct administration of bacteria into the ear canal, normally by injection through the thin bone structures of the cephalad bulla. A thorough review of the histopathology and pathophysiology of experimental models of AOM is available (93).

A gerbil model of bilateral AOM induced by either penicillin-resistant or penicillin-sensitive *S. pneumoniae,* combined with the measurement of ear fluid CFU and drug levels, was used to establish PK/PD parameters for linezolid (279). Following intrabullar injection of *S. pneumoniae,* peak infection occurred at day 2 for the penicillin-resistant strain and at day 3 for the penicillin-sensitive strain. Linezolid, amoxicillin, or vehicle was administered twice per day over 4.5 days. Amoxicillin was effective only against the sensitive strain, whereas linezolid doses of 10 mg/kg or greater produced cure rates above 72% versus both strains. Linezolid efficacy was associated with ear fluid (or plasma) drug levels that provided an AUC_0–24 h/MIC greater than 30, a T > MIC above 42% of the dosing interval, and a C_{max}/MIC ratio greater than 3.1. A similar study (470) demonstrated that, for penicillin-sensitive *S. pneumoniae,* doses of amoxicillin (>2.5 mg/kg) resulting in ear fluid concentrations = 1.4 μg/mL or serum concentrations greater than the MIC for = 14% of the dosing interval were effective in resolving clinical signs and reducing bacterial CFU.

A rat model of otitis media with obstruction was used to profile the inflammatory/immunological response of the ear mucosa to infection with *S. pneumoniae* (270). At various time points postinfection (1 hour to 112 hours), mucosa and effusion fluid were removed, and the mRNA and/or protein levels of IL-1β, TNF-α, IL-6, IL-10, IFN-γ, TGF-β, MCP-I, IL-8, and MIP-2 were determined. On days 1 and 2 postinfection, most of the cytokines/chemokines were detectable. mRNA expression demonstrated the following patterns only in infected ears: early expression, IL-1β, IL-8; late expression, TNF-α, IFN-γ; and biphasic, MCP-1, IL-6, TGF-β. Importantly, this study also showed that up-regulation of cytokine mRNA was not always accompanied by increased protein expression.

Using a model of mixed infection with *S. pneumoniae* and *H. influenzae* (544), amoxicillin/clavulanate and cefuroxime were evaluated as treatment by stratifying the gerbils according to the presence of effusions. Mixed infections had lower effusion rates than AOM due just to *H. influenzae,* and treatment of otitis media with effusions was more difficult. Additionally, the mixed infection model was treatable, but more than 80% of the animals developed culture-negative otitis media with effusions. Furthermore, AOM models have been used to demonstrate the potential of antibiotic treatment to promote a protective immune response (605) and immunization (483). Initiation of penicillin treatment early in *S. pneumoniae* infection in chinchillas produced greater inflammation than late treatment (515). The addition of dexamethasone to antibiotic treatment reduced the structural damage associated with this infection as compared with antibiotics alone (467). However, treatment of experimental AOM in gerbils with antibiotics plus acetaminophen delayed eradication of *H. influenzae* as compared with antibiotics alone, possibly due to a reduction of phagocyte recruitment to the site caused by the antiinflammatory agent (471). In comparing mixed *S. pneumoniae* and *H. influenzae* with mono-infection by *H. influenzae,* it was demonstrated that the exact characteristics of AOM or OME in models depends, at least in part, on the time from the appearance of clinical symptoms until the diagnosis/intervention, on the bacteria involved, and on previous antibiotic treatment. Furthermore, poorer eradication rates occurred with lower levels of inflammation, and PK/PD relationships in middle ear fluid provide better predictive value than serum PK/PD parameters (544). These models have also used β-lactamase–positive *H. influenzae* (478).

Animal Models of Meningitis

Animal models of bacterial meningitis have been considered extremely useful in delineating the pathophysiology of meningitis and elucidating optimal antibiotic and adjunct therapies.

Mouse Models of Meningitis

An increasing number of studies using mouse models of meningitis have been performed recently, in particular with the use of gene-modulated knockout mice. Mice have been infected with various pathogens (e.g., *S. pneumoniae, N. meningitides,* group B streptococci, *E. coli, H. influenzae,* and *C. neoformans*) and using three different routes of inoculation (systemic [641], intracisternal [170], and intracerebral [428]). These models primarily involve evaluating survival and to some degree brain histopathological alterations and have been useful in the study of antibiotic therapy efficacy, adjunctive therapy, and the pathophysiology of meningitis.

Rat Models of Meningitis

A model for the induction of *H. influenzae* type b meningitis in infant rats, which appears to be both simple and reproducible, has been described (424). Five-day-old rats were inoculated intranasally with *H. influenzae* type b, and bacteremic rats and rats with meningitis were identified by sampling of the cerebrospinal fluid (CSF). The rats were sacrificed, the skin and soft tissue over the cisterna magna were removed by dissection for exposure of the dura, and the cisterna magna was entered by puncturing the dura with a sterile dissecting needle. This model system provides a simple method for determining the effectiveness of antibacterials in an acute meningitis infection similar to that seen in human infants (424). However, it apparently has not received much attention as a model for evaluating antibacterial therapy (but see reference 502).

An excellent infant rat model for studying survival, brain damage, and learning deficiency has been described (349). This model, which uses intracisternal inoculation of group B streptococci and *S. pneumoniae,* seems to be able to induce histopathological alterations that mimic the findings in human meningitis and has provided significant knowledge about the pathophysiology of meningitis. Less brain damage seems to develop in the adult rat model of pneumococcal meningitis, but it has been very useful in the study of cerebrovascular alterations, CSF and brain tissue cytochemistry, and hearing loss (324). Because of the limited access for repetitive CSF sampling, the rat meningitis model and the mouse meningitis model have only been used sporadically for the study of antibacterial PKs (168). Excellent technically orientated reviews of the infant rat (591) and adult rat (568) meningitis models are available.

Rabbit Model of Meningitis

The optimal model for studying the PKs and PDs of antibiotics in CNS infections seems to be the rabbit meningitis model, which provides a controlled system for testing antibacterial penetration and efficacy in inflamed and normal CSF (123). Rabbits have been challenged with various pathogens (e.g., *S. pneumoniae, N. meningitides, S. aureus, H. influenzae,* and enterobacteria). The rabbit model allows simultaneous and repetitive sampling of CSF and blood, and it is therefore very useful in kinetic studies of CSF bacterial killing and CSF cytochemistry (463), though less useful in the study of brain damage and survival. For more than 20 years, the rabbit model has yielded considerable information about the PKs and efficacy of antibacterials as well as the pathophysiology of meningitis. The efficacy of antifungals has also been studied using a rabbit model of *C. neoformans* (312a); an excellent technical review of this model has appeared previously (575). Surgical intervention is required to attach a prosthesis to the rabbit's skull, facilitating immobilizing of the deeply anesthetized animal. Blood samples (normally 1–3 mL) and simultaneous CSF samples (normally 0.1 to 0.2 mL) can be collected at frequent intervals (e.g., 0, 2, 4, 6, and 8 hours after initiation of therapy). The rate of removal of CSF should not exceed the rate of its synthesis (approximately 0.4 mL/hour [546]). In this manner, the antibacterial levels in both the blood and CSF and the bactericidal or bacteriostatic titers were determined. This model provides a controlled system for testing antibacterial penetration and efficacy in inflamed and normal meninges (519).

This model yields considerable information about the PKs and efficacy of antibacterials. In one study (392) using the basic model system described, the PK profile and bacteriological efficacy of a single dose or continuous infusion of six antibacterials (penicillin, cefoperazone, ceftriaxone, cefuroxime, moxalactam, and chloramphenicol) were determined in two infections (*S. pneumoniae* and *H. influenzae*). The PK results following continuous infusion allow a comparative determination of the penetration of the antibacterial into the CSF of infected animals. It is evident that the rabbit meningitis model system can provide a great deal of information about the activity of different agents in a very difficult infection. The extrapolation of the results in rabbits to efficacy in humans has generally been good, with one or two exceptions (184).

Animal Models of Infectious Endocarditis

Experimental endocarditis in rabbits and rats has been well studied and been shown to be reliable for the evaluation of the pathogenesis of the disease and the effectiveness of antibacterials (41,73,88,173,258); it is considered highly predictive of the clinical situation. Technical aspects of the rabbit model and some examples of the type of data that can be obtained have been well described (347). Essentially, a polyethylene catheter is inserted into the right carotid artery and advanced toward the heart; after it crosses the aortic valve, it is secured in place by suturing at the site of insertion. The presence of a catheter in the heart results in the development of sterile vegetations consisting of small, rough, whitish nodules 1 to 2 mm in size, usually at points of contact between the catheter and the endocardium. The sterile vegetations were infected by a single injection of bacteria into an ear vein: *S. epidermidis, S. aureus, C. albicans, P. mirabilis,* and *Pseudomonas aeruginosa,* among many other strains, have been used in this model. This basic approach has also been applied to rats (173,512a).

Combinations of antibiotics in most cases are required to effectively treat endocarditis clinically, and this has been largely predicted by animal models (342). In the study by Batard et al. (35), *in vitro* checkerboard assays and time-kill curves showed an indifferent response by various *S. aureus* strains (with different antibiotic-resistance mechanisms) to the combination of quinupristin-dalfopristin and gentamicin. Using a rabbit endocarditis model and simulated human PK, the authors found no benefit from the combination *in vivo,* a result predicted by the *in vitro* testing. An *in vitro* infection model, which uses simulated endocardial vegetations, has been shown to produce results similar to these of the rabbit model when the PK parameters are known (273). Recent studies have used animal models for evaluating prophylaxis, including the use azithromycin or ampicillin (572) and trovafloxacin or ampicillin (313) for *Streptococcus oralis* infection and azithromycin or vancomycin for MRSA (572).

Inflammation of the heart valves occurs in human and experimental endocarditis. The rabbit model was used to evaluate possible benefits of adjunctive dexamethasone regarding the course of experimental aortic valve endocarditis and the degree of valve tissue damage. Using a methicillin-resistant strain of *S. aureus*, researchers found that combining low-dose dexamethasone with an effective dose of vancomycin had no effect on survival, the blood culture sterilization rate, or the valve bacterial CFU. Dexamethasone adjunct treatment did reduce the inflammation and structural damage to the valves; this study also was able to demonstrate an inverse correlation between neutrophil number in vegetations and degree of tissue damage (534).

Animal Models of Eye Infections

Experimental eye infections have received much attention for the evaluation of antiinfective therapy. Animal models of keratitis, endophthalmitis, and eye injury and conjunctivitis are available (485). Technical descriptions of the rabbit model of conjunctivitis (421) and the mouse model of bacterial keratitis (317) have been provided.

Experimental Keratitis

Keratitis can be established by inoculation of the surface of an eye of an anesthetized animal damaged by scratching the surface with a syringe needle (e.g., a 26-g needle) or by direct injection into the cornea. For therapeutic studies, antibacterial therapy by a parenteral or topical (or combined) route could be started within 24 hours after infection. Topical treatment usually is frequently applied to the surface of the eye or administered by less frequent (often only once) intravitreal injection. Normally the concentration of antibiotic in the aqueous humor correlates more closely with therapeutic efficacy than does the concentration in the cornea. Although many antibacterials can extensively reduce the number of bacteria in the cornea, typically by more than 99% in the first 24 hours of therapy, sterilization of the cornea is difficult and may require several additional days of continuous therapy (317).

P. aeruginosa mutants with a lipopolysaccharide core and O antigen defects exhibit reduced viability after internalization by corneal epithelial cells, and a complete core lipopolysaccharide is required for full epithelial invasion (187). Despite effective antibacterial therapy, disease resolution can be delayed with respect to the time of bacterial eradication (346). Ofloxacin (mammalian-cell penetrable) and tobramycin (less cell permeable) have been tested against invasive and noninvasive *P. aeruginosa* in a mouse model of keratitis. Topical ofloxacin and tobramycin, with or without prednisolone acetate, were administered hourly as eye drops for 12 hours postinfection. Tobramycin was less effective than ofloxacin against the invasive strain, but in the other groups, antibiotic treatment was effective against both strains. However, despite effective antibacterial treatment, disease progression continued in all groups, and differences in responses to treatment were not manifest until day 7 (346).

A model of *S. aureus* keratitis after lamellar keratectomy has been described (487). A lamellar flap was created in rabbits using a microkeratome, and an infection was initiated by placing a suspension of *S. aureus* under each flap. The stromal bed was irrigated with 0.3% ofloxacin, with or without additional topical ofloxacin, and topical ofloxacin alone. All regimens were shown to be effective and of low toxicity to the eye, but the combination of topical and stromal bed irrigation treatment was most effective. Lysostaphin appears in this model, being effective against MSSA and MRSA when administered early (4 to 9 hours postinfection), but it loses effectiveness when treatment is delayed (10 to 15 hours) (136,137). Antibodies to lysostaphin appear not to inhibit its activity (138).

Experimental Intraocular Infections

Several methods to obtain reproducible intraocular infections in laboratory animals have been described, and many are modifications of the method discussed here (391). In this method, *S. aureus, E. coli,* or *P. aeruginosa* is inoculated into the center of the rabbit cornea, the anterior chamber, or the vitreous of the eye, and samples of the vitreous humor, irises, and anterior chamber as well as the retina are used to determine the progress of the infection.

The authors (391) found that, when 3×10^6 CFU/0.2 mL of broth were inoculated into the corneas, anterior chamber, and vitreous of rabbit eyes, a virulent panophthalmitis was produced within 24 to 48 hours, and destruction of the eye took place within 72 hours regardless of the site of inoculation. When 5×10^3 CFU/0.2 mL were inoculated into the corneas, anterior chambers, and vitreous, a panophthalmitis resulted in 72 hours. The infections were most severe following intravitreal inoculations and less intense when the anterior chamber was the site of inoculation. When 7×10^2 CFU/0.02 mL were used as the inoculum, the infections were eliminated in the corneas and anterior chambers within 24 hours but not in the vitreous. The anterior chambers were most resistant, the cornea slightly less, and the vitreous the least resistant to virulent infection.

Infectious endophthalmitis is characterized by an inflammatory reaction in a sensitive, normally immune-privileged or protected tissue. Depletion of circulating neutrophils by i.v. administration of specific antibody at 6 or 12 hours after intravitreal injection of *S. aureus* into rats resulted in diminished neutrophil influx, lower and delayed clinical and histopathological evidence of disease, but also a reduction in bacterial clearance from the eye (235). The inflammatory response appears to lag behind bacterial growth of either *S. epidermidis* or *P. aeruginosa,* for a maximum in the number of microorganisms was reached earlier than the influx of leukocytes (320). In *S. epidermidis* endophthalmitis, the number of microorganisms reached a maximum at day 2 after intraviteral inoculation and then declined spontaneously; clinical scores were the worst on day 5 but poor scores persisted in the absence of detectable bacteria. In *P. aeruginosa* endophthalmitis, the number of microorganisms reached a maximum 36 hours after inoculation, and bacteria were detectable for 15 days.

Ravindranath et al. (489) measured the immune response during endophthalmitis. Rats received an intravitreal injection of viable *S. epidermidis* that resolved by day 14. The inflammatory cell content of the vitreous switched from neutrophilic to monoctytic-macrophagic/lymphocytic by day 3 postinfection. B cells (CD45+/CD3−) were also detected, and IgM and IgG antibodies but not IgA antibodies to glycerol teichoic acid were found in the vitreous of injected eyes; IgM antibodies declined by day 7 postinfection. Anti-GTA IgM was observed in vitreous and serum, anti-GTA IgM antibodies were significantly elevated, but a weak IgG response and no IgA response were observed in serum *S. epidermidis*–infected rats (489).

The use of adjunct antiinflammatory agents in endophthalmitis is controversial. Intravitreal vancomycin once plus 7 days of i.m. methylprednisolone was not as effective as vancomycin alone in reducing ocular inflammation and improving retinal function in experimental *S. aureus* endophthalmitis (625). Using a variety of antibiotics in an animal model of *S. aureus* endophthalmitis, researchers found that the combination of vitrectomy and injection of intraocular vancomycin was the most effective regimen and that no improvement resulted from administering adjunct i.v. corticosteroids (85a). The timing of dexamethasone treatment appears to influence outcome (626). Bilateral eye *S. aureus* infection in rabbits was treated once with vancomycin in one eye and vancomycin plus dexamethasone in the other at 24, 36, 48, or 72 hours after intraviteral infection. Early combination treatment (at 24 or 36 hours) produced reduced ocular inflammation as compared with antibiotic alone, but only when treated at 36 hours postinfection did the combination group preserve retinal function better than vancomycin alone; no treatment was able to eradicate infection. However, intravitreal vancomycin and dexamethasone combined did produce a superior outcome than vancomycin alone against MRSE (543) and against *S. pneumoniae* (469). When combined with intravitreal levofloxacin, intravitreal dexamethasone treatment of *S. epidermidis* infection did not affect the clinical scores, but dexamethasone appeared to preserve the ocular architecture (624); this study demonstrated the impact of early treatment on outcome.

Many studies have evaluated the PK of antibiotics in eye tissue. PK modeling of antibiotic eye-blood barrier penetration data has been used to compare different formulations (219) and explain in part why eye penetration in rodents may overestimate antibiotic penetration due to the dependence of larger species on convective fluid flow (617). A single intravenous administration of 5 or 20 mg/kg moxifloxacin demonstrated good penetration into the vitreous, but apparently the penetration was dose-independent and increased when inflammation was present (76). Microdialysis has been used to both measure drugs (e.g., ceftazidime [595] and vancomycin [196]) and dispense drugs (594). Inflammation or eye trauma appears to increase the penetration and residency of many topically applied antibiotics (e.g., levofloxacin [624]; ofloxacin [464], ciprofloxacin [465], and vancomycin [85a]), but apparently not ceftazidime, whose half-life is decreased by inflammation and eye surgery (85a). A 1% vancomycin hydrochloride ophthalmic ointment was administered to the corners of the eyes of rabbits with *Bacillus subtilis* infection. Vancomycin reached effective concentrations in the aqueous humor and extraocular tissues but was not detected in the aqueous humor, iris-ciliary body, vitreous, or serum in uninfected animals; nonetheless, the presence of inflammation permitted concentrations to reach potentially therapeutic levels in these tissues (218).

Systemic treatment with moxifloxacin demonstrated effectiveness against MRSA and MSSA (76), as did treatment with trovafloxacin against *S. epidermidis* (431); this is somewhat surprising, as most antibiotics show poor ocular penetration. Despite inflamed eyes demonstrating improved penetration of i.v. gentamicin or amikacin, aminoglycoside levels in the eye failed to reach therapeutic concentrations sufficient for either *Pseudomonas* spp or *S. epidermidis* (174). However, systemic administration of sparfloxacin, pefloxacin, or imipenem (though not vancomycin or amikacin) was effective as a prophylaxis against intravitreal *S. aureus* challenge (388). Combined topical and oral ofloxacin (465) or ciprofloxacin (464) increased the ocular levels of the drug in a model of posttraumatic endophthalmitis due to *S. aureus* infection (465). Topical treatment with liposomal formulation increased the half-life of fluconazole (256) but was inferior to free fluconazole in the treatment of *C. albicans* endophthalmitis (257; see also 468). Intravitreal treatment with vancomycin plus amikacin was effective against vancomycin-sensitive *E. faecalis,* and intravitreal ampicillin plus gentamicin was effective against vancomycin-resistant *E. faecalis* endophthalmitis (101). Replacement of the vitreous with gas has been studied as an adjunct treatment for *S. aureus* endophthalmitis (383).

Animal Models of Osteomyelitis

Although of relatively low incidence, bone and joint infections are difficult to cure, largely due to limited penetration of antibiotics, coupled with the fact that slow-growing or adherent bacteria are likely to be more resistant to antibiotics. Furthermore, designing and executing clinical trials is difficult due to the likelihood of low recruitment, the heterogeneity of the disease, and the many hard-to-control factors influencing treatment outcome. Consequently, advances in clinical management have heavily relied on the contribution of animal models (131).

The experimental conditions for the rabbit model initially described by Norden (437,438) have recently been reviewed (369). In one study using this procedure, 89% or more of the animals developed osteomyelitis (437,438). The infecting organism was recovered from 91% of rabbits sacrificed 60 to 180 days after infection. If blood samples were taken 6 hours after infection, more than 80% were positive for the infecting organism, but by 24 hours less than 20% were positive. Injection of a bacterial suspension or sodium morrhuate alone did not cause osteomyelitis, as evidenced by radiologic examination or culture of the bone. Antibacterial therapy was initiated 1 to 14 days after infection. Because the radiologic changes of chronic osteomyelitis were present at day 14, treatment at this time was considered to represent therapy of chronic osteomyelitis.

The rat is another commonly used animal for osteomyelitis (455). This model is widely used for experimental chemotherapy, and the practical aspects of this model have been previously described (498). Occasionally overlooked, it is critical to culture at least some remaining crushed bone, initially in broth with subculture on agar plates, in order estimate bone sterility. Typically, single agents are weakly active, and combination chemotherapy generally produces superior results (168a). Serum C_{max}/MICs for ciprofloxacin, pefloxacin, vancomycin, and rifampicin were tested, and the results were 3.40, 6.05, 10.55, and 25.20, respectively. Bone C_{max}/MICs for ciprofloxacin, pefloxacin, vancomycin, and rifampicin were approximately 1.70, 4.15, 2.25, and 38.20, respectively. Although not rigorous, the change in CFU/g bone was correlated with serum C_{max}/MIC ($n = 4$, $r = 0.976$, $p = 0.0245$; Pearson [168a]). More thorough determinations of PK/PD relationships for osteomyelitis are warranted.

These models have also been used to evaluate various drug delivery systems (e.g., a sulbactam-cefoperazone polyhydroxybutyrate-co-hydroxyvalerate depot formulation [620], several depot formulations [331], tobramycin pellets [430], tobramycin fibrin sealant [370], and antibiotic-impregnated hydroxyapatite [532], as reviewed in 309), hyperbaric oxygen combined with antibiotics (401), and adjuvant treatment with GM-CSF (555). An interesting study performed by Nijhof et al. (435) demonstrated that combined tobramycin bone cement and systemic cefazolin was superior to monotherapies, suggesting that combining local and systemic treatments might be a useful approach to treatment of osteomyelitis. Furthermore, this study demonstrated the utility of measuring bacterial DNA, as persistence of DNA may occur despite effective treatment.

Animal Models of Mycobacterium Infections

Models of Disseminated *Mycobacterium avium* Infections

Models of disseminated *M. avium* infection have usually used beige mice (bearing an *Nramp1* mutation), although alternatives include C57BL/6 mice (109), hamsters (622), and immunosuppressed, cyclosporine-treated rats (approximately 0.03 mg cyclosporine/kg [79a]). Reviews of the technical aspects of the beige mouse model of *M. avium* infection have been published (135,226,627).

Several details of the model have been described (e.g., the influence of the route of infection) (225–227). Infections are initiated by intravenous injection of large inocula (10^7 to 10^8 CFU). Although the disease is usually nonfatal, high numbers of *M. avium* are found in the liver, spleen, and lung, and determination of the efficacy of treatment is accomplished by ascertaining the organ bacteria loads. Furthermore, mild chronic CNS infection develops in the mice during sustained systemic *M. avium* infection, similar to what has been reported in most human cases. In one study, *M. avium* was detected initially in the parenchyma of the choroid plexus but also in the ventricles and meninges. However, the mice did not develop clinical signs, nor did they die due to CNS involvement (613). Iron restriction inhibits the *in vitro* and intramacrophagic growth of *M. avium*, and mice fed an iron poor diet experienced reduced *M. avium* proliferation; administration of iron chelators had small effects, as they impacted little on the iron status of mice (240).

In some studies, the beige mouse model demonstrated poor outcome against *M. avium* in the testing of marketed antibiotics (539a). Note that *in vitro* tests do not always accurately predict *in vivo* susceptibility (54). Although previous reports indicated a benefit to infected mice, administration of recombinant G-CSF failed to improve the course of *M. avium* infection in C57Bl/6 or beige mice and did not enhance the activity of the combination of clarithromycin plus ethambutol plus rifabutin (241). A rather extensive combination of antimicrobials was tested by Fattorni et al. (193). The activity of 18 anti–*M. avium* regimens was evaluated. Mice were treated with clarithromycin, ethambutol, amikacin, rifabutin, ciprofloxacin, or clofazimine alone or in combination. Monotherapies were less effective than combinations, and resistant *M. avium* emerged. Some two-drug combinations were active, but none more than clarithromycin alone. The triple combination of clarithromycin, amikacin, and ethambutol was the most effective (193). Moxifloxacin is active against *M. avium* in combination with other agents (53).

Animal Models of *Mycobacterium tuberculosis* Infections

Although animals have long been used to model tuberculosis for experimental chemotherapy, until recently, with the resurgence of tuberculosis (including multidrug-resistant tuberculosis) and the dramatically increased incidence of atypical mycobacteria infections, there has been comparatively little new research to evaluate antibiotic therapy. Experiments involving animal infections with *M. tuberculosis* strains should be carried out in a level-three facility (262a,419). The guinea pig is the historic model for *M. tuberculosis* infections but has been largely supplanted by inbred mice models.

Mouse Model of Tuberculosis

The mouse model of tuberculosis for use in the profiling of new anti–*M. tuberculosis* chemotherapy has been previously reviewed (461) and the technical details and nature of the experiments described (460). Although intravenous infection has been used, the method of choice is aerosol infection, with mice inhaling about 50 bacilli into their lungs. Depending on the virulence of the strain, the bacteria will experience a 4–7 log increase in 20 to 30 days (460).

In a modification of one model, the infection was produced by injection of *M. tuberculosis* H37Rv at a level such that 20 to 21 days after infection all mice died. The compounds to be tested were administered to the mice either subcutaneously or orally by gavage or in a medicated diet, with the mice allowed to feed *ad libitum* from waste-proof mouse feeders. The effectiveness of compounds can be determined in one of two ways: median survival time or 50% effective dose (in mg/kg) (335). A modification of this model induces a dormant *M. tuberculosis* infection (154). Two weeks after intravenous infection, mice are provided antibiotic-supplemented food in such quantities that 25 mg/kg/day isoniazid and 1000 mg/kg/day pyrazinamide are administered for 8 or 14 weeks; this treatment renders the lungs of the mice culture-negative for *M. tuberculosis,* but after a prolonged time on antibiotic-free food, pulmonary infection reemerges. Curative or additional prophylaxis treatments (including vaccination [154]) can be evaluated using mice as hosts.

Mitchison (403) has offered some important comments on the treatment of experimental *M. tuberculosis.* With multidrug combinations, the possibility of drug-drug interaction must be considered. It is known that interactions with isoniazid (and metabolites) can occur and that drug absorption can be altered by coadministration of several compounds (e.g., rifampicin [155]). Careful control of blood (and tissue) PK is essential to ensure no deleterious interactions are occurring, interactions that may in part explain antagonistic results. The iron status of the mice can affect treatment outcome (362). For example, the activity of isoniazid was reduced (and the bactericidal activity of ethambutol was eliminated) in iron-loaded and female BALB/C mice as compared with iron-normal mice. Perhaps surprisingly, relative to other infections, the PK/PD relationships for antimicrobials effective against *M. tuberculosis* are not understood precisely. Using an aerosol infection model, serum AUC/MIC seems to be the best indicator of the activity of rifampicin, with serum C_{max}/MIC and T > MIC also being strong predictors of outcome (286). An interesting model of recrudescence of infection has been described (459).

Animal Models of Sexually Transmitted Diseases

Animal models of human sexually transmitted diseases are problematic, in that the causative microorganisms display a high level of specificity for infections in humans. Consequently, the course of the disease in animals at best only partly mimics that seen in humans.

Disseminated Gonococcal Infection in Mice

In vitro organ culture has been used to demonstrate that sub-MIC levels of antibiotics inhibit adherence of gonococci to rabbit mysentery (285). Subcutaneous chambers in mice (16) or guinea pigs (151,316a) have also been used. The study described in reference 316a demonstrated that *in vitro* growth of *Neisseria gonorrhoeae* under iron-restricted conditions increased virulence (316a). Subcutaneous chambers in rabbits have been used as a system to evaluate the effectiveness of ampicillin against gonococci *in vivo* (175).

Mice have been traditionally considered resistant to gonococcal infection (290), despite some early reports on establishing models (e.g., 323). A mouse model for disseminated gonococcal infections using a gonococcal strain (N24) isolated from a human genital tract has been described (119). This strain was mouse serum–resistant and penicillin-sensitive but predominantly of the T2 colony morphology, which is apparently the morphology associated with human gonococcal infection. For infection, the gonococci were prepared in a combination of 15% mucin and 4% hemoglobin and injected intraperitoneally into 7- to 8-week-old CAW:CF-1 female mice. The mice were monitored for 4 to 7 days after infection. Sublethal infection produced local peritonitis and transient bacteremia, but with larger inocula the local peritoneal infection progressed to fatal septicemia.

Recently, some measure of success has been achieved with mouse models of *N. gonorrhoeae* vaginal infection. A mouse model has recently been established (287) and subsequently used for the study of vaccination efficacy against gonococcal vaginal colonization (476). Mice in diestrus are pretreated with estradiol to facilitate colonization of gonococci and are inoculated intravaginally. Gonococci can be recovered from vaginas for approximately 8.5 days after inoculation from unvaccinated mice and for 4 days from vaccinated mice. Interestingly, a functional MtrCDE multidrug efflux system, but not a functional FarAB-MtrE system, enhances experimental gonococcal genital tract infection in female mice (288). So far, this model has apparently not been used to test antibiotics.

Syphilis in Rabbits and Other Animals

A rabbit model involving dermal lesions caused by *Treponema pallidum* has been used to evaluate the effects of cefetamet on experimental infection (200). Two weeks following intradermal infection with *T. pallidum,* when infection was either subclinical, just clinically evident, or well developed, rabbits received a single intramuscular dose of 23,000 units/kg penicillin G or 1, 15, or 30 mg/kg cefetamet, and the progress of the skin lesions was monitored, as was dissemination of the infection to the CSF; the two higher doses of cefetamet were comparable to the treatment with penicillin G. Ceftizoxime is also comparable to penicillin G (332).

Venereal and congenital syphilis has been described in Syrian hamsters following intraperitoneal or intradermal injection of 10^5 to 10^7 CFU *T. pallidum* subsp *endemicum* (306,307). Symptoms of infection in adults include skin and peroral lesions and, following dissemination of infection, enlarged lymph nodes and thymic atrophy; *T. pallidum* can be demonstrated in lesions and lymph nodes. Infection of females either just before conception or during pregnancy results in the infection of the fetuses (306). Offspring demonstrate rhinitis, skin rash, failure to thrive, and hepatosplenomegaly; *T. pallidum* can be demonstrated in the liver, spleen, and nasal secretions. This model has apparently not been used to evaluate antibiotic therapy. A similar model using guinea pigs has been described (605a). Guinea pigs demonstrate strain-dependent sensitivity to infection (50% infective doses: CD4, 10^2 CFU; Albany strain, 10^9 CFU). Intradermal or intravenous infection 1 to 3 months prior to conception results in an asymptomatic infection; persistence of *T. pallidum* in offspring was inferred by the development of a vigorous humoral immune response and infectivity of guinea pig tissue for rabbits.

Central nervous system syphilis can be induced in rabbits following the intracisternal injection of 10^7 CFU of *T. pallidum* (387). Although apparently self-limiting, in that *T. pallidum* cannot be demonstrated in the brain tissue of rabbits 12 weeks after infection, this infection is accompanied by slowly progressing and self-resolving CSF pleocytosis and ocular involvement (uveitis develops in 6% of infected animals). This model has apparently not been used to evaluate antibiotic therapy.

A model of syphilis in the hamster has also been described (4,5). A *T. pallidum* preparation is injected into the dermis of hamsters in the inguinal region. Skin lesions develop, and the infection spreads to the regional lymph nodes. Penicillin (above 2500 U/kg administered once) and clarithromycin (above 12.5 mg/kg once per day for 6 days) were effective in reducing lymph node contamination below the limit of detectability, while vehicle controls had abundant *T. pallidum* (approximately 2.3×10^6 per lymph node).

Chlamydial Genital Tract Infections

Chlamydia trachomatis is a major cause of sexually transmitted disease worldwide. Although antibiotics are effective in treating infection, reinfection is common. A review from 1982 describes the early *Chlamydia* animal models and their generally poor success (409). Genital inoculation of C3H/He mice with *C. trachomatis* was used to test roxithromycin in a model of acute chlamydial salpingitis (633a). The goal was to determine the efficacy of roxithromycin in preventing irreversible inflammatory damage leading to tubal infertility. Although roxithromycin was effective against *C. trachomatis* in the mouse genital tract, loss of fertility was only partially prevented, and the drug's activity was reduced with delay of treatment.

Intravaginal inoculation of progesterone-treated mice resulted in transient infection with *C. trachomatis* MoPn (42). Vaginal swabs became culture negative after 28 days, but serum antibody titers persisted longer, and upper genital tract inflammation-mediated damage occurred in more than 80% of the animals. Minocycline, doxycycline, amoxicillin-clavulanate, and azithromycin were effective agents when treatment commenced 1 or 7 days postinfection. Early treatment (1 day postinfection) prevented the elevation of antibody titers, in contrast to delayed therapy. Early treatment with amoxicillin-clavulanate or low-dose azithromycin was slightly less effective. Delayed dosing impaired minocycline activity but did not affect the outcome of treatment with amoxicillin-clavulanate; doxycycline and azithromycin were highly effective in restoring fertility. Despite the transience of the infection, murine models of *C. trachomatis* can be used for evaluating chemotherapy.

With the aim of vaccine development, Su et al. (552,553) reported successful treatment of transient infection in progesterone-pretreated mice. They utilized a model of direct vaginal infection that, when left untreated, resolves in about 21 days, following which the mice become resistant to reinfection, likely due to the formation of vigorous CD4(+) T-helper type 1 (Th1) cell-mediated immunity (552). Doxycycline promotes faster rates of elimination of *C. trachomatis,* but its effectiveness is lost somewhat with delay of treatment initiation (38). Although promoting faster resolution of infection of genital tissue and preventing upper genital tract disease (hydrosalpinx), doxycycline-dependent eradication of chlamydia inhibits the development of protective immunity; delayed treatment corresponds with a stronger immune response involving serum IgG, local IgA, and an antigen-specific splenocyte response typical of a Th1 response (552,553). Mice that develop an adequate immune response are resistant to reinfection. Mice that receive early doxycycline intervention are more susceptible to reinfection than those receiving delayed treatment (553).

Animal Models of Peritonitis

Peritonitis can be established in animals either by direct intraperitoneal infection of fecal material (often encased in gelatin capsules) or by puncture of the cecum to provide a focus of infection. These models have been reviewed previously (516).

Intraperitoneal Inoculation

A rat model for simulating intraabdominal sepsis, either with known organisms or with mixed fecal flora cultures, has been developed by Onderdonk et al. (602). A uniform inoculum was prepared from the pooled cecal and large bowel contents of 15 rats that had been maintained on a diet of lean ground meat and water for 2 weeks. The value of this mixed infection model for evaluating agents for effectiveness in preventing mortality and the formation of intraabdominal abscesses was confirmed as follows. Groups of rats were administered clindamycin (80 mg/kg), gentamicin (8 mg/kg), or a combination of both antibiotics intramuscularly every 8 hours for 10 days, starting immediately after implantation. The clindamycin-gentamicin combination reduced mortality rates and the formation of the abscesses, whereas either drug alone reduced mortality rates (gentamicin) or abscess formation (clindamycin) but not both (602).

Cecal Ligation and Puncture

The cecal ligation and puncture (CLP) model has been described for both mice (533) and rats (167). The description given by Hyde et al. (281) is typical of this approach to induction of lethal peritonitis in animals as a model of postsurgical sepsis. This model is amenable to chemotherapy with a variety of antibiotics and biological response modifiers. Combination immunotherapy with soluble tumor necrosis factor receptors plus interleukin 1 receptor antagonist decreases mortality in the CLP model (495). However, the cautionary suggestions by Eichaker and associates (171) need to be heeded when using this model, as it is apparent that more severe sepsis, which is usual for the model, benefits best from chemotherapeutic intervention but may not represent a typical clinical presentation.

The CLP model has been used to evaluate some parameters concerning the differential sensitivity of internal organs to damage during sepsis (614). Increases in microcirculatory permeability were greater in the lung than in the liver 12 hours after CLP, and increases in water mass fraction were greater and occurred earlier in the lung than in the liver. The CLP model has been used to evaluate cardiovascular responses during sepsis characterized by an early hyperdynamic phase followed by a late hypodynamic phase (621). Mice made septic by CLP demonstrated hypotension and a hyperdynamic state that could be monitored using manometric catheters and echocardiography and could be modulated with fluid resuscitation and antibiotics (275).

The administration of the antioxidant phenyl *N*-tert-butyl nitrone (PBN) (150 mg/kg 30 minutes after CLP), followed by the antibiotic imipenem (10 mg/kg 1 hour after CLP), significantly increased survival compared with other single treatment groups. However, the increase in survival found in the PBN plus IMP–treated group was abrogated by anti-IL-10 antibody, indicating that endogenous IL-10 is an effective protective factor (333).

Animal Models of Infected Abscesses

Abscess Formation in Mice

The technical aspects of intraabdominal abscess models have been presented previously (77).

As an example of the formation of abscesses by anaerobes, a model of subcutaneous abscesses in mice caused by *Bacteroides fragilis* has been described (295). Among the advantages of this model are that host factors involved in abscess formation can be studied and that the PK properties of the antimicrobial agents, especially penetration of the abscess, can be assessed. Both the inoculum size and the time of treatment significantly altered the effectiveness of both clindamycin and cefoxitin. At an inoculum of log 7.2 and with treatment beginning at 1 hour postinfection, clindamycin (85 mg/kg) reduced the infection CFU/abscess by log 6.1, and cefoxitin (400 mg/kg) by log 7.4. Delaying treatment to 24 hours reduced the effectiveness of treatment (clindamycin, -1.0 log CFU/abscess; cefoxtin, -0.9 log CFU/abscess). This activity could be related to the PK properties of each antimicrobial. Peak drug levels were measured: clindamycin, 16 ± 2 μg/mL serum, 6.6 ± 1.2 μg/mL abscess fluid (ratio 2.4); cefoxitin, 93 ± 6 μg/mL serum, 15 ± 1.4 μg/mL abscess fluid (ratio 6). In a larger experiment, the rank order of antibiotic efficacy could clearly be determined and related to the peak levels of antimicrobials in serum and abscesses (295).

A model of intraperitoneal abscess formation by *S. aureus* has been described (311).

Animal Models of Gastrointestinal Infections

As with sexually transmitted diseases, animal models of gastrointestinal tract infections are hampered because of the apparent specificity of the causative pathogens for humans, particularly in the case of *Helicobacter* infections.

Clostridium difficile Enterocolitis

Diarrhea following antibiotic chemotherapy can be caused by *C. difficile* and is referred to as *pseudomembranous colitis* or *antibiotic-associated colitis* (549). Proliferation of *C. difficile* following suppression of normal gastrointestinal flora results in an enteric intoxication owing to the release of toxins from *C. difficile*. Current standard treatments include vancomycin (125 to 200 mg/kg orally four times per day) or metronidazole (250 to 500 mg/kg orally four times per day) (379,549,589). Golden Syrian hamsters have often been used to model this disease because they have the causative organism as part of their normal flora, are known to succumb to antibiotic-induced colitis (31,32), and are sensitive to the activity of *C. difficile* toxins (364). Typically, clindamycin (0.8 to 100 mg/kg intraperitoneally or subcutaneously once) is administered, and death attributed to *C. difficile* (by virtue of culture and detection of toxins) ensues rapidly (up to 100% mortality within 1 week), though it is dependent on the clindamycin dose. Modifications of this model include the orogastric infection of clindamycin-treated hamsters with axenic *C. difficile* (4×10^5 spores/clindamycin-treated hamster [606]). Modulation of the diet of hamsters can alter the extent of *C. difficile* disease. As compared with hamsters fed a normal fat and cholesterol diet, hamsters fed an atherogenic (defined high-fat) diet have increased susceptibility to *C. difficile* (62).

Peptidic antibiotics (e.g., vancomycin) appear to be efficacious in this model, but most must be given continuously because regrowth of *C. difficile* occurs following cessation of treatment (162). Following p.o. clindamycin treatment and inoculation with a toxigenic *C. difficile* strain, hamsters developed *C. difficile*–associated ileocecitis and 3 days later were treated with intragastric nitazoxanide (30 to 150 mg/kg), vancomycin (50 mg/kg), or metronidazole (150 mg/kg). All three compounds inhibited the appearance of *C. difficile* gastroenteritis symptoms, but upon treatment cessation, the hamsters relapsed, indicating failure to eradicate *C. difficile*. In a prophylactic mode, only nitazoxanide produced hamsters free of clinical symptoms, histopathology, or residual bacteria (394). *C. diffcle* is affected *in vitro* by sub-MIC levels of antibiotics that establish conditions that precipitate disease (e.g., amoxicillin, clindamycin, cefoxitin, and ceftriaxone) and those antibiotics used for treatment of established infection (vancomycin and metronidazole). The sub-MIC effects are, however complex, strain-dependent and affect both bacterial growth (increasing lag time and overall growth rate) and the timing of initiation of toxin production (faster initiation of production). These effects were observed with clindamycin, metronidazole, and amoxicillin, rarely with vancomycin, and never with cefoxitin (163). However, the *in vivo* significance of the sub-MIC effects remains to be determined.

Models of *Helicobacter* Gastric Infection

The association of *Helicobacter pylori* with gastric ulcers and gastritis has dramatically altered approaches to gastroduodenal disease to now include antimicrobial chemotherapy as a therapeutic modality (345). Normal laboratory animals apparently are difficult to colonize with *H. pylori* but are more susceptible to the related species *H. felis* and *H. mustelae*. Development of a suitable animal model has delayed evaluation of novel antibacterial strategies because *in vitro* antimicrobial susceptibility is apparently not consistently predictive of *in vivo* efficacy (345). Some models have used predisposition of the animals with acetic acid to induce a gastric ulcer, followed by orogastric inoculation; *H. pylori* is capable of efficiently colonizing these heavily damaged areas. Marchetti et al. (384) presented evidence suggesting that passage of clinical *H. pylori* isolates in the gastrointestinal tracts of mice selects for those bacteria with increased colonizing ability while maintaining several of the features of the disease in humans.

Various models have demonstrated that combination chemotherapy is more effective than monotherapy in eradicating *Helicobacter* organisms from gastric tissues. Except for treatment with metronidazole, monotherapy and dual therapies involving amoxicillin, bismuth subcitrate, and clarithromycin (with or without the proton pump inhibitor omeprazole) did not cure mice bearing *H. pylori* Sydney strain gastric infection (587). The triple therapies of OMC (omeprazole, metronidazole, clarithromycin) and BMT (bismuth subcitrate, metronidazole, tetracycline) were more successful in eradicating infection. However, these treatments also produced a different pattern of stomach colonization, suggesting the antrum-body transitional zone is a "sanctuary site" harboring *H. pylori* in cases of treatment failure. The authors concluded that there was good correlation between the Sydney strain mouse model and antibiotic therapy outcome in humans (except for metronidazole monotherapy and OAC triple therapy).

Combination treatments involving proton pump inhibitors or anti-ulcer agents have been evaluated in animal models. The apparent synergic anti–*H. pylori* effects of the proton pump inhibitor lansoprazole are apparently due to enhanced penetration of orally administered amoxicillin in gastric mucus and tissue by lansoprazole-produced increased intragastric pH. Supplemental treatment of rats with clarithromycin did not affect this drug interaction (177). Using a C57BL/6 mouse model, the cytoprotective anti-ulcer agent plaunotol was shown to enhance the activity of clarithromycin or amoxicillin in the treatment of *H. pylori* infection (328).

Animal Models of Infections in Cancer Patients (Infections in Tumor-Bearing Animals)

Cancer patients are more susceptible to infection by virtue of underlying disease as well as severe immunosuppression due to cytotoxic chemotherapy. Development of animal models of infection in tumor-bearing mice received some attention but has not been thoroughly pursued in more recent years. Apparently, there are tumor line– and infecting strain–dependent differences in susceptibility changes caused by tumor growth. Early studies suggested that, as compared with non-tumor-bearing mice, mice bearing L1210 leukemias were similarly susceptible to thigh infections with *C. albicans,* but the presence of tumor rendered mice more susceptible to *C. albicans* infection via the intravenous route (293). Immunosuppression by MethA sarcomas and consequent increased susceptibility to systemic *L. monocytogenes* infection follows an apparently complex pattern over time: decreased resistance occurs soon after subcutaneous tumor implantation, but in tumor-bearing mice resistance increases after 35 days. Adoptive transfer of splenic macrophages from tumor-bearing mice apparently increases resistance to *L. monocytogenes* (436).

In contrast, ascites fluid from tumor-bearing mice promotes resistance to infection with *L. monoctyogenes* (557). Mice bearing sarcoma 180 or MM146 tumors have increased circulating lymphocytes and increased resistance to intravenous *C. albicans* infection (450). Ehrlich ascites tumor promotes the rapid growth of *S. aureus* located in the tumor tissue (427). Recent experimentation demonstrated that the presence of sarcoma 180 tumors delayed mortality due to *Aspergillus fumigatus* sepsis, apparently because of a tumor-dependent reduction of serum iron levels and an increase in serum iron-binding capacity, restricting pathogen growth (450).

Tumor-bearing mice have also been used to profile antiinfective treatment. Mice bearing sarcoma 180 tumors were used to profile the cephamycin antibiotic MT-141, demonstrating it to be superior to cefmetazole and cefoxitin but similar in potency to latamoxef in terms of reduction of liver, spleen, and kidney CFU following intravenous infection with *Proteus morganii* (316). In an extensive multifactorial experiment, mice were injected with P388 leukemia cells intraperitoneally and *K. pneumoniae* intratracheally to establish a model of serious pneumonia in cancer patients (561). Mice were treated with antibiotics (trovafloxacin, ciprofloxacin, or cefazolin) and the immunostimulator G-CSF, with or without anticancer therapy (danorubicin). Tumor presence decreased resistance to infection and reduced the effectiveness of antibiotics. The addition of rG-CSF to trovafloxacin improved outcome in the absence of antitumor therapy. The inclusion of danorubicin promoted the effectiveness of antiinfective therapy, with trovafloxacin being the best therapy, but unlike ciprofloxacin, rG-CSF did not promote the effectiveness of trovafloxacin.

Animal Models for Determining the Effect of Age on Susceptibility to Infection

Age predisposition to infection, in particular the effect of old age on infection, has been long studied. Although many factors are likely to be involved, the focus of research has been on age-related decline in immune function, including both the innate immunity component (e.g., neutrophils [360] and lymphocytes [458]) and the acquired immunity component (559). Pneumonia appears to be the major infection affecting the elderly (194), although immunosenescence is apparently generalized. Animal models of age predisposition are well known, but it is unclear if all studies are carefully controlled for underlying disease, which has been recognized clinically as an important factor (229) and can have serious consequences for data interpretation if not controlled for (14). Antibiotic treatment of the elderly requires careful attention because of their decreased toleration of antibiotics and the increased chance of drug interactions due to concomitant chemotherapy of other diseases (194,353); the elderly also have altered antibiotic PK (194,353).

Young mice may also show differences in susceptibility to infection. In the surgical neonate, infection is a major cause of morbidity and mortality, with relative risk decreasing with age. Lally and Stonum (338) investigated whether there is an age-related susceptibility to intraabdominal abscess formation in C57BL/6 mice. The mice were administered *E. faecalis* and *Bacteroides distasonis* with wheat bran adjuvant intraperitoneally (40 mg/mL injected at 8 μL/g mouse), and intraabdominal abscesses were counted after 7 days. Ten-day-old mice had a similar incidence of abscesses (81%) as adults (91%), but there was a decline from 10 days until weaning (38%). Using newborn (1-day-old) C3H/HEN mice, intraperitoneal injection of *E. coli* was used to evaluate the role of TNFα and IL-10 treatment in neonatal sepsis. The infective inoculum was carefully titrated to produce 30% to 50% mortality, similar to the clinical rate. Anti-TNFα antibody therapy improved survival, but IL-10 at a dose of 25 ng did not. This suggests that the inflammatory response of newborns may be distinct from that of adults (337). A model of neonatal infection with group B streptococci (GBS) has been described by Roewald et al. (501).

Age-related susceptibility to intraperitoneal infection with GBS strain M781 was seen within the first 5 days of life, and infection was made manifest by a rapid increase in bacteremia and clinical and histopathological signs. Passive immunotherapy of pregnant adult mice with rabbit anti–type III GBS polysaccharide passively protected 100% of the offspring. Whereas 8-month-old mice (LD_{50} log 6.6 CFU) appear to be most resistant to mortality produced by *L. monocytogenes* infection, resistance declines with increasing age (24-month-old mice, LD_{50} log 5.2); furthermore, 1-month-old mice appear to be most susceptible (LD_{50} log 4.2). However, for the first 2 days postinfection, the *in vivo* growth rates of *L. monocytogenes* were similar in mice of all ages, suggesting a similar capacity exhibited by the innate mechanisms of antibacterial resistance. After this time, mice showed an age-related decline in bacterial numbers in the spleen and liver. This suggests that the age-related decline in the capacity to acquire specific antibacterial immunity can account (in part) for the increased susceptibility to infection. Old mice demonstrate increased susceptibility to *M. tuberculosis* owing to a decreased capacity to generate mediator T lymphocytes (459). An interesting model of the recrudescence of *M. tuberculosis* has been described (460). Mice exposed to a low, nonfatal aerosol dose of *M. tuberculosis* Erdman at 3 months developed massive infection, to which they succumbed after about 20 months. The capacity of the old mice to maintain acquired immunity to infection declined with age, allowing reemergence of *M. tuberculosis*. Ashman et al. (21) describe a model of old-age predisposition to *C. albicans* infection that involves immunizing one group of CBA/CaH mice at 6 weeks of age and then comparing the susceptibility of previously immunized and nonimmunized mice to subsequent infection. A normally sublethal challenge of systemic candidosis was administered at 16 months of age. Aged nonimmune mice showed rapid progression of the disease, with a marked increase in the number of mycelia in the brain and kidneys and early morbidity. Aged immune mice showed no morbidity after challenge, and both colonization and tissue damage were reduced in comparison with the aged nonimmune animals.

Senescent (24-month-old) mice demonstrated increased sensitivity to CLP sepsis as compared with mature (12-month-old) mice (281). However, 2- to 3-month-old and 19- to 22-month-old Swiss Webster mice showed similar rates of abscess formation following intraperitoneal infection of *B. fragilis* with sterile feces adjuvant (100% and 81%, respectively), similar responses to trovafloxacin (75 mg/kg as the prodrug alatrovafloxacin intraperitoneally 4 times per day for 10 days starting 1 day postinfection; 94% and 73% cure rates), and similar serum trovafloxaxin PK (μg/mL C_{max}, 5.1 and 5.8, respectively; μg/h/mL AUC, 11.7 and 12.4, respectively) and abscess trovafloxacin PK (μg/g C_{max}, 27.1 and 25.0, respectively; μg/g/mL AUC, 204 and 143, respectively). Similar studies were carried out by Turnbull et al. (576).

Fever, which may affect the outcome of infection (e.g., dramatic restriction of the growth of *H. influenzae* during experimental meningitis [457]), can be delayed and reduced in old animals. During experimental *E. coli* peritonitis in rats, the onset of fever was delayed (onset at 2.8 hours for 3-month-olds, 3.9 hours for 12-month-olds, and 5.8 hours for 24-month-olds) and suppressed in older animals (518). Adenylate cyclase activity in brown fat tissue (both receptor and postreceptor stimulated) was reduced in old animals.

TOLERABILITY OF ANTIBIOTICS IN LABORATORY ANIMALS

In comparison with other disease areas (e.g., cancer), anti-infectives are generally exceedingly well tolerated within a wide therapeutic window (the difference between the dosage required for maximal desired pharmacological effect and the dosage at which unwanted effects become apparent). This is likely in part due to the drug substance being directed to targets unique to microorganisms or distinct from mammalian counterparts. Preclinical *in vitro* and *in vivo* toxicity/tolerability testing of novel antibiotics is required prior to initiating clinical trials (34), and although this will reveal toxic effects, they generally occur at doses far in excess of those required for efficacy studies in animal models. There are five main types of toxicity associated with antimicrobials (381): direct effects, where the molecule acts against the host tissues (e.g., anemia caused by chloramphenicol is inhibition of mitochondrial protein synthesis); hypersensitivity, which can include allergic responses (e.g., anaphylactic reaction) or other nonallergic reactions such as diarrhea; disorders resulting from antibiotic-produced changes in bacterial flora (e.g., vaginal yeast infections); drug interactions, where coadministered drugs interact deleteriously together (e.g., ketoconazole interference with cytochrome P450–mediated drug metabolism); and microbial lysis, with the associated massive release of proinflammatory bacterial products that can cause widespread tissue damage, as occurs in bacterial meningitis.

An excellent overview of the use and tolerability of some older (but still clinically used) antibiotics in laboratory animals has been prepared by Morris (418). Experience has indicated that guinea pigs and to a lesser extent rabbits tolerate antibiotic treatment much less well than mice or rats. There are species and strain differences in tolerability to antibiotics (301). Strain is critical to the tolerance of certain compounds; for example, tobramycin is more toxic to Fischer rats than to Sprague-Dawley rats (418). Mice show strain differences in susceptibility to the toxic effects of chloramphenicol (198). Qualitative and quantitative strain differences were observed in the hematological response to chloramphenicol succinate (500–2500 mg/kg administered orally for 7 days). When administered to several inbred mice strains (C3H/He, CBA/Ca, BALB/c, and C57BL/6) and one outbred strain (CD-1), the inbred strains were more susceptible to the toxic effects and produced more variable results. Only the inbred strain developed leukopenia, despite the fact that all strains displayed reticulocytopenia and anemia. The toxicity of chloramphenicol is apparently due to minor metabolites, which may vary due to subtle differences in the metabolism of chloramphenicol, and the levels of antioxidants (e.g., glutathione and vitamin E) may account in part for the differences in tolerability (276).

In a broad sense, animals tolerate drugs better than humans, and in most efficacy studies tolerability issues are not revealed; often relevant effects are simply not observed by the experimenter or the study plan does not facilitate their being observed. This may partly be due to inherent physiological properties of the animal that result in faster elimination of the compound (or deleterious metabolites) from the body, generally short treatment courses because of the fulminant nature of the infection, and the masking of tolerability problems by the symptoms of the infection. Additionally, the psychobehavioral nature of the animal may mask the toxicity of the antibiotic. Anatomical and physiological differences—for example, differences in the gastrointestinal tract resulting in different degrees of exposure, rates of absorption and total fraction of drug absorbed, and drug transit time—may affect tolerability as well as efficacy (312). Antibiotic treatment of rats will change the gastrointestinal bacterial flora and/or composition of the feces but may have little effect on transit time (97). Due to their coprophilic nature, antibiotic treatment of pregnant rats and the resultant changes in intestinal microflora lead to abnormal gastrointestinal flora in suckling rats along with the establishment of potential pathogens in the gastrointestinal tract (80); the same study also found that antibiotic treatment had less impact on skin and vaginal microflora than on gastrointestinal tract microflora (80).

The nephrotoxicity of antiinfectives in animals is often the result of proximal tubule damage, which is related to its relative size and the drug concentration-time profile, the latter being the sum of the effects of drug movement across the lumen and the contraluminal secretory transport processes (574). These processes can be profoundly different in different species. Enhanced renal excretion by rats with streptozotocin-induced diabetes reduces cephaloridine renal toxicity due to higher renal excretion rates (producing lower kidney cephaloridine levels) than normal rats (581); serum PK profiles were similar.

Macrolides possess potential arrhythmogenic properties. The PKS/PDS of the prolongation of the Q-T interval by clarithromycin, roxithromycin, erythromycin, and azithromycin has been determined from electrocardiograms (ECGs) in rats (446). Compounds were administered by infusion in order to override the different PK properties of these compounds and produce controlled serum levels. The data for clarithromycin and erythromycin fit an E_{max} model whereas the data for roxithromycin and azithromycin fit better a linear model. The order of potency of the compounds was erythromycin > clarithromycin > azithromycin > roxithromycin. Futher, the Q-T–prolonging activity of erythromycin and clarithromycin occurred at serum concentrations required for antibacterial effect, whereas such activity occurred only at supraantibacterial levels for azithromycin and roxithromycin.

Norfloxacin was also tested for central nervous system effects in rats. The PK/PD profile was monitored using an electroencephalogram in order to arrive at a PK/PD relationship for norfloxacin (96). Rats received 5 mg/kg norfloxacin over 30 minutes, and the EEG demonstrated a pattern suggestive of eliptogenic potential; in addition, PK/PD modeling indicated that longer diffusion times have a greater eliptogenic potential (96).

Many factors contribute to the tolerability of animals to antimicrobial agents (418). Age, which affects metabolic enzymes and renal function, is another factor. Given that most laboratory animals are nocturnal, time-related functions, such as metabolic rates, food and water intake, and sleep time/activity, may also alter the tolerability (and effectiveness) of antibiotics; for example, exercise can alter the PK profile of mice. The single most important mechanism of antibiotic toxicity in small animals is disruption of the normal bacterial flora. In guinea pigs and hamsters, antibiotic toxicity leading to death is very often due to overgrowth of *C. difficile* and consequent toxin release (418), although *L. monocytogenes, C. perfirngens,* and *C spiroforme* have all been implicated as mediators of toxicity. Induction of overgrowth appears to be most prominent with some macrolides, notably clindamycin and lincomycin. Allergic reactions *senso stricto* do not readily occur in lab animals, and the typical "allergic response" of guinea pigs to penicillin is likely due to enteric overgrowth. Newborn and germ-free guinea pigs are not susceptible to enterocolitis, suggesting the lack of a true allergic response (418). This may also be the case with many of the antibiotics given to laboratory animals.

Commonly, tolerability to compounds is reported without data presentation. Occasionally, some objective measure of tolerability is included. For example, Van Etten et al. (586) reported the maximally tolerated dose of amphotericin B in different formulations and determined renal and liver toxicity based on blood chemistry measurements. Additionally, in rats with subcutaneous staphylococcal abscesses, daptomycin was superior to vancomycin in treating both MSSA and MRSA. No detectable renal damage was elicited by daptomycin. The combination of daptomycin and tobramycin produced less renal injury (as determined by function tests and histology) than tobramycin alone (608). Rarely has observation of the extent of well-being of the experimental animal (i.e., the sum of illness due to infection, toxicity due to the drug substance, and relief from symptoms of infection due to antimicrobial effect) been included in the study design. Radiotelemetry was used to monitor a panel of physiological indices to devise a "sickness behavior" index, which was then applied by Bauhofer et al. (37,38) to monitor the response to antibiotics with or without G-CSF in parallel with more classic indicators of the CLP model such as fever and mortality. Their study indicated a mild improvement from combined treatment over antibiotics alone, prompting their suggestion that the sickness behavior index could serve as the equivalent of a human quality-of-life index.

EVALUATION OF ANTIBODY-BASED THERAPIES IN ANIMAL MODELS OF INFECTION

Use of antibodies has a long history in the therapy of infectious diseases. Polyclonal antibodies, monoclonal antibodies, antibody fragments (Fab), antibody dimers, and antiidiotypic antibodies have been evaluated in experimental models that have, in some instances, led to clinical investigations. Some examples of the testing of antibodies in infection models follow.

Antibodies directed at the core region of bacterial lipopolysaccharide (LPS) have received the most experimental attention. Animal models have usually experienced rapidly fulminant sepsis following parenteral (usually intravenous or intraperitoneal) administration of large numbers of bacteria (or LPS) in a variety of species (e.g., mice, rats, and baboons; for reviews, see references 40,66,120,134,484). Antibodies specific for certain LPS subtypes have also been tested (340,449). Such models should be used with caution, because they may represent models of overwhelming intoxication rather than true infection models mimicking the clinical situation (134).

Interestingly, anti-LPS antibodies may function in other ways besides neutralizing endotoxin. Anti-J5 antisera is raised against *E. coli* and is reactive for LPS. However, anti-J5 also reacts with outer membrane proteins (OMPs) that bind LPS. Incubating the anti-OMP J5 antisera with serum from recovering septic rats indicated that antibody reacts with three outer membrane protein–LPS complexes, especially an 18-kDa OMP. Although considered by many specific to circulating LPS, the anti-J5 antiserum may protect, in part, by reacting with outer membrane proteins (271).

Combinations of passive microbial-directed antibodies and antibiotics have a long history; in 1939, Powel and Jamieson (482) published data on the use of rabbit antipneumococcal antiserum and sulfapyridine in a rat model of *S. pneumoniae* infection. Studies evaluating the combination of such antibodies with antibiotics have also been performed (503). Other examples have utilized antibodies to LPS plus antibiotics in experimental sepsis models (antiflagella plus sparfloxacin [448], anti-LPS plus sparfloxacin [447], antiflagella plus carbapenem or aminoglycoside [577], and anti-LPS plus ciprofloxacin [111]). Combinations of antibodies against microbial antigens (e.g., antibodies against multiple LPS serotypes [340]) or specific anti-LPS antibody, anti-LPS core antibody (antibody J5), and anti-TNF antibody (133) have also been tested in animal models of sepsis.

Using intraperitoneal administration of mouse polyvalent anti–*S. pneumoniae* antisera, researchers demonstrated a beneficial effect of antiserum alone against *S. pneumoniae* sepsis, but they found a dramatic improvement occurred when antiserum was combined with amoxicillin or cefotaxime, as measured by reduction in the minimal antibiotic dose required (91). When combined, the minimally effective antibiotic dose was above the MIC for 3% (amoxicillin) or 5% (cefotaxime) of the dosing interval, as opposed to that occurring in the absence of antiserum (26% and 32% for amoxicillin and cefotaxime, respectively). Locally delivered, prophylactic pooled human polyclonal antibodies (1 mg/mouse) and systemic ceftazidime (0.44 mg/mouse) demonstrated improved outcome (decreased bacteria in wound tissue, reduced bacteremia, and increased survival) in *P. aeruginosa* burn wounds in mice. Monotherapies or combinations involving systemic antibody administration were ineffective (195). Anti–*P. aeruginosa* LPS O-side chain IgM Mab (complement-activating, opsonophagocytic), in combination with ceftazidime, synergistically reduced bacterial density in the thigh muscle of normal and neutropenic mice, as compared with controls or monotherapies (3). Exotoxin A is a major virulence factor of *P. aeruginosa,* and it has been shown that antibodies specific for the exotoxin of *P. aeruginosa* or directed against synthetic peptides encompassing the major epitopes of exotoxin A can be protective to septic mice when administered along with amikacin (176).

EVALUATION OF CYTOKINES AS THERAPEUTIC AGENTS IN ANIMAL MODELS OF INFECTION

Cytokines are (glyco)proteins produced by various cell types (predominately leukocytes) that act as signaling molecules by inducting an intracellular signal cascade via specific cell-surface receptors. Owing to their immunomodulatory properties, their potential therapeutic value in the promotion of resistance to infection has been extensively studied. In the therapy of infectious disease, some cytokines are thought to be largely deleterious when present in high concentrations, particularly systemically (thus necessitating diminution of their activity), and others are thought to be beneficial to the host (implying that supplementation with the specific factor would promote resistance to disease). The therapeutic/prophylactic potential of these proteins has been mostly evaluated in systemic infection models, but models of peritonitis (cecal ligation and puncture), infected burn wounds, pneumonia, foreign body infection, and meningitis have also been used. Most studies have demonstrated that cytokine therapy needs to be initiated prophylactically or early in the infection process in order to demonstrate suitable efficacy (but see ref. 149). Some studies have been done on the use of G-CSF in combination with antibiotics in sepsis models (37,452). Among other findings, it has been discovered that prophylactic IL-2 is protective in the sepsis model due to *E. coli* or *P. aeruginosa* (102), prophylactic IL-1 protects mice against endotoxemia (310), prophylactic G-CSF is protective in postoperative infection (361), IL-10 inhibits mortality and improves overall antibiotic activity in the CLP model (333) and endotoxemia (341), the combination of soluble TNF receptors plus IL-1 receptor antagonist decreases mortality during experimental sepsis (495), and the combination of fluconazole and IL-1 has a beneficial effect on systemic candidiasis in neutropenic mice (336).

DETERMINATION OF THE *IN VIVO* POSTANTIBIOTIC EFFECT

PD parameters such as the rate of bactericidal activity with increasing drug concentrations, the postantibiotic effect (PAE), sub-MIC effects, postantibiotic leukocyte enhancement, and the first-exposure effect more accurately describe the time course of antimicrobial activity than the MIC and MBC (126). The PAE is the persistent inhibition of bacterial growth after a brief exposure to an antibiotic. Most easily demonstrated in the *in vitro* systems, this effect is observable *in vivo* (127,129,130,189,255,367,402,592,593,634), although it is complicated by compounding sub-MIC effects (e.g., the postantibiotic sub-MIC effect [PASME]; 90,442–446,462) and by the enhancement of the phagocytic activity of leukocytes that occurs during the PAE phase and is partially due to sub-MIC effects on bacteria; this effect is termed the postantibiotic leukocyte effect (PALE) (e.g., aminoglycosides and quinolones demonstrate a longer *in vivo* PAE in the presence of neutrophils [127,129,130]).

The PAE may be nonexistent or of varying duration depending on the compound class and target bacterium (126,127). Typically, β-lactams and cephalsporins produce a substantial PAE against streptococci, but a small PAE or none at all against Gram-negative bacteria, although there are exceptions (e.g., imipenem against *P. aeruginosa*) (376). Nucleic acid synthesis inhibitors and protein synthesis inhibitors (notably the aminoglycosides) produce an *in vivo* PAE with many bacteria (e.g., streptococci and Gram-negatives). An *in vivo* PAE occurs with staphylococci treated with many different antibiotics. Furthermore, the use of humanlike PK prolongs the duration of the PAE *in vivo*. Indeed, the expected duration of the PAE (in combination with sub-MIC effects or the PALE) can be incorporated into estimates of clinical treatment regimens (12,60,130). However, Fantin et al. (189) found neither the duration of the PAE *in vitro*, nor the MIC, nor bactericidal activity *in vivo* correlated with the duration of the *in vivo* PAE.

The following are critical for defining the presence and duration of a PAE: the specific microorganism-antimicrobial combination, the antimicrobial combination and the experimental conditions, including the antimicrobial concentration and the length of the antimicrobial exposure (548,635). The PAE is probably also affected by the density of bacteria, their growth rate and metabolic activity, and the extent of inflammation at the site of infection (230). Proposed mechanisms by which the PAE occurs include both nonlethal damage induced by the antimicrobial agent and a limited persistence of the antimicrobial agent at the bacterial binding site (548).

Determination of the PAE *in vivo* is complicated by sub-MIC effects on the bacteria, which can suppress growth and have other physiological effects that contribute to a composite PAE *in vivo* (462). The PA SME is the growth suppression that may occur when a low concentration of antibiotic (typically $\leq 0.3 \times$ MIC) is in the presence of bacteria previously exposed to a suprainhibitory concentration. As low levels of antibiotic are likely still at the infection site at the time of the next treatment, the PA SME probably reflects the *in vivo* situation more closely than the PAE (126,127).

Taken together, dissection of the various components of the protracted effects of drug near the end of the treatment interval, where drug levels fall to the sub-MIC level of activity and then fall still further to the "true" postantibiotic level, is complicated. Required groups include immunocompromised (leukopenic) and immunocompentent animals (to control for the PALE), PK measurements of bloodstream and infected tissue (to determine the duration of the sub-MIC levels and identify the initiation of the "true" PAE phase) in both groups of animals (to control for the influence of neutrophil influx on PK properties), and perhaps a group treated with an antibiotic-inactivating enzyme to further control for sub-MIC effects. Furthermore, groups treated with antibiotic producing a humanlike PK profile would be desirable. With so many groups being followed over time, the mouse thigh infection model is most frequently used for determination of the PAE.

The capability of producing a long PAE facilitates therapy using those antibiotics (e.g., aminoglycosides) to be administered infrequently, and continuous or frequent administration is required for those compounds that lack an *in vivo* PAE (e.g., β-lactams) (635). Extending the dosing interval of an antimicrobial agent that has a PAE has several potential advantages, among them reduced cost, less toxicity, and better compliance among outpatients receiving antimicrobial therapy (126–128,433,520).

IMPACT OF PRETREATMENT INTERVAL ON ANTIMICROBIAL EFFICACY

It is fairly well established that severity of clinical infection, usually associated with a delay in presentation or diagnosis, is related to treatment failure, particularly in the case of neutropenic patients (278,363). Delay in beginning antimicrobial therapy, and hence progression of infection, has been demonstrated to have profound effects on the outcome of antibiotic treatment of experimental infections; however, this issue has not yet been thoroughly studied.

Using the thigh infection model in both leukopenic and normal mice, Gerber et al. (232) found that the age of infection had a profound influence on the outcome of antibacterial therapy of *P. aeruginosa* infection using gentamicin, ticarcillin, and ceftazidime. Antimicrobial treatment was started 0, 1, 2, 4, 6, 8, or 10 hours after infection, and the bacteria were growing exponentially *in vivo* during this entire time period (neutropenic mice: 0 hour, log 6 CFU/g muscle; 10 hours, log 8.5 CFU/g muscle, delta log 2.5 CFU/g muscle; normal mice: 0 hour, log 7 CFU/g muscle; 10 hours, log 8.5 CFU/g muscle; delta log 1.5 CFU/g muscle). The antibiotics were administered to attain humanlike PK (32 mg/kg gentamicin, single bolus; 1000 mg/kg ticarcillin or 225 mg/kg ceftazidime, fractionated dosing), but prolonged serum levels were observed in mice whose treatment was initiated after more than 10 hours, likely due to the influence of shock. Despite sufficient supra-MIC/MBC serum concentrations of antibiotics, delay in gentamicin treatment for 4 hours (normal mice) or 6 hours (leukopenic mice) abrogated the bactericidal effect of the drug, and a delay of more than 2 hours (ticarcillin) or more than 4 hours (ceftazidime) resulted in only bacteriostatic activity of these antibiotics.

Several factors were proposed to account for these observations:

- Alteration of the physiology of the bacteria (e.g., alteration to nongrowing or slowly growing phenotypes typically more resistant to antibiotics or production of an extracellular matrix inhibitory to antibiotics). Note, however, that in the study by Gerber et al. (232), *P. aeruginosa* grew at a constant rate during the entire infection, and therefore slow growth cannot be the only contributing factor.
- The presence of an *in vivo* correlate of the inoculum effect observed *in vitro*. In this case, bacteria within clusters or microcolonies may be protected from the effects of antibiotics or antibiotics may poorly penetrate these foci.
- Pathophysiology at the site of the lesion, resulting in reduction of the activity of antibiotics. For example, low pH and low oxygen at the infected site are nonoptimal for aminoglycosides, and there is reduced penetration of antibiotics in large cardiac vegetations in advanced endocarditis (132).

The effect of delay in treatment of experimental pneumonia due to *S. pneumoniae* with temafloxacin was studied in a mouse model (25). Temafloxacin was administered at 50 mg/kg every 12 hours for 3 days beginning at various times postinfection. The activity of temafloxacin decreased with delay of treatment initiation: survival rates were 100%, 92%, 81%, and 50%, for treatments beginning at 18, 48, 72, and 96 hours postinfection, respectively. However, when C57BL/B6 mice infected with anthrax spores from a doxycycline-sensitive strain were treated with doxycycline, delay in treatment initiation had little effect on survival. Whereas initiation of doxycycline (1.5 mg/kg intraperitoneally once) at 4 hours postinfection was effective (90% survival), initiation of treatment at 24 and 48 hours had no substantial effect on mortality rates, although the onset of death was delayed to 4 days in the 24-hour treatment group and to 2–3 days in the 48-hour treatment group and the control group (308). As death from anthrax infection occurs due to toxin production, it is not surprising that a delay in treatment initiation past a threshold point would have a very small impact on outcome.

DETERMINATION OF *IN VIVO* GENE EXPRESSION IN BACTERIA GROWN IN ANIMAL MODELS OF INFECTION

Determination of Pathogen Presence by DNA Abundance Resulting from PCR

Owing to the very high degree of genetic diversity between pathogenic microorganisms and their hosts, gene amplification techniques have long been used as tools for the clinical diagnosis of infection and the monitoring of the decline of pathogen DNA within humans in response to antimicrobial therapy (582). PCR technologies have also been used as tools for epidemiology and detection of antibiotic resistance. However, their use in the study of infection in animal models has not received much attention. In this case, DNA (host and microbial) is extracted from tissue, and PCR amplification of a pathogen-specific gene is performed. Determination of the residual presence of *B. burgdorferi* by detection of the genes encoding the outer membrane proteins OspA and OspB was strongly correlated with *in vitro* culture of the organism from infected tissues and has demonstrated the effectiveness of ceftriaxone (16 mg/kg every 12 hours for 5 days) in treating infected mice (378). PCR amplification of mitochondrial rRNA of *Pneumocystis carinii* has been used to detect the presence of this organism in the lungs of immunosuppressed rats. PCR strongly correlated with microscopic detection methods and was used to determine the effectiveness of treatment with pentamidine (10 mg/kg subcutaneously 3 times a week for a total of 5, 7, or 18 doses) and co-trimoxizole (250 mg/kg orally every 24 hours for a total of 10, 21, or 42 days) beginning 6 weeks after the start of immunosuppression (451). Amplification of the dihydrofolate reductase gene of *P. carinii* has also been used to monitor the progress of infection in immunosuppressed rats (527). Bowman (71) used PCR to detect *A. fumigatus* during experimental infection. Nijhof et al. (435) measured bacterial DNA during the course of treatment of experimental osteomyelitis, but concluded that the utility of measuring bacterial DNA may be limited due to the persistence of DNA despite effective treatment.

Determination of Genotype Changes in Bacteria Grown *In Vivo* in Animal Models of Infection

The Southern blotting technique has been used to demonstrate genetic rearrangements of the chromosome of *P. aeruginosa* during growth *in vivo* in a model of chronic pulmonary infection in rats (611). During the course of persistence within the lung, *P. aeruginosa* demonstrated a shift from a nonmucoid phenotype to a mucoid one that was associated with a decline in the production of exoenzymes by such bacteria cultured *in vitro*. DNA extracted from the lung isolates grown *in vitro* was subjected to Southern blotting to detect the genes encoding exotoxin A, exoenzyme S, phospholipase C, and elastase and the *algD* gene. This procedure demonstrated that phenotypic change to a mucoid phenotype due to growth *in vivo* was associated with a chromosomal rearrangement upstream from the exotoxin A gene; the other genes studied were of identical size and apparent abundance compared with those of the nonmucoid *P. aeruginosa* used to inoculate the animals (611).

Determination of *In Vivo* Gene Expression in Bacteria Grown in Animal Models of Infection

Growth of bacteria *in vivo* is associated with a phenotypic change to allow adaptation to the *in vivo* environment (395). A novel molecular biology–based technique has been developed that allows identification of genes expressed only *in vivo* (86,372,373,542). This technique has been used to identify five genes expressed *in vivo* during *S. typhimurium* infection of mice (denoted *ivi* for *in vivo*-induced) (372,373). A modification of this technique utilizes the gene for chloramphenicol acetyltransferase as the selection gene, with chloramphenicol treatment of mice infected with transformed *S. typhimurium* as a selection stress (371).

An additional modification of this technique relies on the *in vivo* expression (i.e., being under the control of a bacterial promoter functioning *in vivo*) of the enzyme resolvase (tnpR), which results in the excising of an antibiotic resistance gene present between two DNA sequences recognized by this enzyme. This procedure was used to examine the *in vivo* expression of *igA* (the gene encoding the major iron-regulated outer membrane protein) in *Vibrio cholerae* (86). The authors used this procedure to demonstrate that irgA is not expressed when *V. cholerae* is growing either in the intestinal tract of infant mice or in ligated rabbit ileal loops but is expressed when growing in the peritoneum of mice, suggesting that only the latter site provides an iron-restricted environment; control experiments confirmed the excision of *tet* during growth *in vitro* under conditions of iron limitation (86).

A set of genes is specifically activated during the establishment of a biofilm both *in vitro* and *in vivo* (583). The expression of genes associated with growth as a bioflim were evaluated *in vitro* and *in vivo* using an animal model of foreign body infection. The kinetic pattern of gene expression would indicate that the initial colonization process involves the *ica* gene product, whereas *atlE* was needed for persistence in a biofilm (583).

Moxifloxacin treatment of rabbits with *S. aureus* endophthalmitis was also monitored by RT-PCR in order to determine the *in vivo* expression levels of *luk*-PV (Panton-Valentine leucocidin), *hlgCB* and *hlgA* (γ-hemolysin), *sarA* (staphylococcal accessory regulator), *agr* (accessory gene regulator), and *sigB* (virulence gene regulator) in *S. aureus* growing in the vitreous humor (76). Expression of bacterial genes in the vitreous humor demonstrated that infection was associated with increased levels of *luk*-PV, *hlgCB, sarA,* and *agr* and that a larger increase of *sigB* and *gmk* provides products required during the entire process of biofilm formation. One hour posttreatment with an effective dose of moxifloxacin, a slight decrease occurred in the expression of leucotoxin mRNA and the mRNA encoding the virulence regulatory factors *sarA, agr,* and *sigB*. Moxifloxacin penetrated the eye well (serum into eye, AUC-based, 27% to 46%) and was effective at killing *S. aureus*.

In vivo, in the lungs of C57BL/6 mice, *M. tuberculosis* produces mRNAs associated with iron limitation, alternative carbon metabolism, and cellular hypoxia, genes not normally expressed *in vitro* (564); such genes were also detected in the lungs of tuberculosis patients, but the mouse model and human clinical samples did not always coincide.

Other studies determining *in vivo* expression of genes include *Vibro cholerae* (262) and *S. typhimurium* (298).

Determination of Host Response to Infection

PCR, ELISA, and Western blotting have been used to determine gene expression in infected tissues. Immunohistochemistry has also been used, and this technique has the advantage of providing information on the location of the protein of interest within the site of infection and of identifying of the producing cell type. Immunohistochemistry on frozen lung sections was used to evaluate the distribution and expression of CD40, its ligand CD40L, and the related cytokines IL-12, TNFα, IFN-γ, and TGFβ-1 in mouse lungs during slowly progressing primary tuberculosis (407,599). Further studies delineating the differences in the distribution and expression of these products between mouse strains reveal A/J mice to possess elevated cortisol levels as compared with C57BL/6 mice (2). Again using a bioluminescent PCR method, the differences in pulmonary cytokine responses, possibly linked to serum cortisol levels, indicated that the cytokine pattern produced in the lungs of A/J mice would result in an environment that would not facilitate a protective Th1-type response.

ELISA was used to determine the kinetics of cytokine presence following experimental rat endophthalmitis due to *S. aureus* (236). TNFα, IL-1β, cytokine-induced neutrophil chemoattractant (CINC), and IFN-γ were maximal in vitreous fluid at 24 hours postinfection, but whereas

TNFα, IL-1β, and CINC declined by 48 hours, IFN-γ persisted, not declining until 72 hours postinfection. This shift in the cytokine complement reflected a shift in the composition of the cellular component, which was neutrophil dominated until 48 hours, then shifting to become a more balanced neutrophil-monocyte/macrophage infiltrate.

A rat model of otitis media with obstruction was used to profile the inflammatory/immunological response of the ear mucosa to infection with *S. pneumoniae* (270). At various time points postinfection (1 hour to 112 hours), mucosa and effusion fluid were removed, and the mRNA and/or protein levels of IL-1β, TNFα, IL-6, IL-10, IFN-γ TGF-β, MCP-I, IL-8, and MIP-2 were determined. On days 1 and 2 postinfection, most of the cytokines/chemokines were detectable. mRNA expression demonstrated the following patterns only in infected ears: early expression, IL-1β, IL-8; late expression, TNFα, IFN-γ; and biphasic, MCP-1, IL-6, TGF-β. Importantly, this study also showed that up-regulation of cytokine mRNA was not always accompanied by protein expression. Bloodstream levels of IL-6 and TNFα were measured by ELISA in a rat model of sepsis to provide evidence that ceftazidime can directly modulate proinflammatory cytokine production (6).

Carriage and disease progression of *S. pneumoniae* was linked to induction of cytokine mRNA in the nasopharnyx (356); although activation of the immune system culminated in nonlethal disease, evasion of the immune system was associated with dissemination of infection. Cytokine expression was linked to *L. monocytogenes* virulence (615).

IMAGING TECHNIQUES USED FOR THE EVALUATION OF EXPERIMENTAL INFECTIONS

Noninvasive imaging encompasses a rapidly developing palette of techniques that are continuing to set new standards for clinical diagnosis and disease monitoring. However, such techniques are only slowly becoming established for use in experimental animals and in particular models of infection (113,116,117); a general review of imaging techniques specifically for application in small animals has been published (27). An obvious advantage of the use of noninvasive imaging in animal models is the possibility of a direct comparison of response in animals with that of human patients. As compared with human and human systems, animals require machines with increased resolution before particular techniques can be used really successfully.

Imaging of the Host's Response to Infection

Many imaging techniques are available to noninvasively monitor disease states and their response to therapy. Difficulty in accessing the required equipment and designing of animal-specific imaging systems has perhaps hampered the use of these approaches. Access to specialized reagents may also be limiting (e.g., ^{18}F for use in PET imaging has a short half-life). Labeled cytokines have found use in a variety of imaging techniques for monitoring different leukocyte subsets *in vivo* during infection (536).

Magnetic Resonance Imaging

Using magnetic resonance imaging (MRI) and magnetic resonance spectroscopy (MRS), histopathology and segmentation maps were obtained by the mathematical processing of three-dimensional T_2-weighted MRI data via a neural network. The MRI patterns varied according to the nature and extent of infection with *A. fumigattus*. The MRS results show a statistically significant increase in inorganic phosphate and a significant decrease in phosphocreatine levels in the inflamed region (508). MRI along with contrast agent gadolinium-diethylenetriamine-pentaacetic acid was used to monitor the transient modulation of the blood-brain barrier following intravenous injection of bacterial glycopeptides (547).

The *S. aureus* thigh infection model, including treatment with vancomycin and imipenem/cilastatin, showed that MRI images closely paralleled histological changes occurring as the infection progressed or resolved with antibiotic therapy (390). Therefore, this noninvasive procedure could be used repeatedly on an individual animal to monitor at least some aspects of antimicrobial chemotherapy. Experimental *S. aureus* osteomyelitis in New Zealand white rabbits was examined by MRI, computed tomography (CT), and plain film radiography. MRI detected periostitis despite the absence of periosteal ossification and was more sensitive than CT or PF (545).

Positron Emisson Tomography

Positron emisson tomography (PET) can be used for PK studies as long as the compound can be synthesized to contain the short-lived isotopes used in PET (199a,199b).

Computed Tomography

Contrast material–enhanced CT and MRI were used on rabbits with osteomyelitic *S. aureus* lesions, and the detection rates were similar (95). Three-phase technetium-99m methylene diphosphonate gallium-67 MRI images were obtained from New Zealand rabbits with *S. aureus* osteomyelitis (46). There was no significant difference between radionuclide studies and MRI images in the detection of osteomyelitis, but MRI was significantly more sensitive in the detection of soft-tissue infection, including cellulitis and abscesses. Arthritic knee joints of rabbits have been monitored using CT. The use of the perfluorocarbon macrophage-labeling contrast agent perfluoroctylbromide facilitated discerning the response of rabbits aseptic or septic to tetracycline therapy (513).

Echocardiography

Serial transthoracic echocardiography, during and after treatment of experimental *S. aureus* endocarditis in rabbits, was used as a physiological indicator of the relative benefits of different antibiotic regimens (616). It has also been used with murine CLP models (275).

As for emerging technologies, fluorescence-mediated molecular tomography (FMT) can three-dimensionally image gene expression by resolving fluorescence activation in deep tissues (440).

DETECTION OF BACTERIAL ACTIVITY BY USE OF BIOLUMINESCENCE

Detection of Bacterial Activity by Use of Bacterial Labeling with *lux* Genes

General reviews of the use of cellular labeling by luciferase expression have been published (116,245), and a review of the use of bioluminescence techniques to study gene expression is available (114).

Use of bioluminescence to detect bacteria *in vivo* provides a noninvasive way of monitoring the progress of infection and the response to antiinfective therapies (for reviews, see 85,113,116,117). First described by Contag et al. (115), construction of virulent bacteria bearing lux operons constitutes a sensitive marker of bacterial viability, as the bioluminescence reaction is ATP-dependent. The article by Contag et al. (116) describes the construction and use of this technique in detail.

A thorough description of this approach has been presented by Rocchetta et al. (500), who used *lux*-transformed *E. coli* and a neutropenic mouse thigh infection model. The incorporation of an intensified charge-coupled device (ICCD) camera system facilitated the determination of light emission and therefore the sequential evaluation of individual mice. Dose-dependent bacterial CFU and light emission values were obtained *in vitro* and *in vivo* for controls and the bacteria exposed to ceftazidime, tetracycline, or ciprofloxacin. The detection methods were found to be highly correlated. Similar results were obtained with murine lung infections due to *S. pneumoniae* (207).

Given the extreme differences in the nature of bacterial growth as biofilms or planktonic cultures, bioluminescence may help in understanding the chemotherapy of device-related infections. *lux*-Transposed *S. aureus* and *P. aeruginosa* were used to establish Teflon catheter biofilm infection model mice, with either precolonized or postimplant-infected catheters being used (302). The effectiveness of various antibiotics, the determination of the *in vivo* PAE, and the monitoring of the emergence of antibiotic resistance in this model have also been discussed (303). Seven days after subcutaneous implantation of catheters precolonized with *S. aureus,* treatment with rifampin, tobramycin, or ciprofloxacin was initiated. Tobramycin and ciprofloxacin were poorly active, but rifampin led to an initial decline of bacterial CFU, after which resistance developed as expected.

Detection of Bacterial Activity by Use of Bacterial Labeling with Green Fluorescent Protein

Green fluorescent protein, a 31-kDa gene product of the jellyfish *Aequorea victoria,* has been extensively used to label mammalian and microbial cells. It is capable of "nonspecifically" labeling bacteria (578,579) and of being inserted to act as a reporter gene system (e.g., in organisms [554], *Salmonella Pseudomonas* spp and an *Alcaligenes* sp [65], a *Yersinia* sp [284], *L. pneumoniae* [554], *S. pneumoniae* [1], *Yersina pseudotuberculosis* [580], *C. neoformans* [150], and a *Helicobacter* sp [296]). Care must be taken in the construction of such cell lines in order to optimize the system for *in vivo* activity (525). This technology is advancing, and color variants are being developed (simulation of gene expression [377], profiling of a genetically modified gfp [525], and profiling of a genetically modified gfp [580]). Single-copy gene insertion has been noted for *P. aeruginosa* (554), salmonellae (268), and *S. pneumoniae* (1). Improved data processing (352) and the ability to see single cells have contributed to enhancing this technology. The GFP expression levels of 7000–200,000 copies per cell have been viewed as nondeleterious to the virulence of *S. typhimurium* (604).

SUSCEPTIBILITY TO INFECTION

Inbred Mice Strains

It has been long recognized that some inbred strains of mice possess extreme sensitivity (or resistance) to infection (for reviews, see 84,158,380,381,393,540). For example, C57BL/6, C3H/HeJ, and BALB/cJ mouse strains are all extremely sensitive to *S. typhimurium* infection, whereas A/J and CBA/N are moderately sensitive, and 129S6/SvEvTac is highly resistant (339). Mortality is often used as the end point of susceptibility to infection, but this crude end point may mask more subtle differences in the nature of susceptibility (17). Although T cells play a key role, particularly with respect to intracellular pathogens (410), other cell types are involved.

Interestingly, the C3H/HeJ mouse is also considered highly tolerant to endotoxin (LPS) (339,537). LPS resistance appears to be linked to mutation of TLR-4

(Toll-like receptor), which occurs in C3H/HeJ mice. This mutation occurs in the Toll/interleukin-1 (TIR) signaling domain and inhibits LPS-induced signaling (induced by LPS bound to the LPS-binding protein [LBP]). This cascade requires several accessory proteins to result in (a) "general" TLR signaling via NFkB and MAP kinases to induce cytokine/chemokine responses or (b) TLR-4 to specific signaling via IRAK2 and PKR to induce genes to counteract the invading pathogen (84).

Resistance to *M. tuberculosis* is under simple genetic control in mice: the *Nramp1* gene, which provides natural resistance to associated macrophage protein 1 appears to be the responsible gene (84,158,339). With 12 membrane-traversing segments, *Nramp1* is a putative divalent cation transporter that associates with the phagosome and apparently pumps out divalent cations. Mutation of *Nramp1* is associated with increased susceptibility to infection with intracellular pathogens, notably *M. tuberculosis,* and is characteristic of susceptible inbred mouse strains. Interestingly, *Nramp1* is a member of a gene superfamily of metal-transporting proteins and that orthologous proteins are present in bacteria suggests that a molecular struggle occurs for metal ions within the phagosome (158).

However, the analysis of the susceptibility of inbred mice to *C. albicans* serves as a good example of the complexities of susceptibility to infection. Ashman (17,18) thoroughly examined the reasons behind the differences between inbred mice in their sensitivity to *C. albicans infection.* Mice demonstrate different patterns of mortality, kidney and brain colonization, and tissue damage following systemic infection. The differences unrelated to classical genes involved resistance to infection (e.g., MHC). The highly susceptible A/J and DBA/2 mice, which are both complement component C5 deficient, demonstrate the higher mortality than other mouse strains (AKR, BALB/c, C57BL/6, C57/L, CBA/CaH, C3H, and DBA/1). Further genetic analyses of these strains suggest that a putative gene (*Carg1*) controls the extent of tissue damage; mice with a susceptible allele have increased tissue damage but only a moderate increase in kidney colonization relative to other strains. A second gene (*Carg2*) appears to also regulate susceptibility to kidney colonization and damage, particularly in cases of C5 deficiency (17–19). Nonetheless, passive transfer of C5 to DBA/2 mice reduced the severity of colonization and promoted survival (22). Differences in the colonization of the brain is dependent on the size of the infectious challenge, with A/J and DBA/2 mice being regarded as more susceptible only at high inocula, where the other strains succumb to infection. Therefore, differences in susceptibility may also be related to tissue-specific differences in host protective mechanisms (17,18).

Differences in susceptibility to *C. albicans* infection also are apparently related to the cellular response to infection. Neutrophils are essential in resistance, but macrophages and T cells also contribute. Early cellular responses to infection consist of neutrophilic influx into the tissues, which is reduced in C5-deficient mice (221). Neutrophil depletion increases susceptibility to infection (both systemic and vaginal) and alters the distribution of *C. albicans* and subsequent tissue damage; neutrophil depletion increases brain colonization but without strongly increasing tissue damage, although the heart may manifest severe tissue damage (222).

In the case of the T cell component, it is only with sublethal infections that the role of T cells can be observed (17,18). T cell–deficient nude mice show increased susceptibility to infection, but T cell deficiency does not alter the basal strain–dependent susceptibility differences (223). Antibody-based selective depletion of CD4+ and CD8+ T cells in resistant BALB/c or sensitive CBA/CaH mice demonstrated a role for CD4+ and to a lesser extent for CD8+, T cells in control of tissue damage, which is still dependent on the background of the mouse strain (20). Oral infection demonstrated the need of a balance of a T cell response (involving correct timing of both IFN-γ and IL-4 production): resistant BALB/c mice demonstrated early IFN-γ, IL-12, and IL-4 production in local lymph nodes, whereas sensitive DBA/2 mice demonstrated delayed and reduced IL-4 production (22). The resistance to oral candidiasis appears to involve a functioning neutrophil, macrophage, and CD4+ T cell response (191) and appropriate cytokine production in the oral tissues (e.g., TNFα appears critical for recovery) (172,192). However, the T cell response appears to have a minimal impact on recovery from sublethal systemic infection (22).

Inbred mouse strains also appear to differ in response to chronic *P. aeruginosa* lung infection (416, 550): BALB/c mice are resistant, C57BL/6 and A/J mice are relatively susceptible and experience low mortality, and DBA/2 mice are extremely susceptible and experience high mortality within 3 days of infection. The magnitude and nature of the pulmonary inflammatory response in BALB/c and C57BL/6 mice appeared to correlate with the extent of the bacterial load. Although results of infection studies in cystic fibrosis transmembrane conductance regulator (CFTR) protein–deficient mice have been variable, C57BL/6-Cftr(m1UNC)/Cftr(m1UNC) knockout mice appear highly susceptible to chronic *P. aeruginosa* infection in the lung.

Genetically Modified Hosts in Infectious Disease Models

Knockout mice contain nonfunctional genes due to targeted gene disruption by homologous recombination of modified DNA introduced into germline cells (224,329), and the use of such mice in the study of infectious disease has been reviewed (64,160,314,315,623). Inactivation of genes can lead to loss of expression of proteins that are involved in normal host responses to infection (e.g., cytokines and cytokine receptors). Furthermore, the development and function of cells involved in the inflammatory/immune responses are often dramatically impaired when certain genes are disrupted, possibly altering the susceptibility of the mice to infection (e.g., disruption of certain T cell receptor subtypes results in the loss of specific T cell types). The results obtained to date with knockout mice can be summarized as follows (314,315): (a) the extent of loss of resistance to infection varies considerably with any particular gene deletion; (b) some deletions (e.g., TNF or IFN-α receptors and IFN-γ) are particularly oppressive, resulting in complete loss of resistance; and (c) some deletions (e.g., T cell receptor γ-chain) confer increased susceptibility without the total loss of resistance, indicating redundancy or plasticity of the immune system. For example, two different knockout mice have been used to characterize susceptibility to sepsis following cecal ligation and puncture. Whether IL-10 plays a key role in the controlling the onset of irreversible septic shock after CLP has been examined (341) using IL-10–deficient (IL-10(−/−)) and wild-type (IL-10(+/+)) mice. IL-10–deficient mice demonstrated more rapid onset of mortality, and increased serum TNFα and IL-6 levels, and rescue from shock by surgical intervention ceased 10 hours earlier than in wild-type mice. Furthermore, treatment of both deficient and wild-type mice with exogenous IL-10 promoted survival. However, the beneficial effects of exogenous IL-10 on outcome in a model of hemorrhagic shock preceding CLP have been shown only in CBA/J males and not in females (303a).

The role of CD14 in the inflammatory response to sepsis following CLP was evaluated (169) using knockout (CD14-deficient) and wild-type mice, both groups being treated with antibiotics. Although dependent on the severity of the sepsis, there were no significant differences in survival, temperature, body weight, or motor activity levels between CD14–deficient and wild-type mice. CD14-deficient mice expressed lower bloodstream and peritoneal cavity levels of proinflammatory cytokines (IL-1β, IL-6, TNFα) and MIP-2α chemokine, the antiinflammatory cytokine IL-10, and the cytokine inhibitors IL-1 receptor antagonist and TNF receptors I and II. Despite the central role of the CD14 pathway in the response to CLP, its loss appears to only minimally affect morbidity and mortality resulting from CLP (169).

Although apparently not yet extensively used in conjunction with antimicrobial therapy, these models would appear to be helpful in evaluating biologic response modifiers (e.g., cytokines), with or without conventional chemotherapy, in models of infection in immunodeficiency. Two notable applications of knockout mice in antimicrobial drug profiling include use of the IL-10–deficient mouse for the intestinal parasite *Cryptosporidium parvum* (247) and use of the IFN-γ–deficient mouse for *M. tuberculosis* (350).

PHARMACOGENOMICS IN ANIMAL MODELS OF INFECTION

Genomic approaches utilizing animal models of infection fall into two distinct categories: (a) bacterial genomics, whose goal is to identify bacterial genes involved in the initiation, survival, and propagation of bacteria during pathogenic infection and to uncover the genetic basis of sensitivity (or resistance) to antibiotics; and (b) pharmacogenomics, which in the specialized case of infection concerns itself with understanding the genetics of differences in antibiotic metabolism and disposition and their toxic effects without considering the effects of the drugs on the host physiology as the drugs are targeted to the microorganism. A good overview of the study of microorganism and host genomics using DNA microarrays has been provided by Bryant et al. (83). They outline the use of DNA microarrays in studying the infectious process from the aspect of the pathogen (diagnostics, epidemiology, pathogenicity, and antimicrobial resistance), the host (innate immunity, adoptive or learned immunity, physiological differences related to susceptibility, and drug metabolism and toxicity), and the host-microbe interaction ("normal" and abnormal responses to infectious insult, pathogenic processes such as microbe-induced host cell apoptosis, responses to antibiotic treatment such as inflammatory responses to antibiotic-lysed bacteria, and vaccination).

Pharmacogenomics of Pathogens

Clearly, genomic investigation of the microorganisms' genotype/phenotype during infection will uncover novel genes, perhaps expressed only *in vivo*, that represent potential novel targets for antimicrobial therapy or the means of antimicrobial resistance (94,216,269,325). However, despite the sequencing of entire genomes of several bacteria, exploitation of this new knowledge has perhaps been slower than expected. Despite this, there is great potential for genomics to "customize" clinical treatment of infection, providing information on both the pathogen and the host to aid in drug selection (269). De Backer and Van Dijck (145) have provided a review of the role pharmacogenomics might play in the development of novel antifungal chemotherapeutics.

Pharmacogenomics of the Infected Host

Pharmacogenomics focuses on the host, evaluating genetic-based differences in host drug transport and metabolism, both of which form the basis of PK and tolerability features of any antibiotic (600). For example, polymorphisms occur in P-glycoprotein, an ATP-binding cassette transporter that pumps drugs out of cells and thus affects drug uptake from the gastrointestinal tract as well as tissue distribution. Polymorphisms also occur in drug-metabolizing enzymes that are components of both the "phase I" metabolizing group (e.g., the cytochrome P450 family, which metabolize drugs through oxidation, reduction, or hydrolysis steps) and members of the "phase II" family (e.g., UDP glucuronosyltransferases, glutathione transferases, methyltransferase, and acetyl transferases) and that by conjugating the drug help to facilitate its elimination from the body. In addition to genetic predisposition to infection, inbred mouse strains also carry alterations in drug metabolism, such the differences in tolerability of inbred strains to chloramphenicol toxicity (see 600). Genetic mapping of inbred strains to identify loci and eventually genes that are involved in drug metabolism and display polymorphisms will likely lead to the identification of human homologues. In addition, use of genetically modified mice will aid in identifying drug-metabolizing enzymes (321), and such information can be applied to medicinal chemistry programs to design antibiotics with better PK and metabolic/tolerability profiles. In this regard, the apparent failure or poor activity of antibiotics in some animal models may be due to differences in drug metabolism between different mouse strains or different species.

PREDICTABILITY OF ANIMAL MODELS OF INFECTION FOR HUMAN DISEASE

Perhaps the ultimate question that arises following the preclinical evaluation of an antiinfectives in an animal model of infectious disease is, What is the true utility of the data obtained from the animal model, namely, how predictive is the model for the clinical situation? The answer to this lies in understanding both the model and the clinical situation. In understanding the model, it is as important to know the limitations of the model as much as its advantages and to ask only those questions that the particular model can answer. Few studies have systematically reviewed the correlation of the effect of antibiotics in animal models and clinical outcome. One such a review (455) suggests that the rat osteomyelitis model does have a good measure of predictability. Although discriminative models of infection are designed to mimic the clinical situation more closely than screening models, all models can provide useful information. This is probably due to the mode of action of antibiotics, for they primarily target pathogens of another hierarchical kingdom (prokaryotes). Given this likelihood of high specificity of drug-target interaction, the infecting organism bearing the target remains "constant" irrespective of host, be it an experimental one (mouse, rat, etc.) or one that acquires the infection naturally (humans among other animals) (164). Therefore, the issue of predictability becomes an issue of PK/PD relationship: can the drug attain a sufficient PK profile (and be well tolerated) in the patient and satisfy the PD criteria established during the experimental evaluation (e.g., plasma concentration above the MIC for 80% of the administration interval). Allometry or physiologically based PK/PD modeling can be used to predict dosages for the target patient. But this serves only as a guide to aid decisions; it is on the basis of animal efficacy model data that clinical trials are most often initiated. Such a modeling exercise requires input from many different models to provide a database sufficient for making an educated prediction concerning clinical success.

However, in spite of careful experimentation, clinical failure of a compound effective in preclinical testing, will sometimes occur. In such cases, the researchers will ask, what went wrong?

If only to provide a basis for discussion, consideration should be given to an excellent publication by Eichaker and associates (171). In this study, the authors review clinical data (from 22 trials) and preclinical data (from 95 "trials") concerning the testing of antiinflammatory agents in bacterial sepsis. They argue that the vast amount of preclinical data, do not reflect clinical experience. Using meta-regression techniques to pool the data, they test the hypothesis that a strong relationship exists between risk of death from disease and the effectiveness of antiinflammatory agents in treating disease. If preclinical studies show an exceedingly high risk of death and the clinical trials a more moderate one, then the preclinical data would be misleading; for the findings to be truly comparable, the disease outcomes should be similar in both the preclinical and the clinical trials. The authors show that the mortality rates of control animals (88% [79–96%]; median [25th–75th quartiles]) were highly different from those of the clinical trials (39% [32–43%], $p = 0.0001$). Regression analysis of the animal data indicated that, of the factors evaluated, 70% of the variability of the effect of antiinflammatory agents could be attributed to the risk of death. Normally, the clinical trials did not categorize the patients regarding risk of death, but in two trials that did, the greatest benefit of the antiinflammatory agents was to those at the highest risk of death, similar to the preclinical studies. Plotting the control odds ratio of dying and the odds ratio of the treated group dying for both animal and human studies shows a clustering of the human trial data at a lower risk than in the majority of the animal trials. The authors then modified their animal model to have a range of severity of disease when testing antiinflammatory agents in sepsis and produced data yielding an odds ratio plot very similar to that obtained from the clinical trials. In a reiterative process, the animal model was modified to produce data that better fit the spectrum of disease observed clinically, thus obtaining an animal model of greater predictive quality.

In some cases, definitive clinical trials are difficult, if not impossible, to perform. In such cases, reliance on animal model data is extensive, if not exclusive. For example, endocarditis is a severe, costly infection, and therefore identification of situations invoking prophylaxis against this infection is clearly warranted. Prophylaxis requires the ability to identify clinical procedures that might result in bacteremia, identify the patients at risk, and determine the optimal prophylactic antibiotic regimen, one that maximizes effectiveness and minimizes the risk of side effects. Owing to the difficulty of performing appropriate clinical studies, Moreillon (415) summarizes the information obtained from animal studies of endocarditis and uses it as a basis for a proposal regarding guidelines for clinical prophylaxis of endocarditis. Moreillon observes,

> First, antibiotics do not prevent the early stages of valve colonisation, but rather kill the microorganisms after their attachment to the cardiac lesions. Second, the duration of antibiotic presence in the serum is critical. Under experimental conditions, the drugs must remain above their minimal inhibitory concentration for the organisms for [at least] 10 h, to allow time for bacterial clearance from the valves. Third, antibiotic-induced killing is not the only mechanism allowing bacterial clearance. Other factors, such as platelet microbiocidal proteins, may act in concert with the drugs to sterilize the lesions. (p.)

In such cases, it is likely that collective experience in an "informal setting" (i.e., without a clinical trial) will prove or disprove the principles obtained from the testing of antimicrobial agents in animal models of infection.

In summary, there is a vast amount of information on animal models of infection, but it is likely that only when the models are used wisely and modified to better reflect the clinical situation can predictions based on them be relied upon.

REFERENCES

1. Acebo P, Nieto C, Corrales MA, et al. Quantitative detection of *Streptococcus pneumoniae* cells harbouring single or multiple copies of the gene encoding the green fluorescent protein. *Microbiology* 2000;146:1267–1273.
2. Actor JK. Bioluminescent quantitation and detection of gene expression during infectious disease. *Comb Chem High Throughput Screen* 2000;3:273–288.
3. Akiyama M, Oishi K, Tao M, et al. Antibacterial properties of *Pseudomonas aeruginosa* immunotype 1 lipopolysaccharide-specific monoclonal antibody (MAb) in a murine thigh infection model: combined effects of MAb and ceftazidime. *Microbiol Immunol* 2000;44:629–635.
4. Alder JD. The hamster model of syphilis. In: Zak O, Sande MA, eds. *Handbook of animal models of infection.* San Diego: Academic Press, 1999:285–289.
5. Alder J, Jarvis K, Mitten M, et al. Clarithromycin therapy of experimental *Treponema pallidum* infections in hamsters. *Antimicrob Agents Chemother* 1993;37:864–867.
6. Alkharfy KM, Kellum JA, Frye RF, et al. Effect of ceftazidime on systemic cytokine concentrations in rats. *Antimicrob Agents Chemother* 2000;44:3217–3219.
7. Allen T, Crawford R. Animal care and use committees: an American perspective. In: Zak O, Sande MA, eds. *Handbook of animal models of infection.* San Diego: Academic Press, 1999:19–28.
8. Anaissie EJ, Karyotakis NC, Hachem R, et al. Correlation between in vitro and in vivo activity of antifungal agents against Candida species. *J Infect Dis* 1994;170:384–389.
9. Anderson GG, Palermo JJ, Schilling JD, et al. Intracellular bacterial biofilm-like pods in urinary tract infections. *Science* 2003;301:105–107.
10. Andes D, Craig WA. Animal model pharmacokinetics and pharmacodynamics: a critical review. *Int J Antimicrob Agents* 2002;19:261–268.
11. Andes D, Craig WA. Pharmacodynamics of the new fluoroquinolone gatifloxacin in murine thigh and lung infection models. *Antimicrob Agents Chemother* 2002;46:1665–1670.
12. Andes D, Marchillo K, Lowther J, et al. In vivo pharmacodynamics of HMR 3270, a glucan synthase inhibitor, in a murine candidiasis model. *Antimicrob Agents Chemother* 2003;47:1187–1192.
13. Andes D, Van Ogtrop M. Characterization and quantitation of the pharmacodynamics of fluconazole in a neutropenic murine disseminated candidiasis infection model. *Antimicrob Agents Chemother* 1999;43:2116–2120.
14. Ansfield MJ, Woods DE, Johanson WG. Lung bacterial clearance in murine pneumococcal pneumonia. *Infect Immun* 1977;17:195–204.
15. Anwar H, Strap JL, Chen K, et al. Dynamic interactions of biofilms of mucoid *Pseudomonas aeruginosa* with tobramycin and piperacillin. *Antimicrob Agents Chemother* 1992;36:1208–1214.
16. Arka RJ, Balows A. Animal models of experimental gonococcal infection. In: Zak O, Sande MA, eds. *Experimental models in antimicrobial chemotherapy,* vol. 1. London: Academic Press, 1986:355–369.
17. Ashman RB. *Candida albicans:* pathogenesis, immunity and host defence. *Res Immunol* 1998;149:281–288.
18. Ashman RB. Genetic determination of susceptibility and resistance in the pathogenesis of *Candida albicans* infection. *FEMS Immunol Med Microbiol* 1997;19:183–189.
19. Ashman RB, Fulurija A, Papadimitriou JM. A second *Candida albicans* resistance gene (Carg2) regulates tissue damage, but not fungal clearance, in sub-lethal murine systemic infection. *Microb Pathog* 1998;25:349–352.
20. Ashman RB, Fulurija A, Papadimitriou JM. Both CD4+ and CD8+ lymphocytes reduce the severity of tissue lesions in murine systemic cadidiasis, and CD4+ cells also demonstrate strain-specific immunopathological effects. *Microbiology* 1999;145:1631–1640.
21. Ashman RB, Papadimitriou JM, Fulurija A. Acute susceptibility of aged mice to infection with *Candida albicans. J Med Microbiol* 1999;48:1095–1102.
22. Ashman RB, Papadimitriou JM, Fulurija A, et al. Role of complement C5 and T lymphocytes in pathogenesis of disseminated and mucosal candidiasis in susceptible DBA/2 mice. *Microb Pathog* 2003;34:103–113.
23. Astry CL, Nelson S, Karam GH, et al. Interactions of clindamycin with antibacterial defenses of the lung. *Am Rev Respir Dis* 1987;135:1015–1019.

23a. Attardo Genco C, Arko RJ. Animal chamber models for study of host-parasite interactions. *Methods Enzymol* 1994;235:120–140.

24. Auclair P, Lessard C, Bergeron MG. Renal pharmacokinetic changes of gentamicin during enterococcal pyelonephritis. *Antimicrob Agents Chemother* 1988;32:736–739.
25. Azoulay-Dupuis E, Bedos J-P, Vallee E, et al. Antipneumococcal activity of ciprofloxacin, ofloxacin, and temafloxacin in an experimental mouse pneumonia model

at various stages of disease. *J Infect Dis* 1991;163:319–324.

26. Bagge N, Ciofu O, Skovgaard LT, et al. Rapid development in vitro and in vivo of resistance to ceftazidime in biofilm-growing *Pseudomonas aeruginosa* due to chromosomal beta-lactamase. *APMIS* 2000;108:589–600.
27. Balaban RS, Hampshire VA. Challenges in small animal noninvasive imaging. *ILAR J* 2001;42:248–62.
28. Bakker-Woudenberg IAJM, Jong-Hoenderop YT, Michel MF. Efficacy of antimicrobial therapy in experimental rat pneumonia: effects of impaired phagocytosis. *Infect Immun* 1979;25:366–375.
29. Barbhaiya RH, Knupp CA, Pittman KA. Effects of age and gender on pharmacokinetics of cefepime. *Antimicrob Agents Chemother* 1992;36:1181–1185.
30. Barry B, Muffat-Joly M. Gerbil model of acute otitis media. In: Zak O, Sande MA, eds. *Handbook of animal models of infection.* San Diego: Academic Press, 1999:375–384.
31. Bartlett JG, Chang TW, Onderdonk AB. Comparison of five regimens for treatment of experimental clindamycin-associated colitis. *J Infect Dis* 1977;136:81–86.
32. Bartlett JG, Onderdonk AB, Cisneros RL. Clindamycin-associated colitis due to a toxin-producing species of Clostridium in hamsters. *J Infect Dis* 1977;136:701–705.
33. Barza M. Pharmacokinetics of antibiotics in shallow and deep compartments. *J Antimicrob Chemother* 1993; 31[Suppl D]:17–28.
34. Bass R, Lehnert T. Basic requirements for the toxicity testing of antimicrobial agents. *Eur J Clin Microbiol Infect Dis* 1990;9:488–491.
35. Batard E, Jacqueline C, Boutoille D, et al. Combination of quinupristin-dalfopristin and gentamicin against methicillin-resistant *Staphylococcus aureus*: experimental rabbit endocarditis study. *Antimicrob Agents Chemother* 2002;46:2174–2178.
36. Bateson P. Do animals feel pain? *New Sci* 1992;134(1818): 30–33.
37. Bauhofer A, Witte K, Celik I, et al. Sickness behaviour, an animal equivalent to human quality of life, is improved in septic rats by G-CSF and antibiotic prophylaxis. *Langenbecks Arch Surg* 2001;386:132–140.
38. Bauhofer A, Witte K, Lemmer B, et al. Quality of life in animals as a new outcome for surgical research: G-CSF as a quality of life improving factor. *Eur Surg Res* 2002;34:22–29.
39. Baumans V, ten Berg RGM, Beterns APMG, et al. Experimental procedures. In: van Zutphen LFM, Baumans V, Beyen AC, ed. *Principles of laboratory animal science.* Amsterdam: Elsevier, 1993:299–318.
40. Baumgartner JD, Glauser MP. Immunotherapy of endotoxemia and septicemia. *Immunobiology* 1993;187:464–477.
41. Bayer AS, Greenberg DP, Yih J. Correlates of therapeutic efficacy in experimental methicillin-resistant *Staphylococcus aureus* endocarditis. *Chemotherapy* 1988;34:46–55.
42. Beale AS, Upshon PA. Characteristics of murine model of genital infection with *Chlamydia trachomatis* and effects of therapy with tetracyclines, amoxicillin-clavulanic acid, or azithromycin. *Antimicrob Agents Chemother* 1994;38:1937–1943.
43. Beam TR, Gilbert DN, Kunin CM. General guidelines for the clinical evaluation of anti-infective drug products. *Clin Infect Dis* 1992;15[Suppl 1]:S5–S32.
44. Beauchamp D, Pettigrew M. Influence of hydrocortisone on gentamicin-induced nephrotoxicity in rats. *Antimicrob Agents Chemother* 1988;32:992–996.
45. Beaulac C, Sachetelli S, Lagace J. Aerosolization of low phase transition temperature liposomal tobramycin as a dry powder in an animal model of chronic pulmonary infection caused by *Pseudomonas aeruginosa*. *J Drug Target* 1999;7:33–41.
46. Beltran J, McGhee RB, Shaffer PB, et al. Experimental infections of the musculoskeletal system: evaluation with MR imaging and Tc-99m MDP and Ga-67 scintigraphy. *Radiology* 1988;167:167–172.
47. Beovic B, Mrhar A, Karba R, et al. Influence of fever on cefazolin pharmacokinetics. *J Chemother* 1999;11:40–45.
48. Bergan T. Pharmacokinetic properties of the cephalosporins. *Drugs* 1987;34 [Suppl 2]:89–104.
49. Bergeron MG, Bergeron Y. Influence of endotoxin on the intrarenal distribution of gentamicin, netilmicin, tobramycin, amikacin, and cephalothin. *Antimicrob Agents Chemother* 1986;29:7–12.
50. Bergeron MG, Bergeron Y, Beauchamp D. Influence of hydrocortisone succinate on intrarenal accumulation of gentamicin in endotoxemic rats. *Antimicrob Agents Chemother* 1987;31:1816–1821.
51. Bergeron MG, Marois Y. Benefit from high intraenal levels of gentamicin in the treatment of *E. coli* pyelonephritis. *Kidney Int* 1986;30:481–487.
52. Bergeron MG, Robert J, Beauchamp D. Pharmacodynamics of antibiotics in fibrin clots. *J Antimicrob Chemother* 1993;31[Suppl D]:113–136.
53. Bermudez LE, Inderlied CB, Kolonoski P, et al. Activity of moxifloxacin by itself and in combination with ethambutol, rifabutin, and azithromycin in vitro and in vivo against *Mycobacterium avium*. *Antimicrob Agents Chemother* 2001;45:217–222.
54. Bermudez LE, Inderlied CB, Kolonoski P, et al. Telithromycin is active against *Mycobacterium avium* in mice despite lacking significant activity in standard in vitro and macrophage assays and is associated with low frequency of resistance during treatment. *Antimicrob Agents Chemother* 2001;45:2210–2214.
55. Bernareggi A, Rowland MS. Physiologic modeling of cyclosporine kinetics in rats. *J Pharmacokinet Biopharm* 1991;19:1–19.
56. Beskid G, Christenson JG, Cleeland R, et al. In vivo activity of ceftriaxone (Ro 13–9904), a new broad-spectrum semisynthetic cephalosporin. *Antimicrob Agents Chemother* 1981;20:159–167.
57. Beterns APMG, Booij LHDJ, Flecknell PA, et al. Anaesthesia, analgesia and euthanasia. In: van Zutphen LFM, Baumans V, Beyen AC, eds. *Principles of laboratory animal science.* Amsterdam: Elsevier, 1993:267–298.
58. Beynen AC, Festing MFW. Phases in an animal experiment. In: van Zutphen LFM, Baumans V, Beyen AC, eds. *Principles of laboratory animal science.* Amsterdam: Elsevier, 1993:197–208.
59. Beynen AC, Festing MFW, van Montfort MAJ. Design of animal experiments. In: van Zutphen LFM, Baumans V, Beyen AC, eds. *Principles of laboratory animal science.* Amsterdam: Elsevier, 1993:209–240.
60. Bhardwaj R, Dorr RT, Blanchard J. Approaches to reducing toxicity of parenteral anticancer drug formulations using cyclodextrins. *PDA J Pharm Sci Technol* 2000;54:233–239.
61. Birke L, Michael M. Views from behind the barricade. *New Sci* 1992;1815:29–32.
62. Blankenship-Paris TL, Walton BJ, Hayes YO, et al. Clostridium difficile infection in hamsters fed an atherogenic diet. *Vet Pathol* 1995;32:269–273.
63. Blaser J, Zinner SH. In vitro models for the study of antibiotic activities. *Prog Drug Res* 1987;31:349–381.

64. Bleuthmann H, Rothe J, Schultze N, et al. Establishment of the role of IL-6 and TNF receptor 1 using gene knockout mice. *J Leukocyte Biol* 1994;56:565–570.
65. Bongaerts RJ, Hautefort I, Sidebotham JM, et al. Green fluorescent protein as a marker for conditional gene expression in bacterial cells. *Methods Enzymol* 2002;358:43–66.
66. Boom SJ, Davidson JA, Zhang P, et al. Comparison of HA-1A and E5 monoclonal antibodies to endotoxin in rats with endotoxaemia. *Eur J Surg* 1993;159:559–561.
67. Boswell GW, Bekersky I, Buell D, et al. Toxicological profile and pharmacokinetics of a unilamellar liposomal vesicle formulation of amphotericin B in rats. *Antimicrob Agents Chemother* 1998;42:263–268.
68. Botha T, Ryffel B. Reactivation of latent tuberculosis infection in TNF-deficient mice. *J Immunol* 2003;171:3110–3118.
69. Bottrill K, Combes RD. *Contrib Microbiol* 2001;9:89–117.
70. Bourne DWA. Mathematical modeling of pharmaceutical data. *Encyclopedia of pharmaceutical technology.* New York: Marcel Dekker, 2002:1706–1720.
71. Bowman JC, Abruzzo GK, Anderson JW, et al. Quantitative PCR assay to measure *Aspergillus fumigatus* burden in a murine model of disseminated aspergillosis: demonstration of efficacy of caspofungin acetate. *Antimicrob Agents Chemothers* 2001;45:3474–3481.
72. Boxenbuam H. Interspecies scaling, allometry, physiological time, and the ground plan of pharmacokinetics. *J Pharmacokinet Biopharm* 1982;10:201–227.
73. Braddour LM. Virulence factors among Gram-positive bacteria in experimental endocarditis. *Infect Immun* 1994;62:2143–2148.
74. Brenner D, DeVoe IW, Holbein BE. Increased virulence of *Neisseria meningitidis* after in vitro iron-limited growth at low pH. *Infect Immun* 1981;33:59–66.
75. Brieland J, Essig D, Jackson C, et al. Comparison of pathogenesis and host immune responses to *Candida glabrata* and *Candida albicans* in systemically infected immunocompetant mice. *Infect Immun* 2001;69:5046–5055.
76. Bronner S, Jehl F, Peter JD, et al. Moxifloxacin efficacy and vitreous penetration in a rabbit model of *Staphylococcus aureus* endophthalmitis and effect on gene expression of leucotoxins and virulence regulator factors. *Antimicrob Agents Chemother* 2003;47:1621–1629.
77. Brook I. Intra-abdominal abscess. In: Zak O, Sande MA, eds. *Handbook of animal models of infection.* San Diego: Academic Press, 1999:163–172.
78. Brooks SJD, Lyons JM, Braude AL. Immunization against retrograde pyelonephritis. I. Production of an experimental model of severe ascending *Escherichia coli* pyelonephritis without bacteremia in rats. *Am J Pathol* 1974;74:345–358.
79. Brown MRW, Collier PJ, Gilbert P. Influence of growth rate on susceptibility to antimicrobial agents: modification of the cell envelope and batch and continuous culture studies. *Antimicrob Agents Chemother* 1990;34:1623–1628.
79a. Brown ST, Edwards FF, Bernhard EM, et al. Azithromycin, rifabutin, and rifapentine for treatment and prophylaxis of *Mycobacterium avium* complex in rats treated with cyclosporine. *Antimicrob Agents Chemother* 1993;37:398–402.
80. Brunel A, Gouet P. Influence of the destabilization of the maternal digestive microflora on that of the newborn. *Biol Neonate* 1993;63:236–245.
81. Brunner H, Zeiler HJ. Oral ciprofloxacin treatment for *Salmonella typhimurium* infection of normal and immunocompromised mice. *Antimicrob Agents Chemother* 1988;32:57–62.
82. Bruzzese T, Rimaroli C, Bonabello A, et al. Pharmacokinetics and tissue distribution of rifametane, a new 3-azinomethyl-rifamycin derivative, in several animal species. *Arzneimittelforschung* 2000;50:60–71.
83. Bryant PA, Venter D, Robins-Browne R, et al. Chips with everything: DNA microarrays in infectious diseases. *Lancet Infect Dis* 2004;4:100–111.
84. Buer J, Balling R. Mice, microbes and models of infection. *Nat Rev Genetics* 2003;4:195–199.
85. Burns SM, Jon D, Francis KP, et al. Revealing the spatiotemporal patterns of bacterial infectious diseases using bioluminescent pathogens and whole body imaging. Animal testing in infectology. *Contrib Microbiol* 2001;9:71–88.
85a. Callegan MC, Hill JM, Insler MS, et al. Methicillin-resistant *Staphylococcus aureus* keratitis in the rabbit: therapy with ciprofloxacin, vancomycin and cefazolin. *Curr Eye Res* 1992;11:1111–1119.
86. Camilli A, Beattie DT, Mekalanos JJ. Use of genetic recombination as a reporter of gene expression. *Proc Natl Acad Sci USA* 1994;91:2634–2638.
87. Capilla J, Yustes C, Mayoyo E, et al. Efficacy of albaconazole (UR-9825) in treatment of disseminated *Scedosporium prolificans* infection in rabbits. *Antimicrob Agents Chemother* 2003;47:1948–1951.
88. Carbon C. Experimental endocarditis: a review of its relevance to human endocarditis. *J Antimicrob Chemother* 1993;31[Suppl D]:71–86.
89. Carbon C. Significance of tissue levels for prediction of antibiotic efficacy and determination of dosage. *Eur J Clin Microbiol Infect Dis* 1990;9:510–516.
90. Cars O, Odenholt-Tornqvist I. The post-antibiotic sub-MIC effect in vitro and in vivo. *J Antimicrob Chemother* 1993;31[Suppl D]:159–166.
91. Casal J, Aguilar L, Jado I, et al. Effects of specific antibodies against *Streptococcu pneumoniae* on pharmacodynamic parameters of beta-lactams in a mouse sepsis model. *Antimicrob Agents Chemother* 2002;46:1340–1344.
92. Cash HA, Woods DE, McCullough B, et al. A rat model of chronic respiratory infection with *Pseudomonas aeruginosa. Am Rev Respir Dis* 1979;119:453–459.
93. Caye-Thomasen P, Hermansson A, Tos M, et al. Effect of penicillin on experimental acute otitis media: a histopathological study of goblet cell density, bone modelling dynamics, polyp and adhesion formation. *Acta Otolaryngol [Suppl] (Stockh)* 2000;543:56–57.
94. Chalker AF, Lunsford RD. Rational identification of new antibacterial drug targets that are essential for viability using a genomics-based approach. *Pharmacol Ther* 2002;95:1–20.
95. Chandnani VP, Beltran J, Morris CS, et al. Acute experimental osteomyelitis and abscesses: detection with MR imaging versus CT. *Radiology* 1990;174:233–236.
96. Chenel M, Barbot A, Dupuis A, et al. Pharmacokinetic-pharmacodynamic modeling of the electroencephalogram effect of norfloxacin in rats. *Antimicrob Agents Chemother* 2003;47:1952–1957.
97. Cherbut C, Ferre JP, Corpet DE, et al. Alterations of intestinal microflora by antibiotics: effects on fecal excretion, transit time, and colonic motility in rats. *Dig Dis Sci* 1991;36:1729–1734.
98. Chesa-Jimenez J, Peris JE, Torres-Molina F, et al. Low bioavailablity of amoxicillin in rats as a consequence of presystematic degradation in the intestine. *Antimicrob Agents Chemother* 1994;38:842–847.

99. Chiller TM, Sobel RA, Capilla Luque J, et al. Efficacy of amphotericin B or itraconazole in a murine model of central nervous system Aspergillus infection. *Antimicrob Agents Chemother* 2003;47:813–815.
100. Chmiel JF, Davis PB. State of the art: why do the lungs of patients with cystic fibrosis become infected and why can't they clear the infection? *Respir Res* 2003; 4:8.
101. Choi S, Hahn TW, Osterhout G, et al. Comparative intravitreal antibiotic therapy for experimental *Enterococcus faecalis* endophthalmitis. *Arch Ophthalmol* 1996;114:61–65.
102. Chong K-T. Prophylactic administration of interleukin-2 protects mice from lethal challenge with Gram-negative bacteria. *Infect Immun* 1988;55:668–673.
103. Chuard C, Vaudaux P, Waldvogel FA, et al. Susceptibility of *Staphylococcus aureus* growing on fibronectin-coated surfaces to bactericidal antibiotics. *Antimicrob Agents Chemother* 1993;37:625–632.
104. Ciofu O, Bagge N, Hoiby N. Antibodies against beta-lactamase can improve ceftazidime treatment of lung infection with beta-lactam-resistant *Pseudomonas aeruginosa* in a rat model of chronic lung Infection. *APMIS* 2002;110:881–891.
105. Clark B, Smith DA. *An introduction to pharmacokinetics* 2nd ed. Oxford: Blackwell Scientific Publications, 1986.
106. Clemons KV, Sobel RA, Williams PL, et al. Efficacy of intravenous liposomal amphotericin B (AmBisome) against coccidioidal meningitis in rabbits. *Antimicrob Agents Chemother* 2002;46:2420–2426.
107. Clemons KV, Stevens DA. Efficacy of ravuconazole in treatment of mucosal candidosis in SCID mice. *Antimicrob Agents Chemother* 2001;45:3433–3436.
108. Cohen C. The case for use of animals in biomedical research. *N Engl J Med* 1986;315:865–870.
109. Cohen Y, Perronne C, Lazard T, et al. Use of normal C57BL/6 mice with established *Mycobacterium avium* infections as an alternative model for evaluation of antibiotic activity. *Antimicrob Agents Chemother* 1995;39:735–738.
110. Collins HL, Kaufmann SHE, Schaible UE. Iron chelation via deferoxamine exacerbates experimental salmonellosis via inhibition of the nicotinamide adenine dinucleotide phosphate oxidase-dependent respiratory burst. *J Immunol* 2002;168:3456–3463.
111. Collins MS, Ladehoff D, Mehton NS. Therapy of established experimental *Pseudomonas aeruginosa* infections with oral ciprofloxacin and five human monoclonal antibodies against lipopolysaccharide antigens. *Antibiot Chemother* 1991;44:185–195.
112. Comber KR, Osborne CD, Sutherland R. Comparative effects of amoxicillin and ampicillin in the treatment of experimental mouse infections. *Antimicrob Agents Chemother* 1975;7:179–185.
113. Contag PR. Whole-animal cellular and molecular imaging to accelerate drug development. *Drug Discov Today* 2002;7:555–562.
114. Contag CH, Bachmann MH. Advances in in vivo bioluminescence imaging of gene expression. *Annu Rev Biomed Eng* 2002;4:235–260.
115. Contag CH, Contag PR, Mullins JI, et al. Photonic detection of bacterial pathogens in living hosts. *Mol Microbiol* 1995;18:593–603.
116. Contag PR, Olomu AB, Contag CH. Non-invasive monitoring of infection and gene expression in living animal models. In: Zak O, Sande MA, eds. *Handbook of animal models of infection.* San Diego: Academic Press, 1999: 61–68.
117. Contag PR, Olomu IN, Stevenson DK, et al. Bioluminescent indicators in living mammals. *Nat Med* 1998;4:245–247.
118. Contrepois A, Moulin A-M. Early history of animal models of infection In: Zak O, Sande MA, eds. *Handbook of animal models of infection.* San Diego: Academic Press, 1999:3–8.
119. Corbeil LB, Wunderlich AC, Corbeil RR, et al. Disseminated gonococcal infection in mice. *Infect Immun* 1979;26:984–990.
120. Cornelissen JJ, Schellekens JF, Kraaijeveld CA, et al. Lifesaving immunotherapy with cross-reactive monoclonal antibodies against endotoxin: a critical evaluation of experimental and clinical studies. *Neth J Med* 1991;39:170–176.
121. Costerton JW, Cheng K-J, Geesey GG, et al. Bacterial biofilms in nature and disease. *Annu Rev Microbiol* 1987;41:435–464.
122. Costerton JW, Veeh R, Shirtliff M, et al. The application of biofilm science to the study and control of chronic bacterial infections. *J Clin Invest* 2003;112:1466–1477.
123. Cottagnoud P, Pfister M, Cottagnoud M, et al. Activities of ertapenem, a new long-acting carbapenem, against penicillin-sensitive or -resistant pneumococci in experimental meningitis. *Antimicrob Agents Chemother* 2003;47:1943–1947.
124. Cozens RM. Formulation of compounds and determination of pharmacokinetic parameters. In: Zak O, Sande MA, eds. *Handbook of animal models of infection.* San Diego: Academic Press, 1999:83–92.
125. Cozens RM, Tuomanen E, Tosch W, et al. Evaluation of the bactericidal activity of β-lactam antibiotics on slowly growing bacteria cultured in the chemostat. *Antimicrob Agents Chemother* 1986;29:797–802.
126. Craig W. Pharmacodynamics of antimicrobial agents as a basis for determining dosage regimens. *Eur J Clin Microbiol Infect Dis* 1993;12[Suppl 1]:S6–S8.
127. Craig WA. Post-antibiotic effects in experimental infection models: relationship to in-vitro phenomena and to treatment of infections in man. *J Antimicrob Chemother* 1993;31[Suppl D]:149–158.
128. Craig WA. Pharmacokinetic/pharmacodynamic parameters: rationale for antibacterial dosing of mice and men. *Clin Infect Dis* 1998;26:1–12.
129. Craig WA, Legget J, Totsuka K, et al. Key pharmacokinetic parameters of antibiotic efficacy in experimental animal infections. *J Drug Dev* 1988;1[Suppl 3]:7–15.
130. Craig WA, Redington J, Ebert SC. Pharmacodynamics of amikacin in vitro and in mouse thigh and lung infections. *J Antimicrob Chemother* 1991;27[Suppl C]:29–40.
131. Cremieux AC, Carbon C. Experimental models of bone and prosthetic joint infections. *Clin Infect Dis* 1997;25:1295–1302.
132. Cremieux A-C, Saleh-Mghir A, Vallois J-M, et al. Influence of the pre-treatment duration of infection on the efficacies of various antibiotic regimens in experimental streptococcal endocarditis. *J Antimicrob Chemother* 1993;32:843–852.
133. Cross AS, Opal SM, Palardy JE, et al. The efficacy of combination immunotherapy in experimental *Pseudomonas sepsis. J Infect Dis* 1993;167:112–118.
134. Cross AS, Opal SM, Sadoff JC, et al. Choice of bacteria in animal models of sepsis. *Infect Immun* 1993;61:2741–2747.
135. Cynamon MH, DeStefano MS. Beige mouse model of disseminated Mycobacterium avium complex infection. In: Zak O, Sande MA, eds. *Handbook of animal models of infection.* San Diego: Academic Press, 1999:321–330.

136. Dajcs JJ, Hume EB, Moreau JM, et al. Lysostaphin treatment of methicillin-resistant *Staphylococcus aureus* keratitis in the rabbit. *Invest Ophthalmol Vis Sci* 2000;41:1432–1437.
137. Dajcs JJ, Moreau JM, Stroman DW, et al. The effectiveness of tobramycin and Ocuflox in a prophylaxis model of *Staphylococcus keratitis*. *Curr Eye Res* 2001;23:60–63.
138. Dajcs JJ, Thibodeaux BA, Girgis DO, et al. Immunity to lysostaphin and its therapeutic value for ocular MRSA infections in the rabbit. *Invest Ophthalmol Vis Sci* 2002;43:3712–3716.
139. Dalhoff A, Matuat S, Ullmann U. Effect of quinolones against slowly growing bacteria. *Chemotherapy* 1995;41: 92–99.
140. Dalhoff A, Ullmann U. Correlation between pharmacokinetics, pharmacodynamics and efficacy of antibacterial agents in animal models. *Eur J Clin Microbiol Infect Dis* 1990;9:479–487.
141. Dannaoui E, Mouton JW, Meis JFGM, et al. Efficacy of antifungal therapy in a nonneutropenic murine model of zygomycosis. *Antimicrob Agents Chemother* 2002;46: 1953–1959.
142. Davey PG, Renneberg J, Speller DCE, eds. Bacterial infection models in antimicrobial chemotherapy. *J Antimicrobial Chemother* 1993[Suppl D];31:1–205.
143. Davila D, Kolancy-Babic L. Pharmacokinetics of azithromycin after single oral dosing of experimental animals. *Biopharm Drug Dispos* 1991;12:505–514.
144. Davis CC, Mellencamp MA, Preheim LC. A model of pneumococcal pneumonia in chronically intoxicated rats. *J Infect Dis* 1991;163:799–805.
145. De Backer MD, Van Dijck P. Progress in functional genomics approaches to antifungal drug target discovery. *Trends Microbiol* 2003;11:470–478.
146. Dedrick RL. Animal scale up. *J Pharmacokinet Biopharm* 1973;1:435–461.
147. de Greeve P, de Leeuw W. Ethics committees in Europe: an overview. In: Zak O, Sande MA, eds. *Handbook of animal models of infection*. San Diego: Academic Press, 1999:13–18.
148. de Lalla F. Antimicrobial chemotherapy in the control of surgical infectious complications. *J Chemother* 1999;11:440–445.
149. Deepe GS Jr, Gibbons R. Recombinant murine granulocyte-macrophage colony-stimulating factor modulates the course of pulmonary histoplasmosis in immunocompetent and immunodeficient mice. *Antimicrob Agents Chemother* 2000;44:3328–3336.
150. del Poeta M, Toffaletti DL, Rude TH, et al. *Cryptococcus neoformans* differential gene expression detected in vitro and in vivo with green fluorescent protein. *Infect Immun* 1999;67:1812–1820.
151. Demarco de Hormaeche R, Macpherson A, Bowe F, et al. Alterations of the LPS determine virulence of *Neisseria gonorrhoeae* in guinea-pig subcutaneous chambers. *Microb Pathog* 1991;11:159–170.
152. den Hollander JG, Mouton JW, Verbrugh HA. Use of pharmacodynamic parameters to predict efficacy of combination therapy by using fractional inhibitory concentration kinetics. *Antimicrob Agents Chemother* 1998;42: 744–748.
153. Deshpande LM, Jones RN. Antagonism between penicillin and erythromycin against *Streptococcus pneumoniae*: does it exist? *Diagn Microbiol Infect Dis* 2003;46:223–225.
154. Dhillon J, Mitchison DA. Effect of vaccines in a murine model of dormant tuberculosis. *Tuber Lung Dis* 1994;75:61–64.
155. Dickinson J, Guy A, Mitchison DA. Bioavailability of rifampin in experimental murine tuberculosis. *Antimicrob Agents Chemother* 1992;36:2066–2067.
156. Dickson EW, Doern GV, Trevino L, et al. Prevention of descending pneumonia in rats with perflubron-delivered tobramycin. *Acad Emerg Med* 2003;10:1019–1023.
157. Dickson EW, Heard SO, Tarara TE, et al. Liquid ventilation with perflubron in the treatment of rats with pneumococcal pneumonia. *Crit Care Med* 2002;30:393–395.
158. Dietrich WF. Using mouse genetics to understand infectious disease pathogenesis. *Genome Res* 2001;11:325–331.
159. Dijkstra HM, Manson WL, Klasen HJ, et al. Effect of polymixin B on intestinal bacterial translocation in *Pseudomonas aeruginosa* wound-colonized burned mice. *Eur Surg Res* 1992;24:69–76.
160. Doherty PC, Kaufmann SHE. Novel insights and new models in a time of rapid technological change. *Curr Opin Immunol* 1994;6:515–517.
161. Domingue G, Ellis B, Dasgupta M, Costerton JW. Testing antimicrobial susceptibilities of adherent bacteria by a method that incorporates guidelines of the National Committee for Clinical Laboratory Standards. *J Clin Microbiol* 1994;32:2564–2568.
162. Dong M-Y, Chang T-W, Gorbach SL. Treatment of *Clostridium difficile* colitis in hamsters with a lipopeptide antibiotic, LY146032. *Antimicrob Agents Chemother* 1987;31:1135–1136.
163. Drummond LJ, Smith DG, Poxton IR. Effects of sub-MIC concentrations of antibiotics on growth of and toxin production by *Clostridium difficile*. *J Med Microbiol* 2003;52:1033–1038.
164. Drusano GL. Antimicrobial pharmacodynamics: critical interactions of "bug and drug." *Nat Rev Microbiol* 2004;2:289–300.
165. Dudley MN, Blaser J, Gilbert D, et al. Combination therapy with ciprofloxacin plus azlocillin against *Pseudomonas aeruginosa*: effect of simultaneous versus staggered administration in an in vitro model of infection. *J Infect Dis* 1991;164:499–506.
166. Duguid IG, Evans E, Brown MRW, et al. Growth-rate–independent killing by ciprofloxacin of biofilm-derived *Staphylococcus epidermidis*: evidence for cell-cycle dependency. *J Antimicrob Chemother* 1992;30:791–802.
167. Dupont H, Montravers P. Rat polymicrobial peritonitis infection model. In: Zak O, Sande MA, eds. *Handbook of animal models of infection*. San Diego: Academic Press, 1999:189–194.
168. Dupuis A, Limosin A, Paquereau J, et al. Pharmacokinetic-pharmacodynamic modeling of electroencephalogram effect of imipenem in rats with acute renal failure. *Antimicrob Agents Chemother* 2001;45:3607–3609.
168a. Dworkin R, Modin G, Kunz S, et al. Comparative efficacies of ciprofloxacin, pefloxacin, and vancomycin in combination with rifampin in a rat model of methicillin-resistant *Staphylococcus aureus* chronic osteomyelitis. *Antimicrob Agents Chemother* 1990;34:1014–1016.
169. Ebong SJ, Goyert SM, Nemzek JA, et al. Critical role of CD14 for production of proinflammatory cytokines and cytokine inhibitors during sepsis with failure to alter morbidity or mortality. *Infect Immun* 2001;69:2099–2106.
170. Echchannaoui H, Frei K, Schnell C, et al. Toll-like receptor 2-deficient mice are highly susceptible to *Streptococcus pneumoniae* meningitis because of reduced bacterial clearing and enhanced inflammation. *J Infect Dis* 2002;186:798–806.
171. Eichacker PQ, Parent C, Kalil A, et al. Risk and the efficacy of antiinflammatory agents retrospective and

confirmatory studies of sepsis. *Am J Respir Crit Care Med* 2002;166:1197–1205.

171a. Ehrlich GD, Veeh R, Wang X, et al. Mucosal biofilm formation on middle-ear mucosa in the chinchilla model of otitis media. *JAMA* 2002;287:1710–1715.

172. Elahi S, Pang G, Clancy R, et al. Cellular and cytokine correlates of mucosal protection in murine model of oral candidiasis. *Infect Immun* 2000;68:5771–5777.

173. Eliopoulos GM, Thauvin-Eliopoulos C, Moellering RC. Contribution of animal models in the search for effective therapy for endocarditis due to enterococci with high-level resistance to gentamicin. *Clin Infect Dis* 1992;15:58–62.

174. el-Massry A, Meredith TA, Aguilar HE, et al. Aminoglycoside levels in the rabbit vitreous cavity after intravenous administration. *J Ophthalmol* 1996;122:684–689.

175. Elmros T, Holm SE, Kjellberg E, et al. Ampicillin treatment of *Neisseria gonorrhoeae* in vivo: an experimental study in rabbits. *Acta Pathol Microbiol Scand [B]* 1981;89:43–148.

176. El-Zaim HS, Chopra AK, Peterson JW, et al. Protection against exotoxin A (ETA) and *Pseudomonas aeruginosa* infection in mice with ETA-specific antipeptide antibodies. *Infect Immun* 1998;66:5551–5554.

177. Endo H, Yoshida H, Ohmi N, et al. Effects of lansoprazole, clarithromycin and pH gradient on uptake of [^{14}C]amoxicillin into rat gastric tissue. *J Antimicrob Chemother* 2001;47:405–410.

178. Eng RHK, Hsieh A, Smith SM. Antibiotic killing of bacteria: comparison of bacteria on surfaces and in liquid, growing and nongrowing. *Chemotherapy* 1995;41:113–120.

179. English AR, Girard D, Haskell SL. Pharmacokinetics of sultamicillin in mice, rats, and dogs. *Antimicrob Agents Chemother* 1984;25:599–602.

180. Entenza JM, Blatter M, Glauser MP, et al. Parenteral sparfloxacin compared with ceftriaxone in treatment of experimental endocarditis due to penicillin-susceptible and -resistant streptococci. *Antimicrob Agents Chemother* 1994;38:2638–2688.

181. Entenza JM, Fluckiger U, Glauser MP, et al. Antibiotic treatment of experimental endocarditis due to methicillin-resistant *Staphylococcus epidermidis*. *J Infect Dis* 1994;170:100–109.

182. Erlendsdottir H, Knudsen JD, Odenholt I, et al. Penicillin pharmacodynamics in four experimental pneumococcal infection models. *Antimicrob Agents Chemother* 2001;45:1078–1085.

183. Ernst EJ, Klepser ME, Petzold CR, et al. Evaluation of survival and pharmacodynamic relationships for five fluoroquinolones in a neutropenic murine model of pneumococcal lung Infection. *Pharmacotherapy* 2002;22:463–470.

184. Ernst JD, Sande MA. Selected examples of failure of in vitro testing to predict in vivo response to antibiotics. In: Sabath LD, ed. *Action of antibiotics in patients*. Bern: Hans Huber Publishers, 1982:68–73.

185. Espersen F, Frimdodt-Møller N, Corneliussen L, et al. Experimental foreign body infection in mice. *J Antimicrob Chemother* 1993;31[Suppl D]:103–111.

186. Estrem SA. Bacterial otitis externa in the guinea-pig model. In: Zak O, Sande MA, eds. *Handbook of animal models of infection*. San Diego: Academic Press, 1999:385–387.

187. Evans D, Kuo T, Kwong M, et al. *Pseudomonas aeruginosa* strains with lipopolysaccharide defects exhibit reduced intracellular viability after invasion of corneal epithelial cells. *Exp Eye Res* 2002;75:635–643.

188. Fantin B, Carbon C. In vivo antibiotic synergism: contribution of animal models. *Antimicrob Agents Chemother* 1992;36:907–912.

189. Fantin B, Ebert S, Leggett J, et al. Factors affecting duration of in-vivo postantibiotic effect for aminoglycosides against Gram-negative bacilli. *J Antimicrob Chemother* 1991;27:829–836.

190. Fantin B, Legget J, Ebert S, et al. Correlation between in vitro and in vivo activity of antimicrobial agents against Gram-negative bacilli in a murine infection model. *Antimicrob Agents Chemother* 1991;35:1413–1422.

191. Farah CS, Elahi S, Pang G, et al. T cells augment monocyte and neutrophil function in host resistance against oropharyngeal candidiasis. *Infect Immun* 2001;69:6110–6118.

192. Farah CS, Gotjamanos T, Seymour GJ, et al. Cytokines in the oral mucosa of mice infected with *Candida albicans*. *Oral Microbiol Immunol* 2002;17:375–378.

193. Fattorini L, Xiao Y, Mattei M, et al. Activities of eighteen antimicrobial regimens against *Mycobacterium avium* infection in beige mice. *Microb Drug Resist* 1999;5:227–233.

194. Fein AM. Pneumonia in the elderly: overview of diagnostic and therapeutic approaches. *Clin Infect Dis* 1999;28:726–729.

195. Felts AG, Grainger DW, Slunt JB. Locally delivered antibodies combined with systemic antibiotics confer synergistic protection against antibiotic-resistant burn wound Infection. *J Trauma* 2000;49:873–878.

196. Fernandez de Gatta MM, Fruns I, Calvo MV, et al. Influence of pharmacokinetic model on vancomycin peak concentration targets. *Ther Drug Monit* 1996;18:145–148.

197. Ferrari L, Iavarone L, Braggio S, et al. In vitro and in vivo pharmacokinetics-pharmacodynamics of GV143253A, a novel trinem. *Antimicrob Agents Chemother* 2003;47:770–776.

198. Festing MF, Diamanti P, Turton JA. Strain differences in haematological response to chloramphenicol succinate in mice: implications for toxicological research. *Food Chem Toxicol* 2001;39:375–383.

199. Finney DJ. *Probit analysis*. Cambridge: Cambridge University Press, 1971.

199a. Fischman AJ, Alpert NM, Babich JW, et al. The role of positron emission tomography in pharmacokinetic analysis. *Drug Metab Rev* 1997;29:923–956.

199b. Fischman AJ, Babich JW, Alpert NM, et al. Pharmacokinetics of ^{18}F-labeled trovafloxacin in normal and *Escherichia coli*–infected rats and rabbits studied with positron emission tomography. *Clin Microbiol Infect* 1997;3:63–72.

200. Fitzgerald TJ. Effects of cefetamet (Ro 15–8074) on *Treponema pallidum* and experimental syphilis. *Antimicrob Agents Chemother* 1992;36:598–602.

201. Flaherty JF, Barriere SL, Mordenti J, et al. Effect of dose on pharmacokinetics and serum bactericidal activity of mezlocillin. *Antimicrob Agents Chemother* 1987;31:895–898.

202. Flecknall P, Waterman-Pearson A. *Pain management in animals*. London: WB Saunders, 2000.

203. Fluckiger U, Moreillon P, Blaser J, et al. Simulation of amoxicillin pharmacokinetics in humans for the prevention of streptococcal endocarditis in rats. *Antimicrob Agents Chemother* 1994;38:2846–2849.

204. Fluckiger U, Segessenmann C, Gerber AU. Integration of pharmacokinetics and pharmacodynamics of imipenem in a human-adapted mouse model. *Antimicrob Agents Chemother* 1991;35:1905–1910.

205. Foley I, Brown MRW. Activity of antibiotics against adherent/slow-growing bacteria reflecting the situation in vivo. In: Zak O, Sande MA, eds. *Handbook of animal*

models of infection. San Diego: Academic Press, 1999: 117–123.
206. Francis KP, Joh D, Bellinger-Kawahara C, et al. Monitoring bioluminescent *Staphylococcus aureus* infections in living mice using a novel luxABCDE construct. *Infect Immun* 2000;68:3594–3600.
207. Francis KP, Yu J, Bellinger-Kawahara C, et al. Visualizing pneumococcal infections in the lungs of live mice using bioluminescent *Streptococcus pneumoniae* transformed with a novel Gram-positive. *Infect Immun* 2001;69:3350–3358.
208. Francois P, Tu Quoc PH, Bisognano C, et al. Lack of biofilm contribution to bacterial colonisation in an experimental model of foreign body infection by *Staphylococcus aureus* and *Staphylococcus epidermidis*. *FEMS Immunol Med Microbiol* 2003;35:135–140.
209. Frimodt Møller N. Correlation of in vitro activity and pharmacokinetic parameters with effect in vivo for antibiotics: observations from experimental pneumococcus infection. *Dan Med Bull* 1988;35:422–437.
210. Frimodt Møller N. The mouse peritonitis model: present and future use. *J Antimicrob Chemother* 1993;31[Suppl D]:55–60.
211. Frimodt-Møller N. How predictive is PK/PD for antibacterial agents? *Int J Antimicrob Agents* 2002;19:333–339.
212. Frimodt-Møller N. Correlation between pharmacokinetic/pharmacodynamic parameters and efficacy for antibiotics in the treatment of urinary tract infection. *Int J Antimicrob Agents* 2002;19:546–553.
213. Frimodt Møller N, Knudsen JD, Espersen F. The mouse peritonitis/sepsis model. In: Zak O, Sande MA, eds. *Handbook of animal models of infection*. San Diego: Academic Press, 1999:127–136.
214. Frimodt Møller N, Thomsen VF. The pneumococcus and the mouse protection test: inoculum, dosage and timing. *Acta Path Microbiol Immunol Scand [B]* 1986;94:33–37.
215. Frimodt-Møller N, Thomsen VF. Interaction between beta-lactam antibiotics and gentamicin against *Streptococcus pneumoniae* in vitro and in vivo. *APMIS* 1987;95:269–275.
216. Fritz B, Raczniak GA. Bacterial genomics: potential for antimicrobial drug discovery. *BioDrugs* 2002;16:331–337.
217. Fu KP, Foleno BD, Lafredo SC, et al. In vitro and in vivo antibacterial activities of FK037, a novel parenteral broad-spectrum cephalosporin. *Antimicrob Agents Chemother* 1993;37:301–307.
218. Fukuda M, Hanazome I, Sasaki K. The intraocular dynamics of vancomycin hydrochloride ophthalmic ointment (TN-011) in rabbits. *J Infect Chemother* 2003;9:93–96.
219. Fukuda M, Sasaki K. General purpose antimicrobial ophthalmic solutions evaluated using new pharmacokinetic parameter of maximum drug concentration in aqueous. *Jpn J Ophthalmol* 2002;46:384–390.
220. Fukuoka T, Kawada H, Kitayam A, et al. Efficacy of CS-834 against experimental pneumonia caused by penicillin-susceptible and -resistant *Streptococcus pneumoniae* in mice. *Antimicrob Agents Chemother* 1998;42:23–27.
221. Fulurija A, Ashman RB, Papadimitriou JM. Early inflammatory responses to *Candida albicans* infection in inbred and complement-deficient mice. *FEMS Immunol Med Microbiol* 1996;14:83–94.
222. Fulurija A, Ashman RB, Papadimitriou JM. Neutrophil depletion increases susceptibility to systemic and vaginal candidiasis in mice, and reveals differences between brain and kidney in mechanisms of host resistance. *Microbiology* 1996;142;3487–3496.
223. Fulurija A, Ashman RB, Papadimitriou JM. Increased tissue resistance in the nude mouse against *Candida albicans* without altering strain-dependent differences in susceptibility. *J Med Vet Mycol* 1997;35:197–203.
224. Fung-Leung WP, Mak TW. Embryonic stem cells and homologous recombination. *Curr Opin Immunol* 1992;4:187–194.
225. Gangadharam PR. Beige mouse model for *Mycobacterium avium* complex disease. *Antimicrob Agents Chemother* 1995;30:1647–1654.
226. Gangadharam PRJ, Ashtekar DR, Flasher DL, et al. Therapy of *Mycobacterium avium* complex infections in beige mice with streptomycin encapsulated in sterically stabilized liposomes. *Antimicrob Agents Chemother* 1995;39:725–730.
227. Gangadharam PR, Perumal VK, Farhi DC, et al. The beige mouse model for *Mycobacterium avium* complex (MAC) disease: optimal conditions for the host and parasite. *Tubercule* 1989;70:257–271.
228. Ganzinger U, Haslberger A. Pharmacokinetics of cephalosporins in normal and septicemic rabbits. *Antimicrob Agents Chemother* 1985;28:473–477.
229. Gardner ID. The effect of aging on susceptibility to infection. *Rev Infect Dis* 1980;2:801–810.
229a. Gavalda J, Capdevila JA, Almirante B, et al. Treatment of experimental pneumonia due to penicillin-resistant *Streptococcus pneumoniae* in immunocompetent rats. *Antimicrob Agents Chemother* 1997;41:795–801.
230. Gerber AU. Impact of the antibiotic dosage schedule on efficacy in experimental soft tissue infections. *Scand J Infect Dis Suppl* 1990;74:147–154.
231. Gerber AU, Brugger H-P, Feller C, et al. Antibiotic therapy of infections due to *Pseudomonas aeruginosa* in normal and granulocytopenic mice: comparison of murine and human pharmacokinetics. *J Infect Dis* 1986;153:90–97.
232. Gerber AU, Greter U, Segessenmann C, et al. The impact of pre-treatment interval on antimicrobial efficacy in a biological model. *J Antimicrob Chemother* 1993;31 [Suppl D]:29–39.
233. Gerber AU, Stritzko T, Segessenmann C, et al. Simulation of human pharmacokinetic profiles in mice, and impact on antimicrobial efficacy of netilmicin, ticarcillin and ceftazidime in the peritonitis-septicemia model. *Scand J Infect Dis Suppl* 1990;74:195–203.
234. Giacomini KM, Roberts SM, Levy G. Evaluation of methods for producing renal dysfunction in rats. *J Pharm Sci* 1981;70:117–121.
235. Giese MJ, Rayner SA, Fardin B, et al. Mitigation of neutrophil infiltration in a rat model of early *Staphylococcus aureus* endophthalmitis. *Invest Ophthalmol Vis Sci* 2003;44:3077–3082.
236. Giese MJ, Sumner HL, Berliner JA, et al. Cytokine expression in a rat model of *Staphylococcus aureus* endophthalmitis. *Invest Ophthalmol Vis Sci* 1998;39:2785–2790.
237. Glauser MP, Bonard M. Treatment of experimental ascending *Escherichia coli* pyelonephritis with ceftriaxone alone and in combination with gentamicin. *Chemotherapy* 1982;28:410–416.
238. Glauser MP, Lyons JM, Braude AI. Synergism of ampicillin and gentamicin against obtructive pyelonephritis due to *Escherichia coli* in rats. *J Infect Dis* 1979;139:133–140.
239. Glauser MP, Ransley P, Bille J. Urinary tract infections, pyelonephritic scars, and chemotherapy. In: Zak O, Sande MA, eds. *Experimental models in antimicrobial chemotherapy*, vol. 1. London: Academic Press, 1986: 319–346.

240. Gomes MS, Dom G, Pedrosa J, et al. Effects of iron deprivation on *Mycobacterium avium* growth. *Tuberc Lung Dis* 1999;79:321–328.
241. Goncalves AS, Appelberg R. Effects of recombinant granulocyte-colony stimulating factor administration during *Mycobacterium avium* infection in mice. *Clin Exp Immunol* 2001;124:239–247.
242. Goodman JL, Jurkovich P, Kodner C, et al. Persistent cardiac and urinary tract infections with *Borrelia burgdorferi* in experimentally infected Syrian hamsters. *J Clin Microbiol* 1991;29:894–896.
243. Gordin FM, Rusnak MG, Sande MA. Evaluation of combination chemotherapy in a lightly anesthetized animal model of *Pseudomonas pneumonia*. *Antimicrob Agents Chemother* 1987;31:398–403.
244. Gottstein B. Animal models in parasitology. *Contrib Microbiol* 2001;9:31–44.
245. Greer LF 3rd, Szalay AA. Imaging of light emission from the expression of luciferases in living cells and organisms: a review. *Luminescence* 2002;17:43–74.
246. Griffith DC, Harford L, Williams R, et al. In vivo antibacterial activity of RWJ-54428, a new cephalosporin with activity against Gram-positive bacteria. *Antimicrob Agents Chemother* 2003;47:43–47.
247. Griffiths JK, Theodos C, Paris M, et al. The gamma interferon gene knockout mouse: a highly sensitive model for the evaluation of therapeutic agents against *Cryptosporidium parvum*. *J Clin Microbiol* 1998;36:2503–2508.
248. Grimwood K, To M, Rabin HR, et al. Inhibition of *Pseudomonas aeruginosa* exoenzyme expression by subinhibitory antibiotic concentrations. *Antimicrob Agents Chemother* 1989;33:41–47.
249. Grimwood K, To M, Rabin HR, et al. Subinhibitory antibiotics reduce *Pseudomonas aeruginosa* tissue injury in the rat lung model. *J Antimicrob Chemother* 1989;24:937–945.
250. Grunberg E. The effect of trimethoprim on the activity of sulfonamides and antibiotics in experimental infections. *J Infect Dis* 1973;128[Suppl]:S478–S485
251. Grunberg E, Cleeland R. In vivo activity of the 6-amidinopenicillanic acid derivative, mecillinam, chemically linked or combined in varying ratios with 6-aminopenicillanic acid derivatives. *J Antimicrob Chemother* 1977;3[Suppl B]:59–68.
252. Gudmundsson S, Einarsson S, Erlendsdottir H, et al. The post antibiotic effect of antimicrobial combinations in a neutropenic murine thigh infection model. *J Antimicrob Chemother* 1993;31(Suppl D):177–192.
253. Gudmundsson S, Erlendsdottir H. Murine thigh infection model. In: Zak O, Sande MA, eds. *Handbook of animal models of infection.* San Diego: Academic Press, 1999:137–144.
254. Gudmundsson S, Erlendsdottir H, Gottfredsson M, et al. The postantibiotic effect induced by antimicrobial combinations. *Scand J Infect Dis Suppl* 1990;74:80–93.
255. Gudmundsson S, Vogelman B, Craig WA. The in-vivo postantibiotic effect of imipenem and other new antimicrobials. *J Antimicrob Chemother* 1986;18[Suppl E]: 67–73.
256. Gupta SK, Dhingra N, Velpandian T, et al. Efficacy of fluconazole and liposome entrapped fluconazole for *C. albicans* induced experimental mycotic endophthalmitis in rabbit eyes. *Acta Ophthalmol Scand* 2000;78:448–450.
257. Gupta SK, Velpandian T, Dhingra N, et al. Intravitreal pharmacokinetics of plain and liposome-entrapped fluconazole in rabbit eyes. *J Ocul Pharmacol Ther* 2000;16:511–518.
258. Gutschik E. The *Enterococcus endocarditis* model in experimental animals and its relevance to human infections. *J Antimicrob Chemother* 1993;31[Suppl D]:87–96.
259. Hagberg L, Engberg I, Freter R, et al. Ascending unobstructed urinary tract infection in mice caused by pyelonephritogenic *Escherichia coli* of human origin. *Infect Immun* 1983;40:273–283.
260. Hajek DM, Yuan Z, Quartey MK, et al. Otitis media: the chinchilla model. In: Zak O, Sande MA, eds. *Handbook of animal models of infection.* San Diego: Academic Press, 1999:389–401.
261. Hanfelt JJ. Statistical approaches to experimental design and data analysis of in vivo studies. *Breast Cancer Res Treat* 1997;46:279–302.
262. Hang L, John M, Asaduzzaman M, et al. Use of in vivo-induced antigen technology (IVIAT) to identify genes uniquely expressed during human infection with *Vibrio cholerae*. *Proc Natl Acad Sci USA* 2003;100:8508–8513.
262a. Hansen AK. The impact of general laboratory animal health on experimental models in antimicrobial chemotherapy. In: Zak O, Sande MA, eds. *Handbook of animal models of infection.* San Diego: Academic Press, 1999:49–59.
263. Hansen EJ, Toews GB. Animal models for the study of noninvasive *Haemophilus influenzae* disease: pulmonary clearance systems. *J Infect Dis* 1992;165[Suppl 1]:S185–S187.
264. Haraoka M, Matsumoto T, Takashi K, et al. Suppression of renal scarring by prednisolone combined with ciprofloxacin in ascending pyelonephritis in rats. *J Urol* 1994;151:1078–1080.
265. Harter DH, Petersdorf RG. A consideration of the pathogenesis of bacterial meningitis: review of experimental and clinical studies. *Yale J Biol Med* 1960;32:280–309.
266. Hata K, Kimura J, Miki H, et al. Efficacy of ER-30346, a novel oral triazole antifungal agent, in experimental models of aspergillosis, candidiasis, and cryptococcosis. *Antimicrob Agents Chemother* 1996;40:2243–2247.
267. Hatano K, Wakai Y, Watanabe Y, et al. Simulation of human plasma levels of β-lactams in mice by multiple dosing and the relationship between the therapeutic efficacy and pharmacodynamic parameters. *Chemotherapy* 1994;40:1–7.
268. Hautefort I, Proenca MJ, Hinton JC. Single-copy green fluorescent protein gene fusions allow accurate measurement of Salmonella gene expression in vitro and during infection of mammalian cells. *Appl Environ Microbiol* 2003;69:7480–7491.
269. Hayney MS. Pharmacogenomics and infectious diseases: impact on drug response and applications to disease management. *Am J Health Syst Pharm* 2002;59:1626–1631.
270. Hebda PA, Piltcher OB, Swarts JD, et al. Cytokine profiles in a rat model of otitis media with effusion caused by eustachian tube obstruction with and without *Streptococcus pneumoniae* infection. *Laryngoscope* 2002;112:1657–1662.
271. Hellman J, Loiselle PM, Zanzot EM, et al. Release of Gram-negative outer-membrane proteins into human serum and septic rat blood and their interactions with immunoglobulin in antiserum to *Escherichia coli* J5. *J Infect Dis* 2000;181;1034–1043.
272. Hermans PGC, Fosse RT, van der Gulden WJI, et al. Organisation and management of animal experiments. In: van Zutphen LFM, Baumans V, Beyen AC, eds. *Principles of laboratory animal science.* Amsterdam: Elsevier, 1993:241–254.
273. Hershberger E, Coyle EA, Kaatz GW, et al. Comparison of a rabbit model of bacterial endocarditis and an in vitro

infection model with simulated endocardial vegetations. *Antimicrob Agents Chemother* 2000;44:1921–1924.

274. Hishikawa T, Kusunoki T, Tsushiya K, et al. Application of mathematical model to experimental chemotherapy of fatal murine pneumonia. *Antimicrob Agents Chemother* 1990;34:326–331.
275. Hollenberg SM, Dumasius A, Easington C, et al. Characterization of a hyperdynamic murine model of resuscitated sepsis using echocardiography. *Am J Respir Crit Care Med* 2001;164:891–895.
276. Holt D, Harvey D, Hurley R. Chloramphenicol toxicity. *Adverse Drug React Toxicol Rev* 1993;12:83–95.
277. Hoogeterp JJ, Mattie H, Krul AM, et al. The efficacy of rifampicin against *Staphylococcus aureus* in vitro and in an experimental infection in normal and granulocytopenic mice. *Scand J Infect Dis* 1988;20:649–656.
278. Hughes WT, Armstrong D, Bodey GP, et al. Guidelines for the use of antimicrobial agents in neutropenic patients with unexplained fever. *J Infect Dis* 1990;161:381–396.
279. Humphrey WR, Shattuck MH, Zielinski RJ, et al. Pharmacokinetics and efficacy of linezolid in a gerbil model of *Streptococcus pneumoniae*-induced acute otitis media. *Antimicrob Agents Chemother* 2003;47:1355–1363.
280. Hvidberg H, Struve C, Krogfelt KA, et al. Development of a long-term ascending urinary tract infection mouse model for antibiotic treatment studies. *Antimicrob Agents Chemother* 2000;44:156–163.
281. Hyde SR, Stitih RD, McCallum RE. Mortality and bacteriology of sepsis following cecal ligation and puncture in aged mice. *Infect Immun* 1990;58:619–624.
282. Isenberg HD, Sampson-Scherer J, Cleeland R, et al. Correlation of the results of antibiotic synergy and susceptibility testing in vitro with results in experimental mouse infections. *Crit Rev Microbiol* 1982;10:1–76.
283. Itoyama T, Uchida K, Yamaguchi H. Therapeutic effects of omoconazole nitrate on guinea-pigs experimentally infected with *Trichphyton mentagrophytes*. *J Antimicrob Chemother* 1997;39:825–827.
284. Jacobi CA, Roggenkamp A, Rakin A, et al. In vitro and in vivo expression studies of yopE from *Yersinia enterocolitica* using the gfp reporter gene. *Mol Microbiol* 1998;30:865–882.
285. Jacques M, Turgeon PL, Mathieu LG, et al. Effect of subminimal inhibitory concentrations of antibiotics on adherence of *Neisseria gonorrhoeae* in an experimental model. *Exp Biol* 1985;43:251–256.
286. Jayaram R, Gaonkar S, Kaur P, et al. Pharmacokinetics-pharmacodynamics of rifampin in an aerosol infection model of tuberculosis. *Antimicrob Agents Chemother* 2003;47:2118–2124.
287. Jerse AE. Experimental gonococcal genital tract infection and opacity protein expression in estradiol-treated mice. *Infect Immun* 1999;67:5699–5708.
288. Jerse AE, Sharma ND, Simms AN, et al. A gonococcal efflux pump system enhances bacterial survival in a female mouse model of genital tract infection. *Infect Immun* 2003;71:5576–5582.
289. Johansen HK, Høiby N. Rat model of chronic *Pseudomonas aeruginosa*. In: Zak O, Sande MA, eds. *Handbook of animal models of infection*. San Diego: Academic Press, 1999:517–532.

289a. Johansen HK, Jensen TG, Dessau RB, et al. Antagonism between penicillin and erythromycin against *Streptococcus pneumoniae* in vitro and in vivo. *J Antimicrob Chemother* 2000;46:973–980.

290. Johnson AP, Tuffrey M, Taylor-Robinson D. Resistance of mice to genital infection with *Neisseria gonorrhoeae*. *J Med Microbiol* 1989;30:33–36.
291. Johnson DE, Lockatell CV. Mouse model of ascending UTI involving short- and long-term indwelling catheters. In: Zak O, Sande MA, eds. *Handbook of animal models of infection*. San Diego: Academic Press, 1999:441–445.
292. Johnson DE, Lockatell CV, Hall-Craggs M, et al. Mouse models of short- and long-term foreign body in the urinary bladder: analogies to the bladder segment of urinary catheters. *Lab Anim Sci* 1991;41:451–455.
293. Johnson JA, Lau BH, Nutter RL, et al. Effect of L1210 leukemia on the susceptibility of mice to *Candida albicans* infections. *Infect Immun* 1978;19:146–151.
294. Johnson JR, Brown JJ. Defining inoculation conditions for the mouse model of ascending urinary tract infection that avoid immediate vesicoureteral reflux yet produce renal and bladder infection. *J Infect Dis* 1996;173:1306–1311.
295. Joiner K, Lower B, Dzink J, et al. Comparative efficacy of 10 antimicrobial agents in experimental infections with *Bacteroides fragilis*. *J Infect Dis* 1982;145:561–568.
296. Josenhans C, Friedrich S, Suerbaum S. Green fluorescent protein as a novel marker and reporter system in *Helicobacter* sp. *FEMS Microbiol Lett* 1998;161:263–273.
297. Ju JL, Polhamus C, Marr KA, et al. Efficacies of fluconazole, caspofungin, and amphotericin B in *Candida glabrata*-infected p47 phox−/− knockout mice. *Antimicrob Agents Chemother* 2002;46:1240–1245.
298. Julio SM, Conner CP, Heithoff DM, et al. Directed formation of chromosomal deletions in *Salmonella typhimurium*: targeting of specific genes induced during infection. *Mol Gen Genet* 1998;258:178–181.
299. Jungbluth GL, Jusko WJ. Dose-dependent pharmacokinetics of mezlocillin in rats. *Antimicrob Agents Chemother* 1989;33:839–843.
300. König C, Simmen HP, Blaser J. Effect of pathological changes of pH, pO_2 and pCO_2 on the activity of antimicrobial agents in vitro. *Eur J Clin Microbiol Infect Dis* 1993;12:519–526.
301. Kacew S, Festing MFW. Role of rat strain in the differential sensitivity to pharmaceutical agents and naturally occurring substances. *J Toxicol Environ Health* 1996;47:1–30.
302. Kadurugamuwa JL, Sin L, Albert E, et al. Direct continuous method for monitoring biofilm infection in a mouse model. *Infect Immun* 2003;71:882–890.
303. Kadurugamuwa JL, Sin LV, Yu J, et al. Rapid direct method for monitoring antibiotics in a mouse model of bacterial biofilm infection. *Antimicrob Agents Chemother* 2003;47:3130–3137.

303a. Kahlke V, Dohm C, Mees T, et al. Early interleukin-10 treatment improves survival and enhances immune function only in males after hemorrhage and subsequent sepsis. *Shock* 2002;18:24–28.

304. Kaijser B, Larsson P. Experimental acute pyelonephritis caused by enterobacteria in animals: a review. *J Urol* 1982;127:786–790.
305. Kaiser AB, Kernodle DS. Low-inoculum model of clean wound infection. In: Zak O, Sande MA, eds. *Handbook of animal models of infection*. San Diego: Academic Press, 1999:205–211.
306. Kajdacsy-Balla A, Howeedy A, Bagasra O. Experimental model of congenital syphilis. *Infect Immun* 1993;61:3559–3561.
307. Kajdacsy-Balla A, Howeedy A, Bagasra O. Syphilis in the Syrian hamster: a model of human veneral and congenital syphilis. *Am J Pathol* 1987;126:599–601.
308. Kalns J, Morris J, Eggers J, et al. Delayed treatment with doxycycline has limited effect on anthrax infection in BKL57/B6. *Biochem Biophys Res Commun* 2002;297:506–509.

308a. Kamei K, Miyaji M. Animal models in mycology. *Contrib Microbiol* 2001;9:45–57.

309. Kanellakopoulou K, Giamarellos-Bourboulis EJ. Carrier systems for the local delivery of antibiotics in bone infections. *Drugs* 2000;59:1223–1232.

310. Kaplan E, Dinarello CA, Wakabayachi G, et al. Interleukin-1 pretreatment protects against endotoxin-induced hypotension in rabbits: association with decreased tumor necrosis factor levels. *J Infect Dis* 1993;167:244–247.

311. Kapral FA, Godwin JR, Dye ES. Formation of intraperitoneal abscesses by *Staphylococcus aureus*. *Infect Immun* 1980;30:204–211.

312. Kararli TT. Comparison of the gastrointestinal anatomy, physiology, and biochemistry of humans and commonly used laboratory animals. *Biopharm Drug Dispos* 1995;16:351–380.

312a. Kartalija M, Kaye K, Tureen JH, et al. Treatment of experimental cryptococcal meningitis with fluconazole: impact of dose and addition of flucytosine on mycologic and pathophysiologic outcome. *J Infect Dis* 1996;173:1216–1221.

313. Katsarolis I, Pefanis A, Iliopoulos D, et al. Successful trovafloxacin prophylaxis against experimental streptococcal aortic valve endocarditis. *Antimicrob Agents Chemother* 2000;44:2564–2566.

314. Kaufmann SHE. Bacterial and protozoal infections in genetically disrupted mice. *Curr Opin Immunol* 1994;6:518–525.

315. Kaufmann SHE, Ladel CH. Application of knockout mice to the experimental analysis of infections with bacteria and protozoa. *Trends Microbiol* 1994;2:235–242.

316. Kawaharajo K, Shitoh K, Niizeki M, et al. Therapeutic efficacy of a new cephamycin, MT-141, in compromised mice. *J Antibiot (Tokyo)* 1984;37:1703–1711.

316a. Keevil CW, Davies DB, Spillane BJ, et al. Influence of iron-limited and replete continuous culture on the physiology and virulence of *Neisseria gonorrhoeae*. *J Gen Microbiol* 1989;135:851–863.

317. Kernacki KA, Hobden JA, Hazlett LD. Murine model of bacterial keratitis. In: Zak O, Sande MA, eds. *Handbook of animal models of infection*. San Diego: Academic Press, 1999:361–366.

318. Kerrn MB, Frimodt-Møller N, Espersen F. Effects of sulfamethizole and amdinocillin against *Escherichia coli* strains (with various susceptibilities) in an ascending urinary tract infection mouse model. *Antimicrob Agents Chemother* 2003;47:1002–1009.

319. Khanna PB, Davies I, Faragher EB. Age-related changes in the stomach of the laboratory mouse: a quantitative morphological study. *Age Ageing* 1988;17:257–264.

320. Kim IT, Park SK, Lim JH. Inflammatory response in experimental *Staphylococcus* and *Pseudomonas endophthalmitis*. *Ophthalmologica* 1999;213:305–310.

321. Kimura S, Gonzalez FJ. Applications of genetically manipulated mice in pharmacogenetics and pharmacogenomics. *Pharmacology* 2000;61:147–153.

322. Kirkwood BR. *Essentials of medical statistics*. Oxford: Blackwell Science, 1988.

323. Kita E, Matsuura H, Kashiba S. A mouse model for the study of gonococcal genital infection. *J Infect Dis* 1981;143:67–70.

324. Klein M, Koedel U, Pfister HW, et al. Meningitis-associated hearing loss: protection by adjunctive antioxidant therapy. *Ann Neurol* 2003;54:451–458.

325. Knowles DJ, King F. The impact of bacterial genomics on antibacterial discovery. *Adv Exp Med Biol* 1998;456:183–195.

326. Knudsen JD, Frimodt-Møller N. Animal models in bacteriology. *Contrib Microbiol* 2001;9:1–14.

327. Knudsen JD. The importance of pharmacodynamic properties in treatment of penicillin resistant *Streptococcus pneumoniae Dan Med Bull* 2000;47:313–327.

327a. Knudsen JD, Odenholt I, Erlendsdottir H, et al. Selection of resistant *Streptococcus pneumoniae* during penicillin treatment in vitro and in three animal models. *Antimicrob Agents Chemother* 2003;47:2499–2506.

328. Koga T, Inoue H, Ishii C, et al. Effect of plaunotol in combination with clarithromycin or amoxicillin on *Helicobacter pylori* in vitro and in vivo. *J Antimicrob Chemother* 2002;50:133–136.

329. Koller BH, Smithies O. Altering genes in animals by gene targeting. *Annu Rev Immunol* 1992;10:705–730.

330. Konstan MW, Vargo KM, Davis PB. Ibuprofen attenuates the inflammatory response to *Pseudomonas aeruginosa* in a rat model of chronic pulmonary infection. *Am Rev Respir Dis* 1990;141:186–192.

331. Korkusuz F, Korkusuz P, Eksioglu F, et al. In vivo response to biodegradable controlled antibiotic release systems. *J Biomed Mater Res* 2001;55:217–228.

332. Korting HC, Haag R, Walter D, et al. Efficacy of ceftizoxime in the treatment of incubating syphilis in rabbits. *Chemotherapy* 1993;39:331–335.

333. Kotake Y, Moore DR, Vasquez-Walden A, et al. Antioxidant amplifies antibiotic protection in the cecal ligation and puncture model of microbial sepsis through interleukin-10 production. *Shock* 2003;19:252–256.

334. Kovarik JM, Hoepelman AIM, Smit JM, et al. Steady-state pharmacokinetics and sputum penetration of lomefloxacin in patients with chronic obstructive pulmonary disease and acute respiratory tract infections. *Antimicrob Agents Chemother* 1992;36:2458–2461.

335. Kradolfer F. Models of tuberculosis in mice and guinea pigs. In: Zak O, Sande MA, eds. *Experimental models in antimicrobial chemotherapy*, vol. 2. London: Academic Press, 1986:321–345.

336. Kullberg B-J, van't Wout JW, Poell RJM, et al. Combined effect of fluconazole and recombinant human interleukin-1 on systemic candidiasis in neutropenic mice. *Antimicrob Agents Chemother* 1992;36:1225–1229.

337. Lally KP, Cruz E, Xue H. The role of anti-tumor necrosis factor-alpha and interleukin-10 in protecting murine neonates from *Escherichia coli* sepsis. *J Pediatr Surg* 2000;35:852–854.

338. Lally KP, Stonum TK. Age-dependent susceptibility to intraabdominal abscess formation. *J Pediatr Surg* 1996;31:301–303.

339. Lam-Yuk-Tseung S, Gros P. Genetic control of susceptibility to bacterial infections in mouse models. *Cell Microbiol* 2003;5:299–313.

340. Lang AB, Furer E, Cryz SJ. Feasibility of prophylaxis and therapy against Gram-negative infections by human monoclonal antibodies. *FEMS Immunol Med Microbiol* 1993;7:9–13.

341. Latifi SQ, O'Riordan MA, Levine AD. Interleukin-10 controls the onset of irreversible septic shock. *Infect Immun* 2002;70:4441–4446.

342. Le T, Bayer AS. Combination antibiotic therapy for infective endocarditis. *Clin Infect Dis* 2003;36:615–621.

343. LeBrun M, Grenier L, Gourde P, et al. Effectiveness and toxicity of gentamicin in an experimental model of pyelonephritis: effect of time of administration. *Antimicrob Agents Chemother* 1999;43:1020–1026.

344. Lecamwasam JP, Miller TE. Antimicrobial agents in the management of urinary tract infection: an experimental evaluation. *J Lab Clin Med* 1989;114:510–519.

345. Lee A, Fox J, Hazell S. Pathogenicity of *Helicobacter pylori*: a perspective. *Infect Immun* 1993;61:1601–1610.
346. Lee EJ, Truong TN, Mendoza MN, et al. A comparison of invasive and cytotoxic *Pseudomonas aeruginosa* strain-induced corneal disease responses to therapeutics. *Curr Eye Res* 2003;27:289–299.
347. Lefort A, Fantin B. Rabbit model of bacterial endocarditis. In: Zak O, Sande MA, eds. *Handbook of animal models of infection.* San Diego: Academic Press, 1999:611–618.
348. Legget J. Murine models of pneumonia using aerosol infection In: Zak O, Sande MA, eds. *Handbook of animal models of infection.* San Diego: Academic Press, 1999:533–538.
349. Leib SL, Heimgartner C, Bifrare YD, et al. Dexamethasone aggravates hippocampal apoptosis and learning deficiency in pneumococcal meningitis in infant rats. *Pediatr Res* 2003;353–357.
350. Lenaerts AJ, Gruppo V, Brooks JV, et al. Rapid in vivo screening of experimental drugs for tuberculosis using gamma interferon gene–disrupted mice. *Antimicrob Agents Chemother* 2003;47:783–785.
351. LeVatte MA, Woods DE, Shahrabadi MS, et al. Subinhibitory concentrations of tetracycline inhibit surface expression of the *Pseudomonas aeruginosa* ferripyochelin binding protein in vivo. *J Antimicrob Chemother* 1990;26:215–225.
352. Leveau JH, Lindow SE. Predictive and interpretive simulation of green fluorescent protein expression in reporter bacteria. *J Bacteriol* 2001;183:6752–6762.
353. Lewis DA, Reeves DS. Antibiotics at the extremes of age: choices and constraints. *J Antimicrob Chemother* 1994;34[Suppl A]:11–18.
354. Li X, Zhao H, Lockatell CV, et al. Visualization of *Proteus mirabilis* within the matrix of urease-induced bladder stones during experimental urinary tract infection. *Infect Immun* 2002;70:389–394.
355. Lin JH. Applications and limitations of interspecies scaling and in vitro extrapolation in pharmacokinetics. *Drug Metab Dispos* 1998;26:1202–1212.
356. Ling E, Feldman G, Dagan R, et al. Cytokine mRNA expression in pneumococcal carriage, pneumonia, and sepsis in young mice. *J Infect Dis* 2003;188:1752–1756.
357. Lister PD, Sanders CC. Comparison of ampicillin-sulbactam regimens simulating 1.5- and 3.0-gram doses to humans in treatment of *Escherichia coli* bacteremia in mice. *Antimicrob Agents Chemother* 1995;39:930–936.
358. Ljungberg B, Nilsson-Ehle I. Pharmacokinetics of antimicrobial agents in the elderly. *Rev Infect Dis* 1987;9:250–264.
359. Ljungberg B, Nilsson-Ehle I. Pharmacokinetics of meropenem and its metabolite in young and elderly healthy men. *Antimicrob Agents Chemother* 1992;36:1437–1440.
360. Lord JM, Butcher S, Killampali V, et al. Neutrophil ageing and immunesenescence. *Mech Ageing Dev* 2001;122:1521–1535.
361. Lorenz W, Reimund K-P, Weitzel F, et al. Granulocyte colony-stimulating factor prophylaxis before operation protects against lethal consequences of postoperative peritonitis. *Surgery* 1994;116:925–934.
362. Lounis N, Maslo C, Truffot-Pernot C, et al. Impact of iron loading on the activity of isoniazid or ethambutol in the treatment of murine tuberculosis. *Int J Tuberc Lung Dis* 2003;7:575–579.
363. Love LJ, Schimpff SC, Schiffer CA, et al. Improved prognosis for granulocytopenic patients with Gram-negative bacteremia. *Am J Med* 1980;68:643–647.
364. Lyerly DM, Saum KE, MacDonald DK, et al. Effects of *Clostridium difficile* toxins given intragastrically to animals. *Infect Immun* 1985;47:349–352.
365. MacCallum DM, Odds FC. Influence of grapefruit juice on itraconazole plasma levels in mice and guinea pigs. *J Antimicrob Chemother* 2002;50:219–214.
366. Maciver I, Silverman SJ, Brown MRW, et al. Rat model of chronic lung infections caused by non-typeable *Haemophilus influenzae*. *J Med Microbiol* 1991;35:139–147.
367. MacKenzie FM, Gould IM. The post-antibiotic effect. *J Antimicrob Chemother* 1993;32:519–537.
368. Mackowiak PA. Influence of fever on pharmacokinetics. *Rev Infect Dis* 1989;11:804–807.
369. Mader JT, Shirtliff ME. Rabbit model of bacterial osteomyelitis of the tiba. In: Zak O, Sande MA, eds. *Handbook of animal models of infection.* San Diego: Academic Press, 1999:581–592.
370. Mader JT, Stevens CM, Stevens JH, et al. Treatment of experimental osteomyelitis with a fibrin sealant antibiotic implant. *Clin Orthop* 2002;403:58–72.
371. Mahan MJ. Revealing bacterial infection strategies. *Lancet* 1994;343:869–870.
372. Mahan MJ, Slauch JM, Mekalanos JJ. Selection of bacterial virulence genes that are specifically induced in host tissues. *Science* 1993;259:686–688.
373. Mahan MJ, Tobias JW, Slauch JM, et al. Antibiotic-based selection for bacterial genes that are specifically induced during infection of a host. *Proc Natl Acad Sci USA* 1995;92:669–673.
374. Mahoney E, Reichner J, Bostom LR, et al. Bacterial colonization and the expression of inducible nitric oxide synthase in murine wounds. *Am J Pathol* 2002;161:2143–2152.
375. Maiza A, Daley-Yates PT. Variability in the renal clearance of cephalexin in experimental renal failure. *J Pharmacokinet Biopharm* 1993;21:19–30.
376. Majcherczyk PA, Kunz S, Hattenberger M, et al. Isolation and in-vitro and in-vivo characterisation of a mutant of *Pseudomonas aeruginosa* PA01 that exhibited a reduced postantibiotic effect in response to imipenem. *J Antimicrob Chemother* 1994;34:485–505.
377. Maksimow M, Hakkila K, Karp M, et al. Simultaneous detection of bacteria expressing GFP and DsRed genes with a flow cytometer. *Cytometry* 2002;47:243–247.
378. Malawista SE, Barthold SW, Pershing DH. Fate of *Borrelia burgdoferi* DNA in tissues of infected mice after antibiotic treatment. *J Infect Dis* 1994;170:1312–1316.
379. Malnick SD, Zimhony O. Treatment of *Clostridium difficile*–associated diarrhea. *Ann Pharmacother* 2002;36:1767–1775.
380. Malo D, Skamene E. Genetic control of host resistance to infection. *Trends Genet* 1994;10:365–371.
381. Mandell LA, Ball P, Tillotson G. Antimicrobial safety and tolerability: differences and dilemmas. *Clin Infect Dis* 2001;32:S72–S75.
382. Manson WL, Coenen JMFH, Klasen HJ, et al. Intestinal bacterial transolcation in experimentally burned mice with wounds colonized by *Pseudomonas aeruginosa*. *J Trauma* 1992;33:654–658.
383. Mansour AM, Ferguson E, Lucia H, et al. Vitreous replacement by gas as a therapeutic modality in bacterial endophthalmitis. *Graefe's Arch Ophthalmol* 1991;229:468–472.
384. Marchetti M, Arico B, Burroni D. Development of a mouse model of *Helicobacter pylori* infection that mimics human disease. *Science* 1995;267:1655–1658.

385. Marier JF, Beaudry F, Ducharme MP, et al. A pharmacokinetic study of amoxicillin in febrile beagle dogs following repeated administrations of endotoxin. *J Vet Pharmacol Ther* 2001;24:379–383.
386. Marini RP, Fox JG. Animal models of *Helicobacter* (ferrets). In: Zak O, Sande MA, eds. *Handbook of animal models of infection*. San Diego: Academic Press, 1999:273–284.
387. Marra C, Baker-Zander SA, Hook EW, et al. An experimental model of early central nervous system syphilis. *J Infect Dis* 1991;163:825–829.
388. Marrakchi-Benjaafar S, Cochereau I, Pocidalo JJ, et al. Systemic prophylaxis of experimental staphylococcal endophthalmitis: comparative efficacy of sparfloxacin, pefloxacin, imipenem, vancomycin, and amikacin. *J Infect Dis* 1995;172:1312–1316.
389. Martinez MN, Pedersoli WM, Ravis WR, et al. Feasibility of interspecies extrapolation in determining the bioequivalence of animal products intended for intramuscular administration. *J Vet Pharmacol Ther* 2001;24:125–135.
390. Marzola P, Nicolato E, Di Modugno E, et al. Comparison between MRI, microbiology and histology in evaluation of antibiotics in a murine model of thigh infection. *MAGMA* 1999;9:21–28.
391. Maylath FR, Leopold IH. Study of experimental intraocular infection I. The recoverability of organisms inoculated into ocular tissues and fluids. II. The influence of antibiotics and cortisone, alone and combined, on intraocular growth of these organisms. *Am J Ophthalmol* 1955;40:86–101.
392. McCracken GH, Nelson JD, Grimm L. Pharmacokinetics and bacteriological efficacy of cefoperazone, cefuroxime, ceftriaxone, and moxalactam in experimental *Streptococcus pneumoniae* and *Haemophilus influenzae* meningitis. *Antimicrob Agents Chemother* 1982;21:262–267.
393. McLeod R, Buschman E, Arbuckle LD, et al. Immunogenetics in the analysis of resistance to intracellular pathogens. *Curr Opin Immunol* 1995;7:539–552.
394. McVay CS, Rolfe RD. In vitro and in vivo activities of nitazoxanide against *Clostridium difficile*. *Antimicrob Agents Chemother* 2000;44:2254–2258.
395. Mekalanos JJ. Environmental signals controlling expression of virulence determinants in bacteria. *J Bacteriol* 1992;174:1–7.
396. Mellencamp MA, Preheim LC. Pneumococcal pneumonia in a rat model of cirrhosis: effects of cirrhosis on pulmonary defense mechanisms against *Streptococcus pneumoniae*. *J Infect Dis* 1991;163:102–108.
397. Methner U. The use of animal models in the development of classical vaccines. *Contrib Microbiol* 2001;9:58–70.
398. Meylan PR, Glauser MP. Failure of dexamethasone to prevent polymorphonuclear leukocyte infiltration during experimental acute exudative pyelonephritis and to reduce subsequent chronic scarring. *J Infect Dis* 1988;157:480–485.
399. Miller TE, Findon G, Rainer SP, et al. The pathobiology of subclinical pyelonephritis: an experimental evaluation. *Kidney Int* 1992;41:1356–1365.
400. Mimoz O, Jacolot A, Padoin C, et al. Influence of experimental rat model of multiple organ dysfunction on cefepime and amikacin pharmacokinetics. *Antimicrob Agents Chemother* 1996;40:819–821.
401. Mimoz O, Leotard S, Jacolot A, et al. Efficacies of imipenem, meropenem, cefepime, and ceftazidime in rats with experimental pneumonia due to a carbapenem-hydrolyzing β-lactamase–producing strain of Enterobacter cloacae. *Antimicrob Agents Chemother* 2000;44:885–890.
402. Minguez F, Izquierdo J, Caminero MM, et al. In vivo postantibiotic effect of isepamicin and other aminoglycosides in a thigh infection model in neutropenic mice. *Chemotherapy* 1992;38:179–184.
403. Mitchison DA. Fluoroquinolones in the treatment of tuberculosis: a study in mice. *Am J Respir Crit Care Med* 2004;169:334–335.
404. Miyazaki S, Nunoya T, Matsumoto T, et al. New murine model of bronchopneumonia due to cell-bound *Haemophilus influenzae*. *J Infect Dis* 1997;175:205–209.
405. Mizen L. Methods for obtaining human-like pharmacokinetic patterns in experimental animals. In: Zak O, Sande MA, eds. *Handbook of animal models of infection*. San Diego: Academic Press, 1999:93–103.
406. Mizen L, Woodnutt G, Kernutt I, et al. Simulation of human serum pharmacokinetics of ticarcillin-clavulanic acid and ceftazidime in rabbits, and efficacy against experimental *Klebsiella pneumoniae* meningitis. *Antimicrob Agents Chemother* 1989;33:693–699.
407. Mogga SJ, Mustafa T, Sviland L, et al. In situ expression of CD40, CD40L (CD154), IL-12, TNF-alpha, IFN-gamma and TGF-beta1 in murine lungs during slowly progressive primary tuberculosis. *Scand J Immunol* 2003;58:327–334.
408. Moine P, Mazoit J-X, Bedos J-P, et al. Correlation between in vitro and in vivo activity of amoxicillin against *Streptococcus pneumoniae* in a murine pneumonia model. *J Pharmacol Exp Ther* 1997;280:310–315.
409. Moller BR, Mardh PA. Animal models for the study of chlamydial infections of the urogenital tract. *Scand J Infect Dis Suppl* 1982;32:103–108.
410. Mombaerts P, Arnoldi J, Russ F, et al. Different roles of α/β and γ/δ T cells in immunity against an intracellular bacterial pathogen. *Nature* 1993;365:53–56.
411. Mongodin E, Bajolet O, Cutrona J, et al. Fibronectin-binding proteins of *Staphylococcus aureus* are involved in adherence to human airway epithelium. *Infect Immun* 2002;70:620–630.
412. Montgomerie JZ, Schick DG. Treatment of enterococcal pyelonephritis with trovafloxacin and rifampin: in vitro in vivo contrast. *Antimicrob Agents Chemother* 1998;42:188–189.
413. Mordenti J. Forecasting cephalosporin and monobactam antibiotic half-lives in humans from data collected in laboratory animals. *Antimicrob Agents Chemother* 1985;27:887–891.
414. Mordenti J. Man versus beast: pharmacokinetic scaling in mammals. *J Pharm Sci* 1986;75:1028–1040.
415. Moreillon P. Endocarditis prophylaxis revisited: experimental evidence of efficacy and new Swiss recommendations. Swiss Working Group for Endocarditis Prophylaxis. *Schweiz Med Wochenschr* 2000;130:1013–1026.
416. Morissette C, Skamene E, Gervais F. Endobronchial inflammation following *Pseudomonas aeruginosa* infection in resistant and susceptible strains of mice. *Infect Immun* 1995;63:1718–1724.
417. Morita E, Mizuno N, Nishikata M, et al. Comparison of the pharmacokinetics of five β-lactam antibiotics between neonatal and adult rats. *Dev Pharmacol Ther* 1990;14:223–230.
418. Morris TH. Antibiotic therapeutics in laboratory animals. *Lab Anim* 1995;29:16–36.
419. Morse SA, McDade JE. Recommendations for working with pathogenic bacteria. *Methods Enzymol* 1994;235:126.
420. Morton DB. Ethical aspects of the use of animal models of infection. In: Zak O, Sande MA, eds. *Handbook of animal*

models of infection. San Diego: Academic Press, 1999:29–48.

421. Motschmann M, Behrens Baumann W. Rabbit model of bacterial conjunctivitis. In: Zak O, Sande MA, eds. *Handbook of animal models of infection*. San Diego: Academic Press, 1999:353–359.
422. Mouton JW, Punt N. Use of the t>MIC to choose between different dosing regimens of β-lactam antibiotics. *J Antimicrobial Chemother* 2001;47:500–501.
423. Mouton JW, van Ogtrop ML, Andes D, et al. Use of pharmacodynamic indices to predict efficacy of combination therapy in vivo. *Antimicrob Agents Chemother* 1999;43:2473–2478.
424. Moxon ER, Ostrow PT. *Haemophilus influenzae* meningitis in infant rats: role of bacteremia in pathogenesis of age-dependent inflammatory responses in cerebrospinal fluid. *J Infect Dis* 1977;135:303–307.
425. Mulvey MA, Schilling JD, Hultgren SJ. Establishment of a persistent *Escherichia coli* reservoir during the acute phase of a bladder infection. *Infect Immun* 2001;69:4572–4579.
426. Mulvey MA, Schilling JD, Martinez JJ, et al. Bad bugs and beleaguered bladders: interplay between uropathogenic *Escherichia coli* and innate host defenses. *Proc Natl Acad Sci USA* 2000;97:8829–8835.
427. Murai M, Seki K, Sakurada J, et al. Conspicuous growth of intravenously inoculated *Staphylococcus aureus* in subcutaneously established Ehrlich ascites tumor tissue of mice. *Microbiol Immunol* 1995;39:153–155.
428. Nau R, Wellmer A, Soto A, et al. Rifampin reduces early mortality in experimental *Streptococcus pneumoniae* meningitis. *J Infec Dis* 1999;179:1557–1560.
429. Naziri W, Cheadle WG, Trachtenberg LS, et al. Increased antibiotic effectivness in a model of surgical infection through continuous infusion. *Am Surg* 1995;61: 11–15.
430. Nelson CL, McLaren SG, Skinner RA, et al. The treatment of experimental osteomyelitis by surgical debridement and the implantation of calcium sulfate tobramycin pellets. *J Orthop Res* 2002;20:643–647.
431. Ng EW, Samiy N, Ruoff KL, et al. Treatment of experimental *Staphylococcus epidermidis* endophthalmitis with oral trovafloxacin. *Am J Ophthalmol* 1998;126:278–287.
432. Ngeleka M, Auclair P, Tardif D, et al. Intrarenal distribution of vancomycin in endotoxemic rats. *Antimicrob Agents Chemother* 1989;33:1575–1579.
433. Nicolau DP. Predicting antibacterial response from pharmacodynamic and pharmacokinetic profiles. *Infection* 2001;29[Suppl 2]:11–15.
434. Nicolau DP, Mattoes HM, Banevicius M, et al. Pharmacodynamics of a novel des-F(6)-quinolone, BMS-284756, against *Streptococcus pneumoniae* in the thigh infection model. *Antimicrob Agents Chemother* 2003;47:1630–1635.
435. Nijhof MW, Fleer A, Hardus K, et al. Tobramycin-containing bone cement and systemic cefazolin in a one-stage revision: treatment of infection in a rabbit model. *J Biomed Mater Res* 2001;58:747–753.
436. Nomoto K, Mitsuyama M, Miake S, et al. Augmented nonspecific resistance and simultaneous impairment of specific immunity to *Listeria monocytogenes* in tumor-bearing mice. *J Clin Lab Immunol* 1987;24:75–79.
437. Norden CW. Experimental osteomyelitis. I. A description of the model. *J Infect Dis* 1970;122:410–418.
438. Norden CW. Experimental osteomyelitis. II. Therapeutic trials and measurement of antibiotic levels in bone. *J Infect Dis* 1971;124:565–571.
439. Norrby SR, O'Reilly T, Zak O. Efficacy of antimicrobial agent treatment in relation to treatment regimen: experimental models and clinical evaluation. *J Antimicrob Chemother* 1993;31[Suppl D]: 41–54.
440. Ntziachristos V, Bremer C, Weissleder R. Fluorescence imaging with near-infrared light: new technological advances that enable in vivo molecular imaging. *Eur Radiol* 2003;13:195–208.
441. Obrink KJ. Animal models and ethics. In: Keusch G, Wadstrom T, eds. *Experimental bacterial and parasitic infections*. New York: Elsevier Biomedical, 1982:3–10.
442. Odenholt I. Pharmacodynamic effects of subinhibitory antibiotic concentrations. *Int J Antimicrob Agents* 2001; 17:1–8.
443. Odenholt I, Holm SE, Cars O. An in vivo model for evaluation of the postantibiotic effect. *Scand J Infect Dis* 1988;20:97–103.
444. Odenholt I, Holm SE, Cars O. Effects of supra- and sub-MIC benzylpenicillin concentrations on group A beta-haemolytic streptococci during the postantibiotic phase in vivo. *J Antimicrob Chemother* 1990;26:193–201.
445. Odenholt-Tornqvist I. Pharmacodynamics of beta-lactam antibiotics: studies on the paradoxical and postantibiotic effects in vitro and in an animal model. *Scand J Infect Dis Suppl* 1989;58:1–55.
446. Ohtani H, Taninaka C, Hanada E, et al. Comparative pharmacodynamic analysis of Q-T interval prolongation induced by the macrolides clarithromycin, roxithromycin, and azithromycin in rats. *Antimicrob Agents Chemother* 2000;44:2630–2637.
447. Oishi K, Sonoda F, Iwagaki A, et al. Effects of the combination of lipopolysaccharide-specific monoclonal antibodies and sparfloxacin against *Pseudomonas aeruginosa* pneumonia in neutropenic mice. *Antimicrob Agents Chemother* 1992;36:1352–1357.
448. Oishi K, Sonoda F, Iwagaki A, et al. Therapeutic effects of a human antiflagella monoclonal antibody in a neutropenic murine model of *Pseudomonas aeruginosa* pneumonia. *Antimicrob Agents Chemother* 1993;37:164–170.
449. Oishi K, Sonoda F, Miwa H, et al. Pharmacodynamic and protective properties of a murine lipopolysaccharide-specific monoclonal antibody in experimental *Pseudomonas aeruginosa* pneumonia in mice. *Microbiol Immunol* 1991;35:1131–1141.
450. Okawa Y, Murata Y, Kobayashi M, et al. Augmentation of host resistance to *Candida albicans* infection in ascites tumor-bearing mice. *Microbiol Immunol* 1992;36:517–521.
451. O'Leary TJ, Tsai MM, Wright CF, et al. Use of semiquantiative PCR to assess onset and treatment of *Pneumocystis carinii* infection in a rat model. *J Clin Microbiol* 1995;33:718–724.
452. Onyeji CO, Nicolau DP, Nightingale CH, et al. Modulation of efficacies and pharmacokinetics of antibiotics by granulocyte colony–stimulating factor in neutropenic mice with multidrug-resistant *Enterococcus faecalis* infection. *J Antimicrob Chemother* 2000;46:429–436.
453. O'Reilly T. Relevance of animal models for chronic bacterial airway infections in humans. *Am J Respir Crit Care Med* 1995;151:2101–2108.
454. O'Reilly T, Cleeland R, Squires E. Evaluation of antimicrobials in experimental animal infections. In: Lorian V, ed. *Antibiotics in laboratory medicine,* 4th ed. Baltimore: Williams & Wilkins, 1996:599–759.
455. O'Reilly T, Mader JT. Rat model of osteomyelitis of the tiba. In: Zak O, Sande MA, eds. *Handbook of animal models of infection*. San Diego: Academic Press, 1999:561–576.

456. O'Reilly T, Niven DF. Tryptone-yeast extract broth as a culture medium for *Haemophilus pleuropneumoniae* and *Haemophilus parasuis* to be used as challenge inocula. *Can J Vet Res* 1986;50:441–443.
457. O'Reilly T, Zak O. Elevated body temperature restricts growth of *Haemophilus influenzae* type b during experimental meningitis. *Infect Immun* 1992;60:3448–3451.
458. Orme IM. Aging and immunity to tuberculosis: increased susceptibility of old mice reflects a decreased capacity to generate mediator T lymphocytes. *J Immunol* 1987;138:4414–4418.
459. Orme IM. A mouse model of the recrudescence of latent tuberculosis in the elderly. *Am Rev Respir Dis* 1988;137:716–718.
460. Orme IM. Murine models of tuberculosis. In: Zak O, Sande MA, eds. *Handbook of animal models of infection.* San Diego: Academic Press, 1999:315–319.
461. Orme IM. The mouse as a useful model of tuberculosis. *Tuberculosis (Edinb)* 2003;83:112–115.
462. Oshida T, Onta T, Nakanishi N, et al. Activity of subminimal inhibitory concentrations of aspoxicillin in prolonging the postantibiotic effect against *Staphylococcus aureus*. *J Antimicrob Chemother* 1990;26:29–38.
463. Østergaard C, Benfield T, Gesser B, et al. Pretreatment with granulocyte colony–stimulating factor attenuates the inflammatory response but not the bacterial load in cerebrospinal fluid during experimental pneumococcal meningitis in rabbits. *Infect Immun* 1999;67:3430–3436.
464. Ozturk F, Kortunay S, Kurt E, et al. Effects of trauma and infection on ciprofloxacin levels in the vitreous cavity. *Retina* 1999;19:127–130.
465. Ozturk F, Kurt E, Inan UU, et al. Penetration of topical and oral ofloxacin into the aqueous and vitreous humor of inflamed rabbit eyes. *Int J Pharm* 2000;204:91–95.
466. Pardue RL, White CA. Pharmacokinetic evaluation of liposomal encapsulated ampicillin in male and female rats. *Biopharm Drug Dispos* 1997;18:279–292.
467. Park SN, Yeo SW. Effects of antibiotics and steroid on middle ear mucosa in rats with experimental acute otitis media. *Acta Otolaryngol* 2001;121:808–812.
468. Park SS, D'Amico DJ, Paton B, et al. Treatment of exogenous *Candida endophthlamitis* in rabbits with oral fluconazole. *Antimicrob Agents Chemother* 1995;39:958–963.
469. Park SS, Samiy N, Ruoff K, et al. Effect of intravitreal dexamethasone in treatment of pneumococcal endophthalmitis in rabbits. *Arch Ophthalmol* 1995;113:1324–1329.
470. Parra A, Ponte C, Cenjor C, et al. Optimal dose of amoxicillin in treatment of otitis media caused by a penicillin-resistant pneumococcus strain in the gerbil model. *Antimicrob Agents Chemother* 2002;46:859–862.
471. Parra A, Ponte C, Cenjor C, et al. Is it possible to achieve bacterial eradication in otitis media with effusion by empirical antibiotic high doses and concomitant administration of acetaminophen? A microbiological and pharmacological study in the gerbil model. *Int J Antimicrob Agents* 2003;22:508–515.
472. Pascual A. Pathogenesis of catheter-related infections: lessons for new designs. *Clin Microbiol Infect* 2002;8:256–264.
473. Pennington JE, Dale DC, Reynolds HY, et al. Gentamicin sulfate pharmacokinetics: lower levels of gentamicin in blood during fever. *J Infect Dis* 1975;132:270–275.
474. Perkins RJ, Liu W, Drusano G, et al. Pharmacokinetics of ofloxacin in serum and vitreous humor of albino and pigmented rabbits. *Antimicrob Agents Chemother* 1995;39:1493–1498.
475. Peterson LR. Animal models: the in vivo evaluation of ciprofloxacin. *J Antimicrob Chemother* 1986;18[Suppl D]:55–64.
476. Plante M, Jerse A, Hamel J, et al. Intranasal immunization with gonococcal outer membrane preparations reduces the duration of vaginal colonization of mice by *Neisseria gonorrhoeae*. *J Infect Dis* 2000;182:848–855.
477. Polk HC, Lamont PM, Galland RB. Containment as a mechanism of nonspecific enhancement of defenses against bacterial infection. *Infect Immun* 1990;58:1807–1811.
478. Ponte C, Cenjor C, Parra A, et al. Antimicrobial treatment of an experimental otitis media caused by a beta-lactamase positive isolate of *Haemophilus influenzae*. *J Antimicrob Chemother* 1999;44:85–90.
479. Post JC. Direct evidence of bacterial biofilms in otitis media. *Laryngoscope* 2001;111:2083–2094.
480. Post JC, Aul JJ, White GJ, et al. PCR-based detection of bacterial DNA after antimicrobial treatment is indicative of persistent, viable bacteria in the chinchilla model of otitis media. *Am J Otolaryngol* 1996;17:106–111.
481. Post JC, Preston RA, Aul JJ, et al. Molecular analysis of bacterial pathogens in otitis media with effusion. *JAMA* 1995;273:1598–1604.
482. Powell H, Jamieson W. Combined therapy of pneumococci rat infections with rabbit antipneumococcic serum and sulfapyridine (2-sulfanilaminopyridine). *J Immunol* 1939;36:459–465.
483. Prellner K, Hermansson A, White P, et al. Immunization and protection in pneumococcal otitis media studied in a rat model. *Microb Drug Resist* 1999;5:73–82.
484. Quezado ZM, Natanson C, Alling DW, et al. A controlled trial of HA-1A in a canine model of Gram-negative septic shock. *JAMA* 1993;269:2221–2227.
485. Rank RG, Whittum-Hudson JA. Animal models for ocular infections. *Methods Enzymol* 1994;235:69–83.
486. Rank RG. Animal models for urogenital infections. *Methods Enzymol* 1994;235:83–93.
487. Rao SN, Fong Y, Kampmeier J, et al. The effectiveness of a topical antibiotic irrigating solution in a model of staphylococcal keratitis after lamellar keratectomy. *Am J Ophthalmol* 2000;130:20–24.
488. Rapp RP. Pharmacokinetics and pharmacodynamics of intravenous and oral azithromycin: enhanced tissue activity and minimal drug interactions. *Ann Pharmacother* 1998;32:785–793.
489. Ravindranath RM, Hasan SA, Mondino BJ. Immunopathologic features of *Staphylococcus epidermidis*–induced endophthalmitis in the rat. *Curr Eye Res* 1997;16:1036–1043.
490. Rebuelto M, Ambros L, Rubio M. Daily variations in ceftriaxone pharmacokinetics in rats. *Antimicrob Agents Chemother* 2003;47:809–812.
491. Reed LJ, Muench H. A simple method of estimating fifty percent endpoints. *Am J Hyg* 1938;27:4934–4997.
492. Regan T. The case for animal rights. In: Singer P, ed. *Defense of animals.* New York: Harper & Row, 1985:13–26.
493. Regan T. *The case for animal rights.* London: Routledge, 1988.
494. Reinosos RF, Telfer BA, Rowland M. Tissue water content in rats measured by desiccation. *J Pharmacological Toxicol Methods* 1997;38:87–92.
495. Remick DG, Call DR, Ebong SJ, et al. Combination immunotherapy with soluble tumor necrosis factor receptors plus interleukin 1 receptor antagonist decreases sepsis mortality. *Crit Care Med* 2001;29:473–481.
496. Rex JH, Nelson PW, Paetznick VL, et al. Optimizing the correlation between results of testing in vitro and

therapeutic outcome in vivo for fluconazole by testing critical isolates in a murine model of invasive candidiasis. *Antimicrob Agents Chemother* 1998;42:129–134.

497. Richmond JY, Quimby F. Considerations for working safely with infectious disease agents in research animals. In: Zak O, Sande MA, eds. *Handbook of animal models of infection.* San Diego: Academic Press, 1999:69–73.
498. Rissing JP, Buxton TB, Weinstein RS, et al. Model of experimental osteomyelitis in rats. *Infect Immun* 1985;47:581–586.
499. Roberts JA. Vesicoureteral reflux and pyelonephritis in the monkey: a review. *J Urol* 1992;148:1721–1725.
500. Rocchetta HL, Boylan CJ, Foley JW, et al. Validation of a noninvasive, real-time imaging technology using bioluminescent *Escherichia coli* in the neutropenic mouse thigh model of infection. *Antimicrob Agents Chemother* 2001;45:129–137.
501. Rodewald AK, Onderdonk AB, Warren HB, et al. Neonatal mouse model of group B streptococcal infection. *J Infect Dis* 1992;166:635–639.
502. Rodriguez AF, Kaplan SL, Hawkins EP, et al. Effect of dexamethasone or HWA-138 in combination with antibiotics in experimental *Haemophilus influenzae* type b infection. *Antimicrob Agents Chemother* 1991;53:1980–1984.
503. Romulo RL, Palardy JE, Opal SM. Efficacy of anti-endotoxin monoclonal antibody E5 alone or in combination with ciprofloxacin in neutropenic rats with *Pseudomonas sepsis*. *J Infect Dis* 1993;167:126–130.
504. Roosendaal R, Bakker-Woudenberg IAJM, van den Berghe-van Raffe M, et al. Continuous versus intermittent administration of ceftazidime in experimental *Klebsiella pneumoniae* pneumonia in normal and leukopenic rats. *Antimicrob Agents Chemother* 1986;30:403–408.
505. Roosendaal R, Bakker-Woudenberg IAJM, van den Berghe-van Raffe M, et al. Impact of dosing schedule on the efficacy of ceftazidime, gentamicin and ciprofloxacin in *Klebsiella pneumoniae* pneumonia and septicemia in leukopenic rats. *Eur J Clin Microbiol Infect Dis* 1989;8:878–887.
506. Rouse MS, Wilson WR. General methodologies for animal models. In: Zak O, Sande MA, eds. *Handbook of animal models of infection.* San Diego: Academic Press, 1999: 9–12.
507. Rowlland M, Tozer TN. *Clinical pharmacokinetics: concepts and applications,* 3rd ed. Philadelphia: Williams & Wilkins, 1995.
508. Ruiz-Cabello J, Regadera J, Santisteban C, et al. Monitoring acute inflammatory processes in mouse muscle by MR imaging and spectroscopy: a comparison with pathological results. *NMR Biomed* 2002;15:204–214.
509. Ryan DM. Pharmacokinetics of antibiotics in natural and experimental superficial compartments in animals and humans. *J Antimicrob Chemother* 1993;31[Suppl D]:1–16.
510. Ryan DM. The usefulness of experimental models of urinary tract infections in the assessment of chemotherapeutic compounds. In: Williams JD, Gedes AM, eds. *Chemotherapy,* vol. 2. New York: Plenum, 1976:205–215.
511. Saint S, Chenoweth CE. Biofilms and catheter-associated urinary tract infections. *Infect Dis Clin North Am* 2003;17:411–432.
512. Sapico FL, Ginunas VJ, Montgomerie JZ, et al. Cefpirome, alone and in combination with gentamicin, for enterococcal pyelonephritis in the rodent model. *Diagn Microbiol Infect Dis* 1991;14:297–300.

512a. Santoro J, Levison ME. Rat model of experimental endocarditis. *Infect Immun* 1978;19:915–918.

513. Sartoris DJ, Guerra J Jr, Mattrey RF, et al. Perfluoroctylbromide as a contrast agent for computed tomographic imaging of septic and aseptic arthritis. *Invest Radiol* 1986;21:49–55.
514. Sarwari AR, Mackowiak PA. The pharmacologic consequences of fever. *Infect Dis Clin North Am* 1996;10:21–32.
515. Sato K, Quartey MK, Liebeler CL, et al. Timing of penicillin treatment influences the course of *Streptococcus pneumoniae*–induced middle ear inflammation. *Antimicrob Agents Chemother* 1995;39:1896–1898.
516. Sayek I. Animal models for intra-abdominal infection. *Hepatogastroenterology* 1997;44:923–926.
517. Scaglione F, Mouton JW, Mattina R, et al. Pharmacodynamics of levofloxacin and ciprofloxacin in a murine pneumonia model: peak concentration/MIC versus area under the curve/MIC ratios. *Antimicrob Agents Chemother* 2003;47:2749–2755.
518. Scarpace PJ, Borst SE, Bender BS. The association of *E. coli* peritonitis with an impaired and delayed fever response in senescent rats. *J Gerontol* 1992;47:B142–B145.
519. Scheld WM, Brown RS, Sande MA. Comparison of netilmicin with gentamicin in the therapy of experimental *Escherichia coli* meningitis. *Antimicrob Agents Chemother* 1978;13:899–904.
520. Schentag JJ, Gilliland KK, Paladino JA. What have we learned from pharmacokinetic and pharmacodynamic theories? *Clin Infect Dis* 2001;32[Suppl 1]:S39–S46.
521. Schentag JJ, Goss TF. Quinolone pharmacokinetics in the elderly. *Am J Med* 1992;92[Suppl 4A]:33S–37S.
522. Schentag JJ, Strenkoski-Nix LC, Nix DE, et al. Pharmacodynamic interactions of antibiotics alone and in combination. *Clin Infect Dis* 1998;27:40–46.
523. Schiff JB, Small JG, Pennington JE. Comparative activities of ciprofloxacin, ticarcillin and tobramycin against experimental *Pseudomonas aeruginosa* pneumonia. *Antimicrob Agents Chemother* 1984;26:1–4.
524. Schilling JD, Martin SM, Hung CS, et al. Toll-like receptor 4 on stromal and hematopoietic cells mediates innate resistance to uropathogenic *Escherichia coli. Proc Natl Acad Sci USA* 2003;100:4203–4208.
525. Scholz O, Thiel A, Hillen W, et al. Quantitative analysis of gene expression with an improved green fluorescent protein, p6. *Eur J Biochem* 2000;267:1565–1570.
526. Schwank S, Rajacic Z, Zimmerli W, et al. Impact of bacterial biofilm formation on in vitro and in vivo activities of antibiotics. *Antimicrob Agents Chemother* 1998;42:895–898.
527. Sepkowitz K, Schuler N, Godwin T, et al. DNA amplification in experimental pneumocystosis: characterisation of serum *Pneumocystis carinii* DNA and potential carrier states. *J Infect Dis* 1993;168:421–426.
528. Sharma S, Harjai K, Mittal R. Enhanced siderophore production and mouse kidney pathogenicity in *Escherichia coli* grown in urine. *J Med Microbiol* 1991;35:325–329.
529. Shepard BD, Gilmore MS. Differential expression of virulence-related genes in *Enterococcus faecalis* in response to biological cues in serum and urine. *Infect Immun* 2002;70:4344–4352.
530. Sheppard M, Webb C, Heath F, et al. Dynamics of bacterial growth and distribution within the liver during Salmonella infection. *Cell Microbiol* 2003;5:593–600.
531. Shirbacheh MV, Jones JW, Harralson TA, et al. Pharmacokinetics of intra-arterial delivery of tacrolimus to vascularly isolated rabbit forelimb. *J Pharmacol Exp Ther* 1999;289:1196–1201.
532. Shirtliff ME, Calhoun JH, Mader JT. Experimental osteomyelitis treatment with antibiotic-impregnated hydroxyapatite. *Clin Orthop* 2002;401:239–247.

533. Shrotri M, Peyton JC, Cheadle WG. Mouse peritonitis model using cecal ligation and puncture. In: Zak O, Sande MA, eds. *Handbook of animal models of infection.* San Diego: Academic Press, 1999:173–181.
534. Siaperas P, Pefanis A, Iliopoulos D, et al. Evidence of less severe aortic valve destruction after treatment of experimental staphylococcal endocarditis with vancomycin and dexamethasone. *Antimicrob Agents Chemother* 2001;45:3531–3537.
535. Siefert HM, Domdey-Bette A, Henninger K, et al. Pharmacokinetics of the 8-methoxyquinolone, moxifloxacin: a comparison in humans and other mammalian species. *J Antimicrob Chemother* 1999;43[Suppl B]:69–76.
536. Signore A, Procaccini E, Annovazzi A, et al. The developing role of cytokines for imaging inflammation and infection. *Cytokine* 2000;12:1445–1454.
537. Silvia OJ, Urosevic N. Variations in LPS responsiveness among different mouse substrains of C3H lineage and their congenic derivative sublines. *Immunogenetics* 1999;50:354–357.
538. Singer P. Ethics and the new animal liberation movement. In: Singer P, ed. *Defense of animals.* New York: Harper & Row, 1985:1–10.
539. Singer P. *Animal liberation.* New York: Avon Books, 1990.
539a. Siso JP, Yao Y, Klemper CA, et al. Treatment of *Mycobacterium avium* complex infection: does the beige mouse model predict therapeutic outcome in humans? *J Infect Dis* 1996;173:750–753.
540. Skamene E. Genetic regulation of host resistance to bacterial infection. *Rev Infect Dis* 1983;5:S823–S832.
541. Slater LN. A rat model of prolonged pulmonary infection due to nontypable *Haemophilus influenzae. Am Rev Respir Dis* 1990;142:1429–1435.
542. Slauch JM, Mahan MJ, Mekalanos JJ. In vivo expression technology for selection of bacterial genes specifically induced in host tissues. *Methods Enzymol* 1994;235:481–492.
543. Smith MA, Sorenson JA, D'Aversa G, et al. Treatment of experimental methicillin-resistant *Staphylococcus epidermidis* endophthalmitis with intravitreal vancomycin and intravitreal dexamethasone. *J Infect Dis* 1997;175:462–466.
544. Soriano F, Parra A, Cenjor C, et al. Role of *Streptococcus pneumoniae* and *Haemophilus influenzae* in the development of acute otitis media and otitis media with effusion in a gerbil model. *J Infect Dis* 2000;181:646–652.
545. Spaeth HJ, Chandnani VP, Beltran J, et al. Magnetic resonance imaging detection of early experimental periostitis: comparison of magnetic resonance imaging, computed tomography, and plain radiography with histopathologic correlation. *Invest Radiol* 1991;26:304–308.
546. Spector R, Lorenzo AV. Inhibition of penicillin transport from cerebral spinal fluid after intracisternal inoculation of bacteria. *J Clin Invest* 1974;54:316–325.
547. Spellerberg B, Prasad S, Cabellos C, et al. Penetration of the blood-brain barrier: enhancement of drug delivery and imaging by bacterial glycopeptides. *J Exp Med* 1995;182:1037–1043.
548. Spivey JM. The postantibiotic effect. *Clin Pharm* 1992;11:865–875.
549. Stoddart B, Wilcox MH. *Clostridium difficile. Curr Opin Infect Dis* 2002;15:513–518.
550. Stotland PK, Radzioch D, Stevenson MM. Mouse models of chronic lung infection with *Pseudomonas aeruginosa:* models for the study of cystic fibrosis. *Pediatr Pulmonol* 2000;30:413–424.
551. Stratton CW IV. In vitro testing: correlations between bacterial susceptibility, body fluid levels and effectiveness of antibacterial therapy. In: Lorian V, ed. *Antibiotics in laboratory medicine,* 3rd ed. Baltimore: Williams & Wilkins, 1991;849–879.
552. Su H, Messer R, Whitmire W, et al. Subclinical chlamydial infection of the female mouse genital tract generates a potent protective immune response: implications for development of live attenuated chlamydial vaccine strains. *Infect Immun* 2000;68:192–196.
553. Su H, Morrison R, Messer R, et al. The effect of doxycycline treatment on the development of protective immunity in a murine model of chlamydial genital infection. *J Infect Dis* 1999;180:1252–1258.
554. Suarez A, Guttler A, Stratz M, et al. Green fluorescent protein-based reporter systems for genetic analysis of bacteria including monocopy applications. *Gene* 1997;196:69–74.
555. Subasi M, Kapukaya A, Kesemenli C, et al. Effect of granulocyte-macrophage colony–stimulating factor on treatment of acute osteomyelitis: an experimental investigation in rats. *Arch Orthop Trauma Surg* 2001;121:170–173.
556. Sugawara M, Toda T, Iseki K, et al. Transport characteristics of cephalosporin antibiotics across intestinal brush-border membrane in man, rat and rabbit. *J Pharm Pharmacol* 1992;44:968–972.
557. Takano S, Umenai T, Tanaka K, et al. Isolation of a factor from cancer ascitic fluid increasing susceptibility of mice to *Listeria* infection. *Proc Soc Exp Biol Med* 1983;174:65–73.
558. Tanira MOM, Ali BH, Bashir AK. Effect of endotoxin on gentamicin pharmacokinetics in old and young adult rats. *Life Sci* 1997;60:413–424.
559. Tatara O, Nakahama C, Niki Y. Synergistic effects of romurtide and cefmenoxime against experimental *Klebsiella pneumonia* in mice. *Antimicrob Agents Chemother* 1992;36:167–171.
560. Thadepalli H, Chuah SK, Reddy U, et al. Efficacy of trovafloxacin for treatment of experimental Bacteroides infection in young and senescent mice. *Antimicrob Agents Chemother* 1997;41:1933–1936.
561. Thadepalli H, Reddy U, Chuah SK, et al. Evaluation of trovafloxacin in the treatment of *Klebsiella pneumoniae* lung infection in tumour-bearing mice. *J Antimicrob Chemother* 2000;45:69–75.
562. Thauvin C, Eliopoulos GM, Willey S, et al. Continuous-influsion ampicillin therapy of enterococcal endocarditis in rats. *Antimicrob Agents Chemother* 1987;31:139–143.
563. Thonus IP, de Lange-Macdaniel AV, Otte CJ, et al. Tissue cage infusion: a technique for the achievement of prolonged steady state in experimental animals. *J Pharmacol Methods* 1979;2:63–69.
564. Timm J, Post FA, Bekker LG, et al. Differential expression of iron-, carbon-, and oxygen-responsive mycobacterial genes in the lungs of chronically infected mice and tuberculosis patients. *Proc Natl Acad Sci USA* 2003;100:14321–14326.
565. Toews GB, Gross GN, Pierce AK. The relationship of inoculum size to lung bacterial clearance and phagocytic cell response in mice. *Am Rev Respir Dis* 1979;120:559–566.
566. Torres-Molina F, Peris-Ribera JE, Garcia-Carbonell MC, Nonlinearities in amoxicillin pharmacokinetics. I. Disposition studies in the rat. *Biopharm Drug Dispos* 1992;13:23–38.
567. Torres-Molina F, Peris-Ribera JE, Garcia-Carbonell MC,

et al. Nonlinearities in amoxicillin pharmacokinetics. II. Absorption studies in the rat. *Biopharm Drug Dispos* 1992;13:39–53.

568. Townsend GC, Scheld WM. Adult rat model of bacterial meningitis. In: Zak O, Sande MA, eds. *Handbook of animal models of infection*. San Diego: Academic Press, 1999:631–638.
569. Tran Ba Huy P, Bernard P, Schacht J. Kinetics of gentamicin uptake and release in the rat: comparison of inner ear tissues and fluids with other organs. *J Clin Invest* 1986;77:1492–1500.
570. Tran Ba Huy P, Manuel C, Sterkers O, et al. Pharmacokinetics of gentamicin in perilymph and endolymph of the rat as determined by radioimmunoassay. *J Infect Dis* 1981;143:476–486.
571. Tran Ba Huy P, Meulemans A, Wassef M, et al. Gentamicin persistance in rat endolymph and perilymph after a two-day constant infusion. *Antimicrob Agents Chemother* 1983;23:344–346.
572. Tsitsika A, Pefanis A, Perdikaris GS, et al. Single-oral-dose azithromycin prophylaxis against experimental streptococcal or staphylococcal aortic valve endocarditis. *Antimicrob Agents Chemother* 2000;44:1754–1756.
573. Tsuchimori N, Yamasaki T, Okonogi K. Therapeutic effects of cefozopran against experimental mixed urinary tract infection with *Enterococcus faecalis* and *Pseudomonas aeruginosa* in mice. *J Antimicrob Chemother* 1997;39:423–425.
574. Tune BM. Renal tubular transport and nephrotoxicity of beta lactam antibiotics: structure-activity relationships. *Miner Electrolyte Metab* 1994;20:221–231.
575. Tureen J, Tuomanen E. Rabbit model of bacterial meningitis. In: Zak O, Sande MA, eds. *Handbook of animal models of infection*. San Diego: Academic Press, 1999:631–638.
576. Turnbull IR, Wlzorek JJ, Osborne D, et al. Effects of age on mortality and antibiotic efficacy in cecal ligation and puncture. *Shock* 2003;19:310–313.
577. Uezumi I, Terashima M, Kohzuki T, et al. Effects of a human antiflagellar monoclonal antibody in combination with antibiotics on *Pseudomonas aeruginosa* infection. *Antimicrob Agents Chemother* 1992;36:1290–1295.
578. Valdevia RH, Falkow S. Probing bacterial gene expression within host cells. *Trends Microbiol* 1997;5:360–363.
579. Valdevia RH, Falkow S. Fluorescence-based isolation of bacterial genes expressed within host cells. *Science* 1997; 26:2007–2011.
580. Valdivia RH, Hromockyj AE, Monack D, et al. Applications for green fluorescent protein (GFP) in the study of host-pathogen interactions. *Gene* 1996;173(1 Spec No): 47–52.
581. Valentovic MA, Ball JG, Rogers BA. Comparison of renal accumulation and urinary excretion in normoglycemic and diabetic animals. *Toxicology* 1996;108:93–99.
582. van Belkum A. DNA fingerprinting of medically important microorganisms by use of PCR. *Clin Microbiol Rev* 1994;7:174–184.
583. Vandecasteele SJ, Peetermans WE, Merckx R, et al. Expression of biofilm-associated genes in *Staphylococcus epidermidis* during in vitro and in vivo foreign body infections. *J Infect Dis* 2003;188:730–737.
584. Van der Gulden WJI, Beynen AC, Hau J. Animal models. In: van Zutphen LFM, Baumans V, Beyen AC, eds. *Principles of laboratory animal science*. Amsterdam: Elsevier, 1993:189–196.
585. Van Dongen JJ, Remie R, Rensema JW, et al. *Manual of microsurgery on the laboratory rat*. Part 1. *General information and experimental techniques*. Amsterdam: Elsevier, 1990.
586. Van Etten EWM, ten Kate MT, Stearne LET, et al. Amphotericin B liposomes with prolonged circulation in blood: in vitro antifungal activity, toxicity, nd efficacy in systemic candidiasis in leukopenic mice. *Antimicrob Agents Chemother* 1995;39:1954–1958.
587. Van Zanten SJ, Kolesnikow T, Leung V, et al. Gastric transitional zones, areas where Helicobacter treatment fails: results of a treatment trial using the Sydney strain mouse model. *Antimicrob Agents Chemother* 2003;47:2249–2255.
588. van Zutphen LFM, Baumans V, Beyen AC, eds. *Principles of laboratory animal science*. Amsterdam: Elsevier, 1993.
589. Vasa CV, Glatt AE. Effectiveness and appropriateness of empiric metronidazole for *Clostridium difficile*–associated diarrhea. *Am J Gastroenterol* 2003;98:354–358.
590. Vergeres P, Blaser J. Amikacin, ceftazidime, and flucloxacillin against suspended and adherent *Pseudomonas aeruginosa* and *Staphylococcus epidermidis* in an in vitro model of infection. *J Infect Dis* 1992;165:281–289.
591. Vogel U, Frosch M. Infant rat model of acute meningitis. In: Zak O, Sande MA, eds. *Handbook of animal models of infection*. San Diego: Academic Press, 1999:619–626.
592. Vogelman B, Gudmundsson S, Leggett J, et al. Correlation of antimicrobial pharmacokinetic indices with therapeutic efficacy in an animal model. *J Infect Dis* 1988;158:831–847.
593. Vogelman B, Gudmundsson S, Tumidge J, et al. In vivo postantibiotic effect in a thigh infection in neutropenic mice. *J Infect Dis* 1988;157:287–298.
594. Waga J, Ehinger B. Intravitreal concentrations of some drugs administered with microdialysis. *Acta Ophthalmol Scand* 1997;75:36–40.
595. Waga J, Nilsson-Ehle I, Ljungberg B, et al. Microdialysis for pharmacokinetic studies of ceftazidime in rabbit vitreous. *J Ocul Pharmacol Ther* 1999;15:455–463.
596. Wakebe H, Imada T, Yoneda H, et al. Evaluation of OPC-17116 against important pathogens that cause respiratory tract infections. *Antimicrob Agents Chemother* 1994;38:2340–2345.
597. Walsh TJ, Garrett K, Feuerstein E, et al. Therapeutic monitoring of experimental invasive pulmonary aspergillosis by ultrafast computerized tomography, a novel, noninvasive method for measuring responses to antifungal therapy. *Antimicrob Agents Chemother* 1995;39:1065–1069.

597a. Ward L. Time for talk across the trenches. *New Sci* 1992;1820:28–30.

598. Wardlaw AC. *Practical statistics for experimental biologists*. Chichester, England: John Wiley and Sons, 1985.
599. Watson VE, Hill LL, Owen-Schaub LB, et al. Apoptosis in *Mycobacterium tuberculosis* infection in mice exhibiting varied immunopathology. *J Pathol* 2000;190:211–220.
600. Watters JW, McLeod HL. Using genome-wide mapping in the mouse to identify genes that influence drug response. *Trends Pharmacol Sci* 2003;24:55–58.
601. Weber OF. Animal models in virology. *Contrib Microbiol* 2001;9:15–30.
602. Weinstein WM, Onderdonk AB, Bartlen JC, et al. Antimicrobial therapy of experimental intraabdominal sepsis. *J Infect Dis* 1975;132:282–286.
603. Welkos S, O'Brien A. Determination of median lethal and infectious doses in animal model systems. *Methods Enzymol* 1994;235:29–39.

604. Wendland M, Bumann D. Optimization of GFP levels for analyzing Salmonella gene expression during an infection. *FEBS Lett* 2002;521:105–108.
605. Westman E, Melhus A. The treatment of *Haemophilus influenzae* acute otitis media with amoxicillin protects against reinfection but not against structural changes. *J Antimicrob Chemother* 2002;49:141–147.
605a. Wicher V, Wicher K. Guinea-pig model of acquired and congenital syphilis. In: Zak O, Sande MA, eds. *Handbook of animal models of infection*. San Diego: Academic Press, 1999:291–301.
606. Wilson KH, Sheagren JN, Freter R. Population dynamics of infested *Clostridium difficile* in the gastrointestinal tract of the Syrian hamster. *J Infect Dis* 1985;151:355–361.
607. Wolcott MJ. Advances in nucleic acid–based detection methods. *Clin Microbiol Rev* 1992;5:370–386.
608. Wood CA, Finkbeiner HC, Kohlhepp SJ, et al. Influence of daptomycin on staphylococcal abscesses and experimental tobramycin nephrotoxicity. *Antimicrob Agents Chemother* 1989;33:1280–1285.
609. Woodnutt G, Berry V, Mizen L. Simulation of human serum pharmacokinetics of cefazolin, piperacillin, and BRL 42715 in rats and efficacy against experimental intraperitoneal infections. *Antimicrob Agents Chemother* 1992;36:1427–1431.
610. Woodnutt G, Catherall EJ, Kernutt I, et al. Temocillin efficacy in experimental *Klebsiella pneumoniae* meningitis after infusion into rabbit plasma to simulate antibiotic concentrations in human serum. *Antimicrob Agents Chemother* 1988;32:1705–1709.
611. Woods DE, Sokol PA, Bryan LE, et al. In vivo regulation of virulence in *Pseudomonas aeruginosa* associated with genetic rearrangement. *J Infect Dis* 1991;163:143–149.
612. Woods DE, To M, Sokol PA. *Pseudomonas aeruginosa* exoenzyme S as a pathogenic determinant in respiratory infections. In: Hoiby N, Pedersen SS, Shand GH, et al., eds. *Pseudomonas aeruginosa infection*. Basel: Karger, 1989:27–35.
613. Wu HS, Kolonoski P, Chang YY, et al. Invasion of the brain and chronic central nervous system infection after systemic *Mycobacterium avium* complex infection in mice. *Infect Immun* 2000;68:2979–2984.
614. Wu RQ, Xu YX, Song XH, et al. Relationship between cytokine mRNA expression and organ damage following cecal ligation and puncture. *World J Gastroenterol* 2002;8:131–134.
615. Xiong H, Kawamura I, Nishibori T, et al. Cytokine gene expression in mice at an early stage of infection with various strains of *Listeria* spp. differing in virulence. *Infect Immun* 1994;62:3649–3654.
616. Xiong YQ, Kupferwasser LI, Zack PM, et al. Comparative efficacies of liposomal amikacin (MiKasome) plus oxacillin versus conventional amikacin plus oxacillin in experimental endocarditis induced by *Staphylococcus aureus*: microbiological and echocardiographic analyses. *Antimicrob Agents Chemother* 1999;43:1737–1742.
617. Xu J, Heys JJ, Barocas VH, et al. Permeability and diffusion in vitreous humor: implications for drug delivery. *Pharm Res* 2000;16:664–669.
618. Xuan D, Banevicius M, Capitano B, et al. Pharmacodynamic assessment of ertapenem (MK-0826) against *Streptococcus pneumoniae* in a murine neutropenic thigh infection model. *Antimicrob Agents Chemother* 2002;46:2990–2995.
619. Yagmurlu A, Boleken ME, Ertoy D, et al. Preventive effect of pentoxifylline on renal scarring in rat model of pyelonephritis. *Urology* 2003;61:1037–1041.
620. Yagmurlu MF, Korkusuz F, Gursel I, et al. Sulbactam-cefoperazone polyhydroxybutyrate-co-hydroxyvalerate (PHBV) local antibiotic delivery system: in vivo effectiveness and biocompatibility in the treatment of implant-related experimental osteomyelitis. *J Biomed Mater Res* 1999;46:494–503.
621. Yang S, Chung CS, Ayala A, et al. Differential alterations in cardiovascular responses during the progression of polymicrobial sepsis in the mouse. *Shock* 2002;17:55–60.
622. Yangco BG, Lackman-Smith C, Espinoza CG, et al. The hamster model of chronic *Mycobacterium avium* complex infection. *J Infect Dis* 1989;159:556–561.
623. Yeung RSM, Penninger J, Mak TW. Genetically modified animals and immunodeficiency. *Curr Opin Immunol* 1993;5:585–594.
624. Yildirim O, Oz O, Aslan G, et al. The efficacy of intravitreal levofloxacin and intravitreal dexamethasone in experimental *Staphylococcus epidermidis* endophthalmitis. *Ophthalmic Res* 2002;34:349–356.
625. Yoshizumi MO, Kashani A, Palmer J, et al. High dose intramuscular methylprednisolone in experimental *Staphylococcus aureus* endophthalmitis. *J Ocul Pharmacol Ther* 1999;15:91–96.
626. Yoshizumi MO, Lee GC, Equi RA, et al. Timing of dexamethasone treatment in experimental *Staphylococcus aureus* endophthalmitis. *Retina* 1998;18:130–135.
627. Young LS, Bermudez LE. Perspective on animal models: chronic intracellular infections. *Clin Infect Dis* 2001;33[Suppl 3]:S221–S226.
628. Yuste J, Jado I, Fenoll A, et al. β-lactam modification of the bacteraemic profile and its relationship with mortality in a pneumococcal mouse sepsis model. *J Antimicrob Chemother* 2002;49:331–335.
629. Zak O. Scope and limitations of experimental chemotherapy. *Expertmentia* 1980;36:479–483.
630. Zak O, O'Reilly T. Animal infection models and ethics: the perfect infection model. *J Antimicrob Chemother* 1993;31[Suppl D]:193–205.
631. Zak O, Sande MA. Correlation of in vitro antimicrobial activity of antibiotics with results of treatment in experimental animal models and human infection In: Sabath LD, ed. *Action of antibiotics in patients*. Bern: Hans Huber Publishers, 1982:55–67.
632. Zak O, Sande MA, eds. *Experimental models in antimicrobial chemotherapy*. London, Academic Press, 1986.
633. Zak O, Sande MA, eds. *Handbook of animal models of infection*. San Diego: Academic Press, 1999.
633a. Zana J, Muffat-Joly M, Thomas D, et al. Roxithromycin treatment of mouse chlamydial salpingitis and protective effect on fertility. *Antimicrob Agents Chemother* 1991;35:430–435.
634. Zhanel GG, Craig WA. Pharmacokinetic contributions to postantibiotic effects: focus on aminoglycosides. *Clin Pharmacokinet* 1994;27:377–392.
635. Zhanel GG, Hoban DJ, Harding GK. The postantibiotic effect: a review of in vitro and in vivo data. *DICP* 1991;25:153–163.
636. Zimmerli W. Experimental models in the investigation of device-related infections. *J Antimicrob Chemother* 1993;31[Suppl D]:97–102.
637. Zimmerli W. Tissue cage infection model. In: Zak O, Sande MA, eds. *Handbook of animal models of infection*. San Diego: Academic Press, 1999:409–417.
638. Zimmerli W, Frei R, Widmer AF, et al. Microbiologic tests to predict treatment outcome in experimental

device-related infections due to *Staphyloccus aureus*. *J Antimicrob Chemother* 1994;33:959–967.
639. Zimmerli W, Waldvogel FA, Vaudaux P, et al. Pathogenesis of foreign body infection: description and characteristics of an animal model. *J Infect Dis* 1982;146:487–497.
640. Zini R, Riant P, Barre J, et al. Disease-induced variations in plasma protein levels. I. Implications for drug dosage regimens. *Clin Pharmacokinet* 1990;19:147–159.
641. Zwijnenburg PJ, van der PT, Florquin S, et al. Experimental pneumococcal meningitis in mice: a model of intranasal infection. *J Infect Dis* 2001;183:1143–1146.

CHAPTER 16

Extravascular Antimicrobial Distribution and the Respective Blood and Urine Concentrations in Humans

David M. Bamberger, John W. Foxworth, Darcie L. Bridwell, Christopher S. Shain, Dale N. Gerding

Systemically administered antimicrobials enter the vascular circulation and diffuse or are secreted into a variety of sites in the human body, in widely differing concentrations. The concentration of antimicrobials eventually achieved in a body site is the result of a complex set of factors that includes drug concentration, half-life, protein binding, lipid solubility, ionization, passive diffusion and active transport, extravascular site geometry, and degree of inflammation. Considerable data have been accumulated in the literature about antimicrobial distribution in humans, far more than can be reviewed completely in this chapter. Our purpose is to discuss the principles, models, and methods of assessing antimicrobial distribution in humans and to catalog that distribution in a number of representative extravascular sites.

Parenthetically, the presumed basis for a treatise of this kind, i.e., that the extravascular site antimicrobial concentration correlates with the cure of infection at that site, has been demonstrated for some, but by no means all, infection sites. Obviously, the ultimate cure of an infection entails far more variables than mere attainment of a specific concentration of an antimicrobial agent at the site of infection. Nevertheless, the topic is discussed and the data presented on the assumption that extravascular antimicrobial concentrations within specific sites have at least some importance in the treatment of infection.

TYPES OF EXTRAVASCULAR SITES

Sites of extravascular antimicrobial distribution may be divided into four major categories (195), as shown in Table 16.1. Antibiotic concentrations vary greatly from category to category and from site to site within categories. In general, the highest drug concentrations are found in certain secretory fluids, such as urine or bile, and the lowest in cerebrospinal fluid (CSF) and glandular secretions, such as breast milk and saliva (195).

Fluid-Filled Spaces

These sites provide the most readily interpretable data on extravascular drug distribution. The drug accumulates by means of passive diffusion, specimens rarely are contaminated by blood, and repeated samples can be obtained to profile the drug distribution and determine equilibrium conditions. Sites such as ascitic fluid, joint effusions, pleural effusions, amniotic fluid, pericardial effusions, bursae, blisters, and abscesses are classified in this category. These sites are also characterized by having a relatively small surface area for diffusion, compared with their volume. This results in a slow accumulation of antibiotic with repeated dosing, as well as lower peak and higher trough drug concentrations than those of serum (196,197). In humans, the need to perform an invasive procedure (needle aspiration) to obtain fluid limits the utility of these sites for routine sampling, but cutaneous blister models in humans and tissue cages and semipermeable implanted chambers in animals provide useful models of this type of extravascular site (115,192,418).

Excretory and Secretory Fluids

These fluids provide the greatest variability in achievable drug concentrations of all extravascular sites. Because many antimicrobials are actively secreted into urine or bile, tremendous concentration of drug is possible. In contrast, many glands and organs appear to pose a substantial barrier to penetration by antimicrobials (e.g., milk

TABLE 16.1

Categories of Extravascular Sites in Humans that Have Been Evaluated for Antibiotic Distribution

1. Fluid-filled spaces of relatively large volume into which drug passively diffuses.
   Examples: ascites, pleural effusion, joint effusion, pericardial effusion, amniotic fluid, bursae, blisters, abscesses.
2. Fluids produced by the excretion or secretion of glands or organs.
   Examples: urine, bile, sputum, saliva, tears, sweat, milk, middle ear fluid, sinus fluid, prostatic fluid, semen.
3. Fluid-filled spaces with probable diffusion barriers or active excretory systems.
   Examples: CSF, aqueous humor, vitreous humor.
4. Whole-body tissues.
   Examples: skeletal muscle, skin, bone, cardiac muscle, liver, gallbladder, brain, uterus, ovary, fat, colon, tonsil, adenoid, lung, kidney, prostate, thyroid.

and prostatic fluid). Numerous glandular secretions have been studied for antimicrobial penetration, but bile, urine, sputum, and milk are the most frequently examined. Many of these fluids are readily obtained without the aid of invasive techniques (urine, sputum, milk, and saliva) and thus have been repetitively sampled over time to garner data on secretory rates. As with fluid-filled spaces, secretory fluids usually are free of blood contamination and thus provide the opportunity to determine antimicrobial concentrations quite reliably.

Spaces with Diffusion Barriers

Two body sites, the eye and the CSF, have traditionally been treated as unique because of the low concentration of many antimicrobials achieved there. Other secretory organs, such as breast and prostate, also pose barriers to drug penetration but are included under secretory organs. Although referred to as barriers to diffusion, active transport from CSF to blood or removal, by bulk CSF flow, of certain compounds such as penicillins may be a major reason for the low concentrations in CSF (143). Again, these sites provide reliable data about drug penetration because of their usual lack of blood contamination. However, the invasive nature of procedures used to obtain these fluids limits the number of determinations that can be made in patients.

Whole-Body Tissues

Concentrations of antimicrobials in whole tissues are frequently difficult to interpret because of contamination of the tissues by blood and body fluids. Despite these interpretation difficulties, whole tissue samples are among the specimens most frequently obtained for antimicrobial assay. We have included in this chapter our recommendations for the preparation and assay of whole tissues in order to make these determinations more reliable.

MODELS OF EXTRAVASCULAR ANTIBIOTIC DISTRIBUTION IN HUMANS

The use of human experimental models for extravascular distribution of antimicrobial agents is a potentially important development because it allows the controlled investigation of complex pharmacokinetic relationships seen in humans as intact individuals (444). The proper use and interpretation of these models can lead to a clearer understanding of the nature of drug distribution to sites outside the extravascular space. The primary experimental models currently under investigation include so-called skin-window techniques (both disk and chamber), skin-blister models (created by suction and irritant cantharides), the implantation of subcutaneous threads, and the use of microdialysis probes inserted into muscle or adipose tissue. The most useful models are likely to be the skin-blister models and microdialysis probes. The use of skin blisters provide sufficient volume of locally produced extravascular fluid to enable enough samples to be taken both for evaluation of the chemical composition of the extravascular fluid and for multiple antimicrobial concentration determinations so that a complete drug area under the curve (AUC) for extravascular fluid can be measured. This complete evaluation makes comparison to intravascular kinetic data more meaningful and valid conclusions more likely. Similarly, the use of microdialysis probes is a minimally invasive technique that provides complete pharmacokinetic data, including AUC data, of nonprotein-bound antimicrobial concentrations within the interstial space of a tissue.

Skin-Window Disk

This technique was described by Raeburn (444) as a modification of the skin-window method of Rebuck and Crowley (448). A 25-mm^2 area of skin is abraded using a 25,000-rpm motorized buffer. The abrasion is done (without bleeding) just prior to measurement of the antibiotic. A sterile paper antibiotic disk (6 or 12 mm diameter) is then applied directly to the abraded area and covered with a sterile glass slide, which is secured in position for a selected period of time (usually 1 hour). New applications are made for each additional 1 hour that tissue fluid is to be sampled. Assays are performed by the bioassay technique using paper disks. The amount of tissue fluid on the disk is quantitated by a comparison of disk weight before and after application. Antibiotic standards for the bioassay should contain the same weight of fluid as the unknown specimen (201), a problem of considerable difficulty because disks increase their absorptive capacity with increasing time in contact with fluid, even up to 24 hours (424). The standards should be prepared in a diluent with a protein content similar to that of the tissue fluid (423). The latter point is particularly important for the assay of highly protein-bound drugs and has not been addressed in published studies with this model (201,444). The method allows for measurement of fluid for a relatively short time period at each site and appears to sample tissue fluid that is absorbed from the denuded dermis by the capillary action of the paper disk. However, the limited amount of fluid obtained makes analysis of its composition difficult.

Skin-Window Chamber

This method, described by Tan et al. (534) and used by Tan and Salstrom (531,532), is also a modification of the Rebuck and Crowley (448) skin-window technique. The dermis is exposed by scraping the epidermis with a scalpel blade and placing a tissue-culture chamber, with one glass window removed, over the exposed dermis (533). The chamber is taped in place and filled with 1 mL of sterile saline under slightly negative pressure. During study of a drug, the chamber is periodically emptied and refilled (usually at hourly intervals). The method results in marked dilution of the tissue fluid by saline or buffer. The assumption that equilibration of chamber and tissue fluid occurs within a 1-hour period is likely erroneous, based on the limited diffusing surface area compared with chamber volume. Protein content of the saline fluid is low, as anticipated, and therefore this method is likely to show an apparent reduced penetration of highly bound drugs, compared with systems containing higher levels of albumin (418).

Skin Blister by Suction

This method is based on work by Kiistala and Mustakallio (281), who demonstrated a noninflammatory separation of the epidermis from the dermis by the application of negative pressure. The method used a Perspex block with eight 8-mm holes drilled in it (532). The block is tightly applied to the skin and 0.3 kg/cm^2 of pressure is applied to each bore for approximately 2 hours. A block applied to each forearm yields sixteen 0.15-mL blisters. A different blister is available for evacuation at each sample time. Blisters differ from the skin-window chambers in having fluid with high, rather than low, protein levels. This fluid is produced by the host without the addition of extraneous buffer.

Skin Blister by Cantharides

Cutaneous blisters can also be formed by application of the skin irritant, cantharides, which is prepared from the dried Spanish fly (*Cantharis vesicatoria*) or blister bug. Cantharidin, the most important active ingredient in Spanish fly, has also been used. Simon and Malerczyk (495) were probably the first to use this method. A plaster of 0.2% cantharides (or cantharidin ointment) is applied to the forearms in a 1-cm^2 area 8 to 12 hours before study (584). After formation, the blisters are repeatedly sampled with a fine-bore needle and syringe or capillary tube and the integrity of the blister is maintained by spraying the puncture site with a plastic dressing. The total protein and albumin contents of this inflammatory blister model are the highest of the models currently in use (584).

Subcutaneous Threads

Another method for the study of cutaneous antibiotic penetration in humans (236,237,248) is the subcutaneous thread. An area of the skin is anesthetized locally with lidocaine and multiple umbilical tapes are threaded under the skin with a needle for a distance of 1 to 2 cm. Studies are begun 30 minutes after placement. Tapes are advanced 1 to 2 cm after each time interval to be measured (for long tapes) or removed completely (when multiple short tapes are implanted), and the subcutaneous segment is cut off and assayed. Assay is typically performed by cutting the tape into 1-cm lengths with different concentrations of antibiotic in each piece. Tapes may also be left in place 24 hours prior to antibiotic administration, but this results in a greater inflammatory response (248). The method allows only a limited time for diffusion of tissue fluid at the site when long tapes are continuously advanced, but this problem can be overcome by the implantation of multiple short lengths of umbilical tape. The umbilical tape has a very large surface area exposed for absorption because of the porous cotton weave of the thread. This model poses similar problems for standardization as seen with the paper disk models (424).

Microdialysis Probes

Muller et al. (379a) first described the method of measuring antimicrobial concentrations by use of microdialysis probes. Antimicrobial concentrations within the free interstitial fluid of a tissue is measured by insertion of a microdialysis probe into tissue, usually muscle or subcutaneous adipose tissue. The probe has a semipermeable membrane at its tip and is constantly perfused with a physiologic solution at a flow rate of of 1.5 to 2.0 μL/minute. Antimicrobials within the tissue diffuse out of the extravascular fluid into the probe, resulting in a concentration in the perfusion medium. However, the diffusion may be incomplete and depend on flow rates, temperature, membrane surface and porosity, and may not be constant over time (379b). Therefore, calibration is required, usually using the retrodialysis method, which assumes that the process of diffusion is equal in both directions. The antimicrobial being studied is added to the perfusion medium and its disappearance rate through the membrane is calculated. *In vivo* percent recovery is then defined as

$$100-[100 \bullet (\text{dialysate concentration out}/\text{dialysate concentration in})].$$

In vivo recovery differs markedly among differing antimicrobials (379a). The absolute concentration in the interstitial space is calculated by the following equation:

$$100 \bullet (\text{concentration in the dialysate}/\text{percent in vivo recovery}).$$

Since the semipermeable membrane excludes protein-bound drug, the technique measures free interstitial drug concentrations.

ANTIMICROBIAL ASSAY OF EXTRAVASCULAR FLUIDS AND TISSUE

The determination of antimicrobial agent concentrations contained in tissues can be accomplished by methods that are similar to those used for the determination of antibiotics in body fluids (see Chapter 8). The most readily available assay system at the present time is a microbiological method. This system is based on an indicator organism that is very sensitive to the antibiotic under study and requires no special equipment. It allows for processing of large numbers of samples with minimal expense. An important aspect of this method is preparation of the standard concentration of antibiotic in the same tissue as the unknown sample (275,423). This is necessary so that drug binding to sample constituents is the same in both the unknown sample and the standard curve. Other methods also available for determination of antimicrobial concentrations include (high-pressure) liquid chromatography as well as many specific antibody-based systems such as radioimmunoassay (410) and enzyme immunoassay (562). These other methods, notably liquid chromatography and radioimmunoassay, require extraction of the antimicrobial agent from the specimen prior to assay. Use of these methods necessitates standardization with the tissue and antibiotic under study to ensure that all of the antimicrobial is extracted from the tissue sample or fluid prior to assay.

Microbiological Assay

Antimicrobials can be determined using the bioassay method with only a limited number of organism species and a few selected media. The agar diffusion bioassay method described by Sabath (470) using *Bacillus subtilis* American Type Culture Collection strain 6633 is demonstrative of the technique for assay of antimicrobial compounds. The bioassay relies on an antibiotic-sensitive indicator organism seeded into an agar base on to which paper disks containing antibiotic are placed. Tissue homogenates or body fluids may also be placed on the agar in cylinders or in wells that have been cut into the agar. The cylinder and agar-well techniques usually provide increased sensitivity for the bioassay method. The antibiotic in the sample then diffuses into the agar and inhibits growth of the indicator organism. The diameter of the zone of inhibition is proportional to the concentration of antibiotic in the sample. Multiple variables can affect the diameter of the zone of inhibition. These variables include the indicator organism chosen, the agar base used, and the nature of the sample itself. Most of these variables can be eliminated by preparing the samples for the standard curve determination in the same type of tissue homogenate or body fluid as the specimen to be assayed.

Once the indicator organism and specific medium are selected, the microorganism is grown overnight and added to molten agar at 50 °C. The microorganisms and agar are thoroughly mixed and this mixture is then poured into flat Petri dishes (15 × 100 mm) on a level surface. Each Petri dish contains a measured volume of 6 mL of the bacteria-seeded agar. The plates are left at room temperature on a level surface to harden and are then stored at 4°C until used. Plates should be stored for a maximum of 14 days under these conditions. The standard line is prepared by adding known concentrations of antibiotic to either tissue fluid or tissue homogenate and subsequently making serial dilutions. Samples of both known and unknown antibiotic-containing fluid are then placed on filter paper disks (usually 20 μL per disk) or pipetted (20 to 200 μL) into cylinders or wells cut in the agar surface. If wells or cylinders are used, the sample should be allowed to diffuse into the agar before movement of the plates to the incubator is attempted. The plates are incubated for 24 hours at 37°C and the diameter of the zone of inhibition is read with calipers to the nearest 0.1 mm. All samples should be assayed in triplicate to ensure an error rate of no more than 10%. The standard line is then plotted on semilogarithmic graph paper and the concentration of antimicrobial in the specimen is read from the standard line.

Occasionally, combinations of antimicrobials can be assayed using this method; however, it is not recommended because the influence of combined agents on indicator microorganisms is often unpredictable. Inactivation of aminoglycosides can be accomplished by lowering the agar pH to 5.5 or less. Also, penicillins or cephalosporins can be inactivated by the addition of β-lactamases to the specimen. When this is done, the same procedure should be performed on all standards to ensure the accuracy of the results.

Liquid Chromatography

Liquid chromatography for the measurement of antimicrobial agent concentrations is a specific method for assay of these drugs. The technique measures drugs in a liquid mobile phase by separating them from interferences on a column under high pressure and then using light absorption for agent detection. The technique is able to separate antimicrobials from other compounds in the sample as well as from both serum and tissue interferences. The method has been reviewed by Yoshikawa et al. (608). Extraction of antimicrobial compounds from the specimen is critical for this assay method. Because of the high protein content in most specimens, direct injection onto the liquid chromatography column is not recommended because the proteins plug the column, thus diminishing its efficiency and useful lifetime. Deproteination of samples can be accomplished by use of organic solvents or acids. Methanol, acetonitrile, and trichloroacetic acid are commonly used for this purpose.

After mixing the specimen with these agents, it is necessary to sediment the protein by centrifugation of the specimen and then inject the supernatant into the chromatographic equipment. Extraction has also been performed by adsorption of the specimen with silica gel and by ion-exchange chromatography for aminoglycosides. We have described a method using ion-exchange chromatography for extraction of penicillins and cephalosporins as well (160–162). Liquid chromatography has the advantage of specifically identifying the compounds under study by their pattern of retention on the chromatographic column. The disadvantages are that the extraction procedures and chromatography time required limit the number of specimens that can be assayed in one 24-hour period. The applicability of liquid chromatography for separation of antimicrobial drugs either singly or in combination is extensive. Once extraction techniques and detection methods have been standardized, this method can quantitate virtually any agent. Liquid chromatography is also very precise and highly reproducible, with coefficients of variation usually less than 5%. The sensitivity of liquid chromatography is similar to that of microbiological assays and is satisfactory for both clinical and research use.

Antibody Methods

These methods of antimicrobial assay are based on the availability of specific antibody that binds the drug. The amount of drug bound is then measured either by radioactivity or by the availability for enzymatic reaction (410,562). Antimicrobial detection with radioimmunoassay is generally available for the aminoglycosides. The assays are rapid and specific and are as sensitive as microbiological assays. The radioimmunoassay requires an extraction step; however, the enzyme immunoassay techniques are very rapid and have the advantage of not requiring an extraction. Their usefulness is limited by the availability of specific antisera, and thus far they have been applied to assays of aminoglycosides, vancomycin, and chloramphenicol. The antibody-based methods have been used little for antimicrobial assays of tissue homogenates and, therefore, require considerable standardization before being applied to assays of drugs in tissues.

PREPARATION AND INTERPRETATION OF SAMPLES COLLECTED FROM EXTRAVASCULAR FLUIDS AND TISSUES

The accurate determination and interpretation of antimicrobial assay results from extravascular sites are difficult and often confusing. The tables presented in this chapter illustrate the need for careful sample preparation and standardization in order to avoid conflicting results and possible misinterpretation of data.

Sampling of whole tissues for antibiotic assays in excised tissue should be performed in a carefully controlled manner. The area to be sampled should be identified at operation and easily visible. If possible, the arterial supply should be transiently clamped to allow blood to flow out of the prospective sample area. The specimen is then surgically removed and freed of adherent blood by gentle pressure with sterile gauze. Tissue samples should then be either immediately processed or stored at −70°C until antibiotic assay can be performed. Tissue fluid can be obtained from the tissue sample by homogenization in a phosphate-buffered saline solution at neutral pH. It is usually necessary to dilute the specimen with three volumes of buffer for every one volume of sampled tissue. The homogenization should be done in a hand-homogenizer so that temperature in the specimen is not elevated, which may destroy some drugs. The resulting homogenate can then be assayed directly for antibiotic content as well as for markers of various tissue compartments and blood. The homogenate can also be centrifuged and the supernatant assayed. We suggest preparation of antibiotic solutions for the standard line at the same time as preparation of the unknown sample so that the standards and the unknown are exposed to the tissue for the same amount of time under the same conditions (275).

Rauws and Van Klingeren (447) and Bergan (56) have discussed the difficulty in interpretation of antimicrobial tissue concentrations obtained from homogenized whole tissues. The final amount of detected drug is the sum of the concentrations of the individual components of the tissue as given by:

$$C_T = C_p f_b(1 - Ht) + C_e f_b(Ht) + C_i f_i + C_c f_c + C_s f_s$$

where C is the concentration in whole tissue (C_T), plasma (C_p), erythrocytes (C_e), interstitial fluid (C_i), tissue cells (C_c), and specialized tissue components (C_s) such as secretory fluids, and f is the fraction of the homogenate contributed by blood (f_b), interstitial fluid (f_i), tissue cells (f_c), and specialized tissue components (f_s). Ht is the hematocrit level, a critical determination for most studies. The sum of the homogenate fractions is equal to 1, i.e., $f_b + f_i + f_c + f_s = 1$. Because the contribution of antimicrobial agent in blood is one of the most important potential inaccuracies in the assay of tissue homogenates, correction for blood contamination is essential. We have indicated in the tables whenever this has been done. The formula of Plaue et al. (429) can be used for this correction. Their formula simply states that extravascular concentration = (tissue concentration − serum concentration)/(tissue water volume − blood volume).

Blood contamination can be estimated most simply by measurement of the hemoglobin content of the tissue homogenate and comparison of this with the hemoglobin content of the subject's circulating blood. If estimation of blood contamination is not possible, the significance of this factor can be minimized by obtaining the extravascular fluid or tissue sample at a time when the intravascular antibiotic concentration is expected to be low, or at least lower than that in the extravascular site under study. Rinsing the specimen to remove blood should also be avoided because most antimicrobials at the low concentrations found *in vivo* are readily water-soluble and easily washed out. If desired, the extracellular or interstitial fluid in tissue can also be measured with high-molecular weight dextran, sodium bromide, or sodium thiocyanate, which are excluded from intact cells (e.g., kidney, gallbladder, and prostate). Corrections for antibiotic concentrations of the secretory product also need to be considered because these fluids often contain high concentrations of antimicrobial agent and significantly contaminate tissue specimens. Most published work on tissue distribution of antibiotics fails to make even simple adjustments for blood contamination, making interpretation difficult or impossible.

Finally, because various body tissues bind antimicrobial agents with different capacities (309) and tissue fluid-antibiotic concentration is a combination of bound and unbound drug (419), it is necessary to know the protein binding of an antibiotic to both the tissue or body fluid and plasma or serum in order to interpret correctly the significance of the tissue concentration. Methods for measurement of protein binding to serum, tissues, and body fluids have been published (309,421,422), and measurements should be performed to optimally interpret extravascular fluid and tissue antimicrobial concentrations.

INTERPRETATION OF EXTRAVASCULAR ANTIMICROBIAL DISTRIBUTION

The proper interpretation of an extravascular antimicrobial concentration depends on a series of factors that are often overlooked or ignored (Table 16.2). These factors (with the possible exception of protein concentration) are independent of permeability barriers or effects of inflammation that may influence the amount of antimicrobial that reaches a given site. They also do not take into account the antimicrobial susceptibility of pathogens likely to be found within a given extravascular site. Such comparisons require a higher level of cognition and are left to readers who may wish to correlate minimal inhibitory concentrations for specific organisms found elsewhere in this text with extravascular site drug concentrations found at the end of this chapter (235). Readers who make such an effort are cautioned that expectations of clinical cure or failure should not be made with a high degree of confidence until more clinical studies on this subject are available (141,219).

Administration Method

The method used to administer an antimicrobial can result in marked differences in serum concentration. High concentrations in serum result rapidly from bolus injections and influence the rate at which antimicrobials enter an extravascular site (305,541). Similarly, intermittent administration results in more rapid attainment of high extravascular levels than does constant intravenous infusion (420,556). Furthermore, extravascular drug

TABLE 16.2

Factors that Influence the Interpretation of Extravascular Antimicrobial Concentrations

1. Antimicrobial administration method (oral, intravenous, intramuscular, constant infusion, bolus injection)
2. Single- or multiple-dosage administrations
3. Collection, processing, and assay of specimens
4. Protein (albumin) content of the extravascular site
5. Geometry (ratio of surface area to volume) of the extravascular site
6. Method used to compare serum and extravascular site concentrations
   a. Peak site-to-peak serum concentrations
   b. Simultaneous site and serum concentrations
   c. AUC site-to-AUC serum determination

concentrations are frequently compared with peak serum concentrations. Rapid intravenous infusions can result in very high serum peaks that, when compared with extravascular concentrations, may give the erroneous perception of poor extravascular drug penetration.

Single or Multiple Dosages

The concentration of antimicrobial at an extravascular site is influenced by the number of doses administered, particularly if the administration frequency is short relative to the serum half-life of the drug (123). Multiple doses may result in considerably higher extravascular antibiotic concentrations than do single doses (198), as a drug accumulates over multiple half-lives depending on the dosing interval. This gradient may be reduced if a loading dose is administered, but the level achieved by a loading dose may not equal the result of the multiple half-lives of accumulation required to reach steady-state condition.

Specimen Handling

Different methods of processing and assaying specimens may lead to confusion in interpretation of extravascular levels, particularly in whole tissues. As previously discussed, the method used to remove blood from tissues, the assay method and standards, and blood contamination corrections are all important to the interpretation of extravascular antibiotic concentrations. Comparison of studies that use dissimilar handling methods is extremely difficult.

Extravascular Protein Content

Antibiotics often bind to proteins (usually albumin) at the extravascular site as well as in serum. For highly bound antimicrobials, the amount of drug that accumulates in an extravascular space depends on the protein content of the space. A site with high albumin content binds a substantial amount of a highly bound antibiotic, and the total (free plus protein-bound) antibiotic concentration in the site is greater at equilibrium than it would be for a site with low albumin content (418,419). In contrast, a site that contains little albumin may have a low total antibiotic concentration, but most of the antibiotic present is free (unbound) drug.

Site Geometry

The amount of antibiotic in a fluid-filled space largely depends on diffusion and, in turn, on the surface area available for diffusion compared with the volume of the space, the so-called surface area to volume (SA/V) ratio. It has been shown in experimental models that spaces with high SA/V ratios show fluctuations of antibiotic concentrations that parallel serum fluctuations, while spaces with low SA/V ratios show a damped response with lower peaks and higher troughs than in serum (557). Animal models that use tissue cages and chambers as extravascular sites and human blister models of extravascular distribution are subject to variation in drug penetration because of differences in SA/V ratios (557). This simple ratio of SA/V is the major determinant of peak and trough drug levels in large-volume, fluid-filled spaces that fill mainly by passive diffusion. Experimental data for ascites in dogs clearly support this concept (194).

Method of Serum and Site Comparison

The method used to compare serum and extravascular site antibiotic concentrations can markedly influence the perception of how well a drug enters an extravascular site. Most antimicrobials are administered intermittently, yielding a rapid rise in serum concentration followed by a logarithmic decay in serum levels. Extravascular site concentrations follow a similar pattern, but peak levels are usually lower and occur later than in serum, while trough levels are higher than those in serum (Fig. 16.1). Comparisons of serum and site concentrations are usually done in one of three ways: peak-to-peak comparison, simultaneous-time comparison, or AUC-to-AUC comparison. Peak-to-peak comparisons are difficult to obtain clinically because large numbers of specimens are required to ensure that the peak is obtained. In addition,

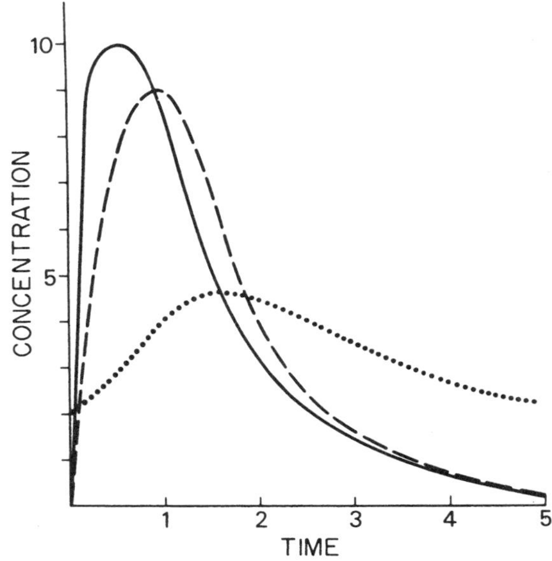

FIGURE 16.1 ● Theoretical concentration versus time profile for an intermittently administered antimicrobial. Serum (——), interstitial fluid (– – –), and a large-volume site with limited surface area for diffusion (. . . .) are shown at equilibrium. AUC values are equal for all sites. (From Cunha and Ristuccia [125a], with permission.)

serum peaks may be very high following rapid intravenous infusion, resulting in an inappropriately low ratio of site-to-serum concentrations. Simultaneous-time determinations are most often employed clinically because it is simpler to obtain a serum specimen at the same time that the site is sampled. Because serum levels are falling at the same time that site levels are rising, the perceived penetration of an antibiotic into an extravascular site may be low if specimens are taken shortly after administration (high serum level and low site level) but appear much higher if sampling is delayed until serum levels have fallen and site levels have risen. Perhaps the best way to compare serum and site antibiotic penetration is by means of AUC data. These studies also require multiple serum and site samples and thus are difficult to perform in certain sites in humans. They are best done following multiple antimicrobial doses to allow equilibrium to occur.

TABLES AND COMMENTS

General Comments

Tables 16.3 to 16.21 have been prepared from published literature for reference purposes to illustrate the concentrations of antimicrobials found in a variety of human extravascular sites. Sites have been selected to be representative of each of the categories listed in Table 16.1. Thus, the sites include fluid-filled spaces such as ascites, pleural effusions, joint fluids, and cutaneous blisters (as well as cutaneous chambers, disks, and threads); secretory fluids such as bile, sputum, breast milk, middle ear fluid, and prostate and sinus secretions; barrier spaces such as aqueous humor and CSF; and the whole-body tissues bone, skeletal muscle, cardiac tissue, gallbladder, lung, and prostate.

Requirements for inclusion of a reference in the tables were that the article supply information about drug dosage, number of doses, concentrations of drug both at the site and in serum, timing of both the site and serum specimens, and, if possible, the range or standard error or standard deviation of the data. Only articles with data from at least three subjects were included. Data from articles were frequently reorganized to include only information for specific sampling times in order to make interpretation easier. Extrapolation of graphical data was occasionally required. Many articles contained far more data than could be included in these concise tables. In such cases, data from specific sampling times (e.g., 1, 2, or 3 hours) were arbitrarily selected to obtain simultaneous-time data for the tables. Certain antimicrobials have been studied numerous times at certain body sites. In these instances, no attempt was made to include every reference in the tables. Rather, emphasis was placed on inclusion of data about as many different drugs as possible. Most citations are from English-language publications. Because much of this work has been done in Europe and Japan, foreign-language data have been included whenever possible within the language limitations of the authors and their ability to obtain references.

Reading the tables should be straightforward. Antimicrobials are grouped into aminoglycosides, cephalosporins and related β-lactams, penicillins, quinolones, tetracyclines, and other antimicrobials. Included under cephalosporins are cephamycins and related β-lactams such as moxalactam, monobactams, and carbapenems. All antimicrobials are listed alphabetically within categories. Method of administration, dose (in grams), and whether single or multiple doses were given are listed after the drug name. The number of subjects studied to obtain the data in the table is given in the column headed n. Serum half-life, if not supplied in the references, was obtained from standard tables (190). The remainder of the table gives the serum concentration (micrograms per milliliter or units per milliliter for penicillin), and time obtained, followed by the site concentration (micrograms per milliliter or micrograms per gram of tissue) and time obtained. The ratio of site concentration to serum concentration is given as a percentage. The "Notes" column includes special information about whether the site was infected or uninfected (if the information is known), whether site assays were corrected for blood contamination (a rarity), and any special information needed to interpret a given study. Specific comments regarding each table are included in the following sections.

Ascites

There are only limited data on antibiotic penetration into ascitic fluid. Data in Table 16.3 are limited to patients from whom ascitic fluid could be aspirated. Only studies that included fluid obtained by aspiration are included. Studies that obtained fluid by placing a paper disk under a loop of bowel at surgery or that measured peritoneal fluid samples from peritoneal drains after abdominal surgery or from patients undergoing peritoneal dialysis were not included. In the majority of studies, antibiotics penetrated into ascitic fluid well, although there was a lag in the ascitic fluid values compared with the serum values in the first few hours after the initial dose. AUC ratios of ascites to serum for several antimicrobial agents of different classes ranged from 30% to greater than 100% (53,152,209,229,426,490,558).

Pleural Fluid

The antibiotic levels in pleural fluid are listed as infected (i.e., empyema) or uninfected (Table 16.4). The uninfected groups consist of patients with congestive heart failure and malignant or parapneumonic effusions; some also included cases of nonpyogenic infection, such as tuberculosis. When specified, most samples were collected

(*text continues on page 731*)

TABLE 16.3

Antimicrobial Concentrations in Ascites

Reference	Antimicrobial	Administration Method[a]	Dose (g) (Multiple or Single)[b]	*n*	Serum Half-life (h)	Serum Concentration Mean (μg/mL) (Range)	Time Serum Obtained (h)	Site Concentration Mean (μg/mL) (Range)	Time Site Specimen Obtained (h)	Ratio of Site/Serum (%)	Notes[c]
Aminoglycosides											
316	Amikacin	IV	7.5 mg/kg (S)	8	2.5	9.5 (4.5–2.0)	4	4.15 (0.56–6.8)	5	58	U
191	Gentamicin	IV or IM	0.06 (M) 0.12 (S)	11	2.0	3.9 (0.6–10)	0.5–30	3.1 (0.7–8.2)	0.5–30	90	I
191	Tobramycin	IM	0.06 (M)	4	2.0	7.0 (2.5–13.6)	1–5	4.5 (1.3–10.8)	1–5	79	I
Cephalosporins and related β-lactams											
23	Aztreonam	IV	0.5 (S)	26	1.8	24.9 (12.6–38.4)	0.5	10.8 (3.4–19.6)	1	43	I
152	Cefdozime	IV	1.0 (S)	6	6.4	17.0	4	10.0	4	59	U
206	Cefonicid	IV	2.0 (M)	9	8.9	83 (37–138)	1	23 (10–16)	1	28	I
558	Cefoperazone	IV	15 mg/kg (S)	7	3.8	25	4	10	4	40	U
467	Cefotaxime	IV	2.0 (S)	41	2.5	22 ± 18	6	23 ± 17	6	120	I
371	Cefotaxime	IM	1.0 (M)	6	2.5	20	2	10.0 (3.8–17.6)	2	50	U
187	Cefoxitin	IV	30 mg/kg (S)	8	1.36	28 (10.3–40.8)	2	32.8 (15.1–54.5)	2	117	U, R
53	Ceftazidime	IV	1.0 (S)	6	5.9	~21	2	9.4	2	45	U
53	Ceftriaxone	IV	1.0 (S)	6	13.6	~35	2	18.4	2	53	U
318	Cefuroxime	IV	2.0 (S)	5	0.8	18	3	16	3	89	U
579	Cephalothin	IV	1.0 (S)	5	0.5	10.22 (± 2.46 SD)	1	3.22 (± 0.71 SD)	1	31	U
458	Imipenem/cilastatin	IV	0.5 (S)	5	0.9	4.7 ± 2.2/3.5 ± 1.9	3	4.0 ± 1.7/2.8 ± 1.6	3	85/71	U

(*continued*)

TABLE 16.3 (Continued)

Antimicrobial Concentrations in Ascites

Reference	Antimicrobial	Administration Method[a]	Dose (g) (Multiple or Single)[b]	n	Serum Half-life (h)	Serum Concentration Mean (μg/mL) (Range)	Time Serum Obtained (h)	Site Concentration Mean (μg/mL) (Range)	Time Site Specimen Obtained (h)	Ratio of Site/Serum (%)	Notes[c]
Penicillins											
209	Amoxicillin/clavulanic acid	IV	1.0 (S)/0.2 (S)	6	1.0	12/1.2	2	10/1	2	83/83	U
191	Ampicillin	IV	1–2 (M)	3	1.1	184 (27–313)	2–3.5	185 (27–313)	2–3.5	100	I
349	Penicillin V	Oral	1 × 10^6 units (M)	3	0.5	6.6 (4.2–8.3)	2	2.6 (0.9–4.7)	2	39	U
229	Piperacillin	IV	4.0 (S)	11	1.95	45	2.5	25	2.5	55	U
Quinolones											
141	Ofloxacin	IV	0.4	7	10.5	2.21	24	1.53	24	69	I
490	Ofloxacin	Oral	0.2 (S)	12	11.6	1.5	8	1.4	8	93	U
Others											
191	Clindamycin	IV	0.4–0.6 (M)	3	2.0	6.5 (5.9–7.6)	1–5.5	2.8 (2.3–3.2)	1–5.5	44	I
361a	Lincomycin	Oral	1.0 (S)	7	4.5	5.7 (1.4–10.4)	4	22.0 (1.6–70)	4	528	U
75	Rifampin	Oral	0.15	4	2.5	1.3 (0.4–7.4)	4	0.3 (0.1–0.5)	4	23	
189	Vancomycin	IV	0.5 (S)	11	6.0	6.9 (6.4–8.0)	1.4	3.6 (1.5–5.2)	1.5	52	U

[a] IV, intravenously; IM, intramuscularly.
[b] S, single dose; M, multiple dose.
[c] U, uninfected; I, infected; R, patients had renal impairment.

TABLE 16.4

Antimicrobial Concentrations in Pleural Fluid

Reference	Antimicrobial	Administration Method[a]	Dose (g) (Multiple or Single)[b]	*n*	Serum Half-life (h)	Serum Concentration Mean (μg/mL) (Range)	Time Serum Obtained (h)	Site Concentration Mean (μg/mL) (Range)	Time Site Specimen Obtained (h)	Ratio of Site/Serum (%)	Notes[c]
Aminoglycosides											
543	Amikacin	IV	7.5 mg/kg (S)	10	2.6	27.6 (±2.0)	0.5	11.0 (±3.1)	0–1	40	U, T, PD
543	Amikacin	IV	7.5 mg/kg (S)	5	2.6	27.6 (±2.0)	0.5	5.7 (±2.2)	7–8	21	I, T, PD
543	Gentamicin	IV	1.5 mg/kg (S)	5	2.9	5.1 (±0.4)	0.5	2.9 (±0.3)	0.5–1	57	U, T, PD
543	Gentamicin	IV	1.5 mg/kg (S)	3	2.9	5.1 (±0.4)	0.5	0	0–8	0	I, T
439	Kanamycin	IM	0.5 (S)	3	2.0	9.3 (4–16)	2	0.8 (0–2.0)	2	9	
543	Netilmicin	IV	2.0 mg/kg (S)	4	3.2	5.4 (±0.5)	0.5	3.7 (±0.8)	1–2	69	U, PD, T
543	Netilmicin	IV	2.0 mg/kg (S)	3	3.2	5.4 (±0.5)	0.5	0	0–8	0	I, T
267	Sisomicin	IM	0.75 (S)	5	2.0	6.7 (±0.6)	1	1.9 (±0.66)	3	28	U
Cephalosporins and related β-lactams											
45	Aztreonam	IV	2 (S)	3	2	64 (±12 SE)	1–3	51 (±31 SE)	1–3	79	
141	Cefadroxil	Oral	0.5 (S)	7	1.3	2.15	8	2.46	8	114	U
118	Cefazolin	IV	1.0 (S)	9	2.0	72.5 (36–112)	0.5–2	21.3 (5–83)	0.5–2	30	U
603	Cefoperazone	IV	2.0 (S)	6	2.9	209 (108–270)	1	15.5 (7–25)	4–6	7	I, U, PD
330	Cefotaxime	IV	1.0 (S)	6	1.2	28	1.0	7.2 (±3.1 SD)	3.0	26	U
269	Cefotaxime	IM/IV	25 mg/kg (M/S)	6	1.2	19.9 (13–34)	0.5	4.8 (2.8–11.2)	3.0	24	I, P
569	Cefoxitin	IV	2.0 (S)	6	0.8	11.8 (4–18)	1–5	3.6 (1–6.4)	1–5	31	U
149	Cefpodoxime	Oral	0.2 (S)	6	1.9–3.2	2.72 (±0.32 SE)	6	1.84 (±0.33 SE)	6	67	U
564a	Ceftazidime	IV	2.0 (S)	5	1.9	80 (±10)	1.0	17 (±3)	1	21	U, E
526	Ceftizoxime	IV	1.0 (S)	5	1.7	24.1 (±4.4 SD)	1.0	7.8 (±2.2 SD)	2–3	32	U
52	Ceftriaxone	IV	1.0 (S)	5	12.4	39.4 (34–50)	4	7.9 (7.0–8.7)	4	20	
318	Cefuroxime	IV	1.0 (S)	6	1.3	24 (14–40)	1.5–4.5	7.3 (5.6–9.1)	1.5–4.5	30	U
536	Cephalothin	IV	1.0 (M)	3	0.5	22.5 (14–34.5)	2.5–4.5	26.0 (21.5–28.5)	2.5–4.5	116	U
603	Moxalactam	IV	2.0 (S)	5	2.4	99 (43–122)	1	20 (9–35)	4–6	20	PD
Quinolones											
265	Ciprofloxacin	IV	0.2 (S)	7	3–5	3.8 (±2.4 SD)	0.1	1.0 (±0.6)	3.25	26	U, PD
265	Ciprofloxacin	Oral	0.75 BID (M)	3	3–5	4.3 (±0.6 SD)	3.5	2.3 (±0.4)	3.5	53	U, PD

(continued)

TABLE 16.4 (Continued)

Antimicrobial Concentrations in Pleural Fluid

Reference	Antimicrobial	Administration Method[a]	Dose (g) (Multiple or Single)[b]	*n*	Serum Half-life (h)	Serum Concentration Mean (μg/mL) (Range)	Time Serum Obtained (h)	Site Concentration Mean (μg/mL) (Range)	Time Site Specimen Obtained (h)	Ratio of Site/Serum (%)	Notes[c]
265	Ciprofloxacin	Oral	0.75 BID (M)	3	3–5	2.3 (± 2.2 SD)	0	2.9 (± 1.5 SD)	2	126	I, PD
282	Lomefloxacin	Oral	0.2 (S)	7	7–8.5	2.16 (1.58–4.34)	1–6	1.36 (0.65–2.18)	6	63	U, PD
604	Ofloxacin	Oral	0.3 QD (M)	21	4–8	4.70 (± 0.63 SD)	2	3.82 (± 0.41 SD)	2	82	U
Penicillins											
131	Amoxicillin	Oral	0.75 (S)	9	2.4	4.5	4	1.6	5.3	36	U, T
328	Ampicillin	Oral	1.0 (S)	6	1.2	21.4 (± 3.7)	1	10.5 (± 1.5)	3	49	U
97	Bacampicillin	Oral	0.8 (M)	9	2.2	7.0 (± 4.3 SD)	1.5	2.9 (± 1.9 SD)	3	41	U, T, PD
293	Mezlocillin	IV	10 (S)	6	1.1	778 (± 270)	0.25	100 (± 38)	1	13	U, T, PD
536	Penicillin	Oral	2–3 × 10^6 units (M)	4	0.5	33 (16–61)	1–3	28.5 (5–56)	1–3	86	I
536	Penicillin	Oral	1–2 × 10^6 units (M)	5	0.5	20.4 (11–25)	1–3	13.6 (3–26)	1–3	67	U
329	Ticarcillin	IV	5.0 (S)	5	1.2	63 (56–70)	1	9 (6–11)	3	14	U, PD
Tetracyclines											
494	Doxycycline	IV	0.2 (S)	16	20	5.0 (± 0.4)	1	1.8 (± 0.2)	10	36	
Others											
409	Clindamycin	Oral	0.15 (M)	3	2	10.1	1–2	9.3 (1.3–22)	1–2	92	U
163	Fosfomycin	IV	30 mg/kg (S)	6	2	195.2 (± 49.2 SD)	0.25	42.6 (± 16 SD)	3.7	22	U, PD
80	Rifampin	Oral	10 mg/kg (S)	8	3.0	6.5 (0.9–11.0)	8–9	2.6 (0.6–6.0)	8–9	40	U
256	Teicoplanin	IV	0.4 (M)	3	40–70	36.2 (± 5.0 SE)	0.5	7.5 (± 1.5)	5	21	PD
189	Vancomycin	IV	0.5 (S)	12	6	7.3 (2.9–10)	1.1–4.0	3.0 (0–8.1)	1.2–4.5	41	U
108a	Vancomycin	IV (CI)	30 mg/kg/day	8	6.3 (± 1.9 SD)	14.0[d] (± 4.3 SD)	4	12.1 (± 2.9 SD)	4	86	U, T
	Vancomycin	IV	15 mg/kg (M)	8	6.3 (± 1.9 SD)	14.4[d] (± 4.9 SD)	4	16 (± 4.5 SD)	4	111	U, T

[a] IV, intravenously; IM, intramuscularly.
[b] S, single dose; M, multiple dose; BID, twice a day; QD, once a day; CI, continuous infusion.
[c] U, uninfected (causes other than empyema); T, tube drainage; PD, peak data; I, infected (empyema).
[d] Measured in the blood.

by chest–tube drainage. Few studies provided data on antibiotic penetration into pleural empyemas. It is notable that the aminoglycosides penetrated poorly into empyema fluid, compared with uninfected pleural fluid, as shown by the study of Thys et al. (543). The quinolones demonstrated good pleural fluid penetration, which appeared to be enhanced by the presence of empyema. Aztreonam also demonstrated excellent penetration into the pleural fluid.

Joint Fluid

In compiling this table of antimicrobial penetration into joint fluid spaces (Table 16.5), single-patient studies were combined when possible to give a better overall reflection of the penetration of individual agents. No attempt at correction for blood contamination was made, and only rarely was there an attempt made to correlate protein content or antimicrobial/tissue fluid protein binding with drug penetration (248). The reported fluid-to-serum antimicrobial concentration ratios are quite high for this group of studies, which is primarily due to the high protein content of the extravascular fluid plus the fact that many of these studies were performed after multiple systemic doses of the antimicrobial agent had been administered. Data from single infected patients treated with cephapirin (481) have not been included in Table 16.5.

Cutaneous Blister/Disks/Threads/ Microdialysis Samples of Interstitial Fluid

Table 16.6 contains a summary of reports of antimicrobial distribution based on models in humans. All sites were done in uninfected patients except the studies done by Tegeder et al. (537) of imipenem. None of the studies have made any attempt to correct for blood contamination other than avoiding gross blood. Data are also available for penicillin (237) and pivampicillin (237) but are not included in Table 16.6 because fewer than three subjects were studied. While only a limited number of multiple-dose studies have been done, even the single-dose studies often demonstrate high ratios of drug concentration in the extravascular site to that in serum, reflecting the small size of the extravascular space under study. One study attempted to correlate protein concentration to drug penetration and found a significant correlation at $r = 0.97$ (236). There was considerable variability in the ratio of extravascular to intravascular antimicrobial concentrations, reflected by ratios as low as 3% for nafcillin in the skin-window model (534) to 238% for FCE22101 in a cantharides blister study (570). Many articles supply data that can provide an AUC for the agent under study in both the intravascular and extravascular spaces. This is a notable achievement in the study of extravascular drug penetration, although more multiple-dose studies are needed as well as more attention to antimicrobial binding at extravascular sites.

Bile

Specimens of bile obtained by three methods are included in Table 16.7: aspirations of gallbladder or common duct bile at surgery, external bile drainage from T-tubes, or bile obtained by endoscopic retrograde cholangiopancreatography. Studies in which bile was obtained by duodenal aspiration were not included because of unknown specimen dilution by gastrointestinal fluids. Several studies in Table 16.7 confirm the observation that bile concentrations are lower or absent in the presence of cystic duct obstruction (390) or common bile duct obstruction (77,100,208). In general, T-tube and common duct bile levels seem to be somewhat higher than gallbladder bile levels (90,95,96,363,364) when comparably timed specimens are obtained. This may be related to partial obstruction of the cystic duct. Multiple antibiotic doses also result in higher bile levels than do single doses (72,364,370).

Ratios of site-to-serum levels are extremely variable, ranging from zero in the presence of obstruction to 18,400% for rifampin (75), with numerous examples of ratios greater than 100%. After relief of biliary obstruction, the excretion of antibiotics (aztreonam, piperacillin, and cefamandole) remains depressed for a prolonged period of time, which may exceed 28 days (77,323). Data on ratios of AUC in bile to AUC in serum were available for a limited number of drugs, and they also showed wide variation: 19% for cephacetrile (91); 38% to 44% for amoxicillin, penicillin G, and oral ampicillin (95,96); 46% for ceftazidime (84); 65% for amikacin (72); 96% for intravenous ampicillin (96); 100% for cefuroxime (94); and 2089% for mezlocillin (93).

Although biliary penetration is often touted as advantageous in the therapy of biliary tract infection, it is not at all clear that this is an important treatment variable in view of the poor penetration in the presence of obstruction. Keighley et al. (279) have shown that biliary antibiotic concentrations have no influence on rates of bacteremia and wound infection associated with biliary tract surgery. Smith and LeFrock (502), Nagar and Berger (385), and Dooley et al. (144) have extensively reviewed biliary antibiotic penetration and clinical use in biliary infection.

Sputum

Both sputum and bronchial secretion specimens are included in Table 16.8. Bronchial secretions were obtained via bronchoscopy or by suction aspiration from patients with endotracheal tubes or tracheostomies. Some articles provide data on antimicrobial concentrations in epithelial lining fluid in the lung, which is indicated in Table 16.8 (242). Most subjects had chronic bronchitis, but some studies were done with children with cystic fibrosis, and occasionally patients had pneumonia. Nearly all studies were done with infected patients. Some studies suggest

(*text continues on page 744*)

TABLE 16.5

Antimicrobial Concentrations in Joint Fluid

Reference	Antimicrobial	Administration Method[a]	Dose (g) (Multiple or Single)[b]	*n*	Serum Half-life (h)	Serum Concentration Mean (μg/mL) (Range)	Time Serum Obtained (h)	Site Concentration Mean (μg/mL) (Range)	Time Site Specimen Obtained (h)	Ratio of Site/Serum (%)	Notes[c]
Aminoglycosides											
241	Amikacin	IM	7.5–15.7 mg/kg/day (M)	4	2.0	15.3 (12.1–21.0)	4.0–7.0	17.0 (12.5–24.4)	4.0–7.0	111	I
137	Gentamicin	IM	1.0–1.5 mg/kg (S)	6	2.0	4.0 (2.4–6.5)	1.0–3.5	3.2 (2.4–4.4)	1.0–3.5	80	
35	Kanamycin	IM	15 mg/kg/day (M)	4	2.0	21.2 (11.0–28.0)	2.0	15.4 (8.7–21.0)	2.0	73	
137	Tobramycin	IM	1.0–1.5 mg/kg (S)	7	2.0	2.7 (1.0–5.6)	1.5–4.0	2.4 (1.3–4.6)	1.5–4.0	89	
Cephalosporins and related β-lactams											
554	Cefadroxil	Oral	0.5 (S)	5	1.3	7.30	2.0	7.14	2.0	98	
552	Cefamandole	IV	2 (S)	29	0.7	66.8	0.5	33.2	0.5	50	
480a	Cefazolin	IV	1.0 (S)	15	1.8	81.4 (56–135)	0.25–0.5	26.2 (7.1–63)	0.25–0.5	32	
226	Cefotaxime	IV	2 (S)	22	1.2	25	2	29	2	116	E, I
389	Cephalexin	Oral	25 mg/kg (M)	5	0.8	17.1 (9.3–20)	2.0	11.3 (5.3–19)	2.0	66	I
Penicillins											
411	Ampicillin	IM	0.5 (M)	14	1.1	8.3 (2.1–19.0)	1.0	4.4 (1.1–12.0)	1.0	53	
35	Ampicillin	Oral	0.5 (M)	19	1.1	2.9 (0.03–10.0)	2.0	1.8 (0.03–5.4)	2.0	62	
552	Cloxacillin	IV	2.0 (S)	29	0.5	120.0	0.75	105.0	0.75	87	
389	Dicloxacillin	Oral	25 mg/kg (M)	6	0.5	13.6 (9.2–28)	2.0	9.5 (3.2–23)	2.0	70	I
388	Methicillin	IV	25–61 mg/kg (M)	6	0.5	23.2 (1.7–60.0)	0.5–4.0	27.8 (3.8–69)	0.5–4.0	120	I
560	Nafcillin	IM	1.5 (S)	20	1.0	15.5 (7.9–26.0)	1.0	2.7 (0.5–7.0)	1.0	17	
36	Penicillin	IM	25–40 × 10^3 units (M)	7	1.0	0.14 (0.06–0.25)	1.0	0.13 (0.09–0.19)	1.0	93	
388	Penicillin G	IV	25 mg/kg (M)	3	0.5	2.6 (0.16–5.1)	1.0–2.0	2.6 (0.08–5.1)	1.0–2.0	100	I
Other											
444b	Linezolid	PO except for last dose which was IV	0.6 (M)	10	4.26–5.4	23 ± 6.5	1.5 h after last dose	20.1 ± 3.4	1.5h after last dose	87.4	
189	Vancomycin	IV	500 mg (M)	6	6.0	7.0 (5.2–8.7)	1.0–1.65	5.7 (4.0–6.4)	1.0–1.65	81	

[a] IM, intramuscularly; IV, intravenously; PO, by mouth.
[b] M, multiple dose; S, single dose; PO, by mouth.
[c] I, infected joint; E, extrapolated from graphical data.

TABLE 16.6

Antimicrobial Concentrations in Cutaneous Blisters, Disks, and Threads

Reference	Antimicrobial	Administration Method[a]	Dose (g) (Multiple or Single)[b]	*n*	Serum Half-life (h)	Serum Concentration Mean (μg/mL) (Range)	Time Serum Obtained (h)	Site Concentration Mean (μg/mL) (Range)	Time Site Specimen Obtained (h)	Ratio of Site/Serum (%)	Notes[c]
Aminoglycosides											
531	Amikacin	IM	7.5 mg/kg (S)	12	2.0	24.6 (±4.72)	2.0	4.2 (±2.1)	2.0	17	W
531	Gentamicin	IM	1.7 mg/kg (S)	12	2.0	5.9 (±2.7)	2.0	1.8 (±0.77)	2.0	31	W
510	Netilmicin	IM	200 mg (S)	3	2.3	5.8 (3.5–9)	2.0	5.6 (3.5–9)	2.0	97	SB
531	Tobramycin	IM	1.7 mg/kg (S)	12	2.0	6.4 (±3.5)	2.0	1.4 (±0.5)	2.0	22	W
Cephalosporins and related β-lactams											
584	Aztreonam	IV	1.0 (S)	6	1.93	24.1 (±3.5)	2.0	21.8 (±3.8)	2.0	90	CB
355b	Cefaclor	Oral	0.5 (S)	8	1.0 (±0.3)	11.1 (±2.3)	2	9.5 (±2.4)	2	85.6	SB
495	Cefadroxil	Oral	1.0 (S)	10	1.5	28.4	1.5–3	20	1.5–3	70	CB
531	Cefamandole	IV	1.0 (S)	12	0.7	5.0 (±1.8)	2.0	1.4 (±0.4)	2.0	28	W
531	Cefazolin	IV	1.0 (S)	12	2.0	40.5 (±0.7)	2.0	4.2 (±1.3)	2.0	11	W
397	Cefepime	IV	2 (S)	6	2.1	58.8 (±9.3)	2	79.1 (±30.5)	2	134	CB
521	Cefixime	Oral	400 mg (S)	6	3.8	3.4 (±1.4)	4	2.3 (±1.5)	4	68	CB, E
301	Cefmenoxime	IM	1 (S)	5	1.4	36	2	21.5	2	60	SB, E
533	Cefmetazole	IV	2.0 (M)	12	1.1	12	1	17.8	1	148	W
302	Cefodizime	IV	1 (S)	6	2.4	34	3	8.4	3	25	SB, E
355a	Cefodizime	IM	1 (S)	4	4.3 (±0.3)	54.2 (±20.6)	1	15.5 (±6.7)	1	28.4	PT
487	Cefonicid	IV	30 mg/kg (S)	6	4.1	140	4	31	4	22	SB, E
236	Cefoperazone	IV	2.0 (S)	14	2.4	47.1 (±8.5)	2.0	6.2 (±1.5)	2.0	13	T
236	Cefotaxime	IV	2.0 (S)	14	0.83	18.2 (±4.5)	2.0	6.3 (±2.4)	2.0	35	T
184	Cefotaxime	IM	1.0 (S)	4	1.2	7.0	2.0	2.0	2.0	29	W
60	Desacetyl-cefotaxime	IV		4	1.5	2.9 (1.2–5.2)	2.0	1.79 (1.06–2.78)	2.0	62	SB
356	Cefotetan	IV	2.0 (S)	4	3.9	65.1	2	57.7	2	87	SB
105	Cefotiam	IV	1 (S)	21	1.5	10.5 (±2.2)	2	11.6 (±2.2)	2	110	SB
236	Cefoxitin	IV	2.0 (S)	14	0.88	13.1 (±3.0)	2.0	5.9 (±1.8)	2.0	45	T

(continued)

TABLE 16.6 (Continued)

Antimicrobial Concentrations in Cutaneous Blisters, Disks, and Threads

Reference	Antimicrobial	Administration Method[a]	Dose (g) (Multiple or Single)[b]	*n*	Serum Half-life (h)	Serum Concentration Mean (μg/mL) (Range)	Time Serum Obtained (h)	Site Concentration Mean (μg/mL) (Range)	Time Site Specimen Obtained (h)	Ratio of Site/Serum (%)	Notes[c]
277	Cefpirome	IV	1.0 (S)	6	2.3	97.4 (70–147)	1.9	39.2 (31–49)	1.9	40	CB
81	Cefpodoxime	Oral	0.2	8	2.1	2.3	2.3	1.6	3.5	70	SB
			0.4	8	2.1	4.2	2.4	2.8	3.5	68	SB
39	Cefprozil	Oral	0.25 (M)	12	1.3	6.1	1.5	3.0	24	49	SB
165	Cefsulodin	IV	1.0 (S)	8	1.5	32	2.0	15.3	2.0	48	CB
238	Ceftazidime	IV	1.0 (M)	4	7.9		2.0		2.0		T, IR, PER
589	Ceftibuten	Oral	0.2 (M)	6	2.5	10	2.0	8.4	2	84	CB
486	Ceftizoxime	IV	30 mg/kg (S)	6	1.4	42	2	35	2	83	SB, E
486	Ceftizoxime	IV	30 mg/kg (S)	6	1.4	37	2	14	2	38	D, E
317	Ceftriaxone	IV	1 (M)	12	7.2	100	4	53	4	53	SB, E
236	Cefuroxime	IV	1.5 (S)	14	0.88	17.8 (±4.2)	2.0	6.7 (±2.1)	2.0	38	T
495	Cephalexin	Oral	1.0 (S)	10	1.0	23.3	1.5–2.0	13.7	1.5–2.0	59	CB
494	Cephalothin	IV	1.0 (S)	17	0.5		1.0		1.0	54	CB, PER
9	Cephalothin	IV	2.0 (M)	3	0.5	45.6	0.33	3.43	0.33	7.5	TC
532	Cephapirin	IV	1.0 (S)	12	0.5	1.2 (±0.4)	2.0	1.1 (±0.4)	2.0	91	W
9	Cephradine	IV	2.0 (M)	3	0.7	84.77	0.33	10.73	0.33	13	TC
201	CGP9000	Oral	1.0 (S)	6	1.0	24	2.0	16.6	2.0	69	D
582	FK-037	IV	2.0 (S)	6	2.0	143	0.5	63	1–2	44	CB
377	Meropenem	IV	30 mg/kg	8	1.0	6.3 (5.4–7.2)	4–12	5.5	4–12	87	SB
537	Imipenem	IV	0.5 (M)	4	0.9–1.3	32 (30–40)	1	2 (1–5)	1	30	MD, SP
			0.5 (S)	5	0.9–1.3	45	1	12	1	47	MD
Penicillins											
585	Amoxicillin	IV	1.0 (S)	6	1.3	15.0	2.0	6.0	2.0	40	CB
583	Amoxicillin/clavulanic acid	Oral	500/250 mg (S)	6	1.2/1.0	4.36 (±1.5)/2.72 (±0.7)	2	3.3 (±3.6)/2.07 (±0.9)	2	76/76	CB
532	Ampicillin	Oral	2.0 (S)	12	1.1	7.5 (±3.6)	2.0	1.0 (±0.6)	2.0	13	W

233	Ampicillin	IV	2.0 (S)	6	0.83	24	1.5	10	1.5	42	T
532	Bacampicillin	Oral	1.6 (S)	12	1.1	13.0 (±5.4)	2.0	2.2 (±0.6)	2.0	17	W
528	Benzylpenicillin	IM	0.5 (S)	9	0.5	3.5 (2–5)	2.0	0.6 (0.4–1.0)	2.0	17	W
531	Carbenicillin	IV	3.0 (S)	12	1.5	48.8 (±15.4 SE)	2.0	10.8 (±5.9 SE)	2.0	22	W
239	Cloxacillin	IV	1.0 (S)	6	0.65	8.0	1.5	1.5	1.5	19	SB
585	Flucloxacillin	IV	1.0 (S)	6	1.1	9.0	2.0	5.0	2.0	56	CB
58	Flucloxacillin	IV	2.0 (S)	5	2.1	24	2.0	3.7	2.0	15	SB, E
534	Nafcillin	IM	0.5 (S)	11	1.0	3 (1.8–40)	2.0	0.1 (0.05–0.2)	2.0	3	W
534	Penicillin V	Oral	1.0 (S)	10	0.5	0.9 (0.4–2.0)	2.0	0.2 (0.1–0.4)	2.0	22	W
588	Piperacillin/	IV	4.0 (S)	6	1.0	224 (136–290)	0.5	77 (43–126)	0.5–3	35	CB
	tazobactam		0.5 (S)	6	1.1	27 (17–36)	0.5	113 (5.0–27)	0.5–3	42	CB
327	Temocillin	IV	1 (S)	6	4.5	95 (±30)	2	40 (±16)	2	42	SB, E
531	Ticarcillin	IV	3.0 (S)	12	1.2	47.1 (±6.4)	2.0	10.9 (±4.6)	2.0	23	W
565	Timentin (ticarcillin/ clavulanic acid)	IV	3.2 (S)	12	1.0/0.9	81 (±19)/1.5 (±0.3)	2	32 (±2.6)/2.6 (±0.8)	2	40/173	SB, E
565	Timentin (ticarcillin/ clavulanic acid)	IV	3.2 (S)	12	1.0/0.9	81 (±19)/1.5 (±0.3)	2	71 (±23)/2.0 (±0.9)	2	88/133	T, E
Quinolones											
317	Ciprofloxacin	Oral	0.5 (S)	12	3.7	2.3 (±0.8)	1.3	1.8 (±0.8)	2.3	80	SB
Ciprofloxacin	Oral	0.5 (M)	12	4.7	3.5 (±1.3)	1.0	1.9 (±0.7)	2.5	57	SB	
587	Enoxacin	Oral	0.6 (S)	6	6.2	3.7 (±0.5)	1.9	2.9 (±0.5)	3.7	78	CB
Enoxacin	IV	0.4 (S)	7	5.1	5.5 (±1.8)	Peak	2.2 (±0.5)	0.5	40	CB	
586	Fleroxacin	Oral	0.4 (S)	6	12.0	6.1 (±2.2)	0.7	3.8 (±0.6)	4.0	62	CB
581a	Gatifloxacin	Oral	0.4 (S)	9	6.8 (±0.72)	4.1 (±0.86) (2.9–5.4 range)	1.8 (±0.94)	3.6 (±1.6) (2.2–7.6 range)	4.2 (±1.9)	87	CB
587	Ofloxacin	Oral	0.6 (S)	6	7.0	10.7 (±6.4)	1.2	5.2 (±6.9)	5.3	49	CB
587	Norfloxacin	Oral	0.4 (S)	6	3.25	1.5 (±0.1)	1.5	1.0 (±0.3)	2.3	67	CB
587	Pefloxacin	IV	0.4 (S)	8	10.5	5.1	Peak	3.3 (±0.7)	1.8	66	CB, E
Others											
121	Azithromycin	Oral	0.5 (S)	6	9.6	0.1 (0.06–15)	6	0.13 (0.1–0.15)	2–4	130	CB
360	Carumonam	IV	2 (S)	6	1.68	36.6 (±8.2)	2	48.1 (±11.4)	2	131	CB
590	CGP31608 (penem)	IV	1 (S)	6	0.5	2.8 (±0.2)	2	5.4 (±1.0)	2	193	CB
444a	Clindamycin	Oral	0.5 (S)	4	2.0	3.75	1.5–2.5		1.5–2.5	9	W, PER
584a	Daptomycin	4 mg/kg	7 (S)	7	7.74 (±0.63)	77.5 (±8.3)	0.5	14.5	2	18.7	CB

(continued)

TABLE 16.6 (Continued)

Antimicrobial Concentrations in Cutaneous Blisters, Disks, and Threads

Reference	Antimicrobial	Administration Method[a]	Dose (g) (Multiple or Single)[b]	*n*	Serum Half-life (h)	Serum Concentration Mean (μg/mL) (Range)	Time Serum Obtained (h)	Site Concentration Mean (μg/mL) (Range)	Time Site Specimen Obtained (h)	Ratio of Site/Serum (%)	Notes[c]
379a	Dirithromycin	Oral	0.25 (S)	6	1.7	0.55 (±0.28)	3.3	0.20 (±0.08)	3.3	42	MD
478	Doxycycline	Oral	100 mg (M)	8	11.7	1.5	2	0.7	2	47	SB, E
545	Erythromycin base	Oral	0.5 (M)	8	1.5	2.92	4–6	1.33	4–6	46	SB, E
545	Erythromycin (EA)	Oral	0.5 (M)	8	1.5	1.24	4–6	0.68	4–6	55	SB, E
59	Erythromycin	Oral	0.5 (M)	4	1.5	1.9	3.0	0.12	3.0	6	SB
570	FCE22101 (penem)	IV	1 (S)	6	0.8	2.1 (±0.4)	2	5.0 (±1.9)	2	238	CB
570	FCE22891 (penem)	Oral	1 (S)	5	0.6	2.0 (±1.5)	2	2.7 (±1.3)	2	135	CB
184a	Fosfomycin	IV	8.0	6	5.7	395 (±46)	1	156 (±16)	1	53	MD, SE
551	Fusidic acid	Oral	0.25 (M)	8	16	39 (13.7–54.9)	3	21 (3.4–35)	6–12	53	SB
57	Methioprim	Oral	320 mg (S)	5	9.3	2.6	4	0.9	4	35	SB, E
57	Methioprim	Oral	160 mg (S)	5	9.3	2.5	4	1.3	4	52	SB, E
509	Rifampin	Oral	450 mg (S)	3	2.5	13.2 (10.0–16.0)	3.0	2.7 (2.7–2.8)	6–9	20	SB
103	Sulfacarbamide	Oral	335 mg (M)	5	4–5	7 (±1)	2.0	4 (±1)	2.0	57	SB
103	Sulfadiazine	Oral	335 mg (M)	5	3–4	39 (±2)	2.0	15 (±2)	2.0	50	SB
103	Sulfadimidine	Oral	335 mg (M)	5	5–7	27 (±3)	2.0	6 (±2)	2.0	22	SB
103	Sulfamethoxazole	Oral	0.8 (M)	5	5–7	115 (±6)	2.0	43 (±4)	2.0	37	SB
361	Teicoplanin	IV	440 mg (S)	6	34.2	21.0 (±4.9)	2	13.2 (±2.1)	2	63	CB
387a	Telithromycin (HMR 3647)	Oral	0.6 (S)	8	9.8 L[d]	0.83 (±0.35)	2.5 (±1.03)	0.44 (±0.23)	10.5 (±5.09)	53	CB
103	Trimethoprim	Oral	320 mg (S)	5	8–10	2.8 (±0.4)	2.0	1.5 (±0.4)	2.0	54	SB
103	Trimethoprim	Oral	160 mg (M)	5	8–10	3.1 (±0.8)	2.0	1.7 (±0.3)	2.0	55	SB

[a] IM, intramuscularly; IV, intravenously.
[b] S, single dose; M, multiple dose;
[c] W, skin window; SB, suction blister; CB, cantharidin blister; E, values extrapolated from graph; PT, plastic template method of Kiistala and Mustakallio (281); T, threads; IR, impaired renal function; PER, actual levels not reported, only percentage penetration data; D, disk; TC, tissue cage; MD, microdialysis probe of interstitial fluid of muscle; SP, septic patients.
[d] Literature value.

TABLE 16.7

Antimicrobial Concentrations in Bile

Reference	Antimicrobial	Administration Method[a]	Dose (g) (Multiple or Single)[b]	*n*	Serum Half-life (h)	Serum Concentration Mean (μg/mL) (Range)	Time Serum Obtained (h)	Site Concentration Mean (μg/mL) (Range)	Time Site Specimen Obtained (h)	Ratio of Site/Serum (%)	Notes[c]
Aminoglycosides											
72	Amikacin	IV	0.5 (M)	10	2.0	13.4 (± 5.4 SD)	2.0	7.2 (± 3.9 SD)	2.0	54	U, T
224	Amikacin	IM	0.5 (S)	7	2.0	14.0 (6–17)	0.75–20	4.2 (<1–7.5)	0.75–2.0	30	U, GB
363	Gentamicin	IM	0.1 (S)	15	2.0	3.2 (2–4.9)	0.8–1.2	1.0 (0–3.9)	0.8–1.2	31	GB
363	Gentamicin	IM	0.12 (S, M)	11	2.0	4.4 (1.5–6.9)	1.0	2.8 (0–10)	1.0	64	T
224	Kanamycin	IM	0.5 (S)	5	2.0	15.4 (10–20)	1.5–2.25	4.6 (<1–12)	1.5–2.25	30	U, GB
438	Streptomycin	IV	0.5 (S)	11	2.5	7.7 (0.6–16)	~1.5–2.0	5.7 (0.5–32)	~1.5–2.0	74	GB
Cephalosporins and related β-lactams											
374	Aztreonam	IV	2.0 (S)	14	1.7	20.0 (± 10 SD)	1–2	32.4 (± 39.7 SD)	1–2	162	U, CD
		IV	2.0 (S)	14	1.7	20.0 (± 10 SD)	1–2	9.3 (± 3.0 SD)	1–2	47	U, GB
398	Cefaclor	Oral	1.0 (S)	6	0.7	8.3 (± 3.7 SD)	2.5	522 (± 342 SD)	2.2	6289	U, E
407	Cefadroxil	Oral	1.0 (S)	4	1.3	20.4 (± 6.7 SE)	3.0	4.5 (± 2.0 SE)	3.0	22	U, T
445	Cefamandole	IV	1.0 (S)	8	0.7	93 (± 5 SD)	0.5	352 (± 64 SD)	0.5	378	U, T
323	Cefamandole	IV	2.0 (S)	6	0.7	37.5 (20–76)	1.0	6.1 (0.5–15)	1.0	16	CD, OD
446	Cefazolin	IV	1.0 (S)	8	2.0	65 (40–88)	0.5	51 (5–168)	1.0	78	U, T
535	Cefbuperazone	IV	1.0 (S)	13	1.7	96.7 (± 12.3)	0.5	6.6 (± 3.0)	0.5	7	U, GB
399	Cefepime	IV	2.0 (M)	20	2.0	7.6 (0.4–62)	8.6	15.5 (0.2–70)	8.6	204	A
504	Cefmenoxime	IV	1.0 (S)	6	1.1	22.4 (17–38)	0.9	117.9 (1.5–204)	0.9	526	U, GB
402	Cefoperazone	IV	1.0 (M)	10	1.9	45.1 (±7.9 SE)	2.9	19.2(± 9.6 SE)	2.9	43	I, GB
280	Ceforanide	IV	1.0 (S)	6	2.7	45 (± 4 SD)	2.0	49 (± 16 SD)	2.0	108	U, GB, PC
280	Ceforanide	IV	1.0 (S)	5	2.7	45 (± 4 SD)	2.0	149 (± 59 SD)	2.0	331	U, CD, PD
513	Cefotaxime	IM	0.5 (M)	5	1.2	12.8 (7.4–17.5)	0.25	2.9 (0.8–7.8)	0–2	23	I, CD
513	Cefotaxime	IV	1.0 (M)	5	1.2	19.4 (8.6–48.2)	1.0	48.9 (34–82)	0.75	252	I, GB
92	Cefpiramide	IV	1.0 (S)	10		106 (±12)	2.0	116 (±392)	2.0	1095	CD, T
566	Ceftazidime	IV	1.0 (S)	20	1.7	24.9 (12.5–37)	1.75	18.5 (10.1–27)	1.75	74	GB
513	Ceftazidime	IV	1.0 (S)	13	1.7	36.1 (24–47)	1.0	31.8 (12.5–55)	1.0	88	CD
195	Ceftizoxime	IV	1.0 (S)	5	1.7	47.6 (±7.4 SD)	1.0	39.0 (±22.4 SD)	0–2	82	U, T
195	Ceftizoxime	IV	1.0 (S)	6	1.7	30.6 (±5.8 SD)	1.0	10.5 (±11.8 SD)	1–3	34	GB

(continued)

TABLE 16.7 (Continued)

Antimicrobial Concentrations in Bile

Reference	Antimicrobial	Administration Method[a]	Dose (g) (Multiple or Single)[b]	n	Serum Half-life (h)	Serum Concentration Mean (μg/mL) (Range)	Time Serum Obtained (h)	Site Concentration Mean (μg/mL) (Range)	Time Site Specimen Obtained (h)	Ratio of Site/Serum (%)	Notes[c]
402	Ceftriazone	IV	1.0 (M)	11	6.5	59.5 (± 13 SE)	2.9	44.5 (± 16 SE)	2.9	75	I, GB
483	Cefuroxime	IV	0.75 (S)	5	1.4	46 (36–69)	0–0.8	10.6 (1.4–19.6)	0.3–1.7	23	CD
91	Cephacetrile	IM	1.0 (S)	5	0.9	11.2 (8.5–17.5)	2.0	0.7 (0–2)	2.0	6	T
446	Cephaloridine	IM	1.0 (S)	7	1.5	32 (23–50)	0.5	17 (1–42)	1.0	53	U, T
364	Cephalothin	IV	1.0 (S)	11	0.5	12.7 (4–46)	0.8–1.2	2.8 (<0.1–10.5)	0.8–1.2	22	GB
364	Cephalothin	IV	1.0 (S)	13	0.5	11.4 (2.2–28)	1.0	5.7 (<0.1–13.1)	1.0	50	T
364	Cephalothin	IV	1.0 (M)	4	0.5	7.2 (3.2–10.3)	1.0	12.0 (0.4–25.7)	1.0	172	U, T
359	Imipenem	IV	1.0 (S)	12	1.2	36.2 (27–49)	0.5	17.5 (3.5–51.3)	0.5	48	T
208	Meropenem	IV	1.0 (S)	11	1.0	14.6 (2.6–44)	1–3.3	14.8 (3.9–20.2)	1–3.3	101	E, CD, PD
		IV	1.0 (S)	13	1.0	20.0 (5.8–40)	1–3.3	8.1 (0.7–25.7)	1–3.3	41	E, CD, OD
119a	Meropenem	IV	1.0 (S)	43	1.2	27.3 (1.9– 87.0)	0.5–1.5 3–5	4.9 (1.5– 16.1)	0.5–1.5	18	
						4.8 (0.3–41.6)		17.7 (1.3–18.9)	3–5	369	
Penicillins											
287	Amoxicillin	IM	1.0 (S)	5	1.1	10.4 (8.6–12)	1.2–1.5	11.6 (9–13.5)	1.2–1.5	110	CD
96	Ampicillin	Oral	0.5 (S)	10	1.1	3.4 (0.5–6.6)	2.0	3.5 (0.6–11)	2.0	103	T
96	Ampicillin	IV	0.5 (S)	5	1.1	16.5 (3.5–28)	1.0	15.7 (8.2–33)	1.0	95	GB
96	Ampicillin	IV	0.5 (S)	5	1.1	16.5 (3.5–28)	1.0	40.7 (13.5–72)	1.0	246	CD
373	Ampicillin/sulbactam	IV	1.0 (S)	14	1.1	20.2 (± 11.3)	0.25–1.5	15.9 (± 12.9)	0.25–1.5	22	GB
		IV	0.5 (S)	14	0.8	19.9 (± 9.6)	0.25–1.5	4.3 (± 5.4)	0.25–1.5	22	
89	Apalcillin	IV	1.0 (S)	10	1.2	38.3 (± 3.1 SEM)	3.0	2,093 (± 859)	3.0	5,464	T
232	Methicillin	IM	1.0 (S)	5	0.5	5.7 (3–12.5)	0.75–2.0	5.5 (<0.8–0)	2.0–2.75	96	GB
93	Mezlocillin	IM	1.0 (S)	10	1.1	23.5 (14.5–38)	2.0	221 (13–680)	2.0	940	T
211	Nafcillin	IM	1.0 (S)	6	1.0	13.5 (9–18)	0.5–1.0	540 (173–1,030)	2–4	4,000	U, T
95	Penicillin G	IV	1×10^6 units (S)	10	0.5	9.9 (4.3–17.5)	1.0	45.7 (2.2–189)	1.0	461	GB

95	Penicillin G	IV	1×10^6 units (S)	10	0.5	9.9 (4.3–17.5)	1.0	93.5 (24–204)	1.0	944	CD
77	Piperacillin	IV	1.0 (S)	11	1.1	43.7 (2.1–120)	0.5	2.9 (0–18)	0.5	7	OD
90	Piperacillin	IV	2.0 (S)	10	1.1	81.7 (± 20.5 SD)	1.0	382 (± 110 SD)	1.0	468	CD
		IV	2.0 (S)	10	1.1	81.7 (± 20.5 SD)	1.0	30.8 (± 2.5 SD)	1.0	38	GB
		IV	2.0 (S)	10	1.1	187 (± 62 SD)	1.0	170 (± 47 SD)	1.0	91	T
591	Temocillin	IV	2.0 (M)	8	3.8	123 (56–168)	2.0	961 (24–2,303)	2.0	782	T
405	Ticarcillin/ clavulanic acid	IV	3.0 (S)	23	1.2	85 (35–210)	2.5	425 (225–700)	2.5	500	CD
		IV	0.2 (S)	23	1.1	2.8	2.5	1.2	2.5	43	CD
Tetracyclines											
438	Chlortetracycline	IV	0.5 (S)	7	9.0	12 (1.2–18)	~1.5–2.0	40 (2.4–72)	~1.5–2.0	333	GB
310	Demethylchlor-tetracycline	IV	0.5 (S)	4	14.0	6.8 (6.2–7.8)	2.0	197 (74–120)	2.0	1,426	U, T
370	Doxycycline	IV	0.2 (S)	5	20.0	3.9 (3.2–4.4)	2.0	12.4 (3.2–18.2)	2.0	318	U, GB
370	Doxycycline	IV	0.2/0.1 (M)	15	20.0	3.0 (0.1–5.0)	20	22.2 (0.1–3)	20	740	U, GB
438	Oxytetracycline	IV	0.5 (S)	12	8.0	10.3 (0.6–18)	~1.5–2.0	45.6 (0.3–144)	~1.5–2.0	443	GB
438	Tetracycline	IV	0.5 (S)	9	10.0	80 (5–160)	~1.5–2.0	200 (40–320)	~1.5–2.0	250	GB
Others											
438	Bacitracin	IV	2.5×10^4 (S)	9		0.75 (0.04–1.3)	~1.5–2.0	1.6 (0.04–5.0)	~1.5–2.0	213	GB
438	Chloramphenicol	IV	0.5 (S)	8	2.5	1.4 (1.25–5)	~1.5–2.0	3.1 (1.3–10)	~1.5–2.0	221	GB
100	Clindamycin	IV	0.6 (S)	7	2.0	14.5 (9–26)	1.0	42 (14–168)	~1.0	290	CD, PD
100	Clindamycin	IV	0.6 (S)	7	2.0	11.3 (6–19)	1.0	0	~1.0	0	CD, OD
438	Erythromycin	Oral	0.4 (S)	5	1.5	1.6 (0.2–5.0)	~1.5–2.0	6.3 (0.1–20)	~1.5–2.0	394	GB
390	Metronidazole	IV	0.5 (S)	14	8.0	12.3 (8.3–16.1)	2.5	0	2.5	0	GB, OC
390	Metronidazole	IV	0.5 (S)	14	8.0	12.3 (8.3–16.1)	2.5	13.2 (10.7–15.1)	2.5	107	CD, PD
390	Metronidazole	IV	0.5 (S)	8	8.0	12.0 (7.7–16.2)	2.5	11.3 (9.8–14.8)	2.5	94	GB, PC
438	Polymyxin	IV	0.1 (S)	7	4.4	3.1 (0.6–8)	~1.5–2.0	2.0 (0.6–9.6)	~1.5–2.0	65	GB
75	Rifampin	Oral	0.15 (S)	4	2.5	1.4 (1.1–1.8)	3–5	258 (41–539)	3–5	18,400	GB
189	Vancomycin	IV	0.5 (S)	9	6.0	7.5 (5.2–10.0)	1.0	3.1 (2.0–3.6)	1.0	41	T

[a] IV, intravenously; IM, intramuscularly.

[b] M, multiple dose; S, single dose.

[c] U, uninfected; T, T-tube drain; GB, gallbladder; CD, common bile duct; E, endoscopic retrograde duct cannulation; OD, obstructed common duct; A, acute cholecystitis; I, infected; PC, patent cystic duct; PD, patent common duct; OC, obstructed cystic duct.

TABLE 16.8

Antimicrobial Concentrations in Sputum and Bronchial Secretions

Reference	Antimicrobial	Administration Method[a]	Dose (g) (Multiple or Single)[b]	*n*	Serum Half-life (h)	Serum Concentration Mean (μg/mL) (Range)	Time Serum Obtained (h)	Site Concentration Mean (μg/mL) (Range)	Time Site Specimen Obtained (h)	Ratio of Site/Serum (%)	Notes[c]
Aminoglycosides											
148	Amikacin	IM	7.5 mg/kg	13	2.8	23.7 (±2.9 SE)	1.5–2.0	5.2 (±1.5 SE)	1.5–2.0	21	U, B
290	Gentamicin	IM	0.08 (M)	8	2.0	6.3 (3–12)	1.0	<0.5	1.0	<8	I, B, P
553	Netilmicin	IV	0.45 (S)	5	2.7	12.0 (±0.7 SE)	2.0	2.0 (±0.3 SE)	2.0	17	I, B
		IV	0.45 (S)	5	2.7	12.0 (±0.7 SE)	2.0	14.7 (±2.2 SE)	2.0	123	I, ELF
289	Sisomicin	IV	1.5 mg/kg (M)	20	2.0	1.0 (±0.25 SE)	1.0	0.5 (±0.1 SE)	1.0	50	I, SP
19	Tobramycin	IM/IV	1.7 mg/kg (M)	10	2.0	8.0 (5.6–12.0)	1–2.2	1.4 (0.5–2.8)	1–2.6	18	U, B
Cephalosporins and related β-lactams											
41	Aztreonam	IV	2.0 (S)	9	1.7	39 (12–69)	2	4.2 (0.04–14.1)	2	21	I, B
329	Cefazolin	IV	1.0 (S)	9	2.0	100 (±30 SD)	0.5	2.3 (±0.5 SD)	0–2	2	I, SP
355b	Cefaclor	Oral	0.75 MR (M)	6	1.2	3.08 (±1.7 SD)	4	2.71 (±0.87 SD)	4	88	ELF
119c	Cefdinir	Oral	0.3 (S)	9		2.00[d]	224[d] min	0.78[d]	224[d] min	41	U, BM
	Cefdinir	Oral	0.6 (S)	8		4.20[d]	223[d] min	1.14[d]	223[d] min	31	U, BM
	Cefdinir	Oral	0.3 (S)	9		2.00[d]	224[d] min	0.29[d]	224[d] min	15	U, ELF
	Cefdinir	Oral	0.6 (S)	8		4.20[d]	223[d] min	0.49[d]	223[d] min	12	U, ELF
112B	Cefepime	IV	2.0 (S)	20		40.4 (±28.1 SD)	4.84	24.1[e] (±17.8 SD)	4.84	60	U, BM
482	Cefmenoxime	IV	1.0 (S)	3	1.4	3.4 (1.4–6.2)	2	0.3 (0.1–0.8)	2	9	I, SP
		IV	1.0 (m)		5	1.4	3.5 (0.6–10)	2	0.3 (0.1–0.5)	2	8
341	Cefotaxime	IM	1.0 (M)	30	1.2	37.5 (±2 SD)	1.0	0.6 (±0.1 SD)	3.0	2	I, SP, PP
66	Cefoxitin	IV	2.0 (S)	36	0.8	13.9	1.0	1.6	1.0	11	I, B
66	Cefoxitin	IV	2.0 (M)	21	0.8	19	1.0	3.0	1.0	16	I, B
37	Cefpirome	IV	1.0 (S)	8	2.0	20.1	0.5–7	7.2 (±1.1 SE)	0.5–7	36	U, ELF
64	Cefsulodin	IV	1.0 (S)	6	1.5	28	2	2.8	2	10	I, B
70	Cefazidime	IV	2.0 (S)	8	1.7	32 (±6.1 SD)	2	5.6 (±4.1 SD)	2	18	I, B

195	Ceftizoxime	IV	2.0 (S)	8	1.7	109 (± 45 SD)	0.5	4.3 (± 4.3 SD)	2.6	4	I, S
253	Ceftriaxone	IV	2.0 (S)	22	6.5	43 (22–80)	3	1.9 (0–6.5)	3	2	I, B
		IV	2.0 (S)	22	6.5	11 (0–46)	24	3.4 (1.0–8.0)	24	33	I, B
		IV	2.0 (M)	12	6.5	34 (11–57)	6	4.5 (2.0–9.5)	6	14	I, B
65	Cefuroxime	IM	0.75 (M)	4	1.4	17.3 (14–25)	1.0	2.4 (1.4–4.8)	1.0	14	I, B
220	Cephalexin	Oral	0.5 (M)	20	0.8			0.3 (0.03–3.4)	0–12		I, P
67	Cephradine	Oral	1.0 (S)	8	0.7	7.8	2–3	1.3	2–3.3	20	I, B
164	Desacetyl cefotaxime	IV	2.0 (M)	7	1.5	9.3 (1.7–15.1)	1.3	5.8 (1.6–9.2)	1.3	62	U, B
380	Imipenem	IV	1.0 (S)	8	1.0	10.5 (± 6.9 SD)	2	2.1 (± 1.0 SD)	2	20	U, B
69	Meropenem	IV	1.0 (S)	8	1.0	2.7 (± 1.3 SD)	3	0.5 (± 0.4 SD)	3	20	U, B
19a	Meropenem	IV	1.0 (S)	6		14.98[f] (± 5.30 SD)	1.0	7.07 (± 2.87 SD)	1.0	47	U, ELF
	Meropenem	IV	1.0 (S)	6		14.98[f] (± 5.30 SD)	1.0	0.086 (± 0.033 SD)	1.0	0.6	U, L
375	Moxalactam	IM	1.0 (M)	20	2.3	54.9	1.0	5.0	1.0	9	I, B
Penicillins											
454	Amoxicillin	Oral	0.5 (M)	12	1.0	30 (± 5.0 SEM)	3	1.3 (± 0.2 SEM)	3	4	I, B, E, MU
85	Amoxicillin	Oral	1.0 (M)	20	1.3	9.4	2	2.2	4	23	I, SP, PP, MU
120	Amoxicillin/ clavulanic acid	Oral	0.5 (S)	15	1.1	6.9 (8.6)	1–2	0.9 (3.5)	1–2	13	U, ELF
		Oral	0.25 (S)	15	1.1	5.3 (9.3)	1–2	1.0 (8.4)	1–2	14	U, ELF
355	Ampicillin	Oral	1.0 (M)	20	1.5	5.5 (3.5–9.8)	2.0	0.25 (0–0.5)	0–24	5	I, S
575	Ampicillin/sulbactam	IV	2.0 (S)	15	1.2	97 (± 95 SE)	0.5	0.6 (± 0.1 SE)	0.5	<1	U, B
		IV	1.0 (S)	15	1.1	38 (± 3.8 SE)	0.5	0.3 (± 0.1 SE)	0.5	<1	U, B
71	Apalcillin	IV	2.1 (S)	6	2.4	27.6	2.0	5.8	2.0	21	I, B, AUC
67	Bacampicillin	Oral	0.8 (S)	11	1.1	9.5	2–3	2.1	2–3.3	22	I, B
218	Benzylpenicillin	IM	10^6 units (M)	29	0.5	10.9 (1–>16)	2–3	0.2 (0–>0.5)	2–3	2	I, S
329	Carbenicillin	IV	5.0 (S)	12	1.5	463 (± 89 SD)	0.5	3.4 (± 0.4 SD)	0–2	1	I, S
471	Cloxacillin	Oral	0.25 (M)	12	0.5	5.6 (3.0–1)	1–2	0.6 (0.01–1.6)	1–2	11	I, C, CF
376	Piperacillin	IV	2.0 (M)	18	1.1	101	2	3.6	2	4	I, B
548	Talampicillin	Oral	0.75 (M)	8		6.8 (4.0–10.9)	1	0.5 (0.3–0.8)	2	7	I, B
329	Ticarcillin	IV	5.0 (S)	11	1.6	469 (± 65 SD)	0.5	4.1 (± 1.0 SD)	0–2	1	I, S

(continued)

TABLE 16.8 (Continued)

Antimicrobial Concentrations in Sputum and Bronchial Secretions

Reference	Antimicrobial	Administration Method[a]	Dose (g) (Multiple or Single)[b]	*n*	Serum Half-life (h)	Serum Concentration Mean (μg/mL) (Range)	Time Serum Obtained (h)	Site Concentration Mean (μg/mL) (Range)	Time Site Specimen Obtained (h)	Ratio of Site/Serum (%)	Notes[c]
Quinolones											
245	Ciprofloxacin	Oral	0.5 (M)	34	4.0	3.80 (2.0–7.5)	2	1.0	2	26	I, SP, AUC
		Oral	0.5 (M)	34	4.0	2.0	4	1.3 (0.7–3.6)	4	65	I, SP, AUC
		Oral	0.5 (M)	34	4.0	1.3	8	0.8	8	62	I, SP, AUC
204a	Ciprofloxacin	Oral	0.5 (M)	4		2.11[f] ($\pm$0.35 SD)	4	1.87 ($\pm$0.91 SD)	4	89	U, ELF
134	Enoxacin	Oral	0.6 (S)	15	5.5	1.8	1	1.1	1	58	UH, I, E
		Oral	0.6 (S)	15	5.5	3.2	3	3.1	3	95	
		Oral	0.6 (S)	15	5.5	2.0	7	2.8	7	140	
48a	Fleroxacin	Oral	0.4 (M)	6	15	8.7[f] ($\pm$1.3 SD)	1.4	10.0 ($\pm$5.3 SD)	2.2	115	I, SP
20a	Garenoxacin	Oral	0.6 (S)	6		10.03[f] ($\pm$2.80 SD)	3.26	6.98[e] ($\pm$1.34 SD)	3.26	72	U, BM
	Garenoxacin	Oral	0.6 (S)	6		10.03[f] ($\pm$2.80 SD)	3.26	9.21 ($\pm$3.62 SD)	3.26	95	U, ELF
243	Gatifloxacin	Oral	0.4 (S)	5		3.96[f] (3.50–4.40)	2	6.24[e] (4.60–8.70)	2	157	U, BM
	Gatifloxacin	Oral	0.4 (S)	5		3.96[f] (3.50–4.40)	2	6.00 (3.90–8.50)	2	151	U, ELF
204a	Levofloxacin	Oral	0.5 (M)	4		5.29[f] ($\pm$1.23 SD)	4	9.94 ($\pm$2.74 SD)	4	188	U, ELF
		Oral	0.75 (M)	4		11.98[f] (2.99 SD)	4	22.12 ($\pm$14.92 SD)	4	185	U, ELF
112a	Lomefloxacin	Oral	0.4 (M)	4		3.2 ($\pm$1.4 SD)	2	2.5 ($\pm$1.2 SD)	2	78	I, B
	Lomefloxacin	Oral	0.4 (M)	4		3.2 ($\pm$1.4 SD)	2	5.9[g] ($\pm$2.1 SD)	2	197	I, BM
	Lomefloxacin	Oral	0.4 (M)	4		3.2 ($\pm$1.4 SD)	2	6.9 ($\pm$2.8 SD)	2	216	I, ELF
511	Moxifloxacin	Oral	0.4 (S)	6		3.22 ($\pm$1.25 SD)	2.2	5.36[e] ($\pm$1.29 SD)	2.2	167	U, BM
	Moxifloxacin	Oral	0.4 (S)	6		3.22 ($\pm$1.25 SD)	2.2	20.7 ($\pm$1.92 SD)	2.2	678	U, ELF
414	Ofloxacin	Oral	0.4 (M)	18	7.0	4.7 ($\pm$2.5 SD)	2.0	2.8 ($\pm$1.5 SD)	2.0	60	I, C, F
135	Pefloxacin	IV	0.4 (S)	20	10.5	4.6	Peak	3.8	Peak	83	E, AUC
		Oral	0.4 (S)	30	10.5	5.1	Peak	4.6	Peak	89	I, E, AUC

Tetracyclines											
465	Doxycycline	Oral	0.1 (S)	10	20	2.3 (1.1–4.4)	2	<0.4 (0.4–0.6)	2–3	17	I, S
465	Minocycline	Oral	0.1 (S)	11	14	4.5 (2.7–8.7)	2	<1.1 (0.4–2.6)	2–3	24	I, S
387	Minocycline	Oral	0.1 (M)	13	14	0.8 (±0.5 SD)	13–20	1.5 (±1.1 SD)	13–20	188	U, B, PT
		Oral	0.1 (M)	10	14	0.8 (±0.4 SD)	13–20	4.5 (±3.2 SD)	13–20	563	U, B, DT
465	Tetracycline	Oral	0.25 (S)	12	10	4.0 (1.2–7.5)	4	<1.2 (<0.4–2.4)	4–5	30	I, S
Others											
38	Azithromycin	Oral	0.5 (S)	20	30	0.13 (±0.05 SD)	12	2.2 (±0.9 SD)	48	1,692	U, ELF
244	Clarithromycin	Oral	0.5 (M)	10	4.9	4.0 (±1.2 SE)	4.25	20.5 (±6.7 SE)	4.25	513	U, ELF
244	14-Hydroxy-Clarithromycin	Oral		10	7.2	0.7 (±0.2 SE)	4.25	1.9 (±0.7 SE)	4.25	271	U, ELF
68	Clindamycin	Oral	0.3 (S)	24	2.0	2.7	2–4	1.6 (0.3–4.8)	2–4	60	B
322	Dirithromycin	Oral	0.5 (M)	13		0.17 (±0.03 SD)	24	1.26 (±0.30 SD)	24	741	I, B
	Dirithromycin	Oral	0.5 (M)	13/10		0.17 (±0.03 SD)	24	6.51[e] (±1.44 SD)	24	3829	I, BM
427	Erythromycin	Oral	1.0 (M)	8	1.5	4.4 (±1.6 SD)	2	1.1 (±0.5 SD)	2	25	I, B
104	Erythromycin ethylsuccinate	Oral	1.0 (M)	19	1.5	0.7 (0.4–1.4)	3	0.6 (0.1–2.5)	3	83	U, B
104	Erythromycin lactobionate	IV	0.5 (S)	11	1.5	1.5 (0.6–1.9)	3	1.3 (0.5–2.5)	3	89	U, B
455	Erythromycin proprionate	Oral	0.5 (M)	30	3.1	3.1 (±0.1 SD)	4	1.2 (±0.1 SD)	4	39	I, B, E
455	Erythromycin stearate	Oral	0.5 (M)	30	3.0	1.9 (±0.1 SD)	4	0.9 (±0.1 SD)	4	47	I, B, E
471	Fusidic acid	Oral	20 mg/kg/day	12	4–12	8.7 (4–14)	1–2	0.5 (0.1–1.6)	1–2	57	I, C, CF
408	Josamycin	Oral	1.0 (M)	10		0.6 (±0.5)	3	0.2 (±0.2)	3	33	U, L
119b	Linezolid	Oral	0.6 (M)	5		15.5[f] (±4.9 SD)	4	64.3 (±33.1 SD)	4	414	U, ELF
280a	Telithromycin	Oral	0.8 (M)	7		1.86[f] (±0.91 SD)	2.45	3.88[e] (±1.87 SD)	2.45	211	U, BM
	Telithromycin	Oral	0.8 (M)	7		1.86[f] (±0.91 SD)	2.45	14.89 (±11.35 SD)	2.45	857	U, ELF

[a] IM, intramuscularly; IV, intravenously.
[b] M, multiple dose; S, single dose; MR, modified release.
[c] U, uninfected; B, bronchial secretions; I, infected; P, pneumonia; ELF, epithelial lining fluid; SP, sputum; BM, bronchial mucosa; PP, peak-to-peak levels; L, lavage fluid; E, extrapolated from graphs; MU, mucolytic agent used; AUC, area under the curve; C, children; CF, cystic fibrosis; DT, distal to tumor.
[d] Value reported as median.
[e] Milligrams per kilogram.
[f] Measured in plasma.
[g] Microgram per gram.

higher sputum antibiotic levels with the use of mucolytic agents (63,85,454). Ratios of sputum-to-serum concentrations are low for most drugs. Data on AUC ratios were limited but showed ratios of 2.7% and 4.5% for cefotaxime (341), 14% for cefuroxime (65), and 19% for netilmicin by both intermittent and continuous intravenous infusions. Sputum concentrations of the cefotaxime metabolite desacetyl-cefotaxime are much higher than those of the parent drug (164).

Some studies have shown a relationship between clinical infection cure and antibiotic concentration in sputum (85,355) and have shown that the antibiotic concentration increases with the degree of sputum purulence for at least some antibiotics (291). Reviews of this topic have differed on the importance of sputum antibiotic concentrations to the cure of infection, with Lambert (315) taking a somewhat skeptical view, while Pennington (415) has taken a supportive stand with which Smith and LeFrock (503) have concurred. Readers are also directed to an excellent study by Wong et al. (601), which could not be included in Table 16.8 because of the graphical presentation of the data. Hitt and Gerding (235) have compiled ratios of sputum antimicrobial levels to the minimal inhibitory concentration for 90% of common bacterial pathogens that cause bronchitis and pneumonia. These ratios may prove predictive of clinical outcome, but good clinical correlation is lacking.

Breast Milk

The studies of breast milk (Table 16.9) were performed in lactating mothers who were normal volunteers or were being treated for nonbreast infections. The results show that the secretion of most antibiotics into breast milk is insignificant. However, a few agents, notably metronidazole, chloramphenicol, tetracycline, and lincomycin, were found in milk at levels approaching the serum levels. Giamarellou et al. (200) reported a study showing that quinolones (ciprofloxacin, ofloxacin, and pefloxacin) also have excellent penetration into breast milk, posing a possible risk to newborn infants. In a single study addressing milk penetration during puerperal mastitis, concentrations of phenoxymethyl-penicillin were higher in the milk from the mastitic breasts than in the nonmastitic breasts, but serum concentrations were not determined for the patients with mastitis (352). Even though only small quantities of most antibiotics reach the breast milk, the potential still exists for allergy or toxicity in the infant.

Middle Ear Fluid

Antibiotic levels were assayed in middle ear fluid from patients categorized as infected (acute otitis media) or uninfected (serous otitis or otitis media with effusion) (Table 16.10). The middle ear fluid samples were usually removed by needle aspiration. Pediatric subjects were studied most often. Most antibiotics penetrated significantly into the middle ear fluid. In the few cases where direct comparison was possible, the presence of acute infection appeared to enhance antibiotic penetration into the middle ear fluid.

Sinus Secretions

The sinus secretion studies were done primarily in patients with either acute or chronic maxillary sinusitis. None of the studies corrected for blood contamination, but this was likely minimal. On the basis of the data presented in Table 16.11, tetracyclines, erythromycin, and trimethoprim seemed to achieve better penetration than the β-lactams. There may be an inverse correlation between degree of purulence and amount of antibiotic penetration (217,332). One clinical correlation showed that an antibiotic concentration higher than the minimal inhibitory concentration of the pathogen was associated with clearance of the bacteria (153).

Prostatic Secretions

There are only a limited number of human studies detailing antibiotic concentrations in human prostatic secretions (Table 16.12). Winningham et al. (581) have determined in a dog model, in which urinary contamination has been excluded, that the major factors controlling antibiotic penetration into the prostatic fluid are the degree of lipid solubility, the pK_a, and the amount of protein binding. Using the dog model, Madsen et al. (339), Meares (357,358), and Gasser et al. (188) have determined that only trimethoprim, erythromycin, rosamicin, oleandomycin, clindamycin, enoxacin, and fleroxacin concentrate into prostatic fluid. The dog model may not necessarily reflect the situation in humans, however, because prostatic secretions in humans with prostatitis are more alkaline than the secretion found in normal dogs (42,426). One study suggested that prostatic fluid concentrations of cephalosporins are increased in patients with acute prostatitis, compared with uninfected controls (276). The higher pH found in humans may favor the penetration of some quinolones that are zwitterions (188). The degree of antibiotic penetration into prostatic fluid may be more important than prostatic tissue concentration because bacteria that cause chronic bacterial prostatitis reside within the prostatic fluid, and the prostatic epithelium acts as a barrier to the passage of most antibiotics into the fluid (515). When prostatic fluid drug levels in normal patients were compared with levels in a patient with ureterosigmoidostomy, it was found that the drug concentrations of nitrofurantoin and ampicillin found in normal patients were almost entirely due to urinary contamination (340,597). One group measured iohexol in the prostatic fluid after intravenous injection to exclude urinary contamination (382–384). Clinical data have revealed that trimethoprim is only partially effective in the treatment of

(*text continues on page 753*)

TABLE 16.9

Antimicrobial Concentrations in Breast Milk

Reference	Antimicrobial	Administration Method[a]	Dose (g) (Multiple or Single)[b]	*n*	Serum Half-life (h)	Serum Concentration Mean (μg/mL) (Range)	Time Serum Obtained (h)	Site Concentration Mean (μg/mL) (Range)	Time Site Specimen Obtained (h)	Ratio of Site/Serum (%)	Notes[c]
Aminoglycosides											
352	Amikacin	IM	0.10 (S)	23	2.0	3.0 (2.9–3.2)	2	0	2	0.0	
117	Kanamycin	IM	1.0 (S)	4	2.0	50	1	18.4	1	37.00	PD
527	Tobramycin	IM	0.08 (S)	5	2.0	2.63	2.5	<0.44 (trace-0.44)	3	<17.0	
Cephalosporins and related β-lactams											
168	Aztreonam	IM	1 (S)	6	1.7–2	40.0 (± 1.8 SE)	1.5	0.34 (± 0.08 SE)	6	1.0	PD
168	Aztreonam	IV	1 (S)	6	1.7–2	126.3 (± 17.1 SE)	0.25	0.22 (± 0.06 SE)	4	0.2	PD
271	Cefadroxil	Oral	1.0 (S)	6	1.3	21.6 (14.6–30.0)	3	1.64 (0.12–2.40)	6	8.0	PD
324	Cefamandole	IV	1.0 (S)	4	0.7	19.1	1	0.46	1	2.0	PD
609	Cefazolin	IV	2.0 (S)	20	2	54.33 (± 15.9 SD)	2	1.51 (± 0.16)	3	3.0	
571	Cefmenoxime	IV	1.0–2.0 (M)	5	0.8–1.2	1.1	12	1.75	12	159.0	
352	Cefmetazole	IV	1.0 (S)	23	1.1	19.2 (17.0–21.4)	2	0-trace	2		
331	Cefonicid	IM	1.0 (S)	10	4.4	67.4 (± 15.8 SD)	1	0.16 (± 0.09 SD)	1	0.2	
530	Cefoperazone	IV	1.0 (S)	4	2	54 (37–88)	0.2–0.6	0.41 (0–0.82)	2	1.0	
271	Cefotaxime	IV	1.0 (S)	12	1.2	9.4 (5.9–18.4)	1	0.32 (0.2–0.5)	2	3.0	PD
352	Cefotetan	IV	1.0 (S)	23	3–4.6	25.0 (21.6–28.5)	2	0.1 (0–0.3)	2	0.4	
352	Cefotiam	IM	0.5 (S)	23	0.7–1.0	5.9 (5.6–6.2)	2	0-trace	2		
146	Cefoxitin	IM	2.0 (S)	5	0.8	40.8 (15.3–77.6)	0.5–1	0.41 (0.31–0.65)	1–7	1.0	PD
529	Cefoxitin	IV	1.0 (S)	4	0.8	18.3 (5.6–25)	0.4–0.5	0.58 (0–1.5)	1	3.0	
488	Cefprozil[d]	Oral	1.0 (S)	9	1.69	14.8 (± 3.2 SD)	2	3.4 (± 2.3 SD)	6	23.0	PD
528	Cefsulodin	IV	1.0 (S)	5	1.2	56.8	1	0.8 (0.7–0.9)	2	1.0	
76	Ceftazidime	IV	2.0 (S)	12	1.8	71.8 (± 47.7 SD)	1	5.2 (± 3.0 SD)	1	7.0	

(continued)

TABLE 16.9 (Continued)

Antimicrobial Concentrations in Breast Milk

Reference	Antimicrobial	Administration Method[a]	Dose (g) (Multiple or Single)[b]	*n*	Serum Half-life (h)	Serum Concentration Mean (μg/mL) (Range)	Time Serum Obtained (h)	Site Concentration Mean (μg/mL) (Range)	Time Site Specimen Obtained (h)	Ratio of Site/Serum (%)	Notes[c]
195	Ceftizoxime	IV	1.0 (S)	6	1.7	22.6 (±6.25 SD)	1	0.3 (±0.1 SD)	1	1.0	
270	Ceftriaxone	IV	1.0 (S)	10	5.3	30	4	0.5 (±0.1 SD)	4	2.0	
270	Ceftriaxone	IM	1.0 (S)	10	5.3	30	4	0.7 (±0.1 SD)	4	2.0	
271	Cephalexin	Oral	1.0 (S)	6	0.8	22.9 (16.9–32.1)	1	0.5 (0.24–0.85)	4	2.0	PD
352	Cephaloridine	IM	1.0 (S)	23	1–1.5	19.0 (18.0–20.0)	1	0.15 (0–0.3)	6	1.0	PD
271	Cephalothin	IV	1.0 (S)	6	0.5	5.9 (3.4–7.8)	1	0.47 (0.32–0.62)	2	8.0	PD
271	Cephapirin	IV	1.0 (S)	6	0.5	6.1 (3.1–8.0)	1	0.43 (0.28–0.64)	2	7.0	PD
368	Cephradine	Oral	0.5 (M)	6	0.7	4.44	2	0.62	2	14.0	
Penicillins											
271	Amoxicillin	Oral	1.0 (S)	6	1.0	14.6 (8.7–18.0)	2	0.81 (0.39–1.3)	5	6.0	PD
352	Ampicillin	Oral	0.5 (S)	23	0.5–1.0	3.3 (2.6–4.0)	2	0.1 (0–0.2)	2	3.0	
352	Bacampicillin	Oral	0.5 (S)	23	1	4.0 (3.2–4.8)	2	0	2	0.0	
352	Carbenicillin	IM	1.0 (S)	23	0.5–1.0	11.6 (7.6–17.0)	2	0.2 (0–0.4)	2	2.0	
352	Cloxacillin	IM	0.5 (S)	23	0.5	2.3 (1.7–2.7)	2	0.1 (0–0.2)	2	4.0	
352	Dicloxacillin	Oral	0.25 (S)	23	0.7	4.7 (4.6–4.8)	2	0.2 (0.2–0.3)	2	4.0	
347	Epicillin	Oral	0.5 (M)	5	1.0	1.1	4	0.16	4	15.0	PD
352	Methicillin	IM	1.0 (S)	23	0.5	5.5 (4.8–6.4)	2	0.26 (0.2–0.3)	2	5.0	
352	Mezlocillin	IM	1.0 (S)	23	1.1	6.8 (6.6–7.0)	2	0	2	0.0	
352	Oxacillin	IM	0.5 (S)	23	0.5	1.0 (0.7–1.3)	2	0.5 (0.23–0.7)	2	50.0	
436	Oxacillin	Oral	0.5 (M)	10	0.5	<1.31 (<0.3–5.6)	1–4	≤0.2	1–4	≤15.0	
212	Penicillin	IM	1×10^5 units (M)	3	0.5	0.80 (0.49–0.96)	1–2	0.05 (0.03–0.06)	1–2	6.0	
460	Penicillin G	IM	3×10^5 units 5×10^5 units (S)	4	0.5	1.08 (0.72–1.92)	2	<0.11 (<0.03–0.24)	2	<10.0	

351	Penicillin V	Oral	1.32 (S)	4	1	4.7 (3.0–6.6)	1–3	0.3 (0.28–0.50)	4–8	6.0	
319	Piperacillin	IV	4.5 (M)	?	1.0	182	1	2	1	1.0	
87	Pivampicillin	Oral	0.35 (M)	9	0.5–1.0	2.13 (0.33–8.20)	1–4.3	0.1 (0.06–0.19)	1–4.5	5.0	
173	Sulbactam	IV	0.5 (S ± M)	6	1.0	2 (0.7–5)	2	0.52 (0–2.2)	0–8	26.0	
116	Ticarcillin	IV	1.0 (S)	5	1.2	52 (29–100)	0.2–1	Trace	2		
352	Ticarcillin	IM	1.0 (S)	23	1.2	8.9 (7.3–10.4)	2	0	2	0.0	
200	Ciprofloxacin	Oral	0.75 BID (M)	10	3–5	2.06 (± 0.68 SD)	2	3.79 (± 1.26 SD)	2	184.0	PD
200	Ofloxacin	Oral	0.4 BID (M)	10	4–8	2.45 (± 0.81 SD)	2	2.41 (± 0.80 SD)	2	98.0	PD
200	Pefloxacin	Oral	0.4 BID (M)	10	8–12	4.75 (± 1.57 SD)	2	3.54 (± 1.25 SD)	2	75.0	PD
Tetracyclines											
216	Chlortetracycline	Oral	2.0–3.0 (M)	8	9	4.13 (1–8)	?	1.25 (1–2)	?	30.0	
435	Tetracycline	Oral	0.5 (M)	5	10	1.84 (0.65–3.2)	0–6	1.14 (0.43–2.58)	0–6	62.0	
372	Doxycline	Oral	0.1 (M)	15	20	2.42 (1.3–4.50)	3	0.77 (0.4–1.40)	3	32.0	PD
Others											
431	Chloramphenicol	Oral	0.5 (S)	4	1.9	5.33 (± 0.39 SE)	2	3.24 (± 0.88 SD)	2	61.0	PD
352	Clindamycin	Oral	0.15 (S)	23	2.4	2.4 (1.8–3.0)	2	0.7 (0.5–1.2)	2	29.0	
517	Clindamycin	Oral	0.15 (M)	5	2	<3.7 (<1–9.9)	6	<1.4 (<0.5–3.1)	6	38.0	
352	Erythromycin	Oral	0.5 (S)	23	1.4	4.3 (3.9–4.7)	1	1.2 (0.9–1.4)	4	28.0	PD
361a	Lincomycin	Oral	0.5 (M)	9	4.5	1.4 (0.4–3.2)	6	1.3 (0.5–2.4)	6	93.0	
230	Metronidazole	Oral	0.2 (M)	11	6–14	5.0 (1.0–11.6)	0–4.5	5.7 (1.6–12.2)	0.3–4.5	99.0	
559	Nitrofurantoin	Oral	0.2 (M)	4	0.3	0.83 (0.2–1.6)	2	0.2 (0–0.5)	2	24.0	
520	Rosaramicin	Oral	0.25 (S)	10	4.4	0.28 (0.165–.485)	2–4	0.03 (0.028–0.045)	2–4	11.0	PD
431	Thiamphenicol	Oral	0.5 (S)	7	2.0	3.64 (± 1.76 SD)	2	2.16 (± 1.04 SD)	4	59.0	PD
345	Tinidazole	IV	0.5 (S)	20	14.0	6.1 (± 0.32 SE)	12	5.8 (± 0.33 SE)	12	95.0	

[a] IM, intramuscularly; IV, intravenously.
[b] S, single dose; M, multiple dose; BID, twice a day.
[c] PD, peak data.

TABLE 16.10

Antimicrobial Concentrations in Middle Ear Fluid

Reference	Antimicrobial	Administration Method[a]	Dose (g) (Multiple or Single)[b]	n^c	Serum Half-life (h)	Serum Concentration Mean (μg/mL) (Range)	Time Serum Obtained (h)	Site Concentration Mean (μg/mL) (Range)	Time Site Specimen Obtained (h)	Ratio of Site/Serum (%)	Notes[d]
Cephalosporins and related β-lactams											
155	Cefaclor	Oral	20 mg/kg (S)	15	0.7	12.3 ($\pm$7.3 SD)	1.5–1.9	2.9 ($\pm$1.5 SD)	1.5–1.9	22.0	P, NS
473	Cefatrizine	Oral	0.5 (S)	3	1.7	6.2 (5.0–7.2)	3	9.5 (8.2–10.5)	3	153.0	I
228	Cefixime	Oral	8 mg/kg (S)	16	2.4–4	2.51 (1.2–4.12)	3–5	1.32 (0.35–2.86)	3–5	52.5	I
228	Cefixime	Oral	8 mg/kg (S)	9	2.4–4	4.21 (2.48–10.7)	3–5	1.51 (0.32–5.69)	3–5	32.5	U
127	Cefotaxime	IV	25 mg/kg (S)	5	1.2	2.1 (2–2.2)	1.0	2.6 (2.0–3.3)	1.0	123.0	P
485	Cefprozil	Oral	20 mg/kg (S)	40	0.9–1.5	9.56 (1.28–21.47)	0.4–6	1.69 (0.17–8.67)	0.4–6	18.0	
311	Loracarbef	Oral	7.5 mg/kg (S)	12	1	4.2 ($\pm$2.0 SD)	1.3–3.3	2.0 ($\pm$2.6 SD)	1.3–3.3	48.0	P
Penicillins											
202	Amoxicillin	Oral	15 mg/kg (S)	12	1.0	4.0 (0.62–6.5)	0.5–3	1.8 (0.3–3.5)	0.5–3	45.0	I, P
307	Amoxicillin	Oral	15 mg/kg (S)	5	1.0	9.4 ($\pm$1.3 SD)	1.5–2	2.3 ($\pm$1.5 SD)	1.5–2	24.0	U, P
314	Ampicillin	Oral	10 mg/kg (S)	15	1.5	4.3 (1.0–9.0)	2	2.17 (0.85–8.0)	2	50.0	I, P
314	Ampicillin	Oral	10 mg/kg (S)	9	1.5	3.6 (1.1–6.6)	2	0.23 (0–0.39)	2	6.0	U, P
314	Azidocillin	Oral	15 mg/kg (S)	15	0.75	7.4 (1.7–27)	2	3.2 (0.58–14)	2	44.0	I, P
314	Azidocillin	Oral	15 mg/kg (S)	18	0.75	4.8 (1.2–12)	2	0.50 (0–1.60)	2	10.0	U, P
313	Penicillin G	IM	4×10^5 units (S)	83	0.5	3.6 (1.2–11.2)	1	1.3 (0–8.2)	1	35.0	I
313	Penicillin G	IM	4×10^5 units (S)	13	0.5	3.2 (1.6–7.1)	1	0-trace	1	0.0	U
273	Penicillin V	Oral	26 mg/kg (S)	6	0.5	13 (8–20)	1.0	6.0 (5–8)	1.0	46.0	I, PD

Tetracyclines											
522	Doxycycline	Oral	0.2 (S)	10	18.5	2.4 (1.0–3.4)	2.3–4.3	1.0 (0–1.7)	2.3–4.3	42.0	
492	Oxytetracycline	IM	0.1 (S)	10	8	2.1 (0.6–7.0)	1–3	0.7 (0.125–1.8)	1–3	33.0	I, P
492	Oxytetracycline	IM	0.1 (S)	4	8	0.74 (0.35–1.3)	1.5–2.8	<0.1	1.5–2.8	<14.0	U
Others											
202	Erythromycin estolate	Oral	15 mg/kg (S)	13	1.5	3.54 (0.6–4.5)	0.5–2	1.66 (0.4–4.0)	0.5–2	47.0	I, P
202	Erythromycin ethylsuccinate	Oral	15 mg/kg (S)	6	1.5	1.55 (0.5–2.6)	1–2	0.6 (0.4–1.0)	1–2	39.0	I, P
261	Metronidazole	Oral	2.4 (S)	12	10	45.2 (±8.3 SD)	2–4	31.8 (±25.65 SD)	2–4	70.0	I
298	Sulfadiazine	Oral	5 mg/kg (M)	24	10–12	18.4 (9.0–30.0)	1.3–4.5	10.5 (0–25)	1.3–4.5	57.0	NS, C
307	Sulfamethoxazole	Oral	20 mg/kg (S)	5	10	62.4 (±15.5)	1.5–2	17.0 (±6.7)	1.5–2	27.0	U, P, C
307	Sulfisoxazole	Oral	37.5 mg/kg (S)	5	5–7	87.4 (±35.2)	1.5–2	3.7 (±0.7)	1.5–2	4.0	U, P, C
307	Trimethoprim	Oral	4 mg/kg (S)	5	10–12	1.6 (±1.1)	1.5–2	1.9 (±1.4)	1.5–2	119.0	U, P, C
202	Trisulfapyrimidine	Oral	80 mg/kg (S)	7	3–4	13.6 (5.5–24)	0.5–1.2	8.1 (4–12)	0.5–1.2	60.0	I, P

[a] IV, intravenously; IM; intramuscularly.
[b] S, single dose; M, multiple dose.
[c] Number of patients studied.
[d] P, pediatric cases; NS, number of site samples is different than number of serum samples; I, infected; U, uninfected; PD, peak data; C, given in combination with another antibiotic.

TABLE 16.11

Antimicrobial Concentrations in Sinus Secretions

Reference	Antimicrobial	Administration Method[a]	Dose (g) (Multiple or Single)[b]	*n*	Serum Half-life (h)	Serum Concentration Mean (μg/mL) (Range)	Time Serum Obtained (h)	Site Concentration Mean (μg/mL) (Range)	Time Site Specimen Obtained (h)	Ratio of Site/Serum (%)	Notes[c]
Cephalosporins and related β-lactams											
473	Cefatrizine	Oral	0.5 (S)	3	1.4	6.0 (5.8–6.2)	3	2.7 (2.1–3.1)	3	45	AC
114	Cefotiam nexetil	Oral	0.2 (M)	8		0.96 (0.5–1.65)	2	1.04 (0.1–1.45)	2	108	CH
297	Cephalexin	Oral	0.5 or 15 mg/kg	9	0.8	8.8 (1.9–19)	2.0	1.1 (<0.1–4.0)	2.0	10	
518a	Loracarbef	Oral	0.4 (M)	20	0.7–1.2	7.9 (4.83–14.0)	2	1.75 (0–5.71)	2		AC
Penicillins											
203a	Ampicillin	Oral	0.5 (M)	4	1.1	3.8 (1.8–8.0)	2–3	0.125 (0–0.3)	2–3	3	
260	Azidocillin	IM	0.75 (M)	15	0.75	4.0	2.5	0.70 (0.16–1.82)	2.5	17.5	CH
260	Azidocillin	IM	1.5 (M)	8	0.75	8.5	2.5	0.34 (0.16–0.8)	2.5	4	
217	Penicillin V	Oral	0.4								
			0.4								
			0.8	17	0.5	2.1 (0–2.4)	2.1	<0.6 (<0.2–1.2)	2.1	<29	AC
332	Penicillin V	Oral	0.4								
			0.4								
			0.8	7	0.5	1.0 (0.4–2.4)	2	<2 (0.2–0.5)	2	<20	P
332	Penicillin V	Oral	0.4								
			0.4								
			0.8	10	0.5	1.0 (<0.1–2.0)	2	0.5 (<0.2–1.2)	2.1	50	M
263	Sultamicillin	Oral	0.75 (S)	3		3.09 (0.67–5.2) (ampicillin)/3.12 (0.57–4.6) (sulbactam)	1.5–2	0.32 (0.1–0.65) (ampicillin)/0.26 (0.2–0.53) (sulbactam)	1.5–2	10	AC
							1.5–2		1.5–2	8	AC

Quinolones											
342	Enoxacin	Oral	0.4 (S)	5	5.5	1.3 (1.0–2.1)	5	1.4 (0.6–2.7)	5	108	AC
Tetracyclines											
154	Doxycycline	Oral	0.1 (M)	24	20	3.5 (1.2–6.0)	2–7	2.0 (0.5–7.5)	2–7	57	
602	Minocycline	Oral	1.0 (M)	8	14	2.5 (0.5–5.1)	2–7	1.06 (0.05–3)	2–7	34	AC, CH
332	Tetracycline HCl	Oral	0.25 (M)	21	10	2.4 (0.9–6.0)	2.1	1.9 (0.5–3.6)	2.1	79	P
332	Tetracycline HCl	Oral	0.25 (M)	14	10	2.9 (1.4–4.8)	2.0	3.0 (1.0–7.0)	2.0	103	M
Others											
272	Erythromycin stearate	Oral	0.5 (M)	10	1.5	2.2 (0.3–5.0)	4.7	1.3 (0.3–2.5)	4.7	59	AC
406	Erythromycin stearate	Oral	0.5 (M)	13	1.5	2.2 (0.2–5.0)	2–3	0.9 (0.1–3.0)	2–3	42	CH
353	Sulfadiazine	Oral	0.5 (M)	10	3.5	42 (24–66)	2–4	6.6 (2.3–15)	2–4	20	AC
353	Trimethoprim	Oral	0.16 (M)	10	9.0	3.0 (2.1–5.6)	2–4	3.9 (1.1–10.8)	2–4	133	AC

[a] IM, intramuscularly.
[b] S, single dose; M, multiple dose.
[c] AC, acute sinusitis; CH, chronic sinusitis; P, purulent; M, mucous.

TABLE 16.12

Antimicrobial Concentrations in Prostatic Secretions

Reference	Antimicrobial	Administration Method[a]	Dose (g) (Multiple or Single)[b]	*n*	Serum Half-life (h)	Serum Concentration Mean (μg/mL) (Range)	Time Serum Obtained (h)	Site Concentration Mean (μg/mL) (Range)	Time Site Specimen Obtained (h)	Ratio of Site/Serum (%)	Notes[c]
Aminoglycosides											
204b	Amikacin	IM	0.20 (S)	10	2–3	12.44 (9.4–18.5)	2.5–3	3.18 (1.24–5.20)	2.5–3	25	U
576	Tobramycin	IM	0.080 (S)	3	2.5	4.0 (4.0–4.0)	1	<0.5	1	<12	U
Cephalosporins and related β-lactams											
276	Cefmenoxime	IV	2.0 (S)	11		39.5 ± 11.7	1	12.8 (2.6–30.8)	1	32	I
				18		52.8 ± 18.0	1	0.7 (0–2.3)	1	2	U
383	Cefpodoxime	Oral	0.2 (S)	3		1.39 (0.3–1.94)	3	0.15 (0–0.42)	3	11	U, UCE
276	Moxalactam	IV	2.0 (S)	11	2.3	84.6 ± 24.1	1	14.0 (1.3–529)	1	17	I
				12		100 ± 20.5	1	1.2 (0.4–2.2)	1	1	U
484	Moxalactam	IV	1.0 (S)	5	2.3	44.6 (26.3–57.9)	1	1.59 (0.33–4.52)	1	4	I
Penicillins											
597	Ampicillin	Oral	0.5 (M)	7	1.5	4.1 (2.9–5.9)	2	4.7 (0.5–10.6)	2	115	U
				9	1.5			17.6 (1.2–61.4)	2	429	I
204b	Piperacillin	IV	1.0 (S)	9	1.3	5.7 (2.0–12.8)	2.5–3	0.30 (0.16–0.78)	2.5–3	5	U
Tetracyclines											
183	Minocycline	Oral	0.2 (S)	5	14	1.19 (± 0.21)	3	2.95 (± 1.29)	3	251	I
		IV	0.2 (S)	3	14	1.61 (± 0.7)	3	2.6 (± 1.66)	3	161	U
83	Tetracycline	IV	0.5 (S)	4	10	6.25 (5.0–10)	1	0.664 (0.156–1.25)	1	11	U
Quinolones											
78	Ciprofloxacin	Oral	0.5 (S)	7	4.3	1.44 (0.27–2.48)	2.4	2.2 (0.02–5.5)	2–4.4	154	U
382	Enoxacin	IV	0.428 (S)	9	4.5	1.26 (1.1–1.71)	2–4	0.57 (0.29–0.96)	2–4	47	U, UCE
278	Fleroxacin	Oral	0.4 (S)	9	12	3.63 (0.44–5.54)	1–4	1.81 (0.53–4.15)	1–4	50	U
380b	Gatifloxacin	Oral	0.4 (S)	7	7.2	1.92 (1.53–2.46)	4	2.35 (2.03–3.10)	4	110	U, UCE
382	Lomefloxacin	Oral	0.4 (S)	5	8	1.81 (1.39–3.0)	4	1.38 (0.6–3.06)	4	48	U, UCE
382	Norfloxacin	Oral	0.8 (S)	8	3.5	1.4 (0.69–2.71)	1–4	0.14 (0.08–0.43)	1–4	12	U, UCE
384	Ofloxacin	IV	0.4 (S)	5	6	2.0 (1.93–2.01)	4	0.66 (0.11–1.31)	4	33	U, UCE
382	Temafloxacin	Oral	0.4 (S)	4	9	2.23 (1.7–2.65)	4	0.78 (0.56–0.92)	4	36	U, UCE
Others											
83	Bacitracin	IV	0.5 (S)	3		0.104 (0.078–1.56)	1	0.104 (<0.039–1.56)	1	100	U
389b	Trimethoprim	Oral	0.005–0.0081/kg (M)	4	14.5	3.1 (2.5–3.7)	9–12	4.2 (2.4–5.6)	9–12	155	

[a] IM, intramuscularly; IV, intravenously.
[b] S, single dose; M, multiple dose.
[c] U, uninfected; I, infected; UCE, urine contamination excluded.

chronic bacterial prostatitis. Quinolones may be of some benefit in the treatment of chronic bacterial prostatitis, but long-term follow-up has often been inadequate (381).

Cerebrospinal Fluid

Table 16.13 lists antimicrobial studies investigating the penetration of various agents into human CSF. There have been several reviews on the same topic that also dealt with the kinetics of central nervous system handling of drugs (40,395). There was no correction for blood contamination in these studies, and the results demonstrated considerable variability in the ratios of antimicrobial concentrations in CSF and serum. Many studies, typified by that of Mullaney and John (378), provide useful information on CSF levels of drugs such as cefotaxime, but make evaluation of drug penetration impossible by not presenting data on concentrations in serum. Similarly, data for ampicillin (540), nafcillin (466), and rifampin (185) are available but include small numbers of patients or lack actual drug levels. The CSF/serum ratio ranged from 0% for rifampin in uninfected controls (498) and 0% for low-dose oxytetracycline (295) to 199% for amoxicillin when measured 4 hours after a single intravenous dose (347). In general, because samples were taken at longer time intervals following the systemic drug administration, serum levels were lower in relation to CSF concentrations and the CSF-to-serum ratios increased. Data for several antimicrobials are included in detail to illustrate changes in CSF concentrations with time after administration, duration of meningitis, and multiple dosing (250,251,347).

Aqueous Humor

In almost all studies, the antibiotic levels in aqueous humor were measured in uninfected patients undergoing cataract surgery (Table 16.14). Under those conditions, most antibiotics penetrated poorly into the aqueous humor when given systemically, resulting in levels that are inadequate for treating endophthalmitis. Data are limited on penetration of antibiotics into infected eyes. One study examined doxycycline levels in acutely inflamed eyes and found levels similar to those in uninflamed eyes (544). Animal studies of bacterial endopthalmitis have shown enhanced penetration into the aqueous and vitreous humors of infected eyes with some antibiotics (15,140).

Skeletal Muscle

The majority of studies measuring antibiotic concentrations in skeletal muscle were done on uninfected normal muscle obtained during surgical procedures (Table 16.15). One study measured drug concentrations in the muscle of a decubitus ulcer (61). The higher concentrations observed for clindamycin and ciprofloxacin (compared with β-lactams) probably reflect the higher intracellular concentrations of lincosamides and quinolones (469).

Bone

A multitude of studies on antibiotic penetration into bone have been published (Table 16.16). Most of the studies were performed on uninfected bone, following antibiotics given prophylactically to patients prior to orthopedic procedures. There is a wide variance in technique, making the results conflicting and difficult to interpret. The majority of studies reported techniques that cut or crushed the bone, suspended the material in a buffer for a variable amount of time, and then measured the antibiotic extracted into the buffer, using a microbiological assay. Many investigators washed or rinsed the bone to remove blood after removing the sample. It is unknown whether this could also remove some of the antibiotic.

The buffer/bone mixture is usually shaken at 4°C to 6°C for 1 to 24 hours. An 8-hour shake/elution technique has resulted in 79.9% recovery of cefazolin and 77% recovery of cephradine, but only 10.8% recovery of cephalothin (125). Schurman et al. (480) found that, when the extraction procedure was performed for more than 3 to 5 hours, the recovery of cephalothin, but not cefamandole, declined by 67% at 24 hours. Rosdahl et al. (461) added several antibiotics to cancellous and cortical bone specimens and then homogenized the specimens before microbiological assay. Recovery of the antibiotic ranged from 4% to 100%. The fall in antibiotic concentration was primarily due to the instability of the antibiotics during the homogenization procedures and was not due to binding of the antibiotic to bone. Adam et al. (12) found that neither ticarcillin nor clavulanate was adsorbed to inorganic bone; however, Wittmann and Kotthaus (592) found that the hydroxyapatite portion of bone acts as a depot carrier for several quinolone antibiotics. Other investigators have found that the quinolones bind to bone samples (169) and require several extraction steps for full extraction of the antibiotic from the bone (592).

Numerous studies noted differences between cortical and cancellous bone antibiotic concentrations, with the cortical bone usually having lower drug levels. This may reflect the fact that many antibiotics do not bind to inorganic bone, or it may be due to a difference in the blood supply. Fitzgerald (166), using data compiled from animal models, concluded that there is no anatomic or physiologic barrier preventing antibiotic diffusion into bone. He concluded that, at least in the case of β-lactams and aminoglycosides, the osseous interstitial fluid concentration of an antibiotic was a reflection of the serum concentration. This agrees with the results of Williams et al. (577), who thought that, although the relationship was not clear-cut, antibiotics with high serum levels and long half-lives usually had higher bone concentrations. Hughes and Anderson (249) thought that the capillary blood

(*text continues on page 767*)

TABLE 16.13

Antimicrobial Concentrations in Cerebrospinal Fluid

Reference	Antimicrobial	Administration Method[a]	Dose (g) (Multiple or Single)[b]	*n*	Serum Half-life (h)	Serum Concentration Mean (μg/mL) (Range)	Time Serum Obtained (h)	Site Concentration Mean (μg/mL) (Range)	Time Site Specimen Obtained (h)	Ratio of Site/Serum (%)	Notes[c]
Aminoglycosides											
606	Amikacin	IV	7.5 mg/kg (M)	5	2.2 ± 1.1	15 (11–18)	2.0	52. (3.8–6.9)	2.0	34.7	I
550	Gentamicin	IM	1.5 mg/kg (S)	16	2.0	1.4 (0.8–3.0)	2.0	0.03 (0–0.10)	2.0	2.5	I
247	Kanamycin	IM	7.5 mg/kg (M)	4	2.0	13	2.0	3.2	2.0	25	I
Cephalosporins and related β-lactams											
213	Aztreonam	IV	2 (S)	6	1.9	44.7 (29.9–74.2)	2.0	2.98 (0.76–6.67)	2.0	6.7	I
303	Cefamandole	IV	125 mg/kg (M)	20	0.7	10–20	1.0–2.0	0.94 (0–3.4)	1.0–2.0	6.5 (0–19)	I
542	Cefazolin	IV	6.0/day (M)	4	2.0	29.1 (± 5.2)	3.0	0	3.0	0	U
542	Cefazolin	IV	6.0/day (M)	4	2.0	52.6 (± 6.5)	6	0	6	0	CI, U
386	Cefixime	IV	8 mg/kg (S)	10	2.6–5.6	2.9 (0.3–4.7)	1–8	0.2	1–5	12	I
250	Cefmenoxime	IV	6.0 (S)	5	1.4	25.09 (15.88–49.22)	1	2.10 (0.43–4.4)	1	8.4	I, CI
250	Cefmenoxime	IV	6.0 (S)	5	1.4	11.71 (7.94–15.88)	2	1.69 (0.65–4.5)	2	14.4	I, CI
250	Cefmenoxime	IV	6.0 (S)	5	1.4	9.08 (0.82–16.12)	4	4.99 (0.52–15)	4	55	I, CI
250	Cefmenoxime	IV	6.0 (S)	5	1.4	2.52 (1.84–4.37)	8	4.28 (0.8–7.7)	8	170	I, CI
111	Cefoperazone	IV	50 mg/kg (S)	6	1.9	85 (60–130)	1.25–3.25	1.53 (<0.8–5.2)	1.25–3.25	1.8	I
51	Cefotaxime	IV	0.15–3.0/day (M)	11	1.2	17 (2.2–42.8)	2.0	8.7 (8.2–27.2)	2.0	51	I
25	Cefotaxime	IV	40 mg/kg (M)	14	1.2	6.6 (1.7–13.6)	14	1.2 (0.63–3.1)	14	18	I, TD 14
250	Cefoxitin	IV	2.0 (M)	17	0.8	9	1.0–2.0	4.7 (± 3.0)	1.0–2.0	52	I
598	Cefpirome	IV	2.0 (S)	9	2.0	20.5 (10.2–43)	4	4.2 (0.5–7.5)	4	20	I
101	Cefsulodin	IV	2.0 (M)	3	1.5	2.97 (1.5 4.4)	6.25–6.67	2.11 (1.31–3.1)	6.25–6.67	71	I
369	Ceftazidime	IV	2.0 (M)	5	1.85	28.2 (21–40)	3.0	7.2 (3–21)	2.0	23.5	I, TD 11–20
516	Ceftriaxone	IV	100 mg/kg/day (M)	15	4.0	128.2 (± 44.2 SE)	2.0	11.0 (± 3.1 SE)	2.0	8.6	I

110	Ceftizoxime	IV	30 mg/kg (S)	12	1.51	22.9 (8.3–60.8)	1.6–3.6	4.9 (0–17.0)	1.6–3.6	21	I
404	Ceftizoxime	IV	200 mg/kg/day (M)	4	1.7	26 (16–50)	3	7.25 (3.6–13)	3	27.9	I, TD 1–14
523	Cefuroxime	IV	3 (M)	9	1.4	5.2 (0.3–21.7)	6.0–8.5	5.6 (0.25–19.8)	6.0–8.5	108	I
321	Cephaloridine	IM	1.0 (S/M)	18	1.5	11.8 (5.9–19.6)	2.0–4.0	0.03 (0–0.26)	2.0–4.0	0.3	I
25	Cephalothin	IV	4.0 (S)	4	0.5	34.0	1.0	"Very low"	1.0	<0.1	U
25	Cephradine	IV	4.0 (S)	14	0.7	136.5	1.0	≤1.5	1.0	≤1	U
136	Imipenem	IV	1.0 (S)	4/10		20.0 (12–41)	1.0–2.0	1.7 (0.65–3.4)	2.0–6.0	8.5	I
136	Cilastatin	IV	1.0 (S)	4/10		19	1.0–2.0	0.9	2.0–6.0	4.7	I
126	Meropenem	IV	40 mg/kg (S)	6	1.0	13.3 (5.7–32)	2–3	2.8 (0.3–6.5)	1–4	21	I
Penicillins											
312	Amoxicillin	IV	1.0 (M)	7	1.1	20.0 (± 10.0)	1.0	2.0 (± 1.4)	1.0	10	1, TD 8–12
548	Ampicillin	IV	15 mg/kg (S)	11	1.1	8.8 (3.2–23.8)	1.0–2.0	0.3 (0–0.9)	1.0–2.0	3.4	I
119	Methicillin	IM	2.0 (M)	3	0.5	50 (27.5–90)	1.0	3.6 (0.78–10.8)	1.0	7	I, P
607	Nafcillin	IV	50 mg/kg (M)	7	1.5–3.2	123.0	0.08–0.5	4.5	2.0–3.0	3.7	I
274	Nafcillin	IV	169–200 mg/kg/day(M)	3	1.0	229 (36–615)	1.0–2.0	33 (2.7–88)	1.0–2.0	14	I
234	Penicillin G	IV	2.5×10^5 units/day (M)	6	0.5	9.5	2.0	0.8	2.0	8	I, TD 5
142	Piperacillin	IV	324–436 mg/kg/day (M)	4	1.1	79 (21–121)	1–10 days	23 (4–35)	1–10	29	I, CI
204	Procaine penicillin	IM	0.6 (M)	10		1.04 (0.49–1.92)	2–3	0.002 (0–0.01)	2–3	0.19	I, TD 14–21
514	Sulbactam	IV	1.0 (S)	7	1	13.0 (5–29)	1.5–7	4.16 (0.65–12)	1.5	32	I
102	Temocillin	IV	2 (S)	4	4.5	86.2 (64.8–113.8)	2	10.15 (<0.5–21.9)	2	11.8	I, TD 1
Quinolones											
193	Ciprofloxacin	IV	0.2 (M)	7	4.0	1.59 (0.85–2.95)	1	0.39 (0.11–0.68)	1	25	I
				5	4.0	1.44 (0.83–2.60)	2	0.56 (0.23–1.20)	2	39	I
				6	4.0	0.24 (0.90–0.40)	8	0.35 (0.07–0.61)	8	146	I

(continued)

TABLE 16.13 (Continued)

Antimicrobial Concentrations in Cerebrospinal Fluid

Reference	Antimicrobial	Administration Method[a]	Dose (g) (Multiple or Single)[b]	*n*	Serum Half-life (h)	Serum Concentration Mean (μg/mL) (Range)	Time Serum Obtained (h)	Site Concentration Mean (μg/mL) (Range)	Time Site Specimen Obtained (h)	Ratio of Site/Serum (%)	Notes[c]
193	Ciprofloxacin	Oral	0.5 (S)	8	4.0	2.41 (±0.8)	2	0.06 (±0.03)	2	3	U
				6	4.0	0.77 (±0.22)	4	0.14 (±0.07)	4	18	U
				7	4.0	0.45 (±0.24)	8	0.08 (±0.02)	8	18	U
193	Ofloxacin	Oral	0.2 (M)	11	7.0	3.1 (0.5–7.75)	1.5	1.3 (0.32–3.60)	1.5	42	I, U, E
				6	7.0	1.16 (0.5–2.3)	12	0.83 (0.49–135)	12	72	I, U, E
193	Pefloxacin	IV	0.5 (M)	6	10.5	10.3 (6.2–16)	1	4.8 (2.40–9.00)	2	47	I
Others											
558a	Chloramphenicol	IV	100 mg/kg/day (M)	11	2.5	15.2 (4.2–29.0)	3.0	5.7 (2.0–15.6)	3.0	38	I, TD 10
79	Dimethylchlor-tetracycline	Oral	1.0 (S)	8	9	3.3 (1.7–7.5)	4.0	0.19 (0.17–0.21)	4.0	5.8	U
605	Doxycycline	Oral	400 mg/day (M)	5		5.8 (3.6–8.6)	4–6	1.3 (0.8–2.0)	4–6	22.4	I
145	Doxycycline	Oral	400 mg/day (M)	10	21	7.5 (4.3–12)	2–3	1.1 (0.6–1.9)	2–3	14.7	I, TD 5–8
549	Lincomycin	IM	20 mg/kg (S)	10	4.5	7.4 (2.3–23.8)	2.0	0.5 (0.14–1.6)	2.0	6.8	I
262	Metronidazole	Oral	2.4 (S)	4	8.0	33.7	1.5	14.5 (6.0–22.7)	1.5	43	U
295	Oxytetracycline	IM	59–100 mg/kg/day (M)	7	8	34.3 (0–80)	24	2.3 (0–5)	24	6.7	I
498	Rifampin	Oral	25 mg/kg (S)	5	3.0	6.8 (4.4–9.3)	3.0	0.27 (0.23–0.33)	3.0	4	I
567	Sulfamethoxazole	IV	25 mg/kg (S)	4	1.0	82.5 (50–150)	1.75–3.0	33 (28–40)	1.75–3.0	40	U
262	Tinidazole	Oral	2.0 (S)	4		35.2	1.5	31 (17.0–39.0)	1.5	88	U
567	Trimethoprim	IV	5 mg/kg (S)	4	8–10	3.7 (3.0–4.1)	1.75–3.0	≤1.1 (≤0.5–1.5)	1.75–3.0	≤41	U
189	Vancomycin	IV	500 mg/kg (M)	9	6.0	6.3 (4.3–10.0)	1.0–2.5	0	1.0–2.5	0	U

[a] IV, intravenously; IM, intramuscularly.
[b] M, multiple dose; S, single dose.
[c] I, infected cerebrospinal fluid; U, uninfected; CI, continuous infusion; TD, treatment day; P, probenecid; E, extrapolated from graphs.

TABLE 16.14

Antimicrobial Concentrations in Aqueous Humor

Reference	Antimicrobial	Administration Method[a]	Dose (g) (Multiple or Single)[b]	*n*	Serum Half-life (h)	Serum Concentration Mean (μg/mL) (Range)	Time Serum Obtained (h)	Site Concentration Mean (μg/mL) (Range)	Time Site Specimen Obtained (h)	Ratio of Site/Serum (%)	Notes[c]
Aminoglycosides											
41	Amikacin	IV	0.5 (S)	5	2	10.6 (±0.58 SE)	2.5	0	2.5	0.5	U
580	Amikacin	IM	7.5 mg/kg (S)	47	2.0	20.85 (5–40)	0.7–7.7	0.85 (0.04–3.1)	0.7–7.7	4.5	U
497	Gentamicin	IV	0.08 (S)	10	2	8.8 (±4.3 SD)	0.25	1.9 (±0.27 SD)	.025	22.5	U
497	Gentamicin	IM	0.08 (S)	9	2	5.2 (±1.2 SD)	1	1.6 (±0.9 SD)	~1	27.5	U
403	Netilmicin	IM	1.5 mg/kg (S)	30	2	6.7	2	<1 (<1–1.4)	0–3.5	<15.5	U
496	Tobramycin	IV	0.08 (S)	6	2	4.9 (±0.5 SD)	1	1.6 (±0.5 SD)	1	32.5	U
425	Tobramycin	IM	0.08 (S)	9	2	4.07 (±2.28)	1	0.3 (±0.26)	1	7.4	U
Cephalosporins and related β-lactams											
227	Aztreonam	IV	2.0 (S)	5	1.3–2.2	90 (±28)	2	1.46 (±1.23)	2	2.5	U
26	Cefaclor	Oral	1.0 (S)	6	0.7	21.0 (7–34)	1–3	0.78 (0.09–1.56)	1–3	4.5	U
74	Cefadroxil	Oral	1.0 (S)	9	1.3	14.77	2	6.15	2	42.5	U
27	Cefamandole	IM	1.0 (S)	7	0.7	17.8 (7–34.4)	1–4.5	0	1–4.5	0.5	U
27	Cefamandole	IV	1.0 (S)	6	0.7	39.3 (31.5–64)	~1	0.59 (0–1.1)	~1	2.5	U
335	Cefazolin	IV	0.5 (S)	3	2.0	35 (32–39)	0.7	<0.6	0.7	<1.7	U
405a	Cefepime	IV	1.0 (S) 2.0 (S)	3 3	2	41.67 (±7.93 SD) 78.34 (±8.66 SD)	1 1	4.87 (±0.06 SD) 5.70 (±1.30 SD)	1 1	11.7 7.3	U, HPC
32	Cefmenoxime	IV	2.0 (S)	4–5	1.1	67 (45–80)	2	3.19 (2.88–3.36)	2	5.5	U
31	Cefonicid	IV	1.0 (S)	7	4.4	89 (70–120)	1–2	0.23 (0.14–0.31)	1–2	0.3	U
199	Cefoperazone	IV	2.0 (M)	6	2	30.5 (16–55)	4–5	1.9 (0.4–3.4)	4–5	6.5	U
440	Cefotaxime	IV	1.0 (S)	17	1.2	58 (3–200)	1–2	0.95 (0.25–4.5)	1–2	2.5	U
28	Cefoxitin	IV	2.0 (S)	5	0.8	48 (40–65)	~1	3.2 (3–3.4)	~1	7.5	U
28	Cefoxitin/probenecid	IV	2.0 (S)	4	?	79.4 (65–90)	~1	2.7 (2.2–3.2)	~1	3.5	U
151a	Cefpirome	IV	2.0 (S)	7	?	57 (±23 SD)	2	2.25 (±0.75 SD)	2	3.9	U, E, HPC

(*continued*)

TABLE 16.14 (Continued)

Antimicrobial Concentrations in Aqueous Humor

Reference	Antimicrobial	Administration Method[a]	Dose (g) (Multiple or Single)[b]	*n*	Serum Half-life (h)	Serum Concentration Mean (μg/mL) (Range)	Time Serum Obtained (h)	Site Concentration Mean (μg/mL) (Range)	Time Site Specimen Obtained (h)	Ratio of Site/Serum (%)	Notes[c]
464	Cefsulodin	IM	0.5 (S)	7	1.5	9.9 (±3.3)	1–1.5	0.36 (±0.38)	1–1.5	4.5	U
199	Cefsulodin	IV	2.0 (M)	6	1.5	31.8 (8–75)	3–5	5.0 (1.8–9.0)	3–5	16.5	U
33	Ceftazidime	IV	2.0 (S)	14	1.8	90.7 (53.2–137.5)	0.5–1	3.3 (2.0–4.5)	0.5–1	4.5	U
199	Ceftazidime	IM	1.0 (M)	5	1.8	21.8 (12–28)	3–5	2.6 (2.0–3.3)	3–5	12.5	U
350	Ceftizoxime	IV	2.0 (S)	6	1.7	48.9 (±21.5)	2	7.9 (±5.7)	2	16.5	U
610	Ceftriaxone	IV	2.0 (S)	10	5.8	198 (90–394)	1–8	1.16 (0.71–1.92)	1–8	1.5	
215	Cefuroxime	IV	2.0 (S)	5	1.3	14.6 (12.5–16.5)	1	1.46 (0.9–2.3)	1	10.5	U
215	Cefuroxime	IM	1.5 (S)	5	1.3	11.9 (8.0–15.5)	1	1.72 (1.0–2.2)	1	14.5	U
452	Cephalexin	Oral	0.5 (S)	10	0.8	17.8 (±3.4)	1	0.35 (±0.14)	1	2.5	U, S
452	Cephalexin/probenicid	Oral	1.0 (S)	13	?	50.0 (±4.7)	1	2.5 (±1.4)	1	5.5	U, NS
456	Cephaloridine	IM	1.0 (S)	6	1.5	28 (25–30)	2–4	1.9 (0.8–4.0)	2–4	7.5	U
451	Cephalothin	IV	1.0 (S)	18	0.5	12.9 (10–14)	0.5	0.48 (0–1.0)	0.5	4.5	U, S
29	Cephradine	Oral	0.5 (S)	8	0.7	9.13 (3.5–18)	0.5–3.4	0.45 (0–1.2)	0.5–3.4	5.5	U
34	Imipenem	IV	1.0 (S)	5	1	37.4 (13.5–56.5)	2	2.99 (2.40–3.90)	2	8.5	U
476a	Meropenem	IV	2.0 (S)	5	1.2	46.11 (37.4–60.4)	0.5	13.39 (12.5–15.8)	0.5	29.0	U, V, HPC
199	Moxalactam	IV	2.0 (M)	5	2.3	26.1(23–32)	3–5	4.1(2.4–9.5)	3–5	16.5	U
30	Moxalactam	IV	2.0 (S)	15	2.3	105 (50–150)	0.5–2	1.26 (0.62–2.3)	0.5–2	1.5	U
Quinolones											
193	Ciprofloxacin	Oral	1.0 (S)	12	4.0	5.7 (1.2–9.2)	1.4–3	0.44 (0.15–0.96)	2.0–3	8.5	U
193	Ciprofloxacin	Oral	0.75 (M)	6	4.0	3.6 (1.6–5.4)	1.4–1.6	0.61 (0.22–0.95)	1.4–1.6	17.5	
193	Ciprofloxacin	IV	0.40 (S)	3	4.0	2.5 (0.9–3.8)	1.5–2.5	0.4 (0.28–0.59)	1.5–2.5	16.5	
225a	Gatifloxacin	Oral	0.40 (M)	11	10.5	5.14 (±1.36 SD)	3.2 (±1.1 SD)	1.08 (±0.54 SD)	3.9 (±1.1 SD)	21.0	U, V, NS, HPC
563	Ofloxacin	Oral	0.2 (S)	12	7.0	2.67 (±0.54 SD)	2	0.38 (±0.15 SD)	2	14.5	U
563	Ofloxacin	IV	0.2 (S)	6	7.0	2.49 (±1.31 SD)	2	0.33 (±0.19 SD)	2	13.5	U
193	Pefloxacin	IV	0.4 (S)	5	12.6	3.4 (2.9–3.5)	6	1.4 (1.20–1.75)	6	41.5	U, E, L
193	Pefloxacin	Oral	0.4 (S)	14	10.5	4.94	3.3	0.89	3.3	18.5	U, E

Penicillins											
259	Azlocillin	IV	4.0 (S)	24	1	151 (±33)	<1	4.44 (±3.05)	<1	3.5	U, PD
546	Cloxacillin	IM	1–4 (S)	4	0.5	11.5	0.7–1.7	<1.0	1.2–1.6	<8.7	
610	Epicillin	IV	2.0 (S)	4	1.0	106 (80–136)	1–2	1.45 (1.09–1.75)	1–2	1.5	
449	Methicillin	IV	4.0 (C)	6	0.5	18.0	24	0	24	0.5	U
449	Methicillin/probenecid	IV	4.0 (C)	16	?	29.7	24	0	24	0.5	U
335	Methicillin	IV	2.0 (S)	5	0.5	76 (50–104)	0.4–1.2	<1.1 (<0.78–2.2)	0.4–1.2	<1.4	U
49	Mezlocillin	IV	4.0 (S)	4	1.1	180 (150–195)	1	4.4 (1.0–7.5)	1	2.5	U, E
335	Nafcillin	IV	2.0 (S)	5	1.0	97 (70–120)	0.5–0.8	<0.84 (<0.4–1.9)	0.5–0.8	<0.9	U
450	Oxacillin	IM	0.5 (M)	9	0.5	4.0	0–4	0	0–4	0.5	U
450	Oxacillin/probenecid	IM	0.5 (M)	10	0.5	5.70	0–4	0	0–4	0.5	U
610	Penicillin G	IV	10×10^6 units	4	0.5	121 (42–222)	2–5	2.94 (0.46–6.86)	2–5	2.5	
600	Piperacillin	IV	4.0 (S)	25	1.5	34	1–7	1.5	1–7	4.5	U, E
Tetracyclines											
544	Doxycycline	Oral	0.1 (M)	10	21	3.56 (1.5–7.96)	4–4.5	0.34 (0.25–0.47)	4–4.5	10.5	U
544	Doxycycline	Oral	0.1 (M)	10	21	4.65 (2.07–7.90)	3.0–4.3	0.60 (0.23–1.45)	3–4.3	13.5	I
433	Minocycline	Oral	0.1 (M)	26	14	6.75 (±1.0)	1	1.15 (±0.05)	1	17.5	U
2	Tetracycline	Oral	3 (S)	3	10	26 (25–28)	3	2.9 (2.5–3.5)	3	11.5	U
2	Tetracycline	IV	7 mg/kg (M)	5	10	63 (34–98)	5	5.5 (3.4–8.6)	5	9.5	U
Macrolides											
525	Azithromycin	Oral	1.0 (S)	5	44	0.58 (±0.31 SD)	3	0.054 (±0.022 SD)	3	9.3	U, C, HPC
19b	Clarithromycin	Oral	0.5 (S)	5	6	1.91 (±0.56 SD)	5.3	0.13 (±0.05 SD)	4.7	6.8	U, V, HPC
Others											
15	Fosfomycin	IV	4.0 (S)	8	2	75.2	2	18.8 (±3.4)	2	25.5	U
48	Lincomycin	IM	0.6 (M)	8	4.5	15.3 (10.2–23)	1–2	1.3 (1.0–2.0)	1–2	8.5	U
354	Metronidazole	IV	0.5 (S)	10	10	15.9 (±2.9 SE)	0.7–1.5	5.2 (±0.5 SE)	0.7–1.5	38.5	U
354	Tinidazole	IV	0.5 (S)	10	14	11.6 (±1.3 SE)	0.7–1.5	5.3 (±0.7 SE)	0.7–1.5	47.5	U
335	Vancomycin	IV	0.5 (S)	5	6	13.8 (11–17)	0.7–1.3	<0.78	0.7–1.3	<5.6	U
512a	Vancomycin	IV	1.0 (M)	7	6	13.51 (±4.96 SD)	6	1.42 (±0.47 SD)	6	10.5	U

[a] IV, intravenously; IM, intramuscularly.
[b] S, single dose; M, multiple dose; C, continuous infusion.
[c] Number of subjects studied.
[d] U, uninfected; HPC, high performance liquid chromatography; E, values extrapolated from graphs; S, secondary aqueous sampled; NS, number of site sample when different from number of serum samples; V, vitreous concentrations measured also; L, lens concentration measured also; PD, peak data, I, infected; C, conjunctival concentrations measured also.

TABLE 16.15

Antimicrobial Concentrations in Skeletal Muscle

Reference	Antimicrobial	Administration Method[a]	Dose (g) (Multiple or Single)[b]	*n*	Serum Half-life (h)	Serum Concentration Mean (μg/mL) (Range)	Time Serum Obtained (h)	Site Concentration Mean (μg/mL) (Range)	Time Site Specimen Obtained (h)	Ratio of Site/Serum (%)	Notes[c]
Aminoglycosides											
129	Amikacin	IM	7.5 mg/kg (S)	6	2.0	14.9 (7–19.3)	1.5	2.2 (0.8–4.5)	1.5	15	U, CHAPTER
61	Gentamicin	IM	0.08 (S)	~9	2.0	5.4 (3.6–7.3)	1.8–3.0	6.5 (<2.8)	1.8–3	111	U
267	Netilmicin	IV	0.0015/kg (S)	6	2.0	2.6 (± 1.2)	2–3	0.8 (0–3.6)	2–3	31	U
Cephalosporins and related β-lactams											
45	Aztreonam	IV	2.0 (S)	6	1.7	108	0.25–0.68	16	0.25–0.68	20	U, C
441	Cefadroxil	Oral	1.0 (M)	12	1.3	20.7 (± 2.9)	2	6.5 (± 0.9)	2	31	U
61	Cefazolin	IM	1.0 (S)	~9	2.0	35 (7.3–82)	1.8–3.8	<6.0 (all)	1.8–3.8	<7–<82	U
457	Cefmenoxime	IV	2.0 (S)	41		52.4	1	12.96	0.75		U, MM
266	Cefotaxime	IV	2.0 (S)	11	1.0	81 (± 10)	0–0.5	3.8 (± 1.3)	0–0.5	5	U
233	Cefoxitin	IV	2.0 (S)	31	0.8	25	1.0	24	1.0	96	U, MM
14	Cefsulodin	IV	2.0 (S)	5	1.5	55.1 (50–90)	1.0	10.2 (5–40)	1.0	19	U
11	Ceftazidime	IV	2.0 (S)	35	1.8	36.5	2	9.4 (3–22)	2	25.8	U, C
46	Cetriaxone	IV	1.0 (S)	53	7.0	90.8	1.3	11.2	1.5		U, C
107	Cephradine	IM	2.0 (S)	10	0.7	119 (49–285)	0.41	21.5 (21–60)	1.5	18	U, P
107	Cephradine	IM	2.0 (S)	10	0.7	119 (49–285)	0.41	14.4 (0.5–26)	1.5	12	D
308	Imipenem	IV	1.0 (S)	10	0.9	47.2	0–1	2.5	0–1	5	U

Penicillins											
264	Dicloxacillin	IV	1 (S)	6	0.7	6	4	3 (2–4)	0.8	13	
176	Flucloxacillin	IV	2.0 (S)	20		125.2	0–1	14.2	0–1	11	U
231	Mezlocillin	IV	5.0 (S)	10	0.99	100 (50–100)	1.5	26.4 (10–40)	1.5	26.4	U
396	Nafcillin	IV or IM	1.0 (S)	14	1.0	2.2 (0.3–10)	4.5	0.58	4.8	26	U
13	Oxacillin	IV	4.0 (S)	6	0.5	94.5 (44–117)	0.58	<2	0.58	<2	U, MM
468	Piperacillin	IV	5.0 (S)	14	1.1	95 (±25)	2.5	30 (±17)	2.5	32	I, C
489	Piperacillin	IV	2.0 (S)	30	1.1	16.4	1–2	8.1	1–2	49	U
205	Temocillin	IV	1.0	7	62.6	2.5–5.5	9.5 (<3.1–17.3)		2.5–5.5	27	U, C
132	Ticarcillin	IV	5.0 (S)	5	1.2	185 (118–242)	1.0–1.5	18 (9–44)	1.0–1.5	10	U
Tetracycline											
443	Tetracycline	Oral	0.5 (M)	5	10	3.7 (2.1–4.6)	3–4	1.9 (0–3.3)	3–4	50	U, C
Quinolones											
169	Ciprofloxacin	Oral	0.5 (S)	7	4.0	1.4 (0.4–2.0)	1.5–4.8	1.1 (0.5–1.9)	1.5–4.8	79	U, C
		Oral	0.75 (S)	7		2.6 (0.9–3.8)	1.5–4.8	1.3 (0.6–2.4)	1.5–4.8	50	U, C
Others											
50	Clindamycin	IV	5 mg/kg	11	2.0	4.9 (1.1–14)	0.8–1.9	6.1 (0–25)	0.5–2.6	124	U, CH
331a	Linezolid	IV	0.6 (S)	12	4–5	15.8 (95% CI[d] 12.5–19.1)	0.33	13.4 (95% CI[d] 10.2–16.5)	0.33	94.3	U
175a	Teicoplanin	IV	12 mg/kg	9		27.5 (±20.3)	1–2	6.7 (±8.8)	1–2		U
130	Vancomycin	IV	0.15 mg	5	6.0	14.2	1–2	3.2	1–2	23	U

[a] IM, intramuscularly; IV, intravenously.
[b] S, single dose; M, multiple dose.
[c] U, uninfected; CH, children; C, corrected; MM, blood contamination measured as minimal; P, proximal muscle; D, distal muscle.
[d] Confidence interval.

TABLE 16.16

Antimicrobial Concentrations in Bone

Reference	Antimicrobial	Administration Method[a]	Dose (g) (Multiple or Single)[b]	*n*	Serum Half-life (h)	Serum Concentration Mean (μg/mL) (Range)	Time Serum Obtained (h)	Site Concentration Mean (μg/mL) (Range)	Time Site Specimen Obtained (h)	Ratio of Site/Serum (%)	Notes[c]
Aminoglycosides											
501	Gentamicin	IM	1.7 mg/kg (M)	3	2.0	5.2 (3.7–7.1)	1–2	1.22 (<2.1–3.6)	1–2	~30.5	U
83a	Isepamicin	IV	15 mg/kg (S)	12		43 (26–57)	1–2	6.3 (1.6–11.9)	1–2	15	U, CO
								8.3 (2.4–20.9)	1–2	19	U, CA
578	Tobramycin	IV	0.0015/kg	5	2.0	6 (2.4–8.3)	0.35	0.8 (0.6–1)	0.35	13.5	U
Cephalosporins and related β-lactams											
336	Aztreonam	IV	2.0 (S)	18	1.7	78 (42–129)	1.5	16 (0–49)	1.5	20.5	U, C, CA
16	Cefaclor	Oral	0.5 (S)	39	0.75	7.5	2	1.59 (0–3.2)	2	18.5	U
554	Cefadroxil	Oral	0.5 (S)	6	1.3	6.33	4	0.4	4	6.3	U, CO
								0.9		14.2	U, CA
441	Cefadroxil	Oral	1.0 (M)	14	1.3	21.5 (±2.3)	2	5.0 (±0.9)	2	23.5	U
417	Cefamandole	IV	1.0–2.0 (S)	7	1.0	47.1 (22–67.5)	0.2–1.3	0.2 (0–1.5)	0.2–1.3		I
480	Cefamandole	IV	2.0 (S)	29	0.7	73.6 (±6.1)	0.85	9.4 (±1.1)	0.85	13.5	U
252	Cefazolin	IV	0.01/kg (S)	10	1.5	32.9 (±10.4)	1.2	3.03 (±1.78)	1.2	6.5	U, CA, C
501	Cefazolin	IM	1.0 (M)	3	2.0	42 (31–50)	0.5–2.0	~5 (<4.1–10)	0.5–2	~12.5	U
538	Cefazolin	IV or IM	50 mg/kg/day (M)	6	1.7	13 (±2)	2	3.8 (3–5)	2–6	29.5	I, CH
125	Cefazolin	IV	1.0 (S)	31	2.0	80	0.67	30	0.67	37.5	U, C
412	Cefazolin	IV	4.0 (S)	7	2.0	101 (74–138)	~1	14.4 (5.6–24.9)	~1	14	U, CO
								29 (3.3–48.9)		29	U, CA

577	Cefazolin	IV	1.0 (S)	17	2.0	51.7	1.15	5.9	1.15	11.4	U, CA
87a	Cefepime	IV	2.0 (S)	10	2	72.9 (32–1270	0.8–1.9	35.6 (22–51)	0.8–1.9	49	U, CO
								52.5 (35–68)	0.8–1.9	72	U, CA
457	Cefmenoxime	IV	2.0	41		52.4	1.0	18.1 (±8.74)	0.83		U, MC, CA
		IV	2.0	41		52.4	1.0	16.5 (±6.23)	0.83	31.5	U, MC, CO
475a	Cefodozime	IV	2.0 (S)	22	3–4	121	2.5	13.42	2.5	11	U, CO
								24.4	2.5	20	U, CA
392	Cefonicid	IV	0.03/kg (S)	12	2.6		1–3	18.7 (5.8–29.6)	1–3	12.5	U, C
86	Cefoperazone	IV	1.0 (M)	5	1.22	46	1.0	5	1.0	11.5	U, CA
		IV	1.0 (M)	5	1.22	46	1.0	4.2	1.0	9.5	U, CO
577	Ceforanide	IV	2.0 (S)	8	2.7	144.0	1.37	13.4	1.37	9.3.5	U, CA
593	Cefotaxime	IV	2.0 (S)	19	1.2	61	0.5–1	5.4	0.5–1	8.8	U, C
137a	Cefotiam	IV	2.0 (S)	10	0.6–1.5	55.2 (±11.5)	1	14.7 (±4.4)	1	27	U
428	Cefoxitin	IV	45 mg/kg (S)	14	0.8	160 (±50)	2	8 (±3)	2	5	U, CO
								16 (±6)		10	U, CA
577	Cefoxitin	IV	2.0 (S)	20	0.8	39.0	1.15	6.3	1.15	16.2	U, CA
320	Ceftazidime	IV	1.0 (S)	12	1.9	49.1 (38.2–59.8)	0.5	14.8 (4.4–21.1)	0.5	30.5	U, C
195	Ceftizoxime	IV	1.0 (M)	5	1.7	33.7 (±6.9)	1	6.3 (±4.6)	1	19.5	U
46	Ceftriaxone	IV	1.0	53	7.0	67.3	1.8	32.4	1.56		U, C
595	Cefuroxime	IV	1.5 (S)	11	1.3	100 (±25)	0.75	5.5 (3–13)	0.75	5.5	U, CO
								12 (7–25)		12	U, CA
18	Cephalexin	Oral	0.5 (S)	36	0.9	11.7 ±2.3	1.5	2.12 ±0.33	2	19.5	U
538	Cephaloridine	IV or IM	100 mg/kg/day (M)	7	1.8	6.5	2	2.0 (0.7–6)	1–3	31.5	I
167	Cephalothin	IV	1.0 (S)	21	0.5	11.9 (6.6–20.8)	1	3.9 (0.9–17.5)	1	33.5	U
577	Cephalothin	IV	1.0 (S)	14	0.5	5.3	1.52	0.5	1.52	9.4	U, CA
481	Cephapirin	IV	1.0 (S)	10	0.28	70.8 (7.1–383)	0.25–1	9.1 (3.8–28.7)	0.25–1	45.5	U, C
133	Cephradine	IV	1.0 (S)	21	0.7	45	0.6	10	0.6	22.5	U, C

(continued)

TABLE 16.16 (Continued)

Antimicrobial Concentrations in Bone

Reference	Antimicrobial	Administration Method[a]	Dose (g) (Multiple or Single)[b]	*n*	Serum Half-life (h)	Serum Concentration Mean (μg/mL) (Range)	Time Serum Obtained (h)	Site Concentration Mean (μg/mL) (Range)	Time Site Specimen Obtained (h)	Ratio of Site/Serum (%)	Notes[c]
98	Cephradine	IM	1.0 (S)	24	0.7	11.7 (6.1–20.4)	1.7	1.79 (±0.98)	1.7	15	U, CA
								3.28 (±1.34)	1.7	28	U, CO
252	Moxalactam	IV	0.01/kg (S)	10	3	33.3 (±7.7)	1.2	2.62 (±2.28)	1.2	7.5	U, CA, C
334	Imipenem	IV	1.0 (M)	10	1.4	35 (±4)	0.25	2.6 (0.4–5.4)	0.5–2.0		I
Penicillins											
214	Amoxycillin/	IV	1.0 (M)	9	1.0	50.1	0.5	3.6	0.5	7.5	U
214	Clavulanic acid	IV	0.2 (M)	9	1.2	9.1	0.5	0.54	0.5	6.5	U
98	Ampicillin	IM	0.5 (S)	24	1.1	10.1 (1.1–34.8)	1.7	0.78 (±1.28)	1.7	8	U, CA
								1.89 (±1.77)	1.7	19	U, CO
137a	Ampicillin/sulbactam	IV	2.0 (S)	10	0.9	46.8 (±27.4)	1	20.7 (±9.6)	1	44	U
		IV	1.0 (S)	10	0.84	13.2 (±8.4)	1	7.7 (±4.1)	1	58	U
109	Azidocillin	Oral	0.75 (S)	6	0.75	12.2 (±5.0)	1	0.8 (±0.4)	1	65.5	U
596	Azlocillin	IV	5.0 (S)	8	1.0	14.3	1	24 (±1.35)	0.8–1.5	17.5	U
306	Carbenicillin	IV	5.0 (S)	15	1.5	281 (155–360)	0.5	32.3	0.5	11.6	U
299	Cloxacillin	Oral	0.5 (S)	10	0.5	3.2 (±0.5)	1	2.0 (±0.4)	1	62.5	U
		Oral	1.0 (S)	5	0.5	17.7 (±2.4)	2	2.9 (±1.3)	2	16	CA, MC, U
538	Dicloxacillin	IM	50 mg/kg/day (M)	8	1.9	6 (±1)	2	6.4 (1.8–21)	2–6	106.5	I
299, 499	Dicloxacillin	Oral	0.5 (S)	10	0.5	13 (±2.5)	1.5	2.0 (±0.5)	1.5	15.5	U
98	Flucloxacillin	IM	0.5 (S)	24		9.3 (2.7–17.8)	1.7	0.87 ±1.28)	1.7	9	U, CA
								1.30 (±1.92)	1.7	13	U, CO
479	Methicillin	IM	1.0 (M)	21	0.5	11.65 (±6.1)	~2	2.6 (0–7)	2	22	U, CO
								2.7 (0–10)		23	U, CA
538	Methicillin	IV	250 mg/kg/day (M)	10	0.8	18 (±8)	2	12.1 (1–46)	1–3	67.5	I
596	Mezlocillin	IV	5.0 (S)	10	1.3	135	1	21 (±2.75)	0.8–1.5	16.5	U

167	Oxacillin	IV	1.0 (S)	22	0.5	18.9 (5–33)	1	2.1 (0.3–14.5)	1	11.5	U
501	Penicillin G	IV	2×10^6 units	3	0.5	5.0 (0.5–9.4)	0.5–1.0	<1	0.5–1.0	<20.5	U
593	Piperacillin	IV	50 mg/kg (S)	12	1.1	46.6	2	15.7	2	33.5	CO, U
254	Piperacillin/tazobactam	IV	3.01	9	1	98.5 ± 19.1	1	21.3 ± 10.1	2	23	U, CA
								18.7 ± 7.8		18	U, CO
			0.375			9.4 ± 2.2	1	2.46 ± 0.96	2	26	U, CA
								2.29 ± 0.93		22	U, CO
3	Ticarcillin	IV	5.0 (S)	20	1.0	127 (28–214)	~1.1	32.4 (13.5–60.2)	~1.1	26	U, C, CO
								30.5 (14–65.1)	~1.1	24	U, C, CA
3	Clavulanic acid	IV	0.2 (S)	20	1.2	8.4 (5–12.5)	~1.1	14.8 (6.7–24.5)	~1.1	176	U, C, CO
								9.6	~1.1	114	U, C, CA
Quinolones											
169	Ciprofloxacin	Oral	0.5 (S)	7	4.0	1.4 (0.4–2.0)	1.5–4.8	0.4 (0.2–0.9)	1.5–4.8	28.5	U, C, CO
		Oral	0.75	7	4.0	2.6 (0.9–3.8)	1.5–4.8	0.7 (0.2–1.4)	1.5–4.8	27.5	U, C, CO
		Oral	0.5	6	4.0	2.0 (0.9–3.2)	2.0–4.5	0.7 (0.2–1.4)	2.0–4.5	35.5	I, C, CO
		Oral	0.75	4	4.0	2.9 (1.0–6.0)	2.0–4.5	1.4 (0.6–2.7)	2.0–4.5	48.5	I, C, CO
170	Enoxacin	Oral	0.4 (S)	5	5.5	2.0 (± 0.4)	1.5–5.5	0.7 (± 0.3)	1.5–5.5	35.5	U, C, CO
		Oral	0.4 (M)	6		2.1 (± 0.3)	1.5–5.5	0.9 (± 0.5)	1.5–5.5	45.5	U, C, CO
		Oral	0.4 (M)	6		2.8 (± 1.6)	1.5–5.5	1.3 (± 1.6)	1.5–5.5	39.5	I, C, CO
		IV	0.4 (S)	6		1.8 (± 0.4)	1.5–5.5	0.9 (± 0.5)	1.5–5.5	48.5	U, C, CO
		IV	0.4 (M)	6		3.1 (± 0.9)	1.5–5.5	1.1 (± 0.5)	1.5–5.5	35.5	U, C, CO
562a	Levofloxacin	IV	0.5 (S)	146	6–7	8.57 (5.25–13.75)	1.5	6.61 (1.95–13.04)	1.5	77	CA
							1.5	3	1.5	35	CO
17	Lomefloxacin	Oral	0.2 (M)	5	8	1.65 ± 0.13	2.5	1.87 ± 0.66	2.5	103.5	U
592	Ofloxacin	Oral	0.4 (S)	10	8.0	2.0 (± 0.88)	4.0	1.22 (± 1.54)	4.5	61.5	U
138	Pefloxacin	IV/Oral	0.4 (M)	15	10.5	9.2 (3.5–17.3)	2.0	4.1 (0.3–10.2)	2.0	44.5	U, C
109	Doxycycline	Oral	0.20 (S)	6	20	3.6 (± 0.8)	3	2.6 (± 2.0)	3	72.5	U
Others											
479	Clindamycin	IM	0.6 (M)	24	2.0	8.5 (± 1.65)	~2	3.87 (1–9.6)	2	45	U, CO
								3.77 (0.7–7)		44	U, CA

(continued)

TABLE 16.16 (Continued)

Antimicrobial Concentrations in Bone

Reference	Antimicrobial	Administration Method[a]	Dose (g) (Multiple or Single)[b]	*n*	Serum Half-life (h)	Serum Concentration Mean (μg/mL) (Range)	Time Serum Obtained (h)	Site Concentration Mean (μg/mL) (Range)	Time Site Specimen Obtained (h)	Ratio of Site/Serum (%)	Notes[c]
109	Clindamycin	Oral	0.3 (S)	6	2.0	2.8 (±1.2)	1.5	0.6 (±0.4)	1.5	21.4	U
109	Erythromycin	Oral	0.5 (S)	6	1.5	1.3 (0.1–2.1)	1	0.2 (±0.1	1.5	18.5	U
512	Erythromycin	IV	1.0 (S)	4	1.5	9.8 (7.6–11)	0.25–2.5	3.8 (1.8–5.5)	0.25–2.5	39.5	U, CA
55	Flurithromycin	Oral	0.5 (M)	8	9.9	1.5	1.5	1.5	1.5	100.5	U, C
547	Lincomycin	Oral	1.0 (M)	8	4.5	0.84 (0.25–1.5)	2–6	0.7 (0.25–1.3)	2–6	83.5	U
547	Lincomycin	IM	0.6 (M)	5	4.5	3.7 (2.6–5.0)	2–6	2.7 (1.0–5.2)	2–6	62.5	U
325	Lincomycin	Oral	1.0 (M)	10	4.5	5.8	~6	2.32	~6	40.5	I
331a	Linezolid	IV	0.6 (S)	12	4–5	19.2 (10.7–38.2)	0.17	9.1 (4.3–13)	0.17	51	U
311a	Linezolid	IV	0.6 (S)	11	4–5	17.1 (11.1–26.6)	0.9	3.9 (1.2–8.3)	0.9	22	I, CO
459	Metronidazole	Rectal	1.0 (S)	13	8.0	9.82 (±4.05)	3	7.45 (±3.85)	3	75.5	U
180	Miokamycin	Oral	0.6 (S)	5		1.0 ±0.48	1	0.88 ±0.13	1	88.5	U
500	Rifampin	Oral	0.3 (M)	8	3.0	6.0 (±2.6)	3–4	0	3–4	19	C, U, CO
								1.2 (±0.5)		19	C, U, CA
500	Rifampin	Oral	0.6 (M)	10	3.0	8.9 (±2.3)	3	1.7 (±1.0)	3	20	C, U, CO
								3.6 (±0.7)		41	C, U, CA
462	Rifampicin	IV	0.6 (S)		1.1	7.4 (3.2–12.8)	4	3.8 (1.9–8.2)	4	51.5	I, C
139	Roxithromycin	Oral	0.15 (M)	24	7.5	6.12	2.75	5.09	4.5	79.5	U, AU
578	Teicoplanin	IV	0.4	10	0.68	29.6 (18–74.4)	0.5	6.6 (2.6–18.4)	0.5	22.5	U
210	Vancomycin	IV	0.015/kg	14	6.0	22.1 (10.5–52.9)	1.3	2.3 (0.5–16)	1.3	13	U, CA, C
				10				0.81 (0–1.58)	1.3	4	U, CO, C
			Variable (M)	5		17.5 (13.6–26.3)	2.5	2.4 (0–8.4)	2.5	14.5	I, CO, C

[a] IM, intramuscularly; IV, intravenously.

[b] M, multiple dose; S, single dose.

[c] U, uninfected; CO, cortical bone; CA, cancellous bone; C, corrected for blood; I, infected; MC, blood contamination was felt to be minimal; CH, children; AUC, ratios of areas under the curve.

supply to the bone was of critical importance in delivering the antibiotic to the bone. In one study in which necrotic bone was sampled, cefamandole concentration was usually not detectable (417). We are not aware of any conclusive studies that attempt to correlate clinical outcome with the degree of antibiotic bone penetration, either in treating osteomyelitis or in preventing postoperative infection.

Cardiac Tissue

Antibiotic levels in cardiac tissue were measured in atrial appendage, valve, or heart muscle (Table 16.17). Virtually all studies were done in uninfected hearts. Study patients received a dose of antibiotic prior to undergoing valve replacements, coronary artery bypass grafting, or repair of congenital heart abnormalities. The cephalosporins were most widely studied and showed moderate penetration into cardiac tissue, with cephalothin and cefonicid having the lowest site-to-serum ratios. Particularly high penetration into cardiac tissue was noted for clindamycin, teicoplanin, and the quinolones. Readers are cautioned to note that cardiac penetration may not correlate with the efficacy of an antibiotic in preventing infection in patients undergoing cardiac surgery.

Gallbladder

Studies of antibiotic concentration in gallbladder tissue (Table 16.18) are difficult to interpret because specimens may be contaminated by bile as well as blood. Only one study cited in Table 16.18 corrected assay results for blood contamination (513). One study failed to show any difference in gallbladder levels of ceforanide when the cystic duct was obstructed or unobstructed (280). Other studies, however, revealed higher gallbladder levels of clindamycin when the common duct was patent than when it was obstructed (100) and higher levels when the gallbladder functioned than when it did not (472).

Lung Tissue

Antimicrobial concentrations in lung tissue (Table 16.19) have been measured almost exclusively following pulmonary resection of lung cancers. An exception involved a unique method of positron emission labeling of erythromycin followed by scanning of the lungs, while increasing numbers of samples of pulmonary tissue were obtained by transbronchial biopsy (599). Correction for blood contamination of specimens was done in only a few studies (416,443,539,568,599). The antimicrobial concentrations achieved in lung tissue were considerably higher than those in sputum (Table 16.8), but far fewer studies of lung tissue have been performed. Several drugs, such as ciprofloxacin (453), erythromycin (103), cefotaxime (186), and trimethoprim (225), showed much higher levels in lung than in blood. These studies were usually done 3 to 15 hours after the last doses of drug, at a time of relatively low serum levels, but nonetheless they showed considerably more activity in lung tissue than in serum. Many of these agents (ciprofloxacin, erythromycin, and rifampin) are concentrated within cells, which may explain their high tissue levels. A few investigators have examined the concentrations of drug in infected or inflamed lung tissue (159,225,286,599). These levels were not substantially different from those in normal lung tissue from the same individuals. We are unaware of good correlation between lung antimicrobial concentrations and clinical therapeutic or prophylactic efficacy in humans. Therefore, clinical inferences from these data should be made with caution.

Prostatic Tissue

Numerous studies have measured antimicrobial concentrations in human prostatic tissue (Table 16.20). Most of the studies were performed with patients without infection, undergoing transurethral or suprapubic prostatectomy. Techniques for tissue preparation were variable. As is the case with prostatic secretions, the prostatic tissue concentrations observed in most of these studies may be due to urinary contamination and therefore must be interpreted with caution (82,339).

Intracellular Penetration

The penetration or entry of antimicrobial agents into human cells has been addressed in a limited number of studies, as outlined in Table 16.21. Several methods have been used in these studies, including hypotonic lysis (344) or freeze-thawing (99) of cells following antimicrobial exposure, as well as routine centrifugation and washing (300) and, more recently, centrifugation of cells through an inert silicon monolayer to separate them from the surrounding aqueous medium (292). This last technique involves layering of antimicrobial-exposed cells over small volumes (0.5 mL) of silicone oil and centrifugation at relatively high speeds (67,000 *g*) for short periods (30 seconds) so that cells are rapidly separated from the medium in which they were originally suspended. This method has been the most widely used and reported in recent publications and it offers promise as a technique that at least provides the capacity to accurately measure cell-associated drug. Laser cytofluorometry is a developing technique that may allow actual determination of drug distribution within cells.

These studies all suffer from problems: using different test media (with and without albumin) affects the study results, using radiolabeled substrates might affect the outcome of the studies, and a definitive demonstration that intracellular antimicrobial concentrations correlate with the clinical outcome of therapy of intracellular infections is generally lacking. Studies such as that by Buggy et al. (106) suggest the clinical importance of intracellular

(*text continues on page 782*)

TABLE 16.17

Antimicrobial Concentrations in Cardiac Tissue

Reference	Antimicrobial	Administration Method[a]	Dose (g) (Multiple or Single)[b]	*n*	Serum Half-life (h)	Serum Concentration Mean (μg/mL) (Range)	Time Serum Obtained (h)	Site Concentration Mean (μg/mL) (Range)	Time Site Specimen Obtained (h)	Ratio of Site/Serum (%)	Notes[c]
Aminoglycosides											
158	Amikacin	IM	0.5 (S)	9	2.0	17.4 (±2.5)	0.6–1.5	4.3 (±0.9)	0.6–1.5	25.5	A
	Gentamicin	IV	1.5 mg/kg (S)	33	2.0	2.7	1–2	0.5	1–2	19.5	V
Cephalosporins and related β-lactams											
45	Aztreonam	IV	2.0 (S)	12	1.7–2	76 (±5 SE)	0.9–1.6	22 (±2 SE)	0.9–1.6	29.5	A
400	Cefamandole	IV	2.0 (S)	23	0.6	78 (25–130)	0.3–2.0	34 (8–70)	0.3–2.0	44.5	A, C
22	Cefamandole	IM	20 mg/kg (S)	15	0.7	47 (22–70)	0.5–2	16 (6–35)	0.5–2	34.5	V
391	Cefazolin	IV	2.0 (S)	16	2	114.1 (50–200)	1	38.9 (25–60)	1	34.1	C
434	Cefazolin	IM	10 mg/kg (S)	9	2	34.0 (21–40)	0.5–1.4	10.1 (±3.2 SD)	0.5–1.4	30.5	A, C
519	Cefonicid	IM	1.0 (S)	7	3.5	85 (48–138)	2	7.5 (2.6–9.5)	2	8.8	
379	Ceforanide	IV	30 mg/kg (S)	11	2.3	127 (40–200)	0.3–1.7	52 (30–80)	0.3–1.7	41.5	A, C
348	Cefoxitin	IV	2.0 (S)	10	0.8	55.8 (29–78.1)	0.75–1	27.3 (18.2–43.2)	0.75–1	49.5	
	Cefsulodin	IV	2.0 (S)	23	1.5	72.1	1–2	10.1	1–2	14.5	V
294	Ceftizoxime	IV	2.0 (S)	22	1.7	80.9 (±7.3)	1	37.0 (±2.8)	1	46.5	A
294	Ceftizoxime	IV	2.0 (S)	7	1.7	56.5 (34.1–92.6)	2	16.9 (9.1–20.7)	2	30.5	MY
46	Ceftriaxone	IV	1.0 (S)	53	15.7	67.3	1.8	30.5	1.9	45.5	A
442	Cephalothin	IV	2.0 (S)	12	0.5	66 (10–140)	0.2–1.7	7.5 (0–17)	0.3–1.9	11.5	A, C
22	Cephalothin	IM	20 mg/kg (S)	15	0.5	30 (20–70)	0.5–1.5	<4 (<1–22)	0.5–1.5	<13.5	V
442	Cephapirin	IV	2.0 (S)	15	0.5	62 (10–140)	0.2–1.7	12 (0–32)	0.3–1.9	19.5	A, C

391	Cephradine	IV	2.0 (S)	17	0.7	40.9 (20–75)	1	18.1 (10–25)	1	44.3	A, C
434	Moxalactam	IV	10 mg/kg (S)	10	2.5	40.1 (± 5.2 SD)	0.5–0.7	19.2 (± 10.4 SD)	0.5–0.7	48.5	A, C
Quinolones											
366	Ciprofloxacin	IV	0.4 (S)	6	3–5	6.19 (± 1.73 SD)	0	31.6 (± 25.0 SD)	0–1	510.5	MY, NS
366	Ciprofloxacin	IV	0.4 (S)	6	3–5	6.19 (± 1.73 SD)	0	5.8 (± 3.2 SD)	0–1	94.5	V, NS
366	Ciprofloxacin	Oral	0.75 (M)	6	3–5	11.59 (± 3.95 SD)	0	21.8 (± 13.0 SD)	0–1	188.5	MY, NS
366	Ciprofloxacin	Oral	0.75 (M)	8	3–5	11.59 (± 3.95 SD)	0	8.3 (± 3.1 SD)	0–1	72.5	V, NS
365	Ofloxacin	IV	0.4 (S)	3	4–8	15.9 (± 2.5 SD)	0	8.89 (± 2.16 SD)	0–1	56.5	MY, NS
365	Ofloxacin	IV	0.4 (S)	3	4–8	15.9 (± 2.5 SD)	0	5.00 (± 0.75 SD)	0–1	31.5	V, NS
88	Pefloxacin	IV	0.8 (S)	9	8–12	7.1 (± 2.02)	4	6.90	4	97.5	V, NS
88	Pefloxacin	IV	0.8 (S)	3	8–12	7.1 (± 2.02)	4	20.1 (± 25.1)	4	284.5	MY, NS
Penicillins											
176	Flucloxacillin	IV	2.0 (S)	9	2.1	125.2 (± 11.7 SE)	0–1	16.5 (± 2.6 SE)	1–2	13.5	V, NS, PD
10	Piperacillin	IV	100 mg/kg (S)	5	1.0	300 (240–400)	0.3–0.5	90 (85–100)	0.3–0.5	30.5	MY
Others											
343	Clindamycin	IV	0.6 (M)	6	2	6.0 (5–8)	1	15.6 (12.5–18)	1	260.5	A
343	Doxycycline	IV	0.1 (M)	11	20	10.3 (8–13)	1	5.9 (5–6.3)	1	57.5	A
561	Lincomycin	IM	0.6 (M)	51	4.5	9.7	1	7.7	1	79.5	
21	Rifampin	Oral	0.6 (S)	10	2–5	15.9	2	3.8	2	24.5	V
171	Teicoplanin	IV	6 mg/kg (S)	32	40–70	22.2 (± 0.7 SE)	1	70.6 (± 1.7 SE)	1	318.5	A
174	Teicoplanin	IV	12 mg/kg (S)	8	40–70	16.2 (± 10.5 SE)	2–3	5.5 (± 5.1 SE)	2–3	34	V, NS
130	Vancomycin	IV	15 mg/kg (S)	7	4–6	14.2 (± 2.0 SE)	1–2	4.2 (± 1.0 SE)	1–2	30.5	V, NS

[a] IM, intramuscularly; IV, intravenously.
[b] S, single dose; M, multiple dose.
[c] A, atrial appendage; V, valve; C, corrected for blood; MY, myocardium; NS, number of site samples is different than number of serum samples; PD, peak data.

TABLE 16.18

Antimicrobial Concentrations in Gallbladder

Reference	Antimicrobial	Administration Method[a]	Dose (g) (Multiple or Single)[b]	*n*	Serum Half-life (h)	Serum Concentration Mean (μg/mL) (Range)	Time Serum Obtained (h)	Site Concentration Mean (μg/mL) (Range)	Time Site Specimen Obtained (h)	Ratio of Site/Serum (%)	Notes[c]
Aminoglycosides											
463	Amikacin	IM	0.5 (S)	8	2.0	31.3 (±8.4 SD)	1–2	2.7 (±2.0 SD)	1–2	9	
Cephalosporins and related β-lactams											
374	Aztreonam	IV	2.0 (S)	14	1.7	20.0 (±10 SD)	1–2	6.6 (±6.0 SD)	1–2	33	U
535	Cefbuperazone	IV	1.0 (S)	13	1.7	96.7 (52–168)	0.5	26.1 (3.2–99)	0.5	27	U
504	Cefmenoxime	IV	1.0 (S)	6	1.1	22.4 (17–38)	0.9	10.1 (2–29)	0.9	45	U
402	Cefoperazone	IV	1.0 (M)	10	1.9	45.1 (±7.9 SE)	2.9	21.7 (±3.25 SE)	2.9	49	A
280	Ceforanide	IV	1.0 (S)	5	2.7	45 (±4 SD)	2.0	20 (±2 SD)	2.0	44	U, OC
280	Ceforanide	IV	1.0 (S)	4	2.7	38 (±4 SD)	2.0	21 (±2 SD)	2.0	55	U
513	Cefotaxime	IM	1.0 (M)	5	1.2	19.4 (9–48)	1.0	2.0 (0.6–5.0)	1.0	10	U, C
91	Cefpiramide	IV	1.0 (S)	10		157 (±21)	1.0	22.6 (±4.2)	1.0	14	
566	Ceftazidime	IV	1.0 (S)	20	1.7	24.9 (12.5–37.3)	1.75	21.3 (8.6–46.5)	1.75	86	U, F
399	Cefepime	IV	2.0 (M)	29	2.0	7.6 (0.4–62)	8.6	5.4 (0.4–28)	8.6	70	A
195	Ceftizoxime	IV	1.0 (S)	6	1.7	31 (±5.8 SD)	1.0	10.5 (±12 SD)	0.5–2.5	34	U
402	Ceftriaxone	IV	1.0 (M)	11	6.5	59.5 (±13 SE)	2.9	25.1 (±8.6 SE)	2.9	42	A
483	Cefuroxime	IV	0.75 (S)	5	1.3	46 (36–69)	0–0.8	12.1 (7.1–16.5)	0.3–1.7	26	F
119a	Meropenem	IV	1.0 (S)	33	1.2	27.3 (1.9–87.0)	0.5–1.5	3.2 (1.3–4.2)	0.5–1.5	12	AD
						4.8 (0.3–41.6)	3–5	0.9 (0.8–1.4)	3–5	19	

Penicillins											
287	Amoxicillin	IM	1.0 (S)	5	1.0	10.4 (8.6–12)	1.2–1.5	4.2 (3–6)	1.2–1.5	40	
573	Ampicillin/	IV	2.0 (S)	8	0.8	18.8 (±4.5 SD)	2	8.7 (±8.3 SD)	2	46	
	sulbactam	IV	1.0 (S)	8	1.0	10.7 (±3.5 SD)	2	4.7 (±1.4 SD)	2	44	
90	Piperacillin	IV	2.0 (S)	10	1.1	81.7 (±20.5 SD)	1.0	10.5 (±2.6 SD)	1.0	13	
591	Temocillin	IV	2.0 (M)	10	3.9	87.5 (34–126)	4	52.5 (28–97)	4	60	U, F
405	Ticarcillin/	IV	3.0 (S)	11	1.2	82 (±30 SD)	1.0–3.8	26 (±12)	1.0–3.8	32	U, F, E
	clavulanic acid	IV	0.2 (S)	11	1.1	2.0 (±1.0)	1.0–3.8	0.9 (±0.7)	1.0–3.8	45	
Tetracyclines											
370	Doxycycline	IV	0.2/0.1 (M)	15	20	3.0 (0.1–5.0)	20	5.4 (1.6–15.2)	20	180	U
157	Doxycycline	Oral	0.1 (M)	31	20	3.4	4–10	3.7 (1.4–8.7)	4–10	110	A
Others											
100	Clindamycin	IV	0.6 (S)	7	2.0	14.5 (9–26)	1.0	12 (5–44)		83	PD
100	Clindamycin	IV	0.6 (S)	5	2.0	11.3 (6–19)	1.0	6 (0–12)		53	OD
472	Clindamycin	Oral	0.3 (M)	6	2.0	1.6	2.0	1.7	2.0	106	F
472	Clindamycin	Oral	0.3 (M)	8	2.0	0.9	2.0	0.3	2.0	35	NF
75	Rifampin	Oral	0.15 (S)	4	2.5	1.4 (1.1–1.8)	3–5	1.8 (0.5–2.6)	3–5	129	
108	Trimethoprim	Oral	1.0 (S)	3	8–10	6.2 (3.0–8.2)	4	13.3 (7.1–19)	4	215	

[a] IM, intramuscularly; IV, intravenously.
[b] S, single dose; M, multiple dose.
[c] U, uninfected; A, acute cholecystitis; OC, obstructed cystic duct; C, corrected for hemoglobin; F, functioning gallbladder; E, extrapolated from graphical data; PD, patent duct; OD, obstructed duct; NF, nonfunctioning gallbladder.

TABLE 16.19

Antimicrobial Concentrations in Lung Tissue

Reference	Antimicrobial	Administration Method[a]	Dose (g) (Multiple or Single)[b]	*n*	Serum Half-life (h)	Serum Concentration Mean (μg/mL) (Range)	Time Serum Obtained (h)	Site Concentration Mean (μg/mL) (Range)	Time Site Specimen Obtained (h)	Ratio of Site/Serum (%)	Notes[c]
Aminoglycosides											
158	Amikacin	IM	0.5 (S)	10	2.0	20.7 (± 1.5 SE)	0.8–1.5	8.3 (± 1.0 SE)	0.8–1.5	40	SR
Cephalosporins and related β-lactams											
441	Cefadroxil	Oral	1.0 (S)	22	1.3	11.5 (± 1.3 SD)	2–4	7.4 (± 0.7 SD)	2–4	64	SR
128	Cefamandole	IV	2.0 (S)	6	0.7	23.1 (± 9.4 SD)	1–2	18.1 (± 9.7 SD)	1–2	78	SR, H
87b	Cefepime	IV	2.0 (M)		2.96	127.85 (± 27.51 SD)	0.5 (± 0.05 SD)	119.29[d] (± 4.89 SD)	0.5 (± 0.05 SD)	94	SR
122	Cefonicid	IM	1.0 (S)	5	4.5	92 (± 14 SD)	2.0	12 (± 2.4 SD)	2.0	13	SR
568	Cefoperazone	IV	2.0 (S)	10	2.4	97 (44–149)	2	45 (21–68)	2	46	SR, C
186	Cefotaxime	IM	1.0 (M)	6	1.2	5.1 (2.6–7.5)	3	19.5 (16.1–20.5)	3	382	SR
181	Cefotetan	IM	2.0 (S)	4	3.2	70.3 (54–84)	3	6.6 (4.2–9.1)	3	9	SR
416	Cefoxitin	IV	1.0 (S)	11	0.8	38.5 (26–55)	1	13.2 (8.8–2.3)	1	35	SR, C
37	Cefpirome	IV	1.0 (S)	37	2.0	34.5 (± 3.3 SE)	0.5–7	19.3 (± 1.9 SE)	0.5–7	56	T
268	Ceftriaxone	IV	2.0 (S)	13	6.5	127 (± 17.6 SD)	1–2	57.4 (± 13.3 SD)	1–2	45	SR
54	Imipenem	IV	1.0 (S)	10		20 (± 4)	1.0	12 (± 9)	1.0	60	SR, E
		IV	1.0 (S)	10	1.0	5.5	2.25	0.3 (± 0.1)	2.25	5	SR, E
Penicillins											
85	Amoxicillin	Oral	1.0 (S)	6	1.0	5.6 (4.9–6.9)	3	2.4 (1.9–2.9)	3	43	SR
104	Amoxicillin	Oral	0.5 (M)	10	1.0	3.3 (2.0–7.1)	3	3.1 (0.6–5.8)	3	94	SR
120	Amoxicillin/	Oral	0.5 (S)	15	1.1	6.9 (8.6)	1–2	3.0 (3.8)	1–2	32	T
	clavulanic acid	Oral	0.25 (S)	15	1.1	5.3 (9.3)	1–2	1.7 (3.7)	1–2	32	T
575	Amoxicillin/	IV	2.0 (S)	15	1.2	97 (± 9.5 SE)	0.5	39 (± 7.2 SE)	0.5	40	T
	sulbactam	IV	1.0 (S)	15	1.1	38 (± 3.8 SE)	0.5	28 (± 5.2 SE)	0.5	74	T
285	Flucloxacillin	IM	0.5 (S)	10	1.1	18.8 (13.2–22)	1.5–2.0	3.9 (3–5)	1.5–2.0	21	SR
285	Flucloxacillin	IM	0.5 (S)	4	1.1	16.2 (11.8–22)	2–2.2	2.4 (0.5–3.6)	2–2.2	15	SR, I

346	Piperacillin	IV	4.0 (M)	6	1.1	196.3 (119–296)	0.5–0.75	55.2 (17.1–98)	0.5–0.75	28	T
283	Piperacillin/	IV	2.0 (S)	6	1.3	36.4	1–2	33.4	1–2	92	SR
	tazobactam	IV	0.5 (S)	6	0.9	10.2	1–2	7.9	1–2	78	SR
284	Oxacillin	IM	0.5 (S)	9	0.5	11.9 (6.6–16.2)	1	2.4 (0.5–4.4)	1	20	SR
Quinolones											
453	Ciprofloxacin	Oral	0.75 (S)	10	4.0	2.0	3.4	4.9 (±1.7 SD)	3.4	275	T
		IV	0.20 (S)	10	4.0	0.9	0.9	4.1 (±1.9 SD)	0.9	624	T
Tetracyclines											
539	Doxycycline	IV	0.1 (M)	12	20	9.3 (3.2–16)	1	6.8 (2.5–12)	1	73	SR, C
387	Minocycline	Oral	0.1 (M)	15	14	0.8 (±0.4 SD)	13–20	3.0 (±1.4 SD)	13–20	364	SR
443	Tetracycline phosphate	Oral	0.5 (M)	6	10	3.9 (1.9–7.6)	>3	2.1 (0–3.6)	>3	54	SR, C
Others											
38	Azithromycin	Oral	0.5 (S)	20	30	0.13 (±0.05 SD)	12	3.9 (±1.2 SD)	48	3000	T
244	Clarithromycin	Oral	0.5 (M)	10	4.9	4.0 (±1.2 SE)	4.25	16.8 (±5.0 SE)	4.25	420	T
244	14-Hydroxy-clarithromycin	Oral		10	7.2	0.7 (±0.2 SE)	4.25	2.7 (±5.0 SE)	4.25	385	T
104	Erythromycin ethylsuccinate	Oral	1.0 (M)	19	1.5	0.7 (0.4–1.4)	3	4.2 (1.3–8.4)	3	547	SR
104	Erythromycin lactobionate	IV	0.5 (M)	11	1.5	1.5 (0.6–1.9)	3	6.5 (3.0–11.1)	3	462	SR
599	Erythromycin lactobionate	IV	0.27 (S)	5	0.7	7.3	0.3	5.5 (±2.2 SD)	02.–0.5	75	SR, I
177	Erythromycin stearate	Oral	0.5 (M)	14	1.5	3.1	2	4.7 (3.3–6.4)	3–4	152	SR
55	Flurithromycin	Oral	0.5 (M)	9	8.6	1.9	4	3.6	4	190	SR
159	Fosfomycin	IM	2.0 (S)	6	1.5	37.6 (±4.5 SE)	1.75–2.3	13.0 (±1.2 SE)	1.75–2.3	34	SR
159	Fosfomycin	IV	2.0 (S)	6	1.5	31.3 (±2.5 SE)	1.3–1.8	16.2 (±2.1 SE)	1.3–1.8	52	SR, I
286	Rifampin	Oral	0.6 (S)	8	3.0	6.4 (3–10)	2–3	2.1 (0.6–3.8)	2–3	33	SR
182	Roxithromycin	Oral	0.15 (M)	53	6.0	4.2 (±0.3 SD)	6	2.1 (±0.9 SD)	6	51	SR
288	Spiramycin	IV	0.5 (M)	6	5.5	0.31 (±0.03 SD)	3.0	1.2 (±0.14 SD)	3.0	371	SR
225	Trimethoprim	Oral	0.2 (M)	31	8–10	2.7 (0.7–11)	11–15	10.9 (2–34)	11–15	403	SR
225	Trimethoprim	Oral	0.2 (M)	14	8–10	3.0 (0.7–8.4)	11–15	16.4 (3.6–42)	11–15	547	SR, I

[a] IM, intramuscularly; IV, intravenously.

[b] S, single dose; M, multiple dose.

[c] SR, surgical resection; H, 2.5 g/100 mL hemoglobin contamination; C, corrected for hemoglobin contamination; T, transbronchial biopsy; E, extrapolated from graphical data; I, infected or inflamed lung tissue.

[d] Micrograms per gram.

TABLE 16.20

Antimicrobial Concentrations in Prostatic Tissue

Reference	Antimicrobial	Administration Method[a]	Dose (g) (Multiple or Single)[b]	n	Serum Half-life (h)	Serum Concentration Mean (μg/mL) (Range)	Time Serum Obtained (h)	Site Concentration Mean (μg/mL) (Range)	Time Site Specimen Obtained (h)	Ratio of Site/Serum (%)	Notes[c]
Aminoglycosides											
204b	Amikacin	IM	0.2 (S)	10	2–3	12.44 (9.4–18.5)	2.5–3	6.09 (2.6–10.8)	2.5–3	49	U, UR
178	Sagamicin	IM	0.060 (S)	4	1.3	3.65 (2.9–4.4)	2.2–2.6	3.08 (2.7–3.3)	2.2–2.6	85	U
576	Tobramycin	IM	0.080 (S)	22	2.0	2.8 (1.5–4.4)	0.75–2	2.7 (0.9–6)	0.75–2	96	U, T, B, UR
Cephalosporins and related β-lactams											
338	Aztreonam	IV	1.0 (S)	8	1.7	31.4 (18–46.3)	0.8–3	8 (1.7–12.1)	0.8–3	25	U, UR
505	Cefaclor	Oral	0.5 (M)	5	0.7	1.87 (0.6–5.0)	2	0.74 (0.24–1.94)	2	39	U, T, O
4	Cefamandole	IV	2.0 (S)	21	0.7	51 (18–70)	1	17.1 (8–43)	1	34	U, T, A
6	Cefazolin	IV	2.0 (S)	14	1.0	139.07 ($\pm$39.68)	0.5	34.63 $\pm$9.75	0.5	25	I, T
255	Cefazolin	IV or IM	1.0 (M or S)	22	2	38 ($\pm$20)	~0.9	14 $\pm$14	~0.9	37	U, T, UR
24	Cefepime	IV	2.0 (S)	5	2.2	60	1	30 (21–38)	1	51	U
474	Cefminoxime	IV	1.0 (S)	15		72.3 $\pm$21.1	1	7.4 $\pm$5.5	1	11	I
				21		72.0 $\pm$55.8	1	6.2 $\pm$3.5	1	9	U
362	Cefoperazone	IM	1.0 (M)	14	2.2	35.8 (4–67)	1.5	23.2 (4.7–44.7)	1.5	65	U
476	Cefotaxime	IV	2.0 (S)	25	1.2	45.2 (30–72)	1.5	22.9 (4–50)	1.5	51	U, T
207	Cefotaxime	IM	1.0 (M)	7	1.2	19.5 (11–30)	1–2	2.8 (1–4)	1–2	15	U, T, UR
475	Cefpirome	IV	1.0 (S)	6	3.0	50 $\pm$8	1–2	12 $\pm$5	1–2	28.5	U
572	Cefpodoxime	Oral	0.2 (S)	8	2.3	1.72 (0.72–2.77)	3	0.68 (0.41–1.23)	3	37	U
9	Cefsulodin	IV	2.0 (S)	10	1.5	55.3 (43–72)	0.5	30.25 (20–40)	0.5	55	U, T, A, UR
1	Ceftazidime	IV	2.0 (S)	4	1.9	73.3 ($\pm$12.3)	0.5–1.5	10.1 ($\pm$2.9)	0.5–1.5	14	U, UR
508	Ceftizoxime	IM	1.0 (S)	5	1.7	33.0 (29–43)	1–1.5	8.7 (5.7–15.1)	1–1.5	26	U
8	Ceftriaxone	IV	2.9 (S)	5	5.3	106.4 (73–158)	1.5	41.4 (11.7–75.4)	1.5	39	U, T, UR
12	Cefuroxime	IV	1.5 (S)	33	1.3	99.6 (40–210)	1	20.1 (6–35)	1	20	U, T, A

5	Cephacetrile	IV	2.0 (S)	19	0.9	65.8 (35.7–117.6)	1	8.5 (5.5–16.7)	1	13	U, T
524	Cephalexin	Oral	0.5 (S)	12	0.8	4.48 (0.17–16.55)	2–7	0.88 (0.09–3)	2–7	20	U, T
326	Cephalexin	Oral	0.5 (M)	17	0.8	∼6–10 (0–715)	0.75–2	<5 (0.5–10)	0.75–2		U, I
5	Cephalothin	IV	2.0 (S)	13	0.5	19.3 (10.4–21.7)	1	4.9 (1.3–7.2)	1	25	U, T
7	Cephapirin	IV	2.0 (S)	13	0.5	50 (20–98)	0.5	20.8 (6.3–56)	0.5	42	U, T, A
507	Moxalactam	IM	0.5 (M)	5	2.3	13.5 (5.1–17.8)	<1	4.0 (2.3–7.3)	<1	30	U, T, O
Penicillins											
339	Ampicillin	Oral	0.5 (M)	12	1.5	8.9 (1.0–20.5)	2–3	4.0 (0.6–6.9)	2–3	75	U, T, B
339	Ampicillin	Oral	0.5 (M)	12	1.5	6.7 (3.0–10.2)	2–3	3.7 (1.0–9.3)	2–3	73	U, T, B, H
292a	Ampicillin	IV	2.0 (S)	19	1.5	118 (± 48.9)	0.5	47.18 (0.4–548)	0.5	40	U, UR
506	Azlocillin	IV	2.9 (M)	8	1.0	64.9 (39.8–97)	1.0–2.0	22.9 (13–37)	1.0–2.0	35	U
506	Mezlocillin	IV	2.0 (M)	8	1.0	36.3 (11.8–49)	1.3–2.5	9.4 (2.4–19)	1.3–3.0	25	U
204b	Piperacillin	IV	1.0 (M)	9	1.3	5.70 (2.0–12.8)	2.5–3	1.28 (0.29–1.20)	2.5–3	21	U, UR
292a	Sulbactam	IV	1.0 (S)	19	1–1.3	32.2 (± 12.2)	0.5	19.7 (0.15–249)	0.5	61	U, UR
Quinolones											
246	Ciprofloxacin	IV	0.1 (S)	25	4.0	1.2 (0.9–1.8)	0.33–0.5	3.0 (1.1–4.6)	0.33	250	U
78	Ciprofloxacin	Oral	0.5 (S)	8	4.3	2.0 (1.1–2.3)	2–5	2.64 (1.1–5.5)	2–5	132	U
			0.5 (M)	8	4.3	1.5 (1.0–2.4)	2–6	3.6 (1.1–9.5)	6	240	U
193	Enoxacin	Oral	0.2 (M)	12	5.5	2.4 (± 0.35)	3.9	4.1 (± 1.18)	3.9	210	
278	Fleroxacin	Oral	0.4 (S)	11	12.0	3.7 (0.4–5.5)	1.3–4	4.4 (0.6–6.8)	1.3–4	112	U, UR
146a	Levofloxacin	Oral then IV	0.5 (M)	20	6–7	8	1	22	1	296	U, E
304	Lomefloxacin	Oral	0.4 (S)	20	8.0	2.4 (0.5–4.8)	3.5	5.4 (1.1–10.1)	3.5	225	U, T, UR
62	Norfloxacin	Oral	0.4 (M)	10	3.3	1.3 (<0.25–5.3)	1–2	1.6 (<0.25–4.65)	1–2	123	U, UR
193	Norfloxacin	Oral	0.4 (M)	9	3.3	1.45 (0.4–5.3)	1–2	1.74 (0.75–4.7)	1–2	120	
193	Ofloxacin	Oral	0.4 (S)	21	7.0	2.04 (± 1.16)	8.5–13	3.47 (± 1.35)	8.5–13	170	
200b	Pefloxacin	IV	0.8 (S)	10	3.8–5.6	5.67 (± 1.98)	6	3.36 (± 1.26)	6	59	U,T, UR

(continued)

TABLE 16.20 (Continued)

Antimicrobial Concentrations in Prostatic Tissue

Reference	Antimicrobial	Administration Method[a]	Dose (g) (Multiple or Single)[b]	*n*	Serum Half-life (h)	Serum Concentration Mean (μg/mL) (Range)	Time Serum Obtained (h)	Site Concentration Mean (μg/mL) (Range)	Time Site Specimen Obtained (h)	Ratio of Site/Serum (%)	Notes[c]
Tetracyclines											
183	Doxycycline	IV	0.200 (M)	5	20	1.1 (±0.27)	3	1.21 (±0.46)	3	110	U, T, B
157	Doxycycline	Oral	0.200 then 0.100	5	20	2.8	4–10	3.1 (1.8–8.2)	4–10	110	U, T
204b	Minocycline	Oral	0.1 (S)	9	11–20	2.05 (1.56–2.55)	2.5–3	1.82 (0.99–1.43)	2.5–3	94	U, UR
Others											
172	Azithromycin	Oral	0.25 (M)	14	56	<0.1	14	2.54	11–18	>2000	U
572	Carumonam	IV	1.0 (S)	4		29.0 (25–33.3)	1.3	5.7 (2.8–8.9)	1.3	20	U
200a	Clarithromycin	Oral	0.75 (M)	45	3–5	1.51 (±0.57)	7	3.83 (±2.14)	7	253	U, O
44	Erythromycin gluceptate	Oral	0.250 (M)	9	1.5	0.42 (0.23–1.16)	2	0.58 (0.14–1.05)	2	138	U, T, B, UR
179	Myocamicin	Oral	0.6 (S)	5		2.6 (1.7–3.4)	1.0	3.8 (2.7–4.2)	1.0	146	U
44	Rosamicin	Oral	0.250 (M)	9	3.1	0.07 (0.06–0.14)	2	2.4 (0.5–3.8)	2	3430	U, T, B, UR
333	Spiramycin	Oral	1.0 (M)	22	0.5	(0.3–0.7)	12–15	~9.0 (7–13)	12–15	1800	U, T
401	Sulfamethoxazole	IM	0.400 (S)	6	11.0	17.8 (12.1–23.2)	4	5.19 (3.2–6.51)	4	29	U, T, O, B
401	Sulfamethoxazole	Oral	0.800 (S)	5	11.0	26.2 (2.3–32.9)	4	7.11 (0.45–13.4)	4	27	U, T, O, B
401	Sulfamethoxazole	Oral	0.800 (M)	8	11.0	65.9 (40–108)	4	34.9 (19–64)	4	53	U, T, O, B
430	Thiamphenicol	IV	1.0 (S)	11	1.5	20.7 (9.6–35)	0.8	32.1 (8.5–64.4)	0.8	191	U, T, O, A
401	Trimethoprim	IM	0.080 (S)	6	14.5	0.40 (0.22–0.51)	4	1.55 (0.81–2.5)	4	387	U, T, O, B
401	Trimethoprim	Oral	0.160 (S)	5	14.5	0.98 (0.4–1.3)	4	2.84 (0.47–5. 0)	4	290	U, T, O, B
401	Trimethoprim	Oral	0.160 (S)	8	14.5	2.39 (0.7–3.0)	4	5.54 (4.1–27)	4	232	U, T, O, B

[a] IM, intramuscularly; IV, intravenously.
[b] S, single dose; M, multiple dose.
[c] U, uninfected; UR, transurethral resection of prostate; T, prostate tissue; B, benign; O, open prostatectomy; A, prostate adenoma; I, infected; H, hetacillin ester given to patients, ampicillin measured in serum and tissue; E, extrapolated from graphs.

TABLE 16.21

Antimicrobial Concentrations within Cells

Reference	Antimicrobial	Cell Type[a]	*n*	Extracellular Concentration (μg/mL)[b]	Time of Incubation (h)	Cellular Concentration (μg/mL)[c]	C/E Ratio (%)	Notes[d]
Aminoglycosides								
222	Gentamicin	PMN	9	25 μmol/L	1–3	R	73–74	SO
555	Gentamicin	PMN		8	1	1.8	21	CW
555	Netilmicin	PMN		10	1	1.8	17	CW
Cephalosporins and related β-lactams								
223	Cefamandole	PMN	2	R	2	R	<1	SO
223	Cefamandole	AM	2	R	2	R	79 ± 49 SE	SO
221	Cefamandole	MN	6	R	0.5	R	130 ± 30 SE	SO
221	Cefazolin	PMN	2	10	2	<1	<10	SO
221	Cefotaxime	MN	3	R	0.5	R	110 ± 30	SO
256	Cefotaxime	PMN	6	R	2	R	34 ± 8 SD	SO
394	Cefoxitin	RBC	1	5 μmol/L	0.3		3	CL
296	Cefpimizole	PMN	4	50	0.5	<0.5[c]	<1	SO
296	Ceftazidime	PMN	4	50	0.5	28[c]	56 + 13 SE	SO
296	Ceftizoxime	PMN	4	50	0.5	45[c] >	90 ± 5 SE	SO
257	Ceftriaxone	PMN	6	R	2	R	38 ± 23 SD	SO
437	Cephalexin	PMN	1	10	2	5.5	55	SO
300	Cephalexin	RBC		R	3	R	1.2–3.7	CW, P
223	Cephalexin	PMN	1	R	2	R	57	SO
300	Cephalothin	RBC		R	3	R	1–1.3	CW, P
257	Imipenem	PMN	6	R	2	R	33 ± 14 SD	SO
Penicillins								
99	Ampicillin	KF	5	31	72	1.8	6	CL
99	Ampicillin	PMN		100	3	7.7	7.7	CL
393	Ampicillin	RBC		100	3	4.1	4.1	CW

(continued)

TABLE 16.21 (Continued)

Antimicrobial Concentrations within Cells

Reference	Antimicrobial	Cell Type[a]	n	Extracellular Concentration (μg/mL)[b]	Time of Incubation (h)	Cellular Concentration (μg/mL)[c]	C/E Ratio (%)	Notes[d]
367	Benzylpenicillin	PMN		10	0.3	<7[c]	<70	SO
393	Cloxacillin	RBC		100	3	32.5	32.5	CW
393	Dicloxacillin	RBC		100	3	35.3	35.3	CW
393	Flucloxacillin	RBC		100	3	37.0	37.0	CW
393	Oxacillin	RBC		100	3	30.5	30.5	CW
555	Oxacillin	PMN		20	1	<2	<10	CW
222	Penicillin G	PMN	9–11	25 μmol/L	1–3	R	37–38	SO
300	Penicillin G	RBC	5	2.5–7.2	3	5–6.3	80–240	CW, P
573	Penicillin G	AM	3	R	0.8	R	58 ± 6 SD	CW
437	Penicillin G	MN	4	R	0.5	R	80 ± 20 SE	SO
296	Piperacillin	PMN	4	50	0.5	<5[c]	<10	SO
393	Propicillin	RBC		100	3	19.4	19.4	CW
Quinolones								
151	Ciprofloxacin	PMN	2	20	1	120–140[c]	600–700	SO
296	Ciprofloxacin	PMN	3	50	0.5	175[c]	349	SO
432	Ciprofloxacin	AM	6	10	0.5	81[c]	810 ± 110 SD	
555	Enoxacin	PMN		20	1	72	360	CW
432	Fleroxacin	PMN	3	10	0.5	20[b]	200 ± 10 SD	
20a	Garenoxacin	AM	6	10.03 (± 2.8)	3.26 (± 0.34)	106.13 (± 60.25)	1,058	
243	Gatifloxacin	AM	5	3.95[c]	2	69.1 (50.8–112.5)	1,749 (approx.)	
204a	Levofloxacin	AM	4	5.29 (± 1.23)	4	97.9 (± 80)	1,850	
511	Moxifloxacin	AM	17	3.22 (± 1.25)	2.2	56.7 (± 1.61)	1,761	
296	Norfloxacin	PMN	3	50	0.5	112[c]	224	SO
296	Ofloxacin	PMN	4	50	0.5	408[c]	815	SO
432	Ofloxacin	AM	3	10	0.5	71[c]	710 ± 30 SD	

296	Pefloxacin	PMN	3	50	0.5	145[c]	290	SO
432	Pefloxacin	AM	6	10	0.5	69[c]	690 ± 170 SD	
491	Pefloxacin	RBC	10	6.0	12	1.7[c]	26	CW, N, E
Others								
555	Ansamycin	PMN		10	1	94.6	940	CW
203	Azithromycin	PMN	4	10	2	790	7,900	CW
574	Azithromycin	PMN	12	4	0.66	1,192[c]	29,800 ± 9,700	SO
574	Azithromycin	MN	3	4	0.66	800[c]	20,000 ± 700 SD	SO
574	Azithromycin	AM	3	4	0.66	2,672[c]	66,800 ± 19,800 SD	SO
574	Azithromycin	RBC	3	4	0.66	16[c]	400 ± 100 SD	SO
296	Chloramphenicol	PMN	4	50	0.5	482[c]	964 ± 59 SE	SO
300	Chloramphenicol	RBC		R	3	R	6.9–40.1	CW, P
223	Chloramphenicol	AM	2	R	2	R	200 ± 30 SE	SO
437	Chloramphenicol	MN	4	R	0.5	R	290 ± 40 SE	SO
300	Chloroquine	RBC		R	3	R	19.6–73.3	CW, P
20	Clarithromycin	PMN	3	2	0.5	18[c]	920 ± 200 SE	SO
437	Clindamycin	PMN	9	10	2	110.8	1,108 ± 108 SE	SO
258	Clindamycin	CGD	2	R	2	R	818 ± 124 SE	SO
518	Clindamycin	PMN	7	10	1	111.5	1,115 ± 120 SE	SO
223	Clindamycin	AM	7	R	1–2	R	2,073–5,610	SO
437	Clindamycin	MN	30	R	0.5	R	610 ± 40 SE	SO
413	Clindamycin	RM	7	10	0.33	69[c]	690 ± 40 SE	SO
292	Clindamycin	RBC	2	10	0.17	10.4	104 ± 24 SE	SO
112	Erythromycin	PMN	19	10	0.5	80[a]	800 ± 100 SD	CW
43	Dirithromycin	AM	9	0.35		0.37	106	CL
223	Erythromycin (nonsmoker)	AM	2	R	2	R	1,770 ± 640 SE	SO
112	Erythromycin	AM	4	10	0.5	460[c]	4,600 ± 400 SD	CW
437	Erythromycin	MN	17	R	0.5	R	420 ± 40 SE	SO
124	Erythromycin	RM	10	2	1	14[c]	700	CL
124	Erythromycin	RM	10	10	1	17[c]	170	CL

(continued)

TABLE 16.21 (Continued)

Antimicrobial Concentrations within Cells

Reference	Antimicrobial	Cell Type[a]	*n*	Extracellular Concentration (μg/mL)[b]	Time of Incubation (h)	Cellular Concentration (μg/mL)[c]	C/E Ratio (%)	Notes[d]
124	Erythromycin	RM	10	20	1	26[a]	130	CL
223	Erythromycin propionate	PMN	5	19.8	2	206.3	1,042 ± 88 SE	SO
223	Erythromycin propionate	AM	8	R	1–2	R	1,588–2,810	SO
223	Ethambutol	AM	8	R	1–2	R	438–486	SO
518	Ethambutol	PMN	6	6.9	2	33.3	483 ± 39 SE	SO
99	Fusidic acid	KF	5	36	72	35.9	99	CL
99	Fusidic acid	PMN		40	3	16	40	CL
296	Isoniazid	PMN	4	50	0.5	53[c]	106 ± 24 SE	SO
223	Isoniazid	AM	7	R	1–2	R	64–155	SO
573	Josamycin	PMN	13	R	0.75	R	2,080 ± 540 SD	CW
573	Josamycin	MN	3	R	0.75	R	2,070 ± 160 SD	CW
573	Josamycin	AM	3	R	0.75	R	2,280 ± 150 SD	CW
573	Josamycin	RBC	3	R	0.75	R	330 ± 50 SD	CW
296	Lincomycin	PMN	3	50	0.5	151[c]	310 ± 34 SE	SO
223	Lincomycin	AM	4	R	1–2	R	285–288	SO
119b	Linezolid	AC	5	10.2 (± 2.3)	12	1.4 (± 1.3)	13.7	C
222	Metronidazole	PMN	3	R	0.02–1	R	85–103	SO
221	Metronidazole	MN	4	R	0.33	R	60 ± 10 SE	SO
300	Minocycline	RBC		R	3	R	212–410	CW
300	Minocycline	RBC		R	3	R	10.2–15	CW, P
300	Nitrofurantoin	RBC		R	3	R	1.8–5.5	CW, P
296	Pipemidic acid	PMN	4	50	0.5	275[c]	550 ± 52 SE	SO
150	Rifampicin	PMN		10	1	7[b]	70	SO
296	Rifampin	PMN	4	50	0.5	412[a]	823 ± 78 SE	SO

240	Rifampin (quinone form)	CGD PMN	2–3	R	0–0.5	R	600–1,376	SO
240	Rifampin (hydroquinone form)	PMN	10–13	R	0–0.5	R	300–882	SO
240	Rifampin (hydroquinone form)	CGD PMN	1	R	0.1–0.5	R	1,150–1,429	SO
223	Rifampin	AM	10	R	1–2	R	522–978	SO
150	Rifapentine	PMN		10	1	37[c]	370	SO
112	Roxithromycin (nonsmoker)	PMN	19	10	0.5	140[c]	1,400 ± 300 SD	CW
112	Roxithromycin (smoker)	AM	3	10	0.5	610[c]	6,100 ± 700 SD	CW
112	Roxithromycin	AM	4	10	0.5	1,900[c]	19,000 ± 2,100 SE	CW
222	Roxithromycin	PMN	13–37	R	0.02–1	R	375–3,383	SO
221	Roxithromycin	MN	18	R	0.5	R	1,390 ± 160 SE	SO
124	Roxithromycin	RM	10	20	1	26[c]	130	CL
73	Sulfonamides	RBC	40	10–30		10–30	80–200	CW
337	Teicoplanin	PMN	5	75	0.33	4,700 ± 300 SE	6,000 ± 1,300 SE	SO
380a	Telithomycin	AM	6	0.63 (0.42–0.72)	8	81 (56–166)	12,857	
413	Teicoplanin (peritoneal)	RM	7	6	0.33	408	4,080 ± 360 SE	SO
99	Tetracycline	KF	5	10	72	35	350	CL
99	Tetracycline	PMN		17.5	3	13	74	CL
300	Tetracycline	RBC		R	3	R	210–248	CW
223	Tetracycline	AM	6	R	1–2	R	241–449	SO
573	Tinidazole	PMN	4	50	0.8	71.5	143 ± 17 SD	CW
258	Trimethoprim	PMN	9	R	2	R	44 ± 11 SE	SO
258	Trimethoprim	CGD PMN	3	R	2	R	38 ± 11 SE	SO
296	Trimethoprim	PMN	3	50	0.33	305[c]	610 ± 63 SE	SO
221	Trimethoprim	MN	9	R	0.5	R	300 ± 50 SE	SO
555	Vancomycin	PMN		20	1	24.6	122	CW

[a] PMN, polymorphonuclear leukocyte; AM, alveolar macrophage; MN, monocyte; RBC, red blood cell; KF, kidney fibroblast; CGD PMN, polymorphonuclear leukocytes from subjects with chronic granulomatous disease; RM, resident macrophage; AC, alveolar cells.
[b] R, radiolabelled drug only.
[c] Calculated values.
[d] SO, centrifugation through silicone oil; R, radiolabeled drug only; CW, centrifugation and washing; CL, cell lysis; P, in plasma medium suspension; N, normal volunteers; E, estimated from 400-mg dose; C, cirrhotic patients.

killing of bacteria by antimicrobials, but more work is needed.

In general, the cephalosporins and penicillins have been shown to have limited access to the intracellular space, with cellular/extracellular (C/E) ratios much less than 1, whereas agents such as clindamycin, azithromycin, clarithromycin, and erythromycin demonstrated C/E ratios of 10:1 to 40:1 and more. However, much of this work was done with a low-protein tissue culture suspension medium, and Berneis and Boguth (73) as well as Kornguth and Kunin (300) demonstrated that addition of protein to the cellular suspension markedly decreased antimicrobial entry into cells. Nishida et al. (393) also correlated the penetration of penicillins into red cells *in vitro* with the extent of protein binding of these agents. Finally, and most contradictory to the *in vitro* studies, Kornguth and Kunin (300) demonstrated much greater penetration of penicillin G (C/E ratio of more than 1) when the drug was given intravenously and exposed to red cells *in vivo* than when the testing was done strictly *in vitro*. Particularly noteworthy is the high C/E ratio of most quinolones rated in these systems. These agents are generally not bound to serum proteins to any significant extent, and the C/E ratio observed may correspond to true accumulation of these agents. Studies of intracellular penetration of drugs must be interpreted cautiously until additional, more-definitive studies are performed, but efficacy of fluoroquinolones and macrolides against intracellular pathogens such as *Legionella* suggests that intracellular drug concentration is an important determinant of clinical success.

INTERPRETATION OF SERUM CONCENTRATIONS OF ANTIMICROBIALS

Interpretation of antimicrobial serum or plasma concentration data requires a basic understanding of the principles that govern pharmacokinetics: absorption, distribution, metabolism, and excretion of drug. In addition, method of administration, number of dosage administrations prior to sample collection, and timing of the sample collection with respect to the previous dose are equally important factors to consider when comparing data (156,463,564). Figure 16.2 depicts theoretical serum concentration data, using a two-compartment open simulation model, following a single 1-g dose of an antimicrobial by four different methods: intravenous bolus (1-minute infusion), 30-minute intravenous infusion, oral, and intramuscular administration. The apparent volume of distribution, bioavailability (100%), rate of elimination, and transfer rate constants between the central and peripheral compartments were all held constant in order to show just how different theoretical concentration-time curves may look when only one of these variables (administration) is altered.

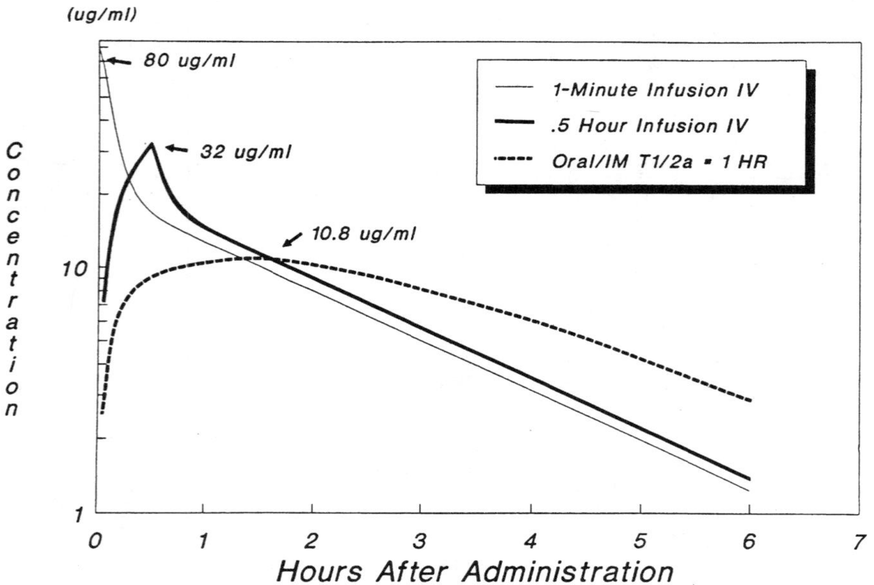

FIGURE 16.2 ● Serum kinetics of a single 1-g dose of an antimicrobial given by intravenous (*IV*) bolus infusion, 0.5-hour IV infusion, oral administration, or intramuscular (*IM*) injection. An absorption half-life ($T_{1/2a}$) of 1 hour was assumed for the oral and intramuscular administrations.

Absorption

Absorption is the process by which antibiotic transfers from the site of administration (such as intravenous, intramuscular, oral, topical) into the general circulation (central compartment) of the body, and it ranges from 0% to 100%. Percentage bioavailability (Table 16.22) is simply 100 times the ratio of the amount of active antibiotic (A) reaching the general circulation to the amount administered (dose).

$$\text{Percentage bioavailability} = 100 \times A/\text{dose}$$

For most antimicrobials administered intravenously or intramuscularly, percentage bioavailability is 100%. However, some, such as chloramphenicol succinate, are in an inactive form when given parenterally and the actual percentage bioavailability may be less than 100% because of partial conversion. Absorption from oral administration is less than 100% for most antimicrobials; therefore, the area under the serum concentration-time curve following oral administration is less than that following parenteral administration, with all other variables held constant. Percentage bioavailability refers only to the extent of absorption; it gives no indication of how rapidly the antimicrobial is absorbed and does not account for protein binding.

Rate of Administration

Difficulty in interpreting differences in concentration with various routes of administration is often attributed to the respective rates of antimicrobial administration. Generally, intravenous administration is achieved through a zero-order process (constant rate of administration over time) and intramuscular and oral administrations are thought to follow a first-order process (Fick's law of passive diffusion). Intramuscular and oral absorption rates are also influenced by a number of local factors, such as pH, gastrointestinal motility, dosage form, food, and muscle perfusion, to mention a few, each of which may be significant. As a result, peak serum concentration following intramuscular or oral administration tends to be lower and less predictable than that after intravenous administration. Again, the simulations in Figure 16.2, in which the oral and intramuscular half-life of drug absorption ($T_{1/2a}$) was held constant (1 hour) and the intravenous rates differ, show the effects observed by simply changing the rate of antibiotic administration.

Distribution

Once the antibiotic reaches the general circulation (central compartment), the antibiotic begins to diffuse into other body spaces and tissues (peripheral compartments) not at equilibrium with the central compartment (Fig. 16.1). This process is often referred to as distribution, and the time period during which this is most evident on the serum concentration-time curve is often referred to as the distribution phase or α-phase. Although distribution takes place following all forms of antimicrobial administration, the distribution phase is most apparent immediately following intravenous bolus or short infusion, which makes timing of sample collection most critical for concentration comparisons. The distribution phase of the serum concentration-time curve is generally short-lived (less than 1 hour); however, minor differences in the time of serum sample collection during the distribution phase may result in major differences in antimicrobial concentrations and therefore interpretation. Because of the difficulty in timing and collecting samples in and around the distribution phase of the curve, peak serum concentration data reported in the literature are often conflicting and misleading. The distribution phase for most antibiotics is of brief duration and is difficult to characterize. In order to avoid confusion and subsequent misinterpretation, many authors choose not to sample during the distribution phase but rather report the time at which serum samples for determination of antibiotic concentration were obtained following antibiotic administration. Data on achievable serum concentrations in Table 16.22 are presented with the time at which samples were obtained. In general, intravenous administration results in serum concentrations that are greater than those following oral or intramuscular administration and are most vulnerable to misinterpretation due to the distribution phase.

Elimination

Elimination is the loss of active antibiotic from the body and is due to excretion and/or metabolism. Excretion is the loss of unchanged antibiotic, and metabolism is the loss due to conversion of the antibiotic to another chemical compound (metabolite). Metabolites may or may not have antimicrobial activity. For most antibiotics, elimination is a first-order process, which simply means that serum concentration declines exponentially with time:

$$C_t = C \times e^{-k}{}_{el} \times t$$

where C is serum concentration, C_t is the serum concentration at some time t after C was determined, and k_{ef} is an elimination rate constant. With first-order elimination, the time for the serum concentration to decline by one half (half-life) is constant:

$$t_{1/2} = (\ln 2)/k_{el}$$

where $t_{1/2}$ is the serum half-life and k_{ef} is the elimination rate constant. Knowing the serum half-life, one can then estimate the fraction of the dose that remains in the body at any time after the dose was given:

$$\text{Fraction remaining} = e^{-0.693n}$$

where n is the number of half-lives that have elapsed since the dose was administered.

(*text continues on page 791*)

TABLE 16.22

Serum Kinetics and Urinary Excretion of Antimicrobials in Humans

Antimicrobial	Dosage/Route[a]	Sampling Time[b]	Serum Concentration (μg/mL)[c]	Half-life (h)		Protein Binding (%)	Renal Excretion Unchanged (%)	Bioavailability (%)[e]
				Normal	ESRD[d]			
Amikacin	7.5 mg/kg IM	1 h	21	2–3	30	0–5	>90	T1
	7.5 mg/kg IV	0.5 h	15–25					
Amoxicillin	0.5 g orally	2 h	8	0.8–2	7–20	20	60–98	80 F
Amoxicillin/clavulanic acid	0.5 g orally/0.5 g orally	1 h	7.6/2.3	0.8–2/0.8–1	7–20	20/22–30	60–98/28–47	80 F
Ampicillin	0.5 g orally	1 h	2	0.8–1.8	7–20	17–20	79–92	50 F
	0.5 g IM	1 h	8					
Ampicillin/sulbactam	0.5 g IV/0.5 g IV	1 h	14/20	0.8–1.8/1–1.3	7–20/21	17–20/21	17–20/38	79–92/75
Azithromycin	0.5 g orally	2–4 h	0.3–0.63	35–60		12–50[f]	4–12	37 F
Azlocillin	2 g IV	5 min	142–363	0.8–1.5	5–6	30–46	50–75	
Aztreonam	1 g IV (0.5-h infusion)		125	1.6–1.7	8.4		65–94	
	1 g IM	1 h	46.5					
Bacampicillin	0.4 g orally	1 h	2.7	0.8–1.5	6–20	17–20	79–92	87–98
Carbenicillin	1 g IM	0.5–2 h	15–20	1.1	10–20	50	80–90	
	1 g IV	0.25 h	71–140					
(Indanyl salt)	0.382 g orally	0.5–1 h	5.1–6.5					30
Cefaclor	1 g orally	0.5–1 h	23	0.5–1	2.8	25	>90	70–100 F
Cefaclor MR	0.75 g orally	2.9 h	9.1 (±1.8 SD)	1.2		25	71	>90
Cefadroxil	1 g orally	1–2	28–35	1.2–1.7	20–25	20	>90	80–100 F
Cefamandole	1 g IM	0.5–2 h	25	0.5–1	7.9–18	56–80	75–100	
	1 g IV	10 min	140					
Cefazolin	1 g IM	1 h	60	1.4–2.5	18–36	70–85	90–96	
	1 g IV	5 min	190					
Cefdinir	0.3 g orally	224* min	2.00*					
	0.6 g orally	223* min	4.20*					

Cefepime	1 g IM	0.5–1.5 h	30–74	2	13.5	16–19	99	
	1 g IV		67					
Cefepime	2 g IV (M)	0.5 h (± 0.05 SD)	127.85 (± 27.51 SD)		2.96			
Cefetamet	1 g orally	3–5 h	5.5–6.5	2–2.5	11–30	22	90	30–50 F
Cefixime	0.2 g orally	2–6 h	1–4	3–9	11.5	65–69	20–50	50
Cefmenoxime	1 g IM	40 h	27	0.9–1.6	6–26	77–84	67–86	
	1 g IV	2 min	100					
Cefmetazole	30 mg/kg IM	0.5–0.75	80	0.8–1.8	15	68	71	
	30 mg/kg IV	h	97					
		1 h						
Cefodizime	1 g IM	1 h	75	2.5–3.7	7.7	81	69–95	88–100
	1 g IV		177–215					
Cefonicid	1 g IM	1 h	99	3.5–4.8	65	95–98	90–99	
	1 g IV	5 min	220					
Cefoperazone	1 g IM	1 h	63	1.6–2.4	2.1–2.5	82–93	75–99	
	1 g IV	5 min	200					
Ceforanide	1 g IM	1 h	70–80	2.2–3.5	25	80	85–95	
	1 g IV	0.25 h	140					
Cefotaxime	1 g IM	0.5 h	21–25	1	2.6	35–51	40–60	
	1 g IV	5 min	100			(active metabolite)		
Cefotetan	1 g IM	1.5 h	75	3–4.6	10–20	78–91	66–100	
	1 g IV	2 min	140–240					
Cefotiam	1 g IV	0.25 h	77.6	0.6–1.5	5.3	62	50–67	
	1 g IM	0.75 h	13.5					
Cefoxitin	1 g IM	0.5 h	24–28	0.7–1	13–22	65–79	85–90	
	1 g IV	5 min	110					
Cefpirome	1 g IM	1.5 h	32	2	14.5	10	80–90	92–98
	1 g IV	5 min	80–100					
Cefpodoxime	0.2 g orally	2–3 h	2.5	2.5	9.8	18–23	80	41–50 FE
Cefprozil	1 g orally	1–2 h	18	1–2	6	35–45	89–95	
Cefsulodin	1 g IM	1.5 h	20	1.7–2	10–13	15–30	50–70	
Ceftazidime	1 g IM	1 h	40	1.4–2	19–24	5–17	75–90	
	1 g IV	5 min	105					

(continued)

TABLE 16.22 (Continued)

Serum Kinetics and Urinary Excretion of Antimicrobials in Humans

Antimicrobial	Dosage/Route[a]	Sampling Time[b]	Serum Concentration (μg/mL)[c]	Half-life (h)		Protein Binding (%)	Renal Excretion Unchanged (%)	Bioavailability (%)[e]
				Normal	ESRD[d]			
Ceftibuten	0.2 g orally	2–3 h	11.6	1.5–2.5	18–29	65–77		80
Ceftizoxime	1 g IM	1 h	40	1.4–1.7	30–36	30–50	85–95	
	1 g IV	5 min	113					
Ceftriaxone	1 g IM	1 h	62–83	7.7–8.6	12–18	83–95	65–95	
	1 g IV (0.5-h infusion)	5 min	100–175					
Cefuroxime	1 g IM	1 h	40	1.1–2.2	15–22	33–50	95	
Cefuroxime	0.5 g IV		42–66					
Cefuroxime axetil	1 g orally	1.8 h	11					36–50 FE
Cephalexin	1 g orally	1 h	32	0.9	20–40	15	91–100	90–100 F
Cephaloridine	1 g IM	0.5–1 h	30	1–1.5	3–11	20	70–85	
Cephalothin	1 g IM	0.5 h	20	0.5–1	3–19	65–80	50–70	
	1 g IV	2 min	30					
Cephapirin	1 g IM	0.5–1 h	10–17	0.3–0.8	1.75–2.5	45–50	30–70	
	1 g IV	5 min	70			(also active metabolite)		
Cephradine	0.5 g orally	1 h	11–16.6	0.6–0.7		8–17	80–100	90–100 F
	1 g IM	1 h	4.4–14					
	1 g IV	5 min	60–86					
Chloramphenicol base	1 g orally	0.5–4 h	10–13	1.6–4	3.2–7	50–60	5–15 (base)	76–93
Chloramphenicol succinate	1 g IV	0.5–1 h	4.9–12					70 IS
Chloramphenicol succinate	1 g IM	5–6						
Chloramphenicol palmitate								80
Cinoxacin	0.5	2–4 h	10.8 ± 5.7	1.1–2.7	8.5–12.1	63–73	60	F
Ciprofloxacin	0.5 g orally	1–2 h	1.9–2.9	3–6	6–8.7	40	30–50	60–80 F
	0.1 g IV							

Clarithromycin	0.25 g orally	2	0.58–0.8	3–5[h]		42–50	20–30	50 F
Clindamycin	0.15 g orally	1 h	2–3	2–4	3–5	60–95		90
	0.3 g IM	1–3 h	6					
	0.6 g IV		10					
Cloxacillin	0.5 g orally	1–2 h	2–9	0.5	1–3	95	70–90	50–77 F
Colistin	2 mg/kg IM	1–2	5–13	2.7–4.8	48–72		>75	
Cyclacillin	0.5 g orally	1 h	11–12	0.5–0.6	8–10	18–25	65–85	95
Daptomycin	4 mg/kg IV	0.5 h	77.5** (± 8.3 SD)**		7.74 (± 0.63 SD)	90%	59.7 (± 10.2 SD)	
Demeclocyline	0.3 g orally	4 h	1–2	10–15		41–90	38–56	F
Dicloxacillin	1 g orally	1 h	10–15	0.5	1–2	88–98	60–90	50
	0.25 g IM	1 h	5					
Dirithromycin[i]	0.5 g orally	4–4.5 h	01–0.5; E,[j] 0.3	E,[j] 20–50		E,[j] 15–30	<5	6–14 FE
Dirithromycin	0.5 g orally (M)	24 h	0.17 (± 0.03 SD)					
Doxycycline	1.2 g orally	2 h	2–3	12–22	16–24	80–95	35–40	90
	0.2 g IV	0.25 h	6.4					
Erythromycin	0.5 g orally		0.3–1.9	1.2–2.6	4–6	75–90	2–15	F
Erythromycin estolate ester	0.5 g orally		4 (80% ester)					
Erythromycin ethylsuccinate ester	0.5 g orally		1.5 (66% ester)					
Erthromycin stearate	0.5 g orally	3 h	0.13–1.3 (base)					F
Erythromycin lactobionate	1 g IV	1 h	10					
Erythromycin gluceptate	1 g IV	1 h	9.9					
Enoxacin	0.4 g orally	1–6 h	2.8–3.6	3.4–6.4	30	18–30	26–72	80–98
Fleroxacin	0.4 g orally	1–2 h	4.4–6.8	8–13		23–32	50–77	>95
Floxacillin	0.5 g orally	1 h	11–20	0.75–1.5		92–94	40–70	50–54 F
Garenoxacin	0.6 g orally	3.26 h	10.03** (2.80 SD)					
Gatifloxacin	0.4 g orally	1.8 h	4.1** (± 0.86 SD)		6.8 (± 0.72 SD)	20%	65 (± 15 SD)	
Gemifloxacin	0.32 g orally	1.2 h	2.31** (± 0.55 SD)		5.9 (+ 0.44 SD)		36.1 (± 7.5 SD)	
Gentamicin	1 mg/kg IM		4	1–3	24–48	0–5	>90	TI
	1.5 mg/kg IV	0.5 h	4–8					
Imipenem/cilastitin	1 g IV (0.5-h infusion)		19–60	0.9–1.3	3	13–25	5–42	
Josamycin	0.5 g orally	1 h	0.65	0.9–2		15	<20	F
Kanamycin	7.5 mg/kg IM	1 h	22	2–3	27–30	0–5	>90	TI
	7.5 mg/kg IV	0.5 h	20–25					

(continued)

TABLE 16.22 (Continued)

Serum Kinetics and Urinary Excretion of Antimicrobials in Humans

Antimicrobial	Dosage/Route[a]	Sampling Time[b]	Serum Concentration (μg/mL)[c]	Half-life (h)		Protein Binding (%)	Renal Excretion Unchanged (%)	Bioavailability (%)[e]
				Normal	ESRD[d]			
Latamoxef	0.5 g IV	15 min	42	2–2.8	19.3	52	67–87	
	1 g IM	0.5–1 h	52					
Levofloxacin	0.1 g orally	1 h	1.4–1.8	6–7		50	61–86	>95 F
Levofloxacin	0.5 g orally (M)	4 h	5.29** (±1.23 SD)					
	0.75 g orally (M)	4 h	11.98** (±2.99 SD)					
Lincomycin	0.5 g orally	2–4 h	6–12	4–5	10–20	70–80	10–70	20–30 F
	0.6 g IM	1–2 h	12–20					
	0.6 g IV							
Linezolid	0.6 g orally (M)	4 h	15.5** (±4.9 SD)	6.9				
Lomefloxacin	0.4 g orally	1–2 h	3.5–4.7	6.4–7.7	21–38	20	57–76	F
Loracarbef	0.2 g orally	1 h	8	0.7–1.2			59–66	90
Mecillinam	10 mg/kg IV	0 h	32–70	1	3–6	5–10	65	
(amdinocillin)	10 mg/kg IM	0.5 h	26					
Meropenem	1 g IV (S)	0.5 h	25.96** (±22.16 SD)					
Methicillin	1 g IM	0.5 h	10–15	0.5–1	4	28–49	62–80	
	1 g IV		60					
Metronidazole	0.5 g orally	1–2 h	12	6–12	8–15	<20	20	>80
Mezlocillin	1 g IM	0.75–1 h	15.4	0.7–1.1	2.5–5.5	45	61–72	
	1 g IV	5 min	64–142					
Minocycline	0.2 g IV (0.5–1-h infusion)	5 min	2.5–6.6	11–20	17–69	60–75	10–13	
	0.2 g orally	1 h	0.7–4.4					90 F
Moxalactam	1 g IM	1–2 h	27	1.7–2.3	18–23	35–50	67–90	
	1 g IV	0.25 h	101					

Moxifloxacin	0.4 g orally (S)	2.2 h	3.22 (± 1.25 SD)					
Nafcillin	1 g IM	1 h	8	0.5–1	1.5	87–90	31–40	10–20
Nalidixic acid	1 g orally	1 h	15–50	6–7	21		0.5–30	F
Netilmicin	1 mg/kg IM		4	2.7	40	0–5	>90	TI
	2 mg/kg IV	0.5 h	7					
Nitrofurantoin	0.1 g orally		<2	0.3–1	1	90	27–56	80–95 D, FE
Norfloxacin	0.4 g orally	1–1.5 h	1.5	2–4	8.34	10–15	12–30	30–40
Ofloxacin	0.3 g orally	1–2 h	2.8–5.3	5–7.5		20	41	96
Oritavancin	0.2 g orally (M)	1.0	46.2** (± 10.7 SD)	151 (± 39 SD)				
	0.8 g orally (S)	1.5	137** (± 28.6 SD)	204 (± 162)				
Oxacillin	1 g orally	1 h	5–10	0.5	1	92–95	39–66	30–88 F
	1 g IV	1 h	15.9					
	0.5 g IM	0.5 h	15					
Oxytetracycline	0.5 g orally	3 h	0.5–2.3	8.5–9.6	50	20–40	60–70	75 F
	0.25 g IM	2 h	1.4					
Pefloxacin	0.4 g orally		3.8–5.6	8–14	16.4	20–30	8–9	80–98
Penicillin G	5×10^6 units IV	10 min	273	0.5	6–20	40–60	70–85	20–30
	1×10^6 units IM	0.5 h	12					
Penicillin V	0.5 g orally		3					60
Piperacillin	2 g IM	0.5 h	36	1.3	3–5	16–22	74–89	
	2 g IV	10 min	164–225					
Piperacillin/tazobactam	4 g IV/0.5 g IV		298/34	0.7–1.3/0.89	3–5	16–48/20–30	74–89	
Pivmecillin	0.4 g orally	1–2 h	2–5.1	1	3–6	5–10	65	F
Polymyxin B	50 mg IM	2 h	1–8	6	48–72	Low	60	
Rosoxacin	0.25 g orally	2–2.5 h	4.9	2–6			4	
Roxithromycin	0.3 g orally	2 h	10	12		85–95	10	F
Sparfloxacin	0.2 g orally	2.7–5.6 h	0.7–1.6	14–18			7–12	
Streptomycin	1 g IM	1 h	25–50	2.5	100	35	>90	TI
Sulfamethoxazole	2 g orally	2–4 h	50–120	9–12	20–50	62–70		95–100
	0.8 g IV (1-h infusion)		46.3					
Sulfisoxazole	2 g IV	Mean concentration	16.7	4.6–8.3	11	85	40–60	96
	2 g IM	1–4 h	16					

(continued)

TABLE 16.22 (Continued)

Serum Kinetics and Urinary Excretion of Antimicrobials in Humans

Antimicrobial	Dosage/Route[a]	Sampling Time[b]	Serum Concentration (μg/mL)[c]	Half-life (h) Normal	Half-life (h) ESRD[d]	Protein Binding (%)	Renal Excretion Unchanged (%)	Bioavailability (%)[e]
Sultamicillin (prodrug of ampicillin/sulbactam)	0.5 g orally	1–2	Ampicillin, 5.6/sulbactam, 4.0	0.8–1.8/1–1.3	7–20/21	17–20/38	79–92/75	80
Telithromycin	0.8 g orally (M)	2 h	1.14** (0.53–1.85)					
Temocillin	1 g IV	5 min	161	4–6	26	63–88	70–85	
Tetracycline	0.5 g orally	2–3 h	3–4	8–10	15–100	25	65	75 F
Ticarcillin	1 g IM	0.5–1 h	21–31	1.2	13–16	45–65	80–99	
	3 g IV	0.25 h	190					
Ticarcillin/clavulanic acid	3 g IV/0.2 g IV	15 min	277/11.4	1.2/0.8–1	13–16	45–65/9	80–99	
Tigecycline	0.1 g IV	1 h	604***				10	
Tobramycin	1 mg/kg IM		4	2.5	56	0–5	>90	TI
	1.5 mg/kg IV	0.5 h	4–8					
Trimethoprim	0.16 g orally	1–4 h	1–3	8–14	24–42	42–46		90 F
	0.16 g IV (1-h infusion)		3.4					
Vancomycin[k]	1 g IV (1-h infusion)	1–2 h	20–25	6–10	200–250	50–60	90–100	

[a] Single-dose studies, except for those denoted (M), which were multiple dose; IM, intramuscularly; intravenous (IV) doses were either bolus or infusions of less than 10-minute duration, except where noted.
[b] Time serum sample was taken after dose administration was completed; chosen to be near the peak level just following the distribution phase.
[c] Serum concentration data reported as a mean or range. *, values reported as median; **, concentrations measured in plasma; ***, ng/mL.
[d] End-stage renal disease.
[e] IS, inactive succinate partially hydrolyzed to base, 30% excreted as inactive succinate by kidneys; TI, therapeutic index is low, serum concentrations are highly variable, recommend monitoring serum concentrations; F, food may alter bioavailability; FE, food may enhance bioavailability; D, bioavailability may be affected by dosage form.
[f] Protein binding is concentration-dependent.
[g] MR, modified release.
[h] Metabolism may be saturable.
[i] Rapidly metabolized torythromyclamine.
[j] E, erythromycylamine-active metabolites.
[k] Timing of samples is critical because of a significant α-phase; serum concentrations are highly variable.

Renal Excretion

Most antimicrobials are eliminated in the urine, either unchanged or as metabolites. The data on achievable urinary concentration are often difficult to interpret. Urinary concentrations are constantly changing as a function of changing serum concentration and urine volume. The fraction of drug in general circulation that is excreted unchanged in the urine, *fe*, is a pharmacokinetic parameter that describes the contribution of urinary elimination to the overall elimination of antibiotic from the body.

$$fe = \text{total drug excreted unchanged/total dose}$$

The percentage of antibiotic excreted unchanged (*fe* 100) is high for antibiotics with renal excretion as the sole or primary route of elimination and low for antibiotics that are not readily excreted in the urine or that undergo significant metabolism. Determination of *fe* requires both an assay that is specific for the parent compound and a sampling time sufficiently long to ensure complete urinary excretion (at least 5 times the half-life).

Appendix 1 shows urinary excretion, metabolites, and reported urine levels for some selected antimicrobial agents.

Disease and Other Factors

A number of diseases are known to influence the absorption, distribution, and elimination of antimicrobials. Absorption may be enhanced or impaired by a number of factors. Gastrointestinal surgery, achlorhydria, malabsorption syndrome, stress, formulation differences, other drugs, and food are some of the more common conditions or factors that may alter drug absorption. Similarly, a number of conditions are associated with altered elimination. The two most readily identifiable conditions are decreased kidney function (renal excretion) and decreased hepatic function (metabolism). Each may be due to intrinsic loss of functional tissue alone or may be due to other causes such as decreased cardiac output, which may result in decreased blood flow to the kidney or liver (156,463,564). Data from human subjects with underlying conditions or disease states or from persons taking any other medications must be interpreted with caution.

Two studies have used the microdialysis method to compare the tissue pharmacokinetics of antimicrobials in healthy individuals with those of critically ill with sepsis. Joukhadar et al. (265a) found that the AUC in serum of piperacillin to be marginally reduced in critically ill patients with sepsis compared with healthy controls. However, the interstitial muscle and subcutaneous skin concentrations of piperacillin were markedly reduced in critically ill patients compared with that of healthy controls, with maximal antimicrobials in tissues in critically ill patients only about 10% of those in healthy controls. Tegeder et al. (537) found the AUC of imipenem in serum to be similar in critically ill patients compared with that of healthy controls, but the AUC in interstitial fluid of muscle and subcutaneous tissue of skin were markedly lower in critically ill patients than in healthy controls. Further, the C_{max} exceeded the usual minimum inhibitory concentration cutoff of 4 μg/mL in only one of four patients after administration of appropriate doses based on renal function.

The data in Table 16.22 have been extracted from published scientific literature and the respective manufacturer's published product information. All data are listed either as a mean value or as a range of values. The purpose of Table 16.22 is to serve as a general reference for the comparative evaluation of the basic pharmacokinetics of antimicrobials. Except where noted, listed serum concentrations and the sampling times, percentage renally excreted, and bioavailability are from single-dose studies. Elimination half-life data are broken into two categories: those from young healthy adults (normal) and those from persons with end-stage renal disease. As previously mentioned, most antimicrobials are eliminated to varying degrees by glomerular filtration or tubular secretion. Percentage renal excretion is that percentage of a single dose that has been reported to be recovered in the urine as the active parent compound. Some antimicrobials have metabolites with significant antimicrobial activity and are noted.

QUALITY CONTROL

The major considerations in quality control of antimicrobial determinations in extravascular sites are proper specimen processing and adequate controls for assay procedures. Blood and body fluid contamination (particularly urine and bile) are the most serious concerns in specimen processing, but care must also be given to possible drug inactivation due to prolonged vigorous specimen preparations such as are often used in assays of bone. These issues have been discussed earlier in the chapter and recommendations were made for optimal handling of specimens.

Problems in quality control of assays center primarily on the use of proper diluents in the preparation of standard curves for biological assays. Again, these principles have been thoroughly discussed earlier in the chapter.

Finally, of major concern is the proper interpretation of extravascular antimicrobial concentrations with regard to any clinical application of this information. Clinical correlations of infection cure as a function of local antimicrobial concentration are still imperfect and probably will remain so until more definitive information becomes available.

Acknowledgments

This chapter was based extensively on the chapters published in previous editions of this text, which included the works of Drs. Lance Peterson, Carolyn Hughes, and Tom Larson. Michelle Beattie provided valued assistance in the literature search for this edition.

REFERENCES

1. Abbas AMA, Taylor MC, DaSilva C, et al. Penetration of ceftazidime into the human prostate gland following intravenous injection. *J Antimicrob Chemother* 1985;15:119–121.
2. Abraham RK, Burnett HH. Tetracycline and chloramphenicol studies on rabbit and human eyes. *Arch Ophthalmol* 1955;54:641–659.
3. Adam D, Heilmann HD, Weismeier K. Concentrations of ticarcillin and clavulanic acid in human bone after prophylactic administration of 5.2 g of Timentin. *Antimicrob Agents Chemother* 1987;31:935–939.
4. Adam D, Hofstetter AG, Eisenberger F. Zur Diffusion von Cefamandol in das Prostatagewebe. *Med Klin* 1979;74:235–238.
5. Adam D, Hofstetter AG, Eisenberger F, et al. Zur Diffusion von Cefacetril in das Prostatagewebe. *Med Welt* 1978;29:1216–1217.
6. Adam D, Hofstetter AG, Reichart B, et al. Zur Diffusion von Cefazedon in das Herzmuskel-, Prostata- und Hautgewebe sowie in die Gallenflussigkeit. *Arzneimittelforschung* 1979;29:1901–1906.
7. Adam D, Hofstetter AG, Staehler G. Studies on diffusion of cephapirin into prostatic tissue. *Fortschr Med* 1977;95:2107–2109.
8. Adam D, Naber KG. Concentrations of ceftriaxone in prostate adenoma tissue. *Chemotherapy* 1984;30:16.
9. Adam D, Reichart B, Beyer J, et al. Diffusion of cephradine and cephalothin into interstitial fluid of human volunteers with tissue cages. *Infection* 1978;6:578–581.
10. Adam D, Reichart B, Rothenfusser B. Diffusion of piperacillin into human heart muscle. In: Nelson JD, Grassi C, eds. *Current chemotherapy and infectious disease: proceedings*. Washington DC: American Society for Microbiology, 1980;307–308.
11. Adam D, Reichart B, Williams KJ. Penetration of ceftazidime into human tissue in patients undergoing cardiac surgery. *J Antimicrob Chemother* 1983;12(Suppl A):269–273.
12. Adam D, Schalkhauser K, Boettger F. Zur Diffusion von Cefuroxim in das Prostata- und andere Gewebe des urogenitalbereichs. *Med Klin* 1979;74:1867–1870.
13. Adam D, Wilhelm K, Chysky V. Antibiotic concentrations in blood and tissue. *Arzneimittelforschung* 1981;31:1972–1976.
14. Adam D, Wittke RR, Eisenberger F. Tissue penetration of cefsulodin, a new antipseudomonas-cephalosporin antibiotic. *Drugs Exp Clin Res* 1981;7:227–231.
15. Adenis JP, Denis F, Frokco JL, et al. Etude de la penetration intraoculaire de la fosfomycine chez l'homme et chez lapin. *J Fr Ophthalmol* 1986;9:533–537.
16. Akimoto Y, Mochizuki Y, Uda A, et al. Cefaclor concentrations in human serum, gingiva, mandibular bone, and dental follicle following a single oral administration. *Gen Pharmacol* 1992;23:639–642.
17. Akimoto Y, Mochizuki Y, Uda A, et al. Concentrations of lomefloxacin in radicular cyst and oral tissues following single or multiple oral administration. *Univ Sch Dent* 1993;35:267–275.
18. Akimoto Y, Uda A, Omata H, et al. Cephalexin concentrations in human serum, gingiva, and mandibular bone following a single oral administration. *Clin Pharmacol* 1990;21:621–623.
19. Alexander M, Schoell S, Hicklin G, et al. Bronchial secretion concentrations of tobramycin. *Am Rev Respir Dis* 1982;125:208–209.
19a. Allegranzi B, Cazzadori A, Di Perri G, et al. Concentrations of single-dose meropenem (1 g IV) in bronchoalveolar lavage and epithelial lining fluid. *J Antimicrob Chemother* 2000;46:319–322.
19b. Al-Sibai MB, Al-Kaff AS, Raines D, et al. Ocular penetration of oral clarithromycin in humans. *J Ocul Pharmacol Ther* 1998;14:575–583.
20. Anderson R, Joone G, Van Rensburg EJ. An in vitro evaluation of the cellular uptake and intraphagocytic bioactivity of clarithromycin (A-56268, TE-031), a new macrolide antimicrobial agent. *J Antimicrob Chemother* 1988;22:923–933.
20a. Andrews J, Honeybourne D, Jevons G, et al. Concentrations of garenoxacin in plasma, bronchial mucosa, alveolar macrophages and epithelial lining fluid following a single oral 600 mg dose in healthy adult subjects. *J Antimicrob Chemother* 2003;51:727–730.
21. Archer GL, Armstrong BC, Kline BJ. Rifampin blood and tissue levels in patients undergoing cardiac valve surgery. *Antimicrob Agents Chemother* 1982;21:800–803.
22. Archer GL, Polk RE, Dumg RJ, et al. Comparison of cephalothin and cefamandole prophylaxis during insertion of prosthetic heart valves. *Antimicrob Agents Chemother* 1978;13:924–929.
23. Ariza J, Xiol X, Esteve M, et al. Aztreonam vs. cefotaxime in the treatment of Gram-negative spontaneous peritonitis in cirrhotic patients. *Hepatology* 1991;14:91–98.
24. Arkell D, Ashrap M, Andrews JM, et al. An evaluation of the penetration of cefepime into prostate tissue in patients undergoing elective prostatectomy. *J Antimicrob Chemother* 1992;29:473–474.
25. Asmar BI, Thirumoorthi MC, Buckley JA, et al. Cefotaxime diffusion into cerebrospinal fluid of children with meningitis. *Antimicrob Agents Chemother* 1985;28:138–140.
26. Axelrod JL, Damask LJ, Kochman RS. Cefaclor levels in human aqueous humor. In: *Program and abstracts of the 17th Interscience Conference on Antimicrobial Agents and Chemotherapy.* Washington, DC: American Society for Microbiology, 1977. Abstract 311.
27. Axelrod JL, Kochman RS. Cefamandole levels in primary aqueous humor in man. *Am J Ophthalmol* 1978;85:342–348.
28. Axelrod JL, Kochman RS. Cefoxitin levels in human aqueous humor. *Am J Ophthalmol* 1980;90:388–393.
29. Axelrod JL, Kochman RS. Cephradine levels in human aqueous humor. *Arch Ophthalmol* 1981;99:2034–2036.
30. Axelrod JL, Kochman RS. Moxalactam concentration in human aqueous humor after intravenous administration. *Arch Ophthalmol* 1982;100:1334–1336.
31. Axelrod JL, Kochman RS. Cefonicid concentrations in human aqueous humor. *Arch Ophthalmol* 1984;102:433–434.
32. Axelrod JL, Kochman RS, Horowitz MA, et al. Comparison of ceftizoxime and cefmenoxime levels in human aqueous humor. In: *Program and abstracts of the 23rd Interscience Conference on Antimicrobial Agents*

and Chemotherapy. Washington, DC: American Society for Microbiology, 1983. Abstract 644.

33. Axelrod JL, Kochman RS, Horowitz MA, et al. Ceftazidime concentrations in human aqueous humor. *Arch Ophthalmol* 1984;102:923–925.
34. Axelrod JL, Newton JC, Klein RM, et al. Penetration of imipenem into human aqueous and vitreous humor. *Am J Ophthalmol* 1987;104:649–653.
35. Baciocco EA, Iles RL. Ampicillin and kanamycin concentrations in joint fluid. *Clin Pharmacol Ther* 1971;12:858–863.
36. Balboni VG, Shapiro IM, Kydd DM. The penetration of penicillin into joint fluid following intramuscular administration. *Am J Med Sci* 1945;210:588–591.
37. Baldwin DR, Maxwell SRJ, Honeybourne D, et al. The penetration of cefpirome into the potential sites of pulmonary infection. *J Antimicrob Chemother* 1991;28:79–86.
38. Baldwin DR, Wise R, Andrews JM, et al. Azithromycin concentrations at the sites of pulmonary Infection. *Eur Respir J* 1990;3:886–890.
39. Barbhaiya RH, Shukla UA, Gleason CR, et al. Comparison of cefprozil and cefaclor pharmacokinetics and tissue penetration. *Antimicrob Agents Chemother* 1990;34:1204–1209.
40. Barling RWA, Selkon JB. The penetration of antibiotics into cerebrospinal fluid and brain tissue. *J Antimicrob Chemother* 1978;4:203–227.
41. Barrera V, Sinues B, Martinez P, et al. Penetration de l'amikacine daus la chambre anterieure de l'oell humain. *J Fr Ophthalmol* 1984;7:539–543.
42. Barza M, Cuchural G. The penetration of antibiotics into the prostate in chronic bacterial prostatitis. *Eur J Clin Microbiol* 1984;3:503–505.
43. Baughman RP, DeSante KA, Lanier TL, et al. The penetration of dirithromycin into bronchoalveolar lavage fluid and alveolar macrophages. *J Antimicrob Chemother* 1994;33:1045–1050.
44. Baumueller A, Hoyme U, Madsen PO. Rosamicin: a new drug for the treatment of bacterial prostatitis. *Antimicrob Agents Chemother* 1977;12:240–242.
45. Beam TR Jr, Galask RP, Friedhoff LT, et al. Aztreonam concentration in human tissues obtained during thoracic and gynecologic surgery. *Antimicrob Agents Chemother* 1986;30:505–507.
46. Beam TR, Raab TA, Spooner JA, et al. Comparison of ceftriaxone and cefazolin prophylaxis against infection in open heart surgery. *Am J Surg* 1984;148(Suppl 4A):8–14.
47. Bechard DL, Hawkins SS, Dhrur R, et al. Penetration of aztreonam into human bronchial secretions. *Antimicrob Agents Chemother* 1985;27:263–264.
48. Becker EF. The intraocular penetration of lincomycin. *Am J Ophthalmol* 1969;67:963–965.

48a. Begg EJ, Robson RA, Saunders DA, et al. The pharmacokinetics of oral fleroxacin and ciprofloxacin in plasma and sputum during acute and chronic dosing. *J Clin Pharmacol* 2000;49:32–38.

49. Behrens-Baumann W, Ansorg R. Mezlocillin concentrations in human aqueous humor after intravenous and subconjunctival administration. *Chemotherapy* 1985;31:169–172.
50. Bell MJ, Shackelford PG, Schroeder KF. Penetration of clindamycin into peritoneal fluid, intestine and muscle in neonates and infants. *Curr Ther Res* 1983;33:751–757.
51. Belohradsky BH, Geiss D, Marget W, et al. Intravenous cefotaxime in children with bacterial meningitis. *Lancet* 1980;1:61–63.
52. Benoni G, Arosio E, Cuzzolin L, et al. Penetration of ceftriaxone into human pleural fluid. *Antimicrob Agents Chemother* 1986;29:906–908.
53. Benoni G, Arosio E, Raimondi MG, et al. Pharmacokinetics of ceftazidime and ceftriaxone and their penetration into the ascitic fluid. *J Antimicrob Chemother* 1985;16:267–273.
54. Benoni G, Cuzzolin L, Bertrand C, et al. Imipenem kinetics in serum, lung tissue and pericardial fluid in patients undergoing thoracotomy. *J Antimicrob Chemother* 1987;20:725–728.
55. Benoni G, Cuzzolin L, Leone R, et al. Pharmacokinetics and human tissue penetration of flurithromycin. *Antimicrob Agents Chemother* 1988;32:1875–1878.
56. Bergan T. Pharmacokinetics of tissue penetration of antibiotics. *Rev Infect Dis* 1981;3:45–66.
57. Bergan T, Bruun JN, Ostby N, et al. Human pharmacokinetics and skin blister levels of sulfonamides and dihydrofolate reductase inhibitors. *Chemotherapy* 1986;32:319–328.
58. Bergan T, Engeset A, Olszewski W, et al. Extravascular penetration of highly protein-bound flucloxacillin. *Antimicrob Agents Chemother* 1986;30:729–732.
59. Bergan T, Hellum KB, Schreiner A, et al. Passage of erythromycin into human suction skin blisters. *Curr Ther Res* 1982;32:597–603.
60. Bergan T, Kalager T, Hellum KB, et al. Penetration of cefotaxime and desacetylcefoxamine into skin blister fluid. *J Antimicrob Chemother* 1982;10:193–196.
61. Berger SA, Barza M, Haher J, et al. Penetration of antibiotics into decubitus ulcers. *J Antimicrob Chemother* 1981;7:193–195.
62. Bergeron MG, Thabet M, Toy R, et al. Norfloxacin penetration into human renal and prostatic tissues. *Antimicrob Agents Chemother* 1985;28:349–350.
63. Bergogne-Berezin E, Berthelot G, Kafe H, et al. Influence of a fluidifying agent (bromhexine) on the penetration of antibiotics into respiratory secretions. *Int J Clin Pharmacol Res* 1985;5:341–344.
64. Bergogne-Berezin E, Berthelot G, Safran D, et al. Penetration of cefsulodin into bronchial secretions. *Chemotherapy* 1984;30:205–210.
65. Bergogne-Berezin E, Even P, Berthelot G, et al. Cefuroxime: pharmacokinetic study in bronchial secretions. *Proc R Soc Med* 1977;70(Suppl 9):34–37.
66. Bergogne Berezin E, Kafe H, Berthelot G, et al. Pharmacokinetic study of cefoxitin in bronchial secretions. In: Siegenthaler W, Luethy R, eds. *Current chemotherapy: proceedings*. Washington, DC: American Society for Microbiology, 1978;758–760.
67. Bergogne-Berezin E, Morel C, Benard Y, et al. Pharmacokinetic study of beta-lactam antibiotics in bronchial secretions. *Scand J Infect Dis* 1978;14(Suppl):267–272.
68. Bergogne-Berezin E, Morel C, Even P, et al. Pharmacocinetique des antibiotiques dans les voies respiratoires. *Nouv Presse Med* 1978;7:2831–2836.
69. Bergogne-Berezin E, Muller-Serieys C, Aubier M, et al. Concentration of meropenem in serum and in bronchial secretions in patients undergoing fiberoptic bronchoscopy. *Eur J Clin Pharmacol* 1994;46:87–88.
70. Bergogne-Berezin E, Pierre J, Berthelot G, et al. Diffusion bronchique des nouvelles beta-lactimes antipseudomonas. *Pathol Biol* 1984;32:421–425.
71. Bergogne-Berezin E, Pierre J, Chastre J, et al. Pharmacokinetics of apalcillin in intensive-care patients: study of penetration into the respiratory tract. *J Antimicrob Chemother* 1984;14:67–73.

72. Bermudez RH, Lugo A, Ramirez-Ronda CH, et al. Amikacin sulfate levels in human serum and bile. *Antimicrob Agents Chemother* 1981;19:352–354.
73. Berneis K, Boguth W. Distribution of sulfonamides and sulfonamide potentiators between red blood cells, proteins and aqueous phases of the blood of different species. *Chemotherapy* 1976;22:390–409.
74. Bidart B, Galindo Hernandez E, Flores Mercado F. Cefadroxil levels in human aqueous humors. In: *Program and abstracts of the 11th International Congress of Chemotherapy and 19th Interscience Conference on Antimicrobial Agents and Chemotherapy.* Washington, DC: American Society for Microbiology, 1979. Abstract 339.
75. Binda GE, Domenichini E, Gottardi A, et al. Rifampicin, a general review. *Arzneimittelforschung* 1971;21:1942–1953.
76. Blanco JD, Jorgensen JH, Castaneda YS, et al. Ceftazidime levels in human breast milk. *Antimicrob Agents Chemother* 1983;23:479–480.
77. Blenkharn JI, Habib N, Mok D, et al. Decreased biliary excretion of piperacillin after percutaneous relief of extrahepatic obstructive jaundice. *Antimicrob Agents Chemother* 1985;28:778–780.
78. Boerma JBJ, Dalhoff A, Debruyne FMY. Ciprofloxacin distribution in prostatic tissue and fluid following oral administration. *Chemotherapy* 1985;31:13–18.
79. Boger WP, Gavin JJ. Demethylchlortetracycline: serum concentration studies and cerebrospinal fluid diffusion. *Antibiot Annu* 1960;1959:393–400.
80. Boman G, Malmberg AS. Rifampin in plasma and pleural fluid after single oral doses. *Eur J Clin Pharmacol* 1974;7:51–58.
81. Borin MT, Hughes GS, Spillers CR, et al. Pharmacokinetics of cefpodoxime in plasma and skin blister fluid following oral dosing of cefpodoxime proxetil. *Antimicrob Agents Chemother* 1990;34:1094–1099.
82. Borrero AJ. Doxycycline levels in serum and prostatic tissue. *Urology* 1973;1:490–491.
83. Borski AA, Pulaski EJ, Kimbrough JC, et al. Prostatic fluid, semen, and prostatic tissue concentrations of the major antibiotics following intravenous administration. *Antibiot Chemother* 1954;4:905–910.
83a. Boselli E, Breilh D, Bel JC, et al. Diffusion of isepamicin into cancellous and cortical bone tissue. *Chemother* 2002;14(4):361–365.
84. Bouza E, Hellin T, Rodriquez-Creixems M, et al. Comparison of ceftazidime concentrations in bile and serum. *Antimicrob Agents Chemother* 1983;24:104–106.
85. Braga PC, Scaglione F, Scarpazza G, et al. Comparison between penetration of amoxicillin combined with carbocysteine and amoxicillin alone in pathological bronchial secretions and pulmonary tissue. *Int J Clin Pharmacol Res* 1985;5:331–340.
86. Braga PC, Scaglione F, Villa S, et al. Cefoperazone pharmacokinetics and sputum levels after single/multiple I.M. injections in bronchopneumopathic patients and bone, pulmonary and prostatic tissue penetration. *Int J Clin Pharmacol Res* 1983;5:349–355.
87. Braneberg PE, Heisterberg L. Blood and milk concentrations of ampicillin in mothers treated with pivampicillin and in their infants. *J Perinatal Med* 1987;15:555–558.
87a. Breilh D, Boselli E, Bel JC, et al. Diffusion of cefepime into cancellous and cortical bone tissue. *J Chemother* 2003;15(2):134–138.
87b. Breilh D, Saux MC, Delaisement C, et al. Pharmacokinetic population study to describe cefepime lung concentrations. *Pulm Pharmacol Ther* 2001;14:69–74.
88. Brion N, Lessana A, Mosset F, et al. Penetration of pefloxacin in human heart valves. *J Antimicrob Chemother* 1986;17(Suppl B):89–92.
89. Brogard JM, Arnaud JP, Blickle JF, et al. Biliary elimination of apalcillin. *Antimicrob Agents Chemother* 1984;26:428–430.
90. Brogard JM, Blickle JF, Dorner M, et al. Biliary pharmacokinetic profile of piperacillin: experimental data and evaluation in man. *Int J Clin Pharmacol* 1990;28:462–470.
91. Brogard JM, Haegele P, Dorner M, et al. Biliary excretion of a new semisynthetic cephalosporin, cephacetrile. *Antimicrob Agents Chemother* 1973;3:19–23.
92. Brogard JM, Jehl F, Blickle JF, et al. Experimental and clinical evaluation of the biliary phamacokinetic profile of cefpiramide, a new cephalosporin with high hepatic elimination. *Drugs Exp Clin Res* 1988;14:519–527.
93. Brogard JM, Kopferschmitt J, Arnaud JP, et al. Biliary elimination of mezlocillin: an experimental and clinical study. *Antimicrob Agents Chemother* 1980;18:69–76.
94. Brogard JM, Kopferschmitt J, Pinget M, et al. Cefuroxime concentrations in serum, urine, and bile: pharmacokinetic profile. *Proc R Soc Med* 1977;70(Suppl 9):42–50.
95. Brogard JM, Pinget M, Doffoel M, et al. Evaluation of the biliary excretion of penicillin G. *Chemotherapy* 1979;25:129–139.
96. Brogard JM, Pinget M, Meyer C, et al. Biliary excretion of ampicillin: experimental and clinical study. *Chemotherapy* 1977;23:213–226.
97. Bronsveld W, Stam J, MacLaren DM. Concentrations of ampicillin in pleural fluid and serum after single and repetitive doses of bacampicillin. *Scand J Infect Dis* 1978;14(Suppl):274–278.
98. Brooks S, Dent AR. Comparison of bone levels after intramuscular administration of cephradine (Velosef) or flucloxacillin/ampicillin in hip replacement. *Pharmatherapeutica* 1984;3:642–649.
99. Brown KN, Percival A. Penetration of antimicrobials into tissue culture cells and leucocytes. *Scand J Infect Dis* 1978;14(Suppl):251–260.
100. Brown RB, Martyak SN, Barza M, et al. Penetration of clindamycin phosphate into the abnormal human biliary tract. *Ann Intern Med* 1976;84:168–170.
101. Bruckner O, Friess D, Schaaf D, et al. Cure of pseudomonal meningitis dependent on levels of cefsulodin in cerebrospinal fluid. *Drugs Exp Clin Res* 1983;9:291–297.
102. Bruckner O, Trautmann M, Borner K. A study of the penetration of temocillin in the cerebrospinal fluid. *Drugs* 1985;29(Suppl 5):162–166.
103. Brun JN, Ostby N, Bredesen JE, et al. Sulfonamide and trimethoprim concentrations in human serum and skin blister fluid. *Antimicrob Agents Chemother* 1981;19:82–85.
104. Brun Y, Forey F, Gamondes JP, et al. Levels of erythromycin in pulmonary tissue and bronchial mucus compared to those of amoxicillin. *J Antimicrob Chemother* 1981;8:459–466.
105. Bryskier A, Elbaz P, Fourtillan JB, et al. Evaluation of the extravascular distribution of cefotiam (SLE 963) by the skin blister technic. *Pathol Biol* 1984;32:506–508.
106. Buggy BP, Schaberg DR, Swartz RD. Intraleukocytic sequestration as a cause of persistent *Staphylococcus aureus* peritonitis in continuous ambulatory peritoneal dialysis. *Am J Med* 1984;76:1035–1040.

107. Bullen BR, Ramsden CT, Kester RC. Tissue levels of cephradine in ischemic limbs, following a single intravenous injection. *Curr Med Res Opin* 1980;6:585–588.
108. Burroughs Wellcome Company. *Septra: a monograph.* Research Triangle Park, NC: Burroughs Wellcome Company, 1973;73.
108a. Byl B, Jacobs F, Wallemacq P, et al. Vancomycin penetration of uninfected pleural fluid exudates after continuous or intermittent infusion. *Antimicrob Agents Chemother* 2003;47:2015–2017.
109. Bystedt H, Dahlback A, Dornbusch K, et al. Concentration of azidocillin, erythromycin, doxycycline plus clindamycin in human mandibular bone. *Int J Oral Surg* 1978;7:442–449.
110. Cable D, Edralin G, Overturf GP. Human cerebrospinal fluid pharmacokinetics and treatment of bacterial meningitis with ceftizoxime. *J Antimicrob Chemother* 1982;10(Suppl C):121–127.
111. Cable D, Overturf G, Edralin G. Concentrations of cefoperazone in cerebrospinal fluid during bacterial meningitis. *Antimicrob Agents Chemother* 1983;23:688–691.
112. Carlier M, Zenebergh A, Tulkens PM. Cellular uptake and subcellular distribution of roxithromycin and erythromycin in phagocytic cells. *J Antimicrob Chemother* 1987;20(Suppl B):47–50.
112a. Cazzola M, Matera MG, Tufano MA, et al. Pulmonary disposition of lomefloxacin in patients with acute exacerbation of chronic obstructive pulmonary disease. A multiple-dose study. *J Chemother* 2001;13:407–412.
113. Chadha D, Wise R, Baldwin DR, et al. Cefepime concentrations in bronchial mucosa and serum following a single 2 gram intravenous dose. *J Antimicrob Chemother* 1990;25:959–963.
114. Cherrier P, Tod M, Le Gros V, et al. Cefotiam concentrations in the sinus fluid of patients with chronic sinusitis after administration of cefotiam hexetil. *Eur J Clin Microbiol Infect Dis* 1993;12:211–215.
115. Chisholm GD, Waterworth PM, Calnan JS, et al. Concentration of antibacterial agents in interstitial tissue fluid. *Br Med J* 1973;1:569–573.
116. Cho N, Nakayama T, Uehara K, et al. Laboratory and clinical evaluation of ticarcillin in the field of obstetrics and gynecology. *Chemotherapy* 1977;25:2911–2923.
117. Chyo N, Sunada H, Nohara S. Clinical studies of kanamycin applied in the field of obstetrics and gynecology. *Asian Med J* 1962;5:293–297.
118. Cole DR, Pung J. Penetration of cefazolin into pleural fluid. *Antimicrob Agents Chemother* 1977;11:1033–1035.
119. Combined Clinical Staff Conference of the National Institutes of Health. A new penicillin derivative resistant to penicillinase, dimethoxyphenyl penicillin. *Antibiot Chemother* 1961;11:537.
119a. Condon RE, Walker AP, Hanna CB, et al. Penetration of meropenem in plasma and abdominal tissues from patients undergoing intraabdominal surgery. *Clin Infect Dis* 1997;24(Suppl 2):S181–S183.
119b. Conte JE Jr, Golden JA, Kipps J, et al. Intrapulmonary pharmacokinetics of linezolid. *Antimicrob Agents Chemother* 2002;46:1475–1480.
119c. Cook PJ, Andrews JM, Wise R, et al. Distribution of cefdinir, a third generation cephalosporin antibiotic, in serum and pulmonary compartments. *J Antimicrob Chemother* 1996;37:331–339.
120. Cook PJ, Andrews JM, Woodcock J, et al. Concentrations of amoxycillin and clavulante in lung compartments in adults without pulmonary infection. *Thorax* 1994;49:1134–1138.
121. Cooper MA, Nye K, Andrews JM, et al. The pharmacokinetics and inflammatory fluid penetration of orally administered azithromycin. *J Antimicrob Chemother* 1990;26:533–538.
122. Cozzola M, Polverino M, Guidetti E, et al. Penetration of cefonicid into human lung tissue and lymph nodes. *Chemotherapy* 1990;36:325–331.
123. Cronberg S. A simple mathematical model of diffusion of drug into an infection site. *Scand J Infect Dis* 1978;14(Suppl):100–104.
124. Cuffini AM, Tullio V, Cimino F, et al. Comparative effects of roxithromycin and erythromycin on cellular immune function in vitro. 1. Uptake of ^{3}H-macrolides by human macrophages. *Microbios* 1989;57:167–178.
125. Cunha BA, Gossling HR, Pasteinak HS, et al. The penetration characteristics of cefazolin, cephalothin, and cephradine into bone in patients undergoing total hip replacement. *J Bone Joint Surg [Am]* 1977;59:856–859.
125a. Cunha BA, Ristuccia AM. *Antimicrobial therapy.* New York: Raven Press, 1984.
126. Dagan R, Velghe L, Rodda JL, et al. Penetration of meropenem into the cerebrospinal fluid of patients with inflamed meninges. *J Antimicrob Chemother* 1994;34:175–179.
127. Danon J. Cefotaxime concentrations in otitis media effusions. *J Antimicrob Chemother* 1980;6(Suppl A):131–132.
128. Daschner F, Blume E, Langmaack H, et al. Cefamandole concentrations in pulmonary and subcutaneous tissue. *J Antimicrob Chemother* 1979;5:474–475.
129. Daschner F, Reiss E, Engert J. Distribution of amikacin in serum, muscle, and fat in children after a single intramuscular injection. *Antimicrob Agents Chemother* 1977;11:1081–1083.
130. Daschner FD, Frank U, Kummel A, et al. Pharmacokinetics of vancomycin in serum and tissue of patients undergoing open heart surgery. *J Antimicrob Chemother* 1987;19:359–362.
131. Daschner FD, Gier E, Lentzen H, et al. Penetration into the pleural fluid after bacampicillin and amoxicillin. *J Antimicrob Chemother* 1981;7:585–588.
132. Daschner FD, Thema G, Langmaack H, et al. Ticarcillin concentrations in serum, muscle, and fat after a single intravenous injection. *Antimicrob Agents Chemother* 1980;17:738–739.
133. Davies AJ, Lockley RM, Jones A, et al. Comparative pharmacokinetics of cefamandole, cefuroxime and cephradine during total hip replacement. *J Antimicrob Chemother* 1986;17:637–640.
134. Davies BI, Maesen FPV, Teengs JP. Serum and sputum concentrations of enoxacin after single oral dosing in a clinical and bacteriological study. *J Antimicrob Chemother* 1984;14(Suppl C):83–89.
135. Davies BI, Maesen FPV, Teengs JP, et al. The quinolones in chronic bronchitis. *Pharm Weekbl (Sci)* 1986;8:53–59.
136. Dealy DH, Duma RJ, Tarktaglione TA, et al. Penetration of primaxin (*N*-formimidoyl thienamicin and cilastatin) into human cerebrospinal fluid. In: *Proceedings of the 14th International Congress of Chemotherapy.* Kyoto, Japan: International Society of Chemotherapy, 1985. Abstract S-78–4.
137. Dee TH, Kozin F. Gentamicin and tobramycin penetration into synovial fluid. *Antimicrob Agents Chemother* 1977;12:548–549.

137a. Dehne MG, Muhling J, Sablotzki A, et al. Pharmacokinetics of antibiotic prophylaxis in major orthopedic surgery and blood-saving techniques. *Orthopedics* 2001;24(7):665–669.
138. Dellamonica P, Bernard E, Etesse H, et al. The diffusion of pefloxacin into bone and the treatment of osteomyelitis. *J Antimicrob Chemother* 1986;17(Suppl B):93–102.
139. Del Tacca M, Danesi R, Bernardini N, et al. Roxithromycin penetration into gingiva and alveolar bone of odontoiatric patients. *Chemotherapy* 1990;36:332–336.
140. Denis F, Adenis JP, Mounier M, et al. Intraocular passage (healthy eye and infected eye) of ceftriaxone in man and rabbit. *Chemioterapia* 1985;4(Suppl 2):338–339.
141. Diaz Gomez ML, Rebora Guiterrez R, Galindo Hernandez E, et al. Cefadroxil, serum, and pleural fluid levels. In: *Program and abstracts of the 18th Interscience Conference on Antimicrobial Agents and Chemotherapy.* Washington, DC: American Society for Microbiology, 1978. Abstract 223.
142. Dickinson GM, Droller DG, Greeman RL, et al. Clinical evaluation of piperacillin with observations on penetrability into cerebrospinal fluid. *Antimicrob Agents Chemother* 1981;20:481–486.
143. Dixon RL, Owens ES, Rall DP. Evidence of active transport of benzyl-^{14}C-penicillin from cerebrospinal fluid to blood. *J Pharm Sci* 1969;58:1106–1109.
144. Dooley JS, Hamilton-Miller JM, Brumfitt W, et al. Antibiotics in the treatment of biliary infection. *Gut* 1984;25:988–998.
145. Dotevall L, Hagberg L. Penetration of doxycycline into cerebrospinal fluid in patients treated for suspected Lyme neuoborreliosis. *Antimicrob Agents Chemother* 1989;33:1078–1080.
146. Dresse A, Lambotte R, Dubois M, et al. Transmammary passage of cefoxitin: additional results. *J Clin Pharmacol* 1983;23:438–440.
147. Drusano GL, Preston SL, Van Guilder M, et al. A population pharmacokinetic analysis of the penetration of the prostate by levofloxacin. *Antimicrab Agents Chemother* 2000;44(8):2046–2051.
148. Dull WL, Alexander MR, Kasik JE. Bronchial secretion levels of amikacin. *Antimicrob Agents Chemother* 1979;16:767–771.
149. Dumont R, Guetat F, Andrews JM, et al. Concentrations of cefpodoxime in plasma and pleural fluid after a single oral dose of cefpodoxime proxetil. *J Antimicrob Chemother* 1990;26(Suppl E):41–46.
150. Easmon CSF, Crane JP. Comparative uptake of rifampicin and rifapentine (DL473) by human neutrophils. *J Antimicrob Chemother* 1984;13:585–591.
151. Easmon CSF, Crane JP. Uptake of cioprofloxacin by human neutrophils. *J Antimicrob Chemother* 1985;16:67–73.
151a. Egger SF, Alzner E, Georgopoulos M, et al. Penetration of cefpirome into the anterior chamber of the human eye after intravenous application. *J Antimicrob Chemother* 2000;45:213–216.
152. el Touny M, el Guinaidy M, Abdel Bary M, et al. Pharmacokinetics of cefodizime in patients with liver cirrhosis and ascites. *Chemotherapy* 1992;38:201–205.
153. Eneroth C-M, Lundberg C. The antibacterial effect of antibiotics in treatment of maxillary sinusitis. *Acta Otolaryngol (Stockh)* 1976;81:475–483.
154. Eneroth C-M, Lundberg C, Wretlind B. Antibiotic concentrations in maxillary sinus secretions and in the sinus mucosa. *Chemotherapy* 1975;21(Suppl 1):1–7.
155. Ernstson S, Anari M, Eden T, et al. Penetration of cefaclor to adenoid tissue and middle ear effusion in chronic OME. *Acta Otolaryngol (Stockh)* 1985;424(Suppl):7–12.
156. Evans WE, Schentag JJ, Jusko JJ. *Applied pharmacokinetics: principles of therapeutic drug monitoring,* 2nd ed. San Francisco: Applied Therapeutics, Inc, 1986.
157. Fabre J, Milek E, Kalfopoulos P, et al. The kinetics of tetracyclines in man. II. Excretion, penetration in normal and inflammatory tissues, behavior in renal insufficiency and hemodialysis. *Schweiz Med Wochenschr* 1971;101:625–633.
158. Farago E, Kiss J, Gomory A, et al. Amikacin: in vitro bacteriologic studies, levels in human serum, lung, and heart tissue, and clinical results. *Int J Clin Pharmacol Biopharm* 1979;17:421–428.
159. Farago E, Kiss IJ, Nabradi Z. Serum and lung tissue levels of fosfomycin in humans. *Int J Clin Pharmacol Ther Toxicol* 1980;18:554–558.
160. Fasching CE, Peterson LR. Anion-exchange extraction of cephapirin, cefotaxime, and cefoxitin from serum for liquid chromatography. *Antimicrob Agents Chemother* 1982;21:628–633.
161. Fasching CE, Peterson LR. High-pressure liquid chromatographic assay of azlocillin and mezlocillin with an anion-exchange extraction technique. *J Liquid Chromatogr* 1983;6:2513–2520.
162. Fasching CE, Peterson LR, Bettin KM, et al. High-pressure liquid chromatographic assay of ceftizoxime with an anion-exchange extraction technique. *Antimicrob Agents Chemother* 1982;22:336–337.
163. Fernandez-Lastra C, Marino EL, Barrueco M, et al. Disposition of phosphomycin in patients with pleural effusion. *Antimicrob Agents Chemother* 1984;25:458–462.
164. Fick RB Jr, Alexander MR, Prince RA, et al. Penetration of cefotaxime into respiratory secretions. *Antimicrob Agents Chemother* 1987;31:815–817.
165. Findlay CD, Wise R, Allcock JE, et al. The tissue penetration, as measured by a blister technique, and pharmacokinetics of cefsulodin compared with carbenicillin and ticarcillin. *J Antimicrob Chemother* 1981;7:637–642.
166. Fitzgerald RH. Antibiotic distribution in normal and osteomyelitic bone. *Orthop Clin North Am* 1984;15:537–546.
167. Fitzgerald RH, Kelly PJ, Snyder RJ, et al. Penetration of methicillin, oxacillin, and cephalothin into bone and synovial tissues. *Antimicrob Agents Chemother* 1978;14:723–726.
168. Fleiss PM, Richward GA, Gordon J, et al. Aztreonam in human serum and breast milk. *Br J Clin Pharmacol* 1985;19:509–511.
169. Fong IW, Ledbetter WH, Vandenbroucke AC, et al. Ciprofloxacin concentrations in bone and muscle after oral dosing. *Antimicrob Agents Chemother* 1986;29:405–408.
170. Fong IW, Rittenhouse BR, Simbul M, et al. Bone penetration of enoxacin in patients with and without osteomyelitis. *Antimicrob Agents Chemother* 1988;32:834–837.
171. Foucault P, Desauliniers D, Saginur R, et al. Concentration of teicoplanin in human heart tissue. In: *Program and abstracts of the 28th Interscience Conference on Antimicrobial Agents and Chemotherapy.* Washington, DC: American Society for Microbiology, 1988. Abstract 937.
172. Foulds G, Madsen P, Cox C, et al. Concentration of azithromycin in human prostatic tissue. *Eur J Clin Microbiol Infect Dis* 1991;10:868–871.

173. Foulds G, Miller RD, Knirsch AK, et al. Sulbactam kinetics and excretion into breast milk in postpartum women. *Clin Pharmacol Ther* 1985;38:692–696.
174. Frank UK, Schmidt-Eisenlohr E, Mlangeni D, et al. Penetration of teicoplanin into heart valves and subcutaneous and muscle tissues of patients undergoing open-heart surgery. *Antimicrob Agents Chemother* 1997;41:2559–2561.
175. Frank U, Schmidt-Eisenlohr E, Schlosser V, et al. Concentrations of flucloxacillin in heart valves and subcutaneous and muscle tissue of patients undergoing open-heart surgery. *Antimicrob Agents Chemother* 1988;32:930–931.
176. Fraschini F, Braĝa PC, Copponi V, et al. Tropism of erythromycin for the respiratory system. In: Nelson JD, Grassi C, eds. *Current chemotherapy and infectious disease: proceedings.* Washington DC: American Society for Microbiology, 1979;659–662.
177. Fraschini F, Braga PC, Scaglione F, et al. Study on pulmonary, prostatic and renal (medulla and cortex) distribution of sagamicin at different time intervals. *Int J Clin Pharmacol Res* 1987;7:51–58.
178. Fraschini F, Scaglione F, Ciccchetti F, et al. Prostatic tissue concentrations and serum levels of myocamicin in human subjects. *Drugs Exp Clin Res* 1988;24:253–255.
179. Fraschini F, Scaglione F, Falchi M, et al. Miokamycin penetration into oral cavity tissues and crevicular fluid. *Int J Clin Pharmacol Res* 1989;9:293–296.
180. Fraschini F, Scaglione F, Mezzetti M, et al. Pharmacokinetic profile of cefotetan in different clinical conditions. *Drugs Exp Clin Res* 1988;14:547–553.
181. Fraschini F, Scaglione F, Pintucci G, et al. The diffusion of clarithromycin and roxithromycin into nasal mucosa, tonsil and lung in humans. *J Antimicrob Chemother* 1991;27(Suppl A):61–65.
182. Friesen VA, Streifinger W, Hofstetter A, et al. Minocyclin-und Doxycyclin-Konzentrationen in Serum, Urin, Prostata-exprimat und -gewebe. *Fortschr Med* 1982;100:605–608.
183. Frongillo RF, Galuppo L, Moretti A. Suction skin blisters, skin window, and skin chamber techniques to determine extravascular passage of cefotaxime in humans. *Antimicrob Agents Chemother* 1981;19:22–28.
184. Frossard M, Joukhadar C, Erovic BM, et al. Distribution and antimicrobial activity of fosfomycin in the interstitial fluid of human soft tissues. *Antimicrob Agents Chemother* 2000;44:2728–2732.
185. Furesz S, Scotti R, Pallanza R, et al. Rifampicin: a new rifamyicin. *Arzneimittelforschung* 1967;17:534–537.
186. Galy J, Mantel O. Concentrations of cefotaxime in tissue and body fluids. *Nouv Presse Med* 1981;10:565–579.
187. Garcia MJ, Dominguez-Gil A, Diaz Perez F. Disposition of cefoxitin in patients with ascites. *Eur J Clin Pharmacol* 1981;20:371–374.
188. Gasser TC, Graversen PH, Madsen PO. Fleroxacin (Ro 23–6240) distribution in canine prostatic tissue and fluids. *Antimicrob Agents Chemother* 1987;31:1010–1013.
189. Geraci JE, Heilman FR, Nichols DR, et al. Some laboratory and clinical experiences with a new antibiotic, vancomycin. *Proc Staff Meet Mayo Clin* 1956;31:564–582.
190. Gerding DN. Principles of antimicrobial therapy. In: Soule BM, ed. *The APIC curriculum for infection control practice.* Dubuque, IA: Kendall/Hunt Publishing Co, 1983;508–509.
191. Gerding DN, Hall WH, Schierl EA. Antibiotic concentrations in ascitic fluid of patients with ascites and bacterial peritonitis. *Ann Intern Med* 1977;86:708–713.
192. Gerding DN, Hall WH, Schierl EA, et al. Cephalosporin and aminoglycoside concentrations in peritoneal capsular fluid in rabbits. *Antimicrob Agents Chemother* 1976;10:902–911.
193. Gerding DN, Hitt JA. Tissue penetration of new quinolones in humans. *Rev Infect Dis* 1989;11(Suppl 5): S1046–S1057.
194. Gerding DN, Kromhout JP, Sullivan JJ, et al. Antibiotic penetrance of ascitic fluid in dogs. *Antimicrob Agents Chemother* 1976;10:850–855.
195. Gerding DN, Peterson LR. Comparative tissue and extravascular fluid concentrations of ceftizoxime. *J Antimicrob Chemother* 1982;10(Suppl C):105–116.
196. Gerding DN, Peterson LR, Legler DC, et al. Ascitic fluid cephalosporin concentrations: influence of protein binding and serum pharmacokinetics. *Antimicrob Agents Chemother* 1978;14:234–239.
197. Gerding DN, Peterson LR, Salomonson JK, et al. Prediction of the concentration of penicillins in ascitic fluid from serum kinetics and protein binding of the antibiotics in serum and ascitic fluid of dogs. *J Infect Dis* 1978;138:166–173.
198. Gerding DN, Van Etta LL, Peterson LR. Role of serum protein binding and multiple antibiotic doses in the extravascular distribution of ceftizoxime and cefotaxime. *Antimicrob Agents Chemother* 1982;22:844–847.
199. Giamarellou H, Kavouklis E, Grammatikou M, et al. Penetration of four-lactam antibiotics with antipseudomonal activity into human aqueous humor. In: Periti P, Grassi G, eds. *Current chemotherapy and immunotherapy: proceedings.* Washington, DC: American Society for Microbiology, 1982;153–155.
200. Giamarellou H, Kolokythas E, Petrikkos G, et al. Pharmacokinetics of three newer quinolones in pregnant and lactating women. *Am J Med* 1989;87(Suppl 5A):49S–51S.
200a. Giannopoulos A, Koratzanis G, Giamarellos-Bourboulis EJ, et al. Pharmacokinetics of clarithromycin in the prostate: implications for the treatment of chronic abacterial prostatitis. *J Urol* 2001;165:97–99.
200b. Giannopoulos A, Koratzanis G, Giamarellos-Bourboulis EJ. Pharmacokinetics of intravenously administered pefloxacin in the prostate; perspectives for its application in surgical prophylaxis. *Int J Antimicrob Agents* 2001;17:221–224.
201. Gillett AP, Wise R. Penetration of four cephalosporins into tissue fluid in man. *Lancet* 1978;1:962–964.
202. Ginsburg CM, McCracken GH, Nelson JD. Pharmacology of oral antibiotics used for treatment of otitis media and tonsillopharyngitis in infants and children. *Ann Otol Rhinol Laryngol* 1981;90(Suppl 84):37–43.
203. Gladue RP, Bright GM, Isaacson RE, et al. In vitro and in vivo uptake of azithromycin (CP-62,993) by phagocytic cells: possible mechanism of delivery and release at sites of infection. *Antimicrob Agents Chemother* 1989;33:277–282.
203a. Gnarpe H, Lundberg C. L-phase organisms in maxillary sinus secretions. *Scand J Infect Dis* 1971;3:257–259.
204. Goh BT, Smith GW, Samarasinghe L, et al. Penicillin concentrations in serum and cerebrospinal fluid after intramuscular injection of aqueous procaine penicillin 0.6 MU with and without probenecid. *Br J Vener Dis* 1984;60:371–373.

204a. Gotfried MH, Danziger LH, Rodvold KA. Steady-state plasma and intrapulmonary concentrations of levofloxacin and ciprofloxacin in healthy adult subjects. *Chest* 2001;119:1114–1122.

204b. Goto T, Makinose S, Ohi Y, et al. Diffusion of piperacillin, cefotiam, minocycline, amikacin and ofloxacin into the prostate. *Int J Urol* 1998;5:243–246.

205. Gould JG, Meikle G, Cooper DL, et al. Temocillin concentrations in human tissues. *Drugs* 1985;29(Suppl 5):167–169.

206. Gomez-Jimenez J, Ribera E, Gasser I, et al. Randomized trial comparing ceftriaxone with cefonicid for treatment of spontaneous bacterial peritonitis in cirrhotic patients. *Antimicrob Agents Chemother* 1993;37:1587–1592.

207. Grabe M, Andersson K-E, Forsgren A, et al. Concentrations of cefotaxime in serum, urine and tissues of urological patients. *Infection* 1981;9:154–158.

208. Granai F, Smart HL, Triger DR. A study of the penetration of meropenem into bile using endoscopic retrograde cholangiography. *J Antimicrob Chemother* 1992;29:711–718.

209. Grange JD, Gouyette A, Gutmann L, et al. Pharmacokinetics of amoxycillin/clavulanic acid in serum and ascitic fluid in cirrhotic patients. *J Antimicrob Chemother* 1989;23:605–611.

210. Graziani AL, Lawson LA, Gibson GA, et al. Vancomycin concentrations in infected and noninfected human bone. *Antimicrob Agents Chemother* 1988;32:1320–1322.

211. Green GR, Geraci JE. A note on the concentration of nafcillin in human bile. *Mayo Clin Proc* 1965;40:700–704.

212. Greene HJ, Burkhart B, Hobby GL. Excretion of penicillin in human milk following parturition. *Am J Obstet Gynecol* 1946;51:732–733.

213. Greenman RL, Arcey SM, Dickenson GM, et al. Penetration of aztreonam into human cerebrospinal fluid in the presence of meningeal inflammation. *J Antimicrob Chemother* 1985;15:637–640.

214. Grimer RJ, Karpinski MRK, Andrews JM, et al. Penetration of amoxycillin and clavulanic acid into bone. *Chemotherapy* 1986;32:185–191.

215. Guerra R, Casu L, Giola K, et al. Penetration of parenteral cefuroxime into the human aqueous humor. *Arzneimittelforschung* 1981;31:861–863.

216. Guilbeau JA, Schoenbach EB, Schaub IG, et al. Aureomycin in obstetrics. *JAMA* 1950;143:520–526.

217. Gullers K, Lundberg C, Malmborg A-S. Penicillin in paranasal sinus secretions. *Chemotherapy* 1969;14:303–307.

218. Hafez FF, Stewart SM, Burnet ME. Penicillin levels in sputum. *Thorax* 1965;20:219–225.

219. Hall WH, Gerding DN, Schierl EA. Penetration of tobramycin into infected extravascular fluids and its therapeutic effectiveness. *J Infect Dis* 1977;135:957–961.

220. Halprin GM, McMahon SM. Cephalexin concentrations in sputum during acute respiratory infections. *Antimicrob Agents Chemother* 1973;3:703–707.

221. Hand WL, King-Thompson NL. The entry of antibiotics into human monocytes. *J Antimicrob Chemother* 1989;23:681–689.

222. Hand WL, King-Thompson NL, Holman JW. Entry of roxithromycin (RU 965), imipenem, cefotaxime, trimethoprim and metronidazole into human polymorphonuclear leukocytes. *Antimicrob Agents Chemother* 1987;31:1553–1557.

223. Hand WL, King-Thompson NL, Steinberg TH. Interactions of antibiotics and phagocytes. *J Antimicrob Chemother* 1983;12(Suppl C):1–11.

224. Hansbrough SF, Clark JE, Reimer LG. Concentrations of kanamycin and amikacin in human gallbladder bile and wall. *Antimicrob Agents Chemother* 1981;20:515–517.

225. Hansen I, Lykkegaard Nielson M, et al. Trimethoprim in normal and pathological human lung tissue. *Chemotherapy* 1973;19:221–234.

225a. Hariprasad SM, Mieler WF, Holz ER. Vitreous and aqueous penetrations of orally administered gatifloxacin in humans. *Arch Ophthalmol* 2003;121:345–350.

226. Harle A, Ritzerfeld W, Kluppelberg FH. Cefotaxime levels in synovial fluid following intravenous administration. *Z Orthop* 1988;126:425–430.

227. Haroche G, Salvanet A, Lafaix C, et al. Pharmacokinetics of aztreonam in the aqueous humor. *J Antimicrob Chemother* 1986;18:195–198.

228. Harrison CJ, Chartrand SA, Rodriguez W, et al. Middle ear fluid concentrations of cefixime in acute otitis media and otitis media with effusion. In: *Program and abstracts of the 34th Interscience Conference on Antimicrobial Agents and Chemotherapy.* Washington, DC: American Society for Microbiology, 1994. Abstract A67.

229. Hary L, Smail A, Ducroix JP, et al. Pharmacokinetics and ascitic fluid penetration of piperacillin in cirrhosis. *Fundam Clin Pharmacol* 1991;5:789–795.

230. Heisterberg L, Branebjerg PE. Blood and milk concentrations of metronidazole in mothers and infants. *J Perinat Med* 1983;11:114–120.

231. Helwing E, Lux M, Duben W, et al. Mezlocillin: Zur Gewebekonzentration und Wirksamkeit. *Med Klin* 1979;74:112–116.

232. Henegar GC, Silverman M, Gardner RJ, et al. Excretion of methicillin in human bile. *Antimicrob Agents Chemother* 1962;1961:348–351.

233. Herlitz V, Langmaack H, Metzger M, et al. Serum and tissue levels of cefoxitin in perioperative prophylaxis. *J Antimicrob Chemother* 1980;6:717–722.

234. Hieber JP, Nelson JD. A pharmacologic evaluation of penicillin in children with purulent meningitis. *N Engl J Med* 1977;197:410–413.

235. Hitt JA, Gerding DN. Sputum antimicrobial levels and clinical outcome in bronchitis. *Semin Respir Infect* 1991;6:122–128.

236. Hoffstedt B, Walder M. Influence of serum protein binding and mode of administration on penetration of five cephalosporins into subcutaneous tissue fluid in humans. *Antimicrob Agents Chemother* 1981;20:783–786.

237. Hoffstedt B, Walder M. Penetration of ampicillin, doxycycline and gentamicin into interstitial fluid in rabbits and of penicillin V and pivampicillin in humans measured with subcutaneously implanted cotton threads. *Infection* 1981;9:7–11.

238. Hoffstedt B, Walder M. Penetration of ceftaxidime into extracellular fluid in patients. *J Antimicrob Chemother* 1981;8(Suppl B):289–292.

239. Hoffstedt B, Walder M, Forsgren A. Comparison of skin blisters and implanted cotton threads for the evaluation of antibiotic tissue concentrations. *Eur J Clin Microbiol* 1982;1:33–37.

240. Hoger PH, Vosbeck K, Seger R, et al. Uptake, intracellular activity and influence of rifampin on normal function of polymorphonuclear leukocytes. *Antimicrob Agents Chemother* 1985;28:667–674.

241. Honda DH, Adams HG, Barriere SL. Amikacin penetration into synovial fluid during treatment of septic arthritis. *Drug Intell Clin Pharm* 1981;15:284–286.

242. Honeybourne D, Baldwin DR. The site concentrations of antimicrobial agents in the lung. *J Antimicrob Chemother* 1992;30:249–260.
243. Honeybourne D, Banerjee D, Andrews J, et al. Concentrations of gatifloxacin in plasma and pulmonary compartments following a single 400 mg oral dose in patients undergoing fibre-optic bronchoscopy. *J Antimicrob Chemother* 2001;48:63–66.
244. Honeybourne D, Kees F, Andrews JM, et al. The levels of clarithormycin and its 14-hydroxy metabolite in the lung. *Eur Respir J* 1994;7:1275–1280.
245. Hoogkamp-Korstanje JAA, Klein SJ. Ciprofloxacin in acute exacerbations of chronic bronchitis. *J Antimicrob Chemother* 1986;18:407–413.
246. Hoogkamp-Korstanje JAA, van Oort HJ, Schipper JJ, et al. Intraprostatic concentration of ciprofloxacin and its activity against urinary pathogens. *J Antimicrob Chemother* 1984;14:641–645.
247. Howard JB, McCracken GH. Reappraisal of kanamycin usage in neonates. *J Pediatr* 1975;86:949–956.
248. Howell A, Sutherland R, Rolinson GN. Effect of protein binding on levels of ampicillin and cloxacillin in synovial fluid. *Clin Pharmacol Ther* 1972;13:724–732.
249. Hughes SPF, Anderson FM. Penetration of antibiotics into bone. *J Antimicrob Chemother* 1985;15:517–519.
250. Humbert G, Leroy A, Rogez J, et al. Cefoxitin concentrations in the cerebrospinal fluids of patients with meningitis. *Antimicrob Agents Chemother* 1980;17:675–678.
251. Humbert G, Veyssier P, Fourtillan JB, et al. Penetration of cefmenoxime into cerebrospinal fluid of patients with bacterial meningitis. *J Antimicrob Chemother* 1986;18:503–506.
252. Hume AL, Polk R, Kline B, et al. Comparative penetration of latamoxef (moxalactam) and cefazolin into human knee following simultaneous administration. *J Antimicrob Chemother* 1983;12:623–627.
253. Husson MO, Debout J, Krivosic-Horber R. Etude de la diffusion bronchique de la ceftriaxone. *Pathol Biol* 1986;34:325–327.
254. Incavo SJ, Ronchetti PJ, Choi JH, et al. Penetration of piperacillin-tazobactam into cancellous and cortical bone tissues. *Antimicrob Agents Chemother* 1994;38:905–907.
255. Iversen P, Madsen PO. Short-term cephalosporin prophylaxis in transurethral surgery. *Clin Ther* 1982;5 (Suppl A):58–66.
256. Jacobs F, Rocmans P, Motte S, et al. Penetration and bactericidal activity of teichoplanin in post-thoracotomy pleural fluids. In: *Program and abstracts of the 26th Interscience Conference on Antimicrobial Agents and Chemotherapy.* Washington, DC: American Society for Microbiology, 1986. Abstract 1251.
257. Jacobs RF, Thompson JW, Kiel DP, et al. Cellular uptake and cell-associated activity of third generation cephalosporins. *Pediatr Res* 1986;20:909–912.
258. Jacobs RF, Wilson CB. Activity of antibiotics in chronic granulomatous disease leukocytes. *Pediatr Res* 1983;17:916–919.
259. Johnson AP, Scoper SV, Woo FL, et al. Azlocillin levels in human tears and aqueous humor. *Am J Ophthalmol* 1985;99:469–472.
260. Jokinen K, Raunto V. Penetration of azidocillin into the secretion and tissues in chronic maxillary sinusitis and tonsilitis. *Acta Otolaryngol (Stockh)* 1975;79:460–465.
261. Jokipii AM, Jokipii L. Metronidazole, tinidazole, ornidazole and anaerobic infections of the middle ear, maxillary sinus and central nervous system. *Scand J Infect Dis* 1981;26(Suppl):123–129.
262. Jokipii AMM, Myllvia VV, Hokkanen E, et al. Penetration of the blood brain barrier by metronidazole and tinidazole. *J Antimicrob Chemother* 1977;3:239–245.
263. Jones S, Yu VL, Johnson JT, et al. Pharmacokinetic and therapeutic trial of sultamicillin in acute sinusitis. *Antimicrob Agents Chemother* 1985;28:832–833.
264. Jorgensen LN, Andreasen JJ, Nielsen PT, et al. Dicloxacillin concentrations in amputation. *Acta Orthop Scand* 1989;60:617–620.
265. Joseph J, Vaughan LM, Basran GS. Penetration of intravenous and oral ciprofloxacin into sterile and empyemic human pleural fluid. *Ann Pharmacother* 1994;28:313–315.
265a. Joukhadar C, Frossard M, Mayer BX, et al. Impaired target site penetration of beta-lactams may account for therapeutic failure in patients with septic shock. *Crit Care Med* 2001;29:385–391.
266. Just HM, Bassler M, Frank U, et al. Penetration of cefotaxime into heart valves, subcutaneous and muscle tissue of patients undergoing open-heart surgery. *J Antimicrob Chemother* 1984;14:431–434.
267. Just HM, Eschenbruch E, Schmuziger M, et al. Penetration of netilmicin into heart valves, subcutaneous and muscular tissue of patients undergoing heart surgery. *Clin Cardiol* 1983;6:217–219.
268. Just HM, Frank U, Simon A, et al. Concentrations of ceftriaxone in serum and lung tissue. *Chemotherapy* 1984;30:81–83.
269. Kafetzis DA. Penetration of cefotaximine into empyema fluid. *J Antimicrob Chemother* 1980;6(Suppl A): 153.
270. Kafetzis DA, Brater DC, Fanourgakis JE, et al. Ceftriaxone distribution between maternal blood and fetal blood and tissues at parturition and between blood and milk postpartum. *Antimicrob Agents Chemother* 1983;23:870–873.
271. Kafetzis DA, Siafas CA, Georgakopoulos PA, et al. Passage of cephalosporins and amoxicillin into the breast milk. *Acta Paediatr Scand* 1981;70:285–288.
272. Kalm O, Kamme C, Bergstrom B, et al. Erythromycin stearate in acute maxillary sinusitis. *Scand J Infect Dis* 1973;7:209–217.
273. Kamme C, Lundgren K, Rundcrantz H. The concentration of penicillin V in serum and middle ear exudate in acute otitis media in children. *Scand J Infect Dis* 1969;1: 77–83.
274. Kane JG, Parker RH, Jordan GW, et al. Nafcillin concentration in cerebrospinal fluid during treatment of staphylococcal infections. *Ann Intern Med* 1977;87:309–311.
275. Kaplan JM, McCracken GH, Snyder E. Influence of methodology upon apparent concentrations of antibiotics in tissues. *Antimicrob Agents Chemother* 1973;3:143–146.
276. Katoh N, Ono Y, Ohshima S, et al. Diffusion of cefmenoxime and latamoxef into prostatic fluid in the patients with acute bacterial prostatitis. *Urol Int* 1992;48:191–194.
277. Kavi J, Andrews JM, Ashby JP, et al. Pharmacokinetics and tissue penetration of cefpirome, a new cephalosporin. *J Antimicrob Chemother* 1988;22:911–916.
278. Kees F, Naber KG, Schumacher H, et al. Penetration of fleroxacin into prostatic secretion and prostatic adenoma tissue. *Chemotherapy* 1988;34:437–443.
279. Keighley MRB, Drysdale RB, Quoraishi AH, et al. Antibiotics in biliary disease: the relative importance of

antibiotic concentrations in bile and serum. *Gut* 1976;17:495–500.

280. Kenady DE, Ram MB. Biliary levels of ceforanide. *Antimicrob Agents Chemother* 1983;23:706–709.

280a. Khair OA, Andrews JM, Honeybourne D, et al. Lung concentrations of telithromycin after oral dosing. *J Antimicrob Chemother* 2001;47:837–840.

281. Kiistala V, Mustakallio KK. Dermo-epidermal separation with suction: electron microscopic and histochemical study of initial events of blistering of human skin. *J Invest Dermatol* 1967;48:466–467.

282. Kimura M, Matsushima T, Nakamura J, et al. Comparative study of penetration of lomefloxacin and ceftriaxone into transudative and exudative pleural effusion. *Antimicrob Agents Chemother* 1992;36:2774–2777.

283. Kinzig M, Sorgel F, Naber KG, et al. Tissue penetration of piperacillin/tazobactam. In: *Proceedings of the 31st Interscience Conference on Antimicrobial Agents and Chemotherapy.* Washington, DC: American Society for Microbiology, 1991. Abstract 862.

284. Kiss IJ, Farago E, Fabian E. Study of oxacillin levels in human serum and lung tissue. *Ther Hung* 1974;22: 55–59.

285. Kiss IJ, Farago E, Gomory A, et al. Investigations on the flucloxacillin levels in human serum, lung tissue, pericardial fluid and heart tissue. *Int J Clin Pharmacol Ther Toxicol* 1980;18:405–411.

286. Kiss IJ, Farago E, Juhasz I, et al. Investigation on the serum and lung tissue level of rifampicin in man. *Int J Clin Pharmacol Biopharm* 1976;13:42–47.

287. Kiss IJ, Farago E, Schnitzler J, et al. Amoxycillin levels in human serum, bile, gallbladder, lung and liver tissue. *Int J Clin Pharmacol Ther Toxicol* 1981;19:69–74.

288. Kitzis M, Desnottes JF, Brunel D, et al. Spiramycin concentrations in lung tissue. *J Antimicrob Chemother* 1988;22(Suppl B):123–126.

289. Klastersky J, Carpentier-Meunier F, Kahan-Coppens L, et al. Endotracheally administered antibiotics for Gram-negative bronchopneumonia. *Chest* 1979;75:586–591.

290. Klastersky J, Greening C, Mouawad E, et al. Endotracheal gentamicin in bronchial infections in patients with tracheostomy. *Chest* 1971;61:117–120.

291. Klastersky J, Thys JP, Mombelli G. Comparative studies of intermittent and continuous administration of aminoglycosides in the treatment of bronchopulmonary infections due to Gram-negative bacteria. *Rev Infect Dis* 1981;3:74–83.

292. Klempner MS, Styrt B. Clindamycin uptake by human neutrophils. *J Infect Dis* 1981;144:472–479.

292a. Klotz T, Braun M, Bin Saleh A, et al. Penetration of a single infusion of ampicillin and sulbactam into prostatic tissue during transurethral prostatectomy. *Int Urol Nephrol* 1999;31:203–209.

293. Knoller J, Schonfeld W, Mayer M, et al. Mezlocillin in pleural effusions: analysis by HPLC. *Zentralbl Bakteriol Hyg[A]* 1988;268:370–375.

294. Kobayashi M, Washio M, Eishin H, et al. Ceftizoxime level in the myocardium (right atrial muscle and mitral papillary muscle) during open heart surgery. *Jpn J Surg* 1988;18:136–141.

295. Koch R. Blood and cerebrospinal fluid levels of intramuscular oxytetracycline. *J Pediatr* 1955;46:44–48.

296. Koga H. High performance liquid chromatography measurement of antimicrobial concentrations in polymorphonuclear leukocytes. *Antimicrob Agents Chemother* 1987;31:1904–1908.

297. Kohonen A, Paavolainen M, Renkonen OV. Concentration of cephalexin in maxillary sinus mucosa and secretion. *Ann Clin Res* 1975;7:50–53.

298. Kohonen A, Palmgren O, Renkonen O. Penetration of trimethoprim-sulfadiazine into middle ear fluid in secretory otitis media. *Int J Pediatr Otorhinolaryngol* 1983;6:89–94.

299. Kondell PA, Nord CE, Nordeniam A. Concentrations of cloxacillin, dicloxacillin, and flucloxacillin in dental alveolar serum and mandibular bone. *Int J Oral Surg* 1982;11:40–43.

300. Kornguth ML, Kunin CM. Uptake of antibiotics by human erythrocytes. *J Infect Dis* 1976;133:175–184.

301. Korting HC. Plasma and skin blister fluid levels of cefotriam and cefmenoxime after single intramuscular application of 1 gm in gonorrhea. *Chemotherapy* 1984;30:277–282.

302. Korting HC, Schafer-Korting M, Maass L, et al. Cefodizime in serum and skin blister fluid after single intravenous and intramuscular doses in healthy volunteers. *Antimicrob Agents Chemother* 1987;31:1822–1825.

303. Korzeniowski OM, Carvalho EM Jr, Rocha H, et al. Evaluation of cefamandole therapy in patients with bacterial meningitis. *J Infect Dis* 1978;137:S169–S179.

304. Kovarik JM, De Hond JAPM, Hoepelman IM, et al. Intraprostatic distribution of lomefloxacin following multiple-dose administration. *Antimicrob Agents Chemother* 1990;34:2398–2401.

305. Kozak AJ, Gerding DN, Peterson LR, et al. Gentamicin intravenous infusion rate: effect on interstitial fluid concentration. *Antimicrob Agents Chemother* 1977;12:606–608.

306. Kramer J, Weuta H. Utersuchungen uber Serum- und Knocheuspiegel nach Injektion von Oxacillin und Carbenicillin. *Z Orthop* 1972;110:216–233.

307. Krause PJ, Owens NJ, Nightingale CH, et al. Penetration of amoxicillin, cefaclor, erythromycin-sulfisoxazole, and trimethoprim-sulfamethoxazole into the middle ear fluid of patients with chronic serous otitis media. *J Infect Dis* 1982;145:815–821.

308. Kummel A, Scholsser V, Petersen E, et al. Pharmacokinetics of imipenem-cilastatin in serum and tissue. *Eur J Clin Microbiol* 1985;4:609–610.

309. Kunin CM. Binding of antibiotics to tissue homogenates. *J Infect Dis* 1970;121:55–64.

310. Kunin CM, Finland M. Excretion of demethylchlortetracycline into the bile. *N Engl J Med* 1959;261:1069–1071.

311. Kusmiesz H, Shelton S, Brown O, et al. Loracarbef concentrations in middle ear fluid. *Antimicrob Agents Chemother* 1990;34:2030–2031.

311a. Kutscha-Lissberg F, Hebler U, Muhr G, et al. Linezolid penetration into bone and joint tissues infected with methicillin-resistant staphylococci. *Antimicrob Agents Chemother* 2003;47:3964–3966.

312. Lacut JY, Humbert G, Aubertin J, et al. Treatment of purulent meningitis in adults with injectable amoxycillin: clinical and pharmacokinetic results. *Curr Ther Res* 1981;29:36–46.

313. Lahikainen EA. Penicillin concentration in middle ear secretion in otitis. *Acta Otolaryngol (Stockh)* 1970;70:358–362.

314. Lahikainen EA, Vuori M, Virtanen S. Azidocillin and ampicillin concentrations in middle ear effusion. *Acta Otolaryngol (Stockh)* 1977;84:227–232.

315. Lambert HP. Clinical significance of tissue penetration of antibiotics in the respiratory tract. *Scand J Infect Dis* 1978;14(Suppl):262–266.

316. Lanao JM, Dominguez A, Mactas JG, et al. The influence of ascites on the pharmacokinetics of amikacin. *Int J Clin Pharmacol Ther Toxicol* 1980;18:57–61.
317. LeBel M, Gregoire S, Caron M, et al. Difference in blister fluid penetration after single and multiple doses of ceftriaxone. *Antimicrob Agents Chemother* 1985;28:123–127.
318. Lechi A, Arosio E, Xerri L, et al. The kinetics of cefuroxime in ascitic and pleural fluid. *Int J Clin Pharmacol Ther Toxicol* 1982;20:493–496.
319. Lederle Laboratories. Piperacil [package insert]. Data on file. Lederle Laboratories, 1982.
320. Leigh DA, Griggs J, Tighe CM, et al. Pharmacokinetic study of ceftazidime in bone and serum of patients undergoing hip and knee arthroplasty. *J Antimicrob Chemother* 1985;16:637–642.
321. Lerner PI. Penetration of cephaloridine into cerebrospinal fluid. *Am J Med Sci* 1971;262:321–326.
322. Leroyer C, Muller-Serieys C, Quiot JJ, et al. Dirithromycin concentrations in bronchial mucosa and secretions. *Respiration* 1998;65:381–385.
323. Levi JU, Martinez OV, Malinin TI, et al. Decreased biliary excretion of cefamandole after percutaneous biliary decompression in patient with total common bile duct obstruction. *Antimicrob Agents Chemother* 1984;26:944–946.
324. Lily and Co. Mandol in lactating mothers. Data on file. Indianapolis, IN: Elilily and Co.
325. Linzenmeier G, Schafer P, Volk H, et al. Determination of lincomycin concentration in chronically inflamed bone and soft tissue of man. *Arzneimittelforschung* 1968;18:204–207.
326. Litvak AS, Franks CD, Vaught SK, et al. Cefazolin and cephalexin levels in prostatic tissue and sera. *Urology* 1976;7:497–498.
327. Lockley MR, Brown RM, Wise R. Pharmacokinetics and tissue penetration of temocillin. *Drugs* 1985;29(Suppl 5):106–108.
328. Lode H, Dzwillo G. Investigation of the diffusion of antibiotics into the human pleural space. In: *Proceedings of the 10th International Congress of Chemotherapy.* Washington, DC: American Society for Microbiology, 1978;1:386–388.
329. Lode H, Gruhlke G, Hallermann W, et al. Significance of pleural and sputum concentrations for antibiotic therapy of bronchopulmonary infections. *Infection* 1980;8(Suppl 1):S49–S53.
330. Lode H, Kemmerich B, Gruhlke G, et al. Cefotaxime in bronchopulmonary infections: a clinical and pharmacological study. *J Antimicrob Chemother* 1980;6(Suppl A):193–198.
331. Lou MA, Wu YH, Jacob LS, et al. Penetration of cefonicid into human breast milk and various body fluids and tissues. *Rev Infect Dis* 1984;6(Suppl 4):5816–5820.
331a. Lovering AM, Zhang J, Bannister GC, et al. Penetration of linezolid into bone, fat, muscle and haematoma of patients undergoing routine hip replacement. *J Antimicrob Chemother* 2002;50:73–77.
332. Lundberg C, Malmborg A-S. Concentration of penicillin V and tetracycline in maxillary sinus secretion after repeated doses. *Scand J Infect Dis* 1973;5:123–133.
333. Macfarlane JA, Walsh JM, Mitchell AAB, et al. Spiramycin in the prevention of postoperative staphylococcal infection. *Lancet* 1968;1:1–4.
334. MacGregor RR, Gibson GA, Bland JA. Imipenem pharmacokinetics and body fluid concentrations in patients receiving high-dose treatment for serious infections. *Antimicrob Agents Chemother* 1986;29:188–192.
335. MacIlwaine WA, Sande MA, Mandell GL. Penetration of antistaphylococcal antibiotics into the human eye. *Am J Ophthalmol* 1974;77:589–592.
336. MacLeod CM, Bartley EA, Galante JO, et al. Aztreonam penetration into synovial fluid and bone. *Antimicrob Agents Chemother* 1986;29:710–712.
337. Maderazo EG, Breaux SP, Woronick CL, et al. High teicoplanin uptake by human neutrophils. *Chemotherapy* 1988;34:248–255.
338. Madsen PO, Dhruv R, Friedhoff LT. Aztreonam concentrations in human prostatic tissue. *Antimicrob Agents Chemother* 1984;26:20–21.
339. Madsen PO, Kjaer TB, Baumueller A, et al. Antimicrobial agents in prostatic fluid and tissue. *Infection* 1976;4 (Suppl 2):154–159.
340. Madsen PO, Wolf H, Barquin OP, Rhodes P. The nitrofurantoin concentration in prostatic fluid of humans and dogs. *J Urol* 1968;100:54–56.
341. Maesen FPV, Davies BI, Drenth BMH, et al. Treatment of acute exacerbations of chronic bronchitis with cefotaxime: a controlled clinical trial. *J Antimicrob Chemother* 1980;6(Suppl A):187–192.
342. Malmborg AS, Kumlien J, Samuelsson A, et al. Concentrations of enoxacin in sinus secretions. *Rev Infect Dis* 1989;11(Suppl 5):S1205–S1206.
343. Mandal AK, Thadepalli H, Bach VT, et al. Antibiotic concentration in the human right atrial appendage. *Curr Ther Res* 1980;28:504–510.
344. Mandell GL. Interaction of intraleukocytic bacteria and antibiotics. *J Clin Invest* 1973;52:1673–1699.
345. Mannisto PT, Karhunen M, Koskela O, et al. Concentrations of tinidazole in breast milk. *Acta Pharmacol Toxicol* 1983;53:254–256.
346. Marlin GE, Burgess KR, Burgoyne J, et al. Penetration of piperacillin into bronchial mucosa and sputum. *Thorax* 1981;36:774–780.
347. Marmo E, Cuppola L, Pempinello R, et al. Levels of amoxycillin in the liquor during continuous intravenous administration. *Chemotherapy* 1982;28:171–175.
348. Martin CM. Tissue levels and body fluid levels of cefoxitin in man after therapeutic doses of the antibiotic. Data on file. Rahway, NJ: Merck Sharp & Dohme, 1979.
349. Martin WJ, Nichols DR, Heilman FR. Penicillin V: further observations. *Proc Staff Meet Mayo Clin* 1955;30:521–526.
350. Martinelli D, Mazzei T, Fallani S, et al. Ceftizoxime concentrations in human aqueous humor following intravenous administration. *Chemioterapia* 1988;7:317–319.
351. Matheson I, Samseth M, Loberg R, et al. Milk transfer of phenoxymethyl-penicillin during puerperal mastitis. *Br J Clin Pharmacol* 1988;25:33–40.
352. Matsuda S. Transfer of antibiotics into maternal milk. *Biol Res Pregnancy* 1984;2:57–60.
353. Mattila J, Mannisto PT, Luodeslampi M. Penetration of trimethoprim and sulfadiazine into sinus secretion in acute maxillary sinusitis. *Chemotherapy* 1983;29:174–177.
354. Mattila J, Nerdrum K, Rouhiainen H, et al. Penetration of metronidazole and tinidazole into the aqueous humor in man. *Chemotherapy* 1983;29:188–191.
355. May JR, Delves DM. Treatment of chronic bronchitis with ampicillin: some pharmacological observations. *Lancet* 1965;1:929–933.
355a. Mazzei T, Novelli A, Esposito S, et al. Cefodizime in skin suction blister fluid and serum following a single intravenous or intramuscular dose in adult patients. *J Chemother* 2000;12:306–313.

355b. Mazzei T, Novelli A, Esposito S, et al. New insight into the clinical pharmacokinetics of cefaclor: tissue penetration. *J Chemother* 2000;12:53–62.

356. Mazzei T, Tonelli F, Novelli A, et al. Penetration of cefotetan into suction skin blister fluid and tissue homogenates in patients undergoing abdominal surgery. *Antimicrob Agents Chemother* 1994;38:2221–2223.

357. Meares EM Jr. Long-term therapy of chronic bacterial prostatitis with trimethoprim-sulfamethoxazole. *Can Med Assoc J* 1975;112:22S–25S.

358. Meares EM Jr. Prostatitis: review of pharmacokinetics and therapy. *Rev Infect Dis* 1982;4:475–483.

359. Mayer M, Tophof C, Opferkuch W. Bile levels of imipenem in patients with T-drain following the administration of imipenem/cilastatin. *Infection* 1988;16:225–228.

360. McNulty CA, Garden GM, Ashby J, et al. Pharmacokinetics and tissue penetration of carumonam, a new synthetic monobactam. *Antimicrob Agents Chemother* 1985;28:425–427.

361. McNulty CA, Garden GM, Wiser R, et al. The pharmacokinetics and tissue penetration of teicoplanin. *J Antimicrob Chemother* 1985;16:743–749.

361a. Medina A, Fiske N, Hjelt-Harvey I, et al. Absorption, diffusion and excretion of a new antibiotic, lincomycin. *Antimicrob Agents Chemother* 1964;1963:189–196.

362. Melloni D, Ammatuna P, Formica P, et al. Pharmacokinetic study on adenomatous prostate tissue concentration of cefoperazone. *Chemotherapy* 1989;35:410–415.

363. Mendelson J, Portnoy J, Sigman H. Pharmacology of gentamicin in the biliary tract of humans. *Antimicrob Agents Chemother* 1973;4:538–541.

364. Mendelson J, Portnoy J, Sigman H, et al. Pharmacology of cephalothin in the biliary tract of humans. *Antimicrob Agents Chemother* 1974;6:659–665.

365. Mertes PM, Jehl F, Burtin P, et al. Penetration of ofloxacin into heart valves, myocardium, mediastinal fat, and sternal bone marrow in humans. *Antimicrob Agents Chemother* 1992;36:2493–2496.

366. Mertes PM, Voiriot P, Dopff C, et al. Penetration of ciprofloxacin into heart valves, myocardium, mediastinal fat, and sternal bone marrow in humans. *Antimicrob Agents Chemother* 1990;34:398–401.

367. Miller MF, Martin JR, Johnson P, et al. Erythromycin uptake and accumulation by human polymorphonuclear leukocytes and efficacy of erythromycin killing of ingested *Legionella pneumophila*. *J Infect Dis* 1984;149:714–718.

368. Mischler TW, Corson SL, Larranaga A, et al. Cephradine and epicillin in body fluids of lactating and pregnant women. *J Reprod Med* 1973;26:130–136.

369. Modai J, Decazes JM, Wolff M, et al. Penetration of ceftazidime into cerebrospinal fluid of patients with bacterial meningitis. *Antimicrob Agents Chemother* 1983;24:126–128.

370. Moorthi K, Wiederholt K. Is the administration of doxycycline still indicated in bacterial infections of the gallbladder and the bile ducts? *Eur J Clin Pharmacol* 1981;20:35–38.

371. Moreau L, Durand H, Biclet P. Cefotaxime concentrations in ascites. *J Antimicrob Chemother* 1980;6(Suppl A):121–122.

372. Morgan G, Ceccarelli G, Ciaffi G. Comparative concentrations of a tetracycline antibiotic in serum and maternal milk. *Antibiotica* 1968;6:216–222.

373. Morris DL, Ubhi CS, Robertson CS, et al. Biliary pharmacokinetics of sulbactam plus ampicillin in humans. *Rev Infect Dis* 1986;8(Suppl 5):S589–S592.

374. Moseley JG, Chaudhuri AK, Desai AL, et al. The distribution of aztreonam in serum, bile, skin and subcutaneous tissues in patients undergoing cholecystectomy. *J Hosp Infect* 1990;15:389–392.

375. Mouton Y, Caillaux M, Beaucaire G, et al. Penetration of moxalactam in bronchial secretions and clinical evaluation in intensive care patients. In: *Program and abstracts of the 21st Interscience Conference on Antimicrobial Agents and Chemotherapy.* Washington, DC: American Society for Microbiology, 1981. Abstract 732.

376. Mouton Y, Caillaux M, Deboscker Y, et al. Etude de la diffusion bronchique de la piperacilline chez dix-huit patients de reanimation. *Pathol Biol* 1985;33:359–362.

377. Mouton JW, Michel MF. Pharmacokinetics of meropenem in serum and suction blister fluid during continuous and intermittent infusion. *J Antimicrob Chemother* 1991;28:911–918.

378. Mullaney DT, John JF. Cefotaxime therapy. *Arch Intern Med* 1983;143:1705–1708.

379. Mullany LD, French MA, Nightingale CH, et al. Penetration of ceforanide and cefamandole into the right atrial appendage, pericardial fluid, sternum, and intercostal muscle of patients undergoing open heart surgery. *Antimicrob Agents Chemother* 1982;21:416–420.

379a. Muller M, Haag O, Burgdorff T, et al. Characterization of peripheral-compartment kinetics of antibiotics by in vivo microdialysis in humans. *Antimicrob Agents Chemother* 1996;40:2703–2709.

379b. Muller M, Rohde B, Kovar A, et al. Relationship between serum and free interstitial concentrations of cefodizime and cefpirome in muscle and subcutaneous adipose tissue of healthy volunteers measured by microdialysis. *J Clin Pharmacol* 1997;37:1108–1113.

380. Muller-Serieys C, Bergogne-Berezin E, Rowan C, et al. Imipenem penetration into bronchial secretions. *J Antimicrob Chemother* 1987;20:618–619.

380a. Muller-Serieys C, Soler P, Cantalloube C, et al. Bronchopulmonary disposition of the ketolide telithromycin (HMR 3647). *Antimicrob Agents Chemother* 2001; 45:3104–3108.

380b. Naber CK, Steghafner M, Kinzig-Schippers M, et al. Concentrations of gatifloxacin in plasma and urine and penetration into prostatic and seminal fluid, ejaculate, and sperm cells after single oral administrations of 400 milligrams to volunteers. *Antimicrob Agents Chemother* 2001;45:293–297.

381. Naber KG. Use of quinolones in urinary tract infections and prostatitis. *Rev Infect Dis* 1989;11(Suppl 5):S1321–S1337.

382. Naber KG. The role of quinolones in the treatment of chronic bacterial prostatitis. *Infection* 1991;19(Suppl 3):S170–S177.

383. Naber KG, Kinzig M, Adam D, et al. Concentrations of cefpodoxime in plasma, ejaculate and in prostatic fluid and adenoma tissue. *Infection* 1991;19:30–35.

384. Naber KG, Kinzig M, Adam D, et al. Penetration of ofloxacin into prostatic fluid, ejaculate and seminal fluid. *Infection* 1993;21:98–100.

385. Nagar H, Berger SA. The excretion of antibiotics by the biliary tract. *Surg Gynecol Obstet* 1984;158:601–607.

386. Nahata MC, Kohlbrenner VM, Barson WJ. Pharmacokinetics and cerebrospinal fluid concentrations of cefixime in infants and young children. *Chemotherapy* 1993;39: 1–5.

387. Naline E, Sanceaume M, Taty L, et al. Penetration of minocycline into lung tissues. *Br J Clin Pharmacol* 1991;32:402–404.

387a. Namour F, Sultan E, Pascual MH, et al. Penetration of telithromycin (HMR 3647) a new ketolide antimicrobial, into inflammatory blister fluid following oral administration. *J Antimicrob Chemother* 2002;49:1035–1038.
388. Nelson JD. Antibiotic concentrations in septic joint effusions. *N Engl J Med* 1971;284:349–353.
389. Nelson JD, Howard JB, Shelton S. Oral antibiotic therapy for skeletal infections of children. *Pediatrics* 1978;92:131–134.
389a. Nicolle LE. Measurement and significance of antibiotic activity in the urine. In: Lorian V, ed. *Antibiotics in laboratory medicine*, 4th ed. Baltimore: Williams & Wilkins, 1996;794–798.
389b. Nielson ML, Hansen IT. Trimethoprim in human prostatic tissue and prostatic fluid. *Scand J Urol Nephrol* 1972;6:244–248.
390. Nielson MW, Justesen T. Excretion of metronidazole in human bile. *Scand J Gastroenterol* 1977;12:1003–1008.
391. Nightingale CH, Klimek JJ, Quintiliani R. Effect of protein binding on the penetration of nonmetabolized cephalosporins into atrial appendage and pericardial fluids in open heart surgical patients. *Antimicrob Agents Chemother* 1980;17:595–598.
392. Nightingale CH, Quintiliani R, Dudley MN, et al. Tissue penetration and half-life of cefonicid. *Rev Infect Dis* 1984;6(Suppl 4):821–828.
393. Nishida MT, Matsubara T, Uemura T, et al. Studies on binding of penicillin and serum protein. II. Relationship between protein binding and incorporation into erythrocytes in vitro. *Jpn J Antibiot* 1970;23:217–222.
394. Nishihata T, Higuchi T, Kamada A. Salicylate-promoted permeation of cefoxitin, insulin and phenylalanine across red cell membrane: possible mechanism. *Life Sci* 1984; 34:437–445.
395. Norrby R. A review of the penetration of antibiotics into CSF and its clinical significance. *Scand J Infect Dis* 1978;14(Suppl):296–309.
396. Nunes HL, Pecora CC, Judy K. Turnover and distribution of nafcillin in tissues and body fluids of surgical patients. *Antimicrob Agents Chemother* 1965;1964:237–249.
397. Nye KJ, Shi YG, Andrews JM, et al. Pharmacokinetics and tissue penetration of cefepime. *J Antimicrob Chemother* 1989;24:23–28.
398. Ohnhaus EE, Halter F, Lebek G. Estimation of the biliary excretion of different cephalosporins utilizing retrograde cholongiopancreatography (ERCP). *Endoscopy* 1981;13:13–32.
399. Okamoto MP, Gill MA, Nakahiro RK, et al. Tissue concentrations of cefepime in acute cholecystitis patients. *Ther Drug Monitor* 1992;14:220–225.
400. Olson NH, Nightingale CH, Quintiliani R. Penetration characteristics of cefamandole into the right atrial appendage and pericardial fluid in patients undergoing open heart surgery. *Ann Thorac Surg* 1979;29:104–108.
401. Oosterlinck W, Defoort R, Renders G. The concentration of sulphamethoxazole and trimethoprim in human prostate gland. *Br J Urol* 1975;47:301–304.
402. Orda R, Berger SA, Levy Y, et al. Penetration of ceftriaxone and cefoperazone into bile and gallbladder tissue in patients with acute cholecystitis. *Dig Dis Sci* 1992;37: 1691–1693.
403. Orr W, Jackson WB, Colden K. Intraocular penetration of netilmicin. *Can J Ophthalmol* 1985;20:171–175.
404. Overturf GD, Cable DC, Forthal DN, et al. Treatment of bacterial meningitis with ceftizoxime. *Antimicrob Agents Chemother* 1984;25:258–262.
405. Owen AWMC, Faragher EB. Biliary pharmacokinetics of ticarcillin and clauvulanic acid. *J Antimicrob Chemother* 1986;17(Suppl C):65–70.
405a. Ozdamar A, Aras C, Ozturk R, et al. Ocular penetration of cefepime following systemic administration in humans. *Ophthalmic Surg Lasers* 2001;32:25–29.
406. Paavolainen M, Kohonen A, Palva T, et al. Penetration of erythromycin stearate into maxillary sinus mucosa and secretion in chronic maxillary sinusitis. *Acta Otolargyngol (Stockh)* 1977;84:292–295.
407. Palmu A, Jarvinen H, Hallynck T, et al. Cefadroxil levels in bile in biliary infection. In: Nelson JD, Grassi C, eds. *Current chemotherapy and infectious disease: proceedings of the 11th International Congress of Chemotherapy and 19th Interscience Conference on Antimicrobial Agents and Chemotherapy.* Washington, DC: American Society for Microbiology, 1979;643–644.
408. Panteix G, Harf R, deMontclos H, et al. Josamycin pulmonary penetration determined by bronchoalveolar lavage in man. *J Antimicrob Chemother* 1988;22:917–921.
409. Panzer JD, Brown DC, Epstein WL, et al. Clindamycin levels in various body tissues and fluids. *J Clin Pharmacol* 1972;12:259–262.
410. Parker CW. Radioimmunoassay. *Annu Rev Pharmacol Toxicol* 1981;21:113–132.
411. Parker RH, Birbara C, Schmid FR. Passage of nafcillin and ampicillin into synovial fluid. *Zentralbl Bakteriol* 1976;(Suppl 5):1115–1123.
412. Parsens RL, Beavis JP, David JA, et al. Plasma, bone, hip capsule, and drain fluid concentrations of cephazolin during total hip replacement. *Br J Clin Pharmacol* 1978;5:331–336.
413. Pascual A, Tsukayama D, Kovarik J, et al. Uptake and activity of rifapentine in human periotoneal macrophages and polymorphonuclear leukocytes. *Eur J Clin Microbiol* 1987;6:152–157.
414. Pedersen SS, Jensen T, Hvidberg EF. Comparative pharmacokinetics of ciprofloxacin and ofloxacin in cystic fibrosis patients. *J Antimicrob Chemother* 1987;20:575–583.
415. Pennington JE. Penetration of antibiotics into respiratory secretions. *Rev Infect Dis* 1981;3:67–73.
416. Perea EJ, Garcia-Iglesias MC, Ayarra J, et al. Comparative concentration of cefoxitin in human lungs and sera. *Antimicrob Agents Chemother* 1983;23:323–324.
417. Perry-Holly BA, Ritterbusch JK, Burdge RE, et al. Cefamandole levels in serum and necrotic bone. *Clin Orthop* 1985;1199:280–281.
418. Peterson LR, Gerding DN. Prediction of cefazolin penetration into high- and low-protein-containing extravascular fluid: new method for performing simultaneous studies. *Antimicrob Agents Chemother* 1978;14:533–538.
419. Peterson LR, Gerding DN. Influence of protein binding of antibiotics on serum pharmacokinetics and extravascular penetration: clinically useful concepts. *Rev Infect Dis* 1980;2:340–348.
420. Peterson LR, Gerding DN, Fasching CE. Effects of method of antibiotic administration on extravascular penetration: crossover study of cefazolin given by intermittent injection or constant infusion. *J Antimicrob Chemother* 1981;7:71–79.
421. Peterson LR, Gerding DN, Zinneman HH, et al. Evaluation of three newer methods for investigating protein interactions of penicillin G. *Antimicrob Agents Chemother* 1977;11:993–998.
422. Peterson LR, Hall WH, Zinneman HH, et al. Standardization of a preparative ultracentrifuge method for

quantitative determination of protein binding of seven antibiotics. *J Infect Dis* 1977;136:778–783.

423. Peterson LR, Schierl EA, Hall WH. Effect of protein concentration and binding on antibiotic assays. *Antimicrob Agents Chemother* 1975;7:540–542.
424. Peterson LR, Van Etta LL, Gerding DN. Interstitial concentration of antibiotics. *J Antimicrob Chemother* 1981;8:425.
425. Petounis A, Papapanos G, Karageorgiou-Makromihelaki C. Penetration of tobryamycin sulfate into the human eye. *Br J Ophthalmol* 1978;62:660–662.
426. Pfau A, Perlberg S, Shapira A. The pH of the prostatic fluid in health and disease: implications of treatment in chronic bacterial prostatitis. *J Urol* 1978;119:384–387.
427. Pierre J, Bergogne-Berezin E, Kafe H, et al. The penetration of macrolides into bronchial secretions. *J Antimicrob Chemother* 1985;16(Suppl A):217–220.
428. Plaue R, Muller O, Fabricius K, et al. Verlaufiger Bericht uber Cefoxitinspiegel-Bestimmungen in menschlichen geweben. *Infection* 1979;7(Suppl 1):S80–S84.
429. Plaue VR, Bethke RO, Fabricius K, et al. Kritische Untersuchungen zur Methodik von Antibiotikaspiegelbestimmungen in Menschlichen Geweben. *Arzneimittelforschung* 1980;30:1–5.
430. Plomp TA, Mattelaer JJ, Maes RAA. The concentration of thiamphenicol in seminal fluid and prostatic tissue. *J Antimicrob Chemother* 1978;4:65–71.
431. Plomp TA, Thiery M, Maes RAA. The passage of thiamphenicol and chloramphenicol into human milk after single and repeated oral administration. *Vet Hum Toxicol* 1983;25:167–172.
432. Pocidalo J. Use of fluoroquinolones for intracellular pathogens. *Rev Infect Dis* 1989;11:S979–S984.
433. Poirier RH, Ellison AC. Ocular penetration of orally administered minocycline. *Ann Ophthalmol* 1979;11:1859–1861.
434. Polk RE, Smith JE, Ducey K, et al. Penetration of moxalactam and cefazolin into atrial appendage after simultaneous intramuscular or intravenous administration. *Antimicrob Agents Chemother* 1982;22:201–203.
435. Posner AC, Prigot A, Konicoff NG. Further observations on the use of tetracycline hydrochloride in prophylaxis and treatment of obstetric infections. *Antibiot Annu* 1955;19541955:594–598.
436. Prigot A, Froix KJ, Rubin E. Absorption, diffusion and excretion of a new penicillin, oxacillin. *Antimicrob Agents Chemother* 1962;1962:402–409.
437. Prokesch RC, Hand WL. Antibiotic entry into human polymorphonuclear leukocytes. *Antimicrob Agents Chemother* 1982;21:373–380.
438. Pulaski EJ, Fusillo MH. Gallbladder bile concentrations of the major antibiotics following intravenous administration. *Surg Gynecol Obstet* 1955;100:571–574.
439. Pulaski EJ, Tubbs RS. Inhibitory effects of kanamycin and diffusion into various body fluids. *Antibiot Med Clin Ther* 1959;6:589–593.
440. Quentin CD, Ansorg R. Penetration of cefotaxime into the aqueous humour after intravenous application. *Graefes Arch Clin Exp Ophthalmol* 1983;220:245–247.
441. Quintiliani R. A review of the penetration of cefadroxil into human tissue. *J Antimicrob Chemother* 1982;19(Suppl B):33–38.
442. Quintiliani R, Klimek J, Nightingale CH. Penetration of cephapirin and cephalothin into the right atrial appendage and pericardial fluid of patients undergoing open heart surgery. *J Infect Dis* 1979;139:348–352.
443. Racz G. Tissue concentration of antibiotic following oral doses of tetracycline phosphate complex. *Curr Ther Res* 1971;13:553–557.
444. Raeburn JA. A review of experimental models for studying the tissue penetration of antibiotics in man. *Scand J Infect Dis* 1978;14(Suppl):225–227.

444a. Raeburn JAA. A method for studying antibiotic concentrations in inflammatory exudate. *J Clin Pathol* 1971;24:633–635.

444b. Rana B, Butcher I, Grigoris P, et al. Linezolid penetration into osteo-articular tissues. *J Antimicron Chemother* 2002;50:747–750.

445. Ratzan KR, Baker HB, Lauredo I. Excretion of cefamandole, cefazolin and cephalothin into T-tube bile. *Antimicrob Agents Chemother* 1978;13:985–987.
446. Ratzan KR, Ruiz C, Irvin GL III. Biliary tract excretion of cefazolin, cephalothin, and cephaloridine in the presence of biliary tract disease. *Antimicrob Agents Chemother* 1974;6:426–431.
447. Rauws AG, Van Klingeren B. Estimation of antibiotic levels of interstitial fluid from whole tissue levels. *Scand J Infect Dis* 1978;14(Suppl):186–188.
448. Rebuck JW, Crowley JH. A method of studying leukocytic functions in vivo. *Ann NY Acad Sci* 1955;59:757–805.
449. Records RE. The human intraocular penetration of methicillin. *Arch Ophthalmol* 1966;76:720–722.
450. Records RE. Human intraocular penetration of sodium oxacillin. *Arch Ophthalmol* 1967;77:693–695.
451. Records RE. Intraocular penetration of cephalothin. *Am J Ophthalmol* 1968;66:441–443.
452. Records RE. The human intraocular penetration of a new orally effective cephalosporin antibiotic, cephalexin. *Ann Ophthalmol* 1971;3:309–313.
453. Reid TMS, Gould IM, Goulder D, et al. Brief report: respiratory tract penetration of ciprofloxacin. *Am J Med* 1989;87(Suppl 5A):60S–61S.
454. Ricevuti G, Mazzone A, Vecilli E, et al. Influence of erdosteine, a mucolytic agent, on amoxycillin penetration into sputum in patients with an infective exacerbation of chronic bronchitis. *Thorax* 1988;43:585–590.
455. Ricevuti G, Pasotti D, Mazzone A, et al. Serum, sputum and bronchial concentrations of erythromycin in chronic bronchitis after single and multiple treatments with either propionate-17-acetylcysteinate or stearate erythromycin. *Chemotherapy* 1988;34:374–379.
456. Riley FC, Boyle GL, Leopold IH. Intraocular penetration of cephaloridine in humans. *Am J Ophthalmol* 1968;66:1042–1049.
457. Robens W. Concentrations of cefmenoxime in human tissues. *Am J Med* 1984;77(Suppl 6A):32–33.
458. Rolando N, Wade JJ, Philpott-Howard JN, et al. The penetration of imipenem/cilastatin into ascitic fluid in patients with chronic liver disease. *J Antimicrob Chemother* 1994;33:163–167.
459. Rood JP, Collier J. Metronidazole levels in alveolar bone. In: *Metronidazole*: Royal Society of Medicine International Congress and Symposium, series 18. 45–47.
460. Rosansky R, Brzczinsky A. The excretion of penicillin in human milk. *J Lab Clin Med* 1949;34:497–500.
461. Rosdahl VT, Sorensen TS, Colding H. Determination of antibiotic concentrations in bone. *J Antimicrob Chemother* 1979;5:275–280.
462. Roth B. Penetration of parenterally administered rifampicin into bone tissue. *Chemotherapy* 1984;30:358–365.
463. Rowland M, Tozer TN. *Clinical pharmacokinetics:*

concepts and applications, 2nd ed. Philadelphia: Lea & Febiger, 1989.

464. Rubinstein E, Avni I, Tuizer H, et al. Cefsulodin levels in the human aqueous humor. *Arch Ophthalmol* 1985;103:426–427.
465. Ruhen RW, Tandon MK. Minocycline, doxycycline and tetracycline levels in serum and bronchial secretions of patients with chronic bronchitis. *Pathology* 1975;7:193–197.
466. Ruiz DE, Warner JF. Nafcillin treatment of *Staphylococcus aureus* meningitis. *Antimicrob Agents Chemother* 1976;9:554–555.
467. Runyon BA, Akriviadis EA, Sattler FR, et al. Ascitic fluid and serum cefotaxime and desacetyl cefotaxime levels in patients treated for bacterial peritonitis. *Dig Dis Sci* 1991;36:1782–1786.
468. Russo J, Thompson MIB, Russo ME. Piperacillin distribution into bile, gallbladder wall, abdominal skeletal muscle, and adipose tissue in surgical patients. *Antimicrob Agents Chemother* 1982;22:488–492.
469. Ryan DM, Cars O. A problem in the interpretation of beta-lactam antibiotic levels in tissue. *J Antimicrob Chemother* 1983;12:281–284.
470. Sabath LD. The assay of antimicrobial compounds. *Hum Pathol* 1976;7:287–295.
471. Saggers BA, Lawson D. In vivo penetration of antibiotics into sputum in cystic fibrosis. *Arch Dis Child* 1968;43:404–409.
472. Sales JE, Sutcliffe M, O'Grady F. Excretion of clindamycin in the bile of patients with biliary tract disease. *Chemotherapy* 1973;19:11–15.
473. Santacroce F, Dainelli B, Mignini F, et al. Determination of cefatrizine levels in blood, tonsils, paranasal sinuses and middle ear. *Drugs Exp Clin Res* 1985;11:453–456.
474. Sasagawa I, Yamaguchi O, Shiraiwa Y. Cefminox sodium penetration into prostatic tissue with and without inflammation. *Int Urol Nephrol* 1991;23:569–572.
475. Saxby MF, Arkell DG, Andrews JM, et al. Penetration of cefpirome into prostatic tissue. *J Antimicrob Chemother* 1990;25:488–490.
475a. Scaglione F, De Martini G, Peretto L, et al. Pharmacokinetic study of cefodizime and ceftriaxone in sera and bones of patients undergoing hip arthroplasty. *Antimicrob Agents Chemother* 1997;41:2292–2294.
476. Schalkhauser K, Adam D. Zur diffusion von Cefotaxim in verschiedene Gewebe des urologischen Bereichs. *Infection* 1980;8(Suppl 3):S327–S329.
477. Schauersberger J, Amon M, Wedrich A, et al. Penetration and decay of meropenem into the human aqueous humor and vitreous. *J Ocul Pharmacol Ther* 1999;15:439–445.
478. Schreiner A, Digranes A. Pharmocokinetics of lymecycline and doxycycline in serum and suction blister fluid. *Chemotherapy* 1985;31:261–265.
479. Schurman DJ, Johnson BL, Finerman G, et al. Antibiotic bone penetration concentration of methicillin and clindamycin phosphate in human bone taken during total hip replacement. *Clin Orthop* 1975;111:142–146.
480. Schurman OJ, Hirshman HP, Burton DS. Cephalothin and cefamandole penetration into bone, synovial fluid, and wound drainage fluid. *J Bone Joint Surg [Am]* 1980;62:981–985.
480a. Schurman OJ, Hirshman HP, Kajiyama G, et al. Cefazolin concentrations in bone and synovial fluid. *J Bone Joint Surg [Am]* 1978;60:359–362.
481. Schurman OJ, Burton DS, Kajiyama G, et al. Sodium cephapirin disposition and distribution into human bone. *Curr Ther Res* 1976;20:194–203.
482. Serieys C, Bergogne-Berezin E, Kafe H, et al. Study of the diffusion of cefmenoxine into the bronchial secretions. *Chemotherapy* 1986;32:1–6.
483. Severn M, Powis SJA. Biliary excretion and tissue levels of cefuroxime: a study in eleven patients undergoing cholecystectomy. *J Antimicrob Chemother* 1979;5:183–188.
484. Shimada J, Ueda Y. Moxalactam: absorption, excretion, distribution, and metabolism. *Rev Infect Dis* 1982;4(Suppl):S569–S580.
485. Shyu WC, Haddad J, Reilly J, et al. Penetration of cefprozil into middle ear fluid of patients with otitis media. *Antimicrob Agents Chemother* 1994;38:2210–2212.
486. Shyu WC, Quintiliani R, Nightingale CH. An improved method to determine interstitial fluid pharmacokinetics. *J Infect Dis* 1985;152:1328–1331.
487. Shyu WC, Quintiliani R, Nightingale CH, et al. Effect of protein binding on drug penetration into blister fluid. *Antimicrob Agents Chemother* 1988;32:128–130.
488. Shyu WC, Shah VR, Campbell DA, et al. Excretion of cefprozil into human breast milk. *Antimicrob Agents Chemother* 1992;36:938–941.
489. Silbermann M, Niederdellmann H, Kluge D, et al. Concentration of piperacillin and cefotaxime in human muscle and fat tissue. In: *Program and abstracts of the 20th Interscience Conference on Antimicrobial Agents and Chemotherapy.* Washington, DC: American Society for Microbiology, 1980. Abstract 755.
490. Silvain C, Bouquet S, Breux JP, et al. Oral pharmacokinetics and ascitic fluid penetration of ofloxacin in cirrhosis. *Eur J Clin Pharmacol* 1989;37:261–265.
491. Silvain C, Breux JP, Rochard E, et al. Decreased erythrocyte penetration of pefloxacin in cirrhotic patients. *J Antimicrob Chemother* 1987;20:290–292.
492. Silverstein H, Bernstein JM, Lerner PI. Antibiotic concentrations in middle ear effusions. *Pediatrics* 1966;38:33–39.
493. Simon C, Malerczyk V, Brahmstaedt E, et al. Cefazolin, Ein Neues Breitspektrum-Antibiotikum. *Dtsch Med Wochenschr* 1973;98:2448–2450.
494. Simon C, Sommerwerck D, Friehoff J. Der Wert von Doxycycloin bei Atemwegsinfektionen (Serum, -Speichel, -Sputum-Lungen, und Pleuraexsudatspiegel). *Prax Klin Pneumol* 1978;32:266–270.
495. Simon VC, Malerczyk V. Serum and skin blister levels of cefadroxil in comparison to cephalexin. In: *Program and abstracts of the 18th Interscience Conference on Antimicrobial Agents and Chemotherapy.* Washington, DC: American Society for Microbiology, 1978. Abstract 225.
496. Sinues B, Martinez P, Barrera V, et al. Taux de la tobramycine dans l'humeur aqueuse et le plasma humains apres administration par voie intraveineuse et sous-conjonctivale. *Therapie* 1983;38:345–353.
497. Sinues B, Martinez P, Palomar A, et al. Niveles de gentamicina en humor acuoso y plasma segun la via de administracion. *Ard Farmacol Toxicol* 1982;8:219–226.
498. Sippel JE, Mikhail IA, Girgis NI, et al. Rifampin concentrations in cerebrospinal fluid of patients with tuberculous meningitis. *Am Rev Respir Dis* 1974;109:579–580.
499. Sirot J, Lopitaux R, Sirot J, et al. Diffusion de la

cloxacilline dans le tissue osseux human apies administration par voie orale. *Pathol Biol* 1982;30:332–335.
500. Sirot J, Prive L, Lopitaux R, et al. Etude de la diffusion de la rifampicine dans le tissu osseux spong ieux et compact au cours de protheses totales de hanches. *Pathol Biol* 1983;31:438–441.
501. Smilak JD, Flittie WH, Williams TW. Bone concentrations of antimicrobial agents after parenteral administration. *Antimicrob Agents Chemother* 1976;9:169–171.
502. Smith BR, LeFrock J. Biliary tree penetration of parenteral antibiotics. *Infect Surg* 1983;2:110–121.
503. Smith BR, LeFrock JL. Bronchial tree penetration of antibiotics. *Chest* 1983;83:904–908.
504. Smith BR, LeFrock J, Carr BB. Cefmenoxime penetration into gallbladder bile and tissue. *Antimicrob Agents Chemother* 1983;23:941–943.
505. Smith RP, Schmid GP, Baltch AL, et al. Concentration of cefaclor in human prostatic tissue. *Am J Med Sci* 1981;281:19–24.
506. Smith R, Wilbur H, Bassey C, et al. Azlocillin and mezolocillin concentration in human prostatic tissue. *Chemotherapy* 1988;34:267–271.
507. Smith RP, Wilbur H, Sutphen NT, et al. Moxalactam concentrations in human prostatic tissue. *Antimicrob Agents Chemother* 1983;24:15–17.
508. Smith Kline & French Laboratories. Data on file. Philadelphia, PA.
509. Solberg CO, Halstensen A, Digranes A, et al. Penetration of antibiotics into human leukocytes and dermal suction blisters. *Rev Infect Dis* 1983;5:S468–S473.
510. Solberg CO, Madsen ST, Digranes A, et al. High dose netilmicin therapy: efficacy, tolerance and tissue penetration. *J Antimicrob Chemother* 1980;6:133–141.
511. Soman A, Honeybourne D, Andrews J, et al. Concentrations of moxifloxacin in serum and pulmonary compartments following a single 400 mg oral dose in patients undergoing fibre-optic bronchoscopy. *J Antimicrob Chemother* 1999;44:835–838.
512. Sorensen TS, Colding H, Schroeder E, et al. The penetration of cefazolin, erythromycin and methicillin into human bone tissue. *Acta Orthop Scand* 1978;49:549–553.
512a. Souli M, Kopsinis G, Kavouklis E, et al. Vancomycin levels in human aqueous humour after intravenous and subconjunctival administration. *Int J Antimicrob Agents* 2001;18:239–243.
513. Soussy CJ, Deforges LP, LeVan Thoi J, et al. Cefotaxime concentration in the bile and wall of the gallbladder. *J Antimicrob Chemother* 1980;6(Suppl A):125–130.
514. Stahl JP, Bru JP, Fredji G, et al. Penetration of sulbactam into the cerebrospinal fluid of patients with bacterial meningitis receiving ampicillin therapy. *Rev Infect Dis* 1986;8(Suppl 5):S612–S616.
515. Stamey TA, Meares EM Jr, Winningham DG. Chronic bacterial prostatitis and the diffusion of drugs into prostatic fluid. *J Urol* 1970;103:187–194.
516. Steele RW, Bradsher RW. Comparison of ceftriaxone with standard therapy for bacterial meningitis. *J Pediatr* 1983;103:138–141.
517. Steen B, Rane A. Clindamycin passage into milk. *Br J Clin Pharmacol* 1982;13:661–664.
518. Steinberg TH, Hand WL. Effects of phagocytosis on antibiotic and nucleoside uptake by human polymorphonuclear leukocytes. *J Infect Dis* 1984;149:397–403.
518a. Stenquist M, Olen L, Jannert M, et al. Penetration of loracarbef into the maxillary sinus: a pharmacokinetic assessment. *Clin Ther* 1996;18:273–284.
519. Sterling RP, Connor DJ, Norman JC, et al. Cefonicid concentration in serum and atrial tissue during open heart surgery. *Antimicrob Agents Chemother* 1983;23:790–792.
520. Stoehr GP, Juhl RP, Veals J, et al. The excretion of rosaramicin into breast milk. *J Clin Pharmacol* 1985;25:89–94.
521. Stone JW, Guan Linong, Andrews JM, et al. Cefixime in-vitro activity, pharmacokinetics and tissue penetration. *J Antimicrob Chemother* 1989;23:221–228.
522. Sundberg L, Eden T, Ernstson S. Penetration of doxycycline in respiratory mucosa. *Acta Otolaryngol (Stockh)* 1983;96:501–508.
523. Swedish Study Group. Cefuroxime versus ampicillin and chloramphenicol for the treatment of bacterial meningitis. *Lancet* 1982;1:295–298.
524. Symes JM, Jarvic JD, Tresidder GC. An appraisal of cephalexin monohydrate levels in semen and prostatic tissue. *Chemotherapy* 1975;20:257–262.
525. Tabbara KF, Al-Kharashi SA, Al-Mansouri SM, et al. Ocular levels of azithromycin. *Arch Ophthalmol* 1998;116:1625–1628.
526. Takamoto M, Ishibashi T, Harada S, et al. Experience with ceftizoxime in respiratory tract infection and its transfer into pleural effusion. *Chemotherapy* 1980;28 (Suppl 5):394–404.
527. Takase Z. Laboratory and clinical studies of tobramycin in the field of obstetrics and gynecology. *Chemotherapy* 1975;23:1390–1403.
528. Takase Z, Obstetrics and Gynecology Research Group. Basic and clinical research on cefsulodin in the field of obstetrics and gynecology. *Jpn J Antibiot* 1982;35:2861–2877.
529. Takase Z, Shirafuji H, Uchida M. Clinical and laboratory studies on cefoxitin in the field of obstetrics and gynecology. *Chemotherapy* 1978;26:502–505.
530. Takase Z, Shirafuji H, Uchida M. Fundamental and clinical studies of cefoperazone in the field of obstetrics and gynecology. *Chemotherapy* 1980;28(Suppl 6):825–836.
531. Tan JS, Salstrom SJ. Levels of carbenicillin, ticarcillin, cephalothin, cefazolin, cefamandole, gentamicin, tobramycin and amikacin in human serum and interstitial fluid. *Antimicrob Agents Chemother* 1977;11:698–700.
532. Tan JS, Salstrom SJ. Bacampicillin, ampicillin, cephalothin and cephapirin levels in human blood and interstitial fluid. *Antimicrob Agents Chemother* 1979; 15:510–512.
533. Tan JS, Salstrom S, Signs SA, et al. Pharmacokinetics of intravenous cefmetazole with emphasis on comparison between predicted theoretical levels in tissue and actual skin window fluid levels. *Antimicrob Agents Chemother* 1989;33:924–927.
534. Tan JS, Trott A, Phair JP, et al. A method for measurement of antibiotics in human interstitial fluid. *J Infect Dis* 1972;126:492–497.
535. Tanaka H, Nishino H, Sawada T, et al. Biliary penetration of cefbuperazone in the presence and absence of obstructive jaundice. *J Antimicrob Chemother* 1987;20:417–420.
536. Taryle DA, Good JT, Morgan EJ, et al. Antibiotic concentrations in human parapneumonic effusions. *J Antimicrob Chemother* 1981;7:171–177.
537. Tegeder I, Schmidtko A, Brautigam L, et al. Tissue

distribution of imipenem in critically ill patients. *Clin Pharmacol Ther* 2002;71:325–333.
538. Tetzlaff TR, Howard JB, McCracken GH, et al. Antibiotic concentrations in pus and bone of children with osteomyelitis. *J Pediatr* 1978;92:135–140.
539. Thadepalli H, Mandal AK, Bach VT, et al. Tissue levels of doxycycline in the human lung and pleura. *Chest* 1980;78:304–305.
540. Thrupp LD, Leedom JM, Ivler D, et al. Ampicillin levels in the cerebrospinal fluid during treatment of bacterial meningitis. *Antimicrob Agents Chemother* 1965;1964:206–213.
541. Thys J, Klastersky J, Mombelli G. Peak or sustained antibiotic serum levels for optimal tissue penetration. *J Antimicrob Chemother* 1981;8(Suppl C):29–36.
542. Thys JP, Vanderkelen B, Klastersky J. Pharmacological study of cefazolin during intermittent and continuous infusion: a crossover investigation in humans. *Antimicrob Agents Chemother* 1976;10:395–398.
543. Thys JP, Vanderhoeft P, Herchuelz A, et al. Penetration of aminoglycosides in uninfected pleural exudates and in pleural empyemas. *Chest* 1988;93:530–532.
544. Tsacopoules M. The penetration of vibramycin (doxycycline) in human aqueous humor. *Ophthalmologica* 1969;159:418–429.
545. Tuominen RK, Mannisto PT, Solkinen A, et al. Antibiotic concentration in suction skin blister fluid and saliva after repeated dosage of erythromycin acistrate and erythromycin base. *J Antimicrob Chemother* 1988;21 (Suppl D):57–65.
546. Uwaydah MM, Faris BM, Samara IN, et al. Cloxacillin penetration. *Am J Ophthalmol* 1976;82:114–116.
547. Vacek V, Hejzlar M, Pavlansky R. Certain problems of rational lincomycin therapy of staphylococcal osteomyelitis. *Rev Czech Med* 1969;15:92–102.
548. Vacek V, Hejzlar M, Skalova M. Penetration of antibiotics into the cerebrospinal fluid in inflammatory conditions. I. Preface and comparative study of ampicillin with hetacillin. *Int J Clin Pharmacol* 1968;1:87–90.
549. Vacek V, Hejzlar M, Skalova M. Penetration of antibiotics into the cerebrospinal fluid in inflammatory conditions. II. Lincomycin. *Int J Clin Pharmacol* 1968;1:501–503.
550. Vacek V, Hejzlar M, Skalova M. Penetration of antibiotics into the cerebrospinal fluid in inflammatory conditions. III. Gentamicin. *Int J Clin Pharmacol* 1969;2:277–279.
551. Vaillant L, Machet L, Taburet AM, et al. Levels of fusidic acid in skin blister fluid and serum after repeated administration of two dosages (250 and 500 mg). *Br J Dermatol* 1992;126:591–595.
552. Vainiopaa S, Wilppula E, Lalla M, et al. Cefamandole and isoxazolyl penicillins in antibiotic prophylaxis of patients undergoing total hip or knee-joint arthroplasty. *Arch Orthop Trauma Surg* 1988;107:228–230.
553. Valcke YJ, Vogelaers DP, Colardyn FA, et al. Penetration of netilmicin in the lower respiratory tract after once-daily dosing. *Chest* 1992;101:1028–1032.
554. Valencia-Chinas A, Galindo-Hernandez F, Reyes-Sanchez J, et al. Concentrations of cefadroxil in osteoarticular tissues. In: *Program and abstracts of the 11th International Congress of Chemotherapy and 19th Interscience Conference on Antimicrobial Agents and Chemotherapy.* Washington, DC: American Society for Microbiology, 1979. Abstract 338.
555. Van der Auwera P, Matsumoto T, Husson M. Intraphagocytic penetration of antibiotics. *J Antimicrob Chemother* 1988;22:185–192.
556. Van Etta LL, Kravitz GR, Russ TE, et al. Effect of method of administration on extravascular penetration of four antibiotics. *Antimicrob Agents Chemother* 1982;21:873–880.
557. Van Etta LL, Peterson LR, Fasching CE, et al. The effect of the ratio of surface area to volume on the penetration of antibiotics into extravascular spaces in an in vitro model. *J Infect Dis* 1982;146:423–428.
558. Van Gossum A, Quenon M, Van Gossum M, et al. Penetration of cefoperazone into ascites. *Eur J Clin Pharmacol* 1989;37:577–580.
558a. Van Niekerk CH, Steyn DL, Davis WG, et al. Chloramphenicol levels in cerebrospinal fluid in meningitis. *S Afr Med J* 1980;58:159–160.
559. Varsano J, Fischl J, Shochet SB. The excretion of orally ingested nitrofurantoin in human milk. *J Pediatr* 1973;82:886–887.
560. Viek P. Concentration of sodium nafcillin in pathological synovial fluid. *Antimicrob Agents Chemother* 1962;1961:379–383.
561. Vitt TG, Panzer JD. Lincomycin at the tissue level following intramuscular lincocin. Kalamazoo, MI: The Upjohn Co. 1973. Lincocin Study C5 034. Data on file.
562. Voller A, Bidwell DE, Bartlett A. Enzyme immunoassays in diagnostic medicine. *Bull WHO* 1976;53:55–65.
562a. von Baum H, Bottcher S, Abel R, et al. Tissue and serum concentrations of levofloxacin in orthopaedic patients. *Int J Antimicr Agents* 2001;18:335–340.
563. Von Gunten S, Lew D, Paccolat F, et al. Aqueous humor penetration of ofloxacin given by various routes. *Am J Ophthalmol* 1994;117:87–89.
564. Wagner JG. *Fundamentals of clinical pharmacokinetics,* 2nd ed. Hamilton, IL: Drug Intelligence Publications, 1979.
564a. Walstad RA, Hellum KB, Blika S, et al. Pharmacokinetics and tissue penetration of ceftazidine: studies on lymph, aqueous humor, skin blister, cerebrospinal fluid and pleural fluid. *J Antimicrob Chemother* 1983;12(Suppl A):275–282.
565. Walstad RA, Hellum KB, Thurmann-Nielsen E, et al. Pharmacokinetics and tissue penetration of timentin: a simultaneous study of serum, urine, lymph, suction blister and subcutaneous thread fluid. *J Antimicrob Chemother* 1986;17(Suppl C):71–80.
566. Walstad RA, Wiig JN, Thurmann-Nielsen E, et al. Pharmacokinetics of ceftazidime in patients with biliary tract disease. *Eur J Clin Pharmacol* 1986;31:327–331.
567. Wang EEL, Prober CG. Ventricular cerebrospinal fluid concentrations of trimethoprim-sulphamethoxazole. *J Antimicrob Chemother* 1983;11:385–389.
568. Warterberg K, Tohak J, Knapp W. Lung tissue concentrations of cefoperazone. *Infection* 1983;11:280–282.
569. Webb D, Thadepalli H, Bach V, et al. Clinical and experimental evaluation of cefoxitin therapy. *Chemotherapy* 1978;26(Suppl 1):306–312.
570. Webberly JM, Wise R, Andrews JM, et al. The pharmacokinetics and tissue penetration of FCE22101 following intravenous and oral administration. *J Antimicrob Chemother* 1988;21:445–450.
571. Weissenbacher ER, Adams D, Gutschow K, et al. Clinical results and concentrations of cefmenoxime in serum, amniotic fluid, mother's milk, and placenta. *Am J Med* 1984;77(Suppl 6A):11–12.

572. Whitby M, Hempenstall J, Gilpin C, et al. Penetration of monobactam antibiotics (aztreonam, carumonam) into human prostatic tissue. *Chemotherapy* 1989;35:7–11.
573. Wildfeuer A, Laufen H, Muller-Wening D, et al. The effect of antibiotics on the intracellular survival of bacteria in human phagocytic cells. *Arzneimittelforschung* 1987;37:1367–1370.
574. Wildfeuer A, Laufen H, Muller-Wening D, et al. Interaction of azithromycin and human phagocytic cells. *Arzneimittelforschung* 1989;39:755–758.
575. Wildfeuer A, Rühle KH, Balk PL, et al. Concentrations of ampicillin and sulbactam in serum and in various compartments of the respiratory tract of patients. *Infection* 1994;22:149–151.
576. Williams CB, Litvak AS, McRoberts JW. Comparison of serum and prostatic levels of tobramycin. *Urology* 1979;13:589–591.
577. Williams DN, Gustilo RB, Bevesley R, et al. Bone and serum concentrations of five cephalosporin drugs: relevance to prophylaxis and treatment in orthopedic surgery. *Clin Orthop* 1983;179:254–265.
578. Wilson APR, Taylor B, Treasure T, et al. Antibiotic prophylaxis in cardiac surgery: serum and tissue levels of teicoplanin, flucloxacillin and tobramycin. *J Antimicrob Chemother* 1988;21:210–212.
579. Wilson DE, Chalmers TC, Medoff MA. The passage of cephalothin into and out of ascitic fluid. *Am J Med Sci* 1967;253:449–452.
580. Wingfield DL, McDougal RL, Roy FH, et al. Ocular penetration of amikacin following intramuscular injection. *Arch Ophthalmol* 1983;101:117–120.
581. Winningham DG, Nemoy MJ, Stamey TA. Diffusion of antibiotics from plasma into prostatic fluid. *Nature* 1968;219:139–143.
581a. Wise R, Andrews JM, Ashby JP, et al. A study to determine the pharmacokinetics and inflammatory fluid penetration of gatifloxacin following a single oral dose. *J Antimicrob Chemother* 1999;44:701–704.
582. Wise R, Andrews JM, O'Neill P, et al. Pharmacokinetics and distribution in tissue of FK-037, a new parenteral cephalosporin. *Antimicrob Agents Chemother* 1994;38:2369–2372.
583. Wise R, Bennett SA, Dent J. The pharmocokinetics of orally absorbed cefuroxime compared with amoxycillin/clavulanic acid. *J Antimicrob Chemother* 1984;13:603–610.
584. Wise R, Dyhs A, Hegarty A, et al. Pharmacokinetics and tissue penetration of aztreonam. *Antimicrob Agents Chemother* 1982;22:969–971.
584a. Wise R, Gee T, Andrews JM, et al. Pharmacokinetics and inflammatory fluid penetration of intravenous daptomycin in volunteers. *Antimicrob Agents Chemother* 2002;46:31–33.
585. Wise R, Gillett AP, Cadge B, et al. The influence of protein binding upon tissue fluid levels of six -lactam antibiotics. *J Infect Dis* 1980;42:77–82.
586. Wise R, Kirkpatrick B, Ashby J, et al. Pharmacokinetics and tissue penetration of Ro 23–6240, a new trifluoroquinolone. *Antimicrob Agents Chemother* 1987;31:161–163.
587. Wise R, Lister D, McNulty CAM, et al. The comparative pharmacokinetics of five quinolones. *J Antimicrob Chemother* 1986;18(Suppl D):71–81.
588. Wise R, Logan M, Cooper M, et al. Pharmacokinetics and tissue penetration of tazobactam administered alone and with piperacillin. *Antimicrob Agents Chemother* 1991;35:1081–1084.
589. Wise R, Nye K, O'Neill P, et al. Pharmacokinetics and tissue penetration of ceftibuten. *Antimicrob Agents Chemother* 1990;34:1053–1055.
590. Wise R, Webberly JM, Andrews JM, et al. The pharmacokinetics and tissue penetration of intravenously administered CGP31608. *J Antimicrob Chemother* 1988;21:85–91.
591. Wittke RR, Adam D, Klein HE. Therapeutic results and tissue concentrations of temocillin in surgical patients. *Drugs* 1985;29(Suppl 5):221–226.
592. Wittmann DH, Kotthaus E. Further methodological improvement in antibiotic bone concentration measurements: penetration of ofloxacin into bone and cartilage. *Infection* 1986;14(Suppl 4):270–273.
593. Wittmann DH, Schassan HH. Bone levels, tissue fluid and peritoneal fluid measurements following piperacillin administration. In: *Program and abstracts of the 20th Interscience Conference on Antimicrobial Agents and Chemotherapy.* Washington, DC: American Society for Microbiology, 1980. Abstract 757.
594. Wittmann DH, Schassan HH Freitag V. Pharmacokinetic studies and results of a clinical trial with cefotaxime (HR-756). In: *Current chemotherapy and infectious disease.* Washington, DC: American Society for Microbiology, 1980;114–116.
595. Wittmann DH, Schassan HH, Seidel H. Untersuchungen uber die Bioverfugbarkeit von Cefuroxim im Knochen und im Wiundsekret. *Med Welt* 1979;30:227–232.
596. Wittmann DH, Schassan HH, Seidel H. Pharmakokinetische Untersuchungen zur Penetration von Azlocillin und Mezlocillin in den Knochen und in die Gewebsflussigkeit. *Arzneimittelforschung* 1981;31:1157–1162.
597. Wolf H, Madsen PO, Rhodes P. The ampicillin concentration in prostatic tissue and prostatic fluid. *Urol Int* 1967;22:453–460.
598. Wolff M, Chavanet P, Kazmierczak A, et al. Diffusion of cefpirome into the cerebrospinal fluid of patients with purulent meningitis. *J Antimicrob Chemother* 1992;29(Suppl A):59–62.
599. Wollmer P, Rhodes CG, Pike VW, et al. Measurement of pulmonary erythromycin concentration in patients with lobar pneumonia by means of positron tomography. *Lancet* 1982;2:1361–1363.
600. Woo FL, Johnson AP, Caldwell DR, et al. Piperacillin levels in human tears and aqueous humor. *Am J Ophthalmol* 1984;98:17–20.
601. Wong GA, Pierce TH, Goldstein E, et al. Penetration of antimicrobial agents into bronchial secretions. *Am J Med* 1975;59:219–223.
602. Worgan D, Daniel RJE. The penetration of minocycline into human sinus secretions. *Scott Med J* 1976;21:197–199.
603. Yamada H, Iwanaga T, Nakanishi H, et al. Penetration and clearance of cefoperazone and moxalactam in pleural fluid. *Antimicrob Agents Chemother* 1985;27:93–95.
604. Yew WW, Lee J, Chan CY, et al. Ofloxacin penetration into tuberculous pleural effusion. *Antimicrob Agents Chemother* 1991;35:2159–2160.
605. Yim CW, Flyan NM, Fitzgerald FT. Penetration of oral doxycycline into the cerebrospinal fluid of patients with latent neurosyphilis. *Antimicrob Agents Chemother* 1985;28:347–348.
606. Yogev R, Kolling WM. Intraventricular levels of amikacin after intravenous administration. *Antimicrob Agents Chemother* 1981;20:583–586.

607. Yogev R, Schultz WE, Rosenman SB. Penetrance of nafcillin into human ventricular fluid: correlation with ventricular pleocytosis and glucose levels. *Antimicrob Agents Chemother* 1981;19:545–548.
608. Yoshikawa TT, Maitra SK, Schotz MC, et al. High-pressure liquid chromatography for quantitation of antimicrobial agents. *Rev Infect Dis* 1980;2:169–181.
609. Yoshioka H, Cho K, Takimoto M, et al. Transfer of cefazolin into human milk. *J Pediatr* 1979;94:151–152.
610. Ziak E, Schuhmann G, Konstantinou D, et al. Levels in aqueous humour of eight relevant antibiotics in humans. In: *Recent advances in chemotherapy: proceedings of the 14th International Congress of Chemotherapy.* Kyoto, Japan. 1985.

APPENDIX 16.1

Urinary Excretion, Metabolites, and Reported Urine Levels (with Normal Renal Function) of Selected Antimicrobials

Drug	Excretion[a]	Metabolites	Urine Levels (μg/mL); Dose[b]
Penicillins			
Natural penicillins			
Penicillin G	TS, GF, some TR	Predominantly parent compound, small amount of inactive penicilloic acid (59)	Mean; 597 in 3 h; 500 mg
Phenoxymethyl-penicillin	TS, GF, some TR	34% penicilloic acid	400–600 units/ml; 500 mg
Aminopenicillins			
Ampicillin	TS, GF	11% penicilloic acid	160–700 in 6 h; 500 mg p.o. 1,000–2,250 in 6 h; 1 g/i.m.
Amoxicillin	TS, GF	20% penicilloic acid	300–1,300 over 6 h; 250–500 mg p.o.
Penicillinase-resistant penicillins			
Cloxacillin, oxacillin, dicloxacillin, flucloxacillin	TS, GF	90% parent compound, <10% bioactive metabolites	>1,000; 1 g i.v.
Methicillin	GF, TS	Parent compound	
Nafcillin	GF, TS,	30% parent compound	285–1,188 for 0–6 h; 500 mg i.m.
Carboxypenicillins			
Carbenicillin	TS, GF	>95% parent compound	5,000–10,000; 5 g i.v. >1,000 for 0–3h; 1 g p.o.
Ticarcillin	TS, GF	Predominantly parent compound, 10%–15% inactive penicilloic acid	600–2,500; 3 g i.v.
Ureidopenicillins			
Piperacillin	TS, GF	Parent compound	Mean, 13,000 over 8 h; 2 g i.v.
Azlocillin	TS, GF	Parent compound	2,240–5,000 in 2 h; 2–4 g i.v.
Mezlocillin	TS, GF	Parent compound	Mean, 3,400 over 6 h; 3 g i.v.
Amdinocillin (mecillinam)	GF, TS	Four metabolites, three bioactive	92–365 for 0-6 h; 400 mg pivmecillinam p.o.
β-Lactamase inhibitors			
Clavulanic acid	GF	Several metabolities	Mean, 403 for 0–4 h; 125 mg
Sulbactam	TS, GF	75% parent compound	
Tazobactam	GF, TS	25% open-ring metabolite	
Cephalosporins			
Cephalothin	GF, TS	33% desacetyl derivative (less active)	707 at 6 h; 500 mg i.m.
Cephalexin	GF, TS	Parent compound	Mean, 2,300 at 1–2 h; 500 mg q.i.d. 5,000–10,000 at 1–2 h; 1.0 g q.i.d.
Cefazolin	GF, TS	Parent compound	700–2,000 in 4–6 h; 1 g i.v.

(continued)

APPENDIX 16.1 (Continued)

Urinary Excretion, Metabolites, and Reported Urine Levels (with Normal Renal Function) of Selected Antimicrobials

Drug	Excretion[a]	Metabolites	Urine Levels (μg/mL); Dose[b]
Cephapirin	GF, TS	40% desacetyl derivatives (active)	300–2,500 over 6 h; 1 g i.v.
Cephradine	GF, TS	Parent compound	Mean, 1.1–3.2 mg/mL first 2 h; 500 mg p.o.
Cefonicid	GF, TR	Parent compound	162–1,017 for 0–2 h; 7.5 mg/kg i.v.
Cephaloridine	GF, some TS	Parent compound	400–1,200 over 6 h; 500 mg i.m.
Cefamandole	GF, TS	Parent compound	1,500–3,100 for 0–2 h; 1 g i.v.
Cefoxitin	GF, TS	About 1% descarbamyl derivative	450–7,200; 1 g i.v. 300–3,600; 500 mg every 6 h over 6 h
Cefotetan	GF, little TS	Parent compound, some bioactive tautomer	1,000 at 1 h; 0.5 g i.m. 2,000 at 1 h; 1 g i.m.
Cefotiam	GF, TS	Insufficient data	>25 at 8–10 h; 2 g i.v.
Ceforanide	GF, TS	Parent compound	
Cefuroxime	GF, TS	Parent compound	1,000–7,000 at 1–2 h; 750 mg to 1 g i.v.
Cefmenoxime	GF, TS	Parent compound	Mean, 3,000; 1 g i.v.
Cefaclor	GF, TS	Some metabolites	1,017 for 0–2 h; 250 mg p.o
Cefadroxil	GF, TS	Parent compound	1,200; 0.5 p.o.
Cefetamet	GF, some TS	Unchanged	832–1,120 at 2–4 h; 1.5 g p.o
Cefpodoxime proxetil	24–36% of dose in 24 h	Little metabolism	19.8 for 8–12 h; 200 mg p.o. for 4 h; 0.25–1 g
Ceprozil	GF, TS	Unchanged	175–658 for 4 h; 0.25–1 g
Cefotaxime	GF, TS	30% parent compound, substantial active desacetyl cefotaxime	250–1,500 for 0–6 h; 500 mg i.m. 1,900–4,000, 0–6 h; 2 g i.v.
Cefoperazone	15–37% excreted by GF, little TS	Parent compound	1,000–2,000 for 0–6 h; 2 g i.v. 120–600 for 0–6 h; 500 mg i.m.
Cefixime	20% excreted	Insufficient data	21–139 at 2–4 h; 400 mg p.o.
Ceftizoxime	GF, TS	Parent compound	$\leq$95 over 18 h; 2–4 g i.v. Mean, 6,150 over 2 h; 1 g i.v.
Ceftazidime	GF	Parent compound	Mean, 526 for 0–2 h; 1 g i.v.
Ceftriaxone	CF	Parent compound	Mean, 855; 1 g i.v.
Cefsulodin	GF, little TS, possible TR	Insufficient data	Mean, 1,400 for 0–2 h; 1 g i.v.
Cefpiramide	23% excreted by GF, little TS	No active metabolities	377–1,087 for 0–2 h; 500–1,000 mg i.v.
Other β-lactams			
Loracabef	GF, TS	Unchanged	12 at 6–12 h; 200 mg
Moxalactam	GF, some TS	Parent compound	565–1,700 for 0–6 h; 500 mg i.m. 1,900–7,500 for 0–6 h; 2 g i.v.

(continued)

APPENDIX 16.1 (Continued)

Urinary Excretion, Metabolites, and Reported Urine Levels (with Normal Renal Function) of Selected Antimicrobials

Drug	Excretion[a]	Metabolites	Urine Levels (μg/mL); Dose[b]
Imipenem/cilastatin	GF, 30% TS	Imipenem: 6%–30% parent without cilastatin, 70% with cilastatin; cilastatin: 76% parent, 14% *N*-acetyl derivative	500 at 2 h; for 500 mg i.v.
Meropenem	GF, TS	80% unchanged 20% open-ring metabolite	
Monobactams			
Aztreonam	GF, some TS	Some hydrolysis	1,000–5,000 for 0–2.5 h; 1 g i.v.
Carumonam	GF	10%–15% inactive opening form	26–792; 2 g i.v.
Aminoglycosides			
Amikacin	GF, some TR	Parent compound	170–1,720; 300 mg/m^2 i.v.
Gentamicin	GF	Parent compound	400–500 at 2–4 h;1.6 mg/kg i.m.
Kanamycin	GF, some TR	Parent compound	250–3,100; 300 mg/m^2 i.v.
Netilmicin	GF (?), some TR	Parent compound	Mean, 110 for 0–8 h; 2 mg/kg i.v.
Tobramycin	GF	Parent compound	94–443 in 1 h; 1 mg/kg i.m.
Macrolides and lincosamides			
Erythromycin	TS (?), TR (?)	5%–10% unchanged, *N*-demethyl metabolite	Mean, 30 for 0–6 h; 1 g every 8 h
Lincomycin	5–25% excreted	Insufficient data	2–255 for 0–4 h; 500 mg p.o
Clindamycin	≤6% excreted	*N*-demethyl and sulfoxide metabolites (both bioactive)	8–20 over 24 h; 150 mg p.o.
Roxithromycin	7–8% excreted	Three major metabolites	
Clarithromycin	40% in 24 h	32% parent compound or 14-OH metabolite (active), several other metabolites	
Azithromycin	6% in 24 h	Parent compound	
Tetracyclines			
Tetracycline	GF	Parent compound	Mean, 273 for 0–8 h; 500 mg
Doxycycline	GF, some TR	Parent compound	Mean, 134 over 4 h; 100 mg p.o.
Minocycline	<10% in urine GF	Uncharacterized metabolites	Mean, 9.4; 150 mg 8.1–19.4 over 12 h; 200 mg
Sulfonamides and trimethoprim			
Sulfadiazine	GF, TS	Substantial inactive acetyl derivative, some glucuronide	13–150 at 8 h; 3 g p.o.
Sulfisoxazole	GF, TS	30%–50% acetyl derivative	65% of 500 mg over 24 h; 4 g i. v. 67% of 2,377 mg over 24 h; 3 g p.o.
Sulfamethoxazole	GF, TS, TR	20%–40% parent compound, glucuronide, hydroxymethyl, and acetyl metabolites	100–600; 500 mg p.o. b.i.d.

(continued)

APPENDIX 16.1 (Continued)

Urinary Excretion, Metabolites, and Reported Urine Levels (with Normal Renal Function) of Selected Antimicrobials

Drug	Excretion[a]	Metabolites	Urine Levels (μg/mL); Dose[b]
Trimethoprim	GF, TS	25%–60% parent compound, several metabolites	70–100 for 0–4 h; 100 mg
Trimethoprim/ sulfamethoxazole			31–165/10–133; 160/800 b.i.d.
Quinolones			
Nalidixic acid	Insufficient data	85% inactive glucuronide, some active hydroxynalidixic acid	63–1,000:1 or 2 g p.o. q.i.d.
Cinoxacin	GF	50%–60% parent compound, four inactive metabolites	Mean, 390 for 0–2 h; 500 mg p.o.
Norfloxacin	GF, TS	25%–40% parent compound, 15%–20% as six metabolites (some active)	168–417 for 0–3 h; 400 mg
Ciprofloxacin	GF, TS	25%–50% parent compound, 10%–15% as four metabolites	>2 at 12–24 h; 500 mg
Enoxacin	GF, TS	40%–60% parent compound, 10%–15% metabolites	>8 at 24–48 h; 600 mg p.o.
Ofloxacin	GF, TS	70%–90% parent compound, 5%–15% as two metabolites	126–438 for 0–3 h; 100 mg i.v.
Pefloxacin	8%–9% excreted unchanged	24%–50% metabolites, major norfloxacin (active), four others	Mean, 42 for 0–24 h; 800 mg p.o.
Fleroxacin	GF	60% unchanged, 7% *N*-demethyl (active), 4.5% *N*-oxide (inactive)	100–200 for 8 h; 200–800 mg p.o.
Lomefloxacin	GF, TS	Small amount of unidentified metabolites	100–250 for 12 h; 200 mg
Levofloxacin	GF	Mainly unchanged	286 at 2–4 h; 200 mg
Other antimicrobials			
Chloramphenicol	GF	<10% parent compound, inactive glucuronide (TS, GF), unhydrolyzed succinate ester	15–200 at 2 h; 1 g p.o.
Colistimethate	Insufficient data	Sulfomethyl derivative	2.6–3.6 for 0–6 h; 30 mg i.m.
Fusidic acid	Not excreted	Insufficient data	<0.8 μg; 500 p.o. t.i.d.
Methenamine mandelate	GF, some TR	Insufficient data	300–3,000 formaldehyde; 1 g q.i.d. p.o.
Metronidazole	GF, TR (?)	15% parent compound, oxidative metabolites (some bioactive) glucuronic acid conjugates	Mean, 15–67 for 4–8 h; 0.25 mg p.o. 76–115 for 4–8 h; 0.50 mg
Nitrofurantoin	GF, TS, TR	30% parent compound	25–300; 100 mg p.o. q.i.d.
Polymyxin B	Insufficient data	60% parent compound	20–100; 2.5–3.0 mg/kg/day
Rifabutin	50% recovered	8% unchanged, >20 metabolites (some bioactive)	
Rifampin	6%–30% excreted GF	Desacetyl derivative (active)	Mean, 34–50 at 12 h; 300 mg p.o. even, 12 h

(continued)

APPENDIX 16.1 (Continued)

Urinary Excretion, Metabolites, and Reported Urine Levels (with Normal Renal Function) of Selected Antimicrobials

Drug	Excretion[a]	Metabolites	Urine Levels (μg/mL); Dose[b]
Spectinomycin	GF	Parent compound	Mean, 1,600 for 0–6 h; 2 g/ day
Teicoplanin	GF	<5% metabolites in rats	Mean, 43 for 0–4 h; 440 mg i.v.
Vancomycin	GF	Parent compound	800; 1 g i.v.
Antifungals			
Amphotercin B	GF, <10% excreted		0.51–4.61 mg/24 h; 5–105 mg
5-Fluorocytocine	GF	99% parent	>2,000 for 0–6 h; 3–5 g
Fluconazole	GF, TR	80% parent compound, 11% metabolites	118 for 0–24 h
Itraconazole	<1%	10 urinary metabolites	

[a] TS, tubular secretion; GF, glomerular filtration; TR, tubular resorption.
[b] p.o., orally; i.m., intramuscularly; i.v., intravenously; b.i.d., twice per day; t.i.d., three times per day; q.i.d., four times per day.
(From Nicolle [389a], with permission.)

CHAPTER 17

Epidemiology of Antimicrobial Resistance: Species Prevalence, Susceptibility Profiles, and Resistance Trends

Thomas R. Fritsche, Helio S. Sader, Ronald N. Jones

INTRODUCTION

The therapy of both nosocomial and community-acquired infections is affected by the continuing evolution of and challenges presented by antimicrobial resistance (1). It is estimated that 50% to 60% of the more than two million nosocomial infections in the United States each year are caused by antimicrobial-resistant bacteria, resulting in increased morbidity and mortality and associated health care costs (1–6). Recent studies tracking the outcomes of inadequately treated patients with bloodstream infections (i.e., patients infected with organisms resistant to the selected therapeutic antimicrobials) have documented greater hospital mortality compared to appropriately treated counterparts (7,8). These studies emphasize the problem of resistance and urge the selection of appropriate broad-spectrum empiric regimens guided by current pathogen prevalences and local, regional, or global resistance patterns.

Although surveillance of organism prevalence and antibiograms should be performed on a local level, data on patient unit populations, specific care units, and infection or specimen type are generally not available to health care providers due to lack of resources, administrative commitment, or recognition of the problem. In response to this situation, surveillance networks have emerged to monitor various aspects of medical practice related to infection therapy and to address current problems associated with antimicrobial resistance (9). While no ideal surveillance system exists, some systems provide meaningful results that can guide empiric antimicrobial regimens and minimize the consequences of antimicrobial resistance (9–11). Surveillance networks such as the Alexander Project, EARSS, ICARE (CDC-NNIS), MYSTIC Programme, PROTEKT, SENTRY Antimicrobial Surveillance Program, and TSN have been established with the support of the pharmaceutical industry or by government agencies to monitor patterns of microbial resistance (11). The most comprehensive programs vary significantly from each other in their stated goals and range from passive repositories of locally generated laboratory data to active surveillance networks utilizing central laboratories that perform organism identification confirmation and standardized reference quality susceptibility testing (12,13).

The MYSTIC Programme (14) and the SENTRY Program (15) were initiated in 1997, and each system contains approximately 100 active sentinel sites located in more than 30 nations around the world. A variety of objectives are pursued as part of the programs' assessment of resistance trends for the most important pathogens responsible for nosocomial and community-acquired infections. The SENTRY Program has reported on pathogen prevalence by site of infection or hospital unit (bloodstream infections; patients hospitalized with pneumonia, skin, and soft tissue infections; urinary tract infections; and intensive care units) and on the patterns of antimicrobial susceptibility to regularly tested and prescribed agents. The following discussion relies heavily on surveillance data generated by such programs and includes data representative of several geographic regions: North America (Canada and United States), Latin America, and Europe. Although medical centers in the Asia–Western Pacific

This chapter is adapted from an article by Dr. Jones published in Seminars in Respiratory and Critical Care Medicine, *vol. 24, no. 1, 2003.*

region participate in many of these studies, results for this region are not presented here.

PATHOGEN PREVALENCE AND SUSCEPTIBILITY PROFILES

Bloodstream Infections (BSIs)

Results from the SENTRY Program examining the epidemiology of BSI pathogens has been summarized previously (16–18) and recent trends in pathogen prevalence for North America over the years 1997–2002 are found in Table 17.1 (19,44). The rank order observed for BSIs over this interval has been remarkably consistent. The widest variation in percentage occurrence has been for *Staphylococcus aureus* (5.8%) because of its increasing prevalence. In contrast, coagulase-negative staphylococci (CoNS) and *Streptococcus pneumoniae* isolations decreased slightly (1% to 2%) over the 6 years. Gram-positive pathogens, including *S. aureus* (22.9% to 28.7%), CoNS (9.3% to 12.9%), and enterococci (9.5% to 10.5%), accounted for 56.5% of BSI isolates in 2002. *Escherichia coli* was the most common Gram-negative organism among the enterobacteria, and *Pseudomonas aeruginosa* (4.1% in 2002) was the most commonly isolated nonfermentative Gram-negative bacillus (19,44).

TABLE 17.1

Consensus Occurrence Rates of Bloodstream Infection (BSI) Pathogens from among 42,857 Episodes Recorded in the SENTRY Program (North America, 1997–2002)

Rank[a]	Pathogen	Percentage Range across Years
1	*S. aureus*	22.9–28.7
2	*E. coli*	16.7–18.6
3	CoNS[b]	9.3–12.9
4	*Enterococcus* spp	9.5–10.5
5	*Klebsiella* spp	7.4–7.9
6	*β* or viridans group streptococci	4.7–5.5
7	*S. pneumoniae*	3.5–5.6
8	*P. aeruginosa*	3.8–4.6
9	*Enterobacter* spp	3.3–4.1
10	*Serratia* spp	1.3–1.8

[a] The top ten ranked pathogens account for 91.5%–92.6% of all BSI over the 6-year period.
[b] CoNS, coagulase-negative staphylococci.
Reprinted from Beidenbach, Moet, Jones (44).

Diekema et al. (20) recently analyzed SENTRY Program BSI results by patient age and nosocomial versus community-acquired infection origin:

> Among nosocomial BSI, CoNS were the most frequently isolated pathogens in infants less than one year of age, but *S. aureus* increased in frequency with increasing age. Among community-onset BSI pathogens, *Streptococcus pneumoniae* was the most frequently reported pathogen causing BSI in patients aged 1–5 years, *S. aureus* among those aged 6–64 years, and *E. coli* predominated at the extremes of age (less than 1 year and ≥65 years of age). (p. 412)

These results for the children are similar to those reported by the CDC-NNIS program (21) and confirms the high risk of cross-transmission of endemic CoNS strains in these young patients (22).

Results from *in vitro* susceptibility testing for the most prevalent Gram-positive and -negative pathogens recovered from bloodstream infections in the United States, Canada, and Latin America for 1998 are summarized in Tables 17.2 and 17.3 (18).

Pneumonias in Hospitalized Patients

The most frequent causes of pneumonias occurring in hospitalized patients are listed in Table 17.4 (23). Similar to the BSI pathogen rank order, *S. aureus* was the most frequently isolated and reported potential cause of pneumonia (28%). *P. aeruginosa* (rank no. 2) and other nonfermentative Gram-negative bacilli were encountered in 26.2% of cases overall. Community-acquired isolates such as *S. pneumoniae* and *Haemophilus influenzae* accounted for 16.4% of cases, and among nosocomial pathogens, *S. aureus* and nonfermentative bacilli were the cause of 54.2% of the cases of pneumonia monitored. A clear majority (59%) of pathogens were Gram-negative. Respiratory pathogens generally display greater resistance to a variety of antimicrobials than do pathogens recovered from other sites, such as the bloodstream (Table 17.5).

The above results for North America stand in contrast to SENTRY Program findings for pneumonias in Latin American medical centers (Table 17.6) (24). In Latin America, *P. aeruginosa* was the most frequently isolated pathogen (26.3%), with *Acinetobacter* spp (9.6%) ranked fourth and *Stenotrophomonas maltophilia* (1.6%) ranked tenth; 37.5% of isolates were nonfermentative Gram-negative bacilli. The types of pathogens encountered (high prevalence of nonfermentative bacilli, enterobacteria, and methicillin-resistant *S. aureus*) indicated that the infections were predominantly nosocomial in origin rather than severe community-acquired pneumonias needing hospitalization. Antibiograms for the

(*text continues on page 825*)

TABLE 17.2

In Vitro Broth Microdilution Susceptibility Results for the Four Most Prevalent Causes of Gram-positive Bacteremia in the USA, Canada, and Latin America (51% of All Bacteremic Episodes)

Organism	Antimicrobial Agent	USA				Canada				Latin America			
		N	MIC Range	$MIC_{50/90}$	% S^a	*N*	MIC Range	$MIC_{50/90}$	% S^a	*N*	MIC Range	$MIC_{50/90}$	% S^a
S. aureus													
Oxacillin-susceptible	Amoxicillin/ Clavulanate	509	≤0.12–>16	1/2	98.6	80	≤0.12–16	1/2	98.8	128	≤0.12–4	1/2	100.0
	Cefazolin	509	≤2–>16	≤2/≤2	98.8	80	≤2–>16	≤2/≤2	98.8	128	≤2–8	≤2/≤2	100.0
	Ceftriaxone	509	1–>32	4/4	98.8	80	1–>32	4/4	98.8	128	1–16	4/4	97.7
	Cefepime	509	0.5–>16	2/4	98.4	80	1–>16	2/4	98.8	128	0.5–8	2/4	100.0
	Imipenem	509	≤0.06–>8	≤0.06/≤0.06	99.4	80	≤0.06–4	≤0.06/≤0.06	100.0	128	≤0.06–0.5	≤0.06/≤0.06	100.0
	Gentamicin	509	≤0.12–>16	0.25/1	99.2	80	≤0.12–4	0.25/1	100.0	128	≤0.12–>16	0.5/2	93.0
	Ciprofloxacin	509	0.03–>2	0.25/1	93.7	80	0.03–>2	0.5/0.5	97.5	128	0.06–>2	0.25/0.5	97.7
	Gatifloxacin	509	≤0.03–>4	0.06/0.12	98.2	80	≤0.03–2	0.06/0.12	100.0	128	≤0.03–2	0.06/0.12	100.0
	Grepafloxacin	509	≤0.25–>2	≤0.25/≤0.25	95.9	80	≤0.25/>2	≤0.25/≤0.25	97.5	128	≤0.25–2	≤0.25/≤0.25	99.2
	Erythromycin	509	≤0.06–>8	0.5/>8	68.6	80	0.25–>8	0.5/1	78.8	128	0.25–>8	0.5/>8	64.1
	Clindamycin	509	0.12–>8	0.25/0.25	96.1	80	≤0.06–0.5	0.25/0.25	100.0	128	≤0.06–>8	0.25/0.5	96.9
	Quinupristin/ dalfopristin	509	0.12–1	0.25/0.5	100.0	80	0.12–0.5	0.25/0.5	100.0	128	0.12–1	0.25/0.5	100.0
	Chloramphenicol	509	1–>16	8/16	74.9	80	2–>16	8/16	76.3	128	2–>16	8/16	63.3
	Rifampicin	509	≤0.25–>2	≤0.25/≤0.25	99.2	80	≤0.25/>2	0.25/≤0.25	97.5	128	≤0.25–>2	≤0.25/≤0.25	95.3
	Tetracycline	509	≤4–>8	≤4/≤4	94.9	80	≤4–>8	≤4/≤4	98.8	128	≤4–>8	≤4/≤4	93.0
	Teicoplanin	509	≤0.12–8	0.5/1	100.0	80	0.25–2	0.5/1	100.0	128	≤0.12–4	0.5/2	100.0
	Vancomycin	509	0.5–4	1/1	100.0	80	0.5–2	1/1	100.0	128	0.25–2	1/1	100.0
Oxacillin-resistant	Gentamicin	233	≤0.12–>16	1/>16	58.6	10	≤0.12–>16	0.5/16	80.0	68	≤0.12–>16	>16/>16	13.2
	Ciprofloxacin	233	0.06–>2	>2/>2	10.3	10	0.25–>2	0.5/>2	60.0	68	0.25–>2	>2/>2	5.9
	Gatifloxacin	233	≤0.03–>4	4/>4	48.3	10	≤0.03–4	0.12/4	60.0	68	0.06–>4	2/4	89.7

(*continued*)

TABLE 17.2 (Continued)

In Vitro Broth Microdilution Susceptibility Results for the Four Most Prevalent Causes of Gram-positive Bacteremia in the USA, Canada, and Latin America (51% of all Bacteremic Episodes)

Organism	Antimicrobial Agent	USA				Canada				Latin America			
		N	MIC Range	$MIC_{50/90}$	% S^a	*N*	MIC Range	$MIC_{50/90}$	% S^a	*N*	MIC Range	$MIC_{50/90}$	% S^a
	Grepafloxacin	233	≤0.25–>2	>2/>2	10.8	10	≤0.25–>2	≤0.25/>2	60.0	68	≤0.25–>2	>2/>2	8.8
	Erythromycin	233	0.25–>8	>8/>8	6.9	10	0.25–>8	>8/>8	20.0	68	0.5–>8	>8/>8	1.5
	Clindamycin	233	0.12–>8	>8/>8	18.5	10	0.12–>8	8/>8	40.0	68	0.25–>8	>8/>8	5.9
	Quinupristin/dalfopristin	233	≤0.06–2	0.5/1	99.1	10	0.12–1	0.5/0.5	100.0	68	0.12–1	0.5/1	100.0
	Chloramphenicol	233	4–>16	16/16	38.8	10	4–16	16/16	40.0	68	≤0.5–>16	16/>16	23.5
	Rifampicin	233	≤0.25–>2	≤0.25/2	88.4	10	≤0.25	≤0.25/≤0.25	100.0	68	≤0.25–>2	2/>2	39.7
	Tetracycline	233	≤4/–>8	≤4/>8	79.3	10	≤4–>8	≤4/≤4	90.0	68	≤4–>8	>8/>8	25.0
	Teicoplanin	233	≤0.12–8	1/2	100.0	10	≤0.12–2	0.5/2	100.0	68	0.25–4	1/2	100.0
	Vancomycin	233	0.25–2	1/2	100.0	10	0.5–1	1/1	100.0	68	0.5–2	1/1	100.0
CoNS[b]													
Oxacillin-susceptible	Amoxicillin/ Clavulanate	84	≤0.12–2	0.25/0.5	100.0	25	0.12–1	0.25/0.5	100.0	25	≤0.12–0.5	0.25/0.5	100.0
	Cefazolin	84	≤2	≤2/≤2	100.0	25	≤2	≤2/≤2	100.0	25	≤2	≤2/≤2	100.0
	Ceftriaxone	84	≤0.25–8	2/4	100.0	25	1–4	2/4	100.0	25	0.5–8	2/4	100.0
	Cefepime	84	0.25–2	1/1	100.0	25	0.25–2	0.5/2	100.0	25	0.25–2	1/2	100.0
	Imipenem	84	≤0.06–>8	≤0.06/≤0.06	98.8	25	≤0.06	≤0.06/≤0.06	100.0	25	≤0.06	≤0.06/≤0.06	100.0
	Gentamicin	84	≤0.12–>16	≤0.12/0.25	96.4	25	≤0.12–>16	≤0.12/>16	88.0	25	≤0.12–8	≤0.12/0.25	96.0
	Ciprofloxacin	84	0.12–>2	0.25/0.5	91.7	26	0.12–0.5	0.25/0.5	100.0	25	0.12–0.25	0.25/0.25	100.0
	Gatifloxacin	84	0.06–2	0.12/0.12	100.0	25	0.06–0.25	0.12/0.12	100.0	25	0.06–0.12	0.12/0.12	100.0
	Grepafloxacin	84	≤0.25–>2	≤0.25/≤0.25	92.9	25	≤0.25	≤0.25/≤0.25	100.0	25	≤0.25–0.5	≤0.25/≤0.25	96.0
	Erythromycin	84	≤0.06–>8	0.5/>8	69.0	25	0.12>8	>8/>8	44.0	25	0.25–>8	0.5/>8	68.0
	Clindamycin	84	≤0.06–>8	0.12/0.25	95.2	25	≤0.06–>8	0.12–>8	84.0	25	0.06–>8	0.12/0.25	92.0
	Quinupristin/dalfopristin	84	≤0.06–0.5	0.12/0.25	100.0	25	≤0.06–1	0.12/0.5	100.0	25	≤0.06–0.25	0.12/0.25	100.0

	Chloramphenicol	84	2–16	8/8	97.6	25	2–8	4/8	100.0	25	1–16	8/8	92.0
	Rifampicin	84	≤0.25–0.5	≤0.25/≤0.25	100.0	25	≤0.25–>2	≤0.25/≤0.25	96.0	25	≤0.25	≤0.25/≤0.25	100.0
	Tetracycline	84	≤4–>8	≤4/>8	88.1	25	≤4–>8	≤4/>8	88.0	25	≤4–>8	≤4/>8	84.0
	Teicoplanin	84	≤0.12–8	1/8	100.0	25	≤0.12–8	2/8	100.0	25	≤0.12–16	1/8	92.0
	Vancomycin	84	≤0.12–2	1/2	100.0	25	0.25–4	1/2	100.0	25	0.25–4	1/2	100.0
Oxacillin-resistant	Gentamicin	283	≤0.12–>16	4/>16	52.7	92	≤0.12–>16	16/>16	22.8	123	≤0.12–>16	16/>16	26.0
	Ciprofloxacin	283	0.06–>2	>2/>2	44.9	92	0.06–>2	0.5/>2	57.6	123	0.12–>2	>2/>2	40.7
	Gatifloxacin	283	≤0.03–>4	1/4	86.9	92	≤0.03–>4	0.12/4	89.1	123	≤0.03–>4	1/2	95.1
	Grepafloxacin	283	≤0.25–>2	2/>2	47.7	92	≤0.25–>2	≤0.25/>2	57.6	123	≤0.25–>2	>2/>2	44.7
	Erythromycin	283	≤0.06–>8	>8/>8	24.0	92	0.12–>8	>8/>8	16.3	123	≤0.06–>8	>8/>8	33.3
	Clindamycin	283	≤0.06–>8	0.5/>8	52.3	92	≤0.06–>8	>8/>8	47.8	123	≤0.06–>8	8/>8	45.5
	Quinupristin/ dalfopristin	283	≤0.06–2	0.25/0.5	98.9	92	0.12–2	0.12/0.5	98.9	123	≤0.06–2	0.12/0.5	98.4
	Chloramphenicol	283	1–>16	8/16	78.8	92	2–>16	8/16	84.8	123	≤0.5–>16	>16/>16	41.5
	Rifampin	283	≤0.25–>2	≤0.25/2	89.4	92	≤0.25–>2	≤0.25/≤0.25	95.7	123	≤0.25–>2	≤0.25/>2	71.5
	Tetracycline	283	≤4–>8	4/>8	75.3	92	≤4–>8	≤4/>8	83.7	123	≤4–>8	≤4/>8	77.2
	Teicoplanin	283	≤0.12–>16	4/8	91.5	92	≤0.12–>16	4/8	92.4	123	≤0.12–>16	4/16	87.8
	Vancomycin	283	0.5–4	2/2	100.0	92	0.25–4	2/2	100.0	123	0.25–4	2/2	100.0
Enterococcus spp	Ampicillin	325	≤0.12–>16	1/>16	72.9	51	0.5–>16	1/>16	82.4	29	≤0.12–>16	1/8	93.1
	Penicillin	325	0.03–>32	4/>32	71.7	51	1–>32	4/>32	78.4	29	0.06–32	2/8	93.1
	Imipenem	325	≤0.06–>8	2/>8	–	51	0.5–>8	2/>8	–	29	≤0.06–>8	2/4	–
	Gentamicin	325	≤500/>1000	≤500/>1000	71.4	51	≤500/>1000	≤500/>1000	52.9	29	≤500–>1000	≤500/>1000	89.7
	Streptomycin	325	≤1000–>2000	≤1000/>2000	54.5	51	≤1000–>2000	2000/>2000	47.1	29	≤1000–>2000	≤1000/>200	75.9
	Ciprofloxacin	325	≤0.015–>2	>2/>2	35.1	51	1–>2	>2/>2	33.3	29	0.5–>2	2/>2	41.4
	Gatifloxacin	325	≤0.03–>4	1/>4	53.5	51	0.25–>4	>4/>4	45.1	29	0.25–>4	0.5/4	89.7
	Grepafloxacin	325	≤0.25–>2	2/>2	–	51	≤0.25–>2	>2/>2	–	29	≤0.25–>2	0.5/>2	–
	Quinupristin/ dalfopristin	325	0.25–>8	8/>8	30.8	51	0.25–>8	4/>8	19.6	29	0.5–>8	4/8	17.2
	Chloramphenicol	325	4–>16	8/>16	80.0	51	4–>16	8/>16	74.5	29	4–>16	8/>16	72.4
	Rifampicin	325	≤0.25–>2	2/>2	–	51	≤0.25–>2	2/>2	–	29	≤0.25–>2	2/>2	–
	Tetracycline	325	≤4–>8	>8/>8	40.3	51	≤4–>8	>8/>8	29.4	29	≤4–>8	>8/>8	37.9

(continued)

TABLE 17.2 (Continued)

In Vitro Broth Microdilution Susceptibility Results for the Four Most Prevalent Causes of Gram-positive Bacteremia in the USA, Canada, and Latin America (51% of all Bacteremic Episodes)

Organism	Antimicrobial Agent	USA				Canada				Latin America			
		N	MIC Range	$MIC_{50/90}$	% *S*[a]	*N*	MIC Range	$MIC_{50/90}$	% *S*[a]	*N*	MIC Range	$MIC_{50/90}$	% *S*[a]
	Teicoplanin	325	≤0.12–>16	0.25/>16	86.8	51	≤0.12–2	0.25/0.5	100.0	29	≤0.12–8	≤0.12/1	100.0
	Vancomycin	325	0.25–>16	1/>16	84.3	51	0.5–>16	1/2	98.0	29	0.5–4	2/2	100.0
S. pneumoniae	Amoxicillin	200	≤0.06–8	≤0.06/1	82.0	45	≤0.06–2	≤0.06/2	88.9	19	≤0.06–2	≤0.06/1	84.2
	Penicillin	200	≤0.03–>4	≤0.03/1	78.5	45	≤0.03–2	≤0.03/2	84.4	19	≤0.03–4	≤0.03/2	78.9
	Cefuroxime	200	≤0.06–>8	≤0.06/4	83.0	45	≤0.06–8	≤0.06/4	82.2	19	≤0.06–4	≤0.06/4	84.2
	Cefotaxime	200	≤0.008–4	0.015/0.5	92.0	45	≤0.008–4	0.015/1	84.4	19	≤0.008–1	0.015/0.5	94.7
	Cefepime	200	≤0.06–4	≤0.06/0.5	92.0	45	≤0.06–2	≤0.06/0.5	91.1	19	≤0.06–1	≤0.06/1	89.5
	Ciprofloxacin	200	0.25–>2	1/2	–	45	0.12–2	1/2	–	19	0.5–2	1/2	–
	Levofloxacin	200	≤0.5–>4	1/1	99.5	45	≤0.5–1	1/1	100.0	19	≤0.5–1	1/1	100.0
	Gatifloxacin[c]	200	0.06–2	0.25/0.25	100.0	45	0.06–0.5	0.25/0.25	100.0	19	0.12–0.25	0.25/0.25	100.0
	Grepafloxacin	200	≤0.12–>1	0.25/0.25	99.5	45	≤0.12–0.5	0.25/0.25	100.0	19	≤0.12–0.25	0.25/0.25	100.0
	Azithromycin	200	≤0.12–>16	≤0.12/1	88.5	45	≤0.12–8	≤0.12/≤0.12	93.3	19	≤0.12–1	≤0.12/≤0.12	94.7
	Clarithromycin	200	≤0.25–>32	≤0.25/1	88.5	45	≤0.25–16	≤0.25/≤0.25	91.1	19	≤0.25–2	≤0.25/≤0.25	94.7
	Erythromycin	200	≤0.25–>32	≤0.25/2	87.5	45	≤0.25–16	≤0.25/≤0.25	93.3	19	≤0.25–2	≤0.25/≤0.25	94.7
	Quinupristin/ dalfopristin	200	≤0.06–1	0.25/0.5	100.0	45	0.25–0.5	0.25/0.5	100.0	19	0.12–0.5	0.25/0.5	100.0
	Vancomycin	200	≤0.12–1	0.25/0.5	100.0	45	≤0.12–1	0.25/0.5	100.0	19	≤0.12–0.5	0.25/0.5	100.0
	Trimethoprim/ Sulfamethoxazole	200	≤0.5–>8	≤0.25/4	80.5	45	≤0.25–8	≤0.25/4	82.2	19	≤0.25–8	0.5/4	52.6

[a] % *S*, percent susceptible determined using NCCLS interpretive criteria. All staphylococci resistant to oxacillin have been reported as resistant to all *β*-lactam agents, irrespective of actual MIC.

[b] All coagulase-negative staphylococci (CoNS).

[c] At the time of publication (18), a provisnal MIC breakpoint for gatifloxacin was ≤2 mg/L; the current NCCLS (13) breakpoint when testing *S. pneumoniae* is ≤1 mg/L.

Reprinted from Diekema et al. (18).

TABLE 17.3

In Vitro Broth Microdilution Susceptibility Results for the Four Most Prevalent Causes of Gram-negative Bacteremia in the USA, Canada, and Latin America (34% of All Bacteremic Episodes)

Organism	Antimicrobial Agent	USA				Canada				Latin America			
		N	MIC Range	$MIC_{50/90}$	% S^a	*N*	MIC Range	$MIC_{50/90}$	% S^a	*N*	MIC Range	$MIC_{50/90}$	% S^a
E. coli	Ampicillin	565	0.5–>16	4/>16	54.2	112	1–>16	4/>16	63.4	192	1–>16	>16/>16	39.6
	Piperacillin	565	≤1–>128	2/>128	57.5	112	≤1–>128	2/>128	64.3	192	≤1–>128	128/>128	42.7
	Ticarcillin	565	≤1–>128	8/>128	55.8	112	≤1–>128	4/>128	63.4	192	≤1–>128	>128/>128	39.6
	Amoxicillin/ clavulanate	565	0.5–>16	4/16	78.9	112	1–>16	4/16	97.3	192	1–>16	8/16	71.9
	Ticarcillin/ clavulanate	565	≤1–>128	8/64	74.7	112	≤1–>128	4/64	77.7	192	≤1–>128	8/128	68.2
	Piperacillin/ tazobactam	565	≤0.5–>64	2/16	92.7	112	1–64	2/16	92.0	192	≤0.5–>64	2/32	88.5
	Cefazolin	565	≤2–>16	≤2/16	88.7	112	≤2–>16	≤2/16	85.7	192	≤2–>16	≤2/>16	81.3
	Cefoxitin	565	≤0.25–>32	4/8	94.9	112	1–>32	4/8	96.4	192	1–>32	4/8	91.7
	Ceftriaxone	565	≤0.25–>32	≤0.25/≤0.25	99.5	112	≤0.25–16	≤0.25/≤0.25	99.1	192	≤0.25–>32	0.25/≤0.25	93.2
	Ceftazidime	565	≤0.12–>16	0.25/0.5	98.4	112	≤0.12–8	0.25/0.5	100.0	192	≤0.12–>16	0.25/0.5	96.4
	Cefepime	565	≤0.12–4	≤0.12/≤0.12	100.0	112	≤0.12–8	≤0.12/≤0.12	100.0	192	≤0.12–>16	≤0.12/0.25	99.5
	Imipenem	565	≤0.06–4	0.12/0.25	100.0	112	≤0.06–1	0.12/0.25	100.0	192	≤0.06–2	0.12/0.25	100.0
	Meropenem	565	≤0.06–0.25	≤0.06/≤0.06	100.0	112	≤0.06–0.12	≤0.06/≤0.06	100.0	192	≤0.06–1	≤0.06/≤0.06	100.0
	Aztreonam	565	≤0.12–>16	≤0.12/0.25	98.4	112	≤0.12–8	≤0.12/≤0.17	100.0	192	≤0.12–>16	≤0.12/0.25	94.3
	Amikacin	565	≤0.25–32	4/8	99.6	112	1–16	2/8	100.0	192	1–>32	4/8	95.8
	Gentamicin	565	≤0.12–>16	1/2	96.8	112	0.5–>16	1/2	96.4	192	0.25–>16	1/4	92.7
	Tobramycin	565	≤0.12–>16	1/2	97.3	112	0.5–>16	1/2	97.3	192	≤0.12–>16	2/4	91.1
	Ciprofloxacin	565	≤0.015–>2	≤0.015/0.03	98.1	112	≤0.015–>2	≤0.015/0.03	96.4	192	≤0.015–>2	≤0.015/>2	85.4
	Ofloxacin	565	≤0.03–>4	0.06/0.12	97.9	112	≤0.03–>4	0.06/0.12	96.4	192	≤0.03–>4	0.06/>4	84.4
	Levofloxacin	565	≤0.5–>4	≤0.5/≤0.5	98.1	112	≤0.5–>4	≤0.5/≤0.5	96.4	192	≤0.5–>4	≤0.5/>4	84.9
	Gatifloxacin	565	≤0.3–>4	≤0.03/0.06	98.1	112	≤0.03–>4	≤0.03/0.06	96.4	192	≤0.03–>4	≤0.03/4	85.9

(continued)

TABLE 17.3 (Continued)

In Vitro Broth Microdilution Susceptibility Results for the Four Most Prevalent Causes of Gram-negative Bacteremia in the USA, Canada, and Latin America (34% of All Bacteremic Episodes)

Organism	Antimicrobial Agent	USA				Canada				Latin America			
		N	MIC Range	$MIC_{50/90}$	% *S*[a]	*N*	MIC Range	$MIC_{50/90}$	% *S*[a]	*N*	MIC Range	$MIC_{50/90}$	% *S*[a]
	Grepafloxacin	565	≤0.25–>2	≤0.25/≤0.25	97.7	112	≤0.25–>2	≤0.25/≤0.25	96.4	192	≤0.25–>2	≤0.25/>2	84.4
	Tetracycline	565	≤4–>8	≤4/>8	73.6	112	≤4–>8	≤4/>8	77.7	192	≤4–>8	>8/>8	45.0
	Trimethoprim/ sulfamethoxazole	565	≤0.5–>1	≤0.5/>1	77.9	112	≤0.5–>1	≤0.5/>1	81.3	192	≤0.5–>1	>1/>1	47.5
Klebsiella spp	Ampicillin	219	1–>16	>16/>16	4.6	29	8–>16	>16/>16	3.4	66	2–>16	>16/>16	3.0
	Piperacillin	219	≤1–>128	8/>128	75.8	29	2–>128	8/>128	65.5	66	2–>128	8/>128	54.5
	Ticarcillin	219	≤1–>128	128/>128	2.7	29	16–>128	>128/>128	3.4	66	4–>128	>128/>128	1.5
	Amoxycillin/ clavulanate	219	1–>16	2/8	91.3	29	1–>16	4/16	89.7	66	1–>16	4/>16	69.7
	Ticarcillin/ clavulanate	219	≤1–>128	4/64	84.9	29	≤1–128	4/32	86.2	66	≤1–>128	8/>128	66.7
	Piperacillin/ tazobactam	219	1–>64	4/32	89.5	29	1–>64	4/32	89.7	66	1–>64	4/>64	69.7
	Cefazolin	219	≤2/>16	≤2/>16	83.1	29	≤2–>16	≤2/>16	79.3	66	≤2–>16	≤2–>16	65.2
	Cefoxitin	219	≤0.25–>32	4/16	86.3	29	1–32	2/8	93.1	66	2–>32	4/16	87.9
	Ceftriaxone	219	≤0.25–>32	≤0.25/1	93.2	29	≤0.25/>32	≤0.25/≤0.25	96.6	66	≤0.25–>32	≤0.25/32	84.8
	Ceftazidime	219	≤0.12/>16	0.25/4	92.2	29	≤0.12–1	0.25/1	100.0	66	≤0.12–>16	0.25/>16	81.8
	Cefepime	219	≤0.12–8	≤0.12/0.5	100.0	29	≤0.12–2	≤0.12/0.25	100.0	66	≤0.12–>16	≤0.12/4	97.0
	Imipenem	219	≤0.06–2	0.25/0.5	100.0	29	≤0.06–1	0.25/0.5	100.0	66	0.12–1	0.25/0.5	100.0
	Meropenem	219	≤0.06–0.25	≤0.06/≤0.06	100.0	29	≤0.06–0.12	≤0.06/≤0.06	100.0	66	≤0.06–0.12	≤0.06/≤0.06	100.0
	Aztreonam	219	≤0.12–>16	≤0.12/4	91.8	29	≤0.12–>16	≤0.12/0.5	96.6	66	≤0.012–>16	0.25/>16	84.8
	Amikacin	219	≤0.25–32	2/2	99.5	29	1–8	2/4	100.0	66	1–>32	2/32	89.4
	Gentamicin	219	≤0.12–>16	0.5/1	92.7	29	0.25–8	0.5/2	93.1	66	0.5–>16	0.5/>16	86.4
	Tobramycin	219	≤0.12–>16	0.5/1	91.8	29	0.25–>16	1/2	93.1	66	0.5–>16	1/>16	75.8
	Ciprofloxacin	219	0.015–>2	0.03/0.25	93.6	29	≤0.015–0.25	0.03/0.12	100.0	66	≤0.015–>2	0.03/1	90.9

	Ofloxacin	219	≤0.03–>4	0.12/1	93.6	29	0.06–1	0.12/0.5	100.0	66	≤0.03–>4	0.12/2	92.4
	Levofloxacin	219	≤0.5–>4	≤0.5/≤0.5	94.1	29	≤0.5–1	≤0.5/≤0.5	100.0	66	≤0.5–>4	≤0.5/1	92.4
	Gatifloxacin	219	≤0.03–>4	0.06/0.5	95.4	29	≤0.03–1	0.06/0.5	100.0	66	≤0.03–>4	0.06/1	92.4
	Grepafloxacin	219	≤0.25–>2	≤0.25/0.5	92.7	29	≤0.25–1	≤0.025/0.5	100.0	66	≤0.25–>2	≤0.25/1	92.4
	Tetracycline	219	≤4–>8	≤4/>8	82.1	29	≤4–>8	≤4/>8	82.8	66	≤4–>8	≤4/>8	78.8
	Trimethprim/ sulphamethoxazole	219	≤0.5–>1	≤0.5/>1	87.7	29	≤0.5–1	≤0.5/>1	86.2	66	≤0.5–>1	≤0.5/>1	81.0
P. aeruginosa	Piperacillin	131	≤1–>128	8/128	87.9	17	2–32	8/16	100.0	75	≤1–>128	16/>128	70.7
	Ticarcillin	131	≤1–>128	32/128	81.7	17	16–128	32/64	94.1	25	≤1–>128	32/>128	61.3
	Ticarcillin/ clavulanate	131	≤1–>128	32/128	82.4	17	16–64	32/64	100.0	75	≤1–>128	32/>128	68.0
	Piperacillin/ tazobactam	131	≤0.5–>64	8/64	90.8	17	2–32	8/16	100.0	75	≤0.5–>64	8/>64	84.0
	Ceftriaxone	131	≤0.25–>32	>32/>32	6.9	17	16–>32	>32/>32	0.0	75	0.5–>32	>32/>32	6.7
	Ceftazidime	131	≤0.12–>16	4/>16	82.4	17	2–16	2/8	94.1	75	1–>16	4/>16	74.7
	Cefepime	131	≤0.12–>16	2/16	88.5	17	1–16	2/8	94.1	75	0.25–>16	4/16	78.7
	Imipenem	131	0.12–>8	2/8	89.3	17	0.5–4	1/4	100.0	75	0.25–>8	2/8	84.0
	Meropenem	131	≤0.06–>8	0.5/2	95.4	17	≤0.06–>8	0.5/2	94.1	75	≤0.06–>8	0.5/8	86.7
	Aztreonam	131	≤0.12–>16	8/>16	72.5	17	2–16	8/16	88.2	75	4–>16	>16/>16	1.3
	Amikacin	131	0.5–32	4/8	98.5	17	1–>32	4/8	94.1	75	1–>32	4/>32	74.7
	Gentamicin	131	0.25–>16	2/4	90.8	17	0.5–>16	2/4	94.1	75	0.5–>16	2/>16	65.3
	Tobramycin	131	≤0.12–>16	0.5/1	96.9	17	0.25–>16	0.5/2	94.1	75	0.25–>16	1/>16	64.0
	Ciprofloxacin	131	≤0.015–>2	0.12/2	86.3	17	0.06–>2	0.12/>2	88.2	75	0.03–>2	0.25/>2	62.7
	Ofloxacin	131	0.06–>4	1/>4	75.6	17	0.5–>4	1/>4	76.5	75	0.25–>4	1/>4	62.7
	Levofloxacin	131	≤0.5–>4	≤0.5/4	83.2	17	≤0.5–>4	≤0.5/>4	82.4	75	≤0.5–>4	1/>4	62.7
	Gatifloxacin	131	≤0.03–>4	1/>4	78.6	17	0.25–>4	0.5/>4	76.5	75	0.12–>4	1/>4	61.3
	Grepafloxacin	131	≤0.25–>2	0.5/>2	80.2	17	0.25–>2	0.5/>2	76.5	75	≤0.25–>2	0.5/>2	61.3
	Tetracycline	131	≤4–>8	>8/>8	3.1	17	8–>8	>8/>8	0.0	75	≤4–>8	>8/>8	1.3
Enterobacter spp	Ampicillin	83	≤0.12–>16	>16/>16	6.0	17	4–>16	>16/>16	5.9	44	2–>16	>16/>16	4.5
	Piperacillin	83	≤1–>128	4/>128	69.9	17	2–128	4/32	82.4	44	≤1–>128	2/>128	59.1
	Ticarcillin	83	2–>128	8/>128	65.1	17	2–>128	8/64	76.5	44	≤1–>128	8/>128	54.5
	Amoxicillin/Clavulanate	83	≤0.12–>16	>16/>16	6.0	17	4–>16	>16/>16	5.9	44	4–>16	>16/>16	9.1

(continued)

TABLE 17.3 (Continued)

In Vitro Broth Microdilution Susceptibility Results for the Four Most Prevalent Causes of Gram-negative Bacteremia in the USA, Canada, and Latin America (34% of All Bacteremic Episodes)

Organism	Antimicrobial Agent	USA				Canada				Latin America			
		N	MIC Range	$MIC_{50/90}$	% S^a	*N*	MIC Range	$MIC_{50/90}$	% S^a	*N*	MIC Range	$MIC_{50/90}$	% S^a
	Ticarcillin/clavulanate	83	≤1–>128	8/>128	66.3	17	2–>128	8/64	70.6	44	≤1–>128	4/>128	56.8
	Piperacillin/tazobactam	83	1–>64	4/64	75.9	17	1–32	4/32	88.2	44	1–>64	2/>64	70.5
	Cefazolin	83	≤2–>16	>16/>16	6.0	17	4–>16	>16/>16	5.9	44	≤2–>16	>16/>16	4.5
	Cefoxitin	83	4–>32	>32/>32	2.4	17	8–>32	>32/>32	5.9	44	4–>32	>32/>32	9.1
	Ceftriaxone	83	≤0.25–>32	≤0.25/>32	75.9	17	≤ 0.25–>32	0.5/>32	88.2	44	≤0.25–>32	≤0.25/>32	70.5
	Ceftazidime	83	≤0.12–>16	0.5/>16	75.9	17	≤0.12–>16	1/16	88.2	44	≤0.12–>16	1/>16	68.2
	Cefepime	83	≤0.12–>16	≤0.12/2	98.8	17	≤0.12–1	≤0.12/0.5	100.0	44	≤0.12–8	≤0.12/4	100.0
	Imipenem	83	0.12–4	0.5/2	100.0	17	0.12–4	0.5/2	100.0	44	0.12–8	0.5/2	97.7
	Meropenem	83	≤0.06–0.25	≤0.06/0.12	100.0	17	≤0.06–0.25	≤0.06/0.12	100.0	44	≤0.06–0.5	≤0.06/0.12	100.0
	Aztreonam	83	≤0.12–>16	0.25/>16	75.9	17	≤0.12–>16	0.25/4	94.1	44	≤0.12–>16	0.25/>16	70.5
	Amikacin	83	0.5–32	2/4	97.6	17	1–2	2/2	100.0	44	1–>32	2/>32	84.1
	Gentamicin	83	≤0.12–>16	1/16	86.7	17	≤0.12–8	0.5/1	94.1	44	0.25–>16	1/>16	79.5
	Tobramycin	83	0.25–>16	1/16	86.7	17	0.5–16	1/1	94.1	44	0.25–>16	1/>16	77.3
	Ciprofloxacin	83	≤0.015–>2	≤0.015/0.12	94.0	17	≤0.015–2	0.03/0.5	94.1	44	≤0.015–>2	0.03/2	88.6
	Ofloxacin	83	≤0.03–>4	0.12/1	94.0	17	0.06–>4	0.12/2	94.1	44	≤0.03–>4	0.12/4	81.8
	Levofloxacin	83	≤0.5–>4	≤0.5/≤0.5	95.2	17	≤0.5–2	≤0.5/	100.0	44	≤0.5–>4	≤ 0.5/4	88.6
	Gatifloxacin	83	≤0.03–>4	0.06/0.5	95.2	17	≤0.03–2	0.06/1	100.0	44	≤0.03–>4	0.06/2	93.2
	Grepafloxacin	83	≤0.25–>2	≤0.25/1	91.6	17	≤0.25–>2	≤0.25/0.5	94.1	44	≤0.25–>2	≤0.25/2	86.4
	Tetracycline	83	≤4–>8	≤4/>8	83.1	17	≤4–8	≤4/8	88.2	44	≤4–>8	≤4/>8	68.2
	Trimethoprim/ sulfamethoxazole	83	≤0.5–>1	≤0.5/>1	83.1	17	≤0.5–>1	≤0.5/1	94.1	44	≤0.5–>1	≤0.5/>1	69.8

[a] % *S*, percent susceptible determined using NCCLS interpretive criteria.
Reprinted from Diekema et al. (18).

TABLE 17.4

Frequency of Occurrence of Bacterial Pathogens Associated with Hospitalized Patients with Suspected Pneumonia in North America (United States and Canada), 2712 Strains (SENTRY, Antimicrobial Surveillance Program, 2000)

Rank	Organism	No. of Isolates (%)
1	*S. aureus*	760 (28.0)
2	*P. aeruginosa*	543 (20.0)
3	*S. pneumoniae*	246 (9.1)
4	*Klebsiella* spp	203 (7.5)
5	*H. influenzae*	199 (7.3)
6	*Enterobacter* spp	156 (5.8)
7	*E. coli*	105 (3.9)
8	*Serratia* spp	96 (3.5)
9	*S. maltophilia*	94 (3.5)
10	*Acinetobacter* spp	72 (2.7)
11	*M. catarrhalis*	64 (2.4)
12	*P. mirabilis*	28 (1.0)
13	*Citrobacter* spp	27 (1.0)
14	*Enterococcus* spp	25 (0.9)
15	Coagulase-negative staphylococci	18 (0.7)
16	Others (14 species)[a]	76 (2.8)

[a] Others include *Alcaligenes* spp (eight strains), *Edwardsiella tarda* (one strain), *Haemophilus* spp (seven strains), *H. alvei* (three strains), *M. morganii* (seven strains), *N. meningitidis* (one strain), *P. agglomerans* (two strains), *Pleisiomonas* spp (one strain), *P. assaccharolytica* (one strain), *P. vulgaris* (two strains), *Providencia* spp (six strains), *Pseudomonas* spp (11 strains), viridans group strep (six strains), and *Streptococcus* spp (20 strains).
Reprinted from Hoban et al. (23).

leading respiratory pathogens seen in Latin America are summarized in Tables 17.7 and 17.8. In general, the pathogen mix includes more species prone to develop resistance, which is reflected in the results. Empiric regimens must consider regional variations in pathogen frequency and the origin (nosocomial versus community) of the organisms. Despite increasing resistance, several compounds for Gram-positive species (vancomycin, quinupristin/dalfopristin, and linezolid) and Gram-negative species (amikacin, tobramycin, carbapenems, cefepime, piperacillin/tazobactam, and the polymyxins) do retain activity against the large majority of such pathogens.

Skin and Soft Tissue Infections (SSTIs)

SENTRY Program listings of the causes of SSTI or wound infections for the year 2000 rank the pathogens for Europe and the Americas in nearly identical order (Table 17.9) (25). Differences for Latin America showed *E. coli* ranked number 3 (12.4%), ahead of enterococci, and *Acinetobacter* spp were almost twice as frequently isolated as in North America (25). For Europe, the ranking of SSTI pathogens was identical to that found in Latin America for positions 1–3, and the occurrence of *S. aureus* was 14.9% less than observed in North America. In contrast, the European rates of isolation were significantly greater (>1.0%) for *P. aeruginosa* (+3.1%), *E. coli* (+6.5%), CoNS (+1.5%), *Proteus* spp (+1.2%), and *Acinetobacter* spp (+1.4%). Antibiograms for the leading pathogens producing SSTI in North America are given in Table 17.10 and for Latin America in Tables 17.11 and 17.12 (26,27). Again, the leading Gram-positive and -negative pathogens tend to be more resistant in Latin America and demonstrate increased resistance to most drug classes.

Urinary Tract Infections (UTIs)

The most frequently isolated pathogen from UTI cultures in the SENTRY Program was the expected *E. coli* (47.3%) (28). The order of isolation ranked by percentage for the remaining organisms is shown in Table 17.13. The top ten pathogens include 96.9% of all isolates in a sample of 2780 strains submitted from sites in North America, Europe, and Latin America in 2000 (28). Regional variations in this order were rare, although Gram-negative species were more predominant in Latin America. Susceptibilities to the four most prevalent species are shown in Table 17.14.

Among the most common species, *E. coli*, cases of resistance to some agents has been identified, and the identification subsequently led to the detection and characterization of clonal outbreaks (29). Molecular epidemiological studies in Latin America (30) have identified the most common mutations in the quinolone-resistance determining region (QRDR) coding for elevated ciprofloxacin MIC results, such as Ser83Leu (six occurrences in four nations), Asp87Gly (two occurrences in two nations), and Asp87Asn (one occurrence). Mutations of the QRDR in *P. aeruginosa* have reduced quinolone activity against UTI isolates, especially for ciprofloxacin (31). Current antibiograms for SENTRY Program isolates from Europe and both American regions demonstrate nearly equal spectrums of activity for ciprofloxacin, gatifloxacin, and levofloxacin, with the most resistant *P. aeruginosa* UTI strains isolated in Latin America (54.5% resistant) (31).

(*text continues on page 828*)

TABLE 17.5

Antimicrobial Activity and Spectrum of Activity of 34 Drugs Tested against the Five Most Prevalent Causes of Pneumonia in Hospitalized Patients in North America (71.9% of All Isolates)

Antimicrobial Class/ Agent Tested (No.)	*S. aureus* (760)		*P. aeruginosa* (543)		*S. pneumoniae* (246)		*Klebsiella* spp (203)		*H. influenzae* (199)	
	$MIC_{50/90}$	% Susc	$MIC_{50/90}$	% Susc	$MIC_{50/90}$	% Susc	$MIC_{50/90}$	% Susc	$MIC_{50/90}$	% Susc
Penicillins (8)										
Ampicillin-amoxicillin	16/>16	9.5	>16/>16	—	≤0.12/2	90.7	>16/>16	5.4	0.25/>16	71.4
Oxacillin	0.5/>8	56.2	NT	—	≤0.06/8	—	NT	—	NT	—
Penicillin	16/>32	8.9	NT	—	≤0.015/2	67.9	NT	—	NT	—
Piperacillin	NT	—[a]	8/>128	82.1	NT	—	8/32	88.7	≤1/32	—
Ticarcillin	NT[a]	—	32/>128	75.6	NT	—	128/>128	8.4	≤1/32	—
Amoxicillin/clavulanate (2:1)	≤2/>16	56.2[b]	>16/>16	—	≤2/≤2	97.2	≤2/8	91.1	≤2/≤2	100.0
Ticarcillin/clavulanate (2 μg/ml)	NT	—	32/>128	74.4	NT	—	4/8	93.1	≤1/≤1	—
Piperacillin/tazobactam (4 μg/ml)	NT	—	8/>64	85.6	NT	—	2/8	97.5	≤0.5/≤0.5	100.0
Cephalosporins (6)										
Cefazolin	≤2/>16	56.2	>16/>16	—	≤2/4	—	≤2/>16	86.2	4/16	—
Cefuroxime	NT	—	>16/>16	—	NT	—	2/16	85.7	1/2	100.0
Cefoxitin	NT	—	>32/>32	—	NT	—	2/16	83.3	2/4	—
Cefotaxime or ceftriaxone	4/>32	56.2	>32/>32	13.6	≤0.25/1	97.2	≤0.25/≤0.25	99.5 (3.4)[c]	≤0.25/≤0.25	100.0
Ceftazidime	8/>16	56.2	4/>16	78.3	0.25/8	—	≤0.12/0.5	96.6 (3.4)[c]	≤0.12/≤0.12	100.0
Cefepime	4/>16	56.2	4/16	80.5	≤0.12/1	98.8	≤0.12/0.25	99.5	≤0.12/≤0.12	100.0
Others (3)										
Aztreonam	NT	—	16/>16	42.0	NT	—	≤0.12/0.5	97.0 (5.4)[c]	≤0.12/≤0.12	100.0
Imipenem	≤0.06/>8	56.2	1/8	85.6	≤0.06/0.25	87.8	0.12/0.25	100.0	0.25/0.5	100.0
Meropenem	NT	—	0.5/8	89.1	NT	—	≤0.06/≤0.06	100.0	≤0.06/≤0.06	100.0

Aminoglycosides (3)										
Amikacin	NT[a]	—	4/8	93.7	NT	—	1/2	100	4/8	—
Gentamicin	≤1/>8	85.7	2/>8	80.8	4/8	—	≤1/≤1	96.1	2/4	—
Tobramycin	NT	—	0.5/4	90.2	NT	—	0.5/1	95.6	4/4	—
Fluoroquinolones (3)										
Ciprofloxacin	0.5/>2	55.7	≤0.25/>2	72.4	1/2	—	≤0.25/≤0.25	97.5	≤0.25/≤0.25	100
Levofloxacin	0.25/4	57.0	1/>4	71.5	1/1	98.8	≤0.03/0.25	97.5	≤0.03/≤0.03	100
Gatifloxacin	0.12/>4	64.7	1/>4	67	0.25/0.5	99.2	≤0.03/0.25	98	≤0.03/≤0.03	100
MLS (3)[d]										
Erythromycin	>8/>8	44.7	NT	—	≤0.06/4	74.8	NT	—	NT	—
Clindamycin	0.12/>8	60.3	NT	—	≤0.06/0.12	90.7	NT	—	NT	—
Quinupristin/dalfopristin (30:70)	0.25/0.5	99.7	NT	—	0.25/0.5	100.0	NT	—	NT	—
Others (8)										
Chloramphenicol	8/16	81.6	NT	—	≤2/4	91.5	NT	—	NT	—
Rifampin	≤0.25/≤0.25	96.4	NT	—	≤0.25/≤0.25	99.2	NT	—	NT	—
Tetracycline	≤4/≤4	91.4	>8/>8	3.9	≤4/>8	80.5	≤4/>8	85.2	≤4/≤4	100.0
Teicoplanin	1/1	100.0	NT	—	≤0.12/≤0.12	—	NT	—	NT	—
Vancomycin	1/1	100.0	NT	—	0.25/0.5	100.0	NT	—	NT	—
Nitrofurantoin	≤32/≤32	100.0	>64/>64	—	≤32/≤32	—	≤32/>64	75.9	≤32/≤32	—
TMP/SMX (1:19)[e]	≤0.5/1	89.9	>1/>1	0	≤0.5/>1	74.0	≤0.5/≤0.5	94.6	≤0.5/>1	82.4
Linezolid	2/2	100.0	NT	—	1/1	100.0	NT	—	NT	—

[a] NT, not tested, and a (—) indicates no interpretative criteria published by the NCCLS (2002).
[b] All β-lactam activity predicted by the oxacillin result.
[c] ESBL phenotype rate taken from the percentage of strains with MIC for ceftazidime or cefotaxime or ceftriaxone, or aztreonam at ≥2 μg/mL (NCCLS, 2002).
[d] MLS, macrolide-lincosamide-streptogramin.
[e] TMP/SMX, trimethoprim/sulfamethoxazole.
Reprinted from Hoban et al. (23).

TABLE 17.6

Frequency of the 2502 Bacterial Pathogens Causing Pneumonia in Patients Hospitalized in the Latin American Medical Centers (SENTRY Antimicrobial Surveillance Program, 1997–2000)

Rank	Organism	No. of Isolates (%)
1	*Pseudomonas aeruginosa*	659 (26.3)
2	*Staphylococcus aureus*	582 (23.3)
3	*Klebsiella pneumoniae*	255 (10.2)
4	*Acinetobacter* spp[a]	239 (9.6)
5	*Enterobacter* spp[b]	134 (5.4)
6	*Streptococcus pneumoniae*	122 (4.9)
7	*Escherichia coli*	114 (4.6)
8	*Haemophilus influenzae*	98 (3.9)
9	*Serratia* spp[c]	71 (2.8)
10	*Stenotrophomonas maltophilia*	41 (1.6)
11	Other 9 species[d]	187 (7.5)

[a] *Acinetobacter* spp: *A. anitratus* (16), *A. baumannii* (181), *A. calcoaceticus* (13), *A. lwoffii* (two strains), and *Acinetobacter* spp (27).
[b] *Enterobacter* spp: *E. cloacae* (69), *E. aerogenes* (40), *E. asburieae* (two strains), *E. gergoviae* (one strain), *E. sakazakii* (one strain), and *Enterobacter* spp (21)
[c] *Serratia* spp: *Serratia marcescens* (64). *Serratia fonticola* (one strain), and *Serratia* spp (6).
[d] Includes *Enterococcus* spp (49 strains); coagulase-negative staphylococci (30 strains); *Proteus* spp (35 strains); *Moraxella catarrhalis* (27 strains); *Citrobacter* spp (20 strains); *Burkholderia cepacia* (15 strains); *Morganella morganii* (eight strains); *Salmonella* spp (two strains); and *Providencia* spp (one strain).
Reprinted from Gales et al. (24).

Pathogens and Resistance Rates in the ICU

A recent survey of bacterial isolates originating from patients in the ICUs of 25 North American medical centers in 2001 has been published (32). For all types of infections, the most common ICU isolates were those listed in Table 17.15. A total of 54.7% of isolates were Gram-negative organisms, although *S. aureus*, *Enterococcus* spp, and CoNS were ranked first, fifth, and sixth in overall frequency of isolation. Antibiogram results from this study are presented in Table 17.16. Although oxacillin resistance among *S. aureus* was 51.4%, no resistance to vancomycin, linezolid or quinupristin/dalfopristin was detected. Cefepime and the carbapenems for the Gram-negative isolates and linezolid for the Gram-positive isolates provided the broadest spectrum of coverage for the recovered isolates.

In an ICU study (33) focusing on Gram-negative pathogens from Europe (6243 strains in 1997–2000), the ranking was as follows: *P. aeruginosa* (22.5%) > *E. coli* (19.8%) > *Klebsiella* spp (13.9%) > *Enterobacter* spp (11.2%) > *Acinetobacter baumannii* (6.8%) > *S. marcescens* (5.1%) > *P. mirabilis* (5.0%). This distribution of organisms was identical to that reported by the SENTRY Program.

Data from these ICU studies are comparable to that of the ICARE (CDC-NNIS) program (34). For BSIs, the ICARE ICU results ranked the prevalence of pathogens as follows: CoNS (37.3%), enterococci (13.5%), *S. aureus* (12.6%), *Enterobacter* spp (4.9%), and *P. aeruginosa* (3.8%). *C. albicans* was noted as causing 5.0% of BSIs. For pneumonias in the ICU, the five most frequently isolated bacteria were *S. aureus* (18.1%), *P. aeruginosa* (17.0%), *Enterobacter* spp (11.2%), *K. pneumoniae* (7.2%), and *H. influenzae* (4.3%). Finally, among the pathogens causing UTI in ICU patients, *E. coli* (17.5%) was most frequently cultured, followed by enterococci (13.8%), *P. aeruginosa* (11.0%), *K. pneumoniae* (6.2%), and *Enterobacter* spp (5.1%). *C. albicans*, at 15.8%, was also very common. Only the frequent occurrence of CoNS in the ICARE Program differed from the rates reported by the SENTRY Program and the MYSTIC Programme.

The SENTRY Program ICU study cited earlier (32) presents resistance rates for the participant ICUs that exceeded the hospital general population results. Table 17.17 compares the rates in this ICU study with those published in the 1999 ICARE study (34). Remarkably similar rates of resistance were observed in the studies. The SENTRY Program resistance rates for the following organisms exceeded those of the ICARE study: vancomycin-resistant enterococci (VRE) (28.4%), *K. pneumoniae* resistant to a third-generation cephalosporin (14.5%), and quinolone-resistant *P. aeruginosa* (24.8%). Streit et al. (32) reported that the following broad-spectrum agents were most effective *in vitro* against pathogens isolated from ICU patients in 2001: carbapenems (imipenem, meropenem), cefepime, piperacillin/tazobactam, aminoglycosides (amikacin, tobramycin), and newer fluoroquinolones (gatifloxacin) for the Gram-negative organisms and linezolid and vancomycin for Gram-positive organisms, (though not enterococci).

Choices of empiric regimens must consider local rates of VRE and multidrug-resistant (MDR) Gram-negative bacilli, which can widely vary.

TRENDS IN ANTIMICROBIAL RESISTANCE RATES

Staphylococcal Resistance

Concerns about antimicrobial resistance in staphylococci have been focused in five areas: (a) continued escalation in oxacillin-resistant *S. aureus* (ORSA); (b) emergence

TABLE 17.7

Antimicrobial Activity and Spectrum of Drugs Tested against the Four Most Prevalent Gram-negative Pathogens Causing Pneumonia in Hospitalized Patients in the Latin American Medical Centers (SENTRY Antimicrobial Surveillance Program 1997–2000)

	Pathogens (No. of Isolates)							
	P. aeruginosa (659)		*K. pneumoniae* (255)		*Acinetobacter* spp (239)		*Enterobacter* spp (134)	
Antimicrobial Class/Agent	$MIC_{50/90}$ (μg/mL)	Percent S^b	$MIC_{50/90}$ (μg/mL)	Percent S^b	$MIC_{50/90}$ (μg/mL)	Percent S^b	$MIC_{50/90}$ (μg/mL)	Percent S^b
β-lactams								
Amoxicilin/clavulanate	—[a]	—[a]	4/>16	62.7	—[a]	—[a]	>16/>16	3.0
Aztreonam	16/>16	42.9	<0.12/>16	60.4	>16/>16	8.1	0.25/>16	64.9
Cefazolin	—[a]	—[a]	8/>16	53.7	—[b]	—[b]	>16/>16	6.0
Cefepime	8/>16	61.2	<0.12/>16	76.1	>16/>16	26.4	0.12/>16	93.3
Cefoxitin	—[a]	—[a]	4/32	81.2	—[a]	—[a]	>32/>32	5.2
Ceftazidime	4/>16	61.2	0.5/>16	63.1	>16/>16	16.7	0.5/>16	63.4
Ceftriaxone	—[a]	—[a]	≤0.5/>32	61.2	>32/>32	8.4	≤0.25/>32	63.4
Cefuroxime	—[a]	—[a]	4/>16	54.1	—[a]	—[a]	>16/>16	40.3
Imipenem	2/>8	69.2	0.25/0.5	99.6	1/>8	84.9	0.5/2	100.0
Meropenem	1/>8	71.6	≤0.06/0.12	99.2	2/>8	84.1	0.06/0.12	100.0
Piperacillin	32/>128	63.9	16/>128	52.2	>128/>128	10.9	8/>128	54.5
Piperacillin/tazobactam	16/>64	70.4	4/>64	68.6	>64/>64	16.7	4/>64	65.7
Ticarcillin	64/>128	53.4	>128/>128	4.7	>128/>128	11.7	8/>128	53.7
Ticarcillin/clavulanate	64/>128	54.3	8/>128	56.5	>128/>128	13.8	16/>128	53.0
Aminoglycosides								
Amikacin	4/>32	71.0	2/32	84.7	>32/>32	20.5	2/32	86.6
Gentamicin	4/>16	60.2	≤1/>16	71.8	>8/>8	23.8	≤1/>16	82.1
Tobramycin	1/>8	60.2	1/>8	59.8	>8/>8	31.1	1/>8	69.4
Fluoroquinolones								
Ciprofloxacin	<0.5/>2	59.5	0.25/>2	86.7	>2/>2	18.8	0.25/>2	83.6
Gatifloxacin	2/>4	54.3	0.06/4	89.4	>4/>4	25.1	0.06/4	86.6
Levofloxacin	1/>4	58.0	≤0.5/4	87.5	>4/>4	21.8	≤0.5/>4	85.8
Others								
Tetracycline	>8/>8	2.0	≤4/>8	69.8	≤4/>8	52.3	≤4/>8	70.9
Trimethoprim/sulfamethoxazole[c]	>1/>1	3.2	≤0.5/>1	72.4	>2/>2	23.4	≤0.5/>1	73.5

[a] Antimicrobial agent with no spectrum of activity against this pathogen.
[b] % S, percentage of susceptibility defined by the NCCLS criteria (2002).
[c] Isolates exhibiting MICs ≤0.5/9.5 μg/mL were classified as susceptible to this association.
Reprinted from Gales et al. (24).

TABLE 17.8

Antimicrobial Activity and Spectrum of Drugs Tested against *Staphylococcus aureus*, the Most Prevalent Gram-positive Pathogen, Causing Pneumonia in Hospitalized Patients in the Latin American Medical Centers (SENTRY Antimicrobial Surveillance Program, 1997–2000)

	***S. aureus* (No. Tested)**					
	Oxacillin-susceptible (268)		Oxacillin-resistant (314)		Total (582)	
Antimicrobial Class/Agent	*MIC* $_{50/90}$ (μg/mL)	*Percent Susc.*	*MIC* $_{50/90}$ (μg/mL)	*Percent Susc.*	*MIC* $_{50/90}$ (μg/mL)	*Percent Susc.*
Oxacillin	0.5/1	100.0	>8/>8	0.0	>8/>8	46.2
Amoxicillin/clavulanate	1/2	100.0	>16/>16	3.2[a]	>16/>16	47.3[a]
Cefazolin	≤2/≤2	99.6	>16/>16	3.2[a]	>16/>16	47.6[a]
Ceftriaxone	4/4	98.9	>32/>32	1.0[a]	>32/>32	46.0[a]
Cefepime	2/4	98.9	>16/>16	2.2[a]	>16/>16	46.7[a]
Gentamicin	0.5/0.5	95.9	>16/>16	3.5	>16/>16	46.0
Ciprofloxacin	0.25/0.5	95.5	>2/>2	2.9	>2/>2	45.5
Gatifloxacin	0.06/0.12	100.0	2/4	72.6	2/4	85.2
Erythromycin	0.5/>8	77.6	>8/>8	1.6	>8/>8	36.6
Clindamycin	0.25/0.25	96.3	>8/>8	3.8	>8/>8	46.4
Quinupristin/dalfopristin	0.25/0.5	100.0	0.5/1	100.0	0.5/1	100.0
Chloramphenicol	8/16	84.0	>16/>16	22.9	8/>16	51.0
Rifampin	0.25/0.25	97.8	2/>2	40.8	≤0.25/>2	67.0
Tetracycline	≤4/8	89.2	>8/>8	37.3	≤4/>8	61.2
Trimethoprim/sulfamethoxazole	≤0.5/≤0.5	99.6	>2/>2	35.5	≤0.5/>2	64.9
Teicoplanin	0.5/1	100.0	1/2	99.7	1/2	99.8
Vancomycin	1/1	100.0	1/2	100.0	1/1	100.0
Linezolid	2/2	100.0	2/2	100.0	2/2	100.0

[a] Oxacillin-resistant strains should be considered resistant to all β-lactams in spite of *in vitro* susceptibility (NCCLS, 2002).
Reprinted from Gales et al. (24).

of vancomycin-intermediate *S. aureus* (VISA) (35–37); (c) reports of single cases of vancomycin-resistant *S. aureus* (38,39); (d) reports of CoNS and *S. aureus* strains resistant to linezolid (40,41) and quinupristin/dalfopristin (42) by well-defined, new mechanisms; and (e) increasing numbers of multi-drug resistant (MDR) strains. Recent trends in several organism-antimicrobial resistance patterns exhibited by bloodstream isolates over the 5 years of the SENTRY Program for North America are shown in Table 17.18. Decreased susceptibilities to oxacillin were observed for each year, with an overall increase of 16.7% in ORSA. Susceptibility of *S. aureus* to the topical agent mupirocin appeared stable at 94.2% to 95.3%; however, emerging resistance has been recorded internationally (43).

Resistance rate trends for ORSA indexed by the geographic region within the SENTRY Program are shown in Table 17.19. As noted in Table 17.18, rates of ORSA increased for North America from (22.4% to 39.1%), a finding also observed for Europe (from 22.1% to 28.5%) and Latin America (from 29.2% to 35.3%). Currently, the ORSA rates are highest for North American participants, although wide variations between medical center rates were noted (data not shown). Among key organism-antimicrobial combinations evaluated by Diekema et al. (20), oxacillin resistance in *S. aureus* increased with increasing age; conversely, oxacillin resistance in CoNS was highest among children 5 years of age or younger. Oxacillin resistance in community-acquired *S. aureus* was less than 10% at ages below 18 years but increased to 30%

TABLE 17.9

Rank Order of Skin and Soft Tissue Infection (SSTI) Isolates from Medical Centers in North America, Latin America, and Europe (2000)

Rank	Organism	Number of Organisms Tested (%) by Region in 2000			Total
		North America	Latin America	Europe	
1	*S. aureus*	645 (45.9)	152 (34.9)	216 (31.0)	1013 (39.9)
2	*P. aeruginosa*	152 (10.8)	58 (13.3)	97 (13.9)	307 (12.1)
3	*E. coli*	98 (7.0)	54 (12.4)	94 (13.5)	246 (9.7)
4	*Enterococcus* spp	115 (8.2)	29 (6.7)	51 (7.3)	195 (7.7)
5	*Klebsiella* spp	71 (5.1)	36 (8.3)	40 (5.7)	147 (5.8)
6	*Enterobacter* spp	81 (5.8)	20 (4.6)	40 (5.7)	141 (5.6)
7	CoNS[a]	48 (3.4)	25 (5.7)	34 (4.9)	107 (4.2)
8	*Proteus* spp	45 (3.2)	18 (4.1)	31 (4.4)	94 (3.7)
9	*Streptococcus* spp	38 (2.7)	8 (1.8)	19 (2.7)	65 (2.6)
10	*Acinetobacter* spp	23 (1.6)	11 (2.5)	21 (3.0)	55 (2.2)
11	*Serratia* spp	28 (2.0)	7 (1.6)	15 (2.2)	50 (2.0)
12	Other species[b]	60 (4.3)	18 (4.1)	39 (5.6)	117 (4.6)
TOTAL		1404	436	697	2537

[a] CoNS, coagulase-negative staphylococci.
[b] Includes isolates from more than 21 different genera.
Reprinted from Kirby et al. (25).

by age 64 years. Generally, nosocomial *S. aureus* isolates were 3% to 16% (average, 11%) more likely to be resistant to oxacillin than community-acquired strains.

Susceptibility profiles for four antimicrobial agents (linezolid, quinupristin/dalfopristin, teicoplanin, and vancomycin) considered to be highly active against oxacillin-resistant staphylococci are shown in Table 17.20 (45). Quinupristin/dalfopristin resistance (5.4%) was highest among oxacillin-resistant *S. aureus* in Europe, where another streptogramin (pristinomycin) had been used in prior years. No resistance to linezolid or vancomycin was noted through 2000 (45). Although some ORSA had vancomycin MIC results at 4 μg/mL, VISA characteristics could not be confirmed in these strains (35,37). Limited numbers of these VISA isolates have been documented in the United States (<10), very different from the rates published by Hiramatsu et al. (36,37) for Japan. A more recent publication (2001) using a 6625-strain ORSA sample from 278 hospitals in Japan refutes the previous reports, and this comprehensive study did not detect heterogeneous vancomycin resistance in ORSA (46). These findings are consistent with the rarity of these VISA strains noted elsewhere. Elevated vancomycin MIC values have also been described in CoNS isolates (47).

Linezolid became the first member of the oxazolidinone class to be licensed for use in clinical practice (48). Although very active against initial native strains of Gram-positive species (49), linezolid resistance (MIC > 32 μg/mL) in an ORSA strain was reported to emerge during therapy (40). Also, another strain of CoNS (*S. epidermidis*) was isolated in the SENTRY Program in early 2002 that possesses a ribosomal target mutation (G2576U) commonly seen in other oxazolidinone-resistant species (41). No single antimicrobial appears to be totally reliable versus ORSA, and the emergence of resistance during chemotherapy may always be a risk, even with these newer antimicrobials.

Enterococcal Resistance

Enterococci have acquired numerous resistances to antimicrobial agents, including strains recently described as having elevated linezolid MIC values (41,50,51). Recognized issues of highest concern include (a) ampicillin resistance, especially in *E. faecium;* (b) high-level resistance to aminoglycosides (gentamicin and streptomycin); and (c) glycopeptide resistance compromising vancomycin chemotherapy (52). The emergence of vancomycin

(*text continues on page 835*)

TABLE 17.10

Antimicrobial Susceptibility of 18 to 26 Antimicrobial Agents Tested against Five of the Six Most Frequent Pathogens Causing Skin and Soft Tissue Infections in North America (SENTRY Program, 2000)

Species (No. Tested)	Antimicrobial Agent	MIC (μg/mL)		
		50%	90%	% Resistant
S. aureus	Ampicillin	16	>16	88.7
	Amoxicillin/clavulanate	≤2	>16	11.0
	Cefazolin	≤2	>16	17.5
	Ceftriaxone	4	>32	16.7
	Ceftazidime	8	>16	25.0
	Cefepime	4	>16	16.1
	Ciprofloxacin	≤0.25	>2	26.5
	Clindamycin	0.12	>8	20.9
	Doxycycline	≤0.5	1	4.2
	Erythromycin	0.5	>8	46.2
	Evernimicin	0.5	1	NA[a]
	Garenoxacin	≤0.03	4	NA
	Gatifloxacin	0.06	4	9.1
	Gentamicin	≤1	≤1	6.8
	Imipenem	≤0.06	4	7.9
	Levofloxacin	0.25	>4	19.7
	Linezolid	2	2	0.0
	Oxacillin	0.5	>8	29.5
	Penicillin	8	>32	89.3
	Quinupristin/dalfopristin	0.5	0.5	0.0
	Rifampin	≤0.25	≤0.25	0.8
	Trimethoprim/sulfamethoxazole	≤0.5	≤0.5	4.8
	Tigecycline	0.25	0.5	NA
	Teicoplanin	1	1	0.0
	Vancomycin	1	1	0.0
P. aeruginosa (152)	Amikacin	4	8	2.0
	Aztreonam	8	>16	23.0
	Ceftriaxone	>32	>32	60.5
	Ceftazidime	2	16	9.9
	Cefepime	2	16	4.6
	Ciprofloxacin	≤0.25	>2	20.4
	Garenoxacin	2	>4	NA
	Gatifloxacin	1	>4	23.0
	Gentamicin	2	>8	10.5
	Imipenem	1	8	8.6
	Isepamicin	4	8	NA
	Levofloxacin	0.5	>4	21.1

(continued)

TABLE 17.10 (Continued)

Antimicrobial Susceptibility of 18 to 26 Antimicrobial Agents Tested against Five of the Six Most Frequent Pathogens Causing Skin and Soft Tissue Infections in North America (SENTRY Program, 2000)

Species (No. Tested)	Antimicrobial Agent	MIC (μg/mL) 50%	MIC (μg/mL) 90%	% Resistant
	Meropenem	1	8	7.2
	Piperacillin	8	128	14.5
	Piperacillin/tazobactam	8	>64	12.5
	Ticarcillin	32	128	21.7
	Ticarcillin/clavulanate	32	128	23.0
	Tobramycin	0.5	4	6.6
E. coli (98)	Amikacin	2	4	0.0
	Ampicillin	4	>16	37.8
	Amoxicillin/clavulanate	4	16	8.2
	Aztreonam	≤0.12	0.25	2.0 (7.1)[b]
	Cefazolin	≤2	>16	10.2
	Cefoxitin	4	16	8.2
	Cefuroxime	4	16	7.1
	Ceftriaxone	≤0.25	≤0.25	0.0 (7.1)[b]
	Ceftazidime	≤0.12	0.5	4.1 (7.1)[b]
	Cefepime	≤0.12	≤0.12	0.0
	Ciprofloxacin	≤0.25	>2	12.2
	Garenoxacin	≤0.03	>4	NA
	Gatifloxacin	≤0.03	>4	10.2
	Gentamicin	≤1	2	7.1
	Imipenem	0.12	0.25	0.0
	Isepamicin	1	2	NA
	Levofloxacin	≤0.03	4	9.2
	Meropenem	≤0.06	≤0.06	0.0
	Nitrofurantoin	≤32	≤32	2.0
	Piperacillin	2	>128	29.6
	Piperacillin/tazobactam	1	4	1.0
	Tetracycline	≤4	>8	23.5
	Ticarcillin	4	>128	36.7
	Ticarcillin/clavulanate	4	128	10.2
	Tobramycin	1	2	1.0
	Trimethoprim/sulfamethoxazole	≤0.5	>1	18.4
Enterobacter spp (81)[c]	Amikacin	1	2	0.0
	Ampicillin	>16	>16	86.4
	Amoxicillin/clavulanate	>16	>16	92.5
	Aztreonam	≤0.12	>16	18.5
	Cefazolin	>16	>16	96.3

(continued)

TABLE 17.10 (Continued)

Antimicrobial Susceptibility of 18 to 26 Antimicrobial Agents Tested against Five of the Six Most Frequent Pathogens Causing Skin and Soft Tissue Infections in North America (SENTRY Program, 2000)

Species (No. Tested)	Antimicrobial Agent	MIC (μg/mL)		
		50%	90%	% Resistant
	Cefoxitin	>32	>32	92.6
	Cefuroxime	16	>16	38.3
	Ceftriaxone	≤0.25	32	7.4
	Ceftazidime	0.25	>16	18.5
	Cefepime	≤0.12	2	0.0
	Ciprofloxacin	≤0.25	0.5	2.5
	Garenoxacin	0.12	2	NA
	Gatifloxacin	≤0.03	0.5	2.5
	Gentamicin	≤1	≤1	7.4
	Imipenem	0.25	0.5	0.0
	Isepamicin	1	1	NA
	Levofloxacin	≤0.03	0.5	2.5
	Meropenem	≤0.06	0.12	0.0
	Nitrofurantoin	≤32	64	11.1
	Piperacillin	4	128	17.3
	Piperacillin/tazobactam	4	64	6.2
	Tetracycline	≤4	8	9.9
	Ticarcillin	8	>128	25.9
	Ticarcillin/clavulanate	4	>128	16.0
	Tobramycin	0.5	1	6.2
	Trimethoprim/sulfamethoxazole	≤0.5	1	9.9
Klebsiella spp (71)[d]	Amikacin	1	2	0.0
	Ampicillin	>16	>16	88.7
	Amoxicillin/clavulanate	≤2	8	5.6
	Aztreonam	≤0.12	4	7.0 (11.3)[b]
	Cefazolin	≤2	>16	12.7
	Cefoxitin	2	16	5.6
	Cefuroxime	2	16	8.5
	Ceftriaxone	≤0.25	1	0.0 (9.9)[b]
	Ceftazidime	≤0.12	2	5.6 (11.3)[b]
	Cefepime	≤0.12	0.5	0.0
	Ciprofloxacin	≤0.25	2	9.9
	Garenoxacin	0.12	2	NA
	Gatifloxacin	0.06	2	2.8
	Gentamicin	≤1	4	2.8
	Imipenem	0.12	0.25	0.0
	Isepamicin	0.5	1	NA

(continued)

TABLE 17.10 (Continued)

Antimicrobial Susceptibility of 18 to 26 Antimicrobial Agents Tested against Five of the Six Most Frequent Pathogens Causing Skin and Soft Tissue Infections in North America (SENTRY Program, 2000)

Species (No. Tested)	Antimicrobial Agent	MIC (μg/mL) 50%	90%	% Resistant
	Levofloxacin	0.06	2	2.8
	Meropenem	≤0.06	≤0.06	0.0
	Nitrofurantoin	≤32	64	9.9
	Piperacillin	8	>128	12.7
	Piperacillin/tazobactam	2	16	4.2
	Tetracycline	≤4	>8	113
	Ticarcillin	128	>128	81.7
	Ticarcillin/clavulanate	4	32	8.5
	Tobramycin	0.5	4	8.5
	Trimethoprim/sulfamethoxazole	≤0.5	1	8.5

[a] NA = not available.
[b] ESBL phenotype rates, MIC at ≥2 μg/mL (NCCLS, 2000).
[c] *Enterobacter* spp: *E. aerogenes* (17), *E. cloacae* (59), and *Enterobacter* spp (5).
[d] *Klebsiella* spp: *K. pneumoniae* (43), *K. oxytoca* (23). *K. ozaenae* (1) and *Klebsiella* spp (4).
Reprinted from Rennie et al. (26).

resistance among enterococci (VRE) has been an alarming development since the first CDC summary reports on the problem appeared in 1993 (53). The highest frequency of occurrence has been in the United States, where the rates continued to increase (52).

Vancomycin appears to remain active against *E. faecalis* bloodstream isolates (96.2% to 99.4% susceptible) in the United States and Canada, and no trend toward increased rates of resistance has been noted since 1997 (Table 17.18) (44). However, for *E. faecium* the rates of vancomycin resistance escalated, leveled off, and may be dropping somewhat, with approximately 40% of contemporary strains being refractory to glycopeptide therapy. Geographic differences in VRE rates are apparent (Table 17.19). Among all enterococci cultured in North America, 17.7% were resistant to vancomycin in 2002. In contrast, Europe has noted a stable rate (1.6% to 5.3% resistance) over the last 6 years. In Latin America, VRE were essentially unknown until 1999, when vancomycin-resistant *E faecalis* strains were first detected in Brazil (54), followed by increasing rates in other nations in the region. When the influence of age on enterococcal and VRE isolation was analyzed by Diekema et al. (20), a significant trend was noted for nosocomial BSI in patients over 50 years of age. The most commonly cited risk factors leading to VRE isolation were identified in a recent matched, case-controlled study: intravenous treatment with third-generation cephalosporins, metronidazole, or fluoroquinolones; coexisting conditions (diabetes mellitus, organ transplant, hepatobiliary disease); infection or colonization with ORSA or *Clostridium difficile* within the past year; and possible contact with wild mammals (55,56).

The *in vitro* efficacy of four possible therapeutic agents tested against VRE from the United States through 2001 is shown in Table 17.20 (44,45). Susceptibility rates ranged from 55.9% (doxycycline) to 97.4% (linezolid) (49). In 2001, reports of linezolid-resistant enterococci emerged (50), and isolates were also discovered in the SENTRY Program (41,49,51) that, in some cases, were not related to prior exposure to oxazolidinone. Such cases may represent nosocomial dissemination, and several of these strains remained susceptible to vancomycin and other therapeutic regimens (41).

These results for VRE, especially for the United States, indicate that prudent physicians should consider the likelihood of VRE when selecting an empiric regimen for a hospital or specialty care unit or an individual patient.

Streptococcal Resistance

The isolation of streptococci (*S. pneumoniae*, viridans group species, and β-haemolytic streptococci) occurs in significant numbers from blood cultures (Table 17.1) and

(*text continues on page 838*)

TABLE 17.11

Antimicrobial Activities and Spectrum of Drugs Tested against the Most Prevalent Gram-positive Pathogens Causing SSTIs in Latin America (SENTRY Program, 1997 to 2000)

	Pathogen (Prevalence Rank/No. Tested)					
	S. aureus (1/584)		CoNS (7/99)		*Enterococcus* spp (4/137)	
Antimicrobial Class/Agent	$MIC_{50/90}$	% Susc.	$MIC_{50/90}$	% Susc.	$MIC_{50/90}$	% Susc.
Cephalosporins						
Cefazolin	<2/>16	71.6[a]	<2/>16	15.2[a]	>16/>16	—
Ceftriaxone	4/>32	71.6[a]	16/>32	15.2[a]	>32/>32	—
Cefepime	4/>16	71.6[a]	4/>16	15.2[a]	>16/>16	—
Ceftazidime	8/>16	61.0	16/>16	15.2[a]	>16/>16	—
Other β-lactams						
Oxacilliin	0.5/>8	71.6	8/>8	15.2	>8/>8	—
Ampicillin	>16/>16	6.2	16/>16	7.1	1/4	97.8
Penicillin	32/>32	5.3	16/>32	4.0	2/8	92.0
Amoxicillin/clavulanate	2/>16	71.6[a]	1/>16	15.2[a]	1/2	92.0[b]
Piperacillin/tazobactam	2/>64	64.7	4/>64	15.2[a]	4/32	92.0[b]
Imipenem	≤0.06/>8	71.6[a]	0.25/>8	15.2[a]	1/8	—
MLS						
Clindamycin	0.25/>8	74.0	0.25/>8	57.6	>8/>8	—
Erythromycin	0.5/>8	54.1	>8/>8	34.3	8/>8	10.9
Quinupristin/dalfopristin	0.25/0.5	99.7	0.12/1	100.0	8/>8	2.2
Fluoroquinolones						
Garenoxacin[c]	≤0.03/1	99.0	0.06/4	84.6	0.25/4	98.3
Gatifloxacin	0.06/2	91.3	0.25/4	87.9	0.5>4	80.3
Levofloxacin[d]	0.12/4	78.3	0.25/4	72.0	1/>4	75.9
Ciprofloxacin	0.5/>2	71.9	0.5/>2	52.5	1/>2	57.7
Others						
Gentamicin	≤1/>16	71.7	16/>16	44.4	16/>16	—
Gentamicin (HL)[e]	<500/<500	—	<500/<500	—	<500/>1000	85.4
Streptomycin (HL)[e]	<1000/2000	—	<1000/>2000	—	<1000/>2000	70.1
Rifampin	≤0.015/2	77.2	1/>2	66.7	>2/>2	19.0
Chloramphenicol	8/>16	65.4	8/>16	68.7	8/>16	75.2
Doxycycline	0.25/8	84.2	1/8	82.8	≤0.5/8	40.1
Tetracycline	≤4/>8	71.2	≤4/>8	69.7	>8/>8	30.7
Trimethoprim/sulfamethoxazole	—	79.1	—	48.5	—	81.0
Vancomycin	1/1	100.0	2/2	100.0	1/2	99.3
Teicoplanin	1/2	99.7	4/16	86.9	0.25/0.5	100.0
Linezolid	2/4	100.0	1/2	100.0	2/2	100.0

[a] Susceptibility is predicted by the oxacillin result.
[b] Susceptibility is predicted by the penicillin result.
[c] Staphylococci with MIC ≤ 2 μg/mL, and enterococci with MIC ≤ 4 μg/mL were considered susceptible to garenoxacin (Fung-Tome et al., 2000). Includes only isolates collected in 1999 and 2000.
[d] Includes only isolates collected in 2000.
[e] HL, high-level aminoglycoside resistance screen.
Reprinted from Sader et al. (27).

TABLE 17.12

Antimicrobial Activities and Spectrum of Drugs Tested against the Five Most Prevalent Gram-negative Pathogens Causing SSTIs in Latin America (SENTRY Program, 1997–2000)

	Pathogen (Prevalence Rank/No. Tested)									
	E. coli (2/233)		*P. aeruginosa* (3/211)		*Klebsiella* spp (5/127)		*Enterobacter* spp (6/100)		*Acinetobacter* spp (8/74)	
Antimicrobial Class/Agent	$MIC_{50/90}$	% Susc.	$MIC_{50/90}$	% Susc.	$MIC_{50/90}$	% Susc.	$MIC_{50/90}$	% Susc.	$MIC_{50/90}$	% Susc.
Cephalosporins										
Cefazolin	2/>16	73.8	>16/>16	0.0	16/>16	45.6	>16/>16	4.0	>16/>16	2.7
Cefuroxime	4/16	84.5	>16>16	0.0	8/>16	52.8	>16/>16	29.0	>16/>16	11.0
Cefoxitin	4/16	85.0	>32/>32	0.0	4/32	82.4	>32/>32	6.0	>32/>32	5.5
Ceftriaxone	≤0.25/0.5	93.6 (8.2)[a]	>32/>32	4.9	≤0.25/>32	62.4 (40.8)[a]	1/>32	63.0	>32/>32	16.4
Ceftazidime	0.25/1	94.4 (9.9)[a]	4/>16	65.9	0.5/>16	70.4 (43.2)[a]	1/>16	59.0	>16/>16	23.3
Cefepime	≤0.12/1	95.7	4/>16	66.2	≤0.12/>16	77.6	0.25/3	91.0	16/>16	30.1
Other β-lactams										
Ampicillin	>16/>16	31.3	>16/>16	0.5	>16/>16	1.6	>16/>16	8.0	>16/>16	—
Aztreonam	≤0.12/1	94.0 (8.6)[a]	16/>16	48.8	0.25/>16	66.4 (39.8)[a]	0.25/>16	56.0	>16/>16	5.5
Amoxicillin/clavulanate	8/>16	64.4	>16/>16	0.0	8/>16	50.3	>16/>16	8.0	16/>16	—
Ticarcillin/clavulanate	16/>128	58.4	32/>128	62.1	32/>128	50.5	32/>128	49.0	>128/>128	23.3
Piperacillin/tazobactam	2/64	87.6	8/>64	76.3	4/>64	60.8	4/>64	59.0	64/>64	20.5
Imipenem	0.12/0.25	99.6	1/>8	74.9	0.25/1	100.0	0.5/1	100.0	1/>8	84.9
Meropenem	≤0.06/≤0.06	99.6	1/>8	80.1	≤0.06/0.12	99.2	≤0.06/0.25	99.0	2/>8	86.3
Aminoglycosides										
Amikacin	4/8	96.1	4/>32	74.9	4/>32	80.8	2/16	91.0	>32/>32	35.6
Gentamicin	1/>16	84.1	2/>16	64.5	1/>16	62.4	0.5/16	77.0	>16/>16	27.4
Tobramycin	1/8	82.8	1/>16	67.8	2/>16	54.4	1/>16	69.0	16/>16	34.2
Fluoroquinolones										
Garenoxacin	≤0.03/>4	77.7	4/>4	56.6	0.12/2	93.8	0.5/>4	65.5	>4/>4	40.1
Gatifloxacin	≤0.03/>4	73.4	2/>4	55.9	0.06/2	36.4	0.12/>4	79.0	>4/>4	30.1
Levofloxacin	≤0.03/>4	73.4	1/>4	57.8	≤0.06/4	89.6	0.12/>4	79.0	>4/>4	27.4
Ciprofloxacin	≤0.015/>2	73.4	0.5/>2	64.5	≤0.06/2	84.8	0.12/>2	76.0	>2/>2	27.4
Others										
Tetracycline	>8/>8	45.4	>8/>8	1.9	≤4/>8	61.4	≤4/>8	64.0	8/>8	36.5
Trimethoprim/sulfamethoxazole	—	52.4	—	1.4	—	66.4	—	76.0	—	27.4

[a] % of strain with MIC ≥2 μg/mL, indicating possible ESBL production.

[b] Susceptibility breakpoint of ≤4 μg/mL was used for aerobic Gram-negative bacilli (Fung-Tome et al., 2000). Only isolates collected in 1999 and 2000 were tested against this compound.

Reprinted by Sader et al. (27).

TABLE 17.13

Rank Order for All Urinary Tract Infection Isolates Processed by the SENTRY Program in 2000

Rank Order	Pathogen	Number by Region			All (%)
		NA	EU	LA	
1	*E. coli*	635	361	320	1,316 (47.3)
2	Enterococci	232	100	19	351 (12.6)
3	*Klebsiella* spp	176	69	61	306 (11.0)
4	*P. aeruginosa*	106	71	33	210 (7.6)
5	*P. mirabilis*	62	56	27	145 (5.2)
6	*Enterobacter* spp	44	33	20	97 (3.5)
7	*Citrobacter* spp	52	17	9	78 (2.8)
8	*S. aureus*	47	13	10	70 (2.5)
9	Indole-positive Proteeae	28	24	11	63 (2.3)
10	CoNS[a]	44	9	6	59 (2.1)
11	*Serratia* spp	18	8	5	31 (1.1)
12	*Acinetabacter* spp	11	15	4	30 (1.1)
13	Other	11	7	6	24 (0.9)
	Total	1,466	783	531	2,780

[a] CoNS, coagulase-negative staphylococci.
Reprinted from Gordon and Jones (28).

pneumonia patients (Table 17.4) but seems less prevalent among ICU patient populations (Table 17.15). Penicillin resistance in community-acquired *S. pneumoniae* strains has been an increasing problem, previously documented by the SENTRY Program and other investigators (57,58). Concurrent with elevated penicillin resistance, the SENTRY Program has documented a significant decline in *S. pneumoniae* susceptibility to macrolides (erythromycin, azithromycin, clarithromycin) and the emergence of fluoroquinolone resistance as indicated by levofloxacin MIC values equal to or greater than 4 μg/mL (57,58). Table 17.18 shows the trends in penicillin and erythromycin resistance among BSI isolates, which increased 0.6% and 4.9%, respectively, between 1997 and 2001. In 2002, resistance to erythromycin again increased, but resistance to penicillin decreased. Of note, the broad-spectrum parenteral cephalosporins remain highly active *in vitro* (97.2% to 98.8% susceptible, Table 17.5) (23), and recently completed clinical trials indicate that some of these β-lactams were reliable for community-acquired pneumonia regardless of the penicillin susceptibility of the strain (59).

Regional variation in the susceptibility of pneumococcal strains has been documented, and local results should be utilized, where available, to guide therapy. Furthermore, Diekema et al. (20) noted that penicillin resistance is related to ages with the highest rates among children younger than 5 years.

Other streptococci of clinical significance in the hospital setting are the viridans group species (VgS), and these can also possess elevated levels of penicillin resistance (60,61). The penicillin resistance rate for VgS isolates was 31.4%, but there was only a 4.2% resistance to ceftriaxone in earlier reports from the SENTRY Program (61). Variation in the utility of newer parenteral quinolones was observed, and resistance to gatifloxacin or levofloxacin was limited to only 1.3% of isolates (61), but the percentage of strains inhibited by ciprofloxacin was only 48% at $\leq$1 μg/mL (13). β-Haemolytic streptococci remain highly susceptible to a wide range of agents, including penicillin (61).

At the current usage levels for orally administered agents that most influence streptococcal resistance patterns, we can expect continued increases in the resistance rates for β-lactams, macrolides, and fluoroquinolones. The parenteral drugs retaining greatest clinical utility against the streptococci will be the newer fluoroquinolones (levofloxacin, gatifloxacin, moxifloxacin), some

TABLE 17.14

Selected Susceptibilities for North American, Latin American, and European Isolates for the Top Four Ranked UTI Isolate Groups Processed by the SENTRY Program in 2000

	% Organism (Rank/No. Tested) Susceptible/Resistant[a]			
Region/Antimicrobial Agent	*E. coli* (1/635)	*Klebsiella* spp (3/176)	*P. aeruginosa* (4/106)	*Enterococci* (2/232)
North America				
Ampicillin	62/37	6/72	0/100	88/12
Amoxicillin/clavulanate	86/5	92/2	0/100	88/12
Cefuroxime axetil	80/2	81/4	0/100	NT[b]
Ciprofloxacin	95/4	96/36	66/29	41/50
Garenoxacin	96/4	98/2	62/38	85/15
Nitrofurantoin	96/1	68/7	0/100	92/1
Trimethoprim/sulfamethoxazole	77/23	86/11	0/100	63/37
Europe				
Ampicillin	48/51	1/80	0/100	84/16
Amoxicillin/clavulanate	81/6	70/16	1/99	86/14
Cefuroxime axetil	73/7	58/29	0/100	NT
Ciprofloxacin	85/15	88/12	55/41	47/43
Garenoxacin	85/15	90/10	52/48	81/19
Nitrofurantoin	91/3	71/20	0/100	87/2
Trimethoprim/sulfamethoxazole	67/33	70/30	1/99	68/32
Latin America				
Ampicillin	45/55	3/84	0/100	100/0
Amoxicillin/clavulanate	79/4	48/23	0/100	100/0
Cefuroxime axetil	81/6	44/41	0/100	NT
Ciprofloxacin	82/18	72/26	42/55	63/21
Garenoxacin	82/18	79/21	42/58	100/0
Nitrofurantoin	93/5	46/34	0/100	100/0
Trimethoprim/sulfamethoxazole	55/45	49/46	0/100	79/21

[a] Susceptibility criteria of the NCCLS (2002).
[b] NT, not tested.
Reprinted from Gordon and Jones (28).

recent generation cephalosporins (cefepime, cefotaxime, ceftriaxone), and meropenem.

Resistance among Enterobacteriaceae

The development of resistance in enteric Gram-negative bacilli includes the recognized decline in their susceptibility to the fluoroquinolones and the third-generation cephalosporins. Fluoroquinolone resistance mechanisms include mutations in the topoisomerase II and III targets. These QRDR modifications of *gyrA* or *gyrB* and *parC* or *parE* can elevate fluoroquinolone MIC values into the resistant range. Table 17.18 shows the trends in *E. coli* and *Klebsiella* spp susceptibility to ciprofloxacin over 6 monitored years. BSI isolates document a slow decline in fluoroquinolone susceptibility that has been more dramatic in other areas of the world (e.g., Latin America and southern Europe). The level of susceptibility to ciprofloxacin, as the representative of other fluoroquinolones, was equal

TABLE 17.15

Frequency of Occurrence for 1321 Bacterial Pathogens from ICU Patient Infections in North American Medical Centers (SENTRY Program, 2001)

Organism	Number of Isolates (% of Total)	Predominant Specimen Source[h]
Staphylococcus aureus	319 (24.1)	Respiratory (52.9)
Pseudomonas aeruginosa	161 (12.2)	Respiratory (59.9)
Escherichia coli	134 (10.1)	Urine (32.1)
Klebsiella spp[a]	117 (8.9)	Respiratory (54.4)
Enterococcus spp[b]	95 (7.2)	Urine (30.2)
Coagulase-negative staphylococci	93 (7.0)	Blood (61.3)
Enterobacter spp[c]	92 (7.0)	Respiratory (56.5)
Acinetobacter spp[d]	53 (4.0)	Respiratory (35.8)
Serratia spp[e]	40 (3.0)	Respiratory (77.5)
Stenotrophomonas maltophilia	40 (3.0)	Respiratory (89.0)
Haemophilus influenzae	37 (2.8)	—
Streptococcus pneumoniae	31 (2.3)	—
Citrobacter spp[f]	26 (2.0)	—
Proteus mirabilis	23 (1.8)	—
Other streptococci[g]	23 (1.8)	—
Other species	37 (2.8)	—

[a] Includes *K. pneumoniae* (96 strains), *K. oxytoca* (16 strains), and *Klebsiella* (not identified to species level; 5 strains).
[b] Includes *E. faecalis* (51 strains), *E. faecium* (38 strains), *E. avium* (1 strain), and *Enterococcus* (not identified to species level; 5 strains).
[c] Includes *E. aerogenes* (29 strains), *E. cloacae* (59 strains), *E. gergoviae* (1 strain), and *Enterobacter* (not identified to species level; 3 strains).
[d] Includes *A. baumannii* (40 strains), *A. anitratus* (3 strains), *A. calcoaceticus* (7 strains), *A. lwoffii* (2 strains), and *Acinetobacter* (not identified to species level; 1 strain).
[e] Includes *S. liquifaciens* (1 strain), *S. marcescens* (37 strains), *S. rubidaea* (1 strain), and *Serratia* (not identified to species level; 1 strain).
[f] Includes *C. amalonaticus* (3 strains), *C. freundii* (11 strains), *C. koseri* (11 strains), and *Citrobacter* (not identified to species level; 1 strain).
[g] Includes β-haemolytic (17 strains) and viridans group (6 strains) species.
[h] Respiratory: broncho-alveolar lavage (BAL), biopsy, fluids, aspirates, and sputum.
Reprinted from Streit et al. (32).

or slightly inferior to the level for a representative aminoglycoside (Table 17.18).

The extended-spectrum β-lactamases (ESBLs) are generally encoded by mobile genes that can be highly prevalent among some enterobacteria, such as *E. coli* and *K. pneumoniae* (62). First detected in the early 1980s, ESBLs have diverse geographic distributions and remarkably variable substrate affinities that can produce confusing susceptibility testing results (62). Contemporary rates of ESBL phenotypes encountered in BSI isolates in North America are shown in Table 17.18 and 17.19 (19,44). The rates of susceptibility for ceftazidime (a representative cephalosporin) when tested against *E. coli* or *Klebsiella* spp declined slightly ($\leq$1.3%) over the 6-year interval ($p > 0.05$). However, if one uses the ESBL-screening criteria of the National Committee for Clinical Laboratory Standards (NCCLS) (13), the ESBL phenotype rates (resistant to cephalosporins) vary from 4.9% to 7.9% for *Klebsiella* spp (Table 17.19). The average ESBL phenotype rates for the 6 years of the SENTRY Program (1997–2002) were highest in Latin America (42.7%), followed by Europe (21.7%) and North America (5.8%). No trend

(*text continues on page 843*)

TABLE 17.16

Potencies and Spectrum of Activity of 20 Antimicrobial Agents Tested against the Six Most Prevalent Causes of Gram-negative ICU Infections in the SENTRY Program (North America; 45% of all Isolates)

Antimicrobial Class/ Agent Tested	Activity by Organism (No. Tested)[a]											
	Pseudomonas aeruginosa (161)		*Escherichia coli* (134)		*Klebsiella* spp (117)		*Enterobacter* spp (92)		*Acinetobacter* spp (53)		*Serratia* spp (40)	
	$MIC_{50/90}$	% S/R	$MIC_{50/90}$	% S/R	$MIC_{50/90}$	% S/R	$MIC_{50/90}$	% S/R	$MIC_{50/90}$	% S/R	$MIC_{50/90}$	% S/R
Penicillins												
Ampicillin	>16/>16	0.0/97.5	>16/>16	46.3/52.2	>16/>16	0.9/82.9	>16/>16	1.1/85.9	>16/>16	5.7/75.5	>16/>16	5.0/80.0
Amoxicillin/ clavulanate	>16/>16	0.6/97.5	8/>16	74.6/13.4	4/16	86.3/6.0	>16/>16	1.1/96.7	>16/>16	22.6/58.5	>16/>16	0.0/100
Piperacillin	8/>128	83.2/16.8	8/>128	56.7/33.6	8/>128	70.9/24.8	2/>128	70.7/19.6	32/>128	35.8/37.7	2/8	97.5/2.5
Piperacillin/ tazobactam	8/>64	87.0/13.0	2/8	95.5/3.0	2/32	89.7/6.0	2/64	73.9/8.7	16/>64	58.5/30.2	2/4	97.5/2.5
Ticarcillin	32/>128	68.9/31.1	32/>128	49.3/46.3	128/>128	2.6/79.5	4/>128	64.8/33.0	32/>128	49.1/35.8	4/>128	85.0/12.5
Ticarcillin/ clavulanate	32/>128	68.3/31.7	8/64	69.4/8.2	4/128	77.8/12.0	4/>128	65.2/29.3	32/>128	49.1/35.8	4/16	95.0/5.0
Cephalosporins												
Cefoxitin	>32/>32	0.0/100.0	4/16	80.6/9.7	4/32	80.3/11.1	>32/>32	3.3/96.7	>32/>32	3.8/96.7	16/>32	10.0/45.0
Cefuroxime	>16/>16	0.0/98.8	4/16	84.3/7.5	4/>16	74.4/17.1	8/>16	50.0/37.0	>16/>16	3.8/88.7	>16/>16	2.5/92.5
Ceftazidime	≤2/>16	77.0/19.3	≤2/≤2	97.0/3.0 (8.2)[b]	≤2/>16	85.5/13.7 (16.2)[b]	≤2/>16	71.7/26.1	8/>16	56.6/37.7	≤2/4	97.5/0.0
Ceftriaxone	>32/>32	10.6/66.5	≤0.25/≤0.25	97.0/1.5 (4.5)[b]	≤0.25/16	89.7/2.6 (15.4)[b]	≤0.25/32	77.2/9.8	16/>32	24.5/35.8	≤0.25/2	92.5/0.0
Cefepime	4/16	80.1/8.1	≤0.12/≤0.12	100.0/0.0	≤0.12/1	98.3/1.7	≤0.12/2	98.9/0.0	8/>16	50.9/35.8	≤0.12/0.5	97.4/0.0

(continued)

TABLE 17.16 (Continued)

Potencies and Spectrum of Activity of 20 Antimicrobial Agents Tested against the Six Most Prevalent Causes of Gram-negative ICU Infections in the SENTRY Program (North America; 45% of all Isolates)

Antimicrobial Class/ Agent Tested	Activity by Organism (No. Tested)[a]											
	Pseudomonas aeruginosa (161)		*Escherichia coli* (134)		*Klebsiella* spp (117)		*Enterobacter* spp (92)		*Acinetobacter* spp (53)		*Serratia* spp (40)	
	$MIC_{50/90}$	% S/R	$MIC_{50/90}$	% S/R	$MIC_{50/90}$	% S/R	$MIC_{50/90}$	% S/R	$MIC_{50/90}$	% S/R	$MIC_{50/90}$	% S/R
Other β-lactams												
Aztreonam	8/>16	60.2/26.7	≤0.12/2	96.3/2.2 (11.2)[b]	≤0.12/>16	86.3/12.8 (15.4)[b]	≤0.12/>16	70.7/17.4	>16/>16	5.7/69.8	≤0.12/0.5	95.0/5.0
Imipenem	1/>8	78.3/16.1	0.12/0.12	100.0/0.0	0.12/0.25	100.0/0.0	0.5/2	97.8/2.2	0.25/>8	81.1/11.3	0.5/1	97.5/2.5
Meropenem	1/>8	79.5/12.4	≤0.06/≤0.05	100.0/0.0	≤0.06/≤0.06	100.0/0.0	≤0.06/0.12	97.8/1.1	1/>8	79.2/20.8	≤0.06/0.12	100.0/0.0
Fluoroquinolones												
Ciprofloxacin	0.25/>2	69.6/24.8	<0.015/>2	87.3/12.7	0.03/>2	84.6/12.8	≤0.015/2	89.1/9.8	1/>2	52.8/45.3	0.06/2	85.0/7.5
Garenoxacin	2/>4	[c]	≤0.03/>4	[c]	0.12/4	[c]	0.12/4	[c]	0.25/>4	[c]	1/>4	[c]
Gatifloxacin	1/>4	62.7/25.5	≤0.03/>4	87.3/11.9	0.06/4	86.3/5.1	≤0.03/2	92.4/3.3	0.5/>4	54.7/37.7	0.25/4	87.5/7
Aminoglycosides												
Amikacin	4/8	96.9/3.1	2/4	99.3/0.0	1/2	95.7/3.4	2/4	97.8/1.1	4/>32	81.1/11.3	2/4	100.0/0.0
Gentamicin	≤2/>8	80.7/13.7	≤2/≤2	92.5/5.3	≤2/8	89.7/6.8	≤2/≤2	95.7/4.3	≤2/>8	52.8/34.0	≤2/≤2	90.0/2.5
Tobramycin	0.5/>16	87.6/12.4	1/2	96.3/3.0	0.5/8	86.3/7.7	0.5/1	94.6/5.4	1/>16	75.5/20.8	2/4	90.0/7.5

[a] MIC_{50} and MIC_{90} in μg/mL at which 50% and 90% of the isolates, respectively, were inhibited. % susceptible (S) and resistant (R) per NCCLS criteria.

[b] Percentage in parenthesis indicates the ESBL phenotype rates using MIC screening concentrations of ≥ 2 μg/mL for aztreonam or ceftazidime or ceftriaxone.

[c] No interpretive criteria have been established.

Reprinted from Streit et al. (32).

TABLE 17.17

Comparisons of Resistance Rates Obtained by Two Surveillance Programs Monitoring ICU Infections in the United States

Organism/Antimicrobial Pair	% Resistance	
	ICARE (34)	SENTRY Program (32)
Vancomycin/enterococci	24.7	28.4
Oxacillin/*S. aureus*	53.5	51.4
Oxacillin/CoNS[a]	88.2	83.9
3GC[b]/*E. coli*	3.9	3.7
3GC[b]/*K. pneumoniae*	10.4	14.5
Imipenem/*P. aeruginosa*	16.4	16.1
Quinolone/*P. aeruginosa*	23.0	24.8
3GC[b]/*P. aeruginosa*	20.6	19.3
3GC[b]/*Enterobacter* spp	33.1	26.1

[a] CoNS, coagulase-negative staphylococci.
[b] 3GC, third-generation cephalosporins.

toward greater ESBL resistance was noted in Europe or Latin America over time.

Potential therapeutic regimens for ESBL-expressing strains are shown in Table 17.20. Only the carbapenems (99.4% to 100% susceptibility) consistently inhibited ESBL-producing strains in all regions over the 5 years. Regional differences in the ESBL type show that cefepime, a fourth-generation cephalosporin, could be used against 88.0% of isolates in North America but not for strains in the other regions (50.0–69.0% susceptible). Piperacillin/tazobactam provided poor coverage for ESBL-*Klebsiella* spp strains (36.6% to 53.6% susceptibility). The prevalence of these ESBL phenotypes can vary widely among medical centers in the same region, and the need for carbapenems as an empiric regimen replacing cephalosporins may not be appropriate for hospitals having rare occurrences of ESBL-producing isolates (<2%). Also when ESBL strains occur, they often exhibit coresistance against the aminoglycosides (tobramycin > gentamicin > amikacin), the tetracyclines, and trimethoprim/sulfamethoxazole (62).

A second type of resistance effecting third-generation cephalosporins and aztreonam (a monobactam) is the hyperproduction of an AmpC cephalosporinase by strains of *Enterobacter aerogenes, Enterobacter cloacae, Citrobacter freundii,* and *Serratia* spp (63). Under normal circumstances, this inducible enzyme is produced in modest amounts and does not significantly destroy the third-generation cephalosporins, but mutations that spontaneously occur (rate 10^{-5} to 10^{-7}) derepress enzyme production, and enough enzyme is generated to hydrolyze these β-lactams (63). Resistances among the species cited were detected before the third-generation cephalosporins were clinically introduced, and overuse in some medical centers has been associated with selection of strains resistant to ceftazidime or similar cephalosporins (63,64).

The susceptibility of ceftazidime and cefepime tested against *Enterobacter* spp isolated from BSIs (North America) is shown in Table 17.18 (19,44). Susceptibility to ceftazidime varied from 75.2% to 82.9% (approximately 20% stably derepressed AmpC-mediated resistances), without a clear trend. Cefepime possesses physico-chemical characteristics that enables clinical use against ceftazidime-resistant enterobacteria (64). The measured rates of cefepime susceptibility have consistently approached 100% (19,44,64). Carbapenems have also been proven to be AmpC β-lactamase stable, and they have near complete activity against these strains (63,64).

Variations in these two resistances (ESBL, AmpC) have been noted in recent years. In these variations, ESBL genes were transferred from strains of *E. coli* or *Klebsiella* spp into *Enterobacter* spp, *C. freundii,* or *S. marcescens.* Conversely, AmpC genomes have been mobilized from parent *Enterobacter* or *Citrobacter* organisms and then transferred into *E. coli* or *Klebsiella* spp. The detection and reporting of these strains remains a challenge to clinical microbiology laboratories, but currently published NCCLS recommendations (12,13) should correctly guide

TABLE 17.18

Antimicrobial Susceptibility of Bloodstream Isolates from SENTRY Program (North America, 1997–2002) for Selected Antimicrobial Pathogens

Organism (No. Tested)	Antimicrobial Agent	% Susceptible by Year					
		1997	1998	1999	2000	2001	2002
S. aureus (11,156)	Oxacillin	77.6	72.2	69.3	65.6	61.3	60.9
	Mupirocin	NT[a]	NT[a]	NT[a]	94.2	94.6	95.3
E. faecium (1044)	Vancomycin	59.9	56.6	49.9	51.9	49.7	39.1
E. faecalis (2764)	Vancomycin	96.2	97.5	99.4	96.6	98.8	97.5
S. pneumoniae (1891)	Penicillin	81.6	84.1	81.7	83.5	81.0	84.9
	Erythromycin	89.3	89.6	88.5	84.7	84.4	82.9
	Ceftriaxone	NT[a]	NT[a]	96.6	97.3	94.9	98.4
	Cefepime	94.6	98.6	98.0	98.1	98.3	98.8
E. coli (7580)	Ceftazidime	99.2	98.6	99.4	99.0	98.7	98.1
	Cefepime	99.9	99.7	99.8	100.0	99.3	99.6
	Ciprofloxacin	97.5	97.4	95.4	95.2	92.3	90.2
	Gentamicin	95.6	96.4	96.9	97.8	96.4	95.0
Klebsiella spp (3268)	Ceftazidime	96.3	95.4	96.3	96.0	95.3	96.2
	Cefepime	98.8	99.4	98.8	98.7	99.8	99.7
	Ciprofloxacin	96.1	95.6	96.5	96.0	95.1	94.6
	Gentamicin	95.6	95.0	96.6	97.2	94.1	95.5
Enterobacter spp (1575)	Ceftazidime	77.9	75.2	77.7	81.2	79.3	82.9
	Cefepime	100.0	99.1	99.0	99.2	98.9	99.6
P. aeruginosa (1851)	Tobramycin	95.0	96.4	97.0	91.5	93.4	93.0
	Ciprofloxacin	88.9	85.9	85.4	78.8	83.3	79.0
	Gatifloxacin	79.9	81.4	79.7	76.8	80.8	76.3
	Ceftazidime	86.9	83.0	85.1	88.2	87.8	88.3
	Cefepime	88.3	87.9	88.1	89.5	88.6	87.7
	Piperacillin/tazobactam	92.8	91.1	89.9	92.4	91.0	91.0
	Imipenem	87.5	91.8	90.7	92.2	88.6	89.0
	Meropenem	95.0	95.4	93.1	92.2	91.8	91.3

[a] Antimicrobial agent not tested.
Adapted from Moet et al. and Biedenbach et al. (19,44).

appropriate therapy following initial broad-spectrum empiric regimens.

Adopted among *P. aeruginosa* Isolates

P. aeruginosa remains the most prevalent pathogen displaying phenotypes highly resistant to contemporary antimicrobial agents (65). In the hospital environment, *P. aeruginosa* causes 3.8% to 4.6% of BSIs, 20% of pneumonias, and 12.2% of infections in the ICU in North America (Tables 17.1, 17.4, and 17.15). Gales et al. (65) previously noted that *P. aeruginosa* isolations appear to be increasing, and distinct differences exist in the frequency by geographic region and site of infections. Examples include generally high rates of occurrence for BSI (6.5%) and pneumonia (25.0%) isolates in Latin America compared to other regions. Also, in the Asia-Pacific region the

TABLE 17.19

SENTRY Program (1997–2002) Bloodstream Infection Isolates from Europe, Latin America, and North America Tested by Four Resistance Phenotypes, Oxacillin-Resistant *S. aureus*, Vancomycin-Resistant Enterococci, ESBL-phenotype *Klebsiella* spp, and Multidrug-resistant *P. aeruginosa*

	% Resistant by Year					
Organisms/Nation (No. Tested)	1997	1998	1999	2000	2001	2002
Oxacillin-resistant *S. aureus*						
Europe (5201)	22.1	25.7	30.2	30.8	30.0	28.5
Latin America (2531)	29.2	36.6	26.9	30.1	36.0	35.3
North America (11,156)	22.4	27.8	30.7	34.4	38.7	39.1
Vancomycin-resistant enterococci						
Europe (1922)	4.1	4.3	1.6	5.3	1.9	4.4
Latin America (382)	0.0	0.0	4.2	6.6	2.9	5.6
North America (4361)	13.0	13.6	14.5	15.8	15.7	17.7
ESBL-phenotype *Klebsiella* spp						
Europe (1941)	14.6	25.1	28.7	31.5	20.5	17.3
Latin America (1183)	46.9	45.8	43.5	46.6	39.5	35.8
North America (3268)	5.7	7.9	5.4	5.5	6.3	4.9
Multidrug-resistant *P. aeruginosa*						
Europe (1620)	5.1	10.1	14.2	9.5	11.7	11.5
Latin America (762)	12.0	14.3	16.0	14.5	17.8	18.7
North America (1851)	2.5	1.6	2.1	2.0	2.0	3.0

Adapted from Beidenbach et al. (44).

percentage of UTIs caused by *P. aeruginosa* (11.1%) was nearly twofold greater than that observed in the United States (6.7%).

Year-on-year trends in *P. aeruginosa* susceptibility to seven agents from five antimicrobial classes are shown in Table 17.18 (19,44). In North America, a slight trend over time toward greater resistance was noted for ciprofloxacin and meropenem. However, the overall susceptibility of the BSI isolates of *P. aeruginosa* was high and ranged from 76.3% to 93.0% in 2002. Table 17.19 illustrates the interregional variation in the occurrence of MDR strains of *P. aeruginosa*. Gales et al. (65) reported in an earlier summary that MDR *P. aeruginosa* strains appear to be most prevalent in Europe and Latin America, with low rates in North America and the Asia-Pacific region. In the results presented here (limited to BSI isolates), the prevalence of MDR *P. aeruginosa* strains in rank order was 12.0% to 18.7% (average, 15.5%) in Latin America, 51.0% to 14.2% (average, 10.4%) in Europe, and 1.6% to 3.0% (average 2.2%) in North America. Although multidrug resistance was defined differently in the two reports, greater resistance among Latin American Gram-negative isolates appears to be persistent through 2002 (19,44).

Figure 17.1 compares the resistance to one antipseudomonal agent (ciprofloxacin) and the resistance rates for five other antimicrobials from four different classes using 5191 *P. aeruginosa* strains from North America. Direct linear correlations were detected between fluoroquinolone susceptibility or resistance and the corresponding patterns for the other agents. These data indicate, regardless of the definition of multidrug resistance, resistance to one agent is likely to be associated with coresistance across several antimicrobial classes. This phenomenon implies the common and increasing occurrence of resistance mechanisms that can affect several drug classes (e.g., drug exclusion by membrane protein alterations or activated efflux pumps). An earlier analysis (65) indicated increasing numbers of MDR strains of *P. aeruginosa*, a trend confirmed in Latin America (Table 17.19). The overall susceptibility rate for ciprofloxacin was only

TABLE 17.20

Most Active Antimicrobial Agents Tested against Isolates from Each Region for the Three Resistance Phenotypes (SENTRY Program, 1997–2001)

Organisms/Antimicrobial Agent	MIC$_{90}$/% Susceptible		
	Europe ($n = 1045$)	Latin America ($n = 654$)	North America ($n = 2803$)
Oxacillin-resistant *S. aureus*			
Vancomycin	2/100.0	2/100.0	2/100.0
Teicoplanin	4/99.8	4/98.6	2/99.8
Linezolid	2/100.0	2/100.0	2/100.0
Quinupristin/dalfopristin	1/94.6	1/99.2	1/99.2
Vancomycin-resistant enterococci			
Linezolid	2/94.4	–/100.0	2/97.4
Quinupristin/dalfopristin	8/46.0	–/0.0	4/82.7
Doxycycline	>4/66.0	–/50.0	>4/55.9
Chloramphenicol	>16/70.0	–/37.5	8/90.2
ESBL-phenotype *Klebsiella* spp			
Meropenem	0.12/99.4	0.25/99.5	0.12/100.0
Imipenem	0.5/99.7	0.5/99.8	0.5/100.0
Piperacillin/tazobactam	>64/40.6	>64/36.6	>64/53.6
Cefepime	>16/69.0	>16/50.0	16/88.0

Reprinted from Rhomberg et al. (45).

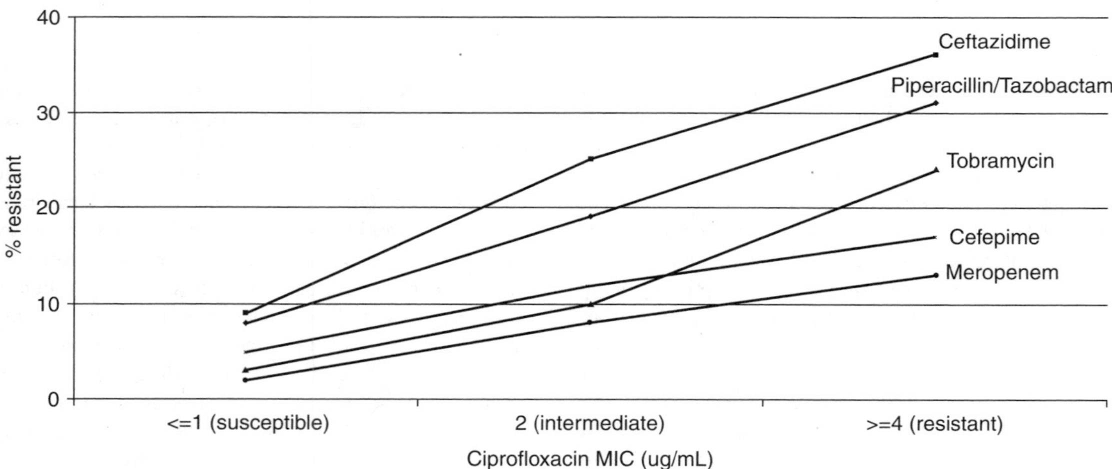

FIGURE 17.1 ● Relationships of ciprofloxacin resistance (17.4%) to the coresistance patterns for carbapenems, cephalosporins, β-lactamase–inhibitor combinations, and aminoglycosides for *P. aeruginosa* strains isolated in the SENTRY Program, 1997–2001 (5191 isolates).

TABLE 17.21

Most Active Antimicrobial Agents Tested against Multidrug-resistant *P. aeruginosa* Isolates[a] for Each Region (SENTRY Program 1997–2001)

	Europe (n = 107)		Latin America (n = 91)		North America (n = 32)	
Antimicrobial Agent	$MIC_{50/90}$[b]	% S[c]	$MIC_{50/90}$[b]	% S[c]	$MIC_{50/90}$[b]	% S[c]
Amikacin	32/>32	41.1	>32/>32	19.8	16/>32	68.8
Tobramycin	>16/>16	6.5	>16/>16	1.1	>16/>16	28.1
Cefepime	>16/>16	5.6	16/>16	4.4	>16/>16	3.1
Imipenem	8/>8	28.0	>8/>8	41.8	>8/>8	37.5
Meropenem	>8/>8	27.1	>8/>8	35.2	8/>8	40.6
Piperacillin/tazobactam	>64/>64	16.8	>64/>64	13.2	>64/>64	9.4

[a] Multidrug resistance defined as coresistances to gentamicin, piperacillin, ciprofloxacin, and ceftazidime.
[b] MIC_{50} and MIC_{90} in μg/mL at which 50% and 90% of the isolates were inhibited, respectively.
[c] Susceptibility (S) rates based on interpretive criteria of the NCCLS (2002).
Reprinted from Rhomberg et al. (45).

79.3%, bringing into question its continued utility in empiric regimens (66).

The susceptibility rates of six broad-spectrum antimicrobials tested against MDR *P. aeruginosa* strains isolated in three geographic regions are displayed in Table 17.21. The most usable agents were the carbapenems (27.1% to 41.8% susceptible) among the β-lactams, and amikacin was best antimicrobial overall (except in Latin America). Other agents useful where these MDR strains have become endemic include the polymyxins (colistin, polymyxin B) (67,68). Favorable responses have been recorded for the polymyxins, but reliable susceptibility testing procedures await further action by the NCCLS (68). Other susceptibility testing issues compromise the accuracy of results for *P. aeruginosa* isolates from cystic fibrosis (CF) patients. Studies by the NCCLS working group (69,70) now direct laboratories to use the agar diffusion methods (disk and Etest [AB Biodisk, Solna, Sweden]) as being most accurate for testing CF isolates. The use of commonly employed commercial systems (Vitek and MicroScan) would likely lead to unacceptable rates of false-susceptible errors (70). More than 90% of MDR *P. aeruginosa* strains worldwide retain susceptibility to polymyxin B using reference methods (12,66–68).

Similar MDR issues affect the therapy of *Acinetobacter* spp in many medical centers (71,72). In these hospitals, susceptibility testing for each MDR *Acinetobacter* spp isolate must guide chemotherapy. Alternative agents have included the carbapenems, amikacin, and ampicillin/sulbactam; in the latter, the inhibitor (sulbactam) has direct antimicrobial potency against *Acinetobacter* spp (73).

Other resistances influencing carbapenem use are the metallo-β-lactamases (74–76) and the chromosomally mediated Bush type 2f enzymes (77). These enzymes are quite rare and beyond current consideration for the selection of empiric antimicrobial regimens.

SUMMARY

When locally derived surveillance results are not available or reliable, prescribers of empiric antimicrobial regimens must utilize current, accurate representative national or global information. ICARE, the SENTRY Program, the MYSTIC Programme and other provide comprehensive data for a wide range of antimicrobials. These data can guide local antimicrobial choices for empiric treatment, but where local data indicate specific resistance problems, corrective interventions must be initiated. Such interventions include (a) infection control policies and measures, (b) formulary changes to reduce selecting agents of resistance (e.g., ceftazidime), (c) consideration of antimicrobial cycling to reduce use pressures, and (d) optimization of antimicrobial dosing by applying pharmacodynamic principals.

The emergence of resistance among pathogens associated with nosocomial infections requires a constant appraisal of susceptibility rates (78). Also, the concept of optimal dosing to attain pharmacokinetic/pharmacodynamic targets has further improved our chances of achieving superior patient outcomes (79–83). Disturbing levels of resistance have been documented worldwide and challenge our ability to select adequate regimens to cover endemic or epidemic resistant strains. Generally, several acceptable choices remain for monotherapy in some hospital environments, such as the carbapenems, cefepime, and piperacillin/tazobactam. Where the resistant population or distribution of pathogens dictates combinations, the addition of an aminoglycoside (amikacin or tobramycin) or a fluoroquinolone to these drugs should be considered. Lastly, the continued utilization of vancomycin may be adequate for many hospital units in the absence of endemic VRE, and where the VRE strains are present, linezolid remains the widest spectrum agent targeting Gram-positive organisms.

As noted in this discussion, no single antimicrobial agent continues to be totally effective in *in vitro* tests because of the escalated discovery of novel resistance mechanisms. The continued evolution of resistance phenomena among clinically important pathogens will persist, and we must be able to adjust our regimens, optimize doses, and encourage the pharmaceutical industry to renew their efforts at developing new antiinfective products.

REFERENCES

1. Jones RN. Resistance patterns among nosocomial pathogens: trends over the past few years. *Chest* 2001;119:397S–404S.
2. Weinstein RA. Nosocomial infection update. *Emerg Infect Dis* 1998;4:416–420.
3. Public Health Initiative Research Institute. *Report from the Bacterial Antibiotic Resistance Group/Infectious Disease Center.* Washington, DC: US Government Printing Office, 1997.
4. US Department of Health and Human Services. *Addressing emerging infectious disease threats: a prevention strategy for the United States.* Washington, DC: US Government Printing Office, 1994.
5. *Impacts of antibiotic-resistant bacteria: thanks to penicillin, he will come home!* Washington, DC: Office of Technology Assessment, 1995. Pub. no. OTA-H-629.
6. Phelps CE. Bug-drug resistance: sometimes less is more. *Med Care* 1989;27:194–203.
7. Ibrahim EH, Sherman G, Ward W, et al. The influence of inadequate antimicrobial treatment of blood stream infections on patient outcomes in the ICU setting. *Chest* 2000;118:146–155.
8. Kollef MH. Antimicrobial therapy of ventilator-associated pneumonia. *Chest* 1999;115:8–11.
9. Jones RN. The emergent needs for basic research, education, and surveillance of antimicrobial resistance: problems facing the report from the American Society for Microbiology Task Force on Antimicrobial Resistance. *Diagn Microbiol Infect Dis* 1996;25:153–161.
10. Bax R, Bywater R, Cornaglia G, et al. Surveillance of antimicrobial resistance: what, how and whither? *Clin Microbiol Infect* 2001;7:316–325.
11. Jones RN, Masterton R. Determining the value of antimicrobial surveillance programs. *Diagn Microbiol Infect Dis* 2001;41:171–175.
12. National Committee for Clinical Laboratory Standards. *Methods for dilution antimicrobial susceptibility tests for bacteria that grow aerobically,* 5th ed. Wayne, PA: National Committee for Clinical Laboratory Standards, 2003. Approved standard M7-A6.
13. National Committee for Clinical Laboratory Standards. *Performance standards for antimicrobial susceptibility testing,* Wayne, PA: National Committee for Clinical Laboratory Standards, 2004. Fourteenth informational supplement M100-S14.
14. Turner PJ, Greenhalgh JM, Edwards JR, et al. The MYSTIC (Meropenem Yearly Susceptibility Test Information Collection) Programme. *Int J Antimicrob Agents* 1999;13:117–125.
15. Global aspects of antimicrobial resistance among key bacterial pathogens: results from the 1997–1999 SENTRY Antimicrobial Surveillance Program. *Clin Infect Dis* 2001;32[Suppl 2]:S81–S167.
16. Pfaller MA, Jones RN, Doern GV, et al. Bacterial pathogens isolated from patients with blood stream infection: frequencies of occurrence and antimicrobial susceptibility patterns from the SENTRY Antimicrobial Surveillance Program (United States and Canada). *Antimicrob Agents Chemother* 1998;42:1762–1770.
17. Pfaller MA, Jones RN, Doern GV, et al. Survey of blood stream infections due to Gram-positive cocci: frequency of occurrence and antimicrobial susceptibility of isolates collected in 1997 in the United States, Canada, and Latin America for the SENTRY Antimicrobial Surveillance Program. *Diagn Microbiol Infect Dis* 1999;33:283–297.
18. Diekema DJ, Pfaller MA, Jones RN, et al. Trends in antimicrobial susceptibility of bacterial pathogens isolated from patients with blood stream infections in the USA, Canada and Latin America. *Int J Antimicrob Agents* 2000;13:257–271.
19. Moet G, Biedenbach D, Pfaller M, et al. Occurrence of blood stream infection (BSI) pathogens and key resistances (R) from the SENTRY Antimicrobial Surveillance Program, a 5-year report. In: Programs and Abstracts of the 42nd Interscience Congress of Antimicrobial Agents and Chemotherapy September 27–30, 2002; San Diego, CA. Abstract C2–299.
20. Diekema DJ, Pfaller MA, Jones RN, et al. Age-related trends in pathogen frequency and antimicrobial susceptibility of blood stream isolates in North America SENTRY Antimicrobial Surveillance Program, 1997–2000. *Int J Antimicrob Agents* 2002;20:412–418.
21. Richards MJ, Edwards JR, Culver DH, et al. Nosocomial infections in pediatric intensive care units in the United States. *Pediatrics* 1999; 103:39–46.
22. Villari P, Sarnataro C, Iacuzio L. Molecular epidemiology of *Staphylococcus epidermidis* in a neonatal intensive care unit over a three year period. *J Clin Microbiol* 2000;38:1740–1746.
23. Hoban DJ, Biedenbach DJ, Mutnick AH, et al. Pathogen of occurrence and susceptibility patterns associated with pneumonia in hospitalized patients in North America: results of the SENTRY Antimicrobial Surveillance Study (2000). *Diagn Microbiol Infect Dis* 2003;45:279–285.
24. Gales AC, Sader HS, Jones RN. Respiratory tract pathogens isolated from patients hospitalized with suspected pneumonia in Latin America: frequency of occurrence and antimicrobial susceptibility profile: results from the SENTRY Antimicrobial Surveillance Program (1997–2000). *Diagn Microbiol Infect Dis* 2002;44:301–311.
25. Kirby JT, Mutnick AH, Jones RN, et al. Geographic variations in garenoxacin (BMS284756) activity tested against pathogens associated with skin and soft tissue infections: report from the SENTRY Antimicrobial Surveillance Program (2000). *Diagn Microbiol Infect Dis* 2002;43:303–309.
26. Rennie RP, Jones RN, Mutnick AH, et al. Occurrence and antimicrobial susceptibility patterns of pathogens isolated from skin and soft tissue infections: report from the SENTRY Antimicrobial Surveillance Program (United States and Canada, 2000). *Diagn Microbiol Infect Dis* 2003;45:287–293.

27. Sader HS, Jones RN, Silva JB, et al. Skin and soft tissue infections in Latin American medical centers: four-year assessment of the pathogen frequency and antimicrobial susceptibility patterns. *Diagn Microbiol Infect Dis* 2002;44:281–288.
28. Gordon KA, Jones RN; SENTRY Participant Groups (Europe, Latin America, North America). Susceptibility patterns of orally administered antimicrobials among urinary tract infection pathogens from hospitalized patients in North America: comparison report to Europe and Latin America: results from the SENTRY Antimicrobial Surveillance Program (2000). *Diagn Microbiol Infect Dis* 2003;45:295–301.
29. Jones RN, Kugler KC, Pfaller MA, et al. Characteristics of pathogens causing urinary tract infections in hospitals in North America: results from the SENTRY Antimicrobial Surveillance Program, 1997. *Diagn Microbiol Infect Dis* 1999;35:55–63.
30. Gales AC, Gordon KA, Wilke WW, et al. Occurrence of single-point *gyr A* mutations among ciprofloxacin-susceptible *Escherichia coli* isolates causing urinary tract infections in Latin America. *Diagn Microbiol Infect Dis* 2000;36:61–64.
31. Jones RN, Beach ML, Pfaller MA. Spectrum and activity of three contemporary fluoroquinolones tested against *Pseudomonas aeruginosa* isolates from urinary tract infections in the SENTRY Antimicrobial Surveillance Program (Europe and the Americas, 2000): more alike than different! *Diagn Microbiol Infect Dis* 2001;41:161–163.
32. Streit J, Jones RN, Sader HS, et al. Assessment of pathogen occurrence and resistance profiles among infected patients in the intensive care unit: report from the SENTRY Antimicrobial Surveillance Program (North America, 2001). *Int J Antimicrob Agents* 2004;24:111–118.
33. Garcia-Rodriguez J-A, Jones RN, MYSTIC Programme Study Group. Antimicrobial resistance in Gram-negative isolates from European intensive care units: data from the Meropenem Yearly Susceptibility Test Information Collection (MYSTIC) Programme. *J Chemother* 2002;14: 25–32.
34. Centers for Disease Control National Nosocomial Infections Surveillance System. National Nosocomial Infections Surveillance (NNIS) System report, data summary from January 1990–May 1999, issued June 1999. *Am J Infect Control* 1999;27:520–532.
35. Centers for Disease Control and Prevention. Update: *Staphylococcus aureus* with reduced susceptibility to vancomycin: United States, 1997. *MMWR* 1997;46:813–815.
36. Hiramatsu K, Aritaka N, Hanaki H, et al. Dissemination in Japanese hospitals of strains of *Staphylococcus aureus* heterogeneously resistant to vancomycin. *Lancet* 1997;350:70–73.
37. Hiramatsu K, Hanaki H, Ino T, et al. Methicillin-resistant *Staphylococcus aureus* clinical strain with reduced vancomycin susceptibility. *J Antimicrob Chemother* 1997;40:135–146.
38. Centers for Disease Control. *Staphylococcus aureus* resistant to vancomycin: United States, 2002. *MMWR* 2002;51:565–567.
39. Whitener CJ, Park SY, Browne FA, et al. Vancomycin-resistant Staphylococcus aureus in the absence of vancomycin exposure. *Clin Infect Dis* 2004;38:1049–1055.
40. Tsiodras S, Godl HS, Sakoulas G, et al. Linezolid resistance in a clinical isolate of *Staphylococcus aureus*. *Lancet* 2001;358:207–208.
41. Mutnick AH, Enne V, Jones RN. Linezolid resistance since 2001: SENTRY Antimicrobial Surveillance Program. *Ann Pharmacother* 2003;37:769–774.
42. Malbruny B, Canu A, Bozdogan B, et al. Resistance to quinupristin/dalfopristin due to mutation of L22 ribosomal protein in *Staphylococcus aureus*. *Antimicrob Agents Chemother* 2002;46:2200–2207.
43. Deshpande LM, Fix AM, Pfaller MA, et al. Emerging elevated mupirocin resistance rates among staphylococcal isolates in the SENTRY Antimicrobial Surveillance Program (2000): correlations of results from disk diffusion, Etest and reference dilution methods. *Diagn Microbiol Infect Dis* 2002;42:283–290.
44. Beidenbach DJ, Moet GJ, Jones RN. Pathogen occurrence and antimicrobial resistance pattern comparisons among bloodstream infection isolates from the SENTRY Antimicrobial Surveillance Program (1997–2002). *Diag Microbiol Infect Dis* 2004;50:59–69.
45. Rhomberg P, Jones RN, Mutnick A. Geographic variations and trends in key bacteremic pathogen resistance (R): report from the SENTRY Antimicrobial Surveillance Program (1997–2001). In: Programs and Abstracts of the 42nd Interscience Congress of Antimicrobial Agents and Chemotherapy; 2002; San Diego, CA. Abstract C2–298.
46. Ike Y, Arakawa Y, Ma X, et al. Nationwide survey shows that methicillin-resistant *Staphylococcus aureus* strains heterogeneously and intermediately resistant to vancomycin are not disseminated throughout Japanese hospitals. *J Clin Microbiol* 2001;39:4445–4451.
47. Schwalbe RS, Stapleton JT, Gilligan PH. Emergence of vancomycin resistance in coagulase-negative staphylococci. *N Engl J Med* 1987;316:927–931.
48. Diekema DJ, Jones RN. Oxazolidinone antibiotics. *Lancet* 2001;358:1975–1982.
49. Mutnick AH, Biedenbach DJ, Turnidge JD, et al. Spectrum and potency evaluation of a new oxazolidinone, linezolid: report from the SENTRY Antimicrobial Surveillance Program, 1998–2000. *Diagn Microbiol Infect Dis* 2002;43:65–73.
50. Gonzales RD, Schreckenberger PC, Graham MG, et al. Infections due to vancomycin-resistant *Enterococcus faecium* resistant to linezolid. *Lancet* 2001;357:1179.
51. Jones RN, Della-Latta PH, Lee LV, et al. Linezolid-resistant *Enterococcus faecium* isolated from a patient without prior exposure to an oxazolidinone: report from the SENTRY Antimicrobial Surveillance Program. *Diagn Microbiol Infect Dis* 2002;2:137–139.
52. Huycke MM, Sahm DF, Gilmore MS. Multiple-drug resistant enterococci: the nature of the problem and an agenda for the future. *Emerg Infect Dis* 1998;4:239–249.
53. Centers for Disease Control. Nosocomial enterococci resistant to vancomycin: United States, 1989–1993: National Nosocomial Infections Surveillance. *MMWR* 1993;42:597–599.
54. Low DE, Keller N, Barth A, et al. Clinical prevalence, antimicrobial susceptibility, and geographic resistance patterns of enterococci: results from the SENTRY Antimicrobial Surveillance Program, 1997–1999. *Clin Infect Dis* 2001;32[Suppl 2]:S133–S145.
55. Carmeli Y, Eliopoulos GM, Samore MH. Antecedent treatment with different antibiotic agents as a risk factor for vancomycin-resistant *Enterococcus*. *Emerg Infect Dis* 2002;8:802–804.
56. Mallon DJP, Corkill JE, Hazel SM, et al. Excretion of vancomycin-resistant enterococci by wild mammals. *Emerg Infect Dis* 2002;8:636–638.
57. Hoban DJ, Doern GV, Fluit AC, et al. Worldwide prevalence of antimicrobial resistance in *Streptococcus pneumoniae, Haemophilus influenzae* and *Moraxella catarrhalis* in the SENTRY Antimicrobial Surveillance Program, 1997–1999. *Clin Infect Dis* 2001;32[Suppl 2]:S81–S93.

58. Jones RN, Pfaller MA. Macrolide and fluoroquinolone (levofloxacin) resistances among *Streptococcus pneumoniae* strains: significant trends from the SENTRY Antimicrobial Surveillance Program (North America, 1997–1999). *J Clin Microbiol* 2000;38:4298–4299.
59. Roson B, Carratala J, Tubau F, et al. Usefulness of β-lactam therapy for community-acquired pneumonia in the era of drug-resistant *Streptococcus pneumoniae:* a randomized study of amoxicillin/clavulanic and ceftriaxone. *Microb Drug Resist* 2001;7:85–96.
60. Jones RN, Pfaller MA. Potencies of newer fluoroquinolones against viridans group streptococci isolated in 637 cases of blood stream infection in the SENTRY Antimicrobial Surveillance Program (1997 to 1999): Beyond Canada! [Letter to the editor]. *Antimicrob Agents Chemother* 2000;44:2922–2923.
61. Gordon KA, Beach ML, Biedenbach DJ, et al. Antimicrobial susceptibility patterns of β-haemolytic and viridans group streptococci: report from the SENTRY Antimicrobial Surveillance Program (1997–2000). *Diagn Microbiol Infect Dis* 2002;43:157–162.
62. Winokur PL, Canton R, Casellas J-M, et al. Variations in the prevalence of strains expressing an extended-spectrum β-lactamase phenotype and characterization of isolates from Europe, the Americas, and the Western Pacific region. *Clin Infect Dis* 2001;32[Suppl 2]:S94–S103.
63. Jones RN, Baquero F, Privitera G, et al. Inducible β-lactamase–mediated resistance to third-generation cephalosporins. *Clin Microbiol Infect* 1997;3[Suppl 1]:S7–S20.
64. Jones RN, Varnam DJ. Antimicrobial activity of broad-spectrum agents tested against Gram-negative bacilli resistant to ceftazidime: report from the SENTRY Antimicrobial Surveillance Program (North America, 2001). *Diagn Microbiol Infect Dis* 2002;44:379–382.
65. Gales AC, Jones RN, Turnidge J, et al. Characterization of *Pseudomonas aeruginosa* isolates: occurrence rates, antimicrobial susceptibility patterns, and molecular typing in the global SENTRY Antimicrobial Surveillance Program, 1997–1999. *Clin Infect Dis* 2001;32[Suppl 2]:S146–S155.
66. Jones RN, Pfaller MA. Ciprofloxacin as broad-spectrum empiric therapy: are fluoroquinolones still viable monotherapeutic agents compared with β-lactams: data from the MYSTIC Program (US)? *Diagn Microbiol Infect Dis* 2002;42:213–215.
67. Evans ME, Feola DJ, Rapp RP. Polymyxin B sulfate and colistin: old antibiotics for emerging multiresistant Gram-negative bacteria. *Ann Pharmacother* 1999;33:960–967.
68. Gales AC, Reis AO, Jones RN. Contemporary assessment of antimicrobial susceptibility testing methods for polymyxin B and colistin: review of available interpretative criteria and quality control guidelines. *J Clin Microbiol* 2001;39:183–190.
69. Burns JL, Saiman L, Whittier S, et al. Comparison of agar diffusion methodologies for antimicrobial susceptibility testing of *Pseudomonas aeruginosa* isolates from cystic fibrosis patients. *J Clin Microbiol* 2000;38:1818–1822.
70. Burns JL, Saiman L, Whittier S, et al. Comparison of two commercial systems (Vitek and MicroScan-WalkAway) for antimicrobial susceptibility testing of *Pseudomonas aeruginosa* isolates from cystic fibrosis patients. *Diagn Microbiol Infect Dis* 2001;39:257–260.
71. Gales AC, Jones RN, Forward KR, et al. Emerging importance of multidrug-resistant *Acinetobacter* species and *Stenotrophomonas maltophilia* as pathogens in serious ill patients: geographic patterns, epidemiological features, and trends in the SENTRY Antimicrobial Surveillance Program (1997–1999). *Clin Infect Dis* 2001;32[Suppl 2]:S104–S113.
72. Wisplinghoff H, Edmond MB, Pfaller MA, et al. Nosocomial blood stream infections caused by *Acinetobacter* species in United States hospitals: clinical features, molecular epidemiology, and antimicrobial susceptibility. *Clin Infect Dis* 2000;31:690–697.
73. Jellison TK, McKinnon PS, Rybak MJ. Epidemiology, resistance, and outcomes of *Acinetobacter baumannii* bacteremia treated with imipenem-cilastatin or ampicillin/sulbactam. *Pharmacotherapy* 2001;21:142–148.
74. Page MI. Understanding metallo-β-lactamases. *ASM News* 2002;68:217–221.
75. Livermore DM, Woodford N. Carbapenems: a problem in waiting? *Curr Opin Microbiol* 2000;3:489–495.
76. Nordmann P, Poirel L. Emerging carbapenemases in Gram-negative aerobes. *Clin Microbiol Infect* 2002;8:321–331.
77. Gales AC, Biedenbach DJ, Winokur P, et al. Carbapenem-resistant *Serratia marcescens* isolated producing Bush Group 2f β-lactamase (SME-1) in the United States: results from the MYSTIC Programme. *Diagn Microbiol Infect Dis* 2001;39:125–127.
78. Kollef MH, Ward S, Sherman G, et al. Inadequate treatment of nosocomial infections is associated with certain empiric antibiotic choices. *Crit Care Med* 2000;28:3458–3464.
79. Ambrose PG, Grasela DM. The use of Monte Carlo simulation to examine the pharmacodynamic variance of drugs: fluoroquinolone pharmacodynamics against *Streptococcus pneumoniae. Diagn Microbiol Infect Dis* 2000;38:151–157.
80. Ambrose PG, Owens RC Jr, Garvey MJ, et al. Pharmacodynamic considerations in the treatment of moderate to severe pseudomonal infections with cefepime. *J Antimicrob Chemother* 2002;49:445–453.
81. Ambrose PG, Owens RC, Grasela DM. Antimicrobial pharmacodynamics. *Med Clinics North Am* 2000;84:1431–1445.
82. Ambrose PG, Richerson MA, Stanton ME, et al. Cost-effective analysis of cefepime compared with ceftazidime in intensive care unit patients with hospital-acquired pneumoniae. *Infect Dis Clin Pract* 1999;8:245–251.
83. Kuti JL, Nightingale CH, Quintiliani R, et al. Pharmacodynamic profiling of continuously infused piperacillin/tazobactam against *Pseudomonas aeruginosa* using Monte Carlo analysis. *Diagn Microbiol Infect Dis* 2002;44:51–57.

Index

Note: Page numbers in italics indicate figures; page numbers followed by t indicate tables.

B

M

P

T

U